Breastfeeding and Human Lactation

FOURTH EDITION

Edited by

Jan Riordan, EdD, RN, IBCLC, FAAN

Professor
School of Nursing
Wichita State University
Wichita, Kansas

Karen Wambach, PhD, RN, IBCLC

Associate Professor
School of Nursing
University of Kansas
Kansas City, Kansas

JONES AND BARTLETT PUBLISHERS

Sudbury, Massachusetts

BOSTON   TORONTO   LONDON   SINGAPORE

World Headquarters

Jones and Bartlett Publishers
40 Tall Pine Drive
Sudbury, MA 01776
978-443-5000
info@jbpub.com
www.jbpub.com

Jones and Bartlett Publishers Canada
6339 Ormindale Way
Mississauga, Ontario L5V 1J2
Canada

Jones and Bartlett Publishers International
Barb House, Barb Mews
London W6 7PA
United Kingdom

Jones and Bartlett's books and products are available through most bookstores and online booksellers. To contact Jones and Bartlett Publishers directly, call 800-832-0034, fax 978-443-8000, or visit our website www.jbpub.com.

Substantial discounts on bulk quantities of Jones and Bartlett's publications are available to corporations, professional associations, and other qualified organizations. For details and specific discount information, contact the special sales department at Jones and Bartlett via the above contact information or send an email to specialsales@jbpub.com.

The authors, editor, and publisher have made every effort to provide accurate information. However, they are not responsible for errors, omissions, or for any outcomes related to the use of the contents of this book and take no responsibility for the use of the products and procedures described. Treatments and side effects described in this book may not be applicable to all people; likewise, some people may require a dose or experience a side effect that is not described herein. Drugs and medical devices are discussed that may have limited availability controlled by the Food and Drug Administration (FDA) for use only in a research study or clinical trial. Research, clinical practice, and government regulations often change the accepted standard in this field. When consideration is being given to use of any drug in the clinical setting, the health care provider or reader is responsible for determining FDA status of the drug, reading the package insert, and reviewing prescribing information for the most up-to-date recommendations on dose, precautions, and contraindications, and determining the appropriate usage for the product. This is especially important in the case of drugs that are new or seldom used.

Additional photographic credits appear on page xxiii, which constitutes a continuation of the copyright page.

Production Credits

Publisher: Kevin Sullivan
Acquisitions Editor: Emily Ekle
Acquisitions Editor: Amy Sibley
Associate Editor: Patricia Donnelly
Editorial Assistant: Rachel Shuster
Senior Production Editor: Carolyn F. Rogers

Marketing Manager: Rebecca Wasley
V.P., Manufacturing and Inventory Control: Therese Connell
Composition: diacriTech, Chennai, India
Cover Design: Brian Moore
Cover Image: Courtesy of Mary-Margaret Coates
Printing and Binding: Replika Press
Cover Printing: Replika Press

Library of Congress Cataloging-in-Publication Data

Breastfeeding and human lactation / [edited by] Jan Riordan, Karen Wambach.–4th ed.
    p. ; cm.
Includes bibliographical references and index.
    ISBN 978-0-7637-5432-7 (pbk.)
    1. Breast feeding. 2. Lactation. I. Riordan, Jan. II. Wambach, Karen.
    [DNLM: 1. Breast Feeding. 2. Infant Nutrition Physiology. 3. Lactation.
4. Milk, Human. WS 125 B8293 2009]
    RJ216.B775 2009
    649'.33–dc22   2008029133

6048

Printed in India
14 13 12 11 10   10 9 8 7 6 5 4 3 2

*This book is dedicated to breastfeeding women
and their babies around the globe.*

Table of Contents

CHAPTER 10

Low Intake in the Breastfed Infant: Maternal and Infant Considerations

SECTION 4
BEYOND POSTPARTUM   495

CHAPTER 15

Maternal Nutrition During Lactation   497

CHAPTER 16

Women's Health and Breastfeeding   519

CHAPTER 24

The Cultural Context of Breastfeeding 799

CHAPTER 25

The Familial and Social Context of Breastfeeding 817

APPENDIXES

Preface

The first notable change in the fourth edition is that the book again has two editors/authors. We both live and work in tallgrass wheatlands of the Midwest and are certified lactation consultants, professors, researchers, mothers, and grandmothers.

The second obvious change in this edition is that we moved the chapter on the lactation consultant/specialist to the first chapter in the book to reflect the worldwide expansion of the lactation specialist role. In 2008, more than 2,000 candidates sat the lactation consultant certification exam.

We mourn the loss of the JoAnne Scott, the founder, champion, and long-time executive of the International Board of Lactation Consultant Examiners. During JoAnne's watch most every United States hospital hired lactation specialists to teach and help mothers to get off to a good start breastfeeding—a world-changing legacy.

On the upside: We are almost there! US breastfeeding rates rose to a record high of 77 percent, surpassing the US government's 75 percent target for initiation of breastfeeding. Now we must work on helping mothers continue to breastfeed for a longer time: exclusive breastfeeding through the first 3 months after birth is 31 percent, only half of the of the US government's goal of 60 percent.

Organizations that teach and promote breastfeeding continue to grow. Physicians formed their own organization, the Academy of Breastfeeding Medicine, and have their own journal. Two university endowed professorships for lactation and breastfeeding research and education have been funded since the last edition, a marker for university acceptance of the importance of this discipline: one in public health at the University of North Carolina and the other in nursing at Wichita State University.

Other innovations affect lactation practice. The explosive growth of Internet-based publishing and online courses is revolutionizing education and ... well, everything else. The Internet has turned us into a "global village" where we chatter back and forth (too) frequently. It holds much promise as an education pathway to teach lactation and, just as important, to make it possible for discussions worldwide.

Can anatomy change? Not really, but it can be better understood with new technology. With ultrasound we can now "look inside" the lactating breast and the infant oral cavity of a suckling baby. This noninvasive procedure has spawned a whole new arm of breastfeeding research and has given us a new view of the anatomy of the lactating breast, crushing cherished beliefs about the structure of the breast.

Birth practices affect lactation and we have long aligned with childbirth educators. Thus, this edition contains considerable content on obstetrical issues, especially the importance of skin-to-skin care. Once a natural event, birthing is now a high-technology procedure of control and convenience. Since 1989, cesarean births have risen 28 percent! Elective labor inductions have risen 125 percent. Mothers are now requesting to have a cesarean section. Are we going backward? And if we are, why?

This text brings together in a single volume the latest clinical techniques and research findings that direct evidence-based clinical practice. We have been fortunate in being able to enlist breastfeeding experts recognized around the world to help with the writing of this extensive volume.

As is true of earlier editions, the fourth edition of this text has a clear clinical focus. More than 2,000 research studies support the clinical recommendations in this book. Nearly every chapter contains a clinical implications section. Important concepts discussed in chapters are summarized at the end of each chapter—a feature that makes studying easier. Throughout the book are new references deemed by the authors to be the most important from the vastly expanded research and clinical literature. Some older references—which introduced then new ideas that are now accepted common knowledge—have been regretfully removed to make room for the new.

Section 1 contrasts the past and present. Chapter 1 concentrates on the work of the present-day health care worker who specializes in lactation and breastfeeding, and it addresses work-related issues of lactation consulting, such as staffing. Chapter 2 presents the history of breastfeeding by placing lactation and breastfeeding in its historical context.

Section 2 focuses on basic anatomic and biologic imperatives of lactation. Researchers continue to find amazing properties in breast milk: stem cells in breast milk, for one. Another: hormones in human milk change according to the emotions of the mother. A breastfed baby with eczema has milder symptoms when his mother laughs. Who would have imagined! Clinical application of techniques must be based on a clear understanding of the relationships between form, function, and biological constructs. Chapter 3 has a new section on basic suck training technique for infants with suckling problems. This section, too, provides the background upon which to understand other aspects of lactation and breastfeeding behavior.

Section 3 is the clinical "heart" of the book that describes the basics of *what* to do, *when* to do it, and *how* to do it when one assists the lactating mother. Section 3 thus concerns itself with the perinatal period in the birth setting and concerns during the postpartum period following the family's return home—notably breast problems, neonatal jaundice, and infant weight gain. This section also addresses special needs of preterm babies and their mothers, and it critically evaluates breastfeeding devices and recommends how and when they are most appropriately used. It concludes with a review of the development and current activities of human milk banking.

The first part of **Section 4** focuses on the mother: maternal nutrition, the mother's health, and returning to work. The topics then turn to the infant and child's health and special health needs. The techniques of infant assessment are explained and demonstrated with photographs. The section ends with a discussion of maternal sexuality and fertility.

Section 5 begins with a careful look at research—how it is conducted, why ongoing research is needed, how research findings can be applied in clinical settings, and what theories are related to lactation practice. The principles of education, the cornerstone of clinical practice, are explored next. The book concludes with chapters on culture's effect on breastfeeding and the sociological context of the breastfeeding family functions.

To avoid linguistic confusion, the book uses the following conventions. The word *nursing* (in italics) in the text refers to the profession. Nursing, meaning breastfeeding, is always shown in ordinary Roman type. The masculine pronoun has been used to denote the infant or child throughout the text as a matter of convenience to distinguish the child from the breastfeeding mother. Nurses, lactation consultants, and other healthcare workers are referred to by feminine pronouns, although we recognize that men serve in all healthcare professions.

Acknowledgments

We gratefully acknowledge the contributions to this book made by the following individuals:

Judy Angeron, BA, RN, IBCLC, Coordinator, Lactation Services, Via Christi Regional Medical Center, Wichita, Kansas

Heather Baker, MSN, ARNP BC, PNP, Clinical Educator, Wichita State University, School of Nursing, Wichita, Kansas

Mary-Margaret Coates, MS, IBCLC, TechEdit, Wheat Ridge, Colorado

Pamela Martin, BSN, MSN, Instructor, Wichita State University, School of Nursing, Wichita, Kansas

Voni Miller, RN, IBCLC, Lactation Consultant, Phoenix Children's Hospital, Phoenix, Arizona

Nancy Powers, MD, FAAP, FABM, Riordan Distinguished Professor, Wichita State University

Christina M. Smillie, MD, FAAP, IBCLC, Breastfeeding Resources, Stratford, Connecticut

Sallie Page Goertz, ARNP, IBCLC, Department of Pediatrics, University of Kansas Medical Center

We are grateful to La Leche League International for providing the foundation for our breastfeeding knowledge and to those institutions which encouraged and supported us in writing the book: the Wichita State University School of Nursing, and Via Christi Regional Medical Center, both of Wichita, Kansas, as well as The University of Kansas School of Nursing in Kansas City, Kansas.

Finally, we would like to thank our families for their help and encouragement over the years. The Riordan family: Michael, Neil and Shirley; Brian, Quinn and Rika; Teresa, Renee and Don Olmstead; and 12 grandchildren. The Wambach family: Bill, Jackie, Nathan and Brandi, and grandson Logan is also recognized and thanked for support and encouragement.

Photo Credits

Section 1 opener: © Sergei Vasilev.

Section 2 opener: Used with permission from WHO/PAHO (1983).

Section 3 opener: © Sergei Vasilev.

Section 4 opener: © Sergei Vasilev.

Section 5 opener: Courtesy of Via Christi Health Systems.

Contributors

Heather Baker, MSN, ARNP BC, PNP
Clinical Educator
School of Nursing
Wichita State University
Wichita, Kansas

Yvonne Bronner, ScD, RD, LD
Professor
School of Community Health and Policy
Morgan State University
Baltimore, Maryland

Mary-Margaret Coates, MS, IBCLC
Technical Editor
TECH Edit
Wheat Ridge, Colorado

Lawrence M. Gartner, MD, FAAP
Professor Emeritus of Pediatrics and OB/GYN
University of Chicago
Chicago, Illinois

Thomas W. Hale, PhD
Department of Pediatrics
Texas Tech University School of Medicine
Amarillo, Texas

Roberta J. Hewat, PhD, RN, IBCLC
Associate Professor Emerita
University of British Columbia
Vancouver, British Columbia, Canada

Kay Hoover, MEd, IBCLC, FILCA
Lactation Consultant
Riddle Memorial Hospital
Media, Pennsylvania

Nancy Hurst, PhD, RN, IBCLC
Lactation Program and Mother's Own Milk Bank
Texas Children's Hospital
Houston, Texas

Frances Jones, RN, MSN, IBCLC
Coordinator Lactation Services and Milk Bank
BC Women's Hospital and Health Centre
Vancouver, British Columbia, Canada

Kathy Irene Kennedy, DrPH, MA, AB
Associate Clinical Professor of Community and
    Behavioral Health
Colorado School of Public Health
University of Colorado, Denver
Denver, Colorado

Mary L. Koehn, PhD, ARNP, FACCE
Associate Professor
School of Nursing
Wichita State University
Wichita, Kansas

Sallie Page-Goertz, MN, ARNP, IBCLC
Clinical Associate Professor
University of Kansas School of Medicine
Kansas City, Kansas

Nancy G. Powers, MD, FAAP, FABM
Janice M. Riordan Distinguished Professor in
    Maternal Child Health
Wichita State University
Wichita, Kansas

Wilaiporn Rojjanasrirat, PhD, RN, IBCLC
Clinical Assistant Professor
University of Kansas School of Nursing
Kansas City, Kansas

Linda Smith, BSE, FACCE, IBCLC
Director
Bright Future Lactation Resource Centre Ltd.
Dayton, Ohio

Mary Rose Tully, MPH, IBCLC
Faculty, Carolina Breastfeeding Institute
Department of Maternal Child Health
School of Public Health
University of North Carolina at Chapel Hill
Chapel Hill, North Carolina

Marsha Walker, RN, IBCLC
Executive Director
National Alliance for Breastfeeding Advocacy
Weston, Massachusetts

Section 1

Historical and Work Perspectives

Just as the course of breastfeeding flows and ebbs in a woman's life, so breastfeeding has experienced flows and ebbs through many millennia. It takes a village to return to breastfeeding, and community-based programs that promote breastfeeding are working to increase the rate of breastfeeding around the world.

Until breastfeeding is again the unremarkable norm, increasing numbers of mothers who begin breastfeeding prompt a need for increasing numbers of specialists who can help those mothers continue breastfeeding. The visibility and acceptance of lactation consulting as an allied health profession offers opportunities for practice in hospitals, the community, and in private practice. Randomized clinical trials conducted around the globe during the past 20 years consistently demonstrate that lactation consultant services lengthen a mother's breastfeeding course and result in healthier mothers and babies.

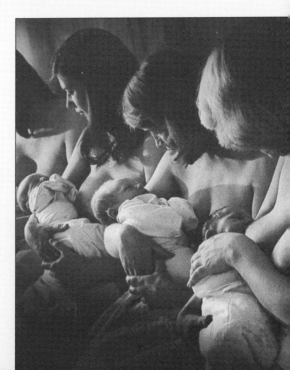

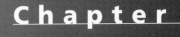
The Lactation Specialist: Roles and Responsibilities

Jan Riordan

A LACTATION CONSULTANT (LC) is a specialist trained to focus on the needs and concerns of the breastfeeding mother-baby pair and to prevent, recognize, and solve breastfeeding difficulties. LC services do not replace those of other healthcare workers; instead, the LC is an extender of maternal–child services. Lactation consultants work with the public in many settings: hospitals, clinics, private medical practices, community health departments, home health agencies, and private practices. Almost all lactation specialists are women; many have educational and clinical backgrounds in the health professions. The majority are registered nurses, although physicians, dietitians, speech therapists, and other health professionals practice as lactation specialists.

Lactation consulting is a rapidly growing new healthcare specialty. Prior to recognition of the LC as a paid specialist in 1985, individuals serving breastfeeding women did so as volunteers or as unrecognized practitioners. The lack of standardization of skills and minimal competencies led to formal development of the specialty practice. This occurred in part through a certification examination, and through the establishment of the International Lactation Consultant Association (ILCA), which publishes the *Journal of Human Lactation* and

other documents relating to lactation consultant education and practice. In 1994, the Academy of Breastfeeding Medicine, an international physician organization, was formed. Their official journal, *Breastfeeding Medicine*, publishes peer-reviewed articles and helpful clinical protocols. La Leche League International and the Australian Breastfeeding Association also publish professional materials that teach and support the LC. This chapter traces the historical roots of lactation professionals and discusses work-related issues.

History

In a cultural setting in which nearly all mothers breastfed, help with breastfeeding was available through the shared knowledge of other family members, neighbors, and friends. As childbirth came to be managed by health professionals in hospital settings, however, knowledge of lactation, which a mother formerly shared with her daughters or a sister with her younger siblings, was set aside.

Thus, during the 1960s (at the nadir of breastfeeding) in the United States and shortly thereafter in other countries (such as Australia and Scandinavia), volunteer breastfeeding support groups became a major source of assistance and information about how to breastfeed (Phillips, 1990). As the numbers of breastfeeding mothers increased, healthcare providers at first denounced these groups; later they came to appreciate them for the important role they played in helping mothers and in forcing the medical profession to consider lactation an integral part of prenatal and postpartum care.

As these volunteers relearned the art of breastfeeding, they also sought more knowledge of the science of lactation. La Leche League responded by providing research information to their group leaders, who serve as mother-to-mother helpers, and by publishing a quarterly newsletter, *Breastfeeding Abstracts,* which focuses exclusively on the scientific literature. Through La Leche League's professional liaison department, key individuals sought to cultivate and maintain communication links to health providers in local communities.

Out of this context, some experienced breastfeeding support group members began to look beyond what they could accomplish as volunteers. Many of these women sought to apply in a paid work setting what they had learned from many years of helping breastfeeding mothers. In 1982 La Leche League formed the Lactation Consultant Department. From this beginning grew the notion

of the need for a new healthcare worker, and in 1985 an independent certification board, the International Board of Lactation Consultant Examiners, was formed. Shortly thereafter, the *Journal of Human Lactation (JHL)* began. Edited by Kathleen Auerbach from 1985 to 1996 when Jan Heinig became editor, *JHL* is peer-reviewed, professionally published, and cited on international indices (Bailey, 2005).

Do Lactation Consultants Make a Difference?

In this day of cost containment in health care, administrators want to know if lactation consultants are effective. Do interventions by lactation specialists and other healthcare providers make a difference in outcomes of breastfeeding? Table 1–1 presents randomized controlled trials, the highest level and most rigorous type of research study, of breastfeeding interventions worldwide. Most of the studies show that the interventions have a positive effect on breastfeeding. Note from the table that even if the results do not reach significance, any intervention (even a booklet given to the mother) results in higher rates of breastfeeding than no intervention. These results hold constant regardless of where the studies were done.

TABLE 1–1	**Controlled Trials on the Effect of Lactation Specialists and Health Providers Intervention on Breastfeeding Outcomes**	
Author	**Intervention Description**	**Outcome: Intervention vs. Control**
Gill, Reifsnider, Lucke, 2007 United States	Convenience sample of women receiving prenatal care at health department Intervention: met with IBCLC prenatally twice; four phone calls postpartum Control: Standard education on benefits of BF	Intervention group had twice the odds of starting BF and twice the odds of continuing BF for 6 months.
Mattar et al., 2007 Singapore	Random sample of low-risk antenatal patients Intervention 1: educational	Exclusive/predominant BF 3 mo, OR 2.6, CI 1.2–5.4* 6 mo, OR 2.5, CI 1.0–6.3*

(Continues)

TABLE 1–1	Controlled Trials on the Effect of Lactation Specialists and Health Providers Intervention on Breastfeeding Outcomes (Continued)	
Author	**Intervention Description**	**Outcome: Intervention vs. Control**
	material and coaching Intervention 2: educational material Control: routine antenatal care Face-to-face encounter most effective	
de Oliveira et al., 2006 Brazil	One 30-minute counseling session on BF techniques No difference in exclusive BF	Exclusive BF at 7 days 70.9% vs. 82.5% Exclusive BF at 30 days 60.8% vs. 53.3%**
Labarere et al., 2005 France	Outpatient visit by 2 wks postpartum to physician who received 5-hour training program	Exclusive BF at 4 wks 83.9% vs. 71.9%* Any BF at 4 wks** 89.3% vs. 81.6%
Kools et al., 2005 The Netherlands	LC services to child care center randomly designated to program care vs. usual care No difference in duration at 3 mo.	Any BF at 3 mo 32% vs. 38%**
Aidam, Perez-Escamilla, Lartey, 2005 Ghana	Intervention 1: pre-peri, postnatal LC support Intervention 2: Peri-postnatal LC support Control: Standard care	Exclusive BF at 6 mo 90%* 74% 47%
Bonuck et al., 2005 United States	Visits: Prenatal, postnatal; hospital, home, telephone No difference in exclusive BF between groups	BF at 20 wks 53% vs. 39%**
Forster et al., 2004 Australia	Intervention 1: 1.5-hour class on practical skills Intervention 2: Two 1-hour classes on attitudes and experiences Control: Standard care	Initiation of BF 97% vs. 95% vs. 96%** Any BF at 6 mo 55% vs. 50% vs. 54%**
Albernaz et al., 2003[§] Brazil	Lactation support visit in the hospital and seven visits at home	Twice as likely to be still BF at 4 mo as control group. No difference in breastmilk intake.
O'Connor et al., 2003 Ontario	Postpartum visit by public health nurses randomized to home visit or telephone call	No differences. Routine home visit not always necessary and more costly than telephone.
Pugh et al., 2002[§] United States	Breastfeeding support visits by community health nurse peer counselor team. Support offered daily when in hospital, and at home during weeks 1, 2 and 4. Telephone support twice weekly through week 8.	Intervention group breastfed longer, had fewer sick visits, and took fewer meds. Intervention cost ($301) was partially offset by savings on formula and health care.

(Continues)

| TABLE 1-1 | Controlled Trials on the Effect of Lactation Specialists and Health Providers Intervention on Breastfeeding Outcomes (Continued) |

Author	Intervention Description	Outcome: Intervention vs. Control
Susin, Guigliana, Kummer et al., 1999 Brazil	Video, explanatory leaflet, discussion, and four home visits N = 400	6.5 times higher exclusive BF at end of 3rd mo than control
Jakobsen et al., 1999 Guinea Bissau	Individual session at 1st prenatal visit and until 9 mo N = 1154	Any BF at 13 wk 29% vs. 18% .003* Full breastfeeding at 4 mo 31% vs. 25%*
Froozani et al., 1999§ Iran	Hospital session, individual counseling in clinic or at home until 4 mo N = 134	Exclusive BF at 4 mo 54% vs. 6%*
Bolam et al., 1998 Nepal	Individual session (20 min), N = 540 Intervention 1: at birth and at 3 mo Intervention 2: at birth Intervention 3: at 3 mo	Exclusive breastfeeding 33% vs. 28%** 24% vs. 28%** 29% vs. 28%**
Pugh & Milligan, 1998 United States	Two home visits to help with in-home tasks at days 3–4. Phone call	Any BF at 6 mo 50% vs. 27%*
Curro et al., 1997 Italy	Booklet: instruction for breastfeeding given during 1st pediatric visit	Full breastfeeding at 6 mo 48% vs. 44%** Any BF at 6 mo 59% vs. 52%**
Duffy, 1997 Australia	Group session 3 times: 2 hr + 25 min video	Any breastfeeding at 6 wk 91% vs. 29%*
Gagnon et al., 1997 Canada	Home visits, early postpartum discharge, phone calls until day 10 postpartum, N = 201	Any BF at 1 mo 55% vs. 39%*
Brent et al., 1995§ United States	Daily round at hospital, 1 phone call, prenatal and postnatal one-on-one consult until 1 yr N = 115	Any BF at 2 mo 37% vs. 9%*
Barros et al., 1994 Brazil	Home visits at days 5, 10, 20 N = 900	Any BF at 2 mo 73% vs. 62%
Hauch & Dimmock, 1994 Australia	33-page breastfeeding booklet sent home shortly after discharge N = 150	Any BF at 6 mo 59% vs. 56%** Any breastfeeding at 12 mo 16% vs. 22%**
Rossiter, 1994 Australia	Groups session 3 times: 2 hr + 25 min video (after 12th week) N = 194	Any BF at 4 wk 50% vs. 26%*

(Continues)

TABLE 1–1	**Controlled Trials on the Effect of Lactation Specialists and Health Providers Intervention on Breastfeeding Outcomes (Continued)**	
Author	**Intervention Description**	**Outcome: Intervention vs. Control**
Serafino-Cross & Donovan, 1992 United States	Five to eight home visits during 2 mo + counselor's phone number available. N = 52	Any BF at 2 mo 62% vs. 35%**
Neyzi et al., 1991 Turkey	Hospital group session + 10-min video, 1 home visit at 5–7 days + booklet N = 941	Any BF at 4 mo 95% vs. 81%** Exclusive BF at 2 mo 4% vs. 2%**
Hill, 1987 United States	Groups session 1 time: 40-min lecture, 5–10 min of questions + pamphlets N = 64	Any breastfeeding at 6 wk 39% vs. 30%**
Frank et al., 1987§ United States	Intervention 1: bedside session in hospital; phone calls until 3 mo + research discharge pack Intervention 2: research discharge pack N = 343	Exclusive BF at 3 mo 20% vs. 6%* Any breastfeeding at 4 mo 71% vs. 54%* Exclusive breastfeeding at 2 mo 15% vs. 6%** Any breastfeeding at 4 mo 56% vs. 54%**
Lynch et al., 1986§ Canada	1 home visit within 5 days of postdischarge + phone calls until 6 mo N = 270	Any breastfeeding at 1, 3, 6, 9 mo**
Bloom et al., 1982 Canada	Phone calls at days 10, 17, 21 + referral to nurse	Any breastfeeding at 6 mo 89% vs. 77%*

* Significant

** Not significant

§ Included in Cochrane List

Source: Adapted from de Oliveira, 2001.

A Cochrane review, the "gold standard" of medical research, studied the effect of any extra support given to breastfeeding women. Lay and professional support together extended duration of breastfeeding, especially that of exclusive breastfeeding (Britton et al., 2007). Face-to-face counseling (Figure 1–1) is the most effective intervention in increasing not only exclusive breastfeeding rates but also the total duration of breastfeeding (Albernaz, 2003).

If the data from the randomized controlled trials in the table were translated to healthcare costs saved by breastfeeding, it would show that lactation services save the healthcare system enormous amounts of money through reduction in illness of both baby and mother. When rates of breastfeeding at hospital discharge were compared between facilities that employed certified lactation consultants and those that did not, those having LCs had a 2.28 times increase in the odds of breastfeeding at hospital discharge (Castrucci, Hoover, Lim, et al., 2006).

Studies show that peer counselor interventions are also effective (see Chapter 25). Clearly lactation services improve the health of our nation, but we have yet to document the extent of this effect in terms of money savings.

Certification

In 1981, experienced La Leche League leaders JoAnne Scott and Linda Smith were asked to develop a certification and training program for lactation consultants. This need derived from (1) an awareness that many healthcare providers discredited the accomplishments of the volunteer

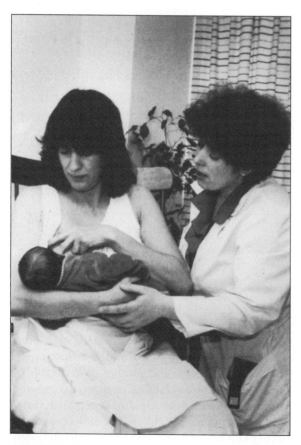

FIGURE 1–1 Early assistance promotes maternal confidence.

because she was unpaid, and (2) a need to establish minimum standards for individuals who were already providing LC services for a fee. A certification program was viewed as a way to recognize the important role of the volunteer and to provide a credential that identified competence.

Scott and Smith assembled a small group of breastfeeding experts who had come to the field of lactation through voluntary service, mostly through La Leche League. In 1984, these individuals gathered and concluded that legitimacy of the field would be heightened if minimal standards of knowledge and skills were recognized through a certification examination. Subsequently, they developed the lactation consultant certification examination based on a three-dimensional content outline or test blueprint and derived from practice analysis.

The first examination was administered in July 1985 under the International Board of Lactation Consultant Examiners (IBLCE). Since 1985, a certification examination has been given annually (Table 1–2). To date, more than 15,000 candidates have been certified, the majority of whom live in Australia, the United States, and Canada. In 2008, IBLCE administered its 23rd annual examination in locations across 36 counties and territories. The test has been administered in English, Dutch, French, German, Italian, Korean, Spanish, Arabic, Japanese, Polish, Swedish, Hebrew, Italian, and Portuguese. The largest numbers of candidates have been in Australia, Canada, Europe, and the United States. Periodic recertification as an LC is required through the acquisition of continuing education credits and by reexamination. This dual-recertification option increases the likelihood that the LC will remain current. Guidelines for becoming certified by IBLCE are found in Appendix D.

IBLCE maintains a current registry of lactation specialists who are certified by the International Board of Lactation Consultant Examiners. Examiners and regulators can thus confirm that an individual is currently certified. For more information on lactation consultant certification, go to the International Board of Lactation Consultant Examiners Web site at www.iblce.org.

Certification, a process by which an individual demonstrates clinical competence in a specialty, is

| TABLE 1–2 | IBLCE Examination Summary Data, 1985–2007 | | | |

Year of Examination	Number of Candidates	Mean Score	Pass-Fail Score	Pass Rate (%)
1985	259	72.8	61.8	94.6
1990	428	72.1	64.6	89.3
1995	1,556	73.8	61.8	94.1
2000	1,862	72.7	60.9	87.8
2001	2,070	76.7	66.7	88.6
2002	2,536	75.4	65.0	90.4
2003	2,094	78.4	67.0	93.3
2004	2,163	77.5	64.0	95.4
2005	2,683	80.4	65	96.8
2006	3,207	77.9	65	95.1
2007	2,941	81.1	67	94.8
2008	3,323	77.8	65	93.5

Source: International Board of Lactation Consultant Examiners (IBLCE), www.iblce.org.

a valued and popular credential, especially in the United States. More than 40 specialty certifications exist in the field of nursing alone, despite the fact that certification is a voluntary credential. Certified nurses and healthcare workers from across a wide variety of specialties consistently place a high value on certification (Niebuhr & Biel, 2007). Nurses in the United States and Canada who earned certification in a specialty area report they felt more confident and experienced fewer errors in patient care since they were certified; thus certification may be a marker for excellence (Cary, 2000; Raudonis & Anderson, 2002).

ILCA

About the same time that IBLCE certification began, the International Lactation Consultant Association (ILCA) formed as the professional organization for LCs. ILCA has played a vital role in continuing education, development and promotion of the LC, and promoting policies to protect and support breastfeeding worldwide. Bailey (2005) points out that ILCA's action have arisen primarily through the grassroots vision and

creativity of its members, such as creation of World Breastfeeding Week Action Kits and the Research Poster Session at the annual conference. ILCA's Web site is a rich and current source for information on conferences and courses. It also contains a listing of LCs and other practical resources such as low-cost professional liability insurance to help aspiring and practicing LCs in their practice (www.ilca.org). In 2006, ILCA divided into separate organizations according to country. For example, USLCA is the professional organization for LCs living in the United States.

Getting a Job as a Lactation Specialist

Most lactation consultants are health professionals who start their career in a job where they work with breastfeeding dyads. They learn about breastfeeding on the job and by personal experience rather than as part of their formal education. Others begin by affiliation with La Leche League and take the necessary courses and gain clinical experience to become certified. Applying for an LC position takes planning to be successful.

Interviewing for a Job

You discover that a position for a lactation consultant is available locally, and you want to apply. Here are some steps to follow to prepare for the interview:

- Research the position. What are the expected skills and experiences needed? Does your background match these skills and experiences? Some state laws limit clinical service to licensed medical or nursing staff, often for legal reasons. A common requirement for a hospital-based job as a lactation consultant is experience working with new mothers and babies, and certification by the IBLCE.
- Research the organization. Is it a clinic, medical office, or small or large hospital? If it is a hospital, how many deliveries does it have each year? Who is its competition? If it does not provide lactation services and a competing hospital does, highlight this lack as a major selling point for your services.
- Identify your strengths and weaknesses. Be ready to highlight skills, experience, personal qualities, and accomplishments you would bring to the healthcare agency.
- Keep in mind that first impressions count. Your appearance tells the interviewer quite a bit about your character. You want the interviewer to see you as a professional in every way including personal hygiene and wardrobe. An expensive outfit is not necessary, but your clothing should fit well and be clean and pressed. A business suit with a knee-length skirt is always appropriate.
- Know what salary to expect before you begin to interview. LCs employed by a hospital or birth center are usually paid on the same scale as staff nurses. Wages will differ according to the region you live in; however, US hospital staff nurses receive an average hourly rate of about $24. Average annual nursing income is listed in Table 1–3. Note that nurses working in a physician's medical office receive the lowest pay.
- Follow the general rule that if an employer does not bring up the subject of salary, don't ask about it until you have a job offer. Until you have that offer, salary doesn't matter. Once

you have the offer, you can negotiate from a position of greater power.
- Evaluate the benefits being offered. Insurance (disability, life, and medical) and a 401(k) or 401(b) retirement plan with matches from your employer must be kept in mind. These extras can make a difference in the total compensation package. Although malpractice is rare with breastfeeding situations, it is not rare in obstetrics, and the LC might become involved in a legal case. Generally, those working in a hospital or community health agency will not need malpractice insurance.

Hafner-Eaton (2000) reported a wide range in hourly wages in her survey of 169 LCs (Table 1–4). She found that nurse practitioners or certified nurse–midwives who are also lactation consultants make the highest annual salary ($61,000).

Gaining Clinical Experience

IBLCE certification requires a considerable number of clinical hours of direct care of the breastfeeding dyad: from 300 to 1,000 clinical hours.

A healthcare professional who needs clinical hours to qualify as an applicant to take the LC certification examination should seek out a job where she will work with breastfeeding mothers to accumulate clinical hours. Working on a mother–baby unit in a hospital is an example.

TABLE 1–3	Average Annual Income of US Nurses

Setting	Average Annual Income ($)
Hospital	53,450
Community/home health	48,990
Physician's office	48,250
Mean annual earnings	52,330
Hourly wages	26.87

Source: Allied Physicians, 2006.

TABLE 1-4	Average Wage and Consult Time of Lactation Consultants		
Practice Setting	**Hourly Wage ($)**	**Initial Consult ($)**	**Length of Consult (min)**
Private	55	79	95
Clinic	43	69	64
Hospital	28	62	74

Source: Hafner-Eaton, 2000.

The individual who is still in a school to become a healthcare professional can investigate the possibility of taking a supervised clinical practicum as a part of a degree. For each hour spent in a clinical practicum, a student can reduce the number of hours needed to take the exam.

Opportunities for clinical experience working with breastfeeding dyads are an issue when the individual who wishes to become an LC does not have access to clinical learning. Not everyone who desires to work as a lactation consultant wishes to become a nurse or other type of health professional. There are other ways to acquire practical experience working with breastfeeding dyads:

- Seek out a formal clinical teaching program in lactation management. The few available programs are of high quality, but you may have to travel to another part of the state (or country) in order to do the clinical practice. Sometimes a clinical arrangement can be made in your own area. For example, some students have completed their clinical requirements by working with a local pediatrician (Smillie, 2000).
- Join La Leche League and become an LLL Leader. The IBLCE will give credit for each year of active practice as a leader. Because the women attending LLL meetings are either pregnant or have breastfed for a long time, it will give you an opportunity to observe the needs and concerns of mothers just learning about breastfeeding and those who have extensive experience.
- Become a WIC peer counselor. As a peer counselor, IBLCE will grant 500 practice hours for each year that you are active in the field.

- Work in a medical office as a breastfeeding specialist teaching breastfeeding classes and counseling mothers.
- Contract with an IBLCE certified health professional to observe and assist in a clinical setting. Sometimes called *shadowing*, observing a qualified practitioner at work can take place in a clinical agency such as a hospital, in a community health clinic, or in a medical office (see Box 1–1). Permission for such an experience will need to be obtained from both the LC and the supervisor or director of the clinical agency.
- Round out your experience by visiting different work settings. For example, if your experience has been in a hospital, visit a WIC clinic to learn about the issues associated with breastfeeding older children or make arrangements to observe a breastfeeding mother in her home environment. Conversely, if your work setting has been a medical office or WIC clinic, go to a hospital setting.
- Keep track of and document the hours spent working with breastfeeding mothers either as paid staff or in a volunteer capacity. Accurate records of contact hours are necessary in order to apply to take the certification examination.

Medical Clinics

A growing number of physicians are emphasizing breastfeeding in their practices. For some this entails advocating for breastfeeding among patients in their general practice (family practice, obstetrics, or pediatrics) and providing staff to assist mothers to be successful. For other physicians, their general

---

BOX 1–1

Shadowing Guidelines

- Seek permission from the preceptor and the client being observed. The facility or LC may welcome you, but the mother may feel uncomfortable. Obey protocols such as wearing scrubs.
- As an observer, introduce yourself and speak only when appropriate.
- Take copious notes on what you've observed.
- Arrange with the preceptor to spend time after the observation period to discuss the cases and ask questions.
- Always thank the client being observed for her willingness to allow you into her "space."

- Do not observe on a day when you have a cold, sore throat, diarrhea, or allergies.
- Thank the preceptor in person and again with a note. Let her know how she has facilitated your education. Stress the positive things you experienced and saw.
- If there were problems during the observation, discuss these with your faculty or mentor.

Source: Smith, 2002.

---

practice also becomes a consulting practice for more complex breastfeeding problems referred by lactation consultants or other physicians. A small number of physicians are developing breastfeeding and lactation specialty clinics or programs either in an academic setting or as a private practice. The specialty clinics serve as tertiary referral practices for complicated medical conditions of mother and baby, for conditions that require prescription medications, or for minor procedures that may be indicated (e.g., frenotomy for tongue-tie). These tertiary centers often rely upon the close working relationships of the physicians with other nonphysician lactation consultants. Some of these offices have retail services that can provide their patients and clients with needed breast pumps, feeding devices, and other accessories. See the section on reimbursement for physicians' breastfeeding services.

Lactation Consultant Education

Most lactation consultants have another healthcare degree in an area such as nursing, medicine, dietetics, or physical therapy, and they obtain certification as an LC as a second credential. Being a health professional who is also a lactation consultant offers greater job security. In addition, this also means you will have already taken many of the courses that are required to be eligible to take the IBLCE certification examination.

As the number of lactation consultants working in health care increases, so does the availability of educational courses on lactation. Although lactation certification by IBLCE is considered the gold standard, other certifications have sprung up, including certification as a "lactation counselor" and as a "lactation educator." These programs are geared toward people, such as WIC personnel, who do not wish to become lactation consultants but want to be more knowledgeable about breastfeeding.

Wilson-Clay (2000) believes that lactation specialists have an identity crisis partly owing to inconsistent professional education. Claiming that a common education creates a sense of shared values, tradition, and practice, she calls for a comprehensive course of study on lactation followed by examination and certification to guarantee consumers that someone with the LC title will be competent. In response to a call for educational standards, ILCA has moved toward a formal accreditation of educational programs that meet criteria for preparing lactation consultants.

Lactation Programs

A New York state law mandated in 1984 that any institution providing care for new mothers and babies had to have at least one person on staff that was designated to serve as a resource for other staff members and to provide breastfeeding assistance to patients. This landmark event helped launch the subsequent growth of the lactation consultant as a clinical specialty.

The 1990s could be characterized as the decade for the emergence of breastfeeding programs and clinics. Only a small number of hospitals in the United States had a lactation program in the early 1990s. But within the past two decades lactation programs have proliferated and most hospitals and birth centers now have lactation services staffed by certified lactation specialists, who have thus grown in numbers and visibility. Although lactation expertise has long been integrated into midwifery practice in countries where midwives predominate, LCs are becoming more common, especially in Australia, Canada, and Europe.

Opportunities for paid positions have increased to the point that hospitals now advertise for lactation consultants (Figure 1–2). Medical centers tend to hire registered nurses into lactation consultant positions because of state practice regulations concerning direct care of patients and because nurses can work in other units of the hospital if the maternity area census is low.

A lactation program may take many guises and offer a variety of services (Box 1–2). A breast pump rental depot, because it is so likely to generate revenue, may serve as a first kind of service for breastfeeding women (Rago, 1987). The Overlake Hospital in Bellevue, Washington, started with a

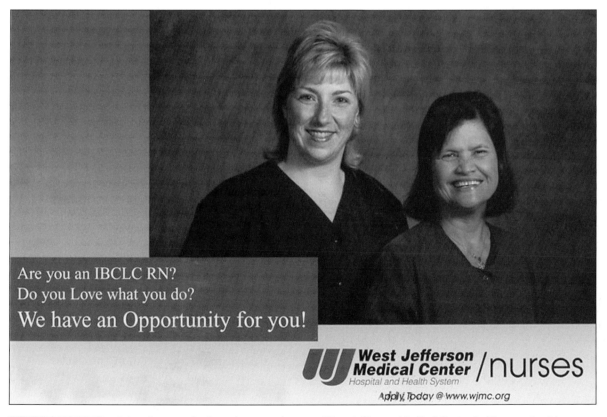

FIGURE **1–2** Advertisement for lactation consultants at West Jefferson Medical Center in Marrero, Louisiana.

Source: Courtesy of West Jefferson Medical Center.

rental station for 10 hospital-grade pumps. It now has 150 pumps, and the majority of these, at any given time, are rented. Their women and infants boutique carries nursing pillows, nursing bras, infant clothing, CDs, books, and much more (Chagnon & Wehmeyer, 2004).

A lactation program may also develop out of a patient education program that began with childbirth preparation and other classes designed to meet the many needs of pregnant and postpartum women and their families. For clientele who have already developed rapport with the patient educator, additional classes may be provided, including prenatal breastfeeding classes and follow-up services after the baby is born.

Other programs may have begun in neonatal intensive care units and later expanded to the rest of the hospital, or they may be the outcome of patient surveys that indicate the need for lactation services. Still others may have developed from a hospital needing to "keep up with the medical Joneses"—meaning, when a competing hospital provides and then publicizes its lactation consultant services, other hospitals compete by providing similar services, such as the lactation clinic seen in Figure 1–3.

How those services are structured varies by the institution. In some programs, the LC sees all new mothers who indicate that they plan to breastfeed. In other cases, she sees all new mothers, identifying her clients when they tell her how they are feeding or planning to feed their babies. A few lactation specialists counsel both breastfeeding and bottle-feeding mothers. Other institutions restrict the LC's contact only to those breastfeeding mothers for whom the referring physician has asked for a consultation and follow-up care. Most of the time hospital-based specialists work on the birthing unit and/or postpartum area and neonatal intensive care, but they also assist breastfeeding mothers who are hospitalized in other areas. Thus their rounds take them to the surgical and medical units and to intensive care. The LC can also consult with women in the hospital for premature labor.

Workload Issues

Whatever system is used, it is wise to estimate the anticipated workload prior to the start of the lactation service. As one hard-working LC notes, "We have one breastfeeding professional each day we work and usually have 12–15 breastfeeding

---

BOX 1–2

Hospital-Based Lactation Programs and Services

- Daily one-on-one mother-baby rounds. Every breastfeeding mother seen by LC without referral or breastfeeding mothers seen only with referral
- Telephone hotline or "warmline"; post-discharge telephone calls
- Prenatal classes on breastfeeding
- Home postpartum visits and assistance with breastfeeding
- Pump rental and sales

- Postpartum breastfeeding consults for problems by appointment or "open clinic" hours
- Continuing education for staff, area seminars, preceptorships, and breastfeeding classes
- Research on lactation and breastfeeding issues (most often at a tertiary-care medical center)
- Evaluation of lactation products, devices, and services

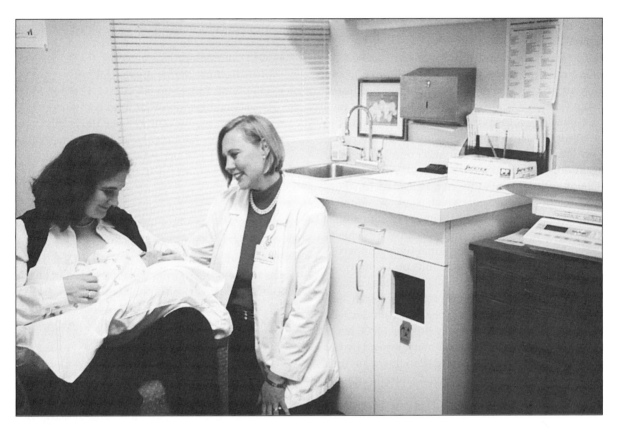

FIGURE 1–3 A hospital-based lactation clinic.

Source: With permission, Pardee Hinson.

women to see, in addition to phone calls, outpatients, pediatric, and NICU patients. We are supposed to be done in 8 hours, but guess what? It's usually 9–10." Most hospital-based programs have been in existence 6 to 10 years and employ two to eight LCs who mostly work part-time. For example, in some hospitals, three part-time LCs share 7 days per week coverage. The actual number of work hours should be based upon the number of births in the institution and the percentage of mothers who are breastfeeding.

I roughly estimate three visits (one 20-minute initial visit and two 15-minute follow-ups) from a lactation consultant for a total 50 minutes per dyad per day. Given these numbers, a lactation specialist would spend about 8 hours each day to see 10 dyads on a mother–baby unit. That does not take into account time spent charting, having lunch, meetings,

planning, and so on. Daily rounds on breastfeeding women may be feasible in a hospital in which the LC sees fewer than 10 patients per day; it may not be feasible if more than 10 breastfeeding mothers are housed in the maternity unit on a given day—unless there is more than one specialist in the service or staff members providing other care are trained to provide optimal lactation-related care as well, thus reserving the LC for mothers and babies needing additional help and as a resource for the staff.

Thus, in a hospital with 200 births per month with an 80% breastfeeding rate, the lactation specialist will see about six to eight patients on weekdays (and fewer on the weekend). A hospital with 3000 deliveries each year should have a minimum of three full-time LC positions or six part-time positions. This staffing produces a bare minimum coverage that usually results in understaffing and/or part-time coverage. The service—to be effective—should be available 7 days a week, on all shifts.

Lactation consultant Pardee Hinson reported 2.6 FTEs (full-time equivalents) LC positions (about 90 hours) for a hospital with 1600 deliveries (Hinson, 2000). These lactation consultants used to see each breastfeeding mother every day but now, in order to be able to keep up with the demand for their services, they see each breastfeeding mother once and see her again only if there is a referral. In an effort to meet patient needs, it is not uncommon for LCs to volunteer additional time for which they are unpaid. Heinig (1998) addressed this issue as "closet consulting," warning that when the caseload is invisible to the employer, the LC's professional time is undervalued and may result in further limits on LC time.

The two reports above are only "educated guesses." Recently Mannel and Mannel (2006) collected data from the hospital's lactation program's productivity reports at a tertiary care teaching hospital (4200 births per year). They measured actual hours worked by LCs over a 2-year period, allocated the hours to their respective activities, and developed ratios for optimal international board-certified lactation consultant (IBCLC) staffing for each component of service. Optimal IBCLC staffing was calculated as follows:

- Mother–baby inpatient care requires 1 full-time equivalent (FTE) per 783 breastfeeding couplets.
- Neonatal intensive care unit (NICU) inpatient care requires 1 FTE per 235 infant admissions.
- Mother–baby outpatient care requires 1 FTE per 1292 breastfeeding couplets discharged.
- NICU outpatient care requires 1 FTE per 818 breastfeeding infants discharged.
- Telephone follow-up requires 1 FTE per 3915 breastfeeding couplets or infants discharged.
- Education requires 0.1 FTE per 1000 deliveries.
- Program development and administration requires 0.1 FTE per 1000 deliveries.
- Research requires 0.1 to 0.2 FTE total.

Using this ratio data, IBCLC staffing needs can be calculated for hospital staffing according to number of deliveries (Box 1–3). All three hospitals have inpatient service, follow-up telephone service and education, administration, and research. Table 1–5 is a calculation of the staffing needs for a hospital with 3000 births per year using the Mannel and Mannel (2006) model. A similar table for hospitals with 1000 and 6000 births per year can be found in the *Journal of Human Lactation* (Mannel & Mannel).

Developing a Lactation Program

In proposing a lactation program, it is essential to realize that such a service will overlap with the interests of several ongoing departments or programs. As a result, it is both politic and appropriate to involve all such departments in the early stages of the proposal process. Touching base with hospital decision makers and developing a working relationship

---

BOX 1–3

Lactation Staffing According to Hospital Size

Hospital Size	FTEs
1. Hospital with 1000 deliveries/yr with a 85% breastfeeding rate, outpatient service. No neonatal services. (Mannel & Mannel, 2006)	2.6
2. Hospital with 3000 deliveries/yr with a 68% breastfeeding rate and neonatal services. No outpatient service. (Angeron & Riordan, 2007)	5.4
3. Hospital with 6000 deliveries/yr with a 70% breastfeeding rate and neonatal services. 50% outpatient service. (Mannel & Mannel, 2006)	13.6

TABLE 1–5 Breakdown of Staffing for Hospital Lactation Program with 3,000 Births per Year

Approx. number of births/yr = 3000 (68% initiate breastfeeding)

Approx. number of NICU admissions/yr = 400 (85% initiate breastfeeding)

One FTE = 1900 work hours (excluding vacations, sick days, etc.)
    1292 hours direct consult time
    608 hours indirect clinical time

FTE ratio is number of available direct consult work hours divided by the amount of hours per dyad.

For example, 1292 hours/FTE divided by 1.65 hrs of direct consult with each dyad = 783 dyads per LC FTE. 2040 births (68% breastfeeding of 3000) divided by 783 = the number of LC FTEs that are needed for direct consult inpatient care.

Category	FTE Ratio	Calculation	Number	FTEs
Inpatient	1:783	3000 × .68 = 2040	2040/783 =	2.6
Outpatient	1:1292	120 couples 120 hours (1 hr each)	1292/120 =	0.1
Telephone	1:3915	3000 × .60	1800/3915 =	0.45
NICU inpatient	1:235	400 × .85 85% initiate BF	340/235 =	1.44
Education	0.1:1000	3000 × .68	2040/1000 =	0.2
Program admin	0.1:1000	3000 × .68	2040/1000 =	0.2
Research/QA	0.2:1000	3000 × .68	2040/1000 =	0.4
Total				about 5.4

Source: Adapted from Mannel & Mannel, 2006.

with them is critical. Without it, any hope of establishing and maintaining a program is seriously undermined, and the likelihood of the program becoming and remaining an integral part of the institution remains low. For example, when planning the postpartum follow-up program at Overlake Hospital, pediatricians were included in the planning to avoid the fear that the program would replace the 10-day physician visit for the newborn (Chagnon & Wehmeyer, 2004).

The hospital-based lactation specialist often creates her own position when hospital administrative personnel respond to patient demands for lactation services. She develops a plan for providing lactation services and then presents a proposal to administration for approval.

No new program will be implemented without someone in power pushing it, especially in a downsizing environment. A sponsor with "clout" is needed to lend momentum beyond the actions of the innovators and to commit resources from the institutional budget. This person can be a high-level administrator, a chief of staff, or department chair.

Department heads particularly critical to securing support for the new program include the director of maternity nursing (who may oversee labor and delivery, postpartum and nursery units, and sometimes the intensive care nursery); the director of the pediatric unit; and the chairman or medical director for obstetrics, pediatrics, and family medicine. If the institution has a midwifery service, the support of its director should also be sought. One option is a lactation service that contracts with the hospital for services. Using the contract services, the hospital saves money because it does not pay for benefits for the lactation consultants who see its patients (Ferrarello, 2001).

If the institution has an employee health service or a women's health clinic, their supervisors should be informed of the proposal and asked for their support. Written proposals or documents that highlight how the new program will assist and support the services that are already being provided helps build their acceptance. For example, the head of employee health may be particularly interested in learning that the lactation program will include services to employees, such as a special place where employees returning to work after the birth of a baby can hand express or pump their breasts or nurse their babies during work hours (Dodgson & Duckett, 1997).

Hospital administrators choose new programs from dozens of possibilities for hospital investment (for example, another magnetic resonance imager versus a new diabetes center). Administration looks at two "bottom-line" factors—revenue and marketing potential—of proposed services before selecting which to offer. In deciding on any new health program, money speaks loudest.

Lactation services are usually provided in a single area that serves as the home base for telephone follow-up and inpatient services, as well as record keeping and as a site for professional resources. LCs can also see mothers who return for outpatient care in this area. In addition to outpatient services, some hospitals offer postpartum home visits as a part of the insurance coverage for the delivery. Nurses can do bilirubin checks to screen for jaundice and newborn hearing screening as well as assess breastfeeding and weight. During a postpartum visit this "perk" differs according to the insurance company with which the hospital contracts for deliveries. Income generated from inpatient care is managed through the regular accounting or finance office and submitted for insurance coverage, as occurs for other hospital-based charges.

Although lactation services generate minimal revenue compared to high-tech medical equipment, they are an effective marketing tool for the hospital. In the United States and many other developed countries, the women most likely to breastfeed are educated and in middle-to-higher income brackets; thus, a lactation service increases the hospital's visibility and credibility with young, educated families who have a high earning potential later on. The income-generating nature of patient care makes such a service attractive, particularly in settings in which several local hospitals are competing for the same patient dollars. The new trend in hospitals is product-line management, an approach that markets a product line of services: lactation services are a "product" that medical centers can offer to their "customers."

Just as the lack of physicians' support can prevent a program from being added to the array of services already offered, physician support can pave the way for the addition of a lactation program. Such support is most likely to be obtained if the key physicians—often chiefs of service or department heads—see that a lactation program will meet needs that they feel are important. In some cases, a female physician who has personal breastfeeding experience champions the need for such a service.

Physicians are still influential figures in the hospital although their power has diminished since managed care; therefore, maintaining positive relations with physicians is critical. Even with managed care, the physician as "gatekeeper" plays a major role in the fiscal health of a hospital. If the physician's patients do not want to go to a particular hospital because it lacks certain amenities—such as a lactation service—the birthing service administrator, with the backing of physicians, may create such a program rather than lose patients to a competing institution. Supportive physicians are more likely to be mothers who breastfed, fathers of breastfed children, those building a new practice, and those from countries where breastfeeding is the norm.

Marketing

Marketing—a discipline used by business to convert people's needs into profitable company opportunities—is still poorly understood and appreciated by health workers; either they need to learn marketing techniques themselves or seek assistance from marketing experts. Nurse entrepreneurs can attend marketing classes, read books on marketing, or seek help from small-business centers at universities that help small businesses at no cost.

The following are basic marketing techniques that LCs may find useful:

- Collect data such as the number and percentage of women giving birth who breastfeed, and survey women who have used lactation services.
- Analyze strengths and weaknesses of competitors and focus on service needs not currently being met.
- Establish a niche within the healthcare market that is ignored by large healthcare providers—for example, a postdischarge visit for a back-to-work consult.
- Promote the practice by advertising and through public relations: brochures, newsletters, letterhead stationery, business cards, fact sheets, and radio and TV interviews all help to inform clients and other health workers about LC services (Gardner & Weinrauch, 1988).

The Unique Characteristics of Counseling Breastfeeding Women

There are unique aspects of working with breastfeeding women that differ from other aspects of health care. Breastfeeding is an emotion-laden subject that may be viewed as an integral part of human sexuality, not just an infant feeding method. It touches deep-seated feelings that people have about themselves and their bodies that reach back to childhood. This emotional content makes breastfeeding counseling, like sex counseling or childbirth education, unusually sensitive. Healthcare workers assisting breastfeeding families must be especially intuitive, caring listeners and advisors.

Working with new mothers and babies is a popular and thus, competitive, activity. Not only are newborns adorable, but also the mothers and fathers are (generally) healthy and happy. By working on the hospital maternity unit or in a birth center, the nurse gets to play a paid, starring role in the usually joyous family dramas of birthing and early breastfeeding. As a result, nurses compete to work there, and the mother–baby unit has a low rate of staff turnover.

Breastfeeding counseling is almost exclusively provided by women who must daily interact and work with other women: mothers and other female health workers. Women interact in the workplace differently than men do. Awareness and understanding of the

typical ways that women interact and compete with each other gives the lactation specialist who comes onto the unit or into the community agency as a "new kid on the block" an advantage (Gilligan, 1982). Table 1–6 summarizes how women tend to work together and how they need to work together. Three characteristics—the emotional quality of breastfeeding, the popularity of caring for babies, and the dysfunctional, covert games that women bring to the work environment—set the stage for potential difficulties between the LC and the nurse, the nurse and the breastfeeding mother, the volunteer counselor and the LC, and the female physician and the LC.

Although workplace standards of behavior tend to follow men's rules, it does not negate feminine elements. Feminine, nurturing qualities help us in working with breastfeeding families. Our best qualities have to do with becoming attached and developing close relationships and friendships with others. These attributes are critical for all healthcare workers, including LCs, if they are to empathize with breastfeeding mothers. However, when women personalize the business or professional setting, it is counterproductive to their professional or business goals.

Survival in the workplace requires that we learn to operate within two concurrent cultures: the culture of nurturing and caring and the culture of the profession's business, which is about accomplishing tasks efficiently. Virginia Woolf noted that the values of women differ from the values of men; yet, she added, "It is the masculine values that prevail" (Woolf, 1929). Women succeed in the workplace when they use their womanly strengths of compassion and intuitiveness in their work, while playing by men's rules.

Roles and Responsibilities

The LC is responsible to the mothers she sees to provide up-to-date and accurate information and appropriate assistance. Quality practice and service are core responsibilities of a profession to the public. ILCA standards of practice are measures or levels of quality that are models for the conduct and evaluation of practice (ILCA, 2008) (See Appendix A). Table 1–7 lists the six competency areas or functions required by an LC practice. Depending upon the setting, however, these will be molded by the other services also provided there.

TABLE 1–6	**Correcting Negative Female Workplace Behaviors**

What Women Tend to Do	**What Women Need to Learn to Do**
Women tend to express anger covertly behind their co-workers' backs rather than openly and confrontationally. Girls learn that they should be "nice" to everyone, not fight, and especially not hit anyone. These concepts are called Mommy's Rules (Davidson-Crews, 1989), and they are deeply embedded female behaviors, especially in white, middle-class, American women.	Be overt, not covert. If there's a problem, confront, forget, and move on.
Women try to avoid being criticized; they often take it personally. Women are socialized to derive their self-worth from external, rather than internal, sources; therefore, they tend to react excessively to others' opinions, whether positive or negative. Women are more likely to hold grudges for long periods.	Communicate. Do not make scenes or public outbursts.
Women tend to become over friendly, one-to-one. Women who work together and become fast friends tell each other their deepest secrets, which are sometimes used against them when the friendship dissolves. Women give away power by giving away too much of themselves. Women are more likely to work for social rewards; men work for money.	Be friendly, but do not strive to be close friends.
Women are less likely than men to have used the give-and-take team concept of "you help me and I'll help you and we'll both get ahead." Women operate on a higher utopian level: what is right and just is more important than any other consideration. Women act as police officers of one another, making sure that what their coworkers do is right and correct and "trashing" them to keep them in their place.	Accept and love yourself. Accept (and appreciate) that some people are not your friends, now or ever.

LCs report that the majority of their time is spent in direct care of clients. The role of the LC closely parallels that of the clinical nurse specialist insofar as it requires in-depth clinical knowledge and expertise in a particular area. Gibbins et al. (2000) describe a model of the nurse practitioner (NP) or clinical nurse specialist (CNS) in the role as a lactation consultant in a breastfeeding clinic. This advanced practice role encompasses the dimensions of the advanced practice model: research, leadership, education, and clinical practice. Like the clinical specialist, the LC does the following:

- Gives direct care
- Teaches
- Consults
- Conducts or assists in conducting research

Giving breastfeeding mothers consistent breastfeeding information is vital. The patient takes for granted that the person to whom she spoke knows exactly what should be done. If confusion or controversy is found among the staff, we cannot expect the patient to become knowledgeable and comfortable with learning mother–infant tasks. Staff in-services on breastfeeding increase the likelihood that the staff will provide consistent information.

Although providing in-service education is an important, perhaps even essential, role of the lactation consultant, one can (like the proverbial horse brought to water) offer but not impel other healthcare workers to drink from the pool of knowledge. Other nursing staff may have fallen into the habit of expecting the LC to take care of all breastfeeding issues. If an LC is not available on all shifts or all days, this person cannot possibly always take care of things. Rather than

TABLE 1–7	**Required Competencies for Lactation Practice**

1. Breastfeeding education and advocacy
2. Clinical management of breastfeeding
3. Technical knowledge
4. Special knowledge and assistance
5. Professional responsibilities and activities
6. Business practices/legal considerations

expecting the LC to do it all, it is more effective for her to teach the staff, so that all healthcare workers are operating from the same frame of reference in how they assist breastfeeding mothers and when they will intervene to resolve a difficulty (Shrago, 1995).

Another function of the LC, whether she is located in a hospital or has a private practice, is to evaluate services and products related to lactation. Evaluating new products and then publishing the results is a professional responsibility. Seeking feedback from patients helps ensure that quality service is being provided (Turner, 1996).

Stages of Role Development

Roles of health professionals have been extensively studied and shown to progress through stages of development. For example, Benner (1984) used the Dreyfus and Dreyfus (1980) model of skill acquisition to describe the progression of skills and competencies of nurses in the clinical setting. This model, a structure for the metamorphosis that occurs as nurses persevere in their practice, can also apply to lactation consultants. According to Benner (1984), there are five stages of role acquisition:

- Novice: Develops technical skills, has narrow scope of practice, needs a mentor
- Advanced beginner: Enhances clinical competencies, develops diagnostic reasoning and clinical decision-making skills, begins to incorporate research findings into practice
- Competent: Expands scope of practice, becomes competent in diagnostic reasoning and clinical skills, senses nuances, develops organizational skills

- Proficient: Achieves highest level of clinical expertise, conducts or directs research projects, acts as change agent, uses holistic approach, interprets nuances
- Expert: Global scope of practice, consults widely, empowers patients and families, serves as mentor

Benner derived these insights from the stories nurses told about their practice and applied them into a logical, orderly progression of skill development. Joel (1997, p. 7) paints a vivid picture of the journey from novice to expert:

> *At first we see situations as tidbits of equal significance; later we move to the idea of a highly complex integrated whole where some pieces are just more important to solving the problem. And, finally the nurse becomes as one with the clinical situation. Rather than looking from the outside in, at the zenith of your practice, you are indivisible from the puzzle you are challenged to solve. You move right to the heart of the matter without responding to distraction.*

Using Benner's model from novice to expert as discussed earlier, LCs—such as experienced clinical nurse specialists—will spend more time as consultant and in scholarly work as they gain experience in the field (Auerbach, Riordan, & Gross, 2000). Because the role of the lactation consultant is relatively new, other health providers may be unclear about what to expect of this new healthcare worker. To clarify areas of expertise that can be expected of such an individual, the International Lactation Consultant Association has developed a set of recommendations and related competencies for LC practice (see Appendix A).

Lactation Consultants in the Community Setting

Because of the heightened awareness of the importance of breastfeeding, community health workers are becoming educated about breastfeeding, and some of them go on to certify as an LC. The 1989 WIC Reauthorization Act that mandated a breastfeeding coordinator in each state accelerated community health workers' interest in breastfeeding.

Most of these coordinators are registered dietitians or registered nurses. Home health nurses are another group of community-based health workers who frequently care for breastfeeding families.

Community-based health care is different from hospital-based care in that the healthcare provider works with the mother over the long term—throughout her pregnancy, childbirth, and postpartum course; thus community-based healthcare workers have an advantage over those working in the hospital in that they see the mother and her family in a total environment. Someone once described this as seeing a whole movie; whereas, in the hospital one sees only one frame. Being in the family home gives a much wider perspective on the mother's needs that are not otherwise apparent. For example, I visited a breastfeeding mother in her home along with a student nurse as a clinical experience. The client was a 15-year-old new mother who recently arrived from Mexico and had no family members here. She was having trouble putting the baby to breast because of extreme engorgement. After we pumped and got the baby on the breast, I suggested that we freeze the milk, since I thought she probably had not thought of this, given her youth and inexperience. She motioned me to her refrigerator and opened the freezer section, which held many bottles of breastmilk that she had expressed and saved. Clearly, this young woman had much more knowledge about lactation than I could have surmised by seeing her one time in the hospital before she was discharged.

Moreover community-based services are organized around a system of interdisciplinary community services and resources. Many times the community health nurse works with mothers who are poor and receive welfare assistance, where breastfeeding problems are but a minor star in a firmament of despairing circumstances.

Worksite Lactation Programs

Corporate lactation programs pay off. Women prefer to work at jobs where the breastfeeding woman is welcomed. Not only that, but breastfeeding mothers miss less work than mothers who are formula feeding (Cohen, Mrtek, & Mrtek, 1995). As a result corporate offices are becoming "breastfeeding friendly" with pumping rooms and hospital-grade pumps. Mothers working full-time spend less than

1 hour over the course of one workday expressing breastmilk. Click (2006) recommends basics for worksite pumping rooms:

- Privacy partitions (to accommodate 1–2 women)
- Breast pumps
- Wastebasket
- Cleaning solution
- Clock
- Sink with running water
- Reading materials

Medical Office

Physicians, especially pediatricians, realize the value of having staff who are knowledgeable about breastfeeding and can quickly and effectively work with breastfeeding women in their practice; thus lactation consultants are employed in the medical office. Their responsibilities include answering phone calls from breastfeeding women, making home visits, and working with the physician during postpartum visits to the medical office and making hospital rounds. The physician office usually pays the lactation consultant a salary; however, advanced practice nurses such as pediatric nurse practitioners may do their own billing.

Lactation Consultants and Volunteer Counselors

The client is apt to obtain more complete services when lactation consultants maintain a congenial, reciprocal relationship with volunteer counselors as well as other healthcare professionals in their community.

The volunteer counselor and the lactation consultant provide similar services. They most often differ about where such service is provided, the nature of clinical assistance, and the degree of follow-up care. For example, volunteer counselors are an excellent source of preventive healthcare information pertaining to breastfeeding and lactation. They also spend more time giving long-term assistance than the LC, particularly if the latter sees clients in a clinic or hospital setting. It is not uncommon for a mother to continue to receive assistance and caring concern from a volunteer counselor through the entire lactation course; only rarely will an LC meet with a client regularly through that entire period. Instead, she is more apt to have sporadic contact, initiated by the client when a specific question or concern arises. The LC is more apt to assist a mother when specific clinical skills are needed to assess or to resolve a problem.

Volunteer breastfeeding helpers and lactation specialists can assist one another (Thorley, 2000). The volunteer may have seen a certain mother in her own home and thus may be able to alert the LC working in a hospital, doctor's office, or clinic to elements about the mother's home life that may bear on her lactation course. The LC may serve as a referral source for persons with complex problems. When the LC works in a medical center where ongoing research is part of her role, she helps generate new knowledge. Both the volunteer and the paid LC can review materials written for clients. The volunteer may be sensitive to ongoing issues that crop up after the mother has left the hospital or does not choose to mention to her healthcare providers. The LC may be aware of aspects of the healthcare system that influence breastfeeding.

Mentoring and Networking

Mentoring and networking serve several purposes. Mentoring plays a major role in any clinically based profession, especially a new specialty. Imagine nurses and physicians without mentors in their clinical training! A mentor is a trusted counselor, guide, or coach over a long period of time. Mentors nurture the novice's growth with advice, information, and support (Lauwers, 2007). As Wiessinger points out, the early pioneers are now the teachers and mentors of novice LCs (2003). Because we are a new specialty, only two decades old, educational programs with a clinical component are rare at this early stage. Moreover, clinical preceptorships are expensive to run and time consuming. Budding LCs take the opportunity to learn where they can. A vacation trip can offer the opportunity to visit the work setting of a colleague. Shadowing lactation specialists in your own home area is an excellent way to learn clinical skills. Since clinical opportunities are scarce it is not uncommon to teach the "see one, do one, teach one" method.

Networking, an established mechanism used by members of groups to exchange information and to get help in solving problems using and learn from one another—is a "good ol' girl" system (see Figure 1–4). When a difficult case arises, they feel more comfortable if they can use the phone to work through the situation with another lactation consultant. Additional assessment of the problem and how to begin moving toward a solution might offer new insights or creative alternatives to the plan of action already considered. Networking also identifies job possibilities, colleagues who will cover for one another, and referrals for clients needing equipment or specialized help. Networks may also be used to change systems and improve methods of providing care.

Opportunities to communicate with others also abound on the Internet. Foremost among these offerings is LACTNET, a worldwide breastfeeding e-mail list. Other networks have started, including one for Spanish-speaking individuals, and one exclusively for private practice. The benefits of electronic contact include ease of communication with persons for whom telephone contact would be too expensive and postal contact would be too slow. In addition, being able to vent and obtain sympathetic electronic "clucks" within minutes or hours or to seek assistance for a troubling case supports the private LC in a way that can be duplicated only by the existence of as many knowledgeable professionals

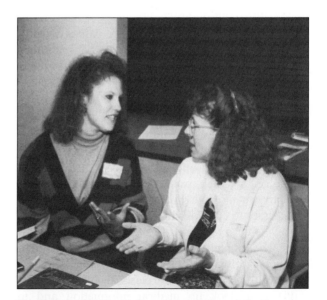

FIGURE **1–4** Making their "net" work for them, two LCs share experiences.

Source: Courtesy of Via Christi Medical Center, Wichita, Kansas.

in the local area. It is the rare setting in which so many colleagues would be gathered in a single place. Electronic networking is here to stay.

In addition to e-mail discussion groups, numerous Web sites also provide information on items of interest to lactation specialists. Exploring the Internet can take hours of time, and new Web sites are created daily. La Leche League International, the Australian Breastfeeding Association, and the International Lactation Consultant Association all have Web sites that describe their purpose, services, and coming events.

Reporting and Charting

It is the responsibility of the lactation specialist, regardless of where she practices, to chart each contact with her clients and to provide complete reports to referring physicians and other healthcare providers (Williams, 1995). Almost all record keeping involves using a computer. Computer skills are a necessity for healthcare workers. As with other healthcare providers, computers can be used to generate records, reports, and charts that do the following:

- Provide other health workers with valuable information.
- Reflect quality of care delivered (quality assurance, continuous quality improvement).
- Highlight sometimes subtle observations or findings.
- Validate health services for insurance companies to determine reimbursement.
- Provide data that can be used for research.
- Serve as evidence in a legal dispute.

In the hospital, the mother's and infant's charts are clinical records that contain information about the hospital stay and all contacts with everyone involved in their care. Because the mother and infant usually have separate charts, it is sometimes necessary to "double chart." At the same time, care plans tend to be geared to the mother, because it is she who is taught and the baby who is the recipient of her learning.

Health professionals use personal digital assistants (PDAs) to look up medical information and to document their interventions by entering coding and diagnosis, among other things. Software for items such as coding and medications can be downloaded from the Internet for a trial period and then purchased if one desires.

The most commonly used methods of charting are narrative charting and problem-oriented charting. Flow sheets and standard care plans that are individualized are becoming more popular. They reduce paperwork and save time (and money).

Narrative Charting

Narrative documentation uses a diary or story format to document client-care events. A simple paragraph describes the client's status and the care that was given. Narrative notes, sometimes called progress notes, are used less now, with the advent of flow sheets and clinical care plans, which capture the routine aspects of care. Narrative notes (Box 1–4) can be easily combined with flow sheets or any other client record.

Problem-Oriented Charting

Charting based on a problem uses a structured problem list and logical format for each entry in the medical record. The format used in problem-oriented charting is called the SOAP or SOAPIE method. Each letter stands for a different phase of the nursing process: subjective data, objective data, assessment and nursing diagnosis, plan, interventions, and evaluation of care (see Box 1–5).

In private practice the completeness of reports also assists the referring healthcare worker to understand the "how" as well as the "why" of an LC's practice and methods. Reporting provides a database for all types of information (e.g., an increase in the number of referrals from a particular physician's practice). Early referrals may be for one or two common problems, whereas tracking over a time period may show that later referrals are for a wider variety of problems.

Electronic Health Records

A patient's lactation information is usually incorporated into existing information systems (IS) in clinics and hospitals. Lactation professionals need to work closely with IS technicians to make sure that the format for electronic healthcare records includes breastfeeding, especially if mother–infant care is

	BOX 1–4

An Example of a Narrative Note

Date	Time	Progress note
05–22–03	0800	Infant alert. Rooting and suckling movements noted. Infant latched on breast and suckled effectively until asleep. Breastfeeding assessment score 9/10.
05–22–03	1500	Discussed basic breastfeeding information including normal infant elimination patterns to watch for after discharge. Mother given written materials on sore nipples, engorgement, use of breast pump, and breastmilk storage.
05–23–03	1100	Explained that a follow-up call will be made 2 to 3 days after discharge. Mother will have the option of a home visit.

involved. Transition to such a system takes significant amounts of time and resources, and often occurs with a good deal of staff frustration. Each facility, outpatient lactation clinic, private lactation practice, medical office, and hospital will have unique needs.

The Cincinnati Children's Center for Breastfeeding Medicine developed a lactation-friendly electronic health record (EHR) at their pediatric facility, which has a breastfeeding clinic. New forms specific to breastfeeding are (1) maternal history, (2) maternal exam, (3) infant feeding history, and (4) breastfeeding assessment. Their computer system includes electronic prescriptions, printed patient handouts, and telephone notes (List et al., 2008). LCs will find the computer pages and drop-down lists in this article to be helpful for developing their own computerized records.

Clinical Care Plans

A clinical care plan provides basic information about client assessment, diagnosis, and planned interventions. It also offers a guide for care, establishes a continuity of care, and represents a means of communication among all caregivers. There are two types of care plans: individual and standard. Individual care plans are developed "from scratch" for each client based on her specific needs. A standard care plan is a preprinted plan of care for a group of patients within the same diagnosis. Because each standard care plan must be tailored according to the needs of a particular client, they are designed to include space for adding information.

The Joint Commission requires a care plan for each patient in the hospital as a necessity for accreditation; however, the plan of care can be computer generated, preprinted, or appear in progress notes or standards of care (American Nurses Association, 1991). Care plans are legal requirements of practice and may also serve as protocols or standards of care.

Traditionally, individual care plans are divided into columns. Column headings change over the years to reflect new ideas in nursing, and some column labels are preferred over others. In this book, for instance, the clinical care plans include assessment, interventions, and rationale. Other commonly used labels are problem, evaluation, nursing diagnosis, patient outcomes, nursing action, or simply intervention-evaluation. An example of a nursing diagnosis and nursing care plan is seen in Box 1–6. The critical care path or

BOX 1–5

Problem-Oriented Medical Records

S = Subjective data. What the mother herself tells you. Example: "My nipples feel sore." Note: If the charting relates to only the infant, there will be no subjective data.

O = Objective data. Concrete data you can observe. Examples: Infant position at breast, temperature, and infant weight.

A = Assessment and nursing diagnosis. An assessment of physical and psychosocial factors based upon subjective and objective data; what you think is going on. Examples: Infant poorly positioned on the breast; breastfeeding at margin of nipple; ineffective breastfeeding; Latch score = 3 (1 low; 10 high).

P = Plan. Organized plan for care. Based upon the assessment, what you plan to do about the problem to help the breastfeeding mother and baby. Example: Will reposition infant on breast at next feeding.

I = Interventions. What you've done to/for the problem or what you plan to do. Includes teaching, referrals, finding the right pump. Example: Infant repositioned on mother's breast so that infant is grasping adequate breast tissue during suckling.

E = Evaluation. Review of outcomes. What happened? Was it effective? Examples: Infant appears to be suckling effectively at the breast. Infant breastfed four times during shift, three times following repositioning. Infant had bowel movement during feeding—appears well hydrated. In some cases in which a nursing care plan with diagnoses is used, evaluation may reflect only the presenting problem. Outcomes are then charted in the flow sheet.

---

clinical path is a commonly used type of care plan in hospitals. These paths, which are abbreviated care plans that focus on the client's length of stay in the hospital, integrate infant feeding into the overall care plan.

Legal Concerns

It is a rare event when a lactation consultant is a defendant in a malpractice suit. But that doesn't mean that it can't happen. The threat of a lawsuit because of excessive jaundice, for example, is a reality. Increased attention to professional liability in health care directly affects nurses and all healthcare workers, especially those in perinatal areas. Liability results from placing the mother and/or baby at risk even if the LC follows a physician's order.

The best way to avoid a lawsuit is by paying attention to these guidelines:

- Keep up to date on new research findings and clinical practices. Read current relevant articles and attend conferences.
- Keep positive relationships with your mother clients. People tend to sue healthcare providers because they feel they were not treated with respect and dignity.
- Document your intervention and the rationale for doing so. Write up assessments, interventions, and outcomes of care notes. Excel, Access, or dBase software programs can be formatted to create a database of your clients to keep track of your clients and record your cases.

BOX **1–6**

Clinical Care Plan

Nursing Interventions·Nursing Care Plan *Lactation Counseling*

COUNTY OF ORANGE • HEALTH CARE AGENCY • FIELD NURSING
NURSING INTERVENTIONS • NURSING CARE PLAN

Client's Name:			Client's Number:					

Lactation Counseling — 5244

DEFINITION: Use of an interactive helping process to assist in maintenance of successful breastfeeding.

ACTIVITIES:	DATE:						
Determine knowledge base about breastfeeding							
Educate parent(s) about infant feeding for informed decision-making							
Provide information about advantages and disadvantages of breastfeeding							
Correct misconceptions, misinformation, and inaccuracies about breastfeeding							
Determine mother's desire and motivation to breastfeed							
Provide support of mother's decisions							
Give parent(s) recommended education material, as needed							
Inform parent(s) about appropriate classes or groups for breastfeeding (e.g., La Leche League)							
Evaluate mother's understanding of infant's feeding cues (e.g., rooting, sucking, and alertness)							
Determine frequency of feedings in relationship to baby's needs							
Monitor maternal skill with latching infant to the nipple							
Evaluate newborn suck/swallow pattern							
Demonstrate suck training, as appropriate							
Teach mother about:							
• Relaxation techniques, including breast massage							
• Ways of increasing rest, including delegation of household tasks and ways of requesting help							
• Record keeping of length and frequency of nursing sessions							
• Infant stool and urination patterns							
• Adequacy of breast emptying with feeding							
• Quality and use of breastfeeding aids							
• Appropriateness of breast pump use							
• Formula information for temporary low supply problems							
• Skin integrity of nipples							
• Nipple care							
• Relieving breast congestion							
• Applying warm compresses							
• Signs of problems to report to health care practitioner							
• How to relactate							
• Continuing lactation upon return to work or school							
• Signs of readiness to wean							
• Options for weaning							
• Alternative methods of feeding							
• Contraception							

Source: With permission, Parris, 1999.

- In the hospital setting, make sure the baby has latched onto the breast before the mother and baby go home. If this has not occurred, first make sure the baby's doctor knows this. Then request that the mother and baby stay a day or two longer (refer this to the appropriate hospital case manager). If the mom and baby are not allowed to stay longer, make sure there is follow-up care: a daily phone call, an early visit to the baby's physician, a home visit—or all three.
- Refer to someone else if the situation calls for expertise you do not have in special situations.

People often sue healthcare workers not because of their clinical actions but because they are angry with them or for some other reason. Therefore, the most effective protection against such actions is establishing a mutually respectful relationship and rapport. The lactation specialist's pattern of practice should avoid causing the mother, the baby, or any other member of the client's family emotional distress as a result of words said, reports written, or other actions.

A clearly written, detailed record of the healthcare provider's actions, initial recommendations, and follow-up assistance (by phone and in person) is one of the most effective ways of avoiding legal action. Referrals increase following a well-written, complete report that is sent in a timely and professional manner. Client records are considered business records of the agency and are admissible as such under legal (court) rules of evidence. Records will often prevent cases from going to court; lawsuits often are won and lost based on what is in the record. Although testimony is another form of evidence, the written health chart is viewed as more accurate and reliable.

The LC who works in a doctor's office, clinic, or hospital is very apt to be part of the staff that are covered in an "umbrella" professional liability policy. The LC in private practice must determine for herself how much coverage she needs and what she can afford. Members of ILCA can get professional liability insurance coverage at a reasonable cost as a membership benefit. Although legal action against an LC is rare, it does occur; therefore, every individual practitioner needs to consider how she will protect herself and her family against a judgment that could ruin her financially.

Confidentiality

Maintain confidentiality about the mother, baby, and family. To fail to do so is an invasion of privacy and a tort (wrongful act) that involves confidential information that is revealed without permission to someone not entitled to know it.

Every LC should be aware of the Health Insurance Portability and Accountability Act (HIPAA) of 1996, which required the US Department of Health and Human Services (US DHHS) to develop a series of rules governing health information. In general, the rules are intended to standardize the communication of electronic health information between healthcare providers and health insurers. In addition, the rules are intended to protect the privacy and security of individually identifiable health information.

Intellectual Property Rights

The IBLCE Code of Ethics contains a tenet that deals with intellectual property rights (IBLCE, 2007). Basic rules for using other people's original materials are the following:

- Attribute the original creator of written material, slides, photographs, Internet sites, blogs, illustrations, online courses, etc. In case of a baby or minor, obtain written permission from parent.
- Seek authorization of the creator/source to reproduce, present, record, broadcast, translate, or adapt materials protected by copyright. A work is considered copyrighted as soon as it exists.
- Credit summaries of research findings, or ideas to authors or copyright owners.
- Limit photocopying of the creator's work to one copy per person/student.
- Quote directly from the original source. Generally a quotation of less than or equal to five typewritten lines should be enclosed in quotation marks, followed by a reference.
- When meaningful efforts fail to resurrect an out-of-print book, you may photocopy materials from the library book as long as the author is credited.

For more detailed information about legal issues and sample forms of consent and other legal documents, see Chapter 31 by Priscilla Bornmann in *Core Curriculum for Lactation Consultant Practice* by Marsha Walker.

Ethics

Why study ethics? Ethical decisions are a routine, inherent part of lactation practice. If we recognize and acknowledge ethical conflicts, then we are more likely to practice ethically. A code of ethics established specifically for LCs covers professional practice and conduct to safeguard interests of clients (Scott, 2002). The code of ethics is a "must," whereas standards of care is a "should" for practice. The purpose of both documents is to provide guidance to LCs in their professional practice. The code of ethics principles, seen in Appendix B, guide the profession and outline commitments and obligations of the LC to self, client, colleagues, society, and the profession. IBLCE mandates that all individuals who take the certification examination must provide evidence of the required 45 continuing education hours, of which five must address professional ethics.

The IBLCE Code of Ethics also states that an IBLCE-certified consultant shall act in a manner that safeguards the interests of individual clients, justifies public trust in her or his competence, and enhances the reputation of the profession. These lofty words look good, but ethical issues are more than the principles put forth in the code of ethics. They range from the broader political issues to those that arise in everyday professional practice. Ethical awareness and values are just as important to an IBCLC as skills and a belief in breastfeeding. Ethical practice is essential for reputation of our profession and necessary if we are to earn public trust (Personal communication, JoAnne Scott, 2004).

Ethical Questions That Come Up in Practice

Different personalities and value systems come into play that complicate making a judgment or finding neutral ground. Many times there is no clear right or wrong but shades of gray in trying to resolve such ethical questions as the following:

- Whether to attend a continuing education boxed lunch sponsored by a formula company. Attendees receive a pen and other goodies.
- Whether to give out gift packs with formula samples and coupons to breastfeeding women being discharged from the birth setting. Do LCs employed at the birth setting have a right to refuse to distribute these items?
- Whether to turn in a colleague who removed client files from the health agency without prior consent or failed to protect a file per HIPAA regulations. Questions: What are the circumstances surrounding this incident? Was it intentional? Was the offender aware of HIPAA regulations?
- Whether to contract with a formula company to write a booklet with quality information on breastfeeding for mothers for publication.
- Whether or not to call oneself a lactation consultant without being certified by the International Board of Lactation Consultant Examiners.

There are several reasons why ethics education is relevant for lactation specialists.

- We are a relatively new profession in health care. As such the public is just now becoming aware of us, our special knowledge and skills, and the role we play in the maternal–child field. How we act will contribute to the acceptance by the public as a welcomed, respected discipline.
- The public has given us tacit approval and trust for a practice that involves touching and manipulating lactating breasts in a society where breasts are blatantly associated with sexuality.
- Birth of a child is a major family event that will be remembered (for good or for bad) by the family for years to come, if not for the rest of their lives.
- The mother (and father) of the baby are emotionally fragile during childbirth and early weeks following birth and vulnerable to suggestions—especially if this is their first child.
- Technologies of lactation practice have expanded dramatically in the last two decades. They

include widespread use of breast pumps, nipple shields, nursing bras, and so on, and include the opportunity for making money at the expense of young families who may not need them.

The WHO Code

LCs are expected to practice within the WHO Code. The WHO Code (International Code of Marketing Breastmilk Substitutes), an international policy, is congruent with the ILCA Code of Ethics. The code acknowledges that there is a legitimate market for formula but mandates that formula companies should not provide promotion to the public, no gifts to health workers or mothers, no free samples, and clear and accurate labeling (Arnold & Blair, 2007).

Moral Dilemmas

Moral dilemmas and ethical issues can be subtle and complex. Noel-Weiss and Walters (2006) remind us that often it is simply a feeling that something is not quite right about a situation, and this uneasy feeling lasts for a long time. Most of us remember an incident in our childhood where our mother (or father) made it very clear that we were doing the wrong thing. Although it was painful at the time, our parents inculcated a moral sense that gave us a behavior compass so that we headed in the right direction as we grew up.

Ethical Dilemmas

An ethical dilemma occurs when two or more morally acceptable courses of action are present and to choose one prevents selecting another. Tension occurs because moral obligations create differing and opposing demands. In some moral dilemmas, the lactation consultant must choose between equally unacceptable alternatives—both may have elements that are morally wrong. The dilemma can also be described as a situation where the patient's rights and professional obligations conflict (Butts & Rich, 2005).

Ethical Dilemmas in Practice

Below are ethical dilemmas most frequently encountered as reported by practicing lactation specialists enrolled in a human lactation course (Unpublished, Riordan, 2007).

- Giving gift bags/discharge packs containing formula to new mothers in the hospital
- Copying original materials (figures, videos) without permission from the author
- Disagreement with physician regarding treatment and advice given to the mother and family
- Receiving gifts (money, jewelry, entertainment tickets) and grants for educational offerings from formula companies
- Selling pumps, nipple cream/gel, breastfeeding pillows, and other gadgets to parents when they are not needed
- Recommending the use of a medication to increase milk supply that is not approved by the FDA although it is being used in other countries

What does a healthcare worker do when her job responsibilities conflict with their ethics—for example giving out gift bags containing formula? When lactation specialists feel that they are being asked to do something they cannot support ethically, it's important for them to acknowledge their personal views and analyze their feelings asking these questions:

- What is the ethical problem, and who are the people involved?
- Are there differences in the values of people involved?
- What are the alternate options for decisions in this situation?
- What is the best way to resolve this dilemma?

Many times, shades of gray complicate the issue, and different belief systems come into play. Most hospitals and large clinics have an ethics committee where the individual can go to help sort out the issues. The committee holds a forum for interdisciplinary review where discussion of the dilemma and answers to questions are addressed.

Ethics vs. Morality

Ethics is an overall set of principles that guide human conduct. Morals, on the other hand, are specific behaviors based on an individual's ideas about what he or she believes is moral and how he or she interprets their own moral experiences. Morality is derived from the Latin word *moralis*, and refers to widely held social consensus about the normal conduct for human beings and society.

Principles of Ethics

Major principles of bioethics include the following (Butts & Rich, 2005):

- Autonomy
- Beneficence
- Nonmaleficence
- Justice
- Professional/client or patient relationship

Autonomy

Being autonomous is to be one's own person without constraints. The principle of autonomy is respect for self-determination and freedom to make one's own decisions.

Example. Autonomy includes the mother's right to choose whether to follow treatment suggestion or to refuse treatment. Autonomy fits well with caring for breastfeeding families because we know so much about the advantages of breastfeeding that it is difficult for us sometimes to stand back and accept the well-informed mother who decides to supplement her baby when she goes back to work even after we suggest ways that she can exclusively breastfeed in this situation. Autonomy for the patient requires the LC to recognize and appreciate the client and family's value choices.

Beneficence

Beneficence is defined as the duty to do good. Beneficence is just what it sounds like: being kind, merciful, and caring about the welfare of other people. It involves promoting the interests and well-being of other people.

Example. Maintain nurturing relationships with your colleagues. That includes those who are in training to become an LC. Seasoned LCs have an obligation to nurture individuals who are in the learning phase. Another example is when some places have out-and-out warfare going on between the nurses in the area and those who are not nurses. The remarks about each other can be vicious.

Nonmaleficence

This is the duty to do no harm. The meaning is obvious but although nonmaleficence is the opposite of beneficence, the two are linked.

Example. A mother who is HIV positive and advised to not breastfeed may deprive her baby of the benefits of her breastmilk but avoid the real potential of transferring HIV to the infant.

Justice

Justice is the right to be treated fairly and equally.

Example. Women who have been told to leave a restaurant or shopping mall because they were breastfeeding their baby. This certainly wasn't a just action.

Professional Client or Patient Relationships

Trust is the foundation of this principle. It includes keeping your word, telling the truth, maintaining privacy, and confidentiality.

Example. Before HIPAA became a law, the names of laboring women (and details) were posted openly on a blackboard in the nursing station. Childbirth and choice of infant feeding was not exactly private!

Ethics and Discipline Committee

IBLCE has an ethics and discipline committee. Members are drawn from IBLCE's board of directors and include a lawyer. The committees' deliberations are confidential and follow strict procedures. The committee reports to the full board. The way to submit a complaint is to do the following:

1. Request a copy of the procedures for making complaint and a copy of the code of ethics from the IBLCE office.
2. Complete the report form identifying which of the 24 tenets of the code were breached.
3. Provide a full explanation with supporting detail and sign it.
4. A designated reviewer will investigate the complaint and present the case to the committee. The committee will make a determination, and the complainant and respondent notified of their decision.

Actual complaints for ethics violations brought to the committee and the outcomes include the following:

- LC was accused of contradicting a physician's order. There was not clear evidence to prove the accusation to be true. Case dismissed because it was unsubstantiated.
- LC suggested a potentially dangerous practice in a published article, which carried her name and IBCLC certification. This was substantiated, but there were mitigating circumstances. Private reprimand was given.

Reimbursement

In most countries lactation services are a part of the national healthcare system, and reimbursement for these services is mainly through salaried positions paid for by government programs. In the United States, reimbursement for lactation services is extremely complex and depends upon the setting where the services are provided, educational qualifications of the provider, and the type of insurance.

Lactation specialists who work in a birthing center, hospital, or medical office are usually salaried employees reimbursed with a set hourly or weekly wage. Hospitals usually include lactation services as part of the total cost of the maternity "package." The cost package is an agreement between the insurance company and the hospital to charge a certain amount of money for healthcare coverage for each birth. This is known as capitation. Managed care companies compete with each other with price bids to win the healthcare contract, the lowest bid gaining the contract.

If postpartum home visits are part of a maternity insurance package, breastfeeding assistance is given as a part of a routine postpartum visit to the mother's home. Nurses providing these home visits are usually salaried by the home health company that employs them. Services above and beyond the packaged LC services are paid for either by a separate insurance claim or by the family themselves.

For the LC in private practice, cash payment for services rendered or for equipment is usually requested from the client at the time of the service. The client in turn seeks reimbursement from her insurance company and provides the third-party

payer with the information it needs. The client may give the LC forms to complete and send to the insurer in the hope of being reimbursed. Insurance companies expect to be sent the HCFA form that can be downloaded from www.medela.com. A "superbill" with ICD-9 codes is displayed in Box 1–7. This form, along with an instruction booklet, is available from Pat Lindsey, IBCLC, at www.patlc.com.

Insurance and Third-Party Payment

Insurance and third-party payment for lactation services is a complex issue. Third-party payment—insurance or payment by another entity besides the patient—varies according to the state (and country) where the services were given. In the United States, third-party payers can be divided into two general categories: government or public health insurance (Medicare, Medicaid) and managed care organizations (MCOs).

Medicare applies to individuals over age 65 and is not applicable for breastfeeding except that insurance companies usually follow Medicare rules for payment. Medicaid is a federal program administered by the states, and state regulations apply to mothers and children who qualify on the basis of poverty. The regulations in various states may differ in billing rules and regulations. About one third of US births are paid for under Medicaid. Medicaid reimbursement for health care is further complicated by the fact that some Medicaid recipients are also enrolled in managed care plans. The plans' policies on reimbursement differ from the state and federal rules governing reimbursement when the patient is not enrolled in managed care.

Insurance policies usually spell out by title who may be reimbursed with third-party payment. Physicians and midlevel providers such as nurse practitioners, certified nurse midwives, and physician assistants, are recognized by third-party payers as providers who can receive direct payment for their services.

To receive reimbursement from Medicaid, the lactation consultant must be accepted as a Medicaid provider by her state Medicaid agency in order to be admitted to the provider panel of an MCO. Generally, providers are accepted on the basis of having a medical or medically related degree and national certification. Lactation consultants can receive direct

BOX 1–7

Superbill (Lactation Visit Receipt)

Pat Lindsey, IBCLC - Lactation Services
Board Certified Lactation Consultant - Registered Lactation Consultant
TAX ID/PROVIDER # 59-3579433
3849 Oakwater Circle, Orlando, FL 32806 - Telephone 407-859-7239 - Fax 407-850-9185 - Email PatIBCLC@aol.com

"Affordable Health Care Begins with Breastfeeding"

© 2002 Pat Lindsey, IBCLC

PATIENT INFORMATION

PATIENT'S LAST NAME	FIRST	INITIAL	PT'S BIRTHDATE	PATIENT: MALE FEMALE	RELATIONSHIP TO SUBSCRIBER

ADDRESS	CITY	STATE	ZIP	REFERRING PHYSICIAN

PHONE ( )	SUBSCRIBER	INSURANCE CARRIER

ADDRESS - IF DIFFERENT	CITY	STATE	INS. ID	COVERAGE CODE	GROUP

LACTATION	ILLNESS	DATE SYMPTOMS APPEARED	OTHER HEATH COVERAGE?	YES	NO	IDENTIFY:
ACCIDENT	PREGNANCY					
INDUSTRIAL						

ASSIGNMENT. I hereby assign my insurance benefits to be paid directly to the undersigned health care provider. I am financially responsible for non-covered services.

RELEASE: I authorize the undersigned health care provider to release any information acquired in the course of my examination or treatment.

SIGNED: (Insured or Authorized Person) _____ Date: _____

SIGNED: (Insured or Authorized Person) _____ Date: _____

DRAFT

NEW	ESTAB	OFFICE SERVICE	FEE
99203 30min	99213 15min	Hx Evaluation and Management	
99204 45min	99214 25min	Hx Evaluation and Management	
99205 60min	99215 40min	Hx Evaluation and Management	

NEW	ESTAB	HOME SERVICE	FEE
99342 30min	99348 25min	Hx Evaluation and Management	
99343 45min	99349 40min	Hx Evaluation and Management	
99344 60min	99350 60min	Hx Evaluation and Management	

NEW	ESTAB	HOSPITAL SERVICE	FEE
99221 30min	99231 15min	Hx Evaluation and Management	
99222 50min	99232 25min	Hx Evaluation and Management	
99223 70min	99233 35min	Hx Evaluation and Management	

NEW	ESTAB	TELEPHONE CONSULT	FEE
99371	99371	Brief	
99372	99372	Intermediate	
99373	99373	Lengthy/complex	

TRAVEL	# Miles @	

SUPPLIES					CPT/MOD	FEE
BREAST PUMPS						
Breast Pump Collection Kit	Single	Double	Conversion		A7002	
Pump In Style	Orginial	Traveler	Companion		E0603	
Purely Yours	with case	w/out case			E0603	
Nurture III	with case	w/out case			E0603	
Mini-Electric					E0603	
Manual Pump	Medela	Ameda	Avent		E0602	
Other Pump					E0603	
SUPPLEMENTAL NURSING SYSTEM	Starter	Regular			A7002	
BREAST SHELLS					99070	
NIPPLE SHIELDS					99070	
BOOKS/PAMPHLETS					99071	
OTHER Feeding Supplies					99070	
Baby Weigh Scale Rental - Serial #	# days @ $				E1399	
ELECTRIC HOSPITAL GRADE PUMP RENTAL					E0604	
Equipment Serial Number						
Rented Date	Return Date					
# days @ $	# months @ $					
Delivery / Extra Cleaning Charge on Rental Pump						
		TOTAL SUPPLIES AND/OR RENTAL				
		SALES TAX IF NO PRESCRIPTION				

LACTATION DX ICD 9 CM CODES

CHILD

BREASTFEEDING PROBLEM
- 783.21 Abnormal Weight Loss
- 775.5 Dehydration Newborn
- 783.41 Failure to Gain Weight
- 779.3 Newborn Feeding Problem
  - Breast Refusal
  - Latch-on Difficulties
  - Regurgitation of food
  - Slow feeding
  - Vomiting
  - Other
- 783.3 Infant Feeding Problem
  - Breast Refusal
  - Latch-on Difficulties
  - Mismanagement of feeding
  - Other
- 783.6 Polyphagia-Overeating
- 783.2 Under weight

SUCKING PROBLEMS
- 796.1 Suck Reflex Abnormal

JAUNDICE   (V12.3)
- 774.39 Breastmilk Jaundice
- 774 Newborn - Physiologic
- 774.2 Newborn - Premature

ABNORMAL FUSSINESS/COLIC
- 777.8 Newborn - Colic
- 789.0 Infant - Colic
- 780.59 Sleep Disturbances Infant

DERMATITIS/INFECTION
- 691.0 Diaper Rash
- 693.1 Due to Food
- 691.8 Eczema
- 771.7 Thrush-Newborn
- 112.0 Thrush-Infant

OTHER
- 750.0 Ankyloglossia - Tongue Tie
- 530.81 GEReflux-NoInflam (V12.7?)
- 530.11 GEReflux-Inflam (V12.7?)
- 750.15 Macroglossia (V12.4?)
- 750.16 Microglossia (V12.4?)
- 520.7 Teething Syndrome

CHILD DIAGNOSIS
PRIMARY DX _____
SECONDARY DX _____
SECONDARY DX _____
SECONDARY DX _____

MOTHER

NIPPLE/AREOLA PROBLEM
- 676.14 Cracked/Fissured
- 692.9 Dermatitis Contact
- 676.04 Dimpled/Folded/Creviced
- 676.34 Flat
- 675.9 Infection (unspecific/Thrush)
- 676.04 Inverted (Retracted)
- 676.34 Sore Nipples
- 676.3 Trauma
- 676.3 Ulceration
- 676.34 Unusual Shape

BREAST PROBLEM
- 676.3 Breast Pain
- 692.9 Dermatitis Contact
- 676.9 Disorder of Lactation
- 676.8 Galactocele
- 757.6 Hypoplasia of Breast
- 611.72 Mass (es) / Lump (s)

ENGORGEMENT, BREAST
- 676.20 After the Perinatal Period
- 676.24 Perinatal, Moderate/Severe

MASTITIS
- 675.14 Breast Abscess
- 675.04 Filled Duct
- 675.20 Non-Purulent Infection
- 675.24 Plugged Duct
- 675.14 Purulent Infection

MILK SUPPLY
- 676.44 Agalactia (No Milk)
- 676.64 Galactorreah
- 676.8 Polygalactia (Over Supply)
- 676.54 Suppressed (Reduced)

LACTATION
- 676.50 Induced (Adoption) (v61.29)
- 676.54 Relactation

OTHER
_____
_____
_____

MOTHER DIAGNOSIS
PRIMARY DX _____
SECONDARY DX _____
SECONDARY DX _____
SECONDARY DX _____

NOTES
_____
_____

INSTRUCTIONS TO PATIENT FOR FILING INSURANCE CLAIMS:	REC'D BY	TODAY'S FEE	
COMPLETE THE PATIENT INFORMATION SECTION AT THE TOP OF THIS FORM. SIGN AND DATE. THEN MAIL THIS FORM DIRECTLY TO YOUR INSURANCE COMPANY. PLEASE ATTACH YOUR OWN INSURANCE CARRIER'S CLAIM FORM.	CHARGE	OLD BALANCE	
	CASH	TOTAL DUE	
PLEASE REMEMBER THAT PAYMENT IS YOUR OBLIGATION.	CHECK	AMT. REC'D	
REGARDLESS OF INSURANCE OR OTHER THIRD PARTY INVOLVEMENT.	# _____	NEW BALANCE	

NEXT APPOINTMENT	PROVIDER'S SIGNATURE	DATE OF SERVICE

Source: With permission, Pat Lindsey, 2003.

reimbursement if they are a physician or an advanced registered nurse practitioner (NP) (including a certified nurse–midwife) who has graduated from an accredited educational program and is certified nationally in a specialty.

Physicians or nurse practitioners can apply for a provider number through the state Medicaid agency by filing a provider application. If accepted as a provider, they can bill the state Medicaid agency on an HCFA 1500 form using the patient's name and identifying information, the ICD-9 code, the Current Procedural Terminology (CPT) code, the charge, and the provider's name, number, and location for services. Fees for CPT codes vary according to locations and providers. For example, in many states in order to receive third-party payment, LC services must be provided in collaboration with a physician. A book by Carolyn Buppert (2008), *Nurse Practitioner's Business Practice and Legal Guide* (3rd ed.), is an excellent resource for learning about reimbursement.

"Incident to" Billing

Lactation services that fall under the category "incident to" can be billed if they are an integral although incidental part of a physician's professional services; however, the physician must personally treat the client on the first visit to the practice and be on site when the service is rendered. So if the LC is a nurse practitioner working in a medical office she can bill for "incident to" services to the breastfeeding dyad if the physician sees the mother and baby first and is in the building (on-site) when the NP sees them. Medicare requires that the claim form for an "incident to" service be filled out with the physician's name and provider number.

Rejection of Billing

If the company rejects a bill, the HCFA 1500 is returned with a short explanation about why it is being rejected. Sometimes several letters back and forth are necessary before the bill will be paid. Persistence is the key, as many claims may not be paid on the first submission. Anyone in a medically related practice quickly learns from trial and error how to best file third-party insurance claims in order to maximize the number of paid claims.

Payers may require documentation to validate that the care was given, the site of the care, and the medical necessity and appropriateness of services provided. Fees for care of breastfeeding women on Medicaid are based on number and type of services provided using the CPT, published in the ninth edition of *International Classification of Diseases* (ICD-9) and the Health Care Financing Administration's Common Procedure Coding System (HCPCS) codes (see Box 1–8).

Major barriers to third-party reimbursement for nonphysician healthcare workers such as lactation consultants have been state licensure laws, opposition by the medical profession, and third-party payers who fear expansion of provider eligibility. The 1997 passage of a provision contained in the budget bill Public Law 105-33 to expand Medicare reimbursement for nurse practitioners allows for reimbursement of NP services including lactation services; however, each state has the option of covering NP services. Even though the law has passed, these nonphysician providers have difficulties in getting third-party payment.

Physicians in the United States are able to obtain reimbursement by using established ICD-9 medical codes for breastfeeding diagnoses, billing for both mother and baby as indicated, and submitting bills for insurance coverage. This often falls into the constraints of contracted fees, managed care, and/or HMO contracts. The American Academy of Pediatrics section on breastfeeding published *Breastfeeding and Lactation, The Pediatrician's Pocket Guide to Coding* in 2006. However, owing to the time-consuming nature of fully evaluating the breastfeeding dyad and observing a feeding, the physician's time will rarely be adequately compensated in full. Creative use of staff is often featured in the physician-led lactation clinic to allow effective time management for the physician.

Coding

Accurate and complete coding for services and supplies is vital to the financial success of a lactation program or service. The HCPCS is a uniform method for health providers to report professional services and supplies. Box 1–9 presents a listing of HCPCS codes for breast pumps. Keep in mind that payment coding requirements and policies vary from payer to payer, and new codes may not be recognized by all payers (International Lactation Consultant

BOX **1–8**

Common Lactation ICD-9 Codes/Diagnosis Codes

Code	Mother	Code	Infant
675.2	Nonpurulent mastitis	276.5	Volume depletion, dehydration, hypovolemia
675.1	Abscess of breast		
676.1	Cracked nipple	524.06	Microgenia; major anomalies of jaw size
676.3	Other and unspecified disorder of breast	783.2	Abnormal loss of weight
675.8	Other specified infection of breast and nipple	750.1	Abnormal tongue position
		774.39	Breastmilk jaundice
692	Dermatitis contact	749	Cleft palate/lip
651.04	Twin pregnancy postpartum condition or complication	750	Tongue tie
		758	Down's syndrome
676.2	Engorgement of breasts	787.2	Dysphagia
676.5	Suppressed lactation	784.41	Failure to thrive, failure to gain weight
676.0	Retracted nipple		
676.4	Failure of lactation	783.3	Feeding difficulty—infant
676.6	Galactorrhea	779.3	Feeding problems in newborn
676.8	Other disorders of lactation	771.7	Neonatal candida infection

Association, 2002). The Reimbursement Tool Kit available from ILCA at www.ilca.org is a valuable source of information. The Healthcare Insurance Guide for Breastfeeding Families can be downloaded free at the Medela Web site (www.medela.com). The best summary of how to bill for lactation services in a pediatric office can be found at www.aap.org/breastfeeding/PDF/coding.pdf.

Private Practice

Rising rates of breastfeeding and short hospital stays have resulted in lactation services as a private practice. Some physicians are successful in building a practice that is limited to breastfeeding families. Both professional health workers and those without a healthcare background are finding they can enjoy the work they love, assisting women with breastfeeding, and still survive.

Auerbach (Riordan & Auerbach, 1999) surveyed lactation consultants in private practice in the United States and Canada to gain information about their experiences. A majority of the private practice LCs reported that they work 4 to 5 hours a day, qualifying for part-time status when seeking professional liability coverage, which all maintained. The number of clients seen in a given week or month varied widely, and was related to several factors, including how long the LC had been in practice, whether she limited herself to home visits (more time consuming and thus less frequent), and whether her practice was located in a rural or more densely populated metropolitan area. LCs in practices for only two to three years reported seeing the fewest number of clients, but their practices grew over time as satisfied customers made referrals to friends, neighbors, and colleagues.

Some LCs started by opening a breast pump rental depot. Others set up a private practice after receiving

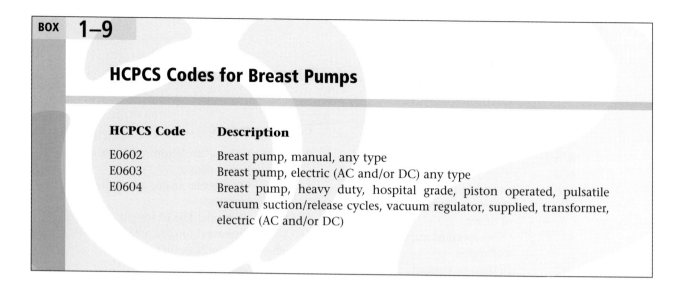

HCPCS Codes for Breast Pumps

HCPCS Code	Description
E0602	Breast pump, manual, any type
E0603	Breast pump, electric (AC and/or DC) any type
E0604	Breast pump, heavy duty, hospital grade, piston operated, pulsatile vacuum suction/release cycles, vacuum regulator, supplied, transformer, electric (AC and/or DC)

numerous calls from mothers who requested their help with breastfeeding. Several had been (or still were) hospital nurses who wanted to do more to help breastfeeding mothers than could be accomplished in the hospital. Still others found that a private practice in lactation consulting was an extension of their previous work as volunteer LLL leaders.

The LC's own home is the most common practice setting for nonhealth professional LCs. For health professionals, practice locations are a clinic, physician's office, or hospital where the LC receives referrals from the staff members of these organizations. Some residential neighborhoods have restrictive covenants that prevent home business or signage that a business is located in a home. Using a post office box for an address avoids neighborhood zoning restrictions. These details must be checked out in advance of opening such a facility. Inadequate road signs in suburban settings or in rural areas will make maps on the backs of flyers and other advertisements a necessity. In North American practices, busy periods clustered in March, April, and May, reflecting the higher birth rates during the warmer months, while slower periods tended to occur in November, December, and January.

The Business of Doing Business

One of the hardest lessons for an LC to learn is that a private practice is a business; if she has no business experience, she must learn about it (Auerbach, 1995). Advertising is essential in establishing and/or maintaining a client pool. Generally, the best advertising is word-of-mouth referral from clients who are satisfied with the LC's services. Other successful advertising includes distributing business cards, flyers, and magnets, and sending personal letters to hospital staff, local physicians (pediatricians, family physicians, obstetricians), community women's groups, childbirth educators, and La Leche League leaders. Teaching a prenatal breastfeeding class is a form of advertising. At the same time, the LC has to make it clear that she charges for later visits. Additional techniques include listings in the telephone book (white or yellow pages), newspaper articles, and press releases for new activities or special events relating to the business.

Lactation consultants disagree about whether to advertise in local newspapers or on the radio. Such visibility has the potential to attract the people merely posing as clients, is expensive, and rarely results in generating clients. The choice of words in advertisements or signs should be considered carefully. In one case, an LC posted a large sign with her name but not the word *breast* or *lactation*, to alert passersby to her business. Using family, parenting, or mother-related phrases works well in lieu of more obvious words. In other communities, inclusion of the words *breastfeeding* or *breast* may not be controversial.

More effective marketing techniques include meeting face to face with local physicians, their office staff, and hospital nurse managers, as well as attending professional meetings, such as hospital grand rounds and continuing education programs for nurses. Presenting a case history to hospital physicians, midwives, doulas, childbirth educators, and other health providers raises the visibility of the LC practice and generates referrals.

Incorporating the private practice should be considered only after carefully reviewing the advantages and disadvantages. The advantages are that the business is a legal entity with possible tax advantages and that the business can be sold or transferred. The disadvantages are the expenses of incorporation and that the business is regulated by state and federal controls.

Payment and Fees

Most clients pay for their visits by cash, check, or credit card at the time of service. Lactation consultants, however, harbor a strong streak of idealism and on occasion refrain from charging a client when it is clear that the client cannot pay. Others establish an informal sliding scale for people for whom a total payment at the time of service is not possible or offer a payment plan for those who cannot pay in full at the time of the visit. Most people prefer to pay something rather than nothing. And when clients pay even a very small amount for the care they receive, they are more inclined to follow through with the suggestions.

Another aspect of doing business is setting fees. This issue seems to generate the greatest concern when lactation specialists first go into practice. Anxiety about how much to charge for their services may stem from having been a volunteer breastfeeding support person for many years and coming to value the helping relationships with the mothers without thinking of charging for the service. This problem is not confined to LCs. Women tend to be reluctant to charge what their services are worth. This undervaluing of skills or services is part of a woman's socialization when she is growing up. In addition, lack of familiarity with running a business results in undervaluing the service provided. Setting fees too low degrades lactation consultant services and lowers expectations for insurance company payments.

The prospective private practice LC needs to set her fees on the basis of what other comparable professionals in her community are charging for similar services (e.g., others in private practice, nurses who make home health visits, and medical office visits). Other factors to consider in setting fees are the length of visits. While well-baby visits to a physician's office may last only 15 to 20 minutes, the usual first LC visit may run 60 to 90 minutes. One lactation clinic charges $29 for 15 minutes; $46 for 30 minutes and $68 for one hour (ILCA, 2002).

If the visits take place in the mother's home, a set time for travel is included in the charge: one lactation consultant adds 1 hour to account for travel time to and from the client's home when she bills the visit. Still others charge a set fee according to the number of miles/kilometers they travel in addition to their usual visit fee. Saturday and Sunday visits are sometimes charged at double the usual rate.

Phone consultations should be considered in establishing a fee structure. Some lactation specialists do not charge for phone consultations at all, preferring instead to limit calls to no more than 10 minutes. If more time is needed, they suggest that a visit for which they will be paid is in order. LCs bill differently for phone consultations. Some bill for a specific amount of time within a set framework, such as up to 1 hour of calls within a week after the first visit. Others bill for each call separately. Still others provide free phone consultation for minor issues.

Overhead costs such as rent, taxes, phone, computers, and traveling should be added to determine fee structure. If the annual cost of overhead is added to annual salary and divided by 52 weeks, the amount should equal weekly income (Ferrarello, 2001).

LCs in private practice are most successful when they have an ongoing, mutually respectful relationship with other healthcare providers in the community who refer clients to them. A physician in private practice found the following:

Initially some physicians raised their eyebrows. They thought breastfeeding was not worthy of a physician's time. However, as I have seen more and more of their patients, and spoken on grand rounds, I have gained their respect and lots of referrals. Once they discover that there is a science behind the art, the breast is as complex and elegant as any other organ system, they are eager to learn more (Smillie, 2000, p. 51).

Relationships with physicians have established rules, one of which is that if a baby is thought to have a medical problem, before proceeding with lactation assistance, the LC refers the family to their baby's own healthcare provider. The LC who is also a nurse practitioner can assess and treat a nursing mother or baby with a medical problem in collaboration with a physician according to the nursing practice laws in her state.

Essential to developing a professional reputation and high ethical standards is sending a written report to the referring physician or calling the physician after the patient has been seen. Referrals increase following a well-written, complete report sent in a timely and professional manner (Williams, 1995).

Partnerships

Partnerships differ in how they are structured. In some cases, each partner sees all clients, and income that is generated is shared equally. In other practices, each partner maintains her own client group. Having a partner to cover for you (as long as the partner is available) is the biggest advantage. Going into a partnership requires that each LC be clear about what she wants from the arrangement at the outset. Complementary ways of working are a plus; it is not necessary for each partner to be a "clone" of the other. However, when very different philosophies exist about how to provide client services, conflicts that cannot be resolved are more likely to arise. Like a marriage, a partnership has its high and low points. Sometimes, partners can simply create a whole new set of problems such as disagreements about workload, methods of practice, and income.

Private practice is clearly not for every lactation consultant. However, those who have done so and have weathered the first 5 years report that it can provide rewards that are rarely found in another occupation. The independence, which is most frightening to persons who are used to a guaranteed salary and set working hours, also offers an opportunity to structure one's workday in a way that may allow the LC more time with her family than is possible otherwise.

Persons already in the field are the best to ask what others entering the field should know. Linda Smith's book, *The Lactation Consultant in Private Practice: The ABCs of Getting Started*, is a valuable resource for starting a private practice. Box 1–10 lists dos and don'ts suggested by LCs in practice—either when establishing a private practice or when initiating an office, clinic, or hospital-based LC service.

BOX 1–10

Dos and Don'ts of Lactation Consulting

DO ...

- Insist on gaining credibility for the profession by passing the IBLCE examination. Ensure that people know this is the minimum credential for any person practicing as an LC in the community.

- From the very first client, behave with the utmost professionalism.
- Charge what you are worth; do not apologize for your fees.
- Set limits immediately, so that people know the boundaries of your availability.

(Continues)

BOX **1–10** **(Continued)**

- Establish your own knowledge and skills boundaries. Do not be afraid to ask for help.
- Develop a network of LCs in the community; they can serve as a sounding board for problems and as back-up when you are not available.
- Avoid repeating problems other LCs have experienced by learning from those with more experience than you have.
- Know what you are doing if you rent or sell equipment. Learn how the equipment works, and who should and should not use it. Be aware that its availability from you may influence what you tell a client to do.
- Use a computer to maintain a database of clients and practice documents and for maintaining your business.
- Learn as much as possible about running a business. It can take years to break even.
- Get a competent business advisor for accounting, marketing, and taxes. Ensure that those advisors understand exactly what you are trying to do.
- Bill the client directly for the service. The client then files a claim to her insurance company. Use standard forms for billing and a letter that the client can use to seek insurance coverage.
- Develop a specialization within the field and make your work visible to others through good care (Brimdyr, 2002).
- Document what you have done and send the original to the primary care

provider, whether or not this individual made the initial referral.
- Recognize that this business is a labor of love. Do not expect to get rich.

DON'T

- Don't get heavily involved in phone consultations, paid or unpaid, without having seen the mother and baby. An overall assessment is needed.
- Don't give away your time without reimbursement.
- Don't waste your money on a lot of expensive advertising. Advertise judiciously and be patient.
- Don't use someone else's opinion as a reason for doing something. Experiment; be creative. What works in one practice may not work in another one.
- Don't get too many partners at the beginning. Knowing how each partner works as an individual will not necessarily predict how each works as part of a group. The more partners one has the greater the number of problems that can arise.
- Never forget that a happy mother and thriving baby are your best advertisements.

Summary

The field of lactation, now into its third decade, is widely accepted as a healthcare specialty. Most hospitals now offer lactation services and employ nurse lactation consultants, and physicians are starting up breastfeeding specialty private practices. And no wonder: of the 4 million women who give birth each year in the United States, approximately three fourths (3 million) start off breastfeeding. The opportunity to work with healthy families and adorable babies—and to enhance early parenting and child health—has made it a popular, satisfying field. Although growth is welcomed, rapid growth causes growing pains. Some health professionals feel threatened by the emergence of new practitioners who expect to share their turf.

The experiences of the lactation consultant in this decade are similar to those of the childbirth educator in the 1960s and 1970s. At that time, it was the childbirth educator who was the innovator and change agent who flew against the prevailing wind and traditional practices in birthing. These two disciplines share more than a common history: both empower mothers and act as change agents for women and for families during an age when technology and defensive medicine rule medical practice.

Those working with breastfeeding families cannot expect to become wealthy. However, they reap the reward of personal fulfillment as they assist other women in becoming empowered by their own breastfeeding experiences. This outcome has no price.

Key Concepts

- A lactation consultant (LC) is a specialist trained to focus on the needs and concerns of the breastfeeding mother–baby pair in hospitals, clinics, private medical practice, health departments, home health agencies, and private practices. LCs usually have educational and clinical backgrounds in the health professions.
- Randomized clinical trials consistently show that interventions by healthcare workers have a positive effect on breastfeeding. Translated to healthcare costs, these studies would show that LC services save the healthcare system enormous amounts of money through reduction in illness of both baby and mother.
- The number of candidates taking the international IBLCE certification examination for lactation consultants has grown steadily since its inception in 1985. Most candidates have been from Australia, Canada, and the United States. Passing rates usually range from 85% to 95%. Periodic recertification is required.
- Salaries for working as a lactation consultant for a clinical agency are similar to those paid to hospital nurses; working in a medical office pays the least. The fee charged for consultation with a mother ranges from about $70 to $95.

- Opportunities to gain clinical experience working with breastfeeding dyads can be obtained through La Leche League, finding a preceptor arrangement with an experienced nurse or physician, serving as a WIC peer counselor, and teaching prenatal classes.
- Certification by the IBLCE is the gold standard for working as a lactation consultant; other certifications with titles have caused confusion to the public and to employers.
- Most hospitals have lactation services. These services usually include mother–baby rounds; telephone hotline and postdischarge telephone calls; prenatal classes on breastfeeding; pump rental or sales; postpartum breastfeeding consults; and continuing education for staff.
- A hospital with 3000 births per year should have at least five full-time LC positions that can be split into part-time positions. The usual time per visit with mothers when doing daily rounds is 15 to 20 minutes. The majority of LC work time is spent in direct care of clients.
- A "prime mover" (i.e., a nursing director, administrator, or physician) who has institutional power is needed in order to develop a lactation program as well as to obtain the

wide support of those who have influence in deciding budget allocations.

- The role of the LC is based on an advanced practice model. Roles develop sequentially according to experience as follows: novice, advanced beginner, competent, proficient, and expert.
- A major responsibility of the LC is documentation through reports and charting. Narrative and problem-oriented charting and clinical care plans are popular methods to organize and chart clinical care. Computer skills are mandatory for getting and keeping a job.

- Ethics is a set of principles that guide human conduct. Morals are specific behaviors based on beliefs. A situation in which an individual feels compelled to make a choice between two or more actions that he or she can reasonably and morally justify, or when evidence or arguments are inconclusive is called an ethical dilemma.
- Physicians and midlevel providers such as nurse practitioners, certified nurse–midwives, and physician assistants are recognized by third-party payers as providers who can receive direct payment for their services.

Internet Resources

Breastfeeding Support Consultants Center for Lactation Education: Offers lactation courses, study modules, products, certification requirements. www.bsccenter.org

International Board for Lactation Consultant Examiners: Provides numerous documents for lactation consultants, including registry of certified lactation consultants and how to become certified. www.iblce.org

International Lactation Consultant Association (ILCA): Offers conferences, courses, professional practice documents, and the Reimbursement Tool Kit. www.ilca.org

United States ILCA: National affiliate that addresses issues important to LCs in the United States. www.uslcaonlline.org

Jones and Bartlett Publishers: Publishes books on breastfeeding. www.jbpub.com

La Leche League International: Provides publications, seminars, and answers to breastfeeding questions. www.lalecheleague.org

Medela: Offers the Insurance Reimbursement Guide. www.medela.com/NewFiles/reburstmt_pro.html

American Academy of Pediatrics: Provides reimbursement guidelines. www.aap.org/breastfeeding/PDF/coding.pdf

References

Aidam BA, Perez-Escamilla R, Lartey A. Lactation counseling increases exclusive breast-feeding rates in Ghana. *J Nutr.* 2005;135:1691–1695.

Albernaz E et al. Lactation counseling increases breast-feeding duration but not breast milk intake as measured by isotopic methods. *J Nutr.* 2003; 133:205–209.

Allied Physicians. Nurse salaries—Nursing salary surveys [Web page]. Rehoboth Beach, DE: Allied Physicians, Inc., 2006. Available at: http://www.allied-physicians.com/salary-surveys/nursing. Accessed December 3, 2008.

Aidam BA, Perez-Escamilla R, Lartey A. Lactation counseling increases exclusive breast-feeding rates in Ghana. *J Nutr.* 135:1691–1695, 2005.

Albernaz E et al. Lactation counseling increases breast-feeding duration but not breast milk intake as measured by isotopic methods. *J Nutr.* 133:205–210, 2003.

American Nurses Association (ANA). Has JCAHO eliminated care plans? *Am Nurse.* 1991; June:6.

Angeron J, Riordan J. Staffing for a lactation program. Via Christi Medical Center, Wichita, Kan. 2007, unpublished.

Arnold LDW, Blair AC. Ethical practice for lactation care providers. La Leche League, International. Unit 12: Lactation Series Two. Schaumburg, IL: La Leche League, International; 2007.

Auerbach KG. Record-keeping: making the business end of doing business work for you. *J Hum Lact.* 1995;11:220–221.

Auerbach KG, Riordan J, Gross A. The lactation consultant: an increasingly visible health care role. *Mother Baby J*. 2000;5(1):41–46.

Bailey D. ILCA: 20 years of building a profession. *J Hum Lact*. 2005;21(3):239–242.

Barros FC et al. A randomized intervention trial to increase breast-feeding prevalence in southern Brazil [in Portuguese]. *Rev Saude Publ*. 1994;28:177–183.

Benner P. *From Novice to Expert: Excellence and Power in Clinical Nursing Practice*. Menlo Park, Calif: Addison-Wesley; 1984.

Bloom I et al. Factors affecting the continuance of breastfeeding. *Acta Paediatr Scand*. 1982;300(suppl):9–14.

Bolam A et al. The effects of postnatal health education for mothers on infant care and family planning practices in Nepal: a randomized controlled trial. *Br Med J*. 1998;316:805–811.

Bonuck KA, Trombley M, Freeman K et al. Randomized controlled trial of a prenatal and postnatal lactation consultant intervention on duration and intensity of breastfeeding up to 12 months. *Pediatrics*. 2005;116:1413–1425.

Bornmann PG. A legal primer for lactation consultants. In: Walker M, ed. *Core Curriculum for Lactation Consultant Practice*. Sudbury, Mass: Jones and Bartlett; 2002:465–516.

Brent NB et al. Breast-feeding in a low-income population: program to increase incidence and duration. *Arch Pediatr Adolesc Med*. 1995;149:798–803.

Brimdyr K. Lactation management: a community of practice. In: Cadwell K, ed. *Reclaiming Breastfeeding for the United States*. Sudbury, Mass: Jones and Bartlett; 2002:51–63.

Britton C et al. Support of breastfeeding mothers (Review). *The Cochrane Collaboration*. Available at: http://www.thecochranelibrary.com. Accessed July 28, 2007.

Buppert C. *Nurse Practitioner's Business Practice and Legal Guide*. 3rd ed. Sudbury, Mass: Jones and Bartlett Publishers; 2008.

Butts J, Rich K. *Nursing ethics*. Sudbury, Mass: Jones and Bartlett Publishers; 2005.

Cary AH. *International Survey of Certified Nurses in the U.S. and Canada*. Washington, DC: Nursing Credentialing Center; 2000.

Castrucci BC, Hoover K, Lim S et al. A comparison of breastfeeding rates in an urban birth cohort among women delivering infants at hospitals that employ and do not employ lactation consultants. *J Pub Health Manage Pract*. 2006;12:577–585.

Chagnon L, Wehmeyer J. Providing comprehensive services in a hospital outpatient center. *AWHONN Lifelines*. 2004;8:336–339.

Chen C-H. Effects of home visits and telephone contacts on breastfeeding compliance in Taiwan. *Maternal Child Nurs J*. 1993;21:82–90.

Click ER. Developing a worksite lactation program. *MCN*. 2006;11:313–317.

Cohen R, Mrtek MB, Mrtek RG. Comparison of maternal absenteeism and infant illness rates among breast-feeding and formula-feeding women in two corporations. *Amer J Health Promotion*. 1995;10:148–153.

Curro V et al. Randomised controlled trial assessing the effectiveness of a booklet on the duration of breast feeding. *Arch Dis Child*. 1997;76:500–504.

de Oliveira LD, Guigliani RG, Santo LC et al. Effect of intervention to improve breastfeeding technique on the frequency of exclusive breastfeeding lactation-related problems. *J Hum Lact*. 2006;22:315–321.

de Oliveira MI. Extending breastfeeding duration through primary care: a systematic review of prenatal and postnatal intervention. *J Hum Lact*. 2001;17:326–343.

Dodgson JE, Duckett L. Breastfeeding in the workplace: building a support program for nursing mothers. *AAOHN J*. 1997;45:290–298.

Dreyfus SE, Dreyfus HO. A five-stage model of the mental activities involved in directed skill acquisition (USAF Contract No. F49620–79–C–0063) Berkeley: University of California; 1980.

Duffy EP, Percival P, Kershaw E. Positive effects of an antenatal group teaching session on postnatal nipple pain, nipple trauma and breastfeeding rates. *Midwifery*. 1997;13:189–196.

Ferrarello DP. The entrepreneurial LC: the mission and the math. Presented at: Annual Meeting and Conference of the ILCA; July 2001; Acapulco, Mexico.

Forster D et al. Two mid-pregnancy interventions to increase the initiation and duration of breast-feeding: a randomized controlled trial. *Birth*. 2004;31:176–182.

Frank DA et al. Commercial discharge packs and breast-feeding counseling effects on infant-feeding practices in a randomized trial. *Pediatrics*. 1987;80:845–854.

Froozani MD et al. Effect of breastfeeding education on the feeding pattern and health of infants in their first 4 months in the Islamic Republic of Iran. *Bull WHO*. 1999;77:381–385.

Gagnon AF et al. A randomized trial of a program of early postpartum discharge with nurse visitation. *Am J Obstet Gynecol*. 1997;176:205–211.

Gardner KL, Weinrauch D. Marketing strategies for nurse entrepreneurs. *Nurse Pract*. 1988;13:46–49.

Gibbins S et al. The role of the clinical nurse specialist/neonatal nurse practitioner in a breastfeeding clinic: a model of advanced practice. *Clin Nurse Special*. 2000;14:56–59.

Gill SL, Reifsnider E, Lucke FL. Effects of support on the initiation and duration of breastfeeding. *Western J Nurs Res*. 2007;29:708–723.

Gilligan C. In a different voice. Cambridge, Mass: Harvard University Press; 1982.

Gross LJ. Statistical report of the 2002 IBLCE examination. Available at: http://www.iblce.org. Accessed November 20, 2008.

Hafner-Eaton C. Lactation consultant reimbursement, consultation, charges/fees, and hours worked: beginning the resource-based relative value scale (RBRVS) method of reimbursement. Presented at: Annual Meeting of the International Lactation Consultant Association; July 2000; Boca Raton, Fla.

Hauch YL, Dimmock JE. Evaluation of an information booklet on breastfeeding duration: a clinical trial. *J Adv Nurs*. 1994;20:836–843.

Heinig MJ. Closet consulting and other enabling behaviors. *J Hum Lact*. 1998;14:181–182.

Hill PD. Effects of education on breastfeeding success. *Maternal Child Nurs J*. 1987;16:145–156.

Hinson P. The business of clinical practice. In: Auerbach KG, ed. *Current Issues in Clinical Lactation 2000*. Sudbury, Mass: Jones and Bartlett; 2000:43–47.

International Board of Lactation Consultant Examiners (IBLCE). Examination data. Available at: http://www.iblce.org. Accessed December, 2007.

International Board of Lactation Consultant Examiners (IBLCE). Code of Ethics. Available at: http://www.iblce.org. Accessed June 5, 2007.

International Lactation Consultant Association (ILCA). Reimbursement tool kit. Raleigh, NC: ILCA; 2002.

International Lactation Consultant Association (ILCA). Standards of practice for international board-certified lactation consultants. Raleigh, NC: ILCA; 2008.

Jakobsen MS et al. Promoting breastfeeding through health education at the time of immunizations: a randomized trial from Guinea Bissau. *Acta Paediatr*. 1999;88:741–747.

Joel LA. An epiphany in retrospect [editorial]. *Amer J Nurs*. 1997;97(11):7.

Labarere J, Gelbert-Baudino N, Ayral A et al. Efficacy of breastfeed support provided by trained clinicians during an early, routine preventive visit: a prospective, randomized open trial of 226 mother-infant pairs. *Pediatrics*. 2005;11:139–146.

Lauwers J. Mentoring and precepting lactation consultants. *J Hum Lact*. 2007;23:10–11.

List BA et al. Electronic health records in an outpatient breastfeeding medicine clinic. *J Hum Lact*. 2008;24:58–68.

Lynch SA et al. Evaluating effect of a breastfeeding consultant on the duration of breastfeeding. *Can J Public Health*. 1986;77:190–195.

Mannel R, Mannel RS. Staffing for hospital lactation programs: recommendations from a tertiary care teaching hospital. *J Hum Lact*. 2006;22:409–417.

Mattar CN et al. Simple antenatal preparation to improve breastfeeding practice: a randomized controlled trial. *Obstet Gynecol*. 2007;109:73–80.

Meier P. Letter to the editor. Concerns regarding industry-funded trials. *J Hum Lact*.

Neyzi O et al. An educational intervention on promotion of breastfeeding. *Paediatr Perinat Epidemio*. 1991;5:286–298.

Niebuhr B, Biel M. The value of specialty certification. *Nursing Outlook*. 2007;55:176–181.

Noel-Weiss J, Walters GJ. Ethics and lactation consultants: Developing knowledge, skills and tools. *J Hum Lact*. 2006;22(2):203–212.

Parris KM. Integrating nursing diagnosis, interventions, and outcomes in public health nursing practice. *Nurs Diag*. 1999;10:49–56.

Phillips V. The Nursing Mother's Association of Australia as a self-help organization. In: Katz AH, Bender EL, eds. *Helping One Another: Self-Help Groups in a Changing World*. Oakland, Calif: Third Party Publishing; 1990.

Pugh LC et al. Breastfeeding duration, costs, and benefits of a support program for low-income breastfeeding women. *Birth*. 2002;29(2):95–100.

Pugh LC, Milligan RA. Nursing intervention to increase the duration of breastfeeding. *Appl Nurs Res*. 1998;11:190–194.

Rago JL. Breast pump rental depot: a way to bridge the gap. *J Hum Lact*. 1987;3:156–157.

Raudonis BM, Anderson CM. A theoretical framework for specialty certification in nursing practice. *Nursing Outlook*. 2002;50:247–252.

Riordan J, Auerbach K. Breastfeeding and human lactation. 2nd ed. Sudbury, Mass: Jones and Bartlett; 1999.

Rossiter JC. The effect of a culture-specific education program to promote breastfeeding among Vietnamese women in Sydney. *Int J Nurs Stud*. 1994;31:369–379.

Scott J. The code of ethics from international board-certified lactation consultant: ethical practice. In: Walker M, ed. *Core Curriculum for Lactation Consultant Practice*. Sudbury, Mass: Jones and Bartlett; 2002:517–527.

Serafino-Cross P, Donovan PR. Effectiveness of professional breastfeeding home-support. *J Nutr Educ*. 1992;24:117–122.

Shrago LC. Fostering collegial relationships among lactation consultants [editorial]. *J Hum Lact*. 1995;11:1–2.

Simpson KC, Creehan, PA. *AWHONN Perinatal Nursing*. 2nd ed. Philadelphia, Pa: Lippincott; 2001.

Smillie C. A specialty practice in breastfeeding. In: Auerbach KG, ed. *Current Issues in Clinical Lactation 2000*. Sudbury, Mass: Jones and Bartlett; 2000:49–54.

Smith L. Shadowing Guidelines. Personal Communication. January 2002.

Susin L et al. Does parental breastfeeding knowledge increase breastfeeding rates? *Birth.* 1999;26: 149–156.

Thorley V. Complementary and competing roles of volunteers and professionals in the breastfeeding field. *Int Self Help Self Care.* 2000;1(2): 171–179.

Turner MR. Twenty questions for the consumer: a quality assurance tool for the lactation consultant. *J Hum Lact.* 1996;12:50–52.

Wiessinger D. Professional responsibility revisited. In: Smith L, ed. The Lactation Consultant in Private Practice. Sudbury, Mass: Jones and Bartlett; 2003:214–226.

Williams EL. Increasing your credibility with physicians: strategies for lactation consultants [editorial]. *J Hum Lact.* 1995;11:3–4.

Wilson-Clay B. Lactation consultants: are we a profession yet? In: Auerbach K, ed. *Clinical Issues in Clinical Lactation.* Sudbury, Mass: Jones and Bartlett; 2000:57–72.

Woolf V. *A room of one's own.* New York, NY: Harcourt, Brace and World; 1929.

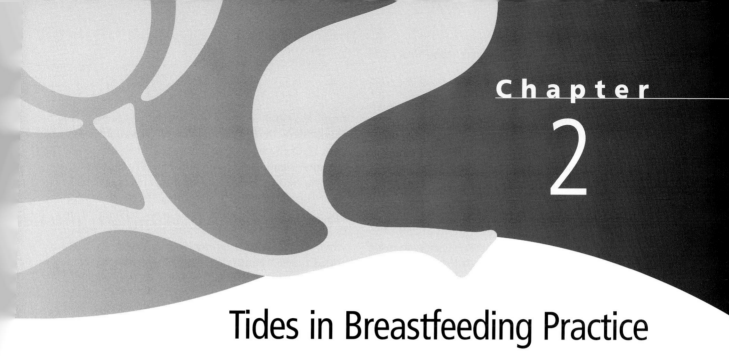

Chapter 2

Tides in Breastfeeding Practice

Mary Margaret Coates

THE NEWS IS ENCOURAGING: Throughout the world today, an infant is apt to receive more breastmilk than during the nadir of breastfeeding in the 1960s and early 1970s. Until the 1940s, the prevalence of breastfeeding was high in nearly all societies. Although the feeding of manufactured milk products (for general use or specifically for infants) had begun before the turn of the century in parts of Europe and North America, the practice spread slowly during the next several decades. It was still generally limited to segments of population elites, and it involved only a small percentage of the world's people. During the post–World War II era, however, the way in which most mothers in industrialized regions fed their infants began to change, and the export of these new practices to developing regions gained speed (for one of many examples, see Schaefer, 1956).

Evidence About Breastfeeding Practices

How do we know what we "know" about the prevalence of breastfeeding? (The word *prevalence* is used here to mean the combined effect of breastfeeding initiation rates and breastfeeding continuance rates.) Before attempting to trace long-term trends in infant feeding practices, let us consider the nature of the evidence available to us in 2007.

Large-Scale Surveys

National surveys that produce the kind of representative data that allow statistical evaluation have become available only recently anywhere in the world; in the United States, they have been available only since 1955. These surveys consist primarily of national fertility or natality surveys and of marketing surveys conducted by manufacturers of artificial baby milk. Some surveys are now (2007) asking not only about any breastfeeding but also about the age of the infant when foods other than breastmilk were introduced and the nature of those foods. A brief description of national surveys conducted in the United States follows (http://www.cdc.gov/nchs/nhis.htm).

During the latter part of the 1900s and earliest years of this century, reliable information about breastfeeding rates in the United States and elsewhere was difficult to obtain. It is a marker of the late interest of public health officials and the medical profession in general in promoting breastfeeding that the earliest and longest continued survey of breastfeeding initiation rates in the United States began in 1956 to provide marketing information for the maker of manufactured substitutes for human milk. Health surveys in the United States or other nations or those sponsored by international organizations only recently began incorporating questions about breastfeeding.

This situation has finally begun to change (Box 2–1). In the United States, various arms of the Centers for Disease Control and Prevention sponsor national surveys that now collect information about breastfeeding: the National Health Interview Survey, National Health and Nutrition Survey, National Immunization Survey, and National Survey of Family Growth, Pediatric Nutrition Surveillance System. With the notable exception of questions in the National Health and Nutrition Examination Survey and the National Immunization Survey, questions in most surveys pertain to "any breastfeeding" and do not distinguish degrees of mixed feeding from exclusive breastfeeding or the age of the infant when other liquids or foods were first regularly added to the infant's diet. Thus, the ability to calculate continuance rates lags well behind our ability to calculate initiation rates.

BOX **2–1**

Large Surveys of Breastfeeding Prevalence and Practices in the United States and Around the World and Selected Reports Using Survey Information

United States

The federal government sponsors several health surveys that include questions about infant feeding.

Surveys Sponsored by the Centers for Disease Control and Prevention (CDC)

This Web address contains links to all CDC surveys listed below:
www.cdc.gov/breastfeeding/data/index.htm:

- Infant Feeding Practices Survey II: Two Infant Feeding Practices Surveys have been undertaken, the first in 1993–1994 (*Infant Feeding Practices Survey I*) and the second in 2005–2007. Both were longitudinal studies that followed women for about 15 months— from the third trimester of pregnancy through their infant's first year. In the second study, about 4000 women began and about 2200 women were expected to finish the study, which required com-

pleting 1 telephone interview and 11 extensive written questionnaires. The survey's goal is to elicit information about what mothers feed their infants and the influences on those feeding choices.
  - www.cdc.gov/breastfeeding/data/ infant_feeding.htm
  - Preliminary results were presented in November 2007 at an American Public Health Association conference (apha.confex.com/apha/135am/tech program/session_22066.htm)

- Maternity Care Practices Survey: The CDC is surveying breastfeeding-related care in labor and delivery units throughout the United States; the first survey occurred 2007 and subsequent surveys are proposed at 2-year intervals.
  - www.cdc.gov/breastfeeding/data/ maternity_care.htm

- National Health and Nutrition Examination Survey: The National Health

(Continues)

BOX **2–1** (Continued)

and Nutrition Examination Survey (NHANES) has as one purpose the gathering of information that will allow researchers to study the relationship between diet, nutrition, and health. It was conducted periodically seven times since its inception in 1959, but beginning in 1999 it was converted to a continuous field survey. About 5000 people drawn from throughout the United States are interviewed in any given 12-month period. The 2005–2006 questionnaire asked seven questions about infant feeding and introduction of non-breastmilk foods.

- Visit www.cdc.gov/nchs/nhanes.htm; then search on NHANES 2005–2006 and then on Survey questionnaires)
- Gibson et al. Prevalence of breastfeeding and acculturation in Hispanics: results from NHANES 1999–2000 study. *Birth*. 2005;32(2):93–98.

- National Immunization Survey: The National Immunization Survey, first used in 1994, completes approximately 36,000 telephone interviews with people in all 50 states and the District of Columbia. All households contacted (by random-digit dialing) contain children aged 19–35 months. Since January 2003, questions about breastfeeding have been asked of all survey respondents. Results of the survey not only provide overall population estimates for the initiation, duration, and exclusivity of breastfeeding, but also provide breastfeeding rates for certain metropolitan areas. As of 2006, data obtained from National Immunization Survey are used to track progress towards the breastfeeding goals outlined in the Surgeon General's report *Healthy People 2010*.

- www.cdc.gov/breastfeeding/data/NIS_data/data_2005.htm
- Li et al. Breastfeeding rates in the United States by characteristics of the child, mother, or family: the 2002 National Immunization Survey. *Pediatrics*. 2005;115(1):e31–e37.
- Ryan. More about the Ross Mothers Survey [letter to the editor]. *Pediatrics*. 2005;115(5):1450.

- National Survey of Family Growth: Face-to-face interviews are conducted at irregular intervals. The 2002 women's questionnaire (a part of cycle 6 of the survey), which obtained information from about 7500 interviewees, contained five questions pertaining to breastfeeding and the introduction of nonbreastmilk foods (www.cdc.gov.nchs/data/nsfg). Cycle 7 of the survey, which is now a continuous survey, began in mid-2006. The first public release of information is projected for late 2009; it will be based on about 11,000 interviews made during 2006–2008.
  - A description of the National Survey of Family Growth can be found at www.cdc.gov/nchs/nsfg.htm.
  - Taylor et al. Duration of breastfeeding among first-time mothers in the United States: results of a national survey. *Acta Paediatr*. 2006;95:980–984.

- National Birth Certificate Data: In 2007, the US Standard Certificate of Live Birth is undergoing revision. For the first time in its history, the proposed birth certificate will include a question on whether the newborn is being breastfed. Two forms will be completed: one reported by the mother, another reported by the birthing health facility.

(*Continues*)

BOX **2–1** (Continued)

Surveys Sponsored by Supplemental Nutrition for Women, Infants, and Children (WIC)

- Pediatric Nutrition Surveillance System (PedNSS): Information about breastfeeding incidence and duration in low-income populations are collected in public health clinics and WIC programs and reported annually. National, state, county, and clinic data are analyzed.
  - www.cdc.gov/pednss/htm
  - The report for 2004, released in 2006, is available at www.cdc.gov/nccdphp/dnpa/pednss.htm.
- Pregnancy Risk Assessment and Monitoring System:
  - www.cdc.gov.prams
  - Ahluwalia et al. Why do women stop breastfeeding? Findings from the Pregnancy Risk Assessment and Monitoring System. *Pediatrics*. 2005;116(6):1408–1412.
- WIC Participant and Program Characteristics: Data on breastfeeding are collected each even-numbered year by the Department of Agriculture about participants in the WIC program. In 2004, approximately 8,500,000 women and children were enrolled in WIC; about a quarter each were mothers and infants under 1 year of age, and about a half were children aged 1 through 4 years. For infants 7–11 months old, data is collected by state about any breastfeeding.
  - www.fns.usda.gov.oane/MENU/Published/WIC/FILES/PC2004ExeSum.pdf

Surveys Sponsored Privately

- Ross Mothers Survey: For marketing purposes, the maker of a manufactured infant milk mails questionnaires to a probability sample of mothers whose names are obtained from a large national database of pregnant or newly delivered women. The survey generates some controversy (Li et al., 2003) in part because the response rate has been as low as 28% (Ryan et al., 2002). Data about the type of milk or milk product fed, but not about exclusive breastfeeding, are collected monthly for up to 12 months for a given cohort and are published on an ad hoc basis. Until 2006, the survey was the source of data used to monitor breastfeeding goals in the U.S. Surgeon General's *Healthy People* programs, the current version of which is *Healthy People 2010*.
  - www.childtrendsdatabank.org/indicators/90Breastfeeding.cfm
  - www.ross.com/images/library/BF_Trends_2003.pdf
- Ryan et al. Regional and sociodemographic variation of breastfeeding in the United States, 2002. *Clin Pediatr*. 2004;43:815–824.
- Ryan et al. Breastfeeding continues to increase into the new millennium. *Pediatrics*. 2002;110:1103–1109.
- Ryan AS. More about the Ross Mothers Survey [letter to the editor]. *Pediatrics*. 2005;115(5):1450.
- Ryan AS, Zhou W. Lower breastfeeding rates persist among the Special Supplemental Nutrition for Women, Infants, and Children participants, 1978–2003. *Pediatrics*. 2006;117(4):1136–1146.

(Continues)

BOX **2–1** (Continued)

- HealthStyles Survey: The HealthStyles Survey is a proprietary (Porter Novelli Consumer Styles) national marketing survey in the United States that asks about health behavior; the survey was first distributed in 1995. It may be the only nationwide survey in the United States that gathers opinion about breastfeeding. The CDC licenses survey results for use in health promotion; it has contributed questions on breastfeeding since 1999. The CDC Web site contains links to those questions and survey results for each year beginning in 1999. This survey is mailed annually to about 5000 persons; the sample is structured so that respondents mirror demographic categories and proportions of United States census data.
  - www.cdc.gov/print; then search on HealthStyles Survey
  - Hannan A, Li R, Benton-Davis S, Grummer-Strawn L. Regional variation in public opinion about breastfeeding in the United States. *J Hum Lact.* 2005;21(3):284–288.

Around the World

Outside the United States, representative data for countries in North America, Latin America, Asia, Africa, and the Middle East can be obtained from the following surveys:

- United Nations International Children's Fund (UNICEF)
  - www.childinfo.org (Worldwide statistics on rate of exclusive breastfeeding, introduction of complementary foods, and continued breastfeeding; data derived from a variety of studies and presented graphically)

- Baby-Friendly Hospital Initiative: Breastfeeding initiation rates in 2001 in United States' hospitals certified as baby-friendly by the Baby-Friendly Hospital Initiative, an international effort sponsored by the World Health Organization and the United Nations Children's Fund.
  - www.unicef.org/programme/breastfeeding/baby.htm
  - Merewood et al. Breastfeeding rates in US Baby-Friendly hospitals: results of a national survey. *Pediatrics.* 2005;116(3):628–634.

- World Health Organization (WHO) Global Databank on Breastfeeding and Complementary Feeding: The World Health Organization places information about breastfeeding and weaning practices obtained from methodologically rigorous local studies into a database that can be searched by country, year, and any of about 30 specific types of information—such as "ever breastfed" or "exclusively breastfed at 3 months." The data bank pools information mainly from national and regional surveys and from studies dealing specifically with the prevalence and duration of breastfeeding and complementary feeding. Data for inclusion are based on two types of indicators: those derived from households and those used to assess health facility practices, which are also part of the Baby-Friendly Hospital Initiative. It is continually updated as new studies and surveys become available.
  - www.who.int/research/iycf/bfcf/bfcf.asp (Links to WHO Global Data Bank on Breastfeeding and Complementary Feeding)

(Continues)

- www.who.int/nutrition/databases/infantfeeding/en/index.html (General information page; links to searchable database on rates of breastfeeding)
- www.who.int/topics/breastfeeding/en/ (Links to WHO publications on breastfeeding)

- Demographic and Health Surveys: The Demographic and Health Surveys are nationally representative household surveys with large sample sizes (usually between 5000 and 30,000 households); they typically are conducted every 5 years. They continue the work of earlier World Fertility Surveys. Now called "Measure DHS," the surveys are part of a US Agency for International Development's program that collects and analyzes information on infant and young child nutrition in some 40 countries. Breastfeeding practices in the newborn period and later and the addition of complementary foods to the diets of breastfed and non-breastfed infants are reported in each country's final report. The most recent update, which was published in 2006, analyzes data collected between 1998 and 2004.
- www.measuredhs.com
- Mukuria et al. Infant and young child feeding update (USAID). Calverton, MD: ORC Macro; 2006. Available at: http://www.measuredhs.com/pubs/pdf/NUT1/NUT1%2Epdf.
- Marriott et al. Preliminary data from Demographic and Health Surveys on infant feeding in 20 developing countries. *J Nutr.* 2007;137:518S–523S.
- Ruel, Menon. Child feeding practices are associated with child nutritional status in Latin America: innovative uses of the Demographic and Health Surveys. *J Nutr.* 2002;132:1180–1187.

Other Evidence

Until the last several decades, breastfeeding was the unremarkable norm. Thus what we "know" about breastfeeding from much earlier times often must be inferred from evidence of other methods of feeding infants. Most historical material available in English-language literature derives from a limited geographic area: Western Europe, Asia Minor, the Middle East, and North Africa. More recently, English-language reviews of ancient breastfeeding practices in other regions and varied religious traditions are beginning to fill this gap (Gartner & Stone, 1994; Laroia & Sharma, 2006; Shaikh & Ahmed, 2006). Written materials, although sparse, extend back to before 2000 BC and include verses, legal statutes, religious tracts, personal correspondence, inscriptions, and medical literature.

Some of the earliest existing medical literature deals at least in passing with infant feeding. An Egyptian medical encyclopedia, the *Papyrus Ebers* (c. 1500 BC), contains recommendations for increasing a mother's milk supply (Fildes, 1986). The first writings to discuss infant feeding in detail are those of the physician Soranus, who practiced in Rome around AD 100; his views were widely repeated by other writers until the mid-1700s. It is not immediately apparent to what degree these early exhortations either reflected or influenced actual practices. Many writings before AD 1800 deal primarily with wet nurses or how to hand-feed infants.

Archeological evidence provides some information about infant feeding prior to 2000 BC. Some of the earliest artifacts are Middle Eastern pottery figurines that depict lactating goddesses, such as Ishtar of Babylon and Isis of Egypt. The abundance of this evidence suggests that lactation was held in high regard (Fildes, 1986). Such artifacts first appear in sites about 3000 BC, when pottery making first became widespread in that region. Information about infant feeding may also be derived from paintings, inscriptions, and infant feeding implements.

Modern ethnography has a place of special importance. By documenting the infant feeding practices of present-day nontechnological hunter–gatherer, herding, and farming societies, ethnographers expand our knowledge of the range of normal breastfeeding practices. At the same time, they provide a richer appreciation of cultural practices that enhance the prevalence of breastfeeding. Such studies are also our best window into breastfeeding practices that may be the biological norm for *Homo sapiens sapiens*.

In summary, the historical aspect of this chapter deals with limited data from a limited social stratum in a limited geographic region. However, the common threads of these data provide a useful context within which we may better understand modern breastfeeding practices, especially in Western cultures.

The Biological Norm in Infant Feeding

Early Human Evolution

The class Mammalia is characterized principally by the presence of breasts (mammae), which secrete and release a fluid that for a time is the sole nourishment of the young. This manner of sustaining newborns is extremely ancient; it dates back to the late Mesozoic era, some 100 million years ago, when the first mammals appeared (see Figure 2–1). Hominid precursors first appeared about 4 million years ago; the genus *Homo* has existed for about 2 million years. Fossil evidence shows that our species, *Homo sapiens*, has existed for approximately 200,000 years and that our species of anatomically modern humans, *Homo sapiens sapiens*, first differentiated about 130,000 years ago in Africa, were in the Near East by 90,000 years ago, and first appeared in what is now southern Europe about 40,000 years ago. Direct information about breastfeeding practices among our earliest ancestors is lacking, although other information about Paleolithic societies that existed 10,000 or more years ago sheds some light on this subject.

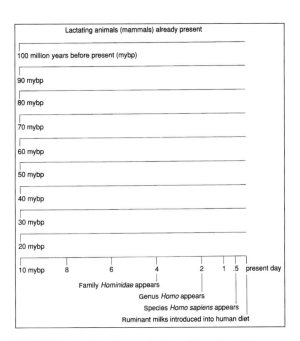

FIGURE 2–1 The antiquity of lactation. The bottom line shows the approximate times of first appearance of lactating precursors of modern humans and of regular use of nonhuman animal milk by humans.

Early Breastfeeding Practices

Diets reconstructed by archeological methods reveal that the Late Paleolithic era, roughly 40,000 to 10,000 years ago, was populated by hunter–gatherer peoples who ate a wide variety of fruits, nuts, vegetables, meat (both large and small game depending on its availability), and in geographically favorable regions, fish and shellfish (Eaton, 1992). This diet closely resembles that of 20th-century hunter–gatherer societies. Therefore, the infant-feeding practices of such societies today may reflect breastfeeding practices of much earlier (prehistoric) times. Consider the breastfeeding practices of the ¡Kung of the Kalahari Desert in southern Africa (Konner & Worthman, 1980) as well as hunter–gatherer societies of Papua New Guinea and elsewhere. Among these people, breastfeeding of young infants is frequent (averaging four feeds per hour) and short (about 2 minutes per feed). It is equally distributed over a 24-hour period and continues, tapering off gradually, for 2 to 6 years (Short, 1984).

Age of weaning (complete cessation of breastfeeding) in this ancient era is more difficult to pin down, but at least two lines of evidence suggest that 2 to 4 years was common in many cultures. First, weaning would be difficult before eruption of a full set of deciduous teeth, about 24 months, that allowed an infant to consume the family diet (Dettwyler, 1995). Second, as is true of other mammals, a human infant must produce lactase, the enzyme that cuts lactose (an otherwise indigestible disaccharide that is the principal sugar in milk) into an easily digestible monosaccharide. In other mammals, the ability to produce lactase attenuates during the nursing interval and is lost after weaning. In most modern human infants, this ability declines steadily after age two years and is rare by age four years (Dettwyler, 1995), suggesting that infants generally were weaned—or consuming only small amounts of breastmilk—by that time. (In those cultures where animal milk is fed throughout childhood and beyond, lactase production may continue longer.) These breastfeeding patterns are considered a direct inheritance of practices that prevailed at the end of a long, and dietetically stable, evolutionary period that began to end about 15,000 BC. This assumption is supported by observations of the human's closest primate relative, the chimpanzee, which secretes a milk quite similar to that of humans, suckles several times per hour, and sleeps with and nurses its young at night (Short, 1984).

Infant Feeding: Alternatives to Maternal Breastfeeding

Infant-feeding practices in most societies commonly have mixed breastfeeding, wet-nursing, and hand-feeding (also called dry-nursing) to one degree or another and at one time or another in the infant's life.

Wet-Nursing

Wet-nursing may not have been the only alternative to maternal breastfeeding, but it was the only one likely to enable the infant to survive. Wet-nursing is common, although not universal, in traditional societies of today and (by inference) among ancient human societies. An already-lactating woman may have been the most obvious choice for a wet nurse, but women who stimulate lactation without a recent pregnancy have been described in many traditional societies (Wieschhoff, 1940; Slome, 1976).

Wet-nursing for hire is mentioned in some of the oldest surviving texts, which implies that the practice was well established even in ancient times. The Babylonian Code of Hammurabi (c. 1700 BC) forbade a wet nurse to substitute a new infant for one who had died. The Old Testament Book of Exodus (Exodus 2:7–9; c. 1250 BC) records the hiring of a wet nurse for the foundling Moses; the fact that the wet nurse was Moses's own mother is incidental. The epic poems of Homer, written down around 900 BC, contain references to wet nurses. A treatise on pediatric care in India, written during the second century AD, contains instructions on how to qualify a wet nurse when the mother could not provide milk. The Koran, set in written form about AD 500, also permits parents to "give your children out to nurse."

Although the history of wet-nursing has continued virtually unbroken from the earliest times to the present, the popularity of the practice among the elite classes who used it most has waxed and waned. In England during the 1600s and 1700s and elsewhere in Europe, the middle classes began to employ wet nurses. The use of less attentive nurses and the sending of infants greater distances from home diminished maternal supervision of either nurse or infant. Often infants were not seen by their parents from the time they were given to the nurse until they were returned home after weaning (providing they lived). However, by the latter part of the 1700s wet-nursing was on the decline in North America and England, except in foundling hospitals, owing to increased public concern regarding the moral character of wet nurses (and in the belief that character was transmitted through the milk) and the quality of the care they provided. In France, government officials and physicians led a campaign against wet-nursing. Throughout this long period, wet nurses were used sometimes because of maternal debility but more often because of the social expectations of the class of women who could afford to hire a wet nurse. Thus the use of wet nurses by social elites foreshadows the demographic pattern later seen in the use of manufactured human-milk substitutes.

Hand-Fed Foods

The Agricultural Revolution

The idea that animal milks are suitable foods for human infants is reflected in such myths as that of Romulus and Remus, the mythical founders of Rome, who are usually depicted as being suckled by a wolf. Surprisingly, the currently most popular hand-fed infant foods—animal milks and cereals—did not become part of the human diet until well along in human history. Cereal grains first appeared in the human diet, in the Near East, only about 15,000 years ago (Eaton, 1992), and animal milks considerably later, perhaps 7000–5000 years ago (McCracken, 1971). The development of agriculture and (later) animal husbandry permitted the widespread adoption of these foods.

Gruels

In much of the world, the soft foods added most commonly to the infant diet have been paps or gruels containing a liquid, a cereal or another starchy food, and other substances common in the family diet that added variety or nutritional value. The liquid might be water, animal milk, or meat broth. The starch might be rice, wheat, or corn; or taro, cassava, or plantain. It might be boiled and mashed, ground and boiled, or—as in the case of bread crumbs—ground, baked, crushed, moistened, and reheated. In some cultures, eggs or butter might also be added.

Animal Milks

Despite the widespread use of animal milks (directly or in manufactured milk products) as a food for infants, animal milks are a relatively recent addition to the human diet. This "newcomer" status is implied genetically, because children beyond weaning age commonly do not produce lactase, an enzyme needed to digest the milk sugar lactose. In cultures that traditionally do not use animal milks, such as those in Mexico or Bangladesh or Thailand, some children may be lactose intolerant before one year of age; in those cultures that use animal milks abundantly, the onset of lactose intolerance occurs considerably later—after age 10, for instance, in Finland (Simoons, 1980). Animal milk thus is a food unknown in the human diet for most of its history

and to which our physiology is incompletely adapted. Such a food should be offered to a young infant as its sole nutriment for several months only with greatest caution.

Feeding Vessels

The earliest "vessel" used to hand-feed an infant was undoubtedly the human hand, and the foods so fed were probably soft or mashed, rather than liquid. The earliest crafted vessels for feeding liquids were probably animal horns pierced by holes in the tips; such horns continued to be used into the 1900s in parts of Europe. The oldest pottery vessel thought to have been used for infant feeding, a small spouted bowl found in an infant's grave in France, is dated c. 2000–1500 BC (Lacaille, 1950). Small spouted or football-shaped bowls have been found in infant burial sites in Germany (c. 900 BC) and in the Sudan in North Africa (c. 400 BC) (Lacaille, 1950). These utensils suggest that hand-feeding of infants has been attempted for more than three millennia (see Figure 2–2).

Age of Infant at Introduction of Hand-Feeding

What archeological evidence cannot tell us is why or how much these infants were hand-fed. Neonates may temporarily be offered certain foods as prelacteal feeds; young infants may be offered occasional tastes of other foods, and they will be offered increasing amounts of soft foods as they make the transition to the adult diet (mixed feeds). Finally, infants may be reared from birth on other foods (artificial feeding).

Prelacteal Feeds

Many of the world's infants, even those who later will be fully breastfed, receive other foods as newborns. Of 120 traditional societies (and, by inference, in many ancient preliterate societies) whose neonatal feeding practices have been described, 50 delay the initial breastfeeding more than 2 days, and some 50 more delay it 1 to 2 days. The stated reason is to avoid the feeding of colostrum, which is described as being dirty, contaminated, bad, bitter, constipating, insufficient, or stale (Morse, Jehle, & Gamble, 1990). For instance, it is reported that up to three quarters of women in

If fed from your breast, be sure that the quantity and quality supply his demands. If you are weak or worn out, your milk cannot contain the nourishment a babe needs.

The Technological Context

Between about 1860 and 1910, scientific advances and technological innovations created many new options in infant feeding that appeared to increase infant survival. The upright feeding bottle and rubber nipple, each of which could be cleaned thoroughly, made artificial feeding easier and safer. New foods to be used with this equipment appeared. Large-scale dairy farming produced abundant supplies of cow milk, which was marketed first as canned evaporated milk and later in condensed (highly sweetened to retard spoilage) or dried forms.

This technological ferment, fueled both by the need for improved infant health care and by a popular belief in the ability of science and technology to provide answers, attracted analytical chemists. Around 1850 chemists had begun to turn their attention to food products. Early investigations (now viewed as rudimentary) into the composition of human and cow milk convinced them that "the combined efforts of the cow and the ingenuity of man" could construct a food the equal of human milk (Gerrard, 1974). Patented foods, such as Liebig's Food and Nestle's Milk Food, were first marketed in Europe and the United States in the 1860s. The Nestle's product was a mixture of flour, cow milk, and sugar that was to be dissolved in milk or water before feeding. Milk modifiers, such as Mellin's Food, and milk foods, such as Horlick's Malted Milk, were popular in the United States by the 1880s.

Extravagant claims for these foods (Liebig's Food was called "the most perfect substitute for mother's milk") were combined with artful advertising that played on fears for the health of the infant and faith in modern science (Apple, 1986) (Figure 2–3). A hundred years later we see these advertising themes played again and again.

In the 1890s, physician Thomas Rotch developed a complex system of modifying cow milk so that it more closely resembled human milk. Rotch

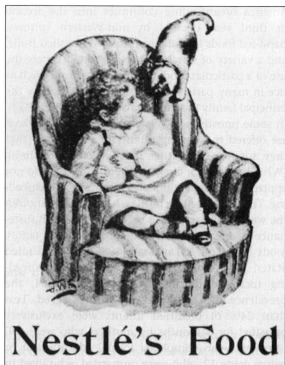

Nestlé's Food

Nestlé's Food is a complete and entire diet for babies. Over all the world Nestlé's Food has been recognized for more than thirty years as possessing great value as a protection against Cholera Infantum and all other forms of Summer Complaint.

Nestlé's Food is safe. It requires only the addition of water to prepare it for use. The great danger always attendant on the use of cow's milk is thus avoided.

Consult your doctor about Nestlé's Food, and send to us for a large sample can and our book, "The Baby," both of which will be sent free on application.

THOMAS LEEMING & CO.
73 Warren Street, New York

FIGURE 2–3 An advertisement for artificial infant milk that appeared in the *Ladies' Home Journal* in 1895.

observed that the composition of human milk varies, as do digestive capacities in infants. He devised mathematical formulas to denote the proportions of fat, sugar, and protein in cow milk that some infants required at a particular age (Rotch, 1907). The result was an exceedingly complex system of feeding that required constant intervention by the physician, who often changed the "formula" weekly. Supervising infant feeding then became a principal focus of the newly emerging specialty of pediatrics.

Commercial advertising promoted the use of manufactured infant milks to both mothers and physicians. Again, the basic themes—a mother's concern for her infant's health and the supposed perfection of the manufactured product and difficulty of breastfeeding—have persisted over the years (Apple, 1986).

The Role of the Medical Community

Breastfeeding may have in fact become more onerous during this interval, as women were impelled to give birth and breastfeed according to externally generated ideas about how those activities should be accomplished.

Regulation of Childbirth

During the early part of the 1900s, childbirth moved largely from home or midwife-attended births to hospitals, where a birthing woman was separated from her family and attended by hospital staff. During the middle part of this century, hospital routines and the widespread use of general anesthesia during labor and delivery separated mother and infant much of the time in the early postpartum period. Bottle-feeding of manufactured human-milk substitutes by nursery staff became increasingly common. Normal postpartum hospital stays in the United States lengthened; during the 1930s and 1940s, they were sometimes as long as 2 weeks. This period, intended to permit the mother to recuperate from a commonly highly medicated childbirth, resulted as well in a return home with an impaired breastmilk supply and a baby who was accustomed to feeding from bottle nipples. Bain (1948) notes that babies who were older than 8 days at discharge were less apt to be breastfed than were younger ones.

Regulation of Breastfeeding

Underlying many changes in the feeding of infants was a "regulatory" frame of mind, the seeds of which had been sown in Europe as early as the 1500s. The advent of book printing about this time permitted a much wider dissemination of works on infant care. Their authors, male physicians, shared a concern for the high incidence of gastrointestinal illness in infants and for high infant-mortality rates.

For reasons not at all clear today, overfeeding was deemed a central factor in both. Writers concerned with child care responded by advocating the regulation of feeding in order to prevent presumed overfeeding. Writing in the mid-1600s, Ettmuller (1703; cited in Wickes, 1953a) was not the first to recommend infrequent feedings:

> *Nothing is more apt to disorder the child than suckling it too often, since large quantities of milk stagnating in the stomach, must needs corrupt ... especially if fresh milk be pour'd in before the preceding be digested.*

Some 250 years later in 1900, Pierre Budin (1907; cited in Wickes, 1953b), a French obstetrician famous for his early interest in premature infants and for his advocacy of breastfeeding, was nonetheless typical of many others in recommending small feedings: "It is better at first to give too little than too much (for an underfed infant failed to gain weight but it was free from digestive troubles)."

Even early medical writers who strongly recommended breastfeeding also recommended highly regulated times for feedings—a fixed number of feedings at fixed times. William Cadogan (1749; cited in Kessen, 1965), whose firm endorsement of breastfeeding and largely sound advice prompted many privileged English women to breastfeed, advocated only four feeds per day at equal intervals, and no night feeds! A prototype mothercraft manual by Hugh Smith (1774; cited in Fildes, 1986) contains excellent advice: to feed colostrum and to allow the newborn to suckle frequently to stimulate lactation. However, it then instructs mothers to limit feeds (beginning at 1 month), to five per day between 7 A.M. and 11 P.M. (although how those feedings were timed in households that generally lacked clocks is difficult to understand). About 50 years later, after recommending ad lib feeds for the first 10 days, Thomas Bull (1849; cited in Wickes, 1953a) instructed mothers to feed for the rest of the first month at regular 4-hour intervals day and night, because he also believed that irregular feeding harmed the infant. After 1 month the night feed was to be eliminated.

These influential publications began to remove the management of infant feeding from the mother (or from the realm of women in general) and placing it in the hands of (usually male) "authorities." Cadogan (1749; cited in Kessen, 1965) commended this change that put "men of sense rather than foolish unlearned women" in charge, and Rotch a century and a half later (1907) deplored that "mothers and nurses … dominated the physicians." The most common explanation among all classes of women in the United States, at least since popular women's magazines became widely distributed in the late 1800s, for feeding artificial products to an infant is that the mother did not have enough milk. It has been observed that "not enough milk" corresponds closely with the widespread implementation of infant feeding schedules (Wolf, 2006). For far too long, women able to consult physicians were thus placed in a double bind, and—as they tried to satisfy both the baby and the authorities directing how she cared for her baby—breastfeeding oftentimes got left behind.

With respect to a newborn's first breastfeed, as late as the 1950s US physicians ordered that newborns be given nothing by mouth for the first 24 hours after birth. In Australia, midwifery texts of the 1940s recommended that the baby not go to the breast until 12 hours after birth (Thorley, 2001). Now (2007) we encourage the newborn to feed at the breast immediately after birth or at least within the first hour after birth (World Health Organization, 1991). One can only wonder which of today's standard recommendations to breastfeeding mothers will be shown, at some time in the future, to be counterproductive.

Many—and perhaps most—of our everyday decisions are influenced by the social norms of our culture, our civic community, and our immediate circle of family and friends (Baranowski et al., 1983; Matich & Sims, 1992). The long-standing need in the United States for breastfeeding "promotion" is rooted in the common perception that the breast functions primarily for sexual gratification and, thus, should not be exposed in public. Legislation in most states in the United States that permits breastfeeding in public notwithstanding, many mothers avoid doing so because of social censure. For instance, a telephone survey in Australia found that almost 83% of respondents favored bottle-feeding rather than breastfeeding in public (McIntyre, Hiller, & Turnbull, 2001). A 2004 HealthStyles survey in the United States reported that about 37% of people questioned agreed that mothers should breastfeed only in private (a nearly equal percentage favored allowing breastfeeding in public; the remainder, about 27%, was undecided) (CDC, 2004). Considerable regional and demographic variation in such attitudes exists in the United States (Ryan, Zhou, & Gaston, 2004; Hannan, Li, Benton-Davis, & Grummer-Strawn, 2005). In general, New England, the mountain West, and Pacific regions were most accepting of breastfeeding in public.

Mass media may also influence perceptions of breastfeeding. One study finds that when the number of commercial advertisements for formula feeding increased in one widely circulated magazine for parents published in the United States, breastfeeding prevalence generally dropped during the following year (Foss & Southwell, 2006). Magazine illustrations depicting breastfeeding may have a decidedly mixed reaction. In 2006, one popular magazine's cover photo depicted a portion of breast with a baby latched on (no nipple visible). In a poll of about 4000 readers, only about a quarter objected to the photo, but those people objected strongly (CBS News, 2006).

Regulation and Industrialization

This "regulatory" frame of mind fit nicely with the needs of the growing industrial sector of the economy, which relied on efficiency and schedules governed by the clock. Societal perceptions of infants' innate characteristics and needs were interpreted in this light (Millard, 1990). Early in the 1900s, infants were seen as needing order imposed onto their characters from the outside (Rossiter, 1908):

> *An infant two days old may be forming either a good or a bad habit. A child that is taken up whenever it cries is trained into a bad habit; the same principle is true in reference to nursing a baby to stop its crying. Both these habits cultivate self-indulgence and a lack of self-control.*

"Good" mothering thus drifted toward meeting the letter of schedules commonly imposed by the medical profession rather than meeting the mutual needs of mother and infant as expressed by and interpreted within the dyad.

Although the use of rigid, externally imposed infant care schedules began diminishing in the 1970s, much "how to" breastfeeding literature assumes that lactation functions better when mother and baby develop feeding routines. The lack of some routine is usually perceived as abnormal by both mother and physician (Millard, 1990). Unfortunately, certain attitudes required of most employees, such as an awareness of time within a hierarchical authority structure, are least apt to enable a mother or a pediatrician to accommodate the normal irregularities of early breastfeeding.

Regulation of Contraception

During the late 1950s and early 1960s, the widespread acceptance of oral contraceptives may have also reinforced the decline in breastfeeding (Meyer, 1968). Contraceptives containing estrogen reduce breastmilk volume and thus contribute to lactation insufficiency, early supplementation, and early weaning from the breast. Moreover, women who planned to use combined estrogen and progestin oral contraceptives were discouraged from breastfeeding in order to avoid passing those hormones to the infant. During this period, several million women per year in the United States alone were thereby removed from the pool of potential breastfeeders. Concurrently, the widespread adoption of manufactured substitutes for human milk led to loss of appreciation for the contraceptive benefit of lactation amenorrhea.

Although low-progestin contraceptives once were thought to pose fewer hazards to the maternal milk supply and the baby (Kelsey, 1996), a more recent review of literature finds the evidence contradictory (Truitt et al., 2003). The Academy of Breastfeeding Medicine currently (2007a) recommends that mothers be advised that all contraceptives that contain any exogenous hormone may reduce breastmilk supply.

Accommodation Between Physicians, Other Health Professionals, and Infant Milk Manufacturers

The relationship between physicians, other health professionals, and infant food manufacturers has in general promoted mothers' dependency on either the manufacturer or the physician for information on infant feeding. In the late 1800s as proprietary infant foods were being developed, manufacturers advertised to both groups. By the 1920s, some preparations were advertised to mothers but could be purchased only by prescription or used only after consulting a physician: the package contained no instructions for use. By 1932 the American Medical Association essentially required baby milk manufacturers to advertise only to the medical profession (Greer & Apple, 1991). The mutual economic benefits of this policy were clearly spelled out in many advertisements placed by formula manufacturers such as Mead Johnson (1930) in medical journals:

> *When mothers in America feed their babies by lay advice, the control of your pediatric cases passes out of your hands, Doctor. Our interest in this important phase of medical economics springs, not from any motives of altruism, philanthropy, or paternalism, but rather from a spirit of enlightened self-interest and cooperation because (our) infant diet materials are advertised only to you, never to the public.*

For several decades this unwritten agreement has extended also to medical education. Formula companies spend about $10,000 per medical student during a student's medical education (Walker, 2001). Many nursing and dietetic professional organizations also accept money from formula companies to fund continuing education, grants, and other projects.

Despite several early studies that showed breastfed infants to be healthier than bottle-fed ones (Howarth, 1905; Woodbury, 1922; Grulee, Sanford, & Herron, 1934), for years many physicians advised mothers that there was little advantage to breastfeeding. This view was expressed persistently up through the 1960s. For instance, Aitken and Hytten (1960) reported that "with modern standards of hygiene artificial feeding on simple mixtures of cow's milk, water, and sugar is a satisfactory substitute for breast feeding." Despite an overwhelming amount of research that shows that infants fed manufactured milk products have higher rates of morbidity, hospitalization, and mortality (Raisler, Alexander, & O'Campo, 1999; International

Ball & Bennett, 2001). Approximately 150 cans of ready-to-feed manufactured baby milk are used during the first 6 months of full artificial feeding. Even mothers who receive free manufactured infant milk from the WIC program (see below) must pay for it after their WIC eligibility expires. In industrial nations, the cost of manufactured baby milk may exceed the cost of additional food for the lactating mother by two or three times (Jarosz, 1993)—and more if a special mixture is required to minimize allergies or other health problems. In developing nations, the ratio is many times higher. In regions where one third to one half of those in large urban areas live in poverty, the cost of manufactured milks required to provide adequate nutrition (and implements with which to feed them) is a significant portion of the family income (Serva et al., 1986). Other members of the family may eat more poorly because the baby is artificially fed.

An equally important consideration is the reduced need for medical care by breastfed infants (particularly those who are exclusively breastfed). The frequency and severity of illnesses in a young infant is often inversely related to the proportion of the diet that comes from breastmilk (Chen et al., 1988; Cattaneo et al., 2006). More breastfeeding increases infant intake of high-quality protein and a variety of other needed nutrients, and it decreases infant exposure to potential pathogens in other foodstuffs (Habicht et al., 1988). In the early 1990s, a large health-maintenance organization in the United States estimated that in one state alone (North Carolina) the cost during the first year of life of treating infants who were breastfed at least 6 months was $1400 less than the cost of treating never-breastfed infants (Kaiser Permanente, 1997). A minimum of $3.6 billion would be saved in the United States alone if breastfeeding were increased from current levels to those recommended by the US Surgeon General (75% initiation and 50% continuation at 6 months) (Ball & Wright, 1999). It is estimated that insurers pay out $1.3 billion more for infants fed manufactured infant milks, as compared with breastfed infants, to treat respiratory infections, ear infections, and diarrhea in the first year of life (Riordan, 1997; Weimer, 2001). These mind-boggling figures likely underestimate the total excess cost of caring for artificially fed infants

because they account for the treatment of only a few types of childhood illnesses.

Consider also some of the ancillary costs of not breastfeeding (US Breastfeeding Committee, 2002).

- If a parent misses 2 hours per year of work for excess illness attributable to formula feeding, greater than 2000 hours—the equivalent of 1 year of employment—are lost per 1000 never-breastfed infants.
- The United States uses 110 billion BTUs of energy (costing about $2 million) each year for processing, packaging, and transporting manufactured infant milks—and even more to either dispose of empty milk containers or to recycle them.

Because full breastfeeding, which includes frequent feeds throughout a 24-hour period, tends to delay resumption of ovulation (Lewis et al., 1991), spacing between births tends to increase. Births spaced less than 2 years apart may increase the mortality risk of both the older and the younger infant (Retherford et al., 1989). Especially in families living at subsistence level, the older a child is when he or she is displaced from the breast and the fewer the number of children in a family, the more likely each child is to be healthy. In malnourished communities, breastfeeding may substantially increase child survival up to 3 years of age (Briend et al., 1988; World Health Organization, 2003).

Thus the breastfed infant stands a significantly greater likelihood of surviving. The mother's physical and emotional investment in pregnancy and lactation and the familial investment in time and money are repaid by the survival of a child; they are lost to the family when that child dies.

Cost to the Community and State
Community or national units that provide health care must respond to the local epidemiology of infant illness, in which feeding may play a major role. Morbidity is more prevalent in artificially fed infants regardless of location. The increase of the infant population, resulting from the loss of the contraceptive effect of breastfeeding, also serves to increase the need for pediatric health care.

The debate on the economic value of breastfeeding has focused on health costs, but the value of the time and energy women expend on breastfeeding is rarely estimated. The value of time spent breastfeeding is neglected (along with all the other unwaged caring work women do, including caring for children who fall ill as a result of not breastfeeding).

Another little-discussed aspect of the replacement of breastfeeding by use of manufactured products is that certain sectors of an economy can become economically dependent on the payrolls met and taxes paid by infant milk manufacturers, especially if capital funds are obtained from outside the country. Once they become a financial presence in a country, those manufacturers may be politically and economically difficult to dislodge, despite increases in health costs elsewhere in the economy. In the United States, infant formula is a $2.5 billion per year industry (United States Breastfeeding Committee, 2002) that generates a large payroll in the community and tax revenues to governmental entities.

Nonetheless, manufactured milk products widely used for infant feeding are subsidized by the diversion of resources (land, dairy cattle, and people to manage both)—and by manufacturing capacity pulled from other possible uses.

When one considers that more than 20 million babies are born annually in Africa alone, it becomes apparent that providing adequate volumes of manufactured milks represents a staggering burden and a largely unnecessary diversion of human and monetary resources from other more beneficial programs. At a time when environmental issues have become paramount, these unnecessary uses of power and raw material, not to mention the disposal of discarded packaging, is an increasing concern.

The Promotion of Breastfeeding

The many ways of encouraging mothers to breastfeed their own infants—breastfeeding promotion—may be considered to lie on a continuum. At one end, in societies where breastfeeding is the cultural norm, "promotion" consists of assuming that mother and infant will breastfeed. This assumption is combined with social arrangements, such as special foods for the mother or lightened duties, especially within the first few weeks after birth, to ensure that breastfeeding becomes well established. At the other end, in societies in which artificial feeding is the norm, promotion often consists of encouragement to breastfeed, sometimes offered by government officials and often

by healthcare professionals or members of elite population groups. These "promoters," unfortunately, are commonly unable to cultivate more accepting attitudes towards breastfeeding or to remove cultural barriers to breastfeeding. Two understandings have become clear: promotion of breastfeeding without support and protection of the breastfeeding mother produces little long-term gain, and the ways in which manufactured infant milks are inferior to human milk—rather than the reverse—must be emphasized.

Breastfeeding Promotion in the United States

Healthy People Statements

National health objectives were first formally defined in 1978 and published the following year as *Healthy People* (US Department of Health and Human Services, 1979). The initial goal for breastfeeding stated that 75% of women should breastfeed at hospital discharge and 35% at 6 months, as opposed to the actual 1978 figures of 45% and 21%. The current report, *Healthy People 2010* (US Department of Health and Human Services, 2000a), calls for the identical rate of newborn breastfeeding, and goal increases at age 6 months to 50% and at age 1 year to 25% (US Department of Health and Human Services, 2000a) (Table 2–2). The same department also published a *Blueprint for Action on Breastfeeding*, a document that affirms breastfeeding and sets goals for federal policies (US Department of Health and Human Services, 2000b). However, it does not recommend specific legislation that would support breastfeeding.

The WIC Program

Although other government agencies in the United States also work to improve infant nutrition, the Special Supplemental Nutrition Program for Women, Infants, and Children—the WIC program—probably directly affects the greatest number of people. Established in 1972, this program provides free nutrition counseling and food supplements, including manufactured baby milk, to low-income mothers and their infants. Clients typically come from the population segment in the United States least likely to breastfeed (Mac-Gowan et al., 1991). Of those infants born in the

TABLE 2–2	**Breastfeeding Rates (Percentages) and US Healthy People 2010 Breastfeeding Objectives for the Nation**		
	1998 Actual	**2005 Actual**	**2010 Goal**
Initiate breastfeeding within the early postpartum period	64	73	75
Breastfeeding at 6 months after birth	29	39	50
Breastfeeding at 12 months of age	16	20	25

Source: Adapted from http://www.ross.com/aboutross/Survey.pdf (accessed March 17, 2002) and National Immunization Survey, http://www.cdc.gov/breastfeeding/data/NIS_data/index.htm (accessed February 25, 2009).

United States in 2005, almost half (48%) were enrolled in WIC (Ryan & Zhou, 2006).

The WIC program follows in the footsteps of United States infant welfare programs of the 1890s and at the turn of the century in France, England, and elsewhere that operated centers where infants could be weighed and examined weekly. These centers also provided cow milk ("fresh and clean" in some cases, sterilized in others) to nonbreastfeeding mothers in an effort to reduce infant illness and death caused by the use of contaminated milk. By 1903, such milk dispensaries were already being accused of discouraging breastfeeding because they seemed to endorse artificial feeding of infants (Wickes, 1953b). Even today, government-sponsored distribution of free milk (as has occurred in Nicaragua since 1970) has been considered one reason for the decline of breastfeeding (Sandiford et al., 1991; Ryan & Zhou, 2006). The WIC program is still the largest purchaser (and distributor, at little cost to the manufacturers (Tuttle, 2000; Kent, 2006) of formula in the United States: $600 million per year. As a result, the direct cost to WIC of supporting mothers who never breastfeed is nearly twice the cost of supporting breastfeeding mothers (United States Breastfeeding Committee, 2002).

The promotion of breastfeeding finally became a goal within WIC in the late 1980s. The Child Nutrition and WIC Reauthorization Act of 1989 required that a certain proportion of WIC's budget be spent on the promotion and support of breastfeeding and that each state health department establish a breastfeeding promotion coordinator. That budget proportion remains small, however: in 2005, only 0.6%—$34 million—of a $5235 million WIC budget was earmarked for promotion and support of breastfeeding (Ryan & Zhou, 2006). Thus, the dollar amount spent to promote breastfeeding is only about 5% of the amount spent for artificial infant milk. Even so, in 2007 breastfeeding women have a higher priority for enrollment in WIC programs than do nonbreastfeeding mothers: they are provided more, and more varied, foods, and their benefits persist longer—1 year, as opposed to 6 months for nonbreastfeeders (USDA, 2007).

Despite these efforts, the increases in breastfeeding rates of WIC enrollees have been minimal. Mothers enrolled in WIC not only initiate breastfeeding at a much lower rate (at least 20% lower at all time points; 2003 data) than mothers at large (Ryan & Zhou, 2006), but initiate at a lower rate than mothers who qualify for WIC aid but are not enrolled (Li et al., 2005). Even women of Hispanic or Asian ethnicity, who traditionally breastfeed, do so at lower rates if they are enrolled in WIC. The conclusion, then, is that WIC participation lowers breastfeeding initiation and duration (Ryan & Zhou, 2006).

US Breastfeeding Committee

In 1998, supported by the Maternal and Child Health Bureau, a national breastfeeding conference was convened to form a breastfeeding committee as had been recommended by the Innocenti Declaration in 1990. The United States Breastfeeding Committee was established, composed of representatives from government and nongovernmental organizations and health professional associations. The committee's goals have been to expand awareness of the value of breastfeeding and to recommend policies to government and corporate organization that increase breastfeeding prevalence (United States Breastfeeding Committee, 2001).

Legislation

Legislation intended to increase the prevalence of breastfeeding may mandate actions that encourage breastfeeding or discourage feeding of artificial baby milk (or use of wet nurses) or both. One of the earliest examples was set in 350 BC by Lycurgus, the king of Sparta: he required not only that mothers nurse their own infants, but that nursing mothers be shown kindness and respect (Hymanson, 1934).

Pressures external to the mother and infant have dictated not only *when* an infant should be breastfed but also *where*. Social censure and in some places the interpretation of statutory laws regarding indecent exposure have limited the public places in which a woman might breastfeed. Although the best situation would be a pervasive social acceptance of breastfeeding such that legislation permitting breastfeeding in public is not needed, legislation protecting the right to breastfeed is for the moment the next best thing. Beginning in 1984 in New York State, American women began to gain the legal right to breastfeed in public places. Ten years later, laws in five states addressed breastfeeding. In the United States, a 1999 federal law makes breastfeeding legal on all federal property where a woman has the right to be (Tiedje et al., 2002). As of August 2007, 42 states (of 50 states plus the District of Columbia) have laws that address breastfeeding in public—either by permitting a woman to breastfeed any place where she is entitled to be or by exempting a woman who is breastfeeding in public from charges of indecent exposure (La Leche League International, 2007a). Wilson-Clay et al. (2005) describe in detail how you can effectively lobby the state legislature to reduce barriers to breastfeeding.

Statements by Health Organizations

In 1997 the American Academy of Pediatrics Work Group on Breastfeeding issued a policy statement endorsing breastfeeding (American Academy of Pediatrics, 1997). The statement received considerable attention from the press, accelerating nationwide interest in breastfeeding. Other professional organizations have published similar public endorsements of breastfeeding: the American College of Obstetricians and Gynecologists (2000; rev. 2002), the American Dietetic Association (1997), the American College of Nurse-Midwives (1992), the American Academy of Family Physicians (2001), the Association of Women's Health, Obstetric, and Neonatal Nurses (1999), National Association of Pediatric Nurse Practitioners (2003), Academy of Breastfeeding Medicine (2007b), and the American Public Health Association, 2008.

International Breastfeeding Promotion

The International Code of Marketing of Breast-Milk Substitutes

In the 1970s, the deleterious effects of manufactured baby milks on infant health and survival became better appreciated, and the role of advertising in spreading the use of these milks became increasingly suspect. In 1981 the World Health Organization, by a vote of 118 to 1 (the United States cast the sole dissenting vote), approved the International Code of Marketing of Breast-Milk Substitutes. The code provides a model of marketing practices that permits the availability of manufactured baby milk but forbids its advertisement or free distribution directly to consumers (Box 2–2).

The code also seeks to balance the information provided by infant milk manufacturers, in both written "educational" material and in the text or pictures on containers of the product (International Baby Food Action Network, 1985; Armstrong, 1988). In 1996, the World Health Assembly passed six resolutions that further clarify the intent of the international code. Of these six, one reaffirms the use of local family foods to complement the diet of breastfeeding infants beyond about 6 months of age. Another reaffirms the need to end the free or low-cost (subsidized) distribution of artificial baby milk to newly parturient women in the hospital. Two other resolutions proscribe receipt of funds from manufacturers or distributors of artificial baby milk or feeding supplies to be used for professional training in infant and child health, or for financial support of any organization that monitors compliance with the international code (United Nations Children's Emergency Fund, 1996).

An individual country may adopt the international code in the manner that best fits the needs of that country. In some, no action has been taken, and formula manufacturers are bound only by voluntary adherence to an industry-written "codes of ethics" that lacks sanctions for noncompliance.

BOX **2–2**

WHO/UNICEF Code for Marketing Breastmilk Substitutes

- No advertising of these products to the public.
- No free samples to mothers.
- No promotion of products in health-care facilities.
- No company mothercraft nurses to advise mothers.
- No gifts or personal samples to health workers.
- No words or pictures idealizing artificial feeding, including pictures of infants, on the products.
- Information to health workers should be scientific and factual.
- All information on artificial feeding, including the labels, should explain the benefits of breastfeeding, and the costs and hazards associated with artificial feeding.
- Unsuitable products, such as condensed milk, should not be promoted for babies.
- All products should be of a high quality and take into account the climatic and storage conditions of the country where they are used.

Source: World Health Organization, 1981b.

A few other countries have adopted and do enforce various aspects of the code.

The international code focuses attention on ways in which the infant formula industry influences both consumers and professionals to increase the use of their products. Direct advertising to consumers may be the most obvious ploy, but what Jelliffe and Jelliffe (1978) called "manipulation by assistance" is also effective. For example, formula manufacturers not only provide free formula to hospital nurseries but also assist in the design of those nurseries, donate equipment and supplies to hospitals and individual physicians (bottles of formula and sterile water, for example), support conferences (including some dealing with breastfeeding), and even entertain hospital staff at company-sponsored events. These gifts are treated by the companies as marketing expenses. Lactation consultants should be watchful in order to avoid succumbing to such "manipulation by assistance" provided by manufacturers of artificial baby milk and of other feeding products banned by the international code.

As individuals and institutions become financially dependent on such gifts and enmeshed in social relationships with company salespeople, they are more likely to tacitly endorse, or even recommend, artificial baby milks. By highlighting such practices as marketing ploys, the code may make healthcare professionals more aware of the intent behind them and thus perhaps more resistant to their allure.

Innocenti Declaration

In 1990, the World Health Organization and the United Nations International Children's Emergency Fund (UNICEF) were instrumental in the development of the Innocenti Declaration, which restated the importance of breastfeeding for maternal and child health. It set forth four goals to be met by 1995: (1) the establishment of national breastfeeding coordinators and a national breastfeeding committee, (2) the practice of Ten Steps to Successful Breastfeeding by maternity services (Box 2–3), (3) the implementation of the WHO International

BOX **2–3**

Ten Steps to Successful Breastfeeding

Every facility providing maternity services and care for newborn infants should

1. Have a written breastfeeding policy that is routinely communicated to all healthcare staff.
2. Train all healthcare staff in skills necessary to implement this policy.
3. Inform all pregnant women about the benefits and management of breastfeeding.
4. Help mothers initiate breastfeeding within 30 minutes after birth.
5. Show mothers how to breastfeed, and how to maintain lactation even if they should be separated from their infants.
6. Give newborn infants no food or drink other than breast milk, unless medically indicated.

7. Practice rooming-in—allow mothers and infants to remain together 24 hours a day.
8. Encourage breastfeeding on demand.
9. Give no artificial teats or pacifiers (also called dummies or soothers) to breastfeeding infants.
10. Foster the establishment of breastfeeding support groups and refer mothers to them on discharge from the hospital or clinic.

Source: World Health Organization, 1989.

Note: These steps and the complete elimination of free and low-cost supplies of breast-milk substitution, bottles, and teats from healthcare facilities form the basis for the Baby-Friendly Hospital Initiative.

Code, and (4) enactment of enforceable laws for protecting the breastfeeding rights of employed women (United Nations Children's Fund, 1990).

An offshoot organization, the World Alliance for Breastfeeding Action (WABA) is a multi-national coalition of individuals and private organizations involved in research and promotion of breastfeeding (World Alliance for Breastfeeding Action, 2007). It works to ensure that the goals of the Innocenti Declaration are met, and it annually supports activities presented during World Breastfeeding Week, the first week in August—an opportunity for people worldwide to celebrate and support breastfeeding. The Texas Breastfeeding Coalition is a helpful resource for building and strengthening a coalition (www.txbfcoalition.org) and for ideas for celebrating World Breastfeeding Week.

Baby-Friendly Hospital Initiative

The World Health Organization and UNICEF launched the Baby-Friendly Hospital Initiative (BFHI) in 1991 to encourage specific birth-center practices in all countries that promote exclusive breastfeeding. To be designated "baby-friendly," a hospital must demonstrate to an external review board that it practices each of the 10 steps to successful breastfeeding outlined in the Innocenti Declaration. With the principal exception of the Scandinavian countries, industrialized nations have moved more slowly than developing nations. Of some 19,000 maternity facilities worldwide that have been designated baby-friendly, 63 are in the United States (Baby-Friendly USA, 2008). The principal stumbling block has been the political and financial difficulty of the requirement that hospitals not accept free artificial infant milk from manufacturers. Breastfeeding advocates in the industrialized world labor against three impediments: an artificial milk industry that is powerful enough, both financially and politically, to avoid most regulation; a pervasive bottle-feeding culture that does not consider breastfeeding important to child or maternal health; and the lack of much precedence for government-mandated health programs. As a result, all industrialized nations together can claim only a small percentage of all baby-friendly hospitals.

Several studies have examined the degree to which the "Ten Steps" are being implemented and their effect on hospital practices and breastfeeding outcomes (DiGirolamo, Grummer-Strawn, & Fein, 2001; Broadfoot et al., 2005; Merewood et al., 2005; Merten et al., 2005). Without exception, these studies show greater initiation and longer duration of breastfeeding, even among populations less likely to breastfeed. A high proportion of mothers delivering in a hospital or birthing center certified as baby-friendly choose to breastfeed because of the consistent support they receive from the staff and from their birth experience in a breastfeeding-friendly environment.

Private Support Movements

During the 1970s, the unthinking acceptance of artificial feeding began to unravel. The reasons are not clear but seem to have been part of a widespread desire of many to include simpler, more natural practices in their lives. In the 1950s and 1960s, voluntary groups that offer information and support to women interested in breastfeeding, such as La Leche League International (LLLI) in the United States, Nursing Mothers' Association of Australia, and Ammenhjelpen of Sweden, had been formed. Such groups assist individual women and have focused national attention on the benefits of breastfeeding. La Leche League is officially recognized as a nongovernmental organization qualified to consult on breastfeeding to organizations such as the United Nations and the United States Agency for International Development. As of 2006, it has a presence—accredited leaders or other ongoing source of LLLI information—in 75 countries (La Leche League International, 2007b). Members of groups such as these, by their demonstration that even "modern" mothers can breastfeed, and by their requests to medical personnel for information about medical practices that support breastfeeding, have been a major force behind the dissemination of technical information concerning lactation, human milk, and breastfeeding.

To better reach low-income women, who are not commonly La Leche League members, LLLI has trained more than 3000 peer counselors—low-income women who have breastfed and have completed a training program. Offering breastfeeding advice and support in clinics that serve low-income populations, such counselors can be very effective (see Chapter 25).

S u m m a r y

Humans evolved within the mammalian lineage, which has provided a species-specific milk for the nourishment and protection of the young of each species. For millennia, the staple of the human infant's diet has been human milk obtained directly from the human breast, commonly in situations where no other food was suitable. Within the last century or so, as breastfeeding became associated with more restrictive aspects of women's lives, as breastmilk was thought by some to be inferior to increasingly available manufactured infant milks, and as use of manufactured milks became a hallmark of privileged segments of society, large portions of both lay and healthcare populations came to believe that there was little reason to persist in traditional breastfeeding practices.

Since the early 1990s, however, it has become increasingly clear that breastfeeding confers health, cognitive, and psychological advantages on the breastfeeding infant and also onto the child and adult into which that infant will grow. Breastfeeding enhances aspects of maternal health as well. Breastfeeding is economically frugal and ecologically sound. Breastfeeding is important at both the family and the community level. The promotion efforts outlined in this chapter are needed because, to some degree in most countries (and particularly those in the United States), the most important requirements are missing: acceptance by society at large of the need for a mother and child to be together, and the right of the breastfeeding dyad to participate in social, civic, and commercial activities outside the home. For many women, the ultimate barrier to breastfeeding is not sore nipples, night-time nursing, or employment outside the home. It is the disapproval they encounter for "wasting" their education and career skills by staying home with their breastfeeding infants, or for being considered disruptive or even obscene for taking their breastfeeding infant with them to work or to worship, or perhaps to a city council or parent-teacher meeting, or simply to a restaurant or to a park. A goal for all women should be to empower mothers so that they are able to attend to all of their duties, maternal as well as civic, religious, and professional.

Those who breastfeed or who promote the reestablishment of breastfeeding as the norm in infant feeding do so not because there are no alternatives but because the alternatives are inferior. Unfortunately, the belief that breastfeeding is the optimal way to nourish an infant may not be enough to empower a woman to breastfeed. Knowledge of beneficial breastfeeding practices and society's acceptance of those practices are also required. Currently, the prevalence of breastfeeding reflects the importance that society places on it, as measured by the degree to which breastfeeding mothers and infants are accepted in the life of the community at large. Returning breastfeeding wisdom to the public domain and reintegrating breastfeeding into the social fabric so that women who wish to breastfeed may do so without hindrance is the challenge that awaits.

Key Concepts

- The class Mammalia is characterized by breasts (mammae) that secrete and release a fluid that for a time is the sole nourishment of the young; breastfeeding dates back some 100 million years.
- Among modern hunter–gatherers, whose breastfeeding practices may be very ancient, breastfeeds tend to be frequent (average 4/hour), short (about 2 minutes), equally distributed throughout a 24-hour day, and persist for 2 to 6 years.
- Beginning in the 1700s, mothercraft manuals began to shift the management of infant feeding from the mother (or women in general) to usually male "authorities," and by the early part of the 1900s, "good mothering" drifted toward meeting feeding and infant-care schedules imposed by authorities.
- Before about 1900, information about breastfeeding incidence, prevalence, and practices came from indirect sources; since the mid-1900s, national surveys and World Health Organization data have been available.
- Before about 1900, wet-nursing was the only alternative to breastfeeding that was likely to allow the infant to survive.
- The currently typical hand-fed infant foods did not become part of the human diet until late in human history; cereal grains were domesticated only about 10,000 years ago and animal milks only about 5000 years ago.
- In the 1890s, physician Thomas Rotch developed a complex system of progressive modifications of cow milk to make it more digestible by infants of various ages; this system required constant intervention by the physician, who might change an infant's "formula" weekly.
- In the decades around 1900, high infant mortality was a major public concern, standards of modesty strictly limited breastfeeding outside the home, and advances in science and technology led to the creation of dry or tinned artificial infant foods.
- In the United States, the proportion of newborns receiving any breastfeeding declined steadily after 1940 to a low of 25% in 1970; the trend then reversed and despite a dip in the late 1980s, has risen steadily since then.
- Infants fed manufactured infant milks suffer more illness because such milks lack the nutritive qualities and immunologic factors of breastmilk. Mothers who use manufactured infant milks are more susceptible to osteoporosis, premenopausal breast cancer, and ovarian cancer.
- Infants who are fed manufactured infant milks are more costly to raise, in part because of the considerable cost of the formula and in part because they suffer more, and more severe, illness as compared with breastfed infants.
- The diversion of land, power, and raw material to the manufacture of artificial infant milks,

and the disposal of discarded packaging, is an increasing ecological concern.

- Especially after World War II, the United States and Western Europe exported hand-feeding practices to countries that they colonized or otherwise influenced.
- Voluntary groups dedicated to promoting breastfeeding, such as La Leche League International in the United States, Nursing Mothers' Association of Australia, and Ammenhjelpen in Sweden, began in the 1960s and 1970s and paved the way for governmental efforts.
- In the United States, national breastfeeding goals were first stated in 1979 in *Healthy People: The Surgeon General's Report on Health Promotion and Disease Prevention.*
- During the 1980s, the promotion of breastfeeding in the United States became an important goal within the Women, Infants, and Children (WIC) program; however, increases in breastfeeding rates of WIC enrollees, who typically come from population segments least likely to breastfeed, have come slowly.
- The International Code of Marketing of Breast-Milk Substitutes was approved in 1981 by the World Health Organization; it permits manufactured infant milks to be available but forbids their advertisement or free distribution directly to consumers.
- The Innocenti Declaration was approved in 1990 by the World Health Organization and the United Nations International Children's Emergency Fund; it encourages specific hospital perinatal practices that promote exclusive breastfeeding.
- Breastfeeding promotion efforts in 2007 are rediscovering that promotion must also include support and protection of the breastfeeding mother and that the harmful outcomes of feeding manufactured infant milks must be addressed as well as the benefits of breastfeeding.

References

Academy of Breastfeeding Medicine. Contraception during breastfeeding: clinical protocol 13. 2005. Available at: http://www.bfmed.org/ace-files/protocol/finalcontraceptionprotocolsent2.pdf. Accessed August 4, 2007a.

Academy of Breastfeeding Medicine. Protocols. Available at: http://www.bfmed.org/index/asp?menuID=139&firstlevelmentuID=139. Accessed October 14, 2007b.

Ackatia-Armah R, Merewood A. State collection of breastfeeding data: who counts what and how? Boston University Medical Center. ILCA Conference and Annual Meeting, "Controversies in Lactation," San Diego, August 15–19, 2007.

Aitken FC, Hytten FE. Infant feeding: comparison of breast and artificial feeding. *Nutr Abstr Rev.* 1960;30:341–371.

American Academy of Family Physicians. AAFP policy and position statement on breastfeeding. Available at: http://www.aafp.org/x633.xml; 2001. Accessed May 2003.

American Academy of Pediatrics, Work Group on Breastfeeding. Breastfeeding and the use of human milk. *Pediatrics.* 1997;100:1035–1039. *Guidelines and Recommendations for Breastfeeding.* Available at: http://www.aap.org/policy/re9729.html.

American College of Nurse-Midwives. *Position Statement on Breastfeeding.* Washington, DC: ACNM; 1992.

American College of Obstetricians and Gynecologists. Breastfeeding: maternal and infant aspects. *ACOG Educat Bull.* 2000;258. Available at: http://www.acog.org/from_homepublications/press_releases/nr07–0100.htm. Accessed July 1, 2002.

American Dietetic Association. Position of the American Dietetic Association: promotion of breastfeeding. *ADA Reports.* 1997;97(6):662–666. Available at: http://www.eatright.org/adar1_101801.html.

American Public Health Association. Policy on breastfeeding and public health. Available at: http://www.apha.org/advocacy/policy. Accessed December 4, 2008.

Apple RD. "Advertised by our loving friends": the infant formula industry and the creation of new pharmaceutical markets, 1870–1910. *J Hist Med Allied Sci.* 1986;41:3–23.

Armstrong H. The International Code of Marketing of Breast-Milk Substitutes (Part 2). *J Hum Lact.* 1988;4:194–199.

Association of Women's Health, Obstetric and Neonatal Nurses (AWHONN). AWHONN position statement. *NAACOG Newsletter.* 1992;19.

Baby-Friendly USA. Baby-friendly hospitals and birth centers. Available at: http://www.babyfriendlyusa.org/idex.html. Accessed October 4, 2007.

Bhale P, Jain S. Is colostrum really discarded by Indian mothers? *Indian Pediatrics.* 1999;36:1069–1070.

Bain K. The incidence of breast feeding in hospitals in the United States. *Pediatrics.* 1948;2:313–320.

Ball TM, Bennett DM. The economic impact of breastfeeding. *Pediatr Clin North Am.* 2001;48:253–262.

Ball TM, Wright AL. Health care costs of formula-feeding in the first year of life. *Pediatrics.* 1999;103:870–876.

Baranowski T, Bee DE, Rassin DK et al. Social support, social influence, ethnicity and the breastfeeding decision. *Soc Sci Med.* 1983;17:1599–1611.

Briend A, Wojtyniak B, Rowland MGM. Breast feeding, nutritional state, and child survival in rural Bangladesh. *Br Med J.* 1988;296:879–882.

Broadfoot M, Britten J, Tappin DM, MacKenzie JM. The Baby Friendly Hospital Initiative and breast feeding rates in Scotland. *Arch Dis Child Fetal Neonat Ed.* 2005;90:F114–F116.

Butte NF et al. Milk composition of insulin-dependent diabetic women. *J Pediatr Gastroenterol Nutr.* 1987;6:936–941.

Butte NF, Wong WW, Hopkinson JM. Energy requirements of lactating women derived from doubly labeled water and milk energy output. *J Nutr.* 2001;131:53–58.

Cattaneo A, Ronfani L, Burmaz T, Quintero-Romero S, Macaluso A, Di Maria S. Infant feeding and cost of health care: a cohort study. *Acta Paediatrica.* 2006;95:540–546.

CBS News. Eyeful of breast-feeding mom sparks outrage. Available at: http://www.cbsnews.com/stories/2006/07/28/national/main1844454_page2.shtml. Accessed September 21, 2007.

Centers for Disease Control and Prevention (CDC). HealthStyles Survey—Breastfeeding practices, 2004. Available at: http://www.cdc.gov/breastfeeding/data/healthstyles_survey/survey_2004.htm#2004. Accessed September 21, 2007.

Centers for Disease Control and Prevention (CDC). Breastfeeding trends and updated national health objectives for exclusive breastfeeding—United States, birth years 2000–2004. *MMWR.* 2007a;56(30):760–763. Available at: http://www.cdc.gov/mmwr/preview/mmwrhtml/mm5630a2.htm. Accessed August 15, 2007a.

Centers for Disease Control and Prevention (CDC). Breastfeeding practices—results from the National Immunization Survey. 2007b. Available at: http://www.cdc.gov/greastfeeding/data/NISdata/data_2004.htm. Accessed October 7, 2007b.

Chen A, Rogan WJ. Breastfeeding and the risk of postneonatal death in the United States. *Pediatrics.* 113(5):e435–e439, 2004.

Chen Y, Yu S, Li W. Artificial feeding and hospitalization in the first 18 months of life. *Pediatrics.* 1988;81:58–62.

Coombs N. 1972. The new Negro, immigration and migration. In: *The Black Experience in America.* Available at: http://www.gale.cengage.com. Accessed September 15, 2007.

Cunningham AS, Jelliffe DB, Jelliffe EFP. Breast-feeding and health in the 1980s: a global epidemiologic review. *J Pediatr.* 1991;118:659–666.

Dearlove JC, Dearlove BM. Prolactin fluid balance and lactation. *Br J Obstet Gynaecol.* 1981;88:652–654.

Deruisseau LG. Infant hygiene in the older medical literature. *Ciba Symposia.* 1940;2:530–560.

Dettwyler KA. A time to wean: the hominid blueprint for the natural age of weaning in modern human populations. In: Stuart-Macadam P, Dettwyler KA, eds. *Breastfeeding—Biocultural Perspectives.* New York, NY: Aldine de Gruyter; 1995:39–73.

DiGirolamo AM, Grummer-Strawn LM, Fein S. Maternity care practices: Implications for breastfeeding. *Birth.* 2001;28(2):94–100.

Dimond HJ, Ashworth A. Infant feeding practices in Kenya, Mexico and Malaysia: the rarity of the exclusively breastfed infant. *Hum Nutr Appl Nutr.* 1987;41A:51–64.

Eaton SB. Humans, lipids and evolution. *Lipids.* 1992;27(10):814–820.

Fildes VA. *Breasts, bottles, and babies: a history of infant feeding.* Edinburgh, Scotland, UK: Edinburgh University Press; 1986.

Foss KA, Southwell BG. Infant feeding and the media: the relationship between *Parents' Magazine* content and breastfeeding, 1972–2000. *Intl Breastfeeding J.* 2006;1:10. Available at: http://www.internationalbreastfeedingjournal.com/content/1/1/10. Accessed August 15, 2007.

Gartner LM, Stone C. Two thousand years of medical advice on breastfeeding: comparison of Chinese and western texts. *Sem Perinatol.* 1994;18(6):532–536.

Gerrard JW. Breast-feeding: second thoughts. *Pediatrics.* 1974;54:757–764.

Greer FR, Apple RD. Physicians, formula companies, and advertising: a historical perspective. *Am J Dis Child.* 1991;145:282–286.

Gregory JN. 1995. The Southern diaspora and the urban dispossessed: demonstrating the census public use microdata samples. *J American History.* 1995;82:111–134. Available at: http://faculty.washington.edu/gregoryj/dispossessed.pdf. Accessed September 15, 2007.

Greiner T. The concept of weaning: definitions and their implications. *J Hum Lact.* 1996;12:123–128.

Grulee CG, Sanford HN, Herron PH. Breast and artificial feeding: influence on morbidity and mortality of twenty thousand infants. *J Am Med Assn.* 1934;103:735–739.

Habicht J-P, DaVanzo J, Butz WP. Mother's milk and sewage: their interactive effect on infant mortality. *Pediatrics.* 1988;88:456–461.

Hannan A, Li R, Benton-Davis S, Grummer-Strawn L. Regional variation in public opinion about breast-feeding in the United States. *J Hum Lact.* 2005;21(3):284–288.

Hastrup K. A question of reason: breastfeeding patterns in seventeenth and eighteenth-century Iceland. In: Maher V, ed. *The Anthropology of Breast-Feeding—Natural Law or Social Construct.* Oxford, UK: Berg Publishers; 1992:91–108.

Howarth WJ. The influence of feeding on the mortality of infants. *Lancet.* 1905;2 (July 22):210–213.

Hymanson A. A short review of the history of infant feeding. *Arch Pediatr*. 1934;51:1–10.

Illingworth PJ. Diminution in energy expenditure during lactation. *Br Med J*. 1986;292:437–441.

International Baby Food Action Network/International Organization of Consumers Unions (IBFAN/IOCU). *Protecting Infant Health: A Health Worker's Guide to the International Code of Marketing of Breast-Milk Substitutes*. Penang, Malaysia: IBFAN/IOCU; 1985.

International Lactation Consultant Association. Position Paper on Infant Feeding (and references therein). Available at: http://www.ilca.org/pubs/pospapers/infantFeeding.pdf. Accessed August 4, 2007.

Ip S, Chung M, Raman G et al. Breastfeeding and maternal and infant health outcomes in developed countries: Evidence Report/Technology Assessment 153. Available at: http://www.ahrq.gov/downloads/pub/evidence/pdf/brfout/brfout.pdf. Accessed August 12, 2007.

Jackson RI. Ecological breastfeeding and child spacing. *Clin Pediatr*. 1988;27:373–377.

Jarosz LA. Breast-feeding versus formula: cost comparison. *Hawaii Med J*. 1993;52:14–16.

Jelliffe DB. Culture, social change and infant feeding: current trends in tropical regions. *Am J Clin Nutr*. 1962;10:19–45, 1962.

Jelliffe DB, Jelliffe EFP. *Human Milk in the Modern World*. Oxford, UK: Oxford University; 1978.

Jethi SC, Shriwastava DK. Knowledge, attitudes and practices regarding infant feeding among mothers. *Indian Pediatr*. 1987;24:921–924.

Kaiser Permanente. Costs of NOT breastfeeding: Kaiser Permanente study. Available at: http://www.visi.com/~artmama/kaiser.htm. Accessed October 8, 2007.

Kelsey JJ. Hormonal contraception and lactation. *J Hum Lact*. 1996;12:315–318.

Kennedy K et al. Consensus statement on the use of breastfeeding as a family planning method. *Contraception*. 1989;39:447–496.

Kent G. WIC's promotion of infant formula in the United States. *International Breastfeeding Journal*. 2006;1(8). Available at: http://www.international breastfeedingjournal.com/content/1/1/8. Accessed October 14, 2007.

Kessen W. *The Child*. New York, NY: Wiley; 1965.

Konner M, Worthman C. Nursing frequency, gonadal function, and birth spacing among Kung hunter-gatherers. *Science*. 1980;207:788–791.

Kusin JA, Kardjati S, van Steenbergen W. Traditional infant feeding practices: right or wrong? *Soc Sci Med*. 1985;21:283–286.

Labbok MH. Effects of breastfeeding on the mother. *Pediatr Clin North America*. 2001;48:143–158.

Lacaille AD. Infant feeding-bottles in prehistoric times. *Proc R Soc Med*. 1950;43:565–568.

La Leche League International. A current summary of breastfeeding legislation in the U.S. Available at: http://www.lalecheleague.org/Law/LawBills.html. Accessed July 14, 2007a.

La Leche League International. Annual report 2005–2006. Available at: http://www.llli.org/docs/2006 Report.pdf. Accessed August 17, 2007b.

Laroia N, Sharma D. The religious and cultural bases for breastfeeding practices among the Hindus. *Breastfeeding Med*. 2006;1(2):94–98.

Latham MC et al. Infant feeding in urban Kenya: a pattern of early triple nipple feeding. *J Trop Pediatr*. 1986;32:276–280.

Levenstein H. "Best for babies" or "Preventable infanticide"? The controversy over artificial feeding of infants in America, 1880–1920. *J Am Hist*. 1983;70:75–94.

Lewis PR et al. The resumption of ovulation and menstruation in a well-nourished population of women breastfeeding for an extended period of time. *Fertil Steril*. 1991;55:529–536.

Li R, Darling N, Maurice E, Barker L, Grummer-Strawn LM. Breastfeeding rates in the United States by characteristics of the child, mother, or family: The 2002 National Immunization Survey. *Pediatrics*. 2005;115(1):e31–e37.

MacGowan RJ et al. Breast-feeding among women attending Women, Infants, and Children clinics in Georgia, 1987. *Pediatrics*. 1991;87:361–366.

Marriott BM, Campbell L, Hirsch E, Wilson D. Preliminary data from Demographic and Health Surveys on infant feeding in 20 developing countries. *J Nutr*. 2007;137:518S–523S.

Martinez GA, Krieger FW. 1984 Milk-feeding patterns in the United States. *Pediatrics*. 1985;76:1004–1008.

Matich JR, Sims LS. A comparison of social support variables between women who intended to breast or bottle-feed. *Soc Sci Med*. 1992;34:919–927.

McCracken RD. Lactase deficiency: an example of dietary evolution. *Curr Anthrop*. 1971;12:479–517.

McDowell MM, Wang CY, Kennedy-Stephenson J. Breastfeeding in the United States: findings from the National Health and Nutrition Examination Surveys 1999–2006. NCHS Data Brief, No. 5, April 2008.

McIntyre E, Hiller JE, Turnbull D. Community attitudes to infant feeding. *Breastfeeding Rev*. 2001;9(3):27–33.

Mead Johnson [advertisement]. *J Am Med Assn*. 1930;95:22.

Merewood A, Mehta SD, Chamberlain LB, Phillipp BL, Bauchner H. Breastfeeding rates in US Baby-Friendly hospitals: results of a national survey. *Pediatrics*. 2005;116(3):628–634.

Merten S, Dratva J, Ackermann-Liebrich U. Do Baby-Friendly Hospitals influence breastfeeding duration on a national level? *Pediatrics*. 2005;116:702–708.

Meyer HF. Breastfeeding in the United States: report of a 1966 national survey with comparable 1946 and 1956 data. *Clin Pediatr*. 1968;7:708–715.

Millard AV. The place of the clock in pediatric advice: rationales, cultural themes, and impediments to breastfeeding. *Soc Sci Med*. 1990;31:211–221.

Millman S. Trends in breastfeeding in a dozen developing countries. *International Family Planning Perspectives*. 1986;12(3):91–95.

Morse JM. "Euch, those are for your husband!" Examination of cultural values and assumptions associated with breast-feeding. *Health Care Women Intl.* 1989;11:223–232.

Morse JM, Jehle C, Gamble D. Initiating breastfeeding: a world survey of the timing of postpartum breast-feeding. *Intl J Nurs Stud.* 1990;27:303–313.

Mukuria AG, Kothari MT, Abderrahim N. Infant and young child feeding update (USAID). Calverton, MD: ORC Macro; 2006.

National Association of Pediatric Nurse Practitioners (NAPNAP). *Position Paper on Breastfeeding.* Available at: http://www.napnap.org/practice/position/breast feeding. Accessed May 2003.

Nestlé's Food [advertisement]. *Ladies' Home Journal.* 1892;9:26.

Nga NT, Weissner P. Breast-feeding and young child nutrition in Uong Bi, Quang Ninh Province, Vietnam. *J Trop Pediatr.* 1986;32:137–139.

Pasternak B, Ching W. Breastfeeding decline in urban China: an exploratory study. *Human Ecol.* 1985;13(4):433–466.

Quigley MA, Cumberland P, Cowden JM, Rodrigues LC. How protective is breast feeding against diarrhoeal disease in infants in 1990s England? A case-control study. *Arch Dis Child.* 2006;91:245–250.

Raisler J, Alexander C, O'Campo P. Breast-feeding and infant illness: a dose-response relationship? *Am J Public Health.* 1999;89(1):25–30.

Retherford RD et al. To what extent does breastfeeding explain birth-interval effects on early childhood mortality? *Demography.* 1989;26:439–450.

Riordan J. Cost of not breastfeeding: A commentary. *J Hum Lact.* 1997;13:93–97.

Rossiter FM. *The practical guide to health, a popular treatise on anatomy, physiology, and hygiene, with a scientific description of diseases, their causes and treatment, designed for nurses and home use.* Pacific Press Publishing; 1908. (Reprinted in part in *J Hum Lact.* 1991;7:89–91.)

Rotch TM. An historical sketch of the development of percentage feeding. *NY Med J.* 1907;85:532–537.

Ryan AS, Zhou W. Lower breastfeeding rates persist among the Special Supplemental Nutrition for Women, Infants, and Children participants, 1978–2003. *Pediatrics.* 2006;117(4):1136–1146.

Ryan AS, Zhou W, Gaston MH. Regional and socio-demographic variation of breastfeeding in the United States. *Clin Pediatr.* 2004;43:815–824.

Saha K. Studies on colostrum: Nutrients and immunologic factors. *Nutr Foundation India Arch.* Available at: http://www.nutritionfoundationofindia.res.in/archives. Accessed August 2, 2007.

Sandiford P et al. Why do child mortality rates fall? An analysis of the Nicaraguan experience. *Am J Public Health.* 1991;81:30–37.

Serva V, Karim H, Ebrahim GJ. Breast-feeding and the urban poor in developing countries. *J Trop Pediatr.* 1986;32:127–129.

Schaefer O. The impact of culture on breastfeeding patterns. *J Perinatology.* 1956;6(1):62–65.

Shaikh U, Ahmed O. Islam and infant feeding. *Breastfeeding Med.* 2006;1(3):164–167.

Short RV. Breast feeding. *Sci Am.* 1984;250:35–41.

Simoons FJ. Age of onset of lactose malabsorption. *Pediatrics.* 1980;66:646–648.

Slome C. Nonpuerperal lactation in grandmothers. *J Pediatr.* 1976;49:550–552.

Stuebe AM, Rich-Edwards JW, Willett WC, Manson JE, Michels KB. Duration of lactation and incidence of type 2 diabetes. *JAMA.* 2005;294(20):2601–2610.

Thorley V. Initiating breastfeeding in postwar Queensland. *Breastfeeding Rev.* 2001;9(3):21–26.

Tiedje LB et al. An ecological approach to breastfeeding. *MCN: Am J Matern Child Nurs.* 2002;27:154–161.

Truitt ST, Fraser AB, Grimes DA, Gallo MF, Schulz KF. Cochrane database systematic review 2003(2) CD003988. Combined hormonal versus nonhormonal versus progestin-only contraception in lactation.

Tuttle CR. An open letter to the WIC program: the time has come to commit to breastfeeding. *J Hum Lact.* 2000;16:99–103.

United Nations Children's Emergency Fund (UNICEF). *Innocenti Declaration on the Protection, Promotion and Support of Breastfeeding, Florence, Italy, August 1990.* New York, NY: UNICEF, Nutrition Cluster (H-8F); 1990.

United States Breastfeeding Committee (USBC). *Breastfeeding in the United States: A national agenda.* Rockville, MD: Health Resources and Services Administration, Maternal and Child Bureau; 2001.

United States Breastfeeding Committee (USBC). *Economic Benefits of Breastfeeding* (issue paper). Raleigh, NC: United States Breastfeeding Committee; 2002. Available at: http://www.usbreast feeding.org/Issues-Papers/Benefits.pdf. Accessed October 7, 2007.

US Department of Agriculture (USDA), Food and Nutrition Service. Breastfeeding promotion and support in WIC. 2007. Available at: http://www.fns.usda,gov/wic/Breastfeeding/breastfeedingmainpage.htm. Accessed October 8, 2007.

US Department of Health and Human Services (USDHHS). *Healthy People: The Surgeon General's Report on Health Promotion and Disease Prevention.* Washington, DC: Government Printing Office; 1979. Available at: http://www.surgeongeneral.gov/library/reports.htm. Accessed June 2002.

US Department of Health and Human Services (USDHHS). *Healthy People 2010.* Vol. II. Washington: Government Printing Office. 2000a. Rev. ed. Available at: http://www.healthypeople.gov/Document/HTML/Volume2/16MICH.htm#_Toc494699668. Accessed October 10, 2007.

US Department of Health and Human Services, Office on Women's Health. Blueprint for action on breastfeeding. 2000b. Available at: http://www.womens health.gov/breastfeeding/bluprntbk2.pdf. Accessed October 14, 2007.

Uvnas-Moberg K et al. Release of GI hormones in mother and infant by sensory stimulation. *Acta Paediatr Scand.* 1987;76:851–860.

Walker M. A fresh look at the risks of artificial infant feeding. *J Hum Lact*. 1993;9:97–107.

Walker M. *Selling Out Mothers and Babies: Marketing of Breast Milk Substitutes*. Weston, MA: National Alliance for Breastfeeding Action; 2001.

Weimer JP. *The economic benefits of breastfeeding: a review and analysis*. Food and Rural Economics Division, Economic Research Service, U.S. Department of Agriculture, Food Assistance and Nutrition Research Report No. 13; March 2001.

Whitehead RG. The human weaning process. *Pediatrics*. 1985;75(suppl 1):189–193.

Wickes IG. A history of infant feeding: III. Eighteenth and nineteenth century writers. *Arch Dis Child*. 1953a;28:332–340.

Wickes IG. A history of infant feeding: V. Nineteenth century concluded and twentieth century. *Arch Dis Child*. 1953b;28:495–502.

Wieschhoff HA. Artificial stimulation of lactation in primitive cultures. *Bull Hist Med*. 1940;8:1403–1415.

Williamson MA. *Infant mortality: Montclair, NJ. A study of infant mortality in a suburban community*. Washington, DC: US Department of Labor, Children's Bureau; 1915.

Wilson-Clay B et al. Learning to lobby for probreastfeeding legislation: the story of a Texas bill to create a breastfeeding-friendly physician designation. *J Hum Lact*. 2005;21:191–198.

Winikoff B, Laukaran VH. Breast feeding and bottle feeding controversies in the developing world: evidence from a study in four countries. *Soc Sci Med*. 1989;29:859–868.

Wolf JH. The first generation of American pediatricians and their inadvertent legacy to breastfeeding. *Breastfeeding Med*. 2006;1(3):172–177.

Woodbury RM. The relation between breast and artificial feeding and infant mortality. *Am J Hyg*. 1922;2:668–687.

Woolridge MW, Greasley V, Silpisornkosol S. The initiation of lactation: the effect of early versus delayed contact for suckling on milk intake in the first week postpartum. A study in Chiang Mai, northern Thailand. *Early Hum Dev*. 1985;12:269–278.

World Alliance for Breastfeeding Action (WABA). Home page. Available at: http://www.waba.org.my. Accessed October 14, 2007.

World Health Organization (WHO). *Contemporary Patterns of Breast-Feeding*. Geneva, Switzerland: WHO; 1981a.

World Health Organization (WHO). *International Code of Marketing Breastmilk Substitutes*. Geneva, Switzerland: WHO; 1981b.

World Health Organization (WHO). *Protecting, Promoting, and Supporting Breastfeeding: The Special Role of Maternity Services*. [A joint WHO/UNICEF statement]. Geneva, Switzerland: WHO; 1989.

World Health Organization (WHO). *Baby-Friendly Hospital Initiative* (A joint WHO/UNICEF statement). International Paediatric Association Meeting, Ankara, Turkey, 1991.

World Health Organization, UNICEF. Global Strategy for Infant and Young Child Feeding. Geneva, Switzerland: WHO, UNICEF; 2003.

Section 2

Anatomical and Biological Imperatives

After pregnancy, the mother continues to nourish her child through breastmilk—energy now synthesized and stored in the breast. Breastmilk, a living fluid that benefits infants, mothers, and society, changes throughout lactation to meet the infant's nutriment needs. No human-made substitute nourishes the infant as well. What drugs and viral infections pose a risk to the breastfeeding baby? Most drugs are compatible with breastfeeding, as this chapter shows. Viruses and bacteria stimulate antibodies in the mother's body, which, except for HIV, protect the vulnerable infant through mother's milk. Scientists are attempting to catch the elusive thread that unravels the tragedy of AIDS and the mystery of the HIV virus within breastmilk cells.

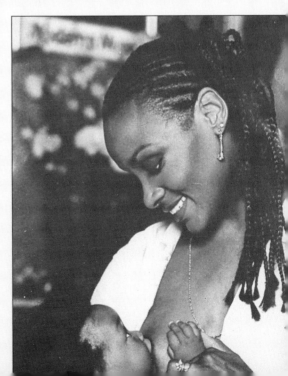

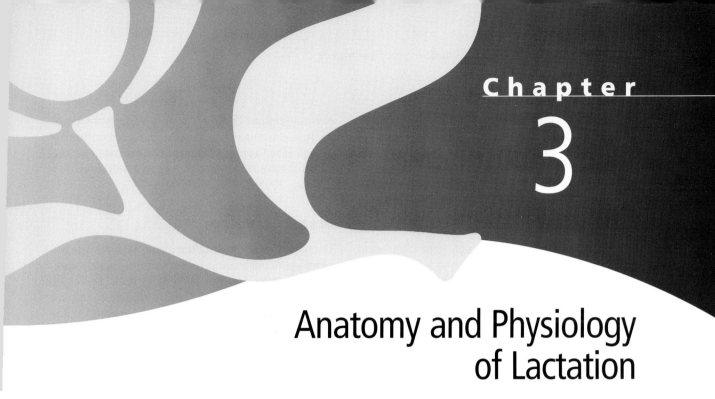

Anatomy and Physiology of Lactation

Jan Riordan

IT IS ESSENTIAL that healthcare providers understand the anatomy of the human female breast and the physiological mechanisms of milk production. It is equally necessary to recognize the unique anatomy of the infant's oral structures and the physiological mechanisms of suckling. Anatomy isn't supposed to change, but it has changed considerably since high-resolution ultrasound has allowed us to look inside the breast. This chapter is divided into two parts: the first focuses on the mother, the second on the infant. In lactation, as in all human biological systems, there is a working relationship between anatomy (form) and physiology (function). Although function changes as form changes, the functional capacity of the human breast is not wholly dictated by form. Breast size, for instance, is a poor predictor of lactational capability. It is the infant's appetite that determines milk yield, rather than the mother's capacity to produce milk. Ultrasound, a simple noninvasive method to observe and measure the lactating breast, has opened the functioning and anatomy of the breast wide open and allows us to look inside. The developmental cycle of the mammary gland has four phases: mammogenesis, lactogenesis (stages I and II), galactopoiesis, and involution.

Mammogenesis

The mammary system is unlike other organ systems. From birth through puberty, pregnancy, and lactation, no other human organ displays such dramatic changes in size, shape, and function as does the breast. The Latin term for breasts, *mammae*, developed from the infant's cry, "mamma," in seeking the breast. In some cultures, female breasts serve more than one function: they attract the sexual attentions of the male adult and then give nourishment and nurturing to the suckling infant. The first part of this chapter, which focuses on the mother, describes breast development from embryo to adulthood, breast anatomy, changes during pregnancy and lactation, and hormones that influence the course of lactogenesis.

Breast development begins early, by the fourth week of gestation when two parallel primitive milk streaks develop from axilla to groin on the trunk of the embryo. These streaks become the mammary ridge or milk line by the fifth week of embryonic life. This ridge or line is actually a thickening of epithelial cells in a localized ventrolateral area on the embryo (the "milk hill" stage) that continues through weeks 7 and 8 and is accompanied by inward growth into the chest wall. Between 12 and 16 weeks' gestation, these specialized cells differentiate further into the smooth muscle of the nipple and areola. Also during this period, epithelial cells continue to develop into mammary buds and then, in a treelike pattern, proliferate to form epithelial branches that eventually become alveoli (Dawson, 1934; Vorherr, 1974).

Placental sex hormones enter fetal circulation and stimulate formation of channels (canalization) of the branched epithelial tissue. This process continues until the fetus is 32 weeks old. From 32 to 40 weeks' gestation, lobular-alveolar structures containing colostrum develop. During this time, the fetal mammary gland mass increases four times over its original mass, and the nipple and areola develop further and become pigmented. After birth, the neonate's mammary tissue may secrete colostral milk (so-called witch's milk).

Mammary gland development during childhood is limited to general growth. However, at puberty, estrogen and a pituitary factor, and probably a growth hormone, become the major influence on breast growth in a girl when, at 10 to 12 years of age, primary and secondary ducts grow and divide and form club-shaped terminal end buds that are associated with beginning function of the hypothalamus-pituitary-ovarian axis. The buds develop into new branches and small ductules of areolar buds, which later become the acini or alveoli in the mature female breast. During each menstrual cycle, proliferation and active growth of duct tissue occurs during the follicular and ovulatory phases, reaching a maximum in the late luteal phase and then regressing. During each ovulatory cycle, peaks of ovarian steroids, primarily progesterone, foster further mammary development that never regresses to its former state of the preceding cycle. Trauma, incisions, or radiation therapy to the breast bud in the prepubertal era can trigger maldevelopment with hypoplasia of the vestigial breast that has future consequences for lactation. For example, radiation during childhood can be associated with an inadequate breast-milk supply as an adult.

Complete development of mammary function occurs only in pregnancy when the breasts increase in size and the nipple pigment darkens. Except for the uterus, no other organ changes so dramatically as the breast does during pregnancy and lactation.

New budding of structures continues until about age 35. In addition to progesterone, prolactin or human placental lactogen is thought to be necessary for the final stages of mammary growth and differentiation (Neville, 2001).

Breast Structure

The basic units of the mature glandular tissue are the *alveoli*, which are composed of secretory acinar units in which the ductules terminate. Each cluster of secretory cells of an alveolus is surrounded by *myoepithelial cells*, a contractile unit responsible for ejecting milk into the *ductules*. Ducts grow inward from the ectodermal layer and canalize by 32 weeks gestation. Each ductule then merges, without communicating with its neighbors, into a larger duct (Figure 3–1). An ultrasound image of a lactating breast is shown in Figure 3–2, where ducts filled with milk can be clearly seen. The ducts intertwine erratically much like tree roots making it difficult to separate them surgically.

Each breast has duct openings, sometimes called nipple "pores." The ducts are lined with stratified squamous epithelium near the nipple, by columnar epithelium at more distal areas, and highly vascular connective tissue.

The alveolus or milk-secreting unit is a single layer of epithelial cells with surrounding supporting structures: myoepithelial cells, contractile cells for milk ejection, and connective tissue. Milk is continuously secreted into the alveolar lumina where it is stored until the letdown reflex triggers the myoepithelial cells to contract and eject the milk (Neville, 2001).

Mammary ducts do not widen into *sinuses* located behind the nipple and the areola as previously thought. Figure 3–3, which shows contrast opacification of a single lactiferous duct, confirms that the duct does not widen before it branches in mammary ducts. In each breast, there are 15 to 20 subdivided *lobes*, each containing between 10 and 100 alveoli. It was believed that each lobe is separate from each other. We now know that there are connections between lobes (Geddes, 2007).

Between and around the uneven edges of the lobes is a thick layer of fat. There is considerable difference in amount of adipose tissue among women—in some, fat composes up to half of the

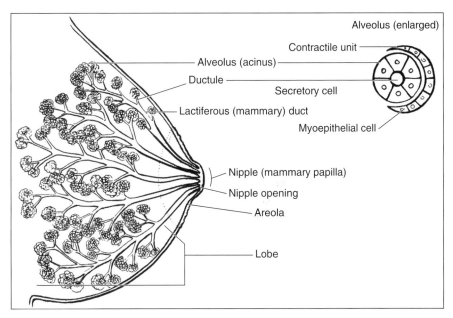

Alveolus (enlarged)

Contractile unit

Alveolus (acinus)

Ductule

Secretory cell

Lactiferous (mammary) duct

Myoepithelial cell

Nipple (mammary papilla)

Nipple opening

Areola

Lobe

FIGURE 3–1   Schematic diagram of a breast.

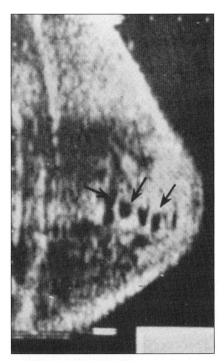

FIGURE 3–2   Ultrasound image showing milk-filled ducts. Mother lactating 10 months.

Source: Telles, 1980.

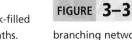

FIGURE 3–3   Contrast opacification of a single lactiferous duct demonstrates a branching network that defines a single lobe of the breast.

Source: Kopans, 1989.

breast. The amount of adipose tissue has affected neither the breast storage capacity nor the milk production (Ramsay et al., 2005a).

Attaching the deep layer of the subcutaneous tissue to the dermis of the skin are the *suspensory ligaments* or *Cooper's ligaments* (Figure 3–4). The breast's structure is mainly the result of fibrous tissues that surround and course through it. Glandular tissue that extends toward the axilla partly under the lateral border of the pectoralis majora is known as the *axillary tail* (Figure 3–5). Each breast of an adult woman weighs, on average, 150 to 200 gm and doubles in weight to 400 to 500 gm (about 1 pound) during lactation. Between 6 and 9 months after the beginning of lactation, breast size decreases slightly. Whether this results from mobilization of breast fatty tissue or greater breast tissue efficiency in making milk, milk production remains constant (Hartmann, Sherriff, & Kent, 1995).

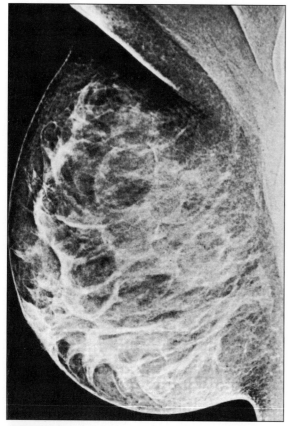

FIGURE 3–4 Curvilinear densities represent Cooper's ligaments.

Source: Kopans, 1989.

The breast is highly vascularized. Blood is supplied to the breast through the internal mammary (60 percent) and lateral thoracic (30 percent) arteries. The lymph vessels of the breast are numerous and, for the most part, join the lymph nodes of the axilla. The majority of lymph vessels follow the lactiferous ducts and thus converge toward the nipple, where they join a plexus situated beneath the areola (subareolar plexus).

The nerve supply of the breast is derived from the second to the sixth intercostal nerves. The fourth intercostal nerve penetrates the posterior aspect of the breast (left breast at 4 o'clock, right breast 8 o'clock) and supplies the greatest amount of sensation to the nipple and to the areola. The breast has uneven patterns of sensation: the areola is the most sensitive part of the breast, the skin adjacent to the areola is less sensitive, and the nipple itself is the least sensitive. Women with larger breasts report less sensation than women with smaller breasts. Of women with small or moderate-sized breasts, those who have never been pregnant report greater sensation in their nipples and areolae. Midway to the nipple and areola, the fourth intercostal nerve becomes more superficial. As it reaches the areola, it divides into five branches: one central, two upper, and two lower. The lowermost branch consistently pierces the areola at 5 o'clock on the left side and 7 o'clock on the right side. Any trauma to this nerve will cause some loss of sensation in the breast (Courtiss & Goldwyn, 1976). If the lowermost nerve branch is severed, the mother loses sensation to the nipple and areola (Farina, Newby, & Alani, 1980).

The covering smooth skin is modified at the center of each breast to form a *mammary papilla* or nipple into which the ducts open. Some of these ducts join so that about 9 openings appear on the nipple surface. It is not known whether these ducts are all open to the outside or patent. Some ducts may be "blind" and not open to the outside. For example, Cooper (1840) found 7–12 patent ducts in a cadaver dissection of a breast from a woman who was lactating before death, although he could cannulate up to 22 ducts.

Milk ducts are small, superficial, easily compressed, and increase in diameter at milk ejection (Geddes, 2007). The nipple projects as a small cylindrical body with pigmented wrinkled skin slightly below the center of each breast at about the level of the fourth intercostal space. Surrounding the

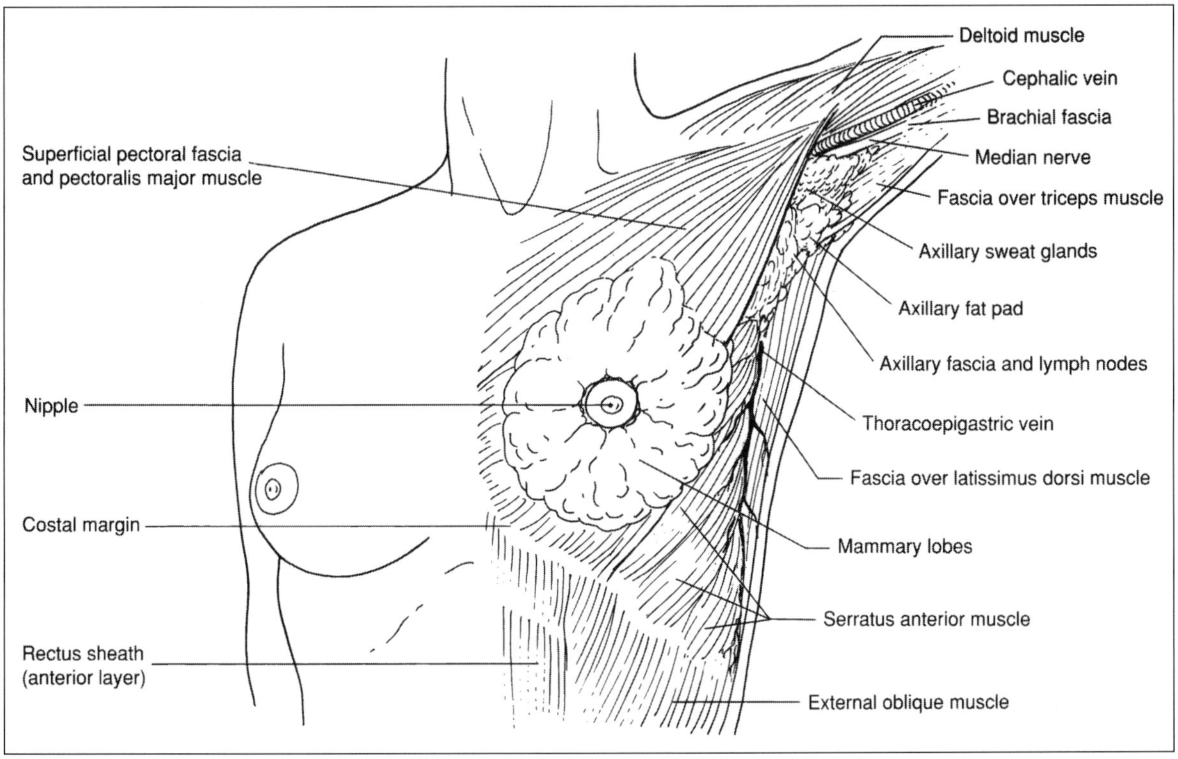

FIGURE **3–5**   Anterior pectoral dissection showing the lobular nature of the mammary gland extending toward the axilla and its location anterior to the pectoralis major muscle. Includes the superficial axillary lymph and sweat glands.

Source: Adapted from Clemente, 1978.

nipple is the *areola*. The nipple and areola contain erectile smooth muscles. Hair follicles surround the nipple and areola but are not within the nipple and areola proper; most women have at least some nipple hair. Contraction of bundles of smooth muscles beneath the nipple and areola cause the nipple to be firm and protruding. These structures are seen in Color Plates 1–3.

Nipple Size

In a lactating mother, the average diameter of the areola is 6.4 cm. The size of the areola increases significantly in the first few days postpartum especially on day 3 with lactogenesis. The average diameter of the erectile portion of the nipple is 1.6 cm and the length is 0.7 cm (Ziemer, 1993). The diameter of the nipple increases during pregnancy approximately from 9.5 to 11.5 mm although the nipple cannot be measured exactly because it varies with the degree of

erection. However, studies of nipple diameter of breastfeeding women show that the sizes are fairly consistent: Ziemer (1993) found an average diameter of 16 mm, Ramsay (2005a) 16 mm, and Hoover 17.5 mm. Wilson-Clay and Hoover (2005) note that women with extra large nipples seem to have more problems with latch on.

Areolar Glands (AG)

Within the areola lie Montgomery's tubercles which consist of mammary milk glands and sebaceous glands; together they are called *areolar glands* (AG) (Smith, 1982; Schaal et al., 2006) (see Figure 3–6). Long a focus of anatomic debate, some of the AG are true mammary glands whose ducts and secretory parenchyma are the same as those of the mammary glands that open at the tip of the nipples. As such, they are an integral part of the mammary structure and total breast tissue (Montagna & MacPherson,

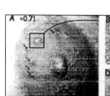

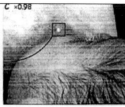

FIGURE 3–6 (A) Photograph of an areola (left breast, postpartum day 3), showing (arrows) skin structures (revealed by relative elevation and pigmental heterogeneity relative to surrounding skin), which were counted as areolar glands. (B) Enlarged (2.5×) view of an areolar gland. (C) An areolar gland giving off a milk-like secretion during a breastfeed. (D) Enlarged (3×) representation of a secretory drop from an areolar gland.

Source: From Schaal B et al. Human breast areolae as scent organs: morphological data and possible involvement in maternal-neonatal coadaptation. *Dev Psychobiol.* 2006;18(2):100–110. Reprinted with permission of John Wiley & Sons, Inc.

1974). From an evolutionary standpoint, it is of interest that the rhesus monkey does not have AGs (MacPherson & Montagna, 1974).

The number of AG present on the areola varies widely among women. Schaal et al. (2006) found that all but one woman in their study (n = 29) had AG. The mean number of glands per each areola was 8.9 (range 0–38). The number of AG is unrelated to the size of the areola and is similar between the left and right breast. More AGs are located on the upper, lateral section of the areola, generally the area in which the baby's nose is most frequently directed. About 1 in 5 lactating women reported seeing a visible fluid emission from their areolar glands (Schaal et al., 2006) (see Figure 3–6).

The presence and number of AG may play a more important role in breastfeeding than we have previously thought. Infants whose mothers have more areolar glands weigh more in the first few days, tend to latch on more rapidly, and suckle more actively after latching. It is possible to conclude that the AG is a scent organ and the fluid from the AG provides a sensory stimulation to the newborn that not only helps guide him to the nipples, but also stimulates the nipples more effectively, increases colostrum intake, and ultimately increases chances for survival.

Variations

From woman to woman, breasts vary in color, size, shape, and placement on the chest wall; these variations are genetically influenced. Lobular size varies within a single breast, from one breast to another, and from woman to woman. Moreover, breast asymmetry is common; the left breast is often larger than the right. Areola and nipple color vary according to complexion: pink in blonds, browner in brunettes, and black in dark-skinned women.

Supernumerary nipples (polymastia) and/or an *accessory nipple* is the spontaneous reappearance of ancestral characteristics in individual members of a species—a reminder of our evolution (Schmidt, 1998). They may occur at any point along the milk line from the axilla to the groin. They occur in about 1 to 5 percent of the population and may be associated with renal or other organ-system anomalies (Berman & Davis, 1994). Polymastia occurs in different forms: breast tissue with a nipple but lacking an areola; breast with a nipple and areola; or breast tissue only. Only rarely does a true or complete accessory mammary gland develop (Grossl, 2000). The most common areas in which a supernumerary nipple might develop are in the axilla and on the thorax (Color Plate 21).

Lack of full protraction of the nipple on the common pinch test (see Figure 3–12, later in this chapter) is fairly common in primigravid women. Poor nipple protractility in women during their first pregnancy has been reported to range from 10 to 35 percent (Alexander et al., 1992; Blaikeley et al., 1953; Hytten & Baird, 1958; Waller, 1946). Protractility of the nipple gradually improves during pregnancy and, by puerperium, most women have good nipple protraction. Generally, nipple protraction continues to improve with each subsequent pregnancy and lactation experience. The relationship between protractility and subsequent breastfeeding difficulty is minimal. Because the infant makes a teat not from the nipple alone but from the surrounding breast tissue, the actual shape of the nipple may be a secondary consideration.

Nipple inversion is found in about 3 percent of women and is usually bilateral (87 percent) (Park, Yoon, & Kim, 1999). Of the total number of inverted nipples, 96 percent are umbilicated and only 4 percent are invaginated (true inversion). Although true inversion is uncommon, its treatment can be difficult. If the inversion is on one breast only, the mother can breastfeed from a single breast and use a silicone breast shield on the other breast. Placing a silicone breast shield over the inverted nipple allows the infant to grasp on to the breast and suckle effectively. When the inversion is bilateral, feedings at the breast may have to be supplemented. The mother's first breastfeeding experience may be more difficult than subsequent ones—frequent suckling by the infant helps to evert the previously inverted tissue.

Pregnancy

During pregnancy, the breasts grow larger, the skin appears thinner, and the veins become more prominent. The diameter of the areola increases from about 34 mm in early pregnancy to 50 mm postpartum (Hytten, 1954), although there is a wide range of areolar width in any population. As the nipples become more erect, pigmentation of the areola increases and the Montgomery's glands enlarge.

Serum hormones stimulate breast growth during pregnancy: nipple growth is related to serum prolactin levels; areolar growth is related to serum placental lactogen (Cregan & Hartmann, 1999). Estrogen and progesterone also exert their specific effect on the breast during pregnancy; the ductal system proliferates and differentiates under the influence of estrogen, whereas progesterone promotes an increase in size of the lobes, lobules, and alveoli. Adrenocorticotropic hormone (ACTH) and growth hormone combine synergistically with prolactin and progesterone to promote mammary growth.

Breast growth during pregnancy varies among women. In a study of eight pregnant women, most had a gradual increase in breast growth throughout their pregnancy; however, one mother had a spurt of breast growth between 10 and 15 weeks and afterward very little growth; another had little or no breast growth (Cregan & Hartmann, 1999).

Lactogenesis

The transition from pregnancy to lactation is called *lactogenesis*. Growth and proliferation of the ductal tree and further formation of lobules characterize the first half of pregnancy. During the second half of pregnancy, secretory activity accelerates and the acini or alveoli become distended by accumulating colostrum (Russo & Russo, 1987). After 16 weeks of pregnancy, lactation occurs even if the pregnancy does not progress. An accessory breast may also swell. Just before and during childbirth, a new wave of mitotic activity increases the total DNA of the mammary gland (Salazar & Tobon, 1974; Vorherr, 1974).

The capacity of the mammary gland to secrete milk from midpregnancy to late pregnancy is called *lactogenesis, stage I* (or *lactogenesis I*) (see Table 3–1). During lactogenesis I, breast size increases as epithelial cells of the alveoli differentiate into secretory cells for milk production. Fat droplets accumulate in these cells and plasma concentration of lactose and α-lactalbumin increase. The milk droplets move through the cell membrane and into the ductules (see Figure 3–7). The onset of copious milk secretion

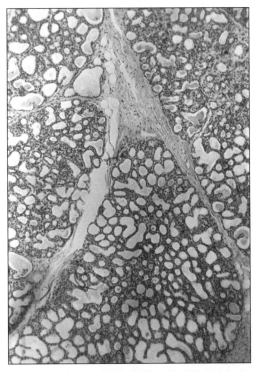

FIGURE 3–7 Milk is secreted from the alveolar cells, where small droplets form and migrate through the cell membrane and into the alveolar ductules. Photomicrograph.

Source: With permission, Victor B. Eichler, PhD.

TABLE 3–1	Stages of Lactation	
Mammogenesis		• Mammary (breast) growth; increased size and weight of breast • Proliferation of ducts and glandular system under estrogen and progesterone
Lactogenesis, stage I (mid-pregnancy to day 2 postpartum)		• Initiation of milk synthesis from mid-pregnancy to late pregnancy • Differentiation of alveolar cells from secretory cells • Prolactin stimulates mammary secretory epithelial cells to produce milk
Lactogenesis, stage II (day 3 to day 8)		• Closure of tight junctions in alveolar cell (Figure 3–6) • Triggered by rapid drop in mother's progesterone levels • Onset of copious secretion of milk • Fullness and warmth in breasts • Switch from endocrine to autocrine control
Galactopoiesis (day 9 to beginning of involution)		• Maintenance of established secretion • Control by autocrine system (supply–demand) • Breast size decreases between 6 and 9 months postpartum
Involution (average 40 days after last breastfeeding)		• Additions of regular supplementation • Decreased milk secretion from build-up of inhibiting peptides • High sodium levels

after birth is *lactogenesis, stage II* (days 2 or 3 to 8 postpartum). During lactogenesis II, milk volume increases rapidly from 38 to 98 hours postpartum and then abruptly levels off.

Lactogenesis II is triggered by a rapid drop of serum progesterone (and possibly estrogen) after the delivery of the placenta. It is also accompanied by a significant fall in breastmilk levels of sodium, chloride, and protein, and a rise in lactose and milk lipids. These changes in cellular metabolism are a result of closure of junction complexes between alveolar cells. Before lactogenesis (first 3 to 4 days), there are large gaps between the alveolar cells. During full lactation, the passage of substances between alveolar cells is stopped by a gasketlike structure called the *tight junction*, which joins the epithelial cells tightly to one another (Figure 3–8). The closure of these tight junctions precedes the onset of copious milk secretion (Neville, 2001).

As lactation begins, these hormonal changes are essential:

• Drop in progesterone levels
• Release of prolactin from the anterior pituitary, which stimulates lactogenesis and initiates milk secretion
• Removal of breastmilk by the infant or pump
• Release of oxytocin from the posterior pituitary (at least by day 3)

Involution of the mammary gland is a process that removes the milk-producing epithelial cells when they become superfluous at weaning. It is a two-step process that involves the death of the secretory epithelium and its replacement by adipocytes. The awesome capacity of the breast to produce milk is matched by the mechanism of apoptosis, a form of programmed cell death (Watson, 2006).

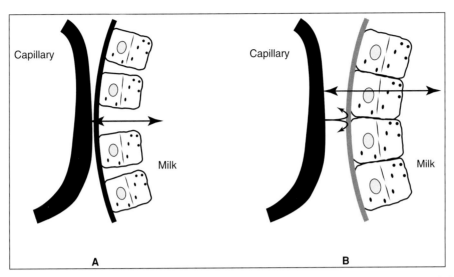

FIGURE 3-8 (A) Gaps between alveolar cells before lactogenesis. (B) Intracellular gaps close tightly to one another following lactogenesis.

Source: Used with permission from Hale TW. *Medications and mother's milk.* 9th ed. Amarillo, TX: Pharmasoft; 2000:6.

Delay in Lactogenesis

Not all women experience the coming in of the milk on the third or fourth day postpartum. A delay or diminishment in lactogenesis, common in certain situations (as listed in Table 3–2), invites us to gain a better understanding of the specific biochemical or hormonal nature of lactogenesis that may lead to a delay in lactogenesis. We do know that high breastmilk sodium levels on or before the third day after birth are significant for impending breastfeeding problems and for lactation involution (Morton, 1994; Humenick et al., 1998). Although the reasons for lactogenesis delay are not always clear, it does appear that lactogenesis is susceptible to outside influence and is thus fragile.

Hormonal Influences

Lactogenesis II is triggered following the expulsion of the placenta by a fall in progesterone levels and the continued presence of prolactin. A great deal of information about these hormonal functions during lactation is now known through radioimmunoassay studies. A programmed transformation of the mammary epithelium mediated by a cascade of hormonal changes leads to a rapid synthesis of breastmilk by day 4 following birth. The postpartum period is characterized hormonally by a drop in progesterone and elevated levels of prolactin, which act synergistically with cortisol, thyroid-stimulating hormone, prolactin-inhibiting factor, and oxytocin to establish and maintain lactation. If the delicate interplay of these hormones are disturbed—for example, by high testosterone levels

TABLE 3-2	**Maternal Conditions That Can Delay or Impair Lactogenesis**
Cesarean birth	Sozmen, 1992
Diabetes, type I	Neubauer et al., 1993
Labor analgesia	Riordan, Gross, & Angeron, 2000
Obesity	Rasmussen et al., 2001
Polycystic ovary syndrome	Marasco et al., 2000
Gestational ovarian theca lutein cysts	Hoover et al., 2002
Placental retention	Neifert, 1981
Stress	Chen, 1998
	Grajeda & Perez-Escamilla, 2002

in the woman with gestational ovarian theca lutein cysts (Hoover, Barbalinardo, & Pia Platia, 2002) or polycystic ovary syndrome (Marasco, Marmet, & Shell, 2000), lactogenesis is delayed and possibly suppressed (see Chapter 16).

Progesterone

Progesterone is required to maintain pregnancy and remains high throughout pregnancy. Lactation during pregnancy is inhibited by high levels of progesterone, which interfere with prolactin action at the alveolar cell receptor level. The inhibiting influence of progesterone is so powerful that lactation is delayed if placental fragments are retained after birth (Neifert, McDonough, & Neville, 1981). Following birth, progesterone decreases about tenfold during the first 4 days. This rapid fall of progesterone in the presence of maintained prolactin levels triggers lactogenesis. Once lactation is initiated, the principal hormone in maintaining milk biosynthesis is prolactin.

Prolactin

Prolactin is essential for both initiating and maintaining milk production. Though oxytocin appears to be keyed more closely to milk ejection, milk is not made if there is an absence of prolactin. During pregnancy, prolactin, which is secreted by the anterior pituitary gland, has an important role in increasing breast mass and cell differentiation. A group of peptides, including angiotensin II, gonadotropin-releasing hormone (GnRH), and vasopressin, stimulate the release of prolactin. The mammary ducts and alveoli mature and proliferate as prolactin levels steadily rise from the normal non-pregnancy level of 10 to 20 ng/ml to a peak of 200 to 400 ng/ml at term (Tyson et al., 1972).

As progesterone and estrogen levels abruptly drop after a woman gives birth, the anterior pituitary gland, no longer inhibited by these two hormones, releases pustile prolactin 7 to 20 times in 24 hours and greater amounts during sleep; thus, for accurate measurement of prolactin, samples should be taken in close intervals around the clock (Madden et al., 1978). Episodic peaks are superimposed on a stable ongoing level of secretion. Because human placental lactogen (HPL) competes with prolactin for breast receptors, the decline of HPL after delivery of the placenta also promotes prolactin action. Figure 3–9 describes the rise and fall of hormones during pregnancy and lactation.

Following lactogenesis II, when milk secretion shifts from endocrine to autocrine control, prolactin secretion continues to be controlled by the hypothalamus. This control is largely inhibitory; that is, whenever the pathway between the hypothalamus and the pituitary is disrupted, prolactin levels rise. During galactopoiesis, the hypothalamus is dependent upon removal of milk in order for lactation to continue. When the nipple is stimulated and milk is removed from the breast, the hypothalamus inhibits the release of dopamine, a prolactin-inhibiting factor; this drop in dopamine stimulates the release of prolactin and causes milk production (Chao, 1987).

Plasma prolactin levels increase the most in the immediate postpartum period but rise and fall in proportion to the frequency, intensity, and duration of nipple stimulation. Prolactin concentration in blood doubles in response to suckling and peaks approximately 45 minutes after the beginning of a breastfeeding session (Noel, Suh, & Frantz, 1974). If lidocaine is applied to the nipples to deaden sensation, prolactin does not increase (Neville, 2001).

Prolactin levels remain elevated throughout the first 6 months postpartum in women who breastfeed at regular intervals. At 6 months postpartum serum

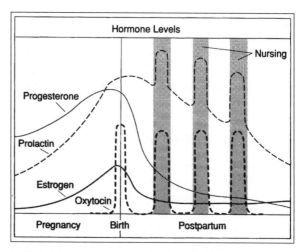

FIGURE 3–9   Hormone levels during pregnancy and lactation.

Source: Adapted from Love, 1990.

prolactin can still more than double in response to suckling (Battin et al., 1985). If a mother does not breastfeed, prolactin levels usually reach nonpregnant levels by 7 days postpartum (Tyson et al., 1972).

During lactation, maternal prolactin levels are described as follows:

- They follow a circadian rhythm; levels during the night (sleep) are higher than during the day.
- They decline slowly over the course of lactation (Battin et al., 1985; Cox, Owens, & Hartmann, 1996) but remain elevated for as long as the mother breastfeeds, even if she breastfeeds for years (Stallings et al., 1996).
- They rise with suckling: the more feedings, the higher the level of serum prolactin. More than eight breastfeedings per 24 hours prevents decline of the concentration of prolactin before the next breastfeeding (Cox, Owens, & Hartmann, 1996; Tay, Glasier, & McNeil, 1996).
- They are not necessarily related to milk yield especially after lactation becomes established (Hill, Chatterton, & Aldag, 1999; Ueda et al., 1994), although feeding two babies simultaneously doubles prolactin surge (Tyson et al., 1972).
- They delay the return of ovulation by inhibiting ovarian response to follicle-stimulating hormone, and prolactin levels are higher in amenorrheic women than in cycling women during the first year postpartum (Battin et al., 1985; Stallings et al., 1996).
- They are not related to the degree of postpartum breast engorgement (West, 1979).
- They drop with cigarette smoking (Baron et al., 1986) and rise with beer drinking (Mennella & Beauchamp, 1993).
- They rise with anxiety and psychological stress (Hill, Chatterton, & Aldag, 1999) even though feeding at the breast and milk ejection reflex are calming (because of oxytocin release).
- Depressed mothers have lower serum prolactin levels (Groer, 2005b).

Normal prolactin levels in nonpregnant or nonlactating women are 20 ng/ml or less. In lactating women, mean baseline prolactin levels are 90 ng/ml at 10 days postpartum; afterward, these levels slowly decline but remained elevated at 180 days postpartum (44.3 ng/ml). Women who remain amenorrheic have higher (about 110.0 ng/ml) baseline prolactin levels as compared to women (about 70.1 ng/ml) who menstruate prior to 180 days (Battin et al., 1985). An overview of prolactin serum levels during pregnancy and breastfeeding is shown in Figure 3–10.

Prolactin also is present in breastmilk. The release of prolactin into intra-alveolar secretions of the breast plays a role in establishing and maintaining lactation. Milk prolactin concentration is lower than its concentration in blood plasma and is highest in early transitional milk (about 43 ng/ml) and the foremilk rather than the hindmilk (Cox, Owens, & Hartmann, 1996). This early transmission of prolactin in the aqueous foremilk is thought to have an effect on intestinal fluid and electrolyte exchange in the newborn (Yuen, 1988). Milk prolactin levels are about the same between left and right breasts and are highest in the morning (Cregan, Mitoulas, & Hartmann, 2002). Breastmilk prolactin steadily declines but remains detectable in mature milk (about 11 ng/ml) until weaning up to 40 weeks postpartum (Yuen, 1988).

De Carvalho et al. (1983) postulated that frequent feeding in early lactation stimulates a faster increase in milk output because suckling stimulates the development of receptors to prolactin in the mammary gland. According to this approach, the number of these receptors per cell increases in early lactation and remains constant thereafter (Hinds & Tyndale-Biscoe, 1982; Sernia & Tyndale-Biscoe, 1979).

Some understanding of the impact of early breastfeeding on prolactin receptors is provided by Zuppa et al. (1988). In this study, although serum prolactin levels were slightly lower in multiparous mothers as compared with primiparous mothers in the first 4 postpartum days, the volume of milk obtained by the infants of the multiparous mothers was significantly higher. The researchers concluded that multiparous women had a greater number of mammary gland receptors for prolactin. The implication here is that the controlling factor in breastmilk output is the number of prolactin receptors rather than the amount of prolactin in serum. More receptors may result in more than adequate milk production, even in the presence of lower prolactin levels. This finding helps to explain why

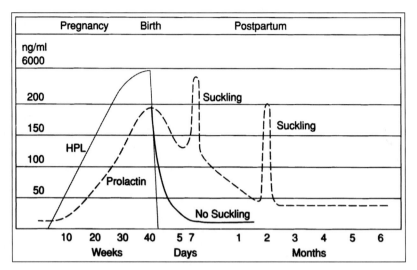

FIGURE 3–10   Fluctuation of human placental lactogen and prolactin serum levels in pregnancy and lactation.

Source: Used with permission from Battin D et al. Effect of suckling on serum prolactin, luteinizing hormone, follicle-stimulating hormone, and estradiol during prolonged lactation. *Obstet Gynecol.* 1985;65:785–788; Tyson JE et al. Studies of prolactin in human pregnancy. *Am J Obstet Gynecol.* 1972;113:14–20; Speroff L, Glass RH, Kase NG. *Clinical gynecology, endocrinology and infertility.* 4th ed. Baltimore, Md: Williams & Wilkins; 1989:283.

infants of multiparous mothers begin gaining weight somewhat faster than do those of primiparous mothers.

Cortisol

Cortisol, a main glucocorticoid, acts synergistically on the mammary system in the presence of prolactin (Neville & Berga, 1983). The final differentiation of the alveolar epithelial cell in a mature milk cell takes place because prolactin is present, but only after prior exposure to cortisol and insulin. Glucocorticoids are hormones secreted by the adrenal glands and help to regulate water transport across the cell membranes during lactation. A high cortisol level is associated with a delay in lactogenesis (Chen et al., 1998).

Thyroid-Stimulating Hormone

The thyroid-stimulating hormone (TSH) promotes mammary growth and lactation through a permissive rather than a regulatory role. Dawood et al. (1981) established a marked and significant increase in plasma thyroid-stimulating hormone level on the third to fifth postpartum days.

Prolactin-Inhibiting Factor

Prolactin-inhibiting factor (PIF) is a hypothalamic substance, either dopamine itself or mediated by dopamine. It stimulates dopamine releases and thus inhibits prolactin secretions (dopamine agonist). Bromocriptine, a drug that suppresses lactation, is an example of a dopamine agonist. Dopamine antagonists have the opposite effect. Nipple stimulation and milk removal suppresses PIF and dopamine, causing prolactin levels to rise and the breast to produce milk. Drugs, such as metoclopramide, phenothiazines, and reserpine derivatives, increase breastmilk production because they inhibit PIF (Bohnet & Kato, 1985).

Oxytocin

In response to suckling, the posterior pituitary hormone oxytocin causes the *milk-ejection reflex* (MER) or *letdown*, a contraction of the myoepithelial cells surrounding the alveoli necessary for the removal of milk from the breast. Oxytocin is released in pulsatile waves and is carried though the bloodstream to the breast where it interacts with receptors on myoepithelial cells, causing contraction and forcing milk from the alveoli into the ducts where it becomes available to the newborn through the nipple openings. Most women feel pressure and a tingling, warm sensation during milk ejection and a significant increase in milk-duct diameter can be observed via ultrasound imaging when the milk ejection is sensed. After lactation becomes established, women will experience multiple milk ejections during a feed. In a study of 45 Australian mothers 88 percent were able to sense the initial milk ejection; however, none sensed subsequent milk ejections (Ramsay, 2005b).

Oxytocin plays a major role in the continuance of lactation. During suckling or breast stimulation, oxytocin is released in discrete pulses. Oxytocin blood levels rise within 1 minute on stimulation, and they return to baseline levels within 6 minutes after the cessation of nipple stimulation. This rise and fall of oxytocin levels continues at each feeding throughout the lactation course, even when the mother breastfeeds for an extended period (Leake et al., 1983). The posterior pituitary contains a surprisingly large store of oxytocin (3000–9000 mU) when compared with the amount required to elicit the ejection reflex (50–100 mU) (Lincoln & Paisley, 1982).

Oxytocin has another important function—to contract the mother's uterus. Uterine contractions help to control postpartum bleeding and to aid in uterine involution. The uterus not only contracts during breastfeeding but also continues to contract rhythmically for as long as 20 minutes after the

feeding. These cramps may be painful during the first few days postpartum. After involution is complete, however, these rhythmical pulsations may be a source of pleasure to the mother. Oxytocin also has peripheral effects, notably dilation of peripheral vascular beds and increased blood flow without increased systemic arterial pressure. As a result, breastfeeding is accompanied by increased skin temperature not unlike that of a menopausal hot flash (Marshall, Cumming, & Fitzsimmons, 1992). New mothers often report an increase in thirst while breastfeeding, which appears to be closely related to the increase in plasma oxytocin (James et al., 1995). Women who have had emergency cesarean births (Nissen et al., 1996) or are under stress (Ueda et al., 1994) have significantly less oxytocin pulses during breastfeeding. Breast massage raises the maternal plasma oxytocin level (Yokoyama et al., 1994).

Through oxytocin mediation, these afferent pathways become so well established that letdown can occur even when the mother merely thinks of her baby. There are many anecdotal reports of spontaneous lactation in mothers who have weaned. Milk synthesis is a complex interplay of the hypothalamic-pituitary-gonadal axis (Figure 3–11) that is susceptible to emotional upheaval and can potentially inhibit the letdown reflex.

The calmness while breastfeeding that mothers report is partly governed by oxytocin. Oxytocin infusion in rats produces sedation, lower blood pressure, and lower levels of corticosteroids

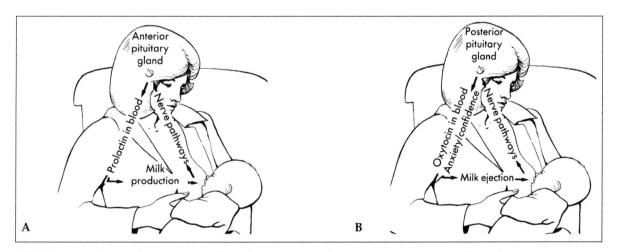

FIGURE 3–11 (A) Release and effect of prolactin on milk ejection. (B) Release and effect of oxytocin.

(Uvnas-Moberg, 1997). Groer and Davis (2002) make the case that breastfeeding women have a diminished response to stressors and to pain. Perceived stress is significantly lower in breastfeeders compared to formula-feeders (Groer, 2005a). When exposed to stress, lactating women had lower levels of ACTH, cortisol, glucose, and norepinephrine than did nonlactating women (Altemus et al., 1996).

Johnstone and Amico (1986) measured the influence of supplemental feedings on oxytocin and prolactin peaks. They discovered that mothers who were exclusively breastfeeding had higher oxytocin levels over time than did women who were giving their babies replacement feedings. The exclusively breastfeeding women's oxytocin levels not only remained higher but also tended to climb over time, so that their oxytocin levels were higher at 15 to 24 weeks than they were at earlier periods (2 to 4 weeks and 5 to 14 weeks). In sharp contrast, the oxytocin levels of the mothers who were supplementing were lower at all times examined, and no rise in oxytocin peaks was noted over time. In both groups of women, prolactin levels tended to decline over time. Among mothers who were not supplementing, however, prolactin levels were consistently higher at all times examined. These data suggest that over time prolactin levels can be expected to fall, but oxytocin levels will continue to climb. However, when a mother supplements with formula-feedings, prolactin levels decline markedly and fall even further over time, and oxytocin levels remain depressed and do not climb.

Milk Production

With closure of tight junctions in the cells of the alveoli (Figure 3–8) and through the mediation of the hypothalamus, the alveolar cells respond with milk secretion at the base of the alveolar cell, where small droplets form and migrate through the cell membrane and into the alveolar ducts for storage (see again Figure 3–7). The rate of milk synthesis after each breastfeeding episode varies, ranging from 17 ml/hr to 33 ml/hr in one study (Arthur et al., 1989). Milk synthesis is related to the degree of breast fullness. For example, a woman who did not breastfeed her baby for 6 hours will have a lower rate of milk synthesis than if she had breastfed every 90 minutes (Cregan & Hartmann, 1999).

The highly vascularized secretory cells extract water, lactose, amino acids, fats, vitamins, minerals, and numerous other substances from the mother's blood, converting them to milk for her infant. Stores of adipose tissue laid down during pregnancy are drawn upon to provide substrate for milk synthesis. When the milk "comes in" or rapidly increases in volume, creating breast fullness 3 to 4 days after birth, closure of the junctional complexes between the mammary alveolar cells prevents direct access of extracellular space to the lumen of the mammary alveoli (Neville, 2001). Thus sodium, chloride, and lactose concentrations are altered. Mothers then begin to feel a tightening in their breasts as the myoepithelial cells contract to expel the milk (Color Plate 3). This physiologic response is known as mammary-ejection reflex (MER) formerly called "letdown."

Autocrine Versus Endocrine

It is at this point that lactation shifts from *endocrine control* (hormone driven) to *autocrine control* (milk removal driven) (Prentice et al., 1989). It follows, then, that the amount of colostrum secreted by non-breastfeeding women during the first few days postpartum is similar to that of breastfeeding women; however, this reverses abruptly after the first few days. Thus breastfeeding is not a major factor for the *initiation* of lactation but it is essential for the *continuation* of lactation (Kulski & Hartmann, 1981). From a clinical standpoint the onset of copious milk secretion after birth or the milk "coming in" will happen whether the baby is being put to the breast or not since it is hormonally driven.

Feedback Inhibitor of Lactation

An autocrine feedback mechanism, the feedback inhibitor of lactation (FIL) appears to locally control milk synthesis. The specific mechanism by which FIL works to inhibit breastmilk synthesis is not clear but it appears to be a compound within the milk, not the distension of the breast that slows the build-up of milk. It is thought that this mechanism of local control of milk synthesis must be a relationship between the filling and emptying cycle of the alveoli. More exact information on how this occurs would be useful to clinicians in treating oversupply or undersupply problems (Cregan & Hartmann, 1999).

Galactopoiesis

Galactopoiesis is the maintenance of the established milk production (Table 3–1). The breast is not a passive container of milk but an organ of active production that is infant rather than hormone driven. The removal of milk from the breasts facilitates continued milk production; conversely, lack of adequate milk removal or stasis tends to limit breastmilk synthesis in the breasts. It is the quantity and quality of infant suckling or milk removal that governs breastmilk synthesis. Milk production reflects the infant's appetite rather than the woman's ability to produce milk, which in fact can be several fold higher (Daly & Hartmann, 1995). As long as milk is removed regularly from the breast, the alveolar cells will continue to secrete milk almost indefinitely.

This phenomenon, the *supply-demand response,* is a feedback control that regulates the production of milk to match the intake of the infant. A common adage that expresses this response is "The more the mother breastfeeds, the more milk there will be" (La Leche League International, 1997). Because lactation is an energy-intensive process, it makes teleological sense that there should be safeguards against wasteful overproduction as well as mechanisms for a prompt response to the infant's need.

A case of a new mother who became pregnant three months after having a pituitary resection supports the concept of autocrine control (de Coopman, 1993). After delivering a healthy infant, this mother had sufficient milk to completely sustain her baby by breastfeeding without supplementation. This unusual situation was attributable to the pituitary abscess that caused milk production to continue through her pregnancy after she weaned her first child; thus her milk yield postpartum was based on milk removal as much as on hormonal stimulation.

Galactorrhea

Galactorrhea is the spontaneous secretion of milk from the breast under nonphysiological circumstances. Small amounts of milk or serous fluid are commonly expressed for weeks, months, or years from women who have previously been pregnant or lactating. Many anecdotal reports of spontaneous lactation present an intriguing enigma. Thyrotoxicosis, certain drugs (reserpine, methyldopa, phenothiazines), and the use of intrauterine devices containing copper (Horn & Scott, 1969) can trigger abnormal milk secretion.

Surprisingly, only 30 percent of women with galactorrhea have higher-than-normal prolactin levels (Frantz, Kleinberg, & Noel, 1972); these women are otherwise healthy and have no history of menstrual irregularity or infertility but may be overly sensitive to normal circulating prolactin levels (Friesen & Cowden, 1989). For other women, galactorrhea is a symptom of a larger problem of hyperprolactinemia; in addition to a spontaneous milk secretion, they may also complain of amenorrhea, difficulty in becoming pregnant, and lack of libido. Any woman with persistent galactorrhea should be referred to a physician for a thorough physical examination and biochemical assessment.

Clinical Implications: Mother

Breast Assessment

Usually little attention is given to prenatal assessment of the breast and nipples because of Western cultural inhibitions about the breast and lack of recognition of its importance. As a consequence, after giving birth, mothers may experience feeding difficulties that could have been prevented. Nurses and lactation consultants practicing as primary caregivers are the ideal people to perform a prenatal breast assessment, particularly because physicians (especially males) are often reluctant to do so.

Ideal for teaching as well as for data gathering, physical assessment of the breast and nipples includes both inspection and palpation. While one is assessing the breasts, the following observations and questions are relevant.

Inspection

Size, symmetry, and shape of the breasts proper have minimal effect on lactation. The assessment provides the opportunity to reassure the woman with small breasts that she will be able to breastfeed and have a sufficient supply of milk. Asymmetry of breast size is usually normal, but marked asymmetry may be an indication of inadequate glandular tissue in a small minority of women (see Color Plate 27). Hypoplasia (lack of breast tissue) accompanied by a wide space between breasts (intramammary space) is another anatomical "red flag" associated with insufficient lactation (Huggins, Petok, & Mireles, 2000). When mothers with possible hypoplasia (underdeveloped breasts) are identified, their newborn baby should be monitored closely for adequate milk intake. Inadequate glandular tissue might prevent the mother from exclusively breastfeeding her baby; however, she can continue to enjoy the breastfeeding relationship if she provides the baby with additional nutrition while feeding from the breast.

For the woman with large breasts, discussing the importance of a support bra and where such a bra may be obtained is helpful. Holding and feeding her infant will not be the same for the large-breasted woman as for mothers with average-sized breasts. Instead of simply holding the breast, the mother with large breasts may need to lift her breast and to hold or push part of the breast back to permit her infant to grasp the nipple and maintain an adequate airway. During prenatal discussions, the mother may talk about some of her deeper feelings about having large breasts and her decision to breastfeed.

The skin of the breast should be inspected for any deviations. Skin turgor and elasticity can be assessed by gently pinching the skin, although the effect of elasticity on lactation is questionable: women who have been pregnant before have more elastic skin because it has been stretched from a previous pregnancy; women pregnant for the first time have firmer tissue.

A lateral incision in the vicinity of the cutaneous branch of the fourth intercostal nerve made during breast augmentation or reduction surgery may mean severed innervation of the nipple and areola (Farina, Newby, & Alani, 1980). Surgery on the breast, especially if it involves an incision at the areolar margin, is likely to interfere to some degree with milk production. However, even having undergone such surgery, most mothers still can breastfeed. Breast-reduction surgery, because of the greater likelihood of the removal of nipple tissue (Hurst, 1996), is more likely than augmentation surgery to negatively influence later lactation performance (Neifert et al., 1990). Scar tissue from injury should be evaluated for its effect on skin elasticity and the degree to which nerve reactivity may have been affected.

Note should also be taken of any skin thickening and dimpling of the breast or nipple tissue. Although rare in a woman of childbearing age, such a change could be an early sign of a tumor and should be promptly referred to a physician for evaluation.

Now is the time to ask questions: "Have your breasts grown during pregnancy?" "Have you had any tenderness and soreness?" An increase in breast size, swelling, and tenderness usually indicates adequately functioning breast tissue responsive to hormonal changes.

Next, the nipple should be carefully inspected. (For the purpose of this discussion, nipple will refer to the areola as well as the nipple shaft and pores.) If the nipples appear small, explain that the size of a woman's nipples is of secondary importance to their functional ability. Likewise, any nipple structural abnormality such as inversion should be assessed only in terms of its function.

The look of the breast does not dictate its ability to function. A case in point may be women who have sustained significant scarring from burns (see Color Plate 25). Second- and third-degree burns rarely extend so deeply into the parenchyma that they destroy the glandular tissue of the breast, even when the burns have occurred in adulthood. Significant scarring of the dermis and epidermis, however, may result in (1) reduced maternal sensation when the infant suckles, (2) minimal tissue elasticity, thus requiring the mother to alter the baby's position at the breast, and (3) reduced milk ejection if a nipple has been surgically reconstructed. Nevertheless, scar tissue on the breast or nipple does not, by itself, preclude breastfeeding.

Palpation

After a thorough washing of the hands, the nurse or lactation consultant should assess the nipple by compressing or palpating the areola between the forefinger and the thumb just behind the base of the nipple (the pinch test). This action simulates the compression that occurs when the infant is at the breast. Because of possible nipple adhesions within the underlying connective tissue, a nipple that initially appears everted may retract inwardly on stimulation. Conversely, a nipple that appears flattened or inverted may, on palpation, evert; therefore, differentiation must be made between structure and function in assessing the nipples.

The classification of nipple function in Table 3–3 is suggested as standard terminology. It must be emphasized that although many primigravidas have nipples that tend to retract during pregnancy, most evert easily by the end of pregnancy and do not interfere with breastfeeding. Thus nipple assessment should be performed periodically through the pregnancy to track changes and to inform the mother how her body is preparing to feed her baby.

Classification of Nipple Function

When the nipple is compressed using the pinch test, it responds in one of the ways identified in Figure 3–12. This response may reflect degree of function.

Flat or retracted nipples may be treatable during pregnancy. Dysfunction may be present in one nipple while the other is perfectly normal, or it may be present in both nipples. Retraction or inversion can prevent the infant from effectively milking milk ducts that lie beneath the areola. Retraction or simple inversion identified in early pregnancy, however, does not necessarily foretell later difficulty. The infant forms a teat not only from the nipple but also from the surrounding breast tissue. When inversion is noted early in pregnancy, time is on the mother's side. As pregnancy progresses, hormonal changes increase the size and protractility of the nipples. The mother also has time to use interventions that help prevent subsequent feeding problems.

Concepts to Practice

Encouraging early and frequent breastfeeding is a simple, low-cost recommendation for breastfeeding initiation. If the infant is able to suckle effectively at the breast soon after birth, there is a direct relationship between the frequency and strength of suckling and subsequent availability of breastmilk. There appears to be an early "window of opportunity" for the infant's suckling to stimulate prolactin receptors (discussed earlier in this chapter), which in turn enhances milk production. A basic knowledge of anatomy and physiology is put to valuable use when the lactation consultant or nurse translates basic concepts into easily understandable teaching materials. If a client realizes a stressful environment may inhibit her milk supply, she may take action to reduce stressful situations over which she has control. If a woman understands that the reason she needs less covering when she breastfeeds is that she literally has "hot flashes" during feedings, she will take measures to "keep cool." Examples of the application of basic biologic principles of maternal lactation are legion and form the basis of many of the chapters that follow.

TABLE 3–3	Classification of Nipple Function	
Protraction	Nipple moves forward; considered a normal functional response. No special interventions are needed.
Retraction	Instead of protracting, the nipple moves inward.
Minimal	An infant with a strong suck exerts sufficient pressure to pull the nipple forward. A weak or premature infant may have difficulties at first.
Moderate to severe	Nipple retracts to a level even with or behind the surrounding areola. Intervention is helpful to stretch the nipple outward and improve protractility.
Inversion	On visual inspection, all or part of the nipple is drawn inward within the folds of the areola.
Simple	The nipple moves outward to protraction with manual pressure or when cold (pseudoinversion).
Complete	The nipple does not respond to manual pressure because adhesions bind the nipple inward; very rarely there is congenital absence of the nipple.

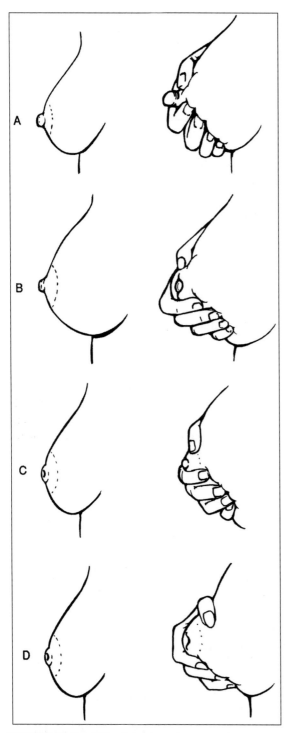

FIGURE 3–12 (A) Protracting normal nipple.
(B) Moderate to severe retraction.
(C) Inverted-appearing nipple which, when compressed using pinch test, will either invert farther inward or will protract forward. (D) True inversion; nipple inverts further.

Newborn Oral Development

Infants perform a series of complex oral movements to obtain sufficient nutriment from their mother's breast to meet daily nutritional requirements and to support rapid growth, especially during the first few months of life. Suckling is a dynamic process, as the infant is continually adjusting to a changing anatomy. The act of suckling is far more than simply obtaining food. The infant's earliest autonomous functions are focused about his mouth and pharynx area. The infant's mouth is the cockpit of his awareness and is the principal site of interaction with his environment.

In the embryo, facial and pharyngeal regions develop from neural-crest cells at about the time of neural-tube closure. Further development is due to tissue differentiation from the endoderm, which later forms the digestive tract. During gestation, the fetus is able to swallow fluid as early as 11 weeks (Miller, 1982) and has a suckle reflex at 24 weeks (Herbst, 1981). Older studies reported that the rooting response and the link between suckling and swallowing was not established until 32 weeks (Amiel-Tison, 1967) and not well coordinated until 37 weeks (Bu'Lock, Woolridge, & Baum, 1990). However, in a study of Swedish preterm infants (Nyqvist, Sjoden, & Ewald, 1999), efficient rooting, areolar grasp, and latching on at the breast were observed at 28 weeks—much earlier than previously thought.

At birth, the infant's mouth is vertically short in comparison with that of the adult. There is so little room that when the newborn's mouth is closed, the tongue is in lateral contact with the gums and with the roof of the mouth. There are other proportional differences in size and shape between the infant and the adult skull (Figures 3–13 and 3–14). The infant's lower jaw (mandible) is small and somewhat receded.

The Palate

Whereas the adult's hard palate is deeply arched and situated on a higher plane relative to the base of the skull, the infant's is short, wide, and only slightly arched at birth. Corrugated transverse folds (rugae) on the hard palate assist the newborn in holding the breast during suckling. While the hard palate works with the tongue to compress the nipple and maintain its position, the soft palate, a muscular flap, elevates forming a seal from the nasal

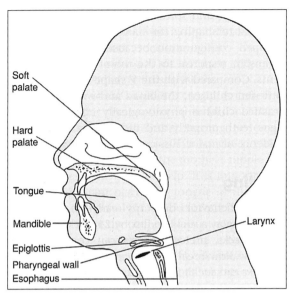

FIGURE 3–13 Midsagittal section of cranial and oral anatomy of an adult while swallowing.

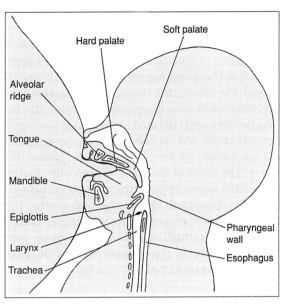

FIGURE 3–14 Midsagittal section of cranial and oral anatomy of an infant while swallowing.

cavity during swallowing that allows passage of the breastmilk bolus (Wolf & Glass, 1992). This momentary action is sometimes called a "pause" in suckling assessment.

Just as infants' ears and noses are shaped differently so too are palates. The most troublesome palate shape for infants is the "bubble" palate. Described by Marmet and Shell (1984) as a concavity in the hard palate, it can cause slow weight gain and sore, abraded nipples if the nipple is pulled into the bubble rather than stay elongated to the juncture of the hard and soft palates. To bring the position of the tongue forward, the mother lies in a supine (on back) position with pillows to support her; the baby placed on the chest to breastfeed (Snyder, 1997). Photographs of prone positions can be found in *Supporting Sucking Skills in Breastfeeding Infants* by Catherine Watson Genna, Chapter 12 (Marmet & Shell, 2008).

The Tongue and Lips

Because the infant's tongue fills the small oral cavity, the extent and the direction of tongue movement is limited. Taste buds on the tongue (mostly on the tongue tip) are present at birth, but the newborn has an increased suckling response only to sweet taste.

The entire surface of the tongue is within the oral cavity. Vacuum increases during the downward motion of the posterior tongue. Peak vacuum occurs when the tongue is in the lowest position at the same time milk flows in the ducts; therefore, vacuum is likely to play a major role in milk removal from the breast (Geddes, 2008). The infant's lips are well adapted to affect an airtight closure around the breast. The lips are partially everted so that the oral mucosa presents slightly externally; they have tiny swellings on the inner surface (eminences of the pars villosa) that facilitate holding the breast and areola in place. The nipple enters a central, grooved trough in the tongue; the baby's lips then close around the nipple.

The Epiglottis

The infant's epiglottis lies just below the soft palate, unlike the adult's, as seen in Figure 3–14. This makes it possible for food to move laterally on the outside of the epiglottis and to pass directly into the esophagus. The epiglottis plays an important role by closing off the pathway to the lungs when the infant swallows. Such closure ensures that the milk will travel into the esophagus rather than into the trachea.

suckling bursts and rests during minimal milk intake). Bowen-Jones, Thompson, and Drewett (1982) challenged the validity of these two categories. The latter study showed that breastfeeding babies *always* suckle in bursts, with resting periods or pauses between bursts. The term *nonnutritive suckling* is now accepted to mean either spontaneous suckling in the absence of anything being introduced into the infant's mouth (common during sleep) or suckling as prompted by something that is not a liquid nutriment (e.g., a pacifier) (McBride & Danner, 1987).

Nonnutritive suckling has important implications for infant development, especially under special circumstances such as prematurity. Nonnutritive suckling in premature infants increases peristalsis, enhances secretion of digestive fluids, and decreases crying in these infants (Measel & Anderson, 1979).

Suckling at the breast has been examined in great detail. With the advent of ultrasonography and other technologies, it is now possible to accurately quantify suckling patterns, replacing earlier descriptions that only inferred what actually occurred. When infants feed from both breasts, milk transfer from the second breast decreases by 58 percent as compared with the first breast, even though there are no significant changes in suckling pressure (Prieto et al., 1996). Jacobs et al. (2007), Marmet and Shell (1984), Woolridge (1986), McBride and Danner (1987), and Smith et al. (1985) described infant suckling mechanics at the breast. The following description of functional suckling is based on the work of these investigators. Figure 3–15 illustrates the complete suck cycle:

1. The nipple and its surrounding areola and underlying breast tissue are drawn deeply into the infant's mouth; the infant's lips and cheeks then form a seal. The infant's lips are flanged outward around the mother's breast and are minimally involved.
2. The tip of the infant's tongue is maintained behind the lower lip and over the lower gum while the rest of the anterior tongue cups the areola of the breast.
3. During the feeding, the mother's highly elastic nipple elongates (two to three times its resting length) into a teat by suction created within the baby's mouth. The nipple extends back as

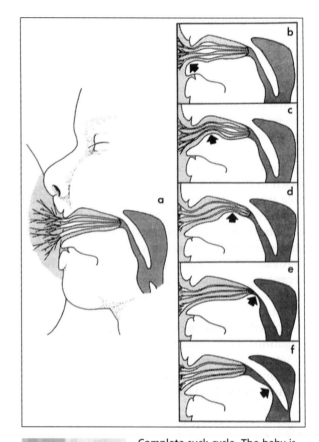

FIGURE 3–15 Complete suck cycle. The baby is shown in median section. The baby exhibits good feeding technique: the nipple is drawn well into the mouth, extending back to the junction of the hard and soft palate (the lactiferous sinuses are depicted within the teat, although these cannot be visualized on scans).

Source: Used with permission from Woolridge MW. The "anatomy" of infant sucking. *Midwifery.* 1986;2:164–167.

far as the posterior tongue junction between the hard and soft palates. At its base, the nipple is held between the upper gum and tongue that covers the lower gum. The mother's nipple and areolar tissue undergo extensive changes during feeding.

4. The jaw moves the tongue up, compressing the maternal areola against the infant's alveolar ridge. The *masseter* is the jaw muscle that is most active during suckling. It raises the jaw and causes it to protrude preparing for compression on the breast (Gomes et al., 2006).

5. As the anterior portion of the tongue is raised, the posterior tongue is depressed and retracted in undulating or peristaltic motions, forming a groove that channels the milk to the back of the oral cavity where it stimulates receptors that initiate the swallowing reflex. This backward movement produces a negative pressure, similar to withdrawing a piston in an airtight syringe.

6. If the volume of milk taken is sufficient to trigger swallowing, the back of the tongue elevates and presses against the posterior pharyngeal wall. New ultrasound videotapes showed that at its most upward position *holding the nipple in contact with the palate does not compress any milk into the mouth.* Instead tongue movement downward posterior to the nipple tip is followed by milk exiting the nipple (Jacobs et al., 2007). The soft palate rises and closes off the nasal passageways. The larynx then moves up and forward to close the trachea, propelling the milk into the esophagus. Afterward, the larynx returns to its previous position.

7. The infant lowers the jaw, and a new cycle begins. A rhythm is created by this sequence of vertical jaw movements and the depression and elevation of the posterior tongue. Each suckle sequence is followed by a swallow.

The differences between bottle-feeding and breastfeeding are shown in Table 3–4. Generally, breastfeeding infants suckle more times per day and maintain a higher level of oxygen pressure (tcPO$_2$) and skin temperature (Mathew, 1988; Meier & Anderson, 1987) than do bottle-feeding infants. The differences between bottle-feeding and breastfeeding premature infants are even greater (Meier & Pugh, 1985).

Breathing, Suckling, and Pacing

In a normal, coordinated, nutritive suckling cycle, breathing appears to continue throughout the sucking cycle; however, at the onset of the swallow, as the bulk of the bolus enters the pharynx, airflow is momentarily interrupted and then immediately restored. Swallowing apnea lasts about 0.5 seconds. In a perfectly coordinated cycle of suckling, swallowing, and breathing, breathing movements appear to be related in a 1:1:1 sequence. The rate of suckling is high for the first 1 or 2 minutes until the milk-ejection reflex occurs, then it slows down. This sequence reoccurs with each milk ejection during a feeding. As the feeding progresses, suckling bursts become shorter with more frequent pauses.

Suckling patterns change as the infant develops. At first it is a reflexive action; however, the infant quickly learns by experimental opportunities, sensory inputs, and neurological maturation so that feeding and swallowing changes from a reflex to a volitional process and the pattern of breathing-swallowing coordination changes (Bronwen et al., 2007). This piece of information is important to keep in mind and to share with parents when working with a baby with feeding problems—things probably will improve as the baby matures.

A prospective study compared the coordination of sucking, swallowing, and breathing and its relationship to oxygen saturation during breastfeeding and two types of bottles: a soft-walled bottle/nipple and a hard-walled bottle/nipple (Goldfield et al., 2006). During breastfeeding, swallowing occurred at regular intervals (nonrandomly) between breaths and did not interfere with breathing. The same distribution of swallowing occurred in infants fed with the soft-walled bottle/nipple, while swallowing occurred randomly in infants fed with the hard-walled bottle/nipple. Oxygen saturation was significantly higher in infants fed with the soft-walled bottle/nipple, suggesting that if a bottle is needed a soft-walled bottle/nipple is preferred. It should be noted that this study was supported by a grant from Playtex Products Int. in addition to an NIH grant.

Although suckling, swallowing, and breathing are generally well coordinated during a feeding, infant cyanosis is a relatively common event, especially in neonates. The neonate almost always recovers spontaneously and often continues to suckle and swallow despite cyanosis. The infant's oxygen saturation normally declines during a feeding. Mean levels drop from 96 percent (during feeding) to 93 percent (postfeeding) in breastfed infants and from 95 percent (during feeding) to 92 percent (postfeeding) in bottle-fed infants (Hammerman & Kaplan, 1995). When term babies were given bottle-feedings with breastmilk, formula, and distilled water, the infants receiving breastmilk had better coordination between swallowing and breathing, which helps prevent subclinical aspiration (Mizuno, Ueda, & Takeuchi, 2002).

TABLE 3–4 Comparisons Between Breastfeeding and Bottle-Feeding in Full-Term Infants

Breastfeeding	Bottle-feeding	References

More frequent suckling/min
  Nutritive: 1 suckle/second
  Nonnutritive: 2 suckles/second
	Less frequent suckling/min	Drewett & Woolridge, 1979;
		  Mathew, 1988; Wolff,
		  1968

Breathing patterns Shortening of expiration Prolonging of inspiration	Breathing patterns Prolonged expiration Shortening of inspiration	Mathew, 1988
Oxygen saturation < 90% 2 of 10 infants	Oxygen saturation < 90% 5 of 10 infants	Mathew, 1988
Bradycardia 0 of 10 infants	Bradycardia 2 of 10 infants	Hammerman & Kaplan, 1995; Mathew, 1988
Extended opening of mouth to grasp mother's nipple	Less extension to grasp rubber teat	Marmet & Shell, 1984

Infant's lips flanged outward, relaxed and
  resting against the breast to make a seal
	Lips closer together and pursed to
	  maintain contact with rubber teat
		McBride & Danner, 1987

Extensive mandibular (jaw) action	Minimal mandibular action	Palmer, 1998

Tongue grooved around nipple; remains
  under nipple throughout feeding. Moves
  in peristaltic, rolling action from front
  to back
	Tongue upward and thrust forward
	  against end of teat, "piston-like," to
	  control milk flow
		Marmet & Shell, 1984;
		  Woolridge, 1986; Weber
		  et al., 1986

Silent, except for soft swallow sounds,
  and (in older infants), cooing or "singing"
	High-pitched squeak at end of intake
	  of air prior to new suck	

Duration of feeding varies from short (few
  minutes) to long (30 minutes or longer)
	Duration of feeding is usually
	  5–10 minutes
		Ardran, Kemp, & Lind,
		  1958

Includes nutritive and nonnutritive
  suckling throughout the feeding but less
  distinct differences
	Involves nearly exclusively nutritive
	  suckling
		Ardran, Kemp, & Lind,
		  1958; Hornell, 1999;
		  Woolridge, 1986

Swallowing occurs nonrandomly between
  breaths and does not interfere with
  breathing
	Swallowing patterns are different
	  according to type of bottle/nipple
	  Soft-walled is most physiological
		Goldfield, 2006

Unless hypoxic, the newborn is usually a nose breather, owing in part to the positioning of the soft palate and to the lack of space in the mouth through which air can travel in and out. Although it is true that babies have ventilatory problems when the nasal passages are occluded, an infant is capable of breathing through the mouth when necessary (Rodenstein, Perlmutter, & Stanescu, 1985). Fatigue is common when beginning to nipple feed, especially with low birth weight babies. Observe the infant's cues for a need for rest. *Pacing* the feeding is removing the nipple at the first sign of disorganized feedings and/or swallowing to allow the infant a breathing break to recover and rest. More

information on pacing feedings of children with neurological disorders will be discussed in later chapters.

Feeding and swallowing are sensitive indicators of the neurological function. Birth injury, congenital defects, or other situations of neurological dysfunction interfere with normal suckling. It may be necessary to bottle-feed until breastfeeding can be initiated. Therefore a basic review of neural control of suckling and swallowing, from either a bottle or breast, is in order. Coordination of more than 20 pairs of muscles and five cranial nerves are required just for swallowing! The cranial nerves involved include the trigeminal (V), facial (VII), glossopharyngeal (IX), vagus (X), and hypoglossal (XII) (see Figure 3–16).

An example of the neural complexity and overlap is described by Wolf and Glass (1992):

> *The motor fibers of the trigeminal nerve (CN V) innervate the muscles of the lower jaw for sucking and the palatal elevator to initiate swallowing. The sensory fibers provide feedback from the mouth during sucking, the soft palate during swallowing, and the nose during respiration.*

A breastfeeding infant who has suckling disorganization should be further evaluated neurologically to help understand the specific reason for the feeding dysfunction.

Wolf and Glass (1992) describe bottle-feeding suckling patterns in Figure 3–17:

- Normal suckling coordination of sucking, swallowing, and breathing in Figure 3–17a is organized into a series of suckling bursts and pauses.
- In feeding-induced apnea (Figure 3–17b) the infant is unable to pace himself and has lengthy suckling bursts without breathing at appropriate intervals. Sucking may cease with infant then compensating with rapid panting breaths. This can lead to fatigue or worse—sputtering and coughing—putting the infant at risk for aspiration.
- In short sucking bursts (Fig 3–17c), the infant takes only one to three sucks before pausing. The pausing is frequent and if too long can lead to apnea and cyanosis. It is most often seen in low birth weight babies and may indicate a swallowing problem. This can be a red flag for future neurological or developmental problems.

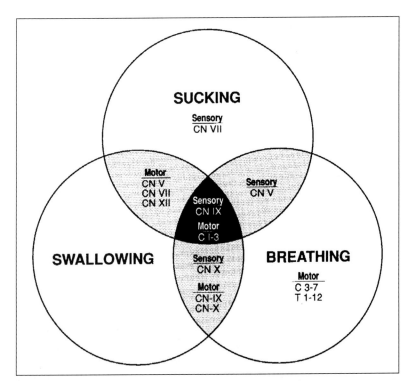

FIGURE 3–16   Overlapping function of cranial nerves in suck-swallow-breathe.

Source: Wolf LS, Glass RP. *Feeding and swallowing disorders in infancy: assessment and management.* Used with permission of Hammill Institute on Disabilities.

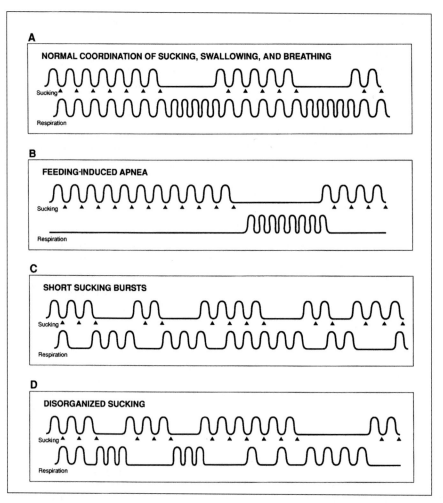

FIGURE **3-17**   Normal coordination of sucking, swallowing, and breathing compared to abnormal patterns. Each ▲ represents a swallow.

Source: Wolf LS, Glass RP. *Feeding and swallowing disorders in infancy: assessment and management.* Used with permission of Hammill Institute on Disabilities.

- Lastly, very disorganized sucking (Fig 3–17d) may reflect general disorganization because of a neurological deficit, respiratory problems, or a too-fast nipple-flow rate.

Frequency of Feedings

How often does the exclusively breastfed infant feed? Hornell et al. (1999) recorded the daily number of feedings of 506 Swedish infants for the first 6 months. These mothers live in a country where breastfeeding is the norm. Each had previously breastfed at least one infant for at least 4 months and considered that they breastfed on demand.

During the first 6 months of life, median frequency of feeds was eight feeds per 24 hours. This is consistent with the data by Howie et al. (1981) and Quandt (1986) but different from the studies by Butte et al. (1985) and de Carvalho et al. (1982) who noted a decline in feeding frequency during the first months. It also differs from a study of La Leche League mothers that showed an average daily number of 15 feedings (Cable & Rothenberger, 1984).

In the Hornell study, the median frequency of daytime feeds of exclusively breastfed infants was slightly below 6 during the first 26 weeks. The median number of night feeds declined from 2.2 at 2 weeks to 1.3 at 12 weeks, after which it increased up to 1.8 at 20 weeks (see Figure 3–18). The frequency and duration of daily feedings varied widely among mothers. For example, at 2 weeks, the frequency of feeds during the day ranged from 2.9 to 10.8 and night feeds from 1.0 to 5.1. Daytime suckling duration ranged from 20 minutes to over 4 hours and nighttime duration from 0 to 2 hours, 8 minutes. Increased feeding frequencies or so-called appetite or growth spurts were not observed in this study.

Australian mothers breastfed in similar patterns: infants exclusively breastfed an average of 11 times in 24 hours (range 6–18) (Kent et al., 2005). As lactation specialists, we teach women to breastfeed more frequently to build their milk supply, but the Kent study found no relationship between the numbers of breastfeedings per day and the 24-hour milk production of the mothers.

The neonate's ability to suckle effectively at the breast takes time and practice. For the first few feedings, even in full-term infants, suckling is usually disorganized. Drugs given to the mother during childbirth can also inhibit early suckling. Usually, after several attempts, the infant latches onto the breast and begins to suckle vigorously and effectively. These first feedings are critical because they imprint a suckling pattern that tends to be repeated in subsequent feedings. A healthy infant unaffected by labor or birth analgesia or anesthesia should be allowed to demonstrate hunger before being offered the breast. Practicing lactation consultants are fully aware that it is difficult, if not impossible to "make" a baby breastfeed when he is in a deep sleep. Forcing the infant to the breast might abolish the rooting reflex and disturb placement of the tongue (Widstrom & Thingstrom-Paulsson, 1993).

Consistent breastfeeding assessment and identification of early problems so that they can be resolved before they worsen is essential. Several breastfeeding assessment tools have been developed over the last decade. While there is not yet general agreement on which is the most valid tool in predicting how well breastfeeding will progress, an evidence-based tool undoubtedly will be developed (Riordan & Koehn, 1997). The more popular

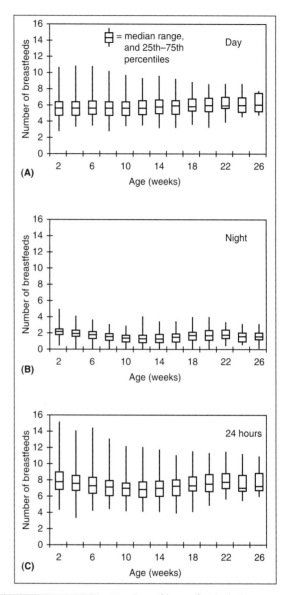

FIGURE 3–18 Number of breastfeeds during (A) daytime, (B) night-time, and (C) 24 hours at different ages. Median, 25th, and 7th percentiles and range.

Source: Used with permission from Hornell A et al. Breastfeeding patterns in exclusively breastfed infants: a longitudinal prospective study in Uppsala, Sweden. *Acta Paediatr.* 1999;88:203–211.

breastfeeding assessment tools are discussed in Chapter 20. The PIBBs breastfeeding tool, developed for assessing preterm infants, can be found as an appendix to Chapter 13.

Summary

Knowledge of maternal breast anatomy and the physiology of lactation are necessary antecedents to clinical practice. The fundamental biological principles of lactation discussed in this chapter are used, although not always consciously, in almost every clinical situation in which lactation is involved. Knowledge of the structure and function of the normal breast and of infant suckling are necessary for assessment; knowing what is normal must precede recognizing the abnormal and recommending actions designed to support an optimal breastfeeding experience. Enabling the natural physiological mechanisms to function optimally is more likely to lead to an uncomplicated breastfeeding experience; interference with these mechanisms can result in difficulty with breastfeeding for mother and infant. For example, restrictive policies in breastfeeding for preterm babies are commonly based on bottle-feeding studies, not on knowledge about the early development of infants' capacity for suckling at the breast (Nyqvist, Aden, & Ewald, 1999).

At the same time, anatomy and physiology are the building blocks in a larger picture of the breastfeeding and lactation experience. Most women are physiologically equipped to produce sufficient milk for their infant or infants. Yet the most commonly cited problem in breastfeeding worldwide is the mother's perception that she has insufficient milk (Hill & Humenick, 1989). Social and cultural influences play a major role in the mother's perceptions of her ability to nourish her infant from her breasts. Succeeding chapters build on the anatomy and physiology of lactation and address the clinical implications as well as its social and cultural aspects.

Key Concepts

- Breastmilk removal (through feeding or pumping) in the first 2 days postpartum is not necessary for lactogenesis II to occur; however, milk removal must begin by day 3 after birth or the likelihood of successful establishment of lactation is decreased.
- Three factors are necessary for lactation: (1) oxytocin released from the posterior pituitary, (2) removal of breastmilk by the infant or pump, and (3) prolactin release from the anterior pituitary, which stimulates lactogenesis and initiates milk secretion.
- Lactogenesis occurs earlier if breastmilk is removed by feeding or pumping within the first 2 to 3 days after birth. Early breastfeeding or pumping is associated with higher milk volume by day 5.
- Short-term rate of milk synthesis is considerably higher when most of the available milk has been removed from the breast.
- Frequency of breastfeedings varies widely; however, exclusively breastfed term infants (living in a country where breastfeeding is the norm) feed a median of 8 times per day (6 times during the day, and twice during the night).

- Mammary ducts do not widen into sinuses behind the nipple as previously thought.
- Suspensory ligaments of the breast are called Cooper's ligaments.
- Each breast of an adult woman weighs, on average 150 to 200 gm. It doubles in weight to 400 to 500 gm (about 1 pound) during lactation.
- Nerves that supply the breast are from the second to the sixth intercostal nerves. The fourth intercostal nerve, which penetrates the left breast at 4 o'clock and right breast at 8 o'clock, supplies the greatest amount of sensation to the nipple and areola.
- If the lowermost nerve branch of the fourth intercostal nerve is severed, the mother loses sensation to the nipple and areola.
- Breast asymmetry is common; the left breast is often larger than the right.
- Marked asymmetry and breast hypoplasia may indicate problems with breastmilk production.
- Areola and nipple color vary according to complexion: pink in blonds, brown in brunettes, and black in dark-skinned women.
- Supernumerary nipples (accessory nipple) occurs in 1 to 5 percent of the population at

any point along the milk line from the axilla to the groin.

- Poor nipple protractility occurs in 10 to 35 percent of women during their first pregnancy.
- Nipple inversion is found in about 3 percent of women, and it is bilateral in 87 percent of these women. Only 4 percent of nipple inversion is true inversion.
- Prolactin influences nipple growth; areolar growth is related to serum placental lactogen; the ductal system proliferates and differentiates under the influence of estrogen; progesterone promotes enlargement of the lobes, lobules, and alveoli.
- Lactogenesis, stage I occurs mid- to late pregnancy when breast size increases as epithelial cells of the alveoli differentiate into secretory cells for milk production.
- Lactogenesis II (days 2 to 8 postpartum) is the onset of copious milk secretion after birth when milk volume increases rapidly and then abruptly levels off.
- Before lactogenesis II large gaps occur between the alveolar epithelial cells. These gaps close suddenly after 3 to 4 days via a gasketlike structure (the tight junction) and trigger the onset of copious milk secretion.
- Maternal conditions that can delay or impair lactogenesis include cesarean birth, type I diabetes, labor analgesia, obesity, polycystic ovary syndrome, gestational ovarian theca lutein cysts, placental retention, and stress.
- The developmental cycle of the mammary gland has four phases: (1) mammogenesis, (2) lactogenesis, (3) galactopoiesis, and (4) involution.
- After delivery, progesterone levels drop and prolactin levels rise; both act synergistically with cortisol, thyroid-stimulating hormone, prolactin-inhibiting factor, and oxytocin to establish and maintain lactation.
- Following lactogenesis II, milk production shifts from endocrine to autocrine control. When the nipple is stimulated and milk removed from the breast, the hypothalamus inhibits dopamine, which in turn stimulates the release of prolactin and causes milk production.
- The basic unit of the breast is the alveolus which is surrounded by a contractile unit of myoepithelial cells responsible for ejecting milk into the ductules. Each ductule merges into a larger duct. The ducts are lined with epithelium and highly vascular connective tissue.
- Milk is secreted into the alveolar lumina where it is stored until the posterior pituitary hormone oxytocin causes the milk-ejection reflex or letdown, a contraction of the myoepithelial cells surrounding the alveoli.
- Oxytocin plays a major role in lactation. Blood levels rise within 1 minute of suckling, remain elevated during the feeding, and return to baseline levels within 6 minutes.
- Oxytocin contracts the mother's uterus, which help to control postpartum bleeding and to aid in uterine involution.
- The supply-demand response is a feedback control that regulates the production of milk to match the intake of the infant.
- Galactorrhea is the spontaneous secretion of milk from the breast from unexpected or unknown circumstances.
- Before lactogenesis, lactation is driven hormonally (endocrine control); after, it is driven by suckling and milk removal (autocrine control).
- Suckling and milk removal is not a major factor for the initiation of lactation but is essential for its continuation.
- If the frenulum—a fold of mucous membrane midline on the undersurface of the baby's tongue—is too short or is too far forward, it can interfere with an infant's ability to suckle.
- The suckling reflex is present at 24 weeks gestation. By 28 weeks preterm, babies can coordinate the suckle/swallow/breathe cycle; by 32 weeks, they can suckle in repeated bursts.
- Forcing a crying baby to the breast evokes a defensive response (tongue to palate) that inhibits suckling and disturbs the rooting-tongue reflex system.
- Nutritive suckling is intake of continuous flow of liquid nutriment; nonnutritive suckling is suckling in the absence of liquid nutriment being introduced into the baby's mouth.
- Breastfeeding infants suckle more times per day and maintain a higher level of oxygen pressure (tcPO$_2$) and skin temperature compared with bottle-fed infants.

- If a bottle/nipple is needed to supplement the baby, use a soft-walled bottle as it is more physiologically like breastfeeding.
- Babies suckle and swallow at a frequency of about once per second. When milk flow increases, the rate of suckling decreases; when milk flow is low, the rate of suckling increases.
- Suck training, an emerging area of lactation practice, involves oral stimulation and manipulation to treat feeding problems in infants.

References

Alexander JM, Grant AM, Campbell MJ. Randomized controlled trial of breast shells and Hoffman's exercises for inverted and non-protractile nipples. *Br Med J.* 1992;304:1030–1032.

Altemus J et al. Suppression hypothalamic-pituitary-adrenal axis responses to stress in lactating women. *J Clin Endocr Metab.* 1996;80:2954–2959.

Amiel-Tison C. Neurological evaluation of the maturity of newborn infant. *Arch Dis Child.* 1967;43:89.

Anderson GC et al. Development of sucking in term infants from birth to four hours postbirth. *Res Nurs Health.* 1982;5:21–27.

Ardran GM, Kemp MB, Lind J. A cineradiographic study of breast feeding. *Br J Radiol.* 1958;31:156–162.

Arthur PG et al. Measuring short-term rates of milk synthesis in breast-feeding mothers. *Q J Exp Physiol.* 1989;74:419–428.

Baron JA et al. Cigarette smoking and prolactin in women. *Br Med J.* 1986;293:482.

Battin D et al. Effect of suckling on serum prolactin, luteinizing hormone, follicle-stimulating hormone, and estradiol during prolonged lactation. *Obstet Gynecol.* 1985;65:785–788.

Berman MA, Davis GD. Lactation from axillary breast tissue in the absence of a supernumerary nipple: a case report. *J Reprod Med.* 1994;39:657–659.

Blaikeley J et al. Breastfeeding—factors affecting success. *J Obstet Gynaecol Br Emp.* 1953;60:657–669.

Blass EM. Behavioral and physiological consequences of suckling in rat and human newborns. *Acta Paediatr Suppl.* 1994;397:71–76.

Bohnet HG, Kato K. Prolactin secretion during pregnancy and puerperium: response to metoclopramide and interactions with placental hormones. *Obstet Gynecol.* 1985;65:789–792.

Bowen-Jones A, Thompson C, Drewett RF. Milk flow and sucking rates during breastfeeding. *Dev Med Child Neurol.* 1982;24:626–633.

Bronwen KN et al. The first year of human life: coordinating respiration and nutritive swallowing. *Dysphagia.* 2007;23:37–43.

Bu'Lock F, Woolridge MW, Baum JD. Development of coordination of sucking, swallowing and breathing: ultrasound study of term and preterm infants. *Dev Med Child Neurol.* 1990;32:669–778.

Butte NF et al. Feeding patterns of exclusively breast-fed infants during the first four months of life. *Early Hum Dev.* 1985;12:291–300.

Cable TA, Rothenberger LA. Breast-feeding behavioral patterns among La Leche League mothers: a descriptive survey. *Pediatrics.* 1984;73:830.

Chao S. The effect of lactation on ovulation and fertility. *Clin Perinatol.* 1987;14:39–49.

Chen DC et al. Stress during labor and delivery and early lactation performance. *Am J Clin Nutr.* 1998;68:335–344.

Clemente CD. *Anatomy: a regional atlas of the human body.* Philadelphia, Pa: Lea & Febiger, 1978.

Cooper AP. *Anatomy of the breast.* London: Longman, Orme, Green, Browne and Longmans; 1840.

Courtiss EH, Goldwyn RM. Breast sensation before and after plastic surgery. *Plast Reconstr Surg.* 1976;58:1–12.

Cox DB, Owens RA, Hartmann PE. Blood and milk prolactin and the rate of milk synthesis in women. *Exp Physiol.* 1996;81:1007–1020.

Cregan M, Hartmann PE. Computerized breast measurement from conception to weaning: clinical implications. *J Hum Lact.* 1999;15:89–95.

Cregan MD, Mitoulas LR, Hartmann PE. Milk prolactin, feed volume, and duration between feeds in women breastfeeding their full-term infants over a 24-hour period. *Exp Physiol.* 2002;87:207–214.

Daly SEJ, Hartmann PE. Infant demand and milk supply. Part 1: Infant demand and milk production in lactating women. *J Hum Lact.* 1995;11:21–23.

Dawood MY et al. Oxytocin release and plasma anterior pituitary and gonadal hormones in women during lactation. *J Clin Endocrinol Metab.* 1981;52:678–683.

Dawson EK. A histological study of the normal mamma in relation to tumour growth: 1. Early development to maturity. *Edinb Med J.* 1934;41:653–682.

de Carvalho M et al. Milk intake and frequency of feeding in breast-fed infants. *Early Hum Dev.* 1982;7:155–163.

de Carvalho M et al. Effect of frequent breast-feeding on early milk production and infant weight gain. *Pediatrics.* 1983;72:307–311.

de Coopman J. Breastfeeding after pituitary resection: support for a theory of autocrine control of milk supply? *J Hum Lact.* 1993;9:35–40.

Drewett RF, Woolridge M. Sucking patterns of human babies on the breast. *Early Hum Dev.* 1979;315:315–321.

Farina MA, Newby BG, Alani HM. Innervation to the nipple-areola complex. *Plast Reconstr Surg.* 1980;66:497–501.

Frantz A, Kleinberg DL, Noel G. Studies on prolactin in man. *Recent Prog Horm Res*. 1972;28:527–534.

Friesen HG, Cowden EA. Lactation and galactorrhea. In: DeGroot LJ, ed. *Endocrinology in pregnancy*. Philadelphia, Pa: Saunders; 1989:2074–2086.

Geddes DT. Inside the lactating breast: the latest anatomy research. *J Midwifery Women's Health*. 2007;52:556–563.

Geddes DT, Kent JC, Mitoulas LB, et al. Tongue movement and intra-oral vacuum in breastfed infants. *Early Hum Dev*. 2008;84(7):471–477.

Goldfield EC et al. Coordination of sucking, swallowing, and breathing and oxygen saturation during early infant breast-feeding and bottle-feeding. *Ped Res*. 2006;60:450–455.

Gomes CF et al. Surface electromyography of facial muscles during natural and artificial feeding of infant. *J Pediatr*. 2006;82:103–109.

Grajeda R, Perez-Escamilla R. Stress during labor and delivery is associated with delayed onset of lactation among urban Guatemalan women. *J Nutr*. 2002;132:3055–3060.

Gray L et al. Breastfeeding is analgesic in healthy newborns. *Pediatrics*. 2002;109:590–593.

Groer M. Neuroendocrine and immune relationships in postpartum fatigue. *Am J Matern Child Nurs*. 2005a;30:133–138.

Groer M. Differences between exclusive breastfeeding, formula-feeders and controls: a study of stress, mood, and endocrine variables. *Biol Res Nurs*. 2005b;7:106.

Groer M, Davis MW. Postpartum stress: current concepts and the possible protective role of breastfeeding. *JOGN Nursing*. 2002;31:411–417.

Grossl NA. Supernumerary tissue: historical perspectives and clinical features. *South Med J*. 2000; 93:29–32.

Hale TW. *Medications and mother's milk*. 9th ed. Amarillo, TX: Pharmasoft; 2000:6.

Hammerman C, Kaplan M. Oxygen saturation during and after feeding in healthy term infants. *Biol Neonate*. 1995;67:94–99.

Hartmann PE, Sherriff JL, Kent JC. Maternal nutrition and milk synthesis. *Proc Nutr Soc*. 1995;54:379–389.

Herbst JJ. Development of suck and swallowing. In: Lebenthal E, ed. *Textbook of gastroenterology and nutrition in infancy*. Vol. 1. New York, NY: Plenum; 1981:97–107.

Hill PD, Chatterton RT, Aldag AC. Serum prolactin in breastfeeding: state of the science. *Biol Res Nurs*. 1999;1:65–75.

Hill PD, Humenick SS. Insufficient milk supply. *Image*. 1989;21:145–148.

Hinds LA, Tyndale-Biscoe CH. Prolactin in the marsupial *Macropus engenii during* the estrous cycle, pregnancy, and lactation. *Biol Reprod*. 1982;26:391–398.

Hoover K, Barbalinardo L, Pia Platia M. Delayed lactogenesis 2 secondary to gestational ovarian theca lutein cysts in two normal singleton pregnancies. *J Hum Lact*. 2002;18:264–268.

Horn HW, Scott JM. IUD insertion and galactorrhea. *Fertil Steril*. 1969;20:400–404.

Hornell A et al. Breastfeeding patterns in exclusively breastfed infants: a longitudinal prospective study in Uppsala, Sweden. *Acta Paediatr*. 1999;88:203–211.

Howie PW et al. Effect of supplementary food on suckling patterns and ovarian activity during lactation. *Br Med J*. 1981;283:757–759.

Huggins K, Petok E, Mireles O. Markers of lactation insufficiency: a study of 34 mothers. In: Auerbach K, ed. *Current issues in clinical lactation*. Sudbury, Mass: Jones and Bartlett; 2000:25–35.

Humenick SS et al. Breast-milk sodium as a predictor of breastfeeding patterns. *Can J Nurs Res*. 1998; 30:67–81.

Hurst N. Lactation after augmentation mammoplasty. *Obstet Gynecol*. 1996;87:30–34.

Hytten FE. Clinical and chemical studies in lactation: IX. Breastfeeding in hospital. *Br Med J*. 1954;18:1447–1452.

Hytten FE, Baird D. The development of the nipple in pregnancy. *Lancet*. June 7, 1958;1:1201–1204.

Inch S, Garforth S. Establishing and maintaining breast-feeding. In: Chalmers I, Enkin M, Keirse M, eds. *Effective care in pregnancy and childbirth*. Oxford, England: Oxford University Press; 1989:1359–1374.

Jacobs LA et al. Normal nipple position in term infants measured on breastfeeding ultrasound. *J Hum Lact*. 2007;23:52–59.

James RJA et al. Thirst induced by a suckling episode during breast feeding and its relation with plasma vasopressin, oxytocin and osmoregulation. *Clin Endocrinol*. 1995;43:277–282.

Johnstone JM, Amico JA. A prospective longitudinal study of the release of oxytocin and prolactin in response to infant suckling in long-term lactation. *J Clin Endocrinol Metab*. 1986;62:653.

Kent JC et al. Volume and frequency of breastfeeding and fat content of breast milk throughout the day. *Pediatrics*. 2005;117:e387–e395.

Kopans DB. *Breast imaging*. Philadelphia, Pa: Lippincott; 1989:20.

Kulski JK, Hartmann PE. Changes in human milk composition during the initiation of lactation. *Aust J Exp Biol Med Sci*. 1981;59:101–114.

La Leche League International. *The womanly art of breast-feeding*. 6th ed. Schaumberg, Ill: La Leche League; 1997.

Leake R et al. Oxytocin and prolactin responses in long-term breast-feeding. *Obstet Gynecol*. 1983;62:565–568.

Lincoln DW, Paisley AC. Neuroendocrine control of milk ejection. *J Reprod Fertil*. 1982;65:571–586.

Love S. *Dr. Susan Love's breast book*. Boston: Addison-Wesley; 1990:34.

MacMullen NJ, Kulski LA. Factors related to suckling ability in healthy newborns. *JOGN Nursing.* 2000;29:390–396.

MacPherson EE, Montagna W. The mammary glands of rhesus monkeys. *J Invest Derm.* 1974;63:17–18.

Madden JD et al. Analysis of secretory patterns of prolactin and gonadotropins during twenty-four hours in a lactating woman before and after resumption of menses. *Am J Obstet Gynecol.* 1978;132:436–441.

Marasco L, Marmet C, Shell E. Polycystic ovary syndrome: a connection to insufficient milk supply? *J Hum Lact.* 2000;16:143–148.

Marmet C, Shell E. Training neonates to suck correctly. *MCN.* 1984;9:401–407.

Marmet C, Shell E. *Lactation forms: a guide to lactation consultant charting.* Encino, Calif: Lactation Institute and Breastfeeding Clinic; 1993:4–7.

Marmet C, Shell E. Therapeutic positioning for breast-feeding. In: Genna CW, ed. *Supporting sucking skills in breastfeeding infants.* Sudbury, Mass: Jones and Bartlett; 2008:305–325.

Marshall WM, Cumming DC, Fitzsimmons GW. Hot flushes during breast feeding? *Fertil Steril.* 1992;57:1349–1350.

Mathew OP. Regulation of breathing patterns during feeding. In: Mathew OP, Sant Ambrogio G, eds. *Respiratory function of the upper airway.* New York, NY: Marcel Dekker; 1988:535–560.

McBride MC, Danner SC. Sucking disorders in neurologically impaired infants: assessment and facilitation of breastfeeding. *Clin Perinatol.* 1987;14:109–130.

Measel CP, Anderson GC. Nonnutritive suckling during tube feedings: effect on clinical course in premature infants. *JOGN Nursing.* 1979;8:265–272.

Meier P, Anderson GC. Responses of small preterm infants to bottle- and breast-feeding. *MCN.* 1987;12:97–105.

Meier P, Pugh EJ. Breastfeeding behavior in small preterm infants. *MCN.* 1985;10:396–401.

Mennella JA, Beauchamp GK. Beer, breastfeeding, and folklore. *Dev Psychobiol.* 1993;26:459–466.

Miller AJ. Deglutition. *Physiol Rev.* 1982;62:129–183.

Mizuno K, Ueda A, Takeuchi T. Effects of different fluids on the relationship between swallowing and breathing during nutritive sucking in neonates. *Bio Neonate.* 2002;81:45–50.

Montagna W, MacPherson EE. Some neglected aspects of the anatomy of the breasts. *J Invest Derm.* 1974;63:10–16.

Montagu A. Breastfeeding and its relation to morphological, behavioral, and psychocultural development. In: Rapheal D, ed. *Breastfeeding and food policy in a hungry world.* New York, NY: Academic; 1979:189–193.

Morton JA. The clinical usefulness of breast milk sodium in the assessment of lactogenesis. *Pediatrics.* 1994;93:802–806.

Neifert MR, McDonough SL, Neville MC. Failure of lactogenesis associated with placental retention. *Am J Obstet Gynecol.* 1981;140:477–478.

Neifert M et al. The influence of breast surgery, breast appearance, and pregnancy-induced breast changes on lactation sufficiency as measured by infant weight gain. *Birth.* 1990;17:31–38.

Neubauer SH et al. Delayed lactogenesis in women with insulin-dependent diabetes mellitus. *Am J Clin Nutr.* 1993;58:54–60.

Neville, MC. Anatomy and physiology of lactation. In: Schanler RJ, ed. Breastfeeding 2001, Part 1: The evidence for breastfeeding. *Pediatr Clin No Amer.* 2001;48:13–34.

Neville MC, Berga SE. Cellular and molecular aspects of the hormonal control of mammary function. In: Neville MC, Neifert MR, eds. *Lactation: physiology, nutrition, and breast-feeding.* New York, NY: Plenum; 1983:141–177.

Nissen E et al. Different patterns of oxytocin, prolactin but not cortisol release during breast-feeding in women delivered by cesarean section or by the vaginal route. *Early Hum Dev.* 1996;45:103–108.

Noel GL, Suh HK, Frantz AG. Prolactin release during nursing and breast stimulation in postpartum and non-postpartum subjects. *J Clin Endocrinol Meta.* 1974;38:413–423.

Notestine GE. The importance of the identification of ankyloglossia (short lingual frenulum) as a cause of breastfeeding problems. *J Hum Lact.* 1990;6:113–115.

Nyqvist K, Sjoden PO, Ewald U. The development of preterm infants' breastfeeding behavior. *Early Hum Dev.* 1999;55:247–264.

Oxford English Dictionary. Vol. 10. Oxford, England: Clarendon Press; 1961.

Palmer B. The influence of breastfeeding on the development of the oral cavity: a commentary. *J Hum Lact.* 1998;14:93–99.

Park HS, Yoon CH, Kim HJ. The prevalence of congenital inverted nipple. *Aesthetic Plast Surg.* 1999;23:1446.

Prentice A et al. Evidence for local feed-back control of human milk secretion. *Biochem Soc Trans.* 1989;17:489–492.

Prieto CR et al. Sucking pressure and its relationship to milk transfer during breastfeeding in humans. *J Reprod Fertil.* 1996;108:69–74.

Quandt SA. Patterns of variation in breast-feeding behaviors. *Soc Sci Med.* 1986;23:445–453.

Ramsay DT et al. Anatomy of the lactating human breast redefined with ultrasound imaging. *J Anat.* 2005a;206:525–534.

Ramsay DT et al. The use of ultrasound to characterize milk ejection in women using an electric breast pump. *J Hum Lact.* 2005b;21:421–428.

Rasmussen KM, Hilson JA, Kjolhede CL. Obesity may impair lactogenesis 2. *J Nutr.* 2001;131:3009S–3011S.

Riordan J, Gross A, Angeron J, et al. The effect of labor pain relief on neonatal suckling and breastfeeding duration. *J Hum Lact.* 2000;16:7–12.

Riordan J, Koehn M. Reliability testing of three breast-feeding assessment tools. *JOGN Nursing.* 1997;26:181–187.

Rodenstein DO, Perlmutter N, Stanescu DC. Infants are not obligatory nose breathers. *Am Rev Respir Dis.* 1985;131:343–347.

Russo J, Russo IH. Development of the human mammary gland. In: Neville MD, Daniel CW, eds. *The mammary gland: development, regulation, and function.* New York, NY: Plenum; 1987:67–93.

Salazar H, Tobon H. Morphologic changes of the mammary gland during development, pregnancy, and lactation. In: Josimovich J, ed. *Lactogenic hormones, fetal nutrition and lactation.* New York, NY: Academic Press; 1974:1–18.

Schaal B et al. Human breast areolae as scent organs: Morphological data and possible involvement in maternal-neonatal coadaptation. *Dev Psychobiol.* 2006;18(2):100–110.

Schmidt H. Supernumerary nipples: prevalence, size, sex and side predilection—a prospective clinical study. *Eur J Pediatr.* 1998;157:821–823.

Sernia C, Tyndale-Biscoe CH. Prolactin receptors in the mammary gland, corpus luteum and other tissues of the Tammar wallaby. *Macropus engenii. J Endocrinol.* 1979;26:391–398.

Smith DM. Montgomery's areolar tubercle: a light microscopic study. *Arch Pathol Lab Med.* 1982;106:60–63.

Smith WL et al. Physiology of sucking in the normal term infant using real-time ultrasound. *Radiology.* 1985;156:379–381.

Snyder JB. Bubble palate and failure-to-thrive: A case report. *J Hum Lact.* 1997;13:139–143.

Sozmen M. Effects of early suckling of cesarean-born babies on lactation. *Biol Neonate.* 1992;62:67–68.

Speroff L, Glass RH, Kase NG. *Clinical gynecology, endocrinology and infertility.* 4th ed. Baltimore, Md: Williams & Wilkins; 1989:283.

Stallings JF et al. Prolactin response to suckling and maintenance of postpartum amenorrhea among intensively breastfeeding Nepali women. *Endocrinol Res.* 1996;22:1–28.

Tay CCK, Glasier AF, McNeil AS. Twenty-four hours patterns of prolactin secretion during lactation and the relationship to suckling and the resumption of fertility in breast-feeding women. *Hum Reprod.* 1996;11:950–955.

Telles, NC, ed. *Atlas of breast ultrasound.* Philadelphia, Pa: Department of Radiology and Department of Pathology, Thomas Jefferson University Medical College and Hospital; 1980:121.

Tyson JE et al. Studies of prolactin in human pregnancy. *Am J Obstet Gynecol.* 1972;113:14–20.

Ueda T, Yokoyama Y, Irahara M, et al. Influence of psychological stress on suckling-induced pulsatile oxytocin release. *Obstet Gynecol.* 1994;84:259–262.

Uvnas-Moberg K. Oxytocin linked antistress effects—the relaxation and growth response. *Acta Physiol Scand Supp.* 1997;640:38–42.

Vorherr H. Development of the female breast. In: Vorherr H, ed. *The breast.* New York, NY: Academic; 1974:1–18.

Waller H. The early failure of breastfeeding. *Arch Dis Child.* 1946;21:1–12.

Watson CJ. Involution: apoptosis and tissue remodeling that convert the mammary gland from milk factory to quiescent organ. BioMed Central Ltd. Available at: http://breast-cancer-research/.com/content/8/2/203. Accessed April 2006.

Weber F, Woolridge MW, Baum JD. An ultrasonographic study of the organization of sucking and swallowing by newborn infants. *Dev Med Child Neurol.* 1986;28:19–24.

West CP. Hormonal profiles in lactating and non-lactating women immediately after delivery and their relationship to breast engorgement. *Am J Obstet Gynecol.* 1979;86:501–506.

Widstrom AM et al. Gastric suction in healthy newborn infants: effects on circulation and developing feeding behaviour. *Acta Paediatr Scand.* 1987;76:566–572.

Widstrom AM, Thingstrom-Paulsson J. The position of the tongue during rooting reflexes elicited in newborn infants before the first suckle. *Acta Paediatr.* 1993;82:281–283.

Wilson-Clay B, Hoover K. *The breastfeeding atlas.* 3rd ed. Manchaca, Tex: LactNews Press; 2005.

Wolf LS, Glass RP. Feeding and swallowing disorders in infancy: assessment and management. San Antonio, Tex: Therapy Skill Builders; 1992:9–10, 133–137.

Wolff PH. The serial organization of sucking in the young infant. *Pediatrics.* 1968;42:943–956.

Woolridge MW. The "anatomy" of infant sucking. *Midwifery.* 1986;2:164–171.

Yokoyama Y et al. Releases of oxytocin and prolactin during breast massage and suckling in puerperal women. *Eur J Obstet Gynecol Reprod Biol.* 1994;53:17–20.

Yuen BH. Prolactin in human milk: the influence of nursing and duration of postpartum lactation. *Am J Obstet Gynecol.* 1988;158:583–586.

Ziemer M. Nipple skin changes and pain during the first week of lactation. *JOGN Nursing.* 1993;22:247–256.

Zuppa AA et al. Relationship between maternal parity, basal prolactin levels and neonatal breast milk intake. *Biol Neonate.* 1988;53:144–147.

Appendix 3-A

Suck Training for Breastfeeding

Suck training is an emerging area of lactation practice for treating feeding problems related to immature and/or abnormal suckling in infants. Suckling problems may be the result of a lack of normal development such as in low birth weight infants and/or an early sign of neurological impairment. Suck training can be as simple as placing one's finger in the neonates mouth to orally stimulate a baby who is "slow" to latch on to the breast—a practice trial whereby he learns how to grasp the mother's nipple. Parents unintentionally perform suck training when they place their "pinky" finger in their baby's mouth while holding him in their crossed arms.

We also might consider finger-feeding, described elsewhere in this book, to be a form of suck training. For example, until the baby matures sufficiently, mothers of preterm infants might first breastfeed then finger-feed the remainder of the breastmilk or formula. Essentially suck training is a method of oral stimulation and manipulation to teach the baby how to effectively suckle bottle nipple or a breast; it is an umbrella term for any therapy used to correct an infant suckling problem.

Most problems can be avoided or corrected by facilitating an effective latch on to the breast. However, for a multitude of reasons described elsewhere in this book, some babies have suckling problems even when the baby has a good latch (Marmet & Shell, 1984).

Practitioners in this area usually are speech and language therapists, occupational therapists, or other specialists with a background in neuro-developmental training (NDT) who understand the anatomy and physiology of the breast and the infant's oral structures. These specialists were trained to help bottle-feed babies; however, a few have subspecialized in breastfeeding sucking problems. If specialists are not available to assist breastfeeding mothers, lactation consultants fill this role, educating themselves by attending continuing education courses, through self-study, and clinical practice.

A form of suck training is used in the neonatal intensive care unit (NICU) to improve suckling ability of low birth weight babies. For example, when introducing first oral feedings to a low birth weight baby, the nurse or LC places a finger in the baby's mouth and slowly introduces one or two drips of expressed breastmilk (EBM) or formula to see how the baby reacts and to observe the baby's ability to swallow and to assess for tongue thrusting and gagging.

The pressure to discharge the baby early because of reimbursement issues generates interest in suck training. Hospital staff are under pressure to discharge low birth weight babies early because of insurance requirements. Suck training, if effective, hastens discharge to home, but there are very few studies that substantiate that when infants receive suck training, they are discharged earlier.

Research on suck training techniques to test their effectiveness is sparse and mostly limited to bottle-feeding, but indicate that suck training is beneficial. Gaebler and Hanzlik (1996) demonstrated that preterm infants receiving peri- and intraoral stimulation just before bottle-feedings scored better on the standardized feeding assessment scale NOMAS (see Chapter 20), had greater weight gain, and fewer days of hospitalization. Fucile, Gisel, and Lau (2002) reaffirmed that preterm infants who received oral stimulation were able to feed significantly earlier. Until studies on suck training of breastfed infants are done, this gap is being filled by clinical experience and opinion of experts.

Some practitioners find suck training techniques helpful; others think they are invasive and controlling and should never be used. Literature on the care of premature infants who required intubation document that the infant oral cavity can cause the baby to avoid having anything further put into the mouth including breast. For those clinicians determined to forge ahead, we emphasize the need for gentleness and close following of infant signals; if the baby doesn't like your finger in its mouth, take it out!

Suck Training Techniques

Therapists use a variety of suck training techniques to improve feedings at the breast. There are probably as many techniques as there are babies with suckling problems. While no standard protocols for suck training for breastfeeding could be found at the time of this writing, other than the Marmet/Shell Basic Suck-training Technique below, several techniques for treating specific sucking dysfunctions exist. Most have evolved from bottle-feeding protocols and then were adapted to breastfeeding. They usually involve oral stimulation in which the baby's mouth, tongue, gums, and palate are massaged and manipulated, as well as involving positioning and cheek and chin support.

Basic Suck Training Technique

The most well-known suck training technique for breastfeeding infants was developed by Chele Marmet and Ellen Shell and published in *Maternal Child Nursing* in 1984. It has become a classic on suck training in the lactation field. They developed the Basic Suck-Training Technique and the Alternate Suck-Training Technique as a result of working with numerous mothers and babies who came to their lactation clinic seeking help with getting their infants to effectively latch and suckle. The basis of their technique is that properly filling the baby's mouth with a finger will teach the baby the correct depth of latch on the breast. This action brings the baby's tongue forward so that the tongue tip covers the alveolar ridge and rests on the lower lip as it troughs and cups. See Figure 3–19.

Technique

1. Stroke the baby's cheek toward the lips.
2. Brush the baby's lips until they relax.
3. Using the pad of the finger, massage the outside of the lower gums, the top of the lower gums, the outside of the upper gums, and the top of the upper gums.
4. Insert the finger into the baby's mouth nail down, pad up. Gently slide the finger to the juncture of hard and soft palate (*S* spot). Women usually use their first finger and men their small "pinky" finger. Only light pressure

is needed. Most babies love to suckle and will quickly draw the finger back to the *S* spot, the place to where the nipple usually extends.

5. Press down and forward with the fingernail portion of the finger as the baby suckles. Alternate rubbing the baby's hard palate with downward and forward pressure. Give praise and encouragement to the baby for the correct motion.

If the baby holds his posterior tongue in a humped position, periodically press down on the humped area with the nail side of the finger for a few seconds then return to light pressure to the *S* spot. The tongue may relax after repeating this exercise several times.

The Jacqui Mouth Model (Figure 3–20) is a tool for teaching position of the tongue in the mouth, placement of the finger and breast in the baby's mouth, for suck assessment, suck training, finger feeding, and for latch. It has four different palates, reference (normal), bubble, high, and channel, to demonstrate differences between types of palatal structure. It is available at www.lactationinstitute.org.

La Leche League ("Walk the Fingers") Technique

Other versions of basic suck training have appeared in the literature since then. La Leche League reported a slightly different technique of basic retraining the infants' tongue using peri- and intra-oral stimulation and a tongue walk (Mohrbacher & Stock, 2003).

Technique

1. Touch the infant's cheek with a finger, moving toward the lips. Then brush the lips a few times with a clean index finger to encourage the infant to open its mouth.
2. Massage the outside of the infant's gum with the index finger, beginning each stroke at the middle of the baby's upper or lower gum and move toward either side.
3. Use the tip of the index finger to press down firmly on the top of the tip of the baby's tongue and count slowly to three before releasing the pressure.

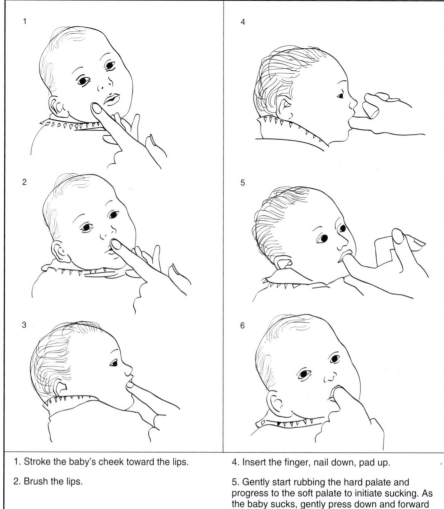

1. Stroke the baby's cheek toward the lips.

2. Brush the lips.

3. Massage the outside of the lower gums, the top of the lower gums, the outside of the upper gums, and the top of the upper gums.

4. Insert the finger, nail down, pad up.

5. Gently start rubbing the hard palate and progress to the soft palate to initiate sucking. As the baby sucks, gently press down and forward with the fingernail portion of the finger. Alternate rubbing the baby's hard palate with downward and forward pressure. Give verbal praise and encouragement to the baby for correct motion.

6. Alternate method. Insert finger, nail side toward the roof of the mouth. Position the pad of the finger at the place where the baby's tongue begins to slant downward toward the pharynx. Use the finger to pull the tongue forward. An eyedropper can be used instead of a finger or in addition to a finger when the baby needs a food reward for behavior modification to occur. The baby is rewarded with expressed breast milk or formula as the tongue is placed into the correct position with the dropper.

FIGURE 3–19 Basic suck-training technique.

Source: Adapted from Marmet C, Shell E. Training neonates to suck correctly. *MCN*. 1984;9:401-407.

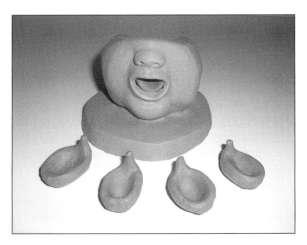

FIGURE 3–20   The Jacqui Mouth Model.

Source: Used with permission of the Lactation Institute/Chele Marmet.

4. Release the pressure keeping the finger in the infant's mouth, and move back slightly on his tongue, pressing again to a count of three.
5. Move back on the tongue one or two more times.
6. If the baby gags, bring the finger forward.
7. Repeat the "tongue walk" three or four times before each breastfeeding.

Sensorial Oral Stimulation in Infants with Suck Feeding Disabilities

The Sensorial Oral Stimulation technique is a feeding program for high-risk infants meant to avoid hospital complications associated with oral gastric feeding, intubation and so on.

Technique

1. Explore the rooting reflex by light contact over the lips and cheeks with five fingertips.
2. Use circular massage on the upper lip and anterior gum side for five minutes.
3. Continue massage towards lateral gum side and inside the cheek for three minutes.
4. Apply tactile stimulus to the lower lip with little pressure.

5. Place pressure on the suckling point (located in the central area of the hard palate behind the upper gum).

A blind study (Rendon-Macias, Perez, Mosco-Peralta, et al., 1999) was done to determine clinical and physiological changes in suck feeding after sensorial oral stimulation in 14 infants. Five of these infants received mother's milk and were described as being breastfed, but it was not clear to what extent the babies fed directly from the mother or if they received the milk by other means. The results showed increased milk intake and significant improvement in suckling using this technique.

Suck Training Methods for Specific Dysfunctions

Techniques below were described by Catherine Watson Genna (2008) as being specifically useful for certain problems.

Tongue Tip Elevation

The tongue tip elevates during suckling and thus the tongue is a physical barrier to the mother's nipple entering the oral cavity. The tongue can be humped or bunched. The tongue may be retracted in addition to being elevated.

1. Calm the baby.
2. Tickle the tongue tip down with a finger just before attachment.
3. Use finger feeding to teach the infant that milk should be at the top of the tongue (Genna, 2008, p. 32).

Tongue Tip Humped

When the tongue tip is humped it blocks the oral cavity. To use this technique, massage the posterior tongue, using finger-feeding counterpressure to the humped area of the tongue (Genna, 2008, p. 34)

Tongue Retracted

This dysfunction occurs when the tongue tip is well behind the alveolar ridges. The retracted tongue is held posteriorly in the mouth with the tongue tip well behind the alveolar ridges and limits contact between it and the retracted tongue. Lack of contact between the nipple and tongue inhibits suction and the ability of the infant to grasp the breast and draw the nipple into his mouth. To remedy this, massage the anterior tongue with a fingertip until it extends over the lower gum. Finger-feed for one or more feedings (Genna, 2008, p. 34).

Suck Training Method for Infant with Neurological Dysfunction

Neurologically impaired infants have immature, damaged, or abnormally developed nervous systems that may cause abnormalities of suckling and swallowing. Suckling abnormalities usually present absence of the suckling response, weakness or incoordination of suckling and swallowing, or some combination of these problems. McBride and Danner (1987) studied the effect of suck training for depressed suckling in a neurologically impaired infant and recommended the following technique.

Technique

1. Place the infant's head and body in a flexed position.
2. Gently stroke or press on the infant's cheeks to encourage suckling.
3. Gently move a finger or another long, soft object in all directions in the infant's mouth, touching the tongue and buccal (cheek) mucosa. Press the finger pad gently onto the hard palate, the tip on the soft palate.
4. If this does not elicit a suckle, encircle the mouth with fingertip several times. Repeat the sequence after tapping with the fingertips using gentle and even pressure around the mouth.
5. Vibrating the laryngopharyngeal musculature with the fingertips beginning under the chin and along either side of the larynx to the sternal notch may be helpful.

Summary

Suck training for breastfeeding babies is in its infancy. Buoyed by rising breastfeeding rates and awareness of the importance of breastmilk, lactation consultants look for effective therapy to help infants to achieve normal suckling function. Other techniques to improve early suckling are described elsewhere in the text. Nonnutritive suckling, for example, which is commonly used to assist breastfeeding skills in low birth weight infants, is addressed in Chapter 13. Thankfully, most infants with a suckling dysfunction improve with time. As the baby grows and develops, the tongue moves back in the mouth and becomes more mobile so the baby can compensate with a greater variety of positions.

Internet Resources

Craniosacral Therapy Association of North America
http://www.craniosacraltherapy.org

Neuro-Development Treatment Association
http://www.ndta.org

References

Fucile S, Gisel EG, Lau C. Oral stimulation accelerates the transition from tube to oral feeding in preterm infants. *J Pediatr*. 2002;141:230–236.

Gaebler CP, Hanzlik JR. The effects of a prefeeding stimulation program on preterm infant. *Am J Occup Ther*. 1996;50:184–192.

Genna CW. *Supporting sucking skills in breastfeeding infants*. Sudbury, Mass: Jones and Bartlett; 2008:32–34.

Marmet C, Shell E. Therapeutic positioning for breastfeeding. In: Genna CW, ed. *Supporting sucking skills in breastfeeding infants*. Sudbury, Mass: Jones and Bartlett; 2008:305–325.

Marmet C, Shell E. Training neonates to suck correctly. *MCN*. 1984;9:401–407.

McBride M, Danner S. Sucking disorders in neurologically impaired infants. *Clin Perinatol*. 1987;14:109–130.

McNeil JS. N-trainer teaches preterm neonates how to suck. *Pediatric News*. 2007;34.

Mohrbacher N, Stock J. *Breastfeeding answer book*. 3rd ed. Schaumburg, Ill: La Leche League International; 2003:80, 92.

Rendon-Macias ME, Perez LA, Mosco-Peralta MR, et al. Assessment of sensorial oral stimulation in infants with suck feeding disabilities. *Indian J Pediatr*. 1999;66:319–329.

Sheppard JJ, Fletcher KR. Evidence-based interventions for breast and bottle feeding in the neonatal intensive care unit. *Semin Speech Lang*. 2007;28:204–212.

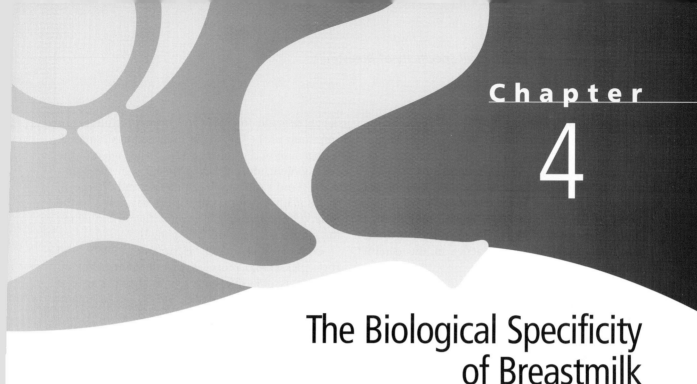

The Biological Specificity of Breastmilk

Jan Riordan

BREASTMILK IS SOMETIMES REFERRED to as *white blood* because it is considered similar to the placental blood of intrauterine life. Indeed, human milk is similar to unstructured living tissue, such as blood, and is capable of transporting nutrients, affecting biochemical systems, enhancing immunity, and destroying pathogens. With the use of sophisticated laboratory techniques, many scientific investigators have substantiated the life-sustaining properties of breastmilk. Organs themselves provide evidence of the profound influence of breastfeeding. For example, the thymus plays a role in the development of the immune system by providing the environment for T-cell differentiation and maturation. At age 4 months, the thymus is about twice as large in exclusively breastfed infants as in infants fed only infant formula. This difference in size continues until the child is at least 10 months old (Hasselbalch et al., 1999). Although thymus size can be influenced by many factors, it would not be unreasonable to generate a variety of hypothetical mechanisms whereby breastfeeding might influence thymic size (Prentice & Collinson, 2000).

Breastmilk, like all other animal milks, is species specific. It has been adapted throughout human existence to meet nutritional and anti-infective requirements of the human infant to ensure optimal growth, development, and survival. At birth the baby's immune system is small but complete. It expands in response to exposure of newly acquired bacteria but takes time before the infant develops full capacity to defend itself (Larsson, 2004). National and international health organizations consistently recommend that mothers breastfeed for the entire first year of life and thereafter as long as it is beneficial to the mother and infant (US Department of Health and Human Services, 2000).

Because an infant's birth weight normally requires about 4 to 6 months to double, the nutritional needs of the human baby must be substantially different from those of other mammals whose birth weight doubles much more rapidly. In addition, breastmilk enhances brain development: breastfed children may be more intelligent than children not breastfed. A meta-analysis of 11 studies in which confounding variables were adjusted showed an average 3.2-point higher cognitive development score among breastfed infants. This advantage was seen early on and continued through childhood (Anderson, Johnstone, & Remley, 1999). Chapter 18 presents a detailed discussion of this topic.

This chapter breaks down the general properties of human milk into specific components and describes for each component species-specific "biochemical messages" that contribute to the well-being of the baby and mother. The chapter also explores the concept that these "messages" can be nutritional programming, triggering an early stimulus or insult during a critical or sensitive period with long-term effects on health and disease (Nommsen-Rivers, 2003; Lucas, 1998). Knowledge of biological constructs of lactation is critical to the clinician because it forms the rationale for effective practice in the clinical setting.

Milk Synthesis and Maturational Changes

Major components of human milk (protein, fat, lactose) are synthesized and secreted by the mammary secretory epithelial cells. Cregan (1999) labeled these cells "lactocytes." During pregnancy these cells further develop under the influence of prolactin. Four of the five milk-secretion pathways necessary for milk secretion are synchronized in the alveolar cell of the mammary gland. In the fifth pathway, the passage of components is between epithelial cells, rather than through them, and is known as the paracellular pathway (Neville, 2001).

Factors that influence milk composition include stage of lactation, gestational age of the infant, stage (beginning or end) of the feeding, frequency of the baby's demand for milk, and degree of fullness or emptiness of the breasts. As discussed in Chapter 3, lactogenesis occurs in two stages. Stage I refers to the development, during late pregnancy, of the mammary gland's capacity to synthesize milk. Stage II, traditionally based on postpartum day, refers to the onset of copious milk secretion or the time at which the mother feels her milk "coming in."

Arthur, Smith, and Hartmann (1989) and Humenick (1987) proposed two different biological markers as objective measures to define stages of breastmilk maturation. Arthur, Smith, and Hartmann hold that in the first stage of lactogenesis, average concentrations of lactose, citrate, and glucose are low. A sudden and rapid increase in concentrations of these components between 24 to 48 hours after birth heralds the transition from stage I to stage II lactogenesis. Stage II lactogenesis markers (lactose, citrate, and total nitrogen) take an additional 24 hours to attain concentration in women who have insulin-dependent diabetes compared with women who do not (Hartmann & Cregan, 2001).

Humenick et al. (1994), on the other hand, consider the breakdown of an emulsion dependent on the ratio of sterols plus phospholipids to fat content of milk (maturation index of colostrum and milk [MICAM]) as the biological marker for breastmilk maturation (Figure 4–1). Both of these methods

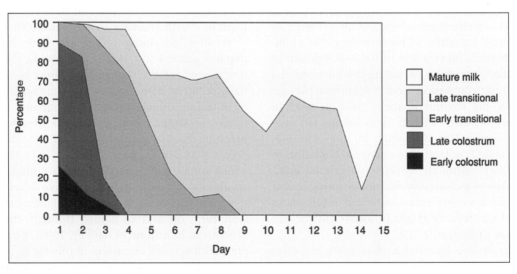

FIGURE 4–1   Milk type by day.

Source: Used with permission from Humenick SS. The clinical significance of breastmilk maturation rates. *Birth*. 1987;14:174-179.

appear to be valid in that they were positively related to greater milk yield (Casey, Hambridge, & Neville, 1985; Saint, Smith, & Hartmann, 1984), infant weight gain, and lower transcutaneous bilimeter readings (Humenick, 1987). These studies also show that breastmilk maturation during lactogenesis proceeds more rapidly in some mothers than in others and is not consistent with the coming in of the milk. Neville (2001) believes that the terms *colostrum* and *transitional milk* used to describe breastmilk during the early postpartum do not define clear-cut changes in milk composition and are not a useful distinction. Instead, they should be viewed as part of a continuum of events where changes in breastmilk occur rapidly during the first few days after birth and are followed by slow changes. The time at which mothers report that their milk comes in is highly variable and ranges from 38 to 98 hours after birth, with an average of 50 to 59 hours (Arthur, Smith, & Hartmann, 1989; Kulski & Hartmann, 1981; Hildebrandt, 1999).

Compared with mature milk, colostrum is richer in protein and minerals and lower in carbohydrates, fat, and some vitamins. This high concentration of total protein and total ash (minerals) and whey in colostrum and early milk gradually changes to reflect the infant's needs over the first two to three weeks as lactation becomes established. The total dose of such key components as immunoglobulin, which the infant receives from breastmilk, remains relatively constant throughout lactation, regardless of the amount of breastmilk provided by the mother. This happens because concentrations decrease as total volume increases as lactation is established; and, at weaning, concentration increases as total volume decreases.

At birth the neonate's intestine is sterile but it is rapidly colonized thereafter. Breastfed infants have an intestinal ecosystem that has a prevalence of bifidobacteria and lactobacilli. A symbiotic substance, human milk has the properties of both a pro- and prebiotic.

Energy, Volume, and Growth

Human milk is rich in nutrient proteins, nonprotein nitrogen compounds, lipids, oligosaccharides, vitamins, and certain minerals. In addition, it contains hormones, enzymes, growth factors, and many types of protective agents. Human milk contains about 10 percent solids for energy and growth; the rest is water, which is vital for maintaining hydration. The pH of early colostrum is 7.45; it falls to a low of 7.0 during the second week of lactation. Thereafter, the pH of milk remains at 7.0 and then rises gradually to 7.4 by 10 months. The significance of these changes is not known (Morriss et al., 1986). Infants can digest breastmilk much more rapidly than formula. The average gastric half-emptying time for breastmilk is substantially less (48 minutes) than for infant formula (78 minutes) (Cavell, 1981).

Healthy infants, even preterm infants, who consume enough breastmilk to satisfy their energy needs receive enough fluid to satisfy their requirements even in hot and dry environments (Almroth & Bidinger, 1990; Brown et al., 1986b; Cohen et al., 2000). Exclusive and prolonged breastfeeding in healthy infants enhances infant growth during the first 3 months of life and growth and does not affect the normal growth pattern during the first year (Kramer et al., 2002).

Caloric Density

The caloric content or energy density of human milk is generally considered to be 65 kcal/dl, although published values differ. Garza et al. (1983) reported 57.7 kcal/dl, Lepage et al. (1984) reported 66.6 kcal/dl, and Lemons et al. (1982) reported 72.2 kcal/dl. Using breastmilk as the "gold standard," the American Academy of Pediatrics (AAP, 1976) recommended a calorie content of 67 kcal/dl for commercial formulas.

Nature abhors waste, and breastmilk is efficiently utilized. During their first 4 months, exclusively breastfed infants attain adequate growth with nutrient intakes substantially less than the current dietary recommendation (Butte, Smith, & Garza, 1990). Energy requirement of breastfed infants is about 20 percent below recommended levels (Butte et al., 2000; Stuff & Nichols, 1989). Breastmilk of women who have been lactating for over 1 year has significantly increased fat and energy compared with breastmilk of women who have been lactating for shorter periods (Mandel et al., 2005). Caloric intake does not increase after solid foods are added to the baby's diet, strongly suggesting that the calorie value of breastmilk feeds is sufficient for the infants' needs.

Kilocalories of breastmilk ingested per kilogram by exclusively breastfed babies decrease significantly during the first few months of life (Table 4–1).

The energy intakes of breastfed and formula-fed infants differ significantly because their energy expenditure differs greatly. Total daily energy expenditure, minimal rates of energy expenditure, metabolic rates during sleep, rectal temperature, and heart rates are all lower in breastfed infants. Total body water and fat-free mass is lower, and body fat is higher in breastfed infants at 4 months of age (Butte et al., 1995). By 8 months, breastfed infants have consumed about 30,000 kcal less than bottle-fed infants (Butte, Smith, & Garza, 1990).

Although this difference in energy intake should result in about a 2.7-kg mean difference of weight, such is not the case. To explain this discrepancy, Garza, Stuff, and Butte (1986) suggested that (1) differences in intake in the general population are not as great as those found in the babies studied; (2) energy expenditure differs substantially between breastfed and bottle-fed infants; or (3) composition of newly acquired tissue differs between these two groups. A possibility is that the energy density of milk taken by a 4-month-old is higher on the average than that taken by the same baby 3 months earlier. The 4-month-old baby's suckle is more active, leading to a higher fat intake that more than compensates for the volumes needed, because breastmilk is used more completely and with less waste than is artificial milk. Differences in energy density among expressed breastmilk, preterm milk, foremilk, and hindmilk can be seen in Figure 4–2.

Milk Volume and Storage Capacity

The volume of milk must provide sufficient caloric energy to permit normal growth and development. Small amounts of colostrum—averaging about 37 ml (range, 7–123)—are yielded in the first 24 hours postpartum (Hartmann, 1987; Hartmann & Prosser, 1984); the infant ingests approximately 7 to 14 ml at each feeding (Houston, Howie, & McNeilly, 1983). This milk yield gradually increases for the first 36 hours, followed by a dramatic increase during the next 49 to 96 hours. By day 5, volume is about

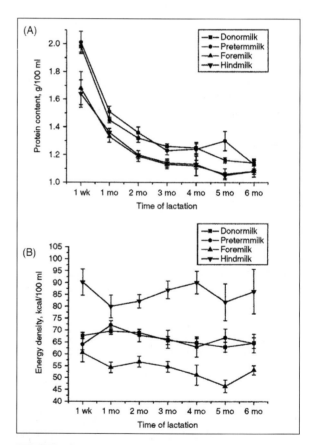

FIGURE 4–2 Mean protein content (A) and energy density (B) of full-term donor and preterm milk and full-term fore- and hindmilk during the first 6 months of lactation. Vertical lines show standard errors of means.

Source: Used with permission from Saarela AT, Kokkonen J, Koivisto M. Macronutrient and energy contents of human milk fractions during the first six months of lactation. *Acta Paediatrica.* 2005;94:1176-1181.

TABLE 4–1 **Kilocalories of Breastmilk Ingested per Kilogram According to Infant Age**

Time Post Birth	kcal per kg
14 days	128
3rd month	70–75
5th month	62.5

Source: Garza, Stuff, & Butte, 1986; Wood et al., 1988.

500 ml/day; it increases more slowly to about 800 ml/day at month 6 of full breastfeeding, with a range between 550 and 1150 (Daly, Owens, & Hartmann, 1993; Cox, Owens, & Hartmann, 1996; Cregan, Mitoulas, & Hartmann, 2002; Neville et al., 1988). These volumes are similar to others established by test-weighing the infant (using prefeeding and postfeeding infant weighings). As seen in Figure 4–3, the volume of milk taken by thriving breastfed infants varies little from 1 to 4 months. Breastmilk intake slowly declines as other foods are added to the baby's diet.

Even if a mother feels that she had insufficient milk to feed her first baby, health professionals should reassure women that it is well worth trying a second time. Multiparous mothers produce more breastmilk (about 140 ml) at 1 week than primiparous women (those giving birth for the first time) (Ingram, Woolridge, & Greenwood, 2001). Breastmilk of adolescent mothers is not different from breastmilk of adult women although adolescents breastfeed fewer times per day (Motil, Krtz, & Thotathuchery, 1997).

It is well established that breastmilk production and intake are related to infant demand. Infants have the capacity to self-regulate their own milk intake. This important concept of lactation has been extensively studied. Australian researchers measured the short-term rates of milk synthesis using a computerized system in which a camera relays video images to a computer that produces a model of the chest by active triangulation (Daly, Owens, & Hartmann, 1993). Their findings and practical applications are summarized in Box 4–1 (Cregan & Hartmann, 1999; Daly & Hartmann, 1995a,b). Breast storage capacity is important in determining how the mother meets the infant's demand for milk. Further discussion on how these research-based principles are used in lactation practice is found in later chapters.

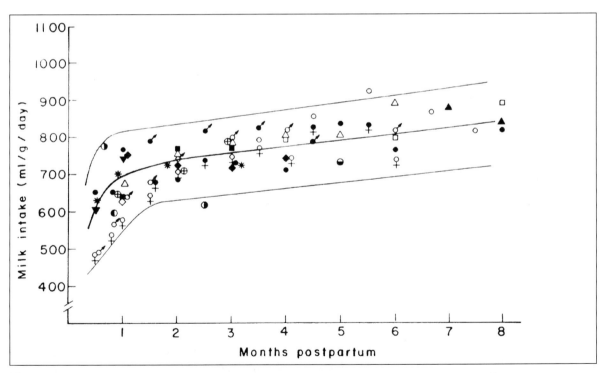

FIGURE 4–3 Milk intakes during established lactation. The lines show the smoothed mean from this study and ± 1 SD. Points are data from the literature obtained by test-weighing of fully breastfed infants.

Source: Used with permission from Neville MC et al. Studies in human lactation: milk volumes in lactating women during the onset of lactation and full lactation. *Am J Clin Nutr.* 1988;48:1375-1386.

BOX 4–1	
Application of Physiological Principles	
Principle from Physiological Research	**Application in Practice**
The breast does balance supply to meet the infant's demand for breastmilk.	Watch the baby for hunger cues.
The breast can rapidly change its rate of milk synthesis from one feed to the next.	Encourage the mother when she thinks she has "run out of milk."
The breasts have the capacity to synthesize more milk than the infant usually requires.	As above.
Breast production varies from one breast to the other; breasts operate independently of each other.	Reassure the mother that infant preference for one breast is normal.
The larger the breasts, the greater the milk storage capacity (i.e., the difference between maximum and minimum breast volumes during a 24-hour period).	Women with large breasts have more flexibility in feeding intervals.
There is no relationship between total milk storage capacity and total 24-hour milk production.	Women with smaller breasts can produce as much milk as women with larger breasts but they must breastfeed more often.
The greater the degree of emptying at a breastfeed, the greater the rate of milk synthesis after that feed.	Advise the mother to avoid fast "switching" from one breast to another and to try to empty one breast as much as possible.
The length of time between feeds (up to 6 hours) does not appear to decrease milk synthesis.	Feeding interval can be flexible once lactation is established.

Differences in Milk Volume Between Breasts

Milk output is more often greater from the right breast versus the left breast (Cox, Owens, & Hartmann, 1996; Daly, Owens, & Hartmann, 1993; Engstrom et al., 2007; Kent et al., 1999; Ramsay et al., 2005) even though right-handed mothers instinctively use the right hand to position the baby and breast, thereby making it easier to feed from the left breast. In addition, in all cultures there is a preference of mothers to hold their babies in their left arm, thus facilitating feeding at the left breast (Engstrom et al., 2007). A likely explanation is that the right breast receives more blood flow than the left breast (Aljazaf, 2004).

Daly, Owens, and Hartmann (1993) were able to determine the rate of synthesis of human milk. Figure 4–4a shows the volume of milk produced by a small-breasted woman who had a storage capacity of 111 ml for her right breast and a capacity of 81 ml for her left breast. Thus the maximum amount of milk that this woman appeared to be able to store

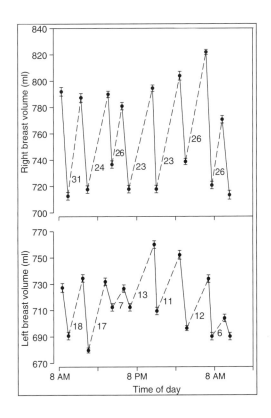

FIGURE 4–4A The right and left breast volume changes of one subject over a period of 24 hours.

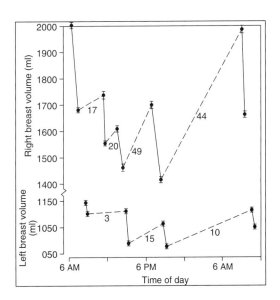

FIGURE 4–4B Breast-volume changes. The right and left breast volume changes of one subject over a period of 28 hours. Each point represents the mean plus or minus the standard error of the mean of replicate breast-volume measurement. Lines link prefeeding and postfeeding mean breast volumes. Dashed lines link postfeeding mean breast volume of a breastfeeding to the prefeeding mean breast volume of the next breast; their slope thus indicates rate of milk synthesis between the two breastfeedings. Rate of milk synthesis also is given by the number of (in milliliters per hour) accompanying each dashed line.

Source: Used with permission from Daly SE, Owens RA, Hartmann PE. The short-term synthesis and infant-regulated removal of milk in lactating women. *Exp Physiol.* 1993;78:209-220.

was about 20 percent of her infant's 24-hour milk intake. From her breast volume changes over time, it appears that her infant met its demand for milk by breastfeeding frequently. Conversely, Figure 4–4b displays a larger-breasted woman who produced similar volumes of milk but with larger storage capacities for her breasts (right breast, 600 ml; left breast, 180 ml), allowing her to store nearly 90 percent of her infant's 24-hour milk intake. Further, there was no relationship between total milk storage capacity and 24-hour milk production. Thus we can conclude that small breast size does not restrict a woman's ability to provide milk for her infant. On the other hand, mothers with a greater storage capacity do have more flexibility with patterns of breastfeeding.

There appear to be wide differences among women in the rate of milk synthesis, which among some women can be double or triple the rate of other women (Arthur et al., 1989; Daly et al., 1992). Milk volume between breasts also differs; left and right breasts rarely produce the same volume of milk (Kent et al., 2006). Milk yield from right breasts appear to be higher than that from left breasts, clearly demonstrating that the rate of milk synthesis within one breast is independent of the rate of milk synthesis in the other breast (Cox, Owens, & Hartmann, 1996; Daly et al., 1993).

At the same time, the amount of milk available in the breast is not necessarily an important determinant of the amount removed by the infant at feedings. Infant intake of breastmilk also varies widely. For example, at 5 months, infant intake of breastmilk can range from 200 ml/day for partial breastfeeding to 3500 ml/day if a wet nurse is used (Neville & Oliva-Rasbach, 1987). These differences appear to be culturally based. Australian women, for example, have been reported to make more breastmilk than do US women. The average daily yield of well-nourished Australian mothers during the first 6 months of lactation was found to be in excess of 1100 ml in one study (Hartmann, 1987) and to range from 535 to 1078 ml in another (Daly et al., 1993). Mothers breastfeeding twins produce in excess of 2100 ml/day in the early months. Breast volume and production decrease in extended lactation. After 6 months of lactation, breast volume, milk production, and storage capacity all decline.

Seasonal changes in breastmilk volume may be influenced by some mothers' need to work during harvest and by their reluctance to introduce supplementary food for fear of diarrheal disease (Serdula, Seward, & Marks, 1986). The nutritional status of the mother does not appear to affect milk volume unless the mother is severely malnourished (Brown et al., 1986a; Forman et al., 1990).

A healthy, breastfeeding, full-term neonate breastfeeds an average of 4.3 times during the first 24 hours (range 0–11) and 7.4 times during the next 24 hours (range 1–22) (Yamauchi & Yamanouchi, 1990), and an overall median of 8 times per day after the first several days (see Hornell, 1999). Breastmilk intake shows little or no correlation with maternal factors, such as weight-for-height, weight gain, nursing frequency, maternal age, and parity (Dewey & Lönnerdal, 1983). Although birth weight is not a strong predictor of milk intake throughout lactation, infant weight at 1 month is. Thus lactation performance during the first 4 weeks postpartum is a strong predictor of milk output during the subsequent period of full lactation (Neville & Oliva-Rasbach, 1987).

Infant Growth

Normal human growth is greatest during infancy. The infant gains about 10 g/kg/day (about 5 to 7 oz/week) until about 4 weeks; then the gain drops to 1 g/kg/day (about 3 oz/week) by the end of the first year.

There are growth differences between breastfed and formula-fed infants. Infants breastfed exclusively have the same or somewhat greater weight gain in the first 3 to 4 months than do bottle-fed or mixed-fed infants (Fawzi et al., 1997; Juex et al., 1983; Motil et al., 1997).

After this time, bottle-fed or mixed-fed infants clearly weigh more. The greatest differences are evident between 6 and 20 months of age, when breastfed infants are lighter than bottle-fed or mixed-fed infants (Dewey et al., 1993, 1995; Yoneyama, Nagata, & Asano, 1994). Increases in length and head circumference growth remain the same for both groups. Length is a reliable indicator for evaluating infant growth and the absence of significant difference in length between breastfed and nonbreastfed infants suggest that formula-fed infants are overfed. Small for gestational age infants who are breastfed show faster postnatal growth and are more likely to have significant catch-up growth than those who are fed a standard term infant formula (Lucas et al., 1997).

Color

Breastmilk comes in several colors. Normally, it is white or yellowish. It can be green if the mother is eating an unusual amount of green vegetables or taking a medication such as nifedipine—or it can be yellow from eating yellow vegetables such as carrots. The "rusty pipe syndrome" where the milk is tinged with pink or red is from old ductal bleeding. A variety of colors of breastmilk are shown in color photos in *The Breastfeeding Atlas* (Wilson-Clay & Hoover, 2005).

Nutritional Values

Around the world, breastmilk is remarkably stable, varying only within a relatively narrow range. Constituents of colostrum and breastmilk and their amounts are shown in Appendix 4-A of this chapter. A profile of lactose protein and lipid concentrations in human milk for the first 30 days of lactation is seen in Figure 4–5. Yet, because breastfeeding is an interactive process, the infant helps to determine composition of the feed. During weaning (involution phase), for example, the concentrations of sodium and protein in breastmilk progressively increase and the milk is saltier; in contrast, concentrations of potassium, glucose, and lactose gradually decrease (Prosser, Saint, & Hartmann, 1984).

Fat

The fat of human milk, which provides about one half of the milk's calories, is its most variable component. Fat varies from one mother to another and from early to late lactation. The total fat content of human milk ranges from 22 to 62 g/L and is independent of breastfeeding frequency (Kent et al., 2006). Hindmilk contains at least twice the amount of fat compared to foremilk (Saarela, Kokkonen & Koivisto, 2005) (Figure 4–2). The energy density of preterm mother's milk is much greater than that of full-term mother's milk, owing to a 30 percent higher fat concentration (Atkinson, Anderson, & Bryan, 1980). Triglycerides, the main constituent (98–99 percent) of milk fat, are readily broken down to free fatty acids and glycerol by the enzyme lipase, which is found not only in an infant's intestine but in the breastmilk itself.

The lipid fraction of human milk provides essential fatty acids. The main concern about fatty acid intake is its effect on brain growth. The rate of brain growth is greatest in the last trimester of pregnancy and continues throughout the first year of life. Tissues of breastfed and formula-fed infants have distinctly different plasma fatty acid compositions. Breastmilk contains a wide range of long-chain polyunsaturated fatty acids (LC-PUFAs), which represent 88 percent of milk fat and are the most variable element in milk (Jensen, 1999). Interestingly, levels of fatty acids are low in lactating women, which indicates that transfer to breastmilk is at the expense of the maternal stores (Koletzko & Rodriquez-Palmero, 1999).

DHA and AA

LC-PUFAs include docosahexanoic acid (DHA) and arachidonic acid (AA), which are associated with higher visual acuity and cognitive ability of the child. An analysis of studies of human-milk feedings, DHA-supplemented, and unsupplemented formula documented advantages of DHA on visual acuity (SanGiovanni et al., 2000). But other studies show that DHA supplementation of the pregnant or breastfeeding woman has no impact on infant development nor visual function (Jensen et al., 1988; Malcolm et al., 2003). AA content in human milk is stable and does not vary widely throughout the world. The content of DHA, on the other hand, varies according to diet; therefore an increased supply of DHA may not always be beneficial. In the case of coastal populations with high intakes of fish, for example, little or no effects will be noted since infants already receive breastmilk with high DHA levels (Brenna et al., 2007).

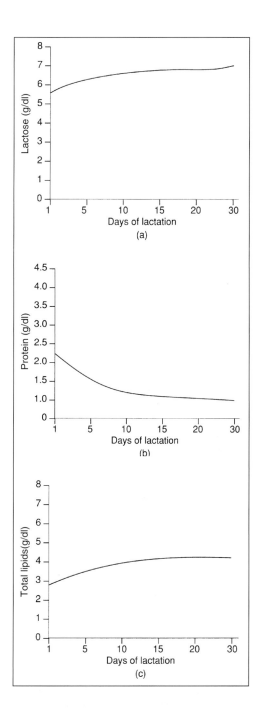

FIGURE 4–5 Lactose protein and total lipid concentration in human milk.

Another reason that not all breastfed infants have higher cognitive development and intelligence is that there are two forms of a gene known as RADS2. In infants who carry the C form of this gene, breastfeeding raises intelligence by producing an enzyme that helps convert fatty acids in breastmilk into components that spur neurons to sprout connections which underlie intelligence, memory, and creativity. The 10 percent of infants who do not carry the C form of the gene lack the enzyme; therefore they derive no cognitive benefit from breastmilk (Caspi, Williams, & Kim-Cohen, 2007).

An essential fatty acid that enhances the developing human visual system, DHA is found in extremely high levels in the photoreceptors and the visual cortex and may ameliorate neurovisual developmental disorders such as the retinopathy of prematurity (Hylander et al., 2001). Breastfed infants accumulate DHA in the cortex, whereas formula-fed infants merely maintain the same amount of DHA present at birth. As a result, breastfed infants have higher levels of DHA than an age-matched group of formula-fed infants (Baur et al., 2000).

DHA and AA Controversy

In years past, commercial infant formula was fortified only with precursor essential fatty acids, α-linolenic acid, and linoleic acid. In an attempt to narrow the "nutrient gap" between formula and breastmilk, formula companies added DHA and AA to their infant formula after the FDA approved it as an additive in 2001. Critics charge that there is insufficient evidence that these additives are safe. DHA is extracted from fermented microalgae and AA from soil fungus. Human fatty acids are structurally different from those manufactured from plant sources and interact with each other in a special matrix that cannot be duplicated. The National Alliance for Breastfeeding Advocacy and the Cornucopia Institute filed a petition with the FDA to require a warning label on infant formula containing DHA and AA believing that parents have the right to know that these oils may be the cause of their infant's diarrhea or other gastrointestinal problems (see http://cornucopia.org/DHA/DHA_FullReport.pdf).

Breastfed infants have a higher proportion of acetic acid in the short-chain fatty acid spectra than do formula-fed infants, which, along with the monoglycerides generated by milk lipases, act against envelope viruses, bacteria, and fungus (Garza et al., 1987; Siigur, Ormission, & Tamm, 1993). The paler color, softer consistency, and milder odor of breastmilk stools, as compared with formula stools, are due in part to a higher concentration of fatty acid soaps

(Quinlan et al., 1995). Fatty acid composition also differs between mothers whose babies develop atopic manifestation during the first year of life and those who remain healthy. Specifically, lower levels of α-linolenic acid and *n*-3 long-chain polyunsaturated fatty acid in mature milk of atopic mothers, especially in those with atopic babies, suggest that the low levels of this fatty acid could be associated with the development of atopy in the infants (Duchen, Yu, & Björkstén, 1999).

Although maternal dietary fat intake does not affect the total amount of fat in a mother's milk, the types of fat in the diet do influence the composition of fatty acids in milk. For example, black mothers in South Africa consuming a traditional maize diet have higher levels of monounsaturated fatty acid in their milk than do their urban counterparts who eat more animal fats (van der Westhuyzen, Chetty, & Atkinson, 1988). If the mother eats a high-carbohydrate, energy-replete diet, the proportion of triglycerides of medium-chain fatty acid increases (Garza et al., 1987).

The effects of breastfeeding can depend on the formerly breastfed individual's age. A prime example is cholesterol. Because cholesterol levels (10–20 mg/dl) in human milk are considerably higher than those of formulas derived from bovine milk (Wagner & Stockhausen, 1988), one would expect cholesterol levels in adulthood to be higher in breastfed individuals. The reverse, however, is true. Exposure to cholesterol in breastmilk may have long-term benefits for cardiovascular health. Coronary artery disease in persons up to 20 years of age is less frequent in individuals who were breastfed (Bergstrom et al., 1995). Serum total cholesterol and LDL levels (1) tend to be higher among breastfed infants compared to nonbreastfed infants, (2) are not different by infant-feeding group by 18 months of age (Demmers et al., 2005) and during childhood, and (3) tend to be lower among adults who were breastfed rather than artificially fed as infants (Owen et al., 2002). In addition to higher cholesterol concentration, adults who were bottle-fed had higher plasma glucose concentrations and impaired glucose tolerance (Ravelli et al., 2000).

Fat content of milk changes throughout a breastfeeding and, generally speaking, increases more steeply as more milk is taken. Fat content varies according to the degree to which the breast is emptied at that breastfeeding, and that fat content increases markedly after most of the milk in the breast has been taken (Daly et al., 1993). The longer the time interval between two breastfeedings, the less likely the infant is to empty the breast and, thus, the lower the fat concentration will be in the subsequent feeding. Although the work of Daly et al. (1993) indicated that the pattern of feedings dictates the infant's fat intake, this is not necessarily the case. Woolridge, Ingram, and Baum (1990) studied mothers who fed in two patterns—either feeding at one breast or at two breasts during a feeding. The infants thus fed were able to regulate their fat intake and to achieve stable fat intakes in spite of disparate patterns of feedings. His findings support flexible "baby-led" feedings.

Lactose

Lactose, a disaccharide, accounts for most of the carbohydrates in human milk, although small quantities of oligosaccharides, galactose, and fructose are also present. Although lactose concentration is relatively constant (7.0 gm/dl) in mature milk, it is affected by maternal diet.

Lactose enhances calcium absorption and metabolizes readily to galactose and glucose, which supply energy to the rapidly growing brain of the infant. Some oligosaccharides promote the growth of *Lactobacillus bifidus*, thus increasing intestinal acidity and stemming the growth of pathogens (Dai et al., 2000).

The enzyme lactase is necessary to convert lactose into simple sugars that can be easily assimilated by the infant. The enzyme is present in the infant's intestinal mucosa from birth. Congenital or primary lactase deficiency is exceedingly rare (Montgomery et al., 1991). Lactose intolerance, however, is common in many mammals as they grow older and is the result of diminishing activity of intestinal lactase after weaning. In humans, lactose intolerance is more prevalent in adults of Asian and African heritage.

Probiotic and Prebiotic Bacteria

There is a current interest in so-called probiotic bacteria, which are certain *Lactobacillus* strains. Probiotic bacteria probably act by competing with other bacteria for nutrients thereby reducing the numbers of potentially pathogenic microbes. For example, certain *Lactobacillus* strains may ameliorate the symptoms of rotavirus infections (Larsson, 2004).

Protein

Protein content of mature human milk from well-nourished mothers is about 0.8 to 0.9 gm of protein per deciliter. Some of the protein in human milk is probably not nutritionally available to the infant; it serves immunological purposes instead. The high quality of protein in human milk and its precisely balanced quantity meet the energy needs of infants (Gaull, 1985; Raiha, 1985). As seen in Figure 4–2, the protein content decreases rapidly during the first several months (Saarela, Kokkonen, & Koivisto, 2005)

Human milk contains casein and whey protein. Casein and whey levels change as lactation progresses to meet the nutritional needs of the infant. Casein is lower in early lactation, then increases rapidly. Whey proteins are at their highest in early lactation and continue to fall. These changes result in a whey/casein ratio of about 90:10 in early lactation, 60:40 in mature milk, and 50:50 in late lactation (Kunz & Lönnerdal, 1992). Whey proteins are acidified in the stomach, forming soft, flocculent curds. These quickly digest, supplying a continuous flow of nutrients to the baby. By contrast, caseins (the primary protein in untreated bovine milk) form a tough, less digestible curd that requires high expenditure of energy for an incomplete digestive process.

Whey protein is composed of five major components: (1) α-lactalbumin, (2) serum albumin, (3) lactoferrin, (4) immunoglobulins, and (5) lysozyme. The latter three elements play important roles in immunological defense. Lactoferrin concentration of milk is higher in iron-deficient women as compared with well-nourished mothers; therefore, milk lactoferrin may also help protect the infant against iron deficiency (Raiha, 1985). A large number of other proteins (enzymes, growth modulators, and hormones) are present in low concentrations.

Nonprotein Nitrogen

Milk proteins are synthesized from amino acids derived from the bloodstream. Nonprotein nitrogen contains a number of free amino acids, including glutamic acid, glycine, alanine, valine, leucine, aspartic acid, serine, threonine, proline, and taurine. When amino acids exist singly or in free form, they are known as *free amino acids*. Of these, leucine, valine, and threonine are essential amino acids; they must be consumed in the diet because the body does not manufacture them.

The percentage of protein in human colostrum is greater than that in mature breastmilk. This high level is due to the fact that in colostrum lactose and water haven't yet flooded the system and also because of the presence of additional amino acids and antibody-rich proteins, especially secretory IgA and lactoferrin. All 10 essential amino acids are present in colostrum and account for approximately 45 percent of its total nitrogen content.

Nucleotides

Nucleotides are low-molecular-weight compounds with a nitrogenous base. Necessary for energy metabolism, enzymatic reactions, and growth and maturation of the developing gastrointestinal tract, they also play several roles in immune function, including enhanced lymphocytic proliferation, stimulation of immunoglobulin production in lymphocytes, and increased natural killer-cell activity. Infant formula manufacturers seek to emulate the many nucleotides of breastmilk in their formulas (Cosgrove, 1998; Leach et al., 1995).

The importance to the baby of available nitrogen cannot be overstated. Atkinson, Anderson, and Bryan (1980) have shown that the concentration of nitrogen in the milk of women who deliver preterm infants is 20 percent greater than that in the milk of women delivering at term. The higher levels of available protein and fat in preterm mother's milk underscore the importance of using the milk of the preterm infant's mother rather than pooled milk from women in other stages of lactation (Table 4–2). Donated milk (not preterm milk), however, can be modified with components from other human milk to make a preterm human milk formula with none of the dangers of commercial bovine-based preterm formulas.

Vitamins and Micronutrients

The amounts of vitamins and micronutrients in human milk vary from one mother to another because of diet and genetic differences. However, it is generally true that human milk will satisfy the micronutrient requirements of a full-term healthy infant and thus can be taken as the primary yardstick of dietary recommendations, or reference values. Generally, as lactation progresses, the level of water-soluble vitamins in breastmilk increases, and the level of fat-soluble vitamins declines. The levels of fat-soluble vitamins (A, D, K, E) in human milk are minimally influenced by recent maternal diet, as these vitamins can be drawn from storage in the body.

Vitamin A

Human milk is a good source of vitamin A (200 IU/dl), which is present mainly as retinol (40–53 ng/dl). Required for vision and maintenance of epithelial structures, vitamin A is at highest levels in the first week after birth and then gradually declines. Deficiency of vitamin A is a serious health problem for young children in many developing countries, leading to blindness through damage to the corneal epithelium (xerophthalmia) and to increased morbidity from infectious diseases. The prolongation of even partial breastfeeding provides an important source of vitamin A to children in developing countries (Bates & Prentice, 1994).

Vitamin D

Human milk has very little fat-soluble vitamin D and breastfed infants can develop rickets, although it is uncommon. The risk of rickets is greatest for dark-skinned children living in inner-city areas, children whose clothing deters skin exposure to the sun, and children of mothers eating vegetarian diets that exclude meat, fish, and dairy products. For example, 10 percent of breastfed infants living in Iowa (41 degrees N) were deficient in vitamin D; most were dark skinned (Ziegler et al., 2006). The child who is adequately exposed to the sun (and thus to radiation-formed precursors of vitamin D) and whose mother consumes adequate nutrients usually does not need routine vitamin D supplements (Greer & Marshall, 1989). Concentrations in human milk range between 5 IU and 20 IU per liter. Increased vitamin D intake results in increased levels in human milk (Specker et al., 1985). Vitamin D may constitute an exception to the general rule that breastmilk micronutrient levels are protected from the effect of maternal deficiency. Scattered reports of rickets led the American Academy of Pediatrics in 2003 to recommend vitamin D supplements not only for children subject to certain conditions but to all infants (Gartner & Greer, 2003).

TABLE 4–2	Composition of Term and Preterm Milk During the First Month of Lactation							
Nutrients	3–5 Days		8–11 Days		15–18 Days		26–29 Days	
	Full Term	Preterm	Full Term	Preterm	Full Term	Preterm	Full Term	Preterm
Energy (kcal/dl)	48	58	59	71	62	71	62	70
Lipid (gm/dl)	1.85	3.00	2.9	4.14	3.06	4.33	3.05	4.09
Protein (gm/dl)	1.87	2.10	1.7	1.86	1.52	1.71	1.29	1.41
Lactose (gm/dl)	5.14	5.04	5.98	5.55	6.00	5.63	6.51	5.97

Source: Adapted from Anderson, 1985.

Vitamin E

Human colostrum is particularly rich in vitamin E (tocopherol). Milk of mothers with preterm and term infants have similar levels of vitamin E (3 IU/100 kcal) and carotenoid levels, which are higher than those in bovine milk (Ostrea et al., 1986) or formula (Sommerburg et al., 2000). A deficiency of vitamin E in infancy can result in hemolytic anemia, especially in the premature infant. Because it is an antioxidant, vitamin E protects cell membranes in the retina and lungs against oxidant-induced injury. The requirement for vitamin E increases with intake of polyunsaturated fatty acids in breastmilk. Mothers who eat foods high in polyunsaturated fats and "fast foods" add to oxidant stress (Guthrie, Picciano, & Sheehe, 1977).

Vitamin K

Vitamin K, which is required for the synthesis of blood-clotting factors, is present in human milk in small amounts. A few days after birth, a baby normally produces vitamin K in sufficient quantities by enteric bacteria. However, neonates are susceptible to vitamin K deficiency until ingestion of copious amounts of breastmilk can promote gastrointestinal bacterial colonization, which enhances their low levels of vitamin K. Vitamin K supplements taken by the mother will increase breastmilk levels and infant plasma levels of the vitamin (Greer, 1999).

Insufficient vitamin K in neonates can lead to vitamin K-responsive hemorrhagic disease. To prevent hemorrhage and to raise prothrombin levels, 1 mg vitamin K is routinely given intramuscularly postpartum. Alternatively, a 1 mg oral dose of vitamin K administered at birth, at 1 to 2 weeks, and at 4 to 6 weeks is absorbed in the intestinal tract in amounts sufficient to prevent bleeding, and the infant is spared the pain of an injection and the risk of nerve damage always possible with any intramuscular injection. Formula-fed infants need not receive vitamin K routinely because formula (other than soy) contains vitamin K (Medves, 2002).

Water-soluble vitamins—ascorbic acid, nicotinic acid, B_{12}, riboflavin, and B_6—are readily influenced by the maternal diet. If maternal supplements are present, the vitamin levels in the milk increase and then plateau. Although supplementation may be beneficial for undernourished women, it is not necessary if the mother is well nourished and eating a diet that contain foods close to their natural state.

Vitamin B_{12}

Vitamin B_{12} is needed for early development of the baby's central nervous system. A mother eating a vegan diet (i.e., without meat or dairy products) may produce milk deficient in B_{12}. A deficiency of B vitamin folate during pregnancy is associated with neural tube defects. The March of Dimes' campaign to educate women on the importance of taking folic acid supplements during preconception and pregnancy has reduced neural tube deformities.

Unlike other micronutrients, folate (which is bound to a folate-binding protein) remains at the same level throughout all stages of lactation. Maternal stores of folate diminish slightly from 3 to 6 months to maintain milk folate levels (Mackey & Picciano, 1999).

Vitamin B₆

High pharmacological doses of vitamin B_6 have been reported to suppress prolactin and thus lactation. However, low nutritionally relevant doses have no effect on plasma prolactin or on breastmilk volume. Doses as high as 4.0 mg of vitamin B_6 taken as part of a vitamin B complex supplement are considered safe for both the lactating mother and the infant (Andon et al., 1985).

Minerals

The total mineral content in human milk is fairly constant. Excepting magnesium, minerals tend to have their highest concentration in human milk in the first few days after birth and decrease slightly in a consistent pattern throughout lactation, with little diurnal variation or variation within feedings. Maternal age, parity, and diet, even when supplemented, usually have minimal influence on mineral concentrations in milk, probably because of their regulation from maternal body stores (Butte et al., 1987; Casey, Neville, & Hambidge, 1989).

Sodium

Breastmilk sodium is elevated in early colostrum but falls dramatically by the third day postpartum and declines at a slower rate for 6 months. Elevated levels of sodium in human milk occur during weaning, in women with mastitis, and during the first months of gestation. A high concentration of sodium has also been found in the milk of mothers whose infants develop malnutrition, dehydration, and hypernatremia. Persistent high levels may be a marker for impaired lactation (Morton, 1994).

Zinc

Zinc is actively transported into the mammary gland. Zinc levels rise to a peak on the second day postpartum and then decline for the duration of lactation (Casey, Neville, & Hambidge, 1989). Zinc is eight times as abundant in human colostrum as in mature milk. Zinc requirements are relatively high in the very young infant and decrease with increasing age of the infant (Krachler, Rossipal, & Irgolic, 1998; Krebs & Hambidge, 1986). For fully breastfed infants, a combination of high absorption and efficient conservation of intestinal endogenous zinc retain enough zinc to meet the demands of infant growth in the face of modest intake (Abrams, Wen, & Stuff, 1996; Krebs et al., 1996). Zinc supplements when taken by women with normal zinc levels, do not affect the infant's growth, morbidity, or motor development (Heinig et al., 2006).

Zinc dramatically improves acrodermatitis enteropathica, a rare but serious congenital metabolic disorder that manifests itself in part in severe dermatitis (Evans & Johnson, 1980). While infants with this disorder continue to receive human milk, they have no symptoms. The high bioavailability of zinc in human milk is brought about by a low-molecular-weight zinc-binding ligand that facilitates zinc absorption. Abnormally low zinc levels in breastmilk are rare but can sometimes occur in mothers of infants with low birth weight or if there is an inherited genetic condition (Chowanadisai, Lönnerdal, & Kelleher, 2006). A slowing growth rate and persistent perioral or perianal rash (with or without diarrhea) in infants fed solely breastmilk may be due to zinc depletion (Atkinson et al., 1989). These infants should continue to breastfeed but they may require zinc supplementation. Maternal diet does not affect breastmilk zinc levels. In the rare case where a woman has low concentrations of breastmilk zinc, she is likely to have delivered her infant prematurely (Lönnerdal, 2000).

Iron

Although human milk has a small amount of iron (0.5–1.0 mg/L), breastfed babies rarely are iron deficient. They maintain their iron status at the same level as that of formula-fed infants receiving iron supplements for up to 9 months (Duncan et al., 1985; Salmenpera et al., 1986; Siimes et al., 1984). Breastfed infants are sustained by sufficient iron stores laid down in utero and by the high lactose and vitamin C levels in human milk, which facilitate iron absorption. Iron in human milk is absorbed five times as well as is a similar amount from cow's milk.

For the first few months of life, healthy, full-term infants draw on extensive iron reserves generally present at birth. Normally, an infant's hemoglobin level is high (16–22 gm/dl) at birth and decreases rapidly as physiological adjustment is made to extrauterine life. At 4 months of age, normal hemoglobin ranges between 10.2 and 15 gm/dl. Iron is well absorbed by older infants and is not affected by mineral intake from solid foods in the diet or by vegetarianism (Abrams, Wen, & Stuff, 1996; Dorea, 2000; Lönnerdal, 2000). Breastmilk iron is only affected by the mother's iron intake when the mother is severely anemic, but not in those with mild to moderate anemia (Kumar et al., 2008).

Unless the infant is anemic, iron supplementation is not usually needed and may in fact be detrimental to the breastfeeding baby during the first 6 months after birth. Excess iron tends to saturate lactoferrin and thereby diminish its anti-infective properties. The authors of a randomized double-blind controlled trial concluded that routine iron supplementation of Swedish and Honduran breastfed infants with normal hemoglobin presented a greater risk of diarrhea (Dewey et al., 2002).

Calcium

Like iron, calcium appears in only small quantities in human milk (20–34 mg/dl). Yet babies absorb 67 percent of the calcium in human milk as compared to only 25 percent of that in cow's milk. Neonatal hypocalcemia and tetany are more commonly seen in the formula-fed infant, because cow's milk has a much higher concentration of phosphorus (calcium/phosphorus ratio of 1.2:1.0 versus 2:1 in human milk), which leads to decreased absorption and increased excretion of calcium. Calcium and phosphorus supplements are sometimes given to breastfed infants with low birth weight who should be monitored for hypercalcemia (calcium > 11 mg/dl) (Steichen, Krug-Wispe, & Tsang, 1987).

Magnesium

Magnesium is present in low levels in breastmilk and decreases in mature milk during 3 to 6 months (Picciano, 2001). Women who have been treated with magnesium sulfate for preeclampsia have high milk magnesium concentrations for the first day postpartum. After that time, levels return to normal (Lönnerdal, 2000).

Other Minerals

Copper levels are highest on the first few days postpartum, decrease for about 5 to 6 months, and then tend to remain stable. The mother's serum levels have no influence on milk concentration (Dorea, 2000). Selenium is usually higher in human milk than in formula (Kumpulainen et al., 1987; Smith,

Picciano, & Milner, 1982). Minute amounts of aluminum, iodine, chromium, and fluorine are also found in breastmilk. Formula-fed infants ingest as much as 80 times more manganese than breastfed infants. Manganese enters the neonatal brain at a much higher rate than in the adult brain. Neonates are therefore at risk of neurotoxicity from excess manganese. High manganese levels in infant formula have been identified as being possibly related to neurocognitive deficits (Tran et al., 2002). Very little is known about the mechanisms or control of the secretion of trace elements into human milk. Table 4–3 lists the major components of human milk and their functions.

Preterm Milk

The milk of a woman who delivers a preterm infant is different from that of a woman who delivers at term, probably to meet the special needs of the low birth weight neonate. Compared with term breastmilk, preterm breastmilk has higher levels of energy, lipids, protein, nitrogen, fatty acids, some vitamins, and minerals (see Table 4–2). In addition, preterm breastmilk has higher levels of immune factors, including cells, immunoglobulins, and anti-inflammatory elements than term breastmilk. In the United States, the extra healthcare cost of not using human milk for preterm infants is estimated to be $9889 per baby (Wight, 2001). Chapter 13 also discusses preterm breastmilk.

Anti-Infective Properties

Breastmilk offers the newborn protection against disease and can reduce the risk of death for infants. When researchers compared CDC records of children who died between 28 days and 1 year, children who were breastfed had 20 percent lower risk of dying between 28 days and 1 year than children who were not breastfed. The longer the breastfeeding, the lower the risk for both black and white children (Chen & Rogan, 2004).

Only in the last few decades have investigators begun to identify the specific anti-infective components of human milk that make it a peerless substance for feeding the human infant. Breastmilk has been viewed from ancient times as living tissue and rightly so. This "white blood" contains enzymes,

TABLE 4-3

Major Components of Human Milk and Their Functions

Cells	Function
Phagocytes (macrophages)	Engulf and absorb pathogens; release IgA; polymorphonuclear and mononuclear.
Lymphocytes	T cells and B cells; essential for cell-mediated immunity; antiviral activity; memory T cells give long-term protection.
Anti-inflammatory Factors	
Prostaglandins PGE1, PGE2	Cytoprotective
Cytokines/chemokines	Immunodulating agents that bind to specific cellular receptors, activate the immune system, promote mammary growth, and move lymphocytes into breastmilk and across neonatal bowel wall. TGF-β is the dominating cytokine in colostrum.
Growth factors	Promote gut maturation, epithelial cell growth. EGF is a type of cytokine.
Enzymes	
Amylase	Facilitates infant digestion of polysaccharides.
Lipase	Hydrolizes fat in infant intestine; bacteriocidal activity.
Growth Factors/Hormones	
Human growth factors	Polypeptides that stimulate proliferation of intestinal mucosa and epithelium; strengthens mucosal barrier to antigens.
Cortisol, insulin, thyroxine cholecystokinin (CCK)	Promotes maturation of the neonate's intestine and intestinal host-defense process. Thyroxin protects against hypothyroidism; CCK enhances digestion.
Prolactin	Enhances development of B and T lymphocytes.
Lipids (Fat)	Major source of calories.
Long-chain polyunsaturated fatty acids (LC-PUFA)	DHA and AA associated with higher visual acuity and cognitive ability; breastmilk content dependent on maternal diet.
Free fatty acids (FFA)	Anti-infective effects.
Triglycerides	Largest source of calories for infant; broken down to free fatty acids and glycerol by lipase; types of fat depend on maternal diet.
Lactose	Carbohydrate, major energy source; breaks down into galactose and glucose; enhances absorption of Ca, Mg, and Mn.
Oligosaccharides	Microbial and viral ligands.
Glycoconjugates	Microbial and viral ligands.
Minerals	Regulates normal body functions; minimal influence by maternal diet.
Protein	
Whey	Contains lactoferrin, lysozyme, and immunoglobulins, alpha-lactalbumin.
Immunoglobulins (SIgA, IgM, IgG)	Immunity response to specific antigens in environment. SIgA pathways to mammary gland called GALT and BALT.

(Continues)

TABLE 4–3	Major Components of Human Milk and Their Functions (Continued)

Cells	Function
Lactoferrin	Antibacterial especially against *E. coli*; iron carrier.
Lysozyme	Bacteriocidal and anti-inflammatory; activity progressively increases starting 6 months after delivery.
Taurine	Abundant amino acid; associated with early brain maturation and retinal development.
Casein	Inhibits microbial adhesion to mucosal membranes.
Vitamins A, C, E	Anti-inflammatory action; scavenges oxygen radicals.
Water	Constitutes 87.5% of human milk volume; provides adequate hydration to infant.

immunoglobulins, and leukocytes in abundance. These components, one frequently enhancing the efficacy of another, account for most of the unique anti-infective properties of human milk. In some cultures, fresh breastmilk is used as eye drops to treat conjunctivitis; elsewhere, it is common practice to apply breastmilk on the skin to heal cracked nipples. Breastmilk provides several tiers of defense against diseases of infants that include a top tier of secretory antibodies against specific pathogens, next a tier of fatty acids and lactoferrin that provide broad-spectrum protection, followed by glyco-conjugates and oligosaccharides, each protecting against one or more specific pathogens (Newburg et al., 1998).

Recent innovations to infant formula have included probiotics as a way of making the flora of formula-fed babies more like that of the breastfed baby. Probiotics are viable nonpathogenic bacteria, so-called healthy bacteria that colonize the intestine and modify the intestinal microflora with less pathogenic bacteria than formula-fed infants. Prebiotics are nondigestible food components that stimulate the growth of bifidobacteria. Oligosaccharides, prebiotic soluble fibers, play an important role in postnatal development of intestinal flora but have not been found in infant formulas until recently.

Infant formula containing probiotics and prebiotics are new on the market as formula companies compete against each other to advertise and sell their new product. Human milk can be called a "symbiotic," a mixture of probiotics and prebiotics that is beneficial to the infant by improving the survival and implantation of live dietary microorganisms in the gastrointestinal tract.

Breastmilk provides a continuous source of microbes to the infant's gastrointestinal tract during the first few weeks after birth. Bacteria commonly isolated include staphylococci, streptococci, micrococci, lactobacilli, and enterococci. Although we tend to think of these bacteria as disease producing, some bacteria are natural microbes, and once in the gastrointestinal tract, such bacteria stimulate the neonate's immune system to grow and, thus, help protect the infant against infectious diseases (Martin et al., 2005a). Microbes that colonize the neonate's gastrointestinal tract during and after birth are safest if they are from the mother because she can provide defense against them. These microbes, especially those in the gastrointestinal tract, are a stimulus for the growth and development of the infant's immune system (Larsson, 2004).

Studies conducted in the later part of the last century measured the protectiveness of human milk to reaffirm its significance in preventing infections (Dewey, Heinig, & Nommsen-Rivers, 1995; Frank et al., 1982; Kovar et al., 1984; Kramer et al., 2001;

Pullan et al., 1980; Rosenberg, 1989; Victora et al., 1987). These studies are joined by increasing numbers of new research. The evidence is strongest for bacterial infections, gastroenteritis, and necrotizing enterocolitis but is less convincing for respiratory infections (Kramer et al., 2001).

Gastroenteritis and Diarrheal Disease

Wherever infant morbidity and mortality are high, breastfeeding conclusively helps to prevent infantile diarrhea and gastrointestinal infections (Almroth & Latham, 1982; Brown et al., 1989; Clavano, 1982; Duffy et al., 1986; Espinoza et al., 1997; Grantham-McGregor & Back, 1972; Habicht, DaVanso, & Butz, 1988; Jason, Niebury, & Marks, 1984; Koopman et al., 1985; Kovar et al., 1984; Mitra & Rabbani, 1995; Perera et al., 1999; Ravelomanana et al., 1995; Ruuska, 1992). Breastfeeding minimizes diarrhea both by providing protective factors and by reducing exposure to other foods or water that may contain enteropathogens (Van Derslice, Popkin, & Briscoe, 1994). As antibiotic resistance becomes a global problem, discoveries about the protective effect of breastfeeding become even more important (Hakansson et al., 2000).

Protection is dose dependent. In a review of field studies conducted to identify the effect of breastfeeding on childhood diarrhea in Bangladesh, children partially breastfed had a greater risk of diarrhea than had those who were exclusively breastfed (Glass & Stoll, 1989). Although breastmilk's protective effect is most easily demonstrated in areas of poverty and malnutrition, evidence of this protection is worldwide. In China, Chen, Yu, and Li (1988) showed that compared with breastfed infants, artificially fed infants are more likely to be admitted to the hospital for gastroenteritis and other conditions. In the Cebu region of the Philippines, giving water, teas, and other liquids to breastfed babies doubled or tripled the likelihood of diarrhea (Popkin et al., 1990). Young Nicaraguan children who develop rotavirus infections very early are partially protected by specific IgA antibodies in their mothers' milk. Rotavirus in stool samples correlated significantly with the concentration of antirotavirus IgA antibodies in colostrum (Espinoza et al., 1997). Canadian infants exclusively breastfed for the first 2 months

had significantly fewer episodes of diarrhea than did infants bottle-fed from birth (Chandra, 1979). Breastfed children in Burma required less oral rehydration solution than did those who were not breastfed during the early acute phase of diarrhea and recovered from diarrhea more quickly (Khin-Maung-U et al., 1985).

A major methodological problem in breastfeeding research on disease is the dose-response effect—the greater the amount of breastmilk the infant receives, the greater the protection against disease; protection improves with the duration of breastfeeding. A lack of a clear consistent definition of breastfeeding is a flaw in many breastfeeding studies given the fact that there is a wide variation in feeding practices and that mothers often erroneously report supplements given to the infant (Aarts, Kylberg, Hornell et al., 2000; Zaman et al., 2002). Moreover, it is neither feasible nor ethical to randomly assign mother–infant dyads to breastfeeding or formula-feeding groups.

Kramer et al. (2001) got around this problem by looking at infant outcomes of hospitals and clinics in Belarus that introduced breastfeeding-friendly hospital initiatives and compared them with hospitals and clinics that continued their traditional practices. Results indicated that infants at the intervention site were more likely to breastfeed to any degree at 12 months and were more likely to be exclusively breastfeeding at 3 and 6 months. The risk of gastrointestinal infections and atopic eczema were significantly lower in the intervention group, but there was not significant reduction in respiratory tract infection. A follow-up study (years 2002–2005) on the children who were in the breastfeeding promotion intervention modeled on the Baby-Friendly Hospital Initiative scored higher means on the Wechsler Intelligence Test (Kramer, Aboud, Mironova et al., 2008).

Epidemiological evidence indicates that human milk continues to confer protection even with supplementation. Partial breastfeeding is better than no breastfeeding at all. This protection is specific to pathogens in the mother's and infant's environment. Moreover, the infant receives protection against the pathogens it is most likely to encounter. Table 4–4 summarizes the ameliorating and protective effects of human milk. We assume that breastfeeding is the norm and that artificial feeding is a deviation from the norm that brings about hazards to infant health. Two infant health problems exacerbated by lack of breastfeeding—respiratory illness and otitis media—are discussed here. Others are discussed throughout this book, especially in Chapters 18 and 19.

Respiratory Illness

Studies of the protective effects of breastfeeding against respiratory tract infections are conflicting and complex because of error in parents' reports and other conditions not related to feeding. Several studies suggest that breastfeeding helps to prevent respiratory illnesses (Abdulmoneim & Al-Gamdi, 2001; Cushing et al., 1998; Lopez-Alarcon, Villalpando, & Fajardo, 1997), and others indicate little protection (Dewey, Heinig, & Nommsen-Rivers, 1995; Kramer et al., 2001). There is, however, strong evidence that breastmilk protects against respiratory syncytial virus (RSV) infection (Bell et al., 1988; Downham et al., 1976; Duffy et al., 1986; Holberg et al., 1991; Naficy et al., 1999; Newburg et al., 1998; Rahman et al., 1987). Downham et al. (1976) compared 115 infants hospitalized with RSV who were younger than 12 months with 162 control infants. Only 7 percent of the hospitalized infants were breastfed, compared with 27.5 percent of the control infants, a statistically significant difference. In the case of pneumonia caused by *Streptococcus*, researchers recently discovered a novel folding variant of α-lactalbumin that is a naturally occurring antibacterial compound in breastmilk (Hakansson et al., 2000).

As with gastroenteritis, the preventive effect of breastmilk is global. When Chen, Yu, and Li (1988) looked for an association between type of feeding and hospitalization of infants in Shanghai, they found that artificial feeding was associated with more frequent hospitalizations for respiratory infections during the first 18 months of life. About one fourth of hospitalizations of United Kingdom infants with lower respiratory tract infection could have been prevented if they had been exclusively breastfed (Quigley, 2007). In Brazil, babies who were not being breastfed were 17 times more likely than those being exclusively breastfed to be admitted to the hospital for pneumonia (Cesar, Victoria, &

Barros, 1999). Similar protection has been established for *Haemophilus influenzae* bacteremia and meningitis (Cochi et al., 1986; Istre et al., 1985; Takala et al., 1989).

Otitis Media

Breastfeeding protects against ear infections (otitis media) for reasons that are not completely clear. However, immunological factors, the feeding position, and lack of irritation from bovine-based formula may explain it. Saarinen et al. (1982) followed healthy term infants for 3 years. Up to 6 months of age, no infant had otitis during the period of exclusive breastfeeding, whereas 10 percent of the babies who were given any cow's milk did. These significant differences persisted up to 3 years of age. Other studies (Aniansson et al., 1994; Dewey, Heinig, & Nommsen-Rivers, 1995) support an inverse relationship between ear infections and breastfeeding.

Controversies and Claims

In contrast to global evidence that breastfeeding helps to protect infants against health problems, Bauchner, Levanthal, and Shapiro (1986), and Leventhal et al. (1986) challenged the claim that breastfeeding protects infants in developed countries, citing lack of control for potentially confounding factors, such as low birth weight, parental smoking, crowding, sanitation, and other characteristics of socioeconomic status.

Howie et al. (1990) settled this controversy by examining the effect of breastfeeding on childhood illness in Scotland in a study using an adequate sample that met the methodological criteria set by Bauchner, Levanthal, and Shapiro (1986). Howie concluded that breastfeeding during the first 13 weeks of life confers protection against gastrointestinal illness beyond the period of breastfeeding itself. A few years later, Fuchs, Victor, and Martines (1996) questioned this long-term protection for diarrhea. They found that children who stopped breastfeeding in the previous 2 months were vulnerable to developing dehydrating diarrhea. Certain supplemental foods such as herbal teas prolonged diarrheal disease in Mexican children (Long et al., 1999).

TABLE 4–4

Amelioration of Disease in Infants and Children By Human Milk

Disease in Child	Ameliorating Properties of Human Milk
Acrodermatitis enteropathica	More efficient zinc absorption (Evans & Johnson, 1980).
Appendicitis	Anti-inflammatory properties (Pisacane et al., 1995b).
Asthma	Introduction of milk other than human milk prior to four months is a risk factor for asthma at age 6 years (Dell & To, 2001; Oddy, 2000). Risk of asthma reduced 4 percent with each additional month of exclusive breast-feeding (Oddy, 2004). Breastfeeding provides protection against asthma in children with family history of atopy (Gdalevich et al., 2001), especially if the child is exposed to tobacco smoke (Chulada et al., 2003).
Atherosclerosis	Having been breastfed is inversely associated with carotid intima-media thickness, carotid plaque, and femoral plaque (Martin et al., 2005).
Bacterial infections, neonatal sepsis	Leukocytes, lactoferrin, immune properties (Ashraf et al., 1991; Fallot, Boyd & Oski, 1980; Leventhal et al., 1986).
Cardiovascular disease	Dietary cholesterol in infancy elevates plasma total cholesterol levels through direct mechanism that persists only until weaning (Demmers et al., 2005). High-adult erythrocyte sedimentation rate, a moderate risk factor for coronary heart disease among those bottle-fed compared to those breastfed (Gunnarsdottir et al., 2007).
Celiac disease	Longer duration and greater exclusivity of breastfeeding associated with later diagnosis. Protects against development of villous atrophy in intestinal mucosa. Later introduction of gluten in breastfeeders (Ascher et al., 1997; Auricchio, 1983; Bouguerra et al., 1998; Greco et al., 1988; Ivarsson et al., 2000; Kelly et al., 1989; Logan, 1990).
Childhood cancer (lymphoma, leukemia neuroblastoma)	Modulates and strengthens defenses against carcinogenic insult by enhancing long-term development of infant immune system (Davis, 1998). Cancer cells undergo apoptosis (destruction) in human milk (Bener, Denic, & Galadari, 2001; Daniels et al., 2002; Davis, Savitz, & Graubard, 1988; Franke, Custer, & Tanaka, 1998; Gimeno & de Suza, 1997; Grufferman et al., 1998; Hakansson et al., 1995; Kwan et al., 2004; Martin et al., 2005; Mathur et al., 1993; Shu et al., 1995; Smulevich et al., 1999; Svanborg et al., 2003); Swartzbaum et al., 1991).
Colitis	Less exposure to cow's milk proteins (Anveden-Hertzberg, 1996; Jenkins et al., 1984; Rigas et al., 1993).
Crohn's disease	Uncertain (Bergstrand & Hellers, 1983; Koletzko et al., 1989; Rigas et al., 1993).
Diabetes, type 1 (IDDM)	Lack of antigenic peptides helps protect against autoimmune disease. Lessens risk 2–26%. Short duration of breastfeeding associated with induction of beta-cell autoantibodies (Borch-Johnson et al., 1984; Gimeno & de Suza, 1997; Kostraba et al., 1993; Mayer et al., 1988; Perez-Bravolt et al., 1996; Rosenbauer, Herzig, & Giani, 2008; Verge et al., 1994; Virtanen et al., 1992; Wahlberg, Vaarala, & Ludvigsson, 2006; Wasmuth & Kolb, 2000) and many more articles.
Dental caries	Less occurrence of dental caries (Erickson, 1999).

(Continues)

TABLE 4–4	**Amelioration of Disease in Infants and Children By Human Milk (Continued)**

Disease in Child	Ameliorating Properties of Human Milk
Gastrointestinal infection/ Diarrheal disease	Humoral and cellular anti-infectious factors (Dewey et al., 1995; Espinoza et al., 1997; Howie et al., 1990; Long et al., 1999; Sadeharju et al., 2007). Numerous other studies discussed throughout this text.
Gastroesophageal reflux	More rapid gastric emptying; lower esophageal pH (Heacock et al., 1992).
Hypertrophic pyloric stenosis	Uncertain; breastfeeding may prevent pyloric spasm and edema (Habbick, Kahnna, & To, 1989).
Hypertension	Children breastfed until at least 6 months have lower systolic blood pressure than those breastfed for a shorter duration (Lawlor, 2004).
Inguinal hernia	Hormones in breastmilk might stimulate neonatal testicular function to close inguinal canal and promote descent of testes. One-fourth incidence (Pisacane et al., 1995a).
Juvenile rheumatoid arthritis	Anti-inflammatory properties protect against autoimmune disease (Mason et al., 1995).
Liver disease	Protease inhibitors (including antitrypsin) protect children with alpha-antitrypsin deficiency (Udall et al., 1985).
Malocclusion	Physiological suckling patterns (Labbok & Hendershot, 1987).
Multiple sclerosis	Protects against autoimmune disease (Pisacane et al., 1994).
Necrotizing entercolitis	Immunological factors, macrophages, osmolarity of human milk, high levels of platelet-activating acetyl-hydrolase; suppression of (IL)-8 (Akisu et al., 1998; Lucas & Cole, 1990; Minekawa et al., 2004).
Otitis media	Antibody, T- and B-cell protection; lack of irritation from cow's milk; upright feeding position (Aniansson et al., 1994; Duncan et al., 1993; Sassen, Brand, & Grote, 1994).
Oral development	Fewer malocclusions and reduced need for orthodontic intervention because breastfed children have well-rounded, U-shaped dental arch. Fewer problems with snoring and sleep apnea in later life (Palmer, 1998).
Respiratory syncytial virus	IgA, IgG antibody transmitted to breastmilk and infant through gut-associated or bronchus-associated lymphoid tissue (GALT & BALT). Lactadherin, a glycoprotein binds to rotavirus and inhibits activity (Bell, 1988; Duffy et al., 1986; Holberg et al., 1991; Naficy et al., 1999; Newburg, et al., 1998; Rahman et al., 1987).
Lower respiratory tract disease	Meta-analysis of 33 studies on healthy infants in developed nations. Severe respiratory tract illnesses with hospitalization were tripled for infants who were not breastfed compared with those who were exclusively breastfed for 4 months (Bachrach, Schwarz, & Bachrach, 2003).
Retinopathy of prematurity	Antioxidants (inositol, vitamin E, beta-carotene) and DHA may protect against the development of retinopathy of prematurity (Hylander et al., 2001).
Sudden infant death syndrome	Uncertain; possibly anti-infectious, antiallergic (Ford et al., 1993; Gilbert et al., 1995; Kum-Nji, 2001).
Urinary tract infections	Antibacterial properties (sIgA) bind to bacteria and prevent them from reaching the urinary tract. Protection is greatest in girls (Marild et al., 2004; Pisacane et al., 1990).

In a prospective multicenter study on the effect of breastmilk in preventing necrotizing enterocolitis in premature infants, Lucas and Cole (1990) found that the disease was 6 to 10 times more common in exclusively formula-fed babies than in exclusively breastfed babies. This held true even though the human milk received was often pooled and not derived from the baby's mother. These findings support the contention that breastfeeding is more than a lifestyle choice; it has profound implications for the health of the child. Parents sometimes ask how long breastmilk protective effects last. Table 4–5 presents research on the length of breastfeeding and expected protection.

Chronic Disease Protection

The protection offered by breastmilk against illness extends beyond infancy to childhood and adulthood. Breastfeeding contributes to prevention of celiac disease, diabetes, multiple sclerosis, sudden infant death syndrome, childhood cancer, and many other health problems that are discussed throughout this book. The longer the duration of breastfeeding and the more complete exclusivity of breastmilk, the greater its protective effect.

Childhood Cancer

Does a mother's milk modulate the interaction between the developing infant immune system and infectious agents that helps protect an infant against carcinogenic insults? The evidence is conflicting. When Davis (1998) reviewed nine case-control studies on the association between infant feeding and childhood cancer, she confirmed that children who are never breastfed or are breastfed for a short term have a higher risk of developing Hodgkin's disease than those breastfed for at least 6 months. It is possible that a type of human α-lactalbumin found in breastmilk lessens the risk of childhood cancer. This alpha-lactalbumin, a protein-lipid complex called HAMLET, induces apoptosis-like death in tumor cells but leaves fully differentiated cells unaffected (Hakansson et al., 1995; Svanborg et al., 2003). A meta-analysis (Martin et al., 2005b) concluded that breastfeeding reduces the risk of childhood acute lymphoblastic leukemia (ALL) and acute myeloblastic leukemia (AML); however, the public health importance may be small. Increasing breastfeeding from 50 percent to 100 percent would prevent at most 5 percent of cases of childhood acute leukemia or lymphoma. In another meta-analysis, Kwan et al. (2004), found that long-term breastfeeding was linked to a 24 percent lower risk of ALL. Breastfeeding for 6 months or less appeared to reduce ALL risk by 12 percent; the next year this same researcher concluded that there was no evidence that breastfeeding affects the occurrence of childhood ALL (Kwan et al., 2005). Evidence showing that breastfeeding is protective against childhood cancer is inconsistent.

TABLE 4–5	**Minimum Length of Breastfeeding for Protection Against Infectious Diseases**		
Health Problem	**Minimum Length of Breastfeeding**	**Length of Protection**	**Source**
Gastroenteritis/diarrheal disease	13 weeks	7 years	Howie, 1990
Otitis media	4 months	3 years	Duncan et al., 1993
Respiratory infections	15 weeks	7 years	Wilson et al., 1998
Wheezing bronchitis	—	6–7 years	Burr et al., 1993; Porro et al., 1993
Haemophilus influenzae, type b	—	10 years	Silfverdal et al., 1997
Hodgkin's disease	6 months	Not specified	Davis, 1998

Allergies and Atopic Disease

The incidence of food-induced allergic disease in children has been estimated to be between 0.3 to 7.5 percent (Metcalfe, 1984). Heredity is a significant predictor of allergic disease, even when the mother is on a milk-free diet during late pregnancy and lactation (Lovegrove, Hampton, & Morgan, 1994). Sixty percent of all those who will develop atopic eczema do so within the first year of life, and 90 percent do so within the first 5 years. Before 6 to 9 months of age, the infant intestinal mucosa is permeable to proteins; moreover, secretory IgA, which will later "paint" the mucosa and bind sensitizing proteins to itself, is not yet functioning effectively. After following 150 infants from birth to 17 years of age, Saarinen and Kajosaari (1995) concluded that breastfeeding is prophylactic against allergies—including eczema, food allergy, and respiratory allergy—throughout childhood and adolescence.

Cow's milk is the most common single allergen affecting infants. Proteins in cow's milk known to act as allergens include lactoglobulin, casein, bovine serum albumin, and lactalbumin. Modern heat treatment of formula has reduced—but certainly not eliminated—the allergic potential of these proteins. The problem is probably increased by the sizable dose of allergens in formula and by the large volume of formula ingested. At 2 to 4 months of age, for example, infants consume their body weight in milk each week. This is the equivalent of nearly 7 quarts per day for an adult—truly a macrodose!

Vomiting, diarrhea, colic, and occult bleeding are symptoms of allergy. It also affects the respiratory tract (runny nose, cough, asthma) and the skin (dermatitis, urticaria). Because the symptoms are varied and nonspecific, the diagnosis is often mistaken or missed.

At birth, the IgE system is defective in the potentially allergic infant, and problems arise if this system is activated by allergens. When the introduction of foreign proteins is delayed for 4 to 6 months, the baby's own IgA system is permitted to become more fully functional; thus allergic responses may be minimized or entirely avoided. Exclusive consumption of breastmilk facilitates the early maturation of the intestinal barrier and provides a passive barrier to potentially antigenic molecules until the baby's own natural barriers develop.

Chemokines IL-8 are higher in the breastmilk of allergic women who also have significantly more IL-4 in their milk, needed for the production of IgE. High levels of neonatal blood IgE are thought to predict later development of atopic symptoms. When the relationship between fecal IgE levels (a reliable indicator of serum IgE levels) was compared in infants 1 month old, formula-fed babies showed a higher incidence of high fecal IgE levels than did the breastfed infants (Furukawa et al., 1994).

A few breastfed infants develop atopic eczema. Of those who do, the culprit is often foods ingested by the mother—especially cow's milk. Cow's milk antigen can be detected in breastmilk (Axelsson et al., 1986; Cavagni et al., 1988; Odze et al., 1995; Paganelli, Cavagni, & Pallone, 1986). Early and occasional exposure to cow's milk protein sensitizes neonates so that even minute amounts of bovine milk protein in human milk may later act as booster doses that elicit allergic reactions (Host, Husby, & Osterballe, 1988). Prolonged breastfeeding exclusively or combined with infrequent exposure to small amounts of cow's milk during the first 8 weeks induces the development of IgE-mediated cow's milk allergy (Saarinen et al., 2000). By almost completely excluding milk, other dairy products, eggs, fish, beef, and peanuts throughout pregnancy and lactation, Chandra et al. (1986) documented a significant reduction in the incidence and severity of atopic eczema among breastfed infants of these mothers.

The "hygiene hypothesis" maintains that early exposure to microbes helps prevent allergies in children. As Larsson explains it, normal bacteria in the gut is important for the maturation of the immune system so that it learns to react against microbes rather than its own tissue. The infant develops an immunological tolerance to food, pollen, mites and other structures instead of reacting against them causing allergic reactions. Thus, having pets such as cats or dogs and ingestion or inhalation of endotoxin-containing material appears to help prevent allergies (Larsson, 2004).

Problems in conducting research on allergies and breastfeeding are manifold. Because it is not possible to classify mothers randomly into breastfeeding and nonbreastfeeding groups, are those infants with a family history of atopic eczema more likely to be breastfed because the parents are aware that it has a protective effect? When the infant is identified as breastfed, does that mean that the baby received no other nutriments? If so, for how long was breastfeeding continued? After conducting a meta-analysis of 22 original research reports on infant feeding and atopic disease, Kramer (1988) decided that errors in research methods are conflicting and seriously flawed, which thus, precludes definitive conclusions.

Asthma

Outcomes of epidemiological and clinical studies on asthma and breastfeeding are inconsistent, and the longstanding question of whether breastfeeding prevents or reduces the incidence of asthma has been controversial. To help settle the question Gdalevich, Mimouni, and Mimouni (2001) conducted a meta-analysis of research on the effect of breastfeeding on bronchial asthma. They found 41 studies that showed a protective effect, five studies that had no association, and two studies that had a positive association. Twelve of these studies were prospective and met the standards for study methodology as determined by Kramer (1988). Meta-analysis of these 12 showed that exclusive breastfeeding during the first months after birth is associated with lower asthma rates during childhood (OR 0.70, 95% CI 0.60 to 0.81). Oddy (2000, 2004) has carefully researched the effect of breastfeeding on asthma in children in Western Australia and found an association with less exclusive breastfeeding and asthma.

Finally, in regard to breastfeeding's protective effect against chronic disease, Palmer (1998) makes a convincing case that artificial feedings alter normal early oral cavity development so much that it can cause later problems such as snoring, sleep apnea, and malocclusion. For the mother herself, breastfeeding promotes health because it helps to prevent breast and ovarian cancer (see Chapter 16).

The Immune System

The notion of a separate immune system as an integral part of a body capable of fighting disease at all of the body's surfaces is relatively new, starting in the mid 1900s. Although it had long appeared that breastfeeding enhances immunity, a cause-effect relationship was not acknowledged as a scientific fact until more was known about the existence of an immune system outside of the bloodstream. (Koerber, 2006). Because the human immune system is not fully developed at birth, infants are particularly vulnerable to infections and gastrointestinal illnesses. Breastmilk stimulates and supplements the infant's developing immune system.

The body's overall immune system is known as the *systemic immune system*. Another immune system, the *secretory immune system*, involves surfaces of the body (such as the breast) and acts locally. Lymphocytes in the secretory immune system are different from other lymphocytes. Sensitized to antigens found in the gastrointestinal or the respiratory tracts, these lymphocytes travel through mucosal lymphoid tissues (e.g., breasts, salivary glands, bronchi, intestines, and genitourinary tract) where they secrete antibodies.

Most antigens to which a mother has been exposed sensitize lymphocytes migrating to the breast. There they secrete immunoglobulins into the milk—hence, the term *secretory IgA* or *sIgA*. These components are described later in this chapter where immunoglobulins are discussed. Lawrence and Pane (2007) have presented a recent extensive review of the immunology of human milk.

Active Versus Passive Immunity

Immunity occurs actively and passively. Maternal antibodies passed to the fetus through the placenta before birth present an example of passive immunity. Passive immunological protection is only temporary, as the infant's immune system has not itself responded. Breastfeeding can also confer long-term protection by stimulating an active immune response. Active immunity is a specific immunity whereby the immune system formulates a long-term memory of exposure to a certain antigen. Later exposure to the same antigen will produce an immune response. Poliovirus or rubella immunization of women or any attenuated virus immunization of the mother provides active immunity to the infant, as the virus will likely appear in her milk and thus immunize the infant. Reports indicate enhanced vaccine responses in breastfed infants compared with those not breastfeeding. After being vaccinated for measles-mumps-rubella (MMR), only breastfed children had increased production of interferon-gamma (Pabst et al., 1997). Another example of active immunity is the breastfed infant's immune response to cytomegalovirus in human milk.

Cells

Human milk contains two main types of white cells (leukocytes): phagocytes and lymphocytes (Figures 4–6 and 4–7). Although phagocytes (mostly macrophages) are most abundant (90 percent), the lymphocyte population (10 percent) provides significant protective effects to the recipient infant. The concentration of these cells and the predominant cell type vary with the duration of lactation. After birth, the number of these cells is higher than at any other time; they decline progressively thereafter.

Phagocytes

Macrophages, a type of leukocyte, are the dominant phagocyte in human milk. They engulf and absorb pathogens. Macrophages release IgA, although they probably do not synthesize it. Macrophages are both polymorphonuclear (PMN) and mononuclear. Because PMN numbers increase dramatically during inflammation of the breast, they may function to protect the mammary tissue per se rather than to impart protection to the newborn (Buescher & Pickering, 1986). Macrophages also produce complement, lactoferrin and lysozyme (discussed later in this chapter). Neutrophils are yet another phagocytic leukocyte. Short lived but effective, they are first to arrive at an inflamed site, such as that which may occur during mastitis.

Lymphocytes

Lymphocytes are also leukocytes and include T cells, B cells, and assorted T-cell subsets. Lymphocytes compose about 4 percent of the total leukocytes in early lactation; about 83 percent of the lymphocytes are T cells that appear to transfer through human milk to infants (Wirt et al., 1992). The various ways in which lymphocytes recognize and help to destroy antigens are called *cell-mediated immunity*. Such immunity is important in the destruction of viruses because the cells within which viruses live shield them from the action of antibodies. Formula-fed and breastfed infants have different types of lymphocyte subsets (Hawkes & Gibson, 2001).

Decreasing rapidly in the first week after birth and continuing to decline steadily, T cells are a special and separate immune component that can be activated into memory T cells (Wirt et al., 1992).

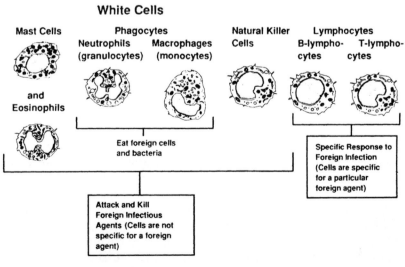

Cells of the Blood

FIGURE **4–6**   White cells of the blood.

Source: Fan, Conner, & Villareal, 1989.

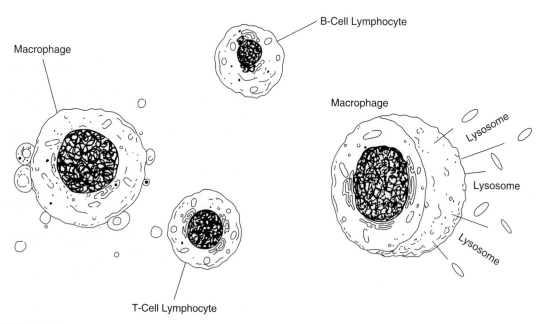

FIGURE 4–7 Microscope view of living cells in human milk. The 4,000 cells per centimeter of human milk consist mainly of macrophages and T-cell and B-cell lymphocytes. Macrophages secrete lysozyme, which help destroy the cell walls of bacteria.

These memory cells are the key to active immunity. Antibodies persist for only a few weeks before breaking down; however, memory cells can live for years, providing long-lasting protection. It is not clear whether T cells are activated in human milk or whether there is a specific homing of activated and memory T lymphocytes to the breast. B cells have functional capabilities similar to those of T cells. They mature into plasmalike cells that travel to epithelial tissues in the breast and release antibodies (Bellig, 1995; Newman, 1995) that reflect exposure to pathogens encountered in their environment. For example, milk from mothers living in Nigeria and exposed to malaria was compared with milk from a control population of mothers living in Washington, DC. The Nigerian mothers carried a high IgA level of antimalaria antibodies compared with the Washington mothers (Kassim et al., 2000).

Stem Cells

Human mammary tissue contains stem cells—an exciting new discovery. The discovery of stem cells in mammary tissue has led to research to determine whether mammary stem cells are present in expressed breastmilk (Cregan et al., 2007). The presence of nestin-positive putative mammary stem cells suggest that breastmilk is a readily available and noninvasive source of mammary stem cells that could be used to treat a multitude of health problems (see Figure 4–8). If so, they promise to provide an ethical means of harvesting stem cells.

Antibodies and Immunoglobulins

Antibodies are immunoglobulins that recognize and act on a particular antigen. Immunoglobulins are proteins produced by plasma cells in response to an immunogen. There are five types of immunoglobulins: (1) IgG, (2) IgA, (3) IgM, (4) IgE, and (5) IgD. Both IgA and IgE play a critical role in biological specificity of human milk on the recipient infant.

Secretory IgA (sIgA) is the major immunoglobulin in all human secretions. sIgA provides the initial bolus that supplements immunoglobulins transferred earlier across the placenta to the fetus. It is the immunoglobulin most frequently noted in medical literature as having immense immunological value to the neonate. sIgA, which is both synthesized and stored in the breast, reaches levels up to 5 mg/ml in colostrum; then it decreases to 1 mg/ml in mature milk. Interleukin-6 in human milk may be partly responsible for the genesis of IgA- and IgM-producing cells in the mammary gland (Rudloff et al., 1993). As the mother yields more milk, the infant receives more sIgA so that the total dose of sIgA the baby receives throughout lactation is constant or even increases (depending on the milk intake). Mothers of infants with a systemic infection and poor suckling have higher IgA levels in their breastmilk (Feist, Berger, & Speer, 2000) as well as women with a low income who have nearly three times the milk sIgA of high-income women (Groer, Davis & Steele, 2004).

sIgA synthesis via the secretory immune system described is an elegant lymphocyte traffic pathway called *gut-associated lymphoid tissue* (GALT) or *bronchus-associated lymphoid tissue* (BALT). This pathway leads to the development of lymphoid cells in the mammary gland, which produce IgA antibodies after exposure to specific microbial or environmental antigens on the intestinal or the respiratory mucosa (Goldman et al., 1983; Okamoto & Ogra, 1989). This migration of immunological responsiveness from both BALT and GALT to the mammary glands supports the unique concept of a common mucosal immune system (see Color Plate 4).

Because the infant's own IgA is deficient and only slowly increases during the first several months after birth, sIgA in human milk provides important passive immunological protection to the digestive tract of newborn infants. sIgA protects the newborn's entire intestinal tract. It is only minimally absorbed from the intestine because it is bound to the human milk fat globule membrane, travels through the newborn's entire intestinal tract, and is found unaltered in the newborn feces (Schroten et al., 1999).

A number of IgA antibodies in human milk that act upon viruses or bacteria that cause respiratory and gastrointestinal tract infections have been reported. These infecting agents include *E. coli, V. cholerae, Clostridium difficile, Salmonella, G. lamblia, E. histolytica, Campylobacter,* rotavirus, and poliovirus (Pickering & Kohl, 1986; Ruiz-Palacios et al., 1990). As stated earlier, immunizing breastfeeding women with poliovirus or rubella creates IgA antibodies in milk that specifically target these agents. IgA4 may also play a role in host defense of mucosal surfaces; in some women IgA4 is produced locally in the mammary gland (Keller et al., 1988).

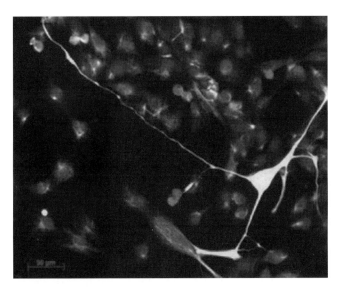

In addition to IgA, other Ig classes, including IgD, may be involved in local immunity of the breast. Several investigators (Litwin, Zehr, & Insel, 1990; Steel & Leslie, 1985) have demonstrated high levels of locally produced IgD in breast tissues and breastmilk. Another immune messenger, sCD14, has been found in significant quantities in breastmilk (25,100 ng/ml) versus formula (0.6 ng/ml). sCD14 plays an important role in enabling intestinal epithelial cells to prevent gastrointestinal gram-negative infections and stimulating the newborn immune system (Blais, Harrold & Altosaar, 2006).

As shown in Figure 4–9, clear biological rhythms of protective factors predictably rise and fall as lactation progresses. The reasons for waxing and waning of various anti-infective components are not always clear but are assumed to be adapted to the needs of the infant.

Nonantibody Antibacterial Protection

Nonantibody factors in human milk make up an elegant and intricate system that protects the infant against bacterial infection. These factors include lactoferrin, the bifidus factor, lactoperoxidase, and oligosaccharides.

Lactoferrin

Lactoferrin, a potent bacteriostatic iron-binding protein, is abundant in human milk (1–6 mg/ml) but is not present in bovine milk. It is present in higher proportions relative to total protein in preterm milk (de Ferrer et al., 2000). Lactoferrin inhibits adhesion of *Escherichia coli* to cells and helps prevent diarrheal disease (de Araujo & Giugliano, 2001). In the presence of IgA antibody and bicarbonate, lactoferrin readily absorbs enteric iron and thus prevents pathogenic organisms, particularly *Escherichia coli* and *Candida albicans* (Borgnolo et al., 1996; Kirkpatrick et al., 1971), from obtaining the iron needed for survival. Because exogenous iron may well interfere with the protective effects of lactoferrin, giving iron supplements to the healthy breastfed infant must be carefully weighed. Lactoferrin also has been shown to be an essential growth factor for human B and T lymphocytes (Hashizume, Kuroda, & Murakami, 1983) and to inhibit fungal growth.

The Bifidus Factor

The intestinal flora of breastfed infants is dominated by gram-positive lactobacilli, especially *Lactobacillus bifidus*. This bifidus factor in human milk, first recognized by Gyorgy (1953), promotes the growth of these beneficial bacteria. The buffering capacities of milk (bifidus factor), together with the low protein and phosphate levels, contribute to the low pH (5–6) of stools. This acid environment, present even in the first days of life of the breastfeeding infant (Rubaltelli et al., 1998) discourages replication of enteropathogens such as *Shigella*, *Salmonella*, and some *E. coli*. This protection does not appear to be complete, however. Although breastmilk inhibits bacterial-cellular adhesion to intestinal epithelial cells, a sign of the beginning of the infectious process, it does not prevent loss of the epithelial barrier (Kohler, 2002). Whether the breastfed infants in the study were fed other liquids and foods was not addressed.

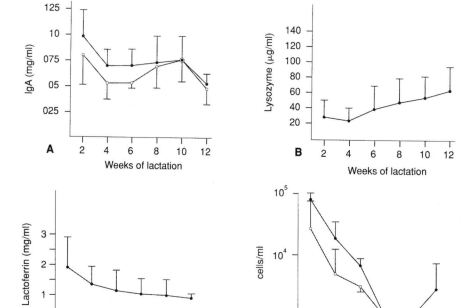

FIGURE 4–9   A longitudinal study of selected resistance factors in human milk. (A) Total (•) and secretory (○) IgA. (B) Lysozyme. (C) Lactoferrin. (D) Macrophages-neutrophils (•-•) and lymphocytes (○-○).

Source: Adapted from Goldman et al., 1982.

Lactoperoxidase

Although levels of the enzyme lactoperoxidase are low, substantial amounts are present in the newborn's saliva. It is thought that IgA in milk enhances the ability of lactoperoxidase to kill streptococci.

Oligosaccharides

Oligosaccharides (carbohydrates composed of a few monosaccharides) in human milk help to block antigens from adhering to the epithelium of the gastrointestinal tract. This blocking mechanism prevents the attachment of *Pneumococcus*, which is particularly adhesive (Goldman et al., 1986). There are about 130 different oligosaccharides in human milk. Breastmilk contains many times the amount of oligosaccharides that are found in bovine milk or formula. A few formula companies are adding a limited number of simple oligosaccharides to infant formula; yet the oligosaccharides found in human milk can be thought of as 130 reasons to breastfeed (McVeagh & Miller, 1997). Because of their complexity, oligosaccharides with structures identical to human milk oligosaccharides are not yet available; instead non-milk-derived oligosaccharides are being used in formula and other foods.

Cytokines and Chemokines

Cytokines are protein signals secreted by lymphocytes, monocytes, macrophages and other cells. Proinflammatory cytokines are responsible for body responses of swelling, tenderness, and fever. Chemokines are proinflammatory cytokines that signal to bring in more phagocytic cells to an infected or inflamed site (Larsson, 2004). Chemokines are also called immunomodulators in that they operate in networks and orchestrate activation of the immune system (Goldman et al., 1996) probably by moving lymphocytes into breastmilk and across the neonatal bowel wall (Michie et al., 1998). Several different cytokines and chemokines have been discovered in human milk recently, and the list is growing rapidly (Garofalo & Goldman, 1998). In addition to activating the immune system to protect the infant against infection (Wallace et al., 1997), these biologically active molecules also appear to play a role in growth and differentiation of the mammary gland (Goldman et al., 1996). Groer (2005, 2006) measured cytokines Th1/Th2 and stress levels in breastfeeding and formula-feeding women. Formula-feeding women

had decreased cytokines and other immunologic factors suggesting that breastfeeding was more protective against stress. Much has yet to be learned about cytokines.

Anti-Inflammatory and Immunomodulating Components

Many host defense agents in human milk have more than one function. Secretory IgA, lactoferrin, and lysozyme are examples. Human milk, rich in anti-inflammatory agents, supplies key protection during the vulnerable period of infancy. Major biochemical pathways of inflammations are either absent or poorly represented in breastmilk. Garofalo and Goldman (1999) have identified several anti-inflammatory factors in breastmilk, such as antioxidants (vitamins A, C, and E, and enzymes), alpha$_1$-antitrypsin, cortisol, epidermal growth factor, IgA, lysozyme, prostaglandins, and cytokines. The anti-inflammatory effects of these components have not as yet been directly demonstrated in the nursing infant, but they are thought to modulate cytokine responses to infection and facilitate defense mechanisms while minimizing tissue damage (Kelleher & Lönnerdal, 2001).

Goldman et al. (1996) suggest that the immunomodulating properties of human milk have a long-term influence on the development of the immune system and explain why the long-term risk for many diseases are lessened by breastfeeding. An immunomodulator changes the function of another defense agent and thus changes the quality or magnitude of the immune response. Fibronectin in human milk is an example of an immunomodulator that acts by augmenting the clearance of bacteria and intravascular debris. Interferon-alpha is not in human milk; yet breastfed infants with respiratory syncytial virus infection have higher blood levels of this element than nonbreastfed infants. Cytokines are also thought to immunomodulate the immune system. For example, interleukin-18, which is activated by macrophages, is higher in colostrum compared with early milk and mature milk. Interleukin-10 increases the development of IgA antibody production, thus playing an important role in host defense of neonates (Takahata et al., 2001). Other anti-inflammatory properties of human milk such as sIgA are more indirect.

Bioactive Components

Hamosh (2001) designates a special group of substances in human milk as *bioactive components*. These substances promote growth and development of the newborn by special activities that continue after the infant ingests breastmilk. Many are not available to the infant in commercial infant formula. Research on bioactive components is a growing area of investigation. These bioactive components may play a significant role in child health.

Enzymes

Mammalian milk contains a large number of enzymes, some of which appear to have a beneficial effect on the development of the newborn. The enzyme content of human milk and bovine milk differ substantially (Hamosh, 1996). For example, lysozyme activity is several thousand times greater in human milk than in bovine milk. The alkaline pH of the human infant's stomach has a limited effect on the antitrypsin activity of breastmilk, thereby protecting children with alpha$_1$-antitrypsin deficiency against severe liver disease and early death (Udall et al., 1985). Most mammal milks contain many enzymes that appear to be species specific because of their varying level of activity in different species. The enzymes discussed next serve a digestive function in the infant or may be important to neonatal development.

Lysozyme

Lysozyme, a major component of human milk whey fraction, produces both bacteriocidal and anti-inflammatory action. It acts with peroxide and ascorbate to destroy *E. coli* and some *Salmonella* strains (Pickering & Kohl, 1986). Lysozyme is much more abundant in human milk (400 ug/ml) than in bovine milk. Rather than slowly declining as lactation progresses, lysozyme activity increases progressively, beginning about 6 months after delivery (Goldman et al., 1982; Prentice et al., 1984). The lysozyme differs from other protective factors in this respect because babies begin receiving solid foods around 6 months, and high levels of lysozyme may be a teleological, practical safeguard against the greater risk from pathogens and diarrheal disease at this time.

Lipase

For human infants to digest fat, adequate lipase activity and bile salt levels must be present. The bile salt-stimulated lipase and lipoprotein lipase present in human milk compensate for immature pancreatic function and for the absence of amylase in neonates, especially in the premature infant. When human milk is frozen or refrigerated (Hamosh et al., 1997), lipase is not affected; however, heating severely reduces lipase activity. Several protozoa—*Giardia lamblia*, *Entamoeba histolytica*, and *Trichomonas vaginalis*—have been shown in vitro to be killed rapidly by exposure to salt-stimulated lipase, which is found only in the milk of humans and mountain gorillas (Blackberg et al., 1980).

Amylase

Amylase is necessary for the digestion of starch. Although amylase is synthesized and stored in the pancreas of the newborn, the infant is around 6 months old before amylase is released into the duodenum. Human milk contains about 10 to 60 times as much alpha-amylase as does normal human serum, thus providing an alternate source of this starch-digestive substance. No alpha-amylase is present in bovine, goat, or swine milk, suggesting that this enzyme appeared late in the evolutionary continuum. Breastfed infants have fewer problems digesting solid foods than do formula-fed infants, even if these foods are introduced early, because of the alpha-amylase provided by breastmilk. Amylase is stable when refrigerated (95–100 percent activity after 24 hours storage at 15 to 25°C) (Hamosh et al., 1997).

Leptin

Leptin, a hormone that regulates appetite, food intake, and energy metabolism, is present in breastmilk but not in formula. Leptin is produced mainly by the adipose tissue and varies significantly between people. Leptin concentrations in breastmilk decrease with time during lactation and show significant relationships with other maternal hormones. A recent study (Miralles et al., 2006) showed that leptin in breastmilk may regulate body weight during infancy. The higher the milk leptin concentration the lower the infants' BMI indicating that milk leptin could explain, at least partially, the greater risk of obesity in formula-fed infants compared with breastfed infants.

Growth Factors and Hormones

Human milk contains growth-promoting components also known as *growth factors* or *growth modulators*. As with the anti-infective properties of breastmilk, these substances are more pronounced in colostrum than in mature milk. Neither their biological significance nor their method of action is yet clear, but it appears that they have a greater synergistic effect when combined with each other. The source of growth factors is epithelial and stromal cells, and macrophages in the breast. These factors exert growth-promoting and protective effects on the neonatal gastrointestinal tract that cannot be provided by commercial formula (Kobata et al., 2008). Different growth factors may have overlapping functions, both stimulating cell growth and indirectly affecting the infant's defense mechanisms against disease (Morriss et al., 1986).

Epidermal Growth Factor

Epidermal growth factor (EGF), a type of cytokine, is a major growth-promoting agent in breastmilk that stimulates proliferation of intestinal mucosa and epithelium and strengthens the mucosal barrier to antigens (Carpenter, 1980; Petschow et al., 1993). A polypeptide that contains 53 amino acids, EGF is highest in human milk after delivery and decreases rapidly thereafter (Matsuoka & Idota, 1995). There is no diurnal variation or variation between preterm and term milk. EGF is also present in plasma, saliva, and amniotic fluid, but human milk contains a higher concentration. EGF may also be involved in the development of low-density lipoprotein receptors and in cholesterol metabolism.

Human Milk Growth Factors I, II, and III

Three polypeptides—called *human milk growth factors* (HMGF) I, II, and III—have been isolated (Shing & Klagsburn, 1984). HMGF III stimulates DNA synthesis and cellular proliferation, suggesting that it is an epidermal growth factor. In vivo studies (Heird, Schward, & Hansen, 1984; Widdowson, Colombo, & Artavanis, 1996) on growth factors in animal milk have shown striking increases in the mass of intestinal mucosa. Growth factors in human milk influence the growth of target tissues in the breastfed infant by provoking an endogenous hormonal response that is different from that provoked by formula—a possible stimulus of nutritional programming.

Insulin-Like Growth Factor

An insulin-like growth factor (IGF-I) in human milk is thought to have a growth-promoting role. The concentration of this factor in colostrum is about 30 times that in human serum, significantly higher than cow's milk, and very low to almost absent in formula (Shehadeh et al., 2001). These high levels (4.1 nmol/L) decrease rapidly (to 1.3 nmol/L) as colostrum alters to transitional milk (Read et al., 1984) but do not decline further. In fact, Corps et al. (1988) found that the concentration of an insulin-like growth factor in human milk increased (2.5 nmol/L) by the sixth week postpartum.

Thyroxine and Thyrotropin-Releasing Hormone

Thyroxine is present in human milk in small quantities but is not found in commercial formulas. The concentration in colostrum is low, increases by the first week postpartum, and gradually declines thereafter. It has been suggested that thyroxine may stimulate the maturation of the infant's intestine (Morriss, 1985).

Although the thyroxine level is significantly higher in breastfed children than in formula-fed children at 1 and 2 months of age (Rovet, 1990), it is unclear whether breastfeeding protects breastfed infants against clinical evidence of congenital hypothyroidism (Latarte et al., 1980; Rovet, 1990). Some infants receive sufficient thyroxine in their mother's milk to compensate for hypothyroidism; thus the symptoms may be masked for several months. Although this does not appear to be true for all infants, the results of thyroid studies after the first week of life should be interpreted with caution in breastfed infants and should include measurements of both thyroxine and thyroid-stimulating hormone (TSH) concentrations.

Cortisol

Cortisol is present in relatively high concentrations in colostrum, declines rapidly by the second day, and remains low thereafter. Its role in infant physiology is not clear. Three theories have been presented concerning the function of cortisol in infants. The first is that it may control the transport of fluids and salts in an infant's gastrointestinal tract

(Kulski & Hartmann, 1981). Another theory is that it may play a role in the growth of an infant's pancreas (Morrisset & Jolicoeur, 1980). Or cortisol may serve as a hormone released during chronic stress. A mother's higher level of satisfaction with breast-feeding is associated with lower levels of cortisol in her milk. The amount of cortisol in milk is inversely related to sIgA, suggesting that cortisol may suppress the function of immunoglobulin-producing cells in milk (Groer, Humenick, & Hill, 1994).

Cholecystokinin

Cholecystokinin (CCK) is a gastrointestinal hormone that enhances digestion, sedation, and a feeling of satiation and well-being. During suckling, vagal stimulation causes CCK release in both mother and infant, producing a sleepy feeling. The infant's CCK level peaks twice after suckling. The first peak occurs immediately after the feeding. It peaks again 30 to 60 minutes later. The first CCK rise is probably induced by suckling; the second by the presence of milk in the gastrointestinal tract (Marchini & Linden, 1992; Uvnas-Moberg, Marchini, & Windberg, 1993).

Beta-Endorphins

Beta-endorphins are higher in the colostrum of women who delivered (1) prematurely, (2) vaginally and, (3) without epidural analgesia. It is hypothesized that elevated beta-endorphin concentrations in colostrum may contribute to postnatal fetal adaptation to overcoming birth stress of natural labor and delivery, and at the same time contribute to the postnatal development of several related biological functions of the growing newborn (Zanardo et al., 2001).

Prostaglandins

Prostaglandins, a special group of lipids, are present in most mammal cells and tissues and affect almost every biological system. Formed by numerous body tissues, prostaglandins affect many physiological functions, including local circulation, gastric and mucous secretion, electrolyte balance, zinc absorption, and the release of brush border enzymes. The protective activity of milk lipids is thought to be due to the presence of prostaglandins PGE_2 and PGF_{2a}, present both in colostrum and in mature milk. Concentrations there are about 100 times as great as their levels in adult plasma (Lucas & Mitchell, 1980). PGE_2 particularly is thought to exert a cytoprotective action (protection against inflammation and necrosis) on the gastric mucosa by promoting the accumulation of phospholipids in the neonatal stomach (Reid, Smith, & Friedman, 1980). The full extent of the beneficial effects of prostaglandins in human milk awaits future scientific investigation.

Taurine

Taurine, absent in bovine milk, is the second most abundant amino acid in human milk (Raiha, 1985). This unusual amino acid, which may function as a neurotransmitter, plays an important role in early brain maturation (Gaull, 1985). Before 1983, taurine was thought to act only in the conjugation of bile acids. Infants who do not receive taurine in their diet conjugate bile acids with glycine, which less effectively assists in absorbing dietary fats. Although deleterious effects of low taurine levels are not known in humans, deficiencies have caused retinal problems in cats and monkeys (Jensen et al., 1988). Taurine was added to most commercial formulas when formula-fed infants were found to have plasma taurine levels only half as high as those of breastfed infants.

Implications for Clinical Practice

Human milk is a species-specific fluid of diverse composition that includes both nutrient and non-nutrient substances, all of which protect the infant. Although the significance to young infants of these components is well known, the influence of their nutritional programming on the subsequent health of infants is a relatively new field.

A thorough understanding of the biological components of human and bovine milks and of manufactured formulas is essential for the healthcare specialist who is providing lactation assistance. When prenatal discussion with the parents and prenatal classes include information about the immunological protection available from breastmilk but absent from formula, parents can then make an informed choice of infant feeding method.

This chapter objectively describes human milk components—but what about mothers' views of their breastmilk? Bottorff and Morse (1990) revealed that mothers clearly recognize the difference between colostrum and mature breastmilk. Because of the relative thickness of colostrum, some mothers believe it is the "strongest" milk, significant for its "rich" supply of antibodies rather than for its nutritional properties. Breastmilk was frequently described by using fat-related terms (e.g., lean, creamy, rich) and evaluated by drawing comparisons to cow's milk and infant formula, as if some similarities should exist between the two.

Knowledge of lactation physiology and breastmilk components provides us direction for lactation practice and advice to mothers. For example, the high fat (and thus calories) in hindmilk—the milk that appears when the breast is nearly empty—imply caution in routinely recommending "switch" nursing (repeatedly switching feedings from breast to breast during a breastfeeding) (Woolridge & Fisher, 1988). On the other hand, infants whose requirements may fluctuate with time are amazingly adept at self-regulating their nutrient intake (Woolridge, Ingram, & Baum, 1990). Thus we can encourage women to be flexible about breastfeedings and to be led by infants' cues that tell mothers when to continue and when to stop a feeding.

Given the differences between the growth patterns of breastfed infants and infants fed human-milk substitutes, practitioners need to evaluate infant growth using standardized growth charts based on breastfed infants. Otherwise, breastfeeding mothers might be told that their babies are gaining too slowly and that their milk production must be insufficient, when their babies are healthy in all respects. (See Chapter 10 on slow weight gain for a more detailed discussion of this issue.)

The drop of infant CCK levels 10 minutes after a feeding implies a "window" within which the infant can be awakened to feed from the second breast or to reattach to the first side for additional fat-rich milk. Waiting 30 minutes after the feeding before laying the baby down takes advantage of the second CCK peak to help the infant to stay asleep.

The studies cited here support giving fresh, rather than heat-treated or frozen, human milk whenever possible. Some living cells are killed by both of these treatments. Pasteurization significantly decreases concentrations of IgM, IgA, IgG and lysozymes (Koenig et al., 2005). Also, due to the action of the bile salt-stimulated lipase, fat in fresh human milk is absorbed more completely than that in pasteurized milk. Mixing mother's milk with formula is acceptable. It is particularly important for premature infants, who lack digestive enzymes, and mixing fresh human milk with formula improves fat absorption. Ideally, preterm infants will be receiving high volumes of their own mother's milk or mother's milk enriched with human milk components, both of which sustain excellent growth without the risks of bovine milk.

During the assessment phase of working with a breastfeeding family, the practitioner needs to ask if there is a family history of allergies. If so, the mother should be encouraged to breastfeed for a minimum of 12 months and to delay feeding the infant solid foods until the baby shows signs of readiness. Because of the risk of sensitization to allergenic proteins, particularly in babies who have a family history of allergies, even occasional formula supplements can trigger an allergic reaction and should be avoided as long as possible. In addition to preventing allergies, infant malabsorption problems, such as celiac disease, are lessened when the baby is breastfed and solid foods are delayed. Solid foods are usually started around 6 months of age as a baby's intestinal enzymes mature and become increasingly capable of digesting complex proteins and starches. After 6 months, babies can eat whatever they like and in any order they want.

In the maternal diet, dairy products are particularly potential allergens to the breastfeeding baby. If the mother notices that a particular food seems to cause an allergic response in her infant, she needs to consider eliminating it from her diet. A case report (Wilson, Self, & Hamburger, 1990) describes rectal bleeding in a 4-day-old infant who was exclusively breastfed: Her mother was drinking four to five glasses of cow's milk per day. Although this case is extreme and rare, it demonstrates the potential for problems when a breastfeeding mother drinks large quantities of cow's milk. Discussion of diet and appropriate substitution should be part of the care provided the mother by the healthcare worker offering lactation consultation and support.

Summary

The nutritional components of human milk, combined with its immune and antiallergic properties, make it the ideal foundation for optimal infant health. Immunological and allergy protection are obvious, but it is more difficult to substantiate the protection by breastfeeding against inflammatory and immunologically determined disorders that emerge later in life. There appears to be a threshold level for passive immunity conferred by breastmilk that is related to the amount of breastmilk a baby receives—a dose-response effect where exclusively breastfed infants benefit far more than infants who receive minimum amounts of breastmilk (Raisler, 1999).

Allowed to breastfeed at will in response to their own needs, infants generally obtain milk in amounts that satisfy their energy needs and maintain normal growth. Practical experience clearly supports the benefits of breastfeeding. In recent years, scientific data from all parts of the world confirm what the practitioner has long observed. It is ironic that many of the complex properties of human milk described in this chapter have been identified through research funded by formula companies, which stand to make large sums of money if they can develop products for which they can claim a close resemblance to human milk.

With the advent of managed care that rewards prevention of health problems and avoidance of using health services, healthcare corporations look for cost-effective ways to keep their insured clients healthy. Studies discussed in Chapter 2 show additional billions of dollars in healthcare costs for not breastfeeding.

Human milk has a remarkable fitness in terms of the demands and needs of the infant. The configuration of elements in breastmilk is nutritional programming with a reciprocal fitness between the mother and the infant. In special cases, such as the accelerated energy needs of the premature infant, this adaptability is seen in the greater availability of energy in preterm milk. Human milk is a carrier of important physiological messages to the recipient infant.

Key Concepts

- Human milk—the gold standard for infant nutriment—has between 57 to 65 kcal per deciliter.
- Breastfed infants ingest less volume than formula-fed infants because human milk is more energy efficient.
- Babies do not usually remove all the milk available in the breast during a single feeding.
- Small amounts of colostrum are produced in the first day or two after delivery followed by rapid increases to about 500 ml at five days postpartum.
- Differences in milk output from the right and left breasts are common. Milk output is often greater from the right breast.
- Milk storage capacity differs among women. Women with larger breasts have a greater milk storage capacity and may breastfeed less often; women with small breasts may need to breastfeed more often; otherwise, breast size does not affect the ability to breastfeed.
- Milk synthesis and volume differs between breasts.
- The nutritional status of a lactating mother has a minimal effect on milk volume unless she is malnourished.
- Multiparous women produce more breastmilk than primiparous women; mothers produce significantly more breastmilk with their second baby.
- Breastfed infants grow at about the same rate as those not breastfed for the first 3 to 4 months.
- Fat in human milk varies according to the degree to which the breast is emptied; high volume is associated with low milk fat content; accordingly, fat content progressively increases during a single feeding.
- Breastfeeding should be early and frequent; the longer the interval between feedings, the lower the fat content.
- The type of fat the mother eats affects the type of fatty acids present in her milk.
- Primary or congenital lactose deficiency or intolerance in infants is rare or nonexistent.

- Lactose in human milk supplies quick energy to the infant's rapidly growing brain.
- Human milk contains two main proteins: casein and whey. Casein is tough and less digestible curd; whey is soft and flocculent, and it digests rapidly.
- The amount of protein in colostrum is greater than that in mature milk because of the immune factors (IgA, lactoferrin) present in colostrum.
- Preterm mother's milk contains high levels of protein and fat compared with nonpreterm milk; thus using the milk of the preterm infant's mother is preferred.
- Generally speaking, human milk contains sufficient amounts of vitamins and minerals to meet the needs of full-term infants. Exceptions are premature infants and vitamin D supplementation for dark-skinned babies living in northern climates.
- Mineral content in human milk is fairly constant, tending to be highest right after birth and decreasing slightly throughout lactation.
- Healthy infants who consume enough breastmilk to satisfy their energy needs receive enough fluid to satisfy their requirements even in hot and dry environments.
- In the first 1 to 2 days after birth, the infant ingests small amounts, approximately 7 to 14 ml of colostrum at each feeding. Milk yield gradually increases for the first 36 hours, then rapidly increases. By day 5, volume is about 500 ml/day and 800 ml/day (range 550 and 1150) during months 1 and 6 of full breastfeeding.
- Immunity occurs actively and passively. Colostrum is densely packed with antibodies and immunoglobulins.
- Human milk contains two types of white cells: phagocytes and lymphocytes. Phagocytes (1) engulf and absorb pathogens and (2) release IgA. Lymphocytes (83 percent are T cells) protect an infant by destroying cell walls of viruses in a process called cell-mediated immunity.
- Antibodies are immunoglobulins that act against specific antigens or pathogens. Secretory IgA is the major immunoglobulin. Total sIgA remains relatively constant throughout lactation.
- sIgA passes from the mother's mucosa (intestinal, respiratory) to the mammary gland/breastmilk through lymphocyte traffic pathways (GALT and BALT).
- Immunity has a dose-response effect—the more breastmilk the infant ingests, the greater the immunity.

Internet Resources

CDC growth charts based on both breastfed and formula-fed infants:
http://www.cdc.gov/growthcharts

Report on DHA and AA in infant formula:
http://cornucopia.org/DHA/DHA_FullReport.pdf

References

Aarts E, Kylberg A, Hornell A, et al. How exclusive is breastfeeding? A comparison data since birth with current status data. *Int J Epidemiol*. 2000;29:1041–1046.

Abrams SA, Wen H, Stuff JE. Absorption of calcium, zinc, and iron from breast milk by five to seven-month-old infants. *Pediatr Res*. 1996;39:384–390.

Abdulmoneim I, Al-Gamdi SA. Relationship between breastfeeding duration and acute respiratory infections in infant. *Saudi Med J*. 2001;22:347–350.

Akisu M, Kultursay N, Ozkayin N, et al. Platelet-activating factor levels in term and pre-term milk. *Biol Neonate*. 1998;74:289–283.

Aljazaf KMNH. Ultrasound imaging in the analysis of the blood supply and blood flow in the human lactating breast [dissertation]. Perth, Australia, Medical Imaging Science, Curtin University of Technology; 2004.

Almroth S, Bidinger PD. No need for water supplementation for exclusively breast-fed infants under hot and arid conditions. *Trans Roy Soc Trop Med Hyg*. 1990;84:602–604.

Almroth SG, Latham MC. Breast feeding practices in rural Jamaica. *J Trop Pediatr*. 1982;28:103–109.

American Academy of Pediatrics, Committee on Nutrition. Commentary on breastfeeding and infant formulas, including standards for formulas. *Pediatrics*. 1976;57:278–285.

Anderson CH. Human milk feeding. *Pediatr Clin No Amer*. 1985;32:335–352.

Anderson JW, Johnstone BM, Remley DT. Breastfeeding and cognitive development: a meta-analysis. *Am J Clin Nutr*. 1999;70:25–35.

Andon MB et al. Nutritionally relevant supplementation of vitamin B_6 in lactating women: effect on plasma prolactin. *Pediatrics*. 1985;76:769–773.

Aniansson G et al. A prospective cohort study on breast-feeding and otitis media in Swedish infants. *Pediatr Infect Dis J*. 1994;13:183–188.

Anveden-Hertzberg L. Proctocolitis in exclusively breast-fed infants. *Eur J Pediatr*. 1996;155:464–467.

Arthur PG et al. Measuring short-term rates of milk synthesis in breast-feeding mothers. *Q J Exp Physiology*. 1989;47:419–428.

Arthur PG, Smith M, Hartmann PE. Milk lactose, citrate, and glucose as markers of lactogenesis in normal and diabetic women. *J Pediatr Gastroenterol Nutr*. 1989;9:488–496.

Ascher H et al. Influence of infant feeding and gluten intake on celiac disease. *Arch Dis Child*. 1997;76:113.

Ashraf RN et al. Breast feeding and protection against neonatal sepsis in a high-risk population. *Arch Dis Child*. 1991;66:488–490.

Atkinson SA, Anderson G, Bryan MH. Human milk: comparison of the nitrogen composition of milk from mothers of premature infants. *Am J Clin Nutr*. 1980;33:811–815.

Atkinson SA et al. Abnormal zinc content in human milk: risk for development of nutritional zinc deficiency in infants. *Am J Dis Child*. 1989;143:608–611.

Auricchio S et al. Does breast feeding protect against the development of clinical symptoms of celiac disease in children? *J Pediatr Gastroenterol Nutr*. 1983;2:428–433.

Axelsson I et al. Bovine beta-lactoglobulin in the human milk. *Acta Pediatr Scand*. 1986;75:702.

Bachrach VR, Schwarz E, Bachrach LR. Breastfeeding and the risk of hospitalization for respiratory disease in infancy: a meta-analysis. *Arch Pediatr Adolesc Med*. 2003;157:237–243.

Bates CJ, Prentice A. Breast milk as a source of vitamins, essential minerals and trace elements. *Pharmacol Ther*. 1994;62:193–220.

Bauchner J, Levanthal JM, Shapiro ED. Studies of breastfeeding and infections: how good is the evidence? *JAMA*. 1986;256:887–892.

Baur LA et al. Relationships between the fatty acid composition of muscle and erythrocyte membrane phospholipid in young children and the effect of type of infant feeding. *Lipids*. 2000;35:77–82.

Bell LM et al. Rotavirus serotype-specific neutralizing activity in human milk. *Am J Dis Child*. 1988;142:275–278.

Bellig LL. Immunization and the prevention of childhood diseases. *J Obstet Gynecol Neonatal Nurs*. 1995;24:469–477.

Bener A, Denic S, Galadari S. Longer breast-feeding and protection against childhood leukaemia and lymphomas. *European J Cancer*. 2001;37:234–238.

Bergstrand O, Hellers G. Breast-feeding during infancy in patients who develop Crohn's disease. *Scand J Gastroenterol*. 1983;18:903–906.

Bergstrom O et al. Serum lipid values in adolescents are related to family history, infant feeding, and physical growth. *Atherosclerosis*. 1995;17:1–13.

Blackberg LD et al. The bile salt-stimulated lipase in human milk is an evolutionary newcomer derived from a non-milk protein. *FEBS Lett*. 1980;112:151.

Blais DR, Harrold J, Altosaar I. Killing the messenger in the nick of time: persistence of breastmilk sCD14 in the neonatal gastrointestinal tract. *Pediatric Res*. 2006;59:371–376.

Borch-Johnson K et al. Relation between breast-feeding and incidence rates of insulin-dependent diabetes mellitus. *Lancet*. 1984;2:1083–1086.

Borgnolo G et al. A case-control study of Salmonella gastrointestinal infection in Italian children. *Acta Paediatr*. 1996;85:804–808.

Bottorff JL, Morse JM. Mother's perceptions of breast milk. *JOGN Nursing*. 1990;19:518–527.

Bouguerra F et al. Effect of breastfeeding relative to the age at onset of celiac disease. *Arch Pediatr*. 1998;5:621.

Brenna JT et al. Docosahexaenoic and arachidonic acid concentrations in human breastmilk worldwide. *Am J Clin Nutr*. 2007;85:1457–1464.

Brown KH et al. Lactational capacity of marginally nourished mothers: relationships between maternal nutritional status and quantity and proximate composition of milk. *Pediatrics*. 1986a;78:909–919.

Brown KH et al. Milk consumption and hydration status of exclusively breast-fed infants in a warm climate. *J Pediatr*. 1986b;108:677–680.

Brown KH et al. Infant-feeding practices and their relationship with diarrheal and other diseases in Huascar (Lima), Peru. *Pediatrics*. 1989;83:31–40.

Buescher ES, Pickering LK. Polymorphonuclear leukocytes in human colostrum and milk. In: Howell RR, Morriss FH, Pickering LK, eds. *Human milk in infant nutrition and health*. Springfield, Ill: Thomas; 1986:160–173.

Burr ML et al. Infant feeding, wheezing, and allergy: a prospective study. *Arch Dis Child*. 1993;68:724–728.

Butte NF, Smith EO, Garza C. Energy utilization of breast-fed and formula-fed infants. *Am J Clin Nutr*. 1990;51:350–358.

Butte NF et al. Macro- and trace-mineral intakes of exclusively breast-fed infants. *Am J Clin Nutr*. 1987;45:42–47.

Butte NF et al. Influence of early feeding mode on body composition of infants. *Biol Neonate*. 1995;67:414–424.

Butte NF et al. Energy requirements derived from total energy expenditure and energy deposition during the first 2 years of life. *Am J Clin Nutr*. 2000;72:1558–1569.

Carpenter G. Epidermal growth factor is a major growth-promoting agent in human milk. *Science.* 1980;210:198–199.

Casey CE, Hambidge KM, Neville MC. Studies in human lactation: zinc, copper, manganese and chromium in human milk in the first month of lactation. *Am J Clin Nutr.* 1985;41:1193–1200.

Casey CE, Neville MC, Hambidge KM. Studies in human lactation: secretion of zinc, copper, and manganese in human milk. *Am J Clin Nutr.* 1989;49: 773–785.

Caspi A, Williams B, Kim-Cohen J. Moderation of breastfeeding effect on the IQ by genetic variation in fatty acid metabolism. *Proc Natl Acad Sci USA.* 2007;104(47):188860–188865.

Cavagni G et al. Passage of food antigens into circulation of breast-fed infants with atopic dermatitis. *Ann Allergy.* 1988;61:361–365.

Cavell B. Gastric emptying in infants fed human or infant formula. *Acta Paediatr Scand.* 1981;70: 639–641.

Cesar JA, Victoria CG, Barros FC. Impact of breastfeeding on admission for pneumonia during postneonatal period in Brazil: nested case-control study. *Br Med J.* 1999;318:1316–1320.

Chandra RK. Prospective studies of the effect of breastfeeding on incidence of infection and allergy. *Acta Paediatr Scand.* 1979;68:691–694.

Chandra RK et al. Influence of maternal food antigen avoidance during pregnancy and lactation on incidence of atopic eczema in infants. *Clin Allergy.* 1986;16:563–569.

Chen A, Rogan WJ. Breastfeeding and the risk of post neonatal death in the United States. *Pediatrics.* 2004;113:435–439.

Chen Y, Yu S, Li W. Artificial feeding and hospitalization in the first 18 months of life. *Pediatrics.* 1988; 81:58–62.

Chowanadisai W, Lönnerdal B, Kelleher SL. Identification of a mutation in SLC30A2 (ZnT-2) in women with low milk zinc concentration that results in transient neonatal zinc deficiency. *J Biol Chem.* 2006;281: 39699–39707.

Chulada PC et al. Breast-feeding and the prevalence of asthma and wheeze in children: analyses from the third national health and nutrition examination survey, 1988–1994. *J Allergy Clin Immunol.* 2003;111: 328–336.

Clavano NR. Mode of feeding and its effect on infant mortality and morbidity. *J Trop Pediatr.* 1982;28: 287–293.

Cochi SL et al. Primary invasive *Haemophilus influenzae* type b disease: a population-based assessment of risk factors. *J Pediatr.* 1986;108:87–96.

Cohen RJ et al. Exclusively breastfed, low birth weight term infants do not need supplemental water. *Acta Paediatr.* 2000;89:550–552.

Corps AN et al. The insulin-like growth factor I content in human milk increases between early and full lactation. *J Clin Endocrinol Metab.* 1988;67:25–29.

Cosgrove M. Perinatal and infant nutrition: nucleotides. *Nutrition.* 1998;14:748.

Cox DB, Owens RA, Hartmann PE. Blood and milk prolactin and the rate of milk synthesis in women. *Exp Physiol.* 1996;81:1007–1020.

Cregan MD, Hartmann PE. Computerized breast measurement from conception to weaning: clinical implications. *J Hum Lact.* 1999;15:89–95.

Cregan MD et al. Identification of nestin-positive putative mammary stem cells in human breastmilk. *Cell Tissue Res.* 2007;329:129.

Cregan MD, Mitoulas LR, Hartmann PE. Milk prolactin, feed volume, and duration between feeds in women breastfeeding their full-term infants over a 24-hour period. *Exp Physiol.* 2002;87:207–214.

Cushing AH et al. Breastfeeding reduces the risk of respiratory illness in infants. *Am J Epidemiol.* 1998; 147:863–870.

Dai D et al. Role of oligosaccharides and glycoconjugates in intestinal host defense. *J Pediatr Gastroenterol Nutr.* 2000;30(suppl):23.

Daly SE, Hartmann PE. Infant demand and milk supply. Part 1: Infant demand and milk production in lactating women. *J Hum Lact.* 1995a;11:21–26.

Daly SE, Hartmann PE. Infant demand and milk supply. Part 2: The short-term control of milk synthesis in lactating women. *J Hum Lact.* 1995b;11:27–36.

Daly SE, Owens RA, Hartmann PE. The short-term synthesis and infant-regulated removal of milk in lactating women. *Exp Physiol.* 1993;78:209–220.

Daly SE et al. The determination of short-term breast volume changes and the rate of synthesis of human milk using computerized breast measurement. *Exp Physiol.* 1992;77:79–87.

Daly SE et al. Degree of breast emptying explains changes in the fat content, but not fatty acid composition of human milk. *Exp Physiol.* 1993;78:741–755.

Daniels JL et al. Breast-feeding and neuroblastoma, USA and Canada. *Cancer Causes Control.* 2002;13:401–405.

Davis MK. Review of the evidence for an association between infant feeding and childhood cancer. *Int J Cancer.* 1998;S11:29–33.

Davis MK, Savitz DA, Graubard B. Infant feeding and childhood cancer. *Lancet.* 1988;2(8607):365–368.

de Araujo AN, Giugliano LG. Lactoferrin and free secretory component of human milk inhibits the adhesion of enteropathic *Escherichia coli* to HeLa cells. *BMC Microbiol.* 2001;1:25.

de Ferrer PA et al. Lactoferrin levels in term and preterm milk. *J Amer College Nutr.* 2000;19:370–373.

Dell S, To T. Breastfeeding and asthma in young children: findings from a population-based study. *Arch Pediatr Adolesc Med.* 2001;155:1261–1265.

Demmers TA et al. Effects of early cholesterol intake on cholesterol biosynthesis and plasma lipids among infants until 28 months of age. *Pediatrics.* 2005;115: 1594–1601.

Dewey KG, Heinig J, Nommsen-Rivers LA. Differences in morbidity between breast-fed and formula-fed infants. *J Pediatr.* 1995;126:697–702.

Dewey KG, Lönnerdal B. Milk and nutrient intake of breast-fed infants from 1 to 6 months: relation to growth and fatness. *J Pediatr Gastroenterol Nutr.* 1983; 2:497–506.

Dewey KG et al. Breast-fed infants are leaner than formula-fed infants at 1 year of age: the DARLING study. *Am J Clin Nutr.* 1993;57:140–145.

Dewey KG et al. Growth of breast-fed infants deviates from current reference data: a pooled analysis of US, Canadian, and European data sets. *Pediatrics.* 1995; 96:495–503.

Dewey KG et al. Iron supplementation affects growth and morbidity of breast-fed infants: results of a randomized trial in Sweden and Honduras. *J Nutr.* 2002; 132:3249–3255.

Dorea JG. Iron and copper in human milk. *Nutrition.* 2000;16:209–220.

Downham MA et al. Breast-feeding protects against respiratory syncytial virus infection. *Br Med J.* 1976; 2:274–276.

Duchen K, Yu G, Björkstén B. Polyunsaturated fatty acids in breast milk in relation to atopy in the mother and her child. *Int Arch Allergy Immunol.* 1999;118:321–323.

Duffy LC et al. The effects of infant feeding on rotavirus-induced gastroenteritis: a prospective study. *Am J Public Health.* 1986;76:259–263.

Duncan B et al. Iron and the exclusively breast-fed infant from birth to six months. *J Pediatr Gastroenterol Nutr.* 1985;4:412–425.

Duncan J et al. Exclusive breast-feeding for at least 4 months protects against otitis media. *Pediatrics.* 1993;91:867–872.

Engstrom JL et al. Comparison of milk output from the right and left breasts during simultaneous pumping in mothers of very low birth weight infants. *Breastfeeding Medicine.* 2007;2:83–91.

Erickson PR, Mazhari E. Investigation of the role of human breast milk in caries development. *Pediatr Dent.* 1999;21:86–90.

Espinoza E et al. Rotavirus infections in young Nicaraguan children. *Pediatr Infect Dis.* 1997;16:564–571.

Evans GS, Johnson PE. Characterization and quantitation of a zinc-binding ligand and human milk. *Pediatr Res.* 1980;14:876–880.

Fallot MB et al. Breast-feeding reduces incidence of hospital admissions for infections in infants. *Pediatrics.* 1980;65:1121–1124.

Fan H, Conner R, Villareal L. *The Biology of AIDS.* Boston, Mass: Jones and Bartlett; 1989:28.

Fawzi WW et al. Maternal anthropometry and infant feeding practices in Israel in relation to growth in infancy: the North African Infant Feeding Study. *Am J Clin Nutr.* 1997;65:1731–1737.

Feist N, Berger D, Speer CP. Anti-endotoxin antibodies in human milk: correlation with infection of the newborn. *Acta Paediatr.* 2000;89:1087–1092.

Ford RPK et al. Breastfeeding and the risk of sudden infant death syndrome. *Int J Epidemiol.* 1993;22: 885–890.

Forman MR et al. Undernutrition among Bedouin Arab infants: the Bedouin Infant Feeding Study. *Am J Clin Nutr.* 1990;51:339–343.

Frank AL et al. Breast-feeding and respiratory virus infection. *Pediatrics.* 1982;70:239–245.

Franke AA, Custer LJ, Tanaka Y. Isoflavones in human breast milk and other biological fluids. *Am J Clin Nutr.* 1998;68(suppl):1466S–1473S.

Fuchs SC, Victor CG, Martines J. Case-control study of risk of dehydrating diarrhoea in infants in vulnerable period after full weaning. *BMJ.* 1996;313:391–394.

Furukawa SK et al. Fecal IgE in infants at 1 month of age as indicator of atopic disease. *Allergy.* 1994;49: 791–794.

Garofalo RP, Goldman AS. Cytokines, chemokines, and colony-stimulating factors in human milk. *Biol Neonate.* 1998;74:134–142.

Garofalo RP, Goldman AS. Expression of functional immunomodulating and anti-inflammatory factors in human milk. *Clin Perinatol.* 1999;26:361.

Gartner LM, Greer FR. Prevention of rickets and vitamin D deficiency: new guidelines for vitamin D intake. *Pediatrics.* 2003;111(Part 1):908–910.

Garza C, Stuff J, Butte N. Growth of the breast-fed infant. In: Goldman AS, Atkinson SA, Hanson LA, eds. *Human Lactation: The Effects of Human Milk on the Recipient Infant.* New York, NY: Plenum; 1986: 109–121.

Garza C et al. Changes in the nutrient composition of human milk during gradual weaning. *Am J Clin Nutr.* 1983;37:61–65.

Garza C et al. Special properties of human milk. *Clin Perinatol.* 1987;14:11–31.

Gaull GE. Significance of growth modulators in human milk. *Pediatrics.* 1985;75(suppl):142–145.

Gdalevich M, Mimouni D, Mimouni M. Breast-feeding and the risk of bronchial asthma in childhood: a systematic review with meta-analysis of prospective studies. *J Pediatr.* 2001;139:261–266.

Gilbert RE et al. Bottle-feeding and the sudden infant death syndrome. *BMJ.* 1995;310:88–90.

Gimeno SGA, de Suza JMP. IDDM and milk consumption. *Diabetes Care.* 1997;20:1256–1260.

Glass RI, Stoll BJ. The protective effect of human milk against diarrhea: a review of studies from Bangladesh. *Acta Paediatr Scand.* 1989;351(suppl):131–136.

Goldman AS et al. Immunologic factors in human milk during the first year of lactation. *J Pediatr.* 1982; 100:563–567.

Goldman AS et al. Immunologic components in human milk during gradual weaning. *Acta Paediatr Scand.* 1983;72:133–134.

Goldman AS et al. Anti-inflammatory properties of human milk. *Acta Paediatr Scand.* 1986;75:689–695.

Goldman AS et al. Cytokines in human milk: properties and potential effects upon the mammary gland and the neonate. *J Mammary Gland Biol Neoplasia.* 1996;1:251–258.

Grantham-McGregor SM, Back EH. Breast feeding in Kingston, Jamaica. *Arch Dis Child.* 1972;45:404–409.

Greco L et al. Case control study on nutritional risk factors in celiac disease. *J Pediar Gastroenterol Nutr.* 1983;7:395–399.

Greer FR. Vitamin K status of lactating mothers and their infants. *Acta Paediatr.* 1999;88(suppl):95.

Greer FR Marshall S. Bone mineral content, serum vitamin D metabolite concentrations and ultraviolet B light exposure in infants fed human milk with and without vitamin D2 supplements. *J Pediatr.* 1989;114:204–212.

Groer M, Davis M, Steele K. Associations between human milk sIgA and maternal immune, infections, endocrine, and stress variables. *J Hum Lact.* 2004;20:153–158.

Groer MW, Humenick S, Hill P. Characterizations and psychoneuroimmunologic implications of secretory immunoglobulin A and cortisol in preterm and term breast milk. *J Perinat Neonatal Nurs.* 1994;7:42–51.

Gulick EE. The effect of breast-feeding on toddler health. *Pediatr Nurs.* 1986;12:51–54.

Gunnarsdottir I et al. Infant feeding patterns and midlife erythrocyte sedimentation rate. *Acta Paediatrica.* 2007;96:852–856.

Guthrie HA, Picciano MF, Sheehe D. Fatty acid patterns of human milk. *J Pediatr.* 1977;90:39–41.

Gyorgy P. A hitherto unrecognized biochemical difference between human milk and cow's milk. *Pediatrics.* 1953;11:98–104.

Habbick BF, Kahnna C, To T. Infantile hypertropic pyloric stenosis: a study of feeding practices and other possible causes. *Can Med Assoc J.* 1989;140:401–404.

Habicht JP, DaVanso J, Butz WP. Mother's milk and sewage: their interactive effects on infant mortality. *Pediatrics.* 1988;81:456–460.

Hakansson A, Svensson M, Mossberg A-K et al. A folding variant of α-lactalbumin with bactericidal activity against *Streptococcus pneumoniae*. *Molec Microbiol.* 2000;35:589–600.

Hakansson A et al. Apoptosis induced by a human protein. *Proc Natl Acad Sci.* 1995;92:8064.

Hamosh M. Human milk. Digestion in the neonate. *Clin Perinatol.* 1996;23:191.

Hamosh M. Bioactive factors in human milk. In: Schanler, RJ, ed. *The Evidence for Breastfeeding*. Breastfeeding 2001, Part I. *Ped Clin N Amer.* 2001;48:69–86.

Hamosh M et al. Digestive enzymes in human milk: stability at suboptimal storage temperatures. *J Pediatr Gastroenterol Nutr.* 1997;24:38–43.

Hartmann PE. Lactation and reproduction in Western Australian women. *J Reprod Med.* 1987;32:543–557.

Hartmann PE, Cregan M. Lactogenesis and the effects of insulin-dependent diabetes mellitus and prematurity. *J Nutrition.* 2001;131:3016S–3020S.

Hartmann PE, Prosser CG. Physiological basis of longitudinal changes in human milk yield and composition. *Fed Proc.* 1984;43:2448–2453.

Hashizume S, Kuroda K, Murakami H. Identification of lactoferrin as an essential growth factor for human lymphocytic cell lines in serum-free medium. *Biochem Biophys Acta.* 1983;763:377.

Hasselbalch H et al. Breastfeeding influences thymic size in late infancy. *Eur J Pediatr.* 1999;158:964–967.

Hawkes JS, Gibson RA. Lymphocyte subpopulations in breast-fed and formula-fed infants at six months of age. *Adv Exp Med Biol.* 2001;501:497–504.

Heacock H et al. Influence of breast versus formula milk on physiological gastroesophageal reflux in healthy, newborn infants. *J Pediatr Gastroenterol.* 1992;14:41–46.

Heinig J et al. Zinc supplementation does not affect growth, morbidity, or motor development of US term breastfed infants at 4–10 mo of age. *Am J Clin Nutr.* 2006;84:594–601.

Heird WC, Schward SM, Hansen IH. Colostrum-induced enteric mucosal growth in beagle puppies. *Pediatr Res.* 1984;18:512.

Hildebrandt HM. Maternal perception of lactogenesis time: a clinical report. *J Hum Lact.* 1999;15:317–323.

Holberg CJ et al. Risk factors for respiratory syncytial virus-associated lower respiratory illnesses in the first year of life. *Am J Epidemiol.* 1991;133:1135–1151.

Host A, Husby S, Osterballe O. A prospective study of cow's milk allergy in exclusively breast-fed infants. *Acta Paediatr Scand.* 1988;77:663–670.

Hornell A et al. Breastfeeding patterns in exclusively breastfed infants: a longitudinal prospective study in Uppsala, Sweden. *Acta Paediatr.* 1999;88:203–211.

Houston MJ, Howie PW, McNeilly AS. Factors affecting the duration of breast feeding: 1. measurement of breast milk intake in the first week of life. *Early Hum Dev.* 1983;8:49–54.

Howie PW et al. Protective effect of breast feeding against infection. *Br Med J.* 1990;300:11–16.

Humenick SS. The clinical significance of breastmilk maturation rates. *Birth.* 1987;14:174–179.

Humenick SS et al. The maturation index of colostrum and milk (MICAM): a measurement of breast milk maturation. *J Nurs Measurement.* 1994;2:16-86.

Hylander MA et al. Association of human milk feedings with a reduction in retinopathy of prematurity among very low birth weight infants. *J Perinatology.* 2001;21:356–362.

Ingram JC, Woolridge MS, Greenwood RJ. Breastfeeding: it is worth trying with the second baby. *Lancet.* 2001;358:986–987.

Istre GR et al. Risk factors for primary *Haemophilus influenzae* disease: increased risk from day care attendance and school-aged household members. *J Pediatr.* 1985;106:190–195.

Ivarsson A et al. Epidemic of celiac disease in Swedish children. *Acta Pediatr.* 2000;89:165.

Jason JM, Niebury P, Marks JS. Mortality and infectious disease associated with infant-feeding practices in developing countries. *Pediatrics.* 1984;74(suppl):702–727.

Jenkins HR et al. Food allergy: the major cause of infantile colitis. *Arch Dis Child.* 1984;59:326–329.

Jensen CL. Effects of maternal docosahexaenoic acid intake on visual function and neurodevelopment in breastfed term infants. *Am J Clin Nutr.* 2005;82:125–132.

Jensen RG. Lipids in human milk. *Lipids*. 1999;34:1243.

Jensen RG et al. Human milk as a carrier of messages to the nursing infant. *Nutr Today*. 1988;23:20–25.

Juex G et al. Growth pattern of selected urban Chilean infants during exclusive breast feeding. *Am J Clin Nutr*. 1983;38:462–468.

Kassim OO et al. Inhibitory factors in breast milk, maternal and infant sera against in vitro growth of *Plasmodium falciparum* malaria parasite. *J Trop Pediatr*. 2000;46:92–96.

Kelleher SL, Lönnerdal B. Immunological activities associated with milk. *Adv Nutr Res*. 2001;10:39–65.

Keller MA et al. IgAG$_4$ in human colostrum and human milk: continued local production or selective transport form serum. *Acta Paediatr Scand*. 1988;77:24–29.

Kelly DW et al. Rise and fall of coeliac disease 1960–1985. *Arch Dis Child*. 1989;64:1157–1160.

Kent JC et al. Volume and frequency of breastfeedings and fat content of breastmilk throughout the day. *Pediatrics*. 2006;117:387–395.

Kent et al. Breast volume and milk production during extended lactation in women. *Exp Physiol*. 1999; 82:435–447.

Khin-Maung-U J et al. Effect of clinical outcome of breastfeeding during acute diarrhea. *Br Med J*. 1985; 290:587–589.

Kirkpatrick CH et al. Inhibition of growth of *Candida albicans* by iron-unsaturated lactoferrin: relation to host defense mechanisms in chronic mucocutaneous candidiasis. *J Infect Dis*. 1971;124:539.

Kobata R et al. High levels of growth factors in human breast milk. *Early Hum Dev*. 2008;84:67–9.

Koenig A et al. Immunologic factors in human milk: the effects of gestational age and pasteurization. *J Hum Lact*. 2005;21(4):439–443.

Kohler H et al. Antibacterial characteristics in the feces of breast-fed and formula-fed infants during the first year of life. *J Pediatr Gastroenterol Nutr*. 2002;34: 188–193.

Koletzko B, Rodriquez-Palmero M. Polyunsaturated fatty acids in human milk and their role in early human development. *J Mammary Gland Biol Neoplasia*. 1999;4:269.

Koletzko S et al. Role of infant feeding practices in development of Crohn's disease in childhood. *Br Med J*. 1989;298:1617–1618.

Koopman JS et al. Infant formulas and gastrointestinal illness. *Am J Public Health*. 1985;75:477–480.

Koerber A. From folklore to fact: the rhetorical history of breastfeeding immunity, 1950–1997. *J Med Humanity*. 2006;27:151–166.

Kostraba JN et al. Early exposure to cow's milk and solid foods in infancy, genetic predisposition and risk of IDDM. *Diabetes*. 1993;42:288–295.

Kovar MG et al. Review of the epidemiologic evidence for an association between infant feeding and infant health. *Pediatrics*. 1984;74(suppl):615–638.

Krachler M, Rossipal SE, Irgolic KJ. Changes in the concentrations of trace elements in human milk during lactation. *J Trace Elements Biol*. 1998;12: 159–176.

Kramer MS, Aboud F, Mironova E, et al. Breastfeeding and child cognitive development: new evidence from a large randomized trial. *Arch Gen Psychiatry*. 2008;65:578–584.

Kramer MS. Infant feeding, infection, and public health. *Pediatrics*. 1988;81:164–166.

Kramer MS et al. Promotion of breastfeeding intervention trial (PROBIT): a randomized trial in the Republic of Belarus. *JAMA*. 2001;285:413–420.

Kramer MS et al. Breastfeeding and infant growth: biology or bias? *Pediatrics*. 2002;110:343–347.

Krebs NF, Hambidge KM. Zinc requirements and zinc intakes of breast-fed infants. *Am J Clin Nutr*. 1986;43:288–292.

Krebs NF et al. Zinc homeostasis in breast-fed infant. *Pediatr Res*. 1996;39:661–665.

Kulski JK, Hartmann PE. Changes in the concentration of cortisol in milk during different stages of human lactation. *Aust J Exp Biol Med Sci*. 1981;59:769.

Kumar A et al. Cord blood and breast milk iron status in maternal anemia. *Pediatrics*. 2008;121:e673–e677.

Kum-Nji et al. Reducing the incidence of sudden infant death syndrome in the delta region of Mississippi: a three-pronged approach. *South Med J*. 2001;94: 704–710.

Kumpulainen J et al. Formula feeding results in lower selenium status than breast-feeding or selenium-supplemented formula feeding: a longitudinal study. *Am J Clin Nutr*. 1987;45:49–53.

Kunz C, Lönnerdal B. Re–evaluation of the whey protein/casein ratio of human milk. *Acta Paediatr*. 1992;81:107–112.

Kwan ML et al. Breastfeeding patterns and risk of childhood acute lymphoblastic leukaemia. Br J *Cancer*. 2005;93:379–384.

Kwan ML et al. Breastfeeding and the risk of childhood leukemia: a meta-analysis. *Public Health Rep*. 2004;119:521–535.

Labbok M, Hendershot GE. Does breast-feeding protect against malocclusion? An analysis of the 1981 Child Health Supplement to the National Health Interview survey. *Am J Priv Med*. 1987;3:227–232.

Larsson LA. *Immunobiology of Human Milk*. Amarillo, Tex: Pharmasoft; 2004:32.

Latarte J et al. Lack of protective effect of breast-feeding in congenital hypothyroidism: report of 12 cases. *Pediatrics*. 1980;65:703–705.

Lawlor DA et al. Associations of parental, birth, and early life characteristics with systolic blood pressure at 5 years of age. *Circulation*. 2004;110:2417–2423.

Lawrence RM, Pane CA. Human breast milk: current concepts of immunology and infectious diseases. *Curr Probl Pediatr Adolesc Health Care*. 2007;37:7–36.

Leach JL et al. Total potentially available nucleotides of human milk by stage of lactation. *Am J Clin Nutr.* 1995;61:1224–1230.

Lemons JA et al. Differences in the composition of preterm and term human milk during early lactation. *Pediatr Res.* 1982;16:113–117.

Lepage G et al. The composition of preterm milk in relation to the degree of prematurity. *Am J Clin Nutr.* 1984;40:1042–1049.

Leventhal JM et al. Does breastfeeding protect against infection in infants less than 3 months of age? *Pediatrics.* 1986;78:896–903.

Litwin SD, Zehr BD, Insel RA. Selective concentration of IgD class-specific antibodies in human milk. *Clin Exp Immunol.* 1990;80:262–267.

Long K et al. The impact of infant feeding patterns on infection and diarrheal disease due to enterotoxigenic *Escherichia coli. Salud Publica Mex.* 1999;41:263–270.

Lönnerdal B. Regulation of mineral and trace elements in human milk: exogenous and endogenous factors. *Nutr Review.* 2000;58:223–229.

Lopez-Alarcon M, Villalpando S, Fajardo A. Breast-feeding lowers the frequency and duration of acute respiratory infection and diarrhea in infants under six months of age. *J Nutr.* 1997;127:436–443.

Lovegrove JA, Hampton SM, Morgan JB. The immunological and long-term atopic outcome of infants born to women following a milk-free diet during late pregnancy and lactation: a pilot study. *Br J Nutr.* 1994;71:223–238.

Lucas A. Programming by early nutrition: an experimental approach. *J Nutr.* 1998;128:401S–406S.

Lucas A, Cole TJ. Breast milk and neonatal necrotizing enterocolitis. *Lancet.* 1990;336:1519–1523.

Lucas A, Mitchell MD. Prostaglandins in human milk. *Arch Dis Child.* 1980;55:950.

Lucas A et al. Breastfeeding and catch-up growth in infants born small for gestational age. *Acta Paediatr.* 1997;86:564–569.

Mackey AD, Picciano MF. Maternal folate status during extended lactation and the effect of supplemental folic acid. *Am J Clin Nutr.* 1999;69:285.

Malcolm CA et al. Maternal docosahexaenoic acid supplementation during pregnancy and visual evoked potential development in term infants: a double blind, prospective, randomised trial. *Arch Dis Child.* 2003;88:F383.

Mandel D et al. Fat and energy contents of expressed human breast milk in prolonged lactation. *Pediatrics.* 2005;116:e432–e435.

Marchini G, Linden A. Cholecystokinin, a satiety signal in newborn infants? *J Dev Physiol.* 1992;17:215–219.

Marild S et al. Protective effect of breastfeeding against urinary tract infection. *Acta Paediatr.* 2004;93:164–167.

Martin R et al. Probiotic potential of 3 lactobacilli strains isolated from breast milk. *J Hum Lact.* 2005a;21:8–17.

Martin RM et al. Breast-feeding and childhood cancer: a systematic review with meta-analysis. *Int. J Cancer.* 2005b;117:1020–1031.

Martin RM et al. Breastfeeding and atherosclerosis: intima-media thickness and plaques at 65-year follow-up of the Boyd Orr Cohort. *Arterioscler Thrombo Vasc Biol.* 2005c;25:1482–1488.

Mason T et al. Breast feeding and the development of juvenile rheumatoid arthritis. *J Rheumatol.* 1995;22:1166–1170.

Mathur GP et al. Breastfeeding and childhood cancer. *Indian Pediatr.* 1993;30:651–657.

Matsuoka Y, Idota T. The concentration of epidermal growth factor in Japanese mother's milk. *J Nutr Sci Vitaminol.* 1995;41:24–51.

Mayer EJ et al. Reduced risk of IDDM among breast-fed children. *Diabetes.* 1988;37:1625–1632.

McVeagh P, Miller JB. Human milk oligosaccharides: only the breast. *J Paediatr Child Health.* 1997;33:281–286.

Medves JM. Three infant care interventions: reconsidering the evidence. *JOGNN.* 2002;31:563–569.

Metcalfe DD. Food hypersensitivity. *J Allergy Clin Immunol.* 1984;73:749–762.

Michie et al. Physiological secretion of chemokines in human breast milk. *Eur Cytokine Netw.* 1998;9:123–129.

Minekawa R et al. Human breast milk suppresses the transcriptional regulation of IL-1(beta)-induced NF-(kappa)B signaling in human intestinal cells. *Am J Physiol.* 2004;287:C1404–C1411.

Miralles O et al. A physiological role of breast milk leptin in body weight control in developing infants. *Obesity.* 2006;14:1371–1377.

Mitra AK, Rabbani F. The importance of breastfeeding in minimizing mortality and morbidity from diarrhoeal diseases: the Bangladesh perspective. *J Diarrhoeal Dis Res.* 1995;13:1–7.

Montgomery RK et al. Lactose intolerance and the genetic regulation of intestinal lactose-phlorizin hydrotase. *Fed Am Soc Exp Biol J.* 1991;5:2824–2832.

Morriss FH. Method for investigating the presence and physiologic role of growth factors in milk. In: Jensen RG, Neville MC, eds. *Human Lactation: Milk Components and Methodologies.* New York, NY: Plenum; 1985:193–200.

Morriss FH et al. Relationship of human milk pH during course of lactation to concentrations of citrate and fatty acids. *Pediatrics.* 1986;78:458–464.

Morrisset J, Jolicoeur L. Effect of hydrocortisone on pancreatic growth in rats. *Am J Physiol.* 1980;239:295.

Morton JA. The clinical usefulness of breast milk sodium in the assessment of lactogenesis. *Pediatrics.* 1994;93:802–806.

Motil KJ, Krtz B, Thotathuchery M. Lactation performance of adolescent mothers show preliminary differences from that of adult women. *J Adolescent Med.* 1997;20:442–449.

Motil KJ et al. Human milk protein does not limit growth of breast-fed infants. *J Pediatr Gastroenterol Nutr.* 1997;24:10–17.

Naficy AB et al. Epidemiology of rotavirus diarrhea in Egyptian children and implications for disease control. *Am J Epidemiol.* 1999;150:770–777.

Neville MC. Lactogenesis. In: Schanler RJ, ed. *Breastfeeding 2001. Part I. The Evidence for Breastfeeding. Ped Clin N Amer.* 2001;48:69–86.

Neville MC, Oliva-Rasbach J. Is maternal milk production limiting for infant growth during the first year of life in breast-fed infants? In: Goldman AS, Atkinson SA, Hanson LA, eds. *Human Lactation.* Vol. 3. New York, NY: Plenum; 1987:123–133.

Neville MC et al. Studies in human lactation: milk volumes in lactating women during the onset of lactation and full lactation. *Am J Clin Nutr.* 1988;48:1375–1386.

Newburg DS et al. Role of human-milk lactadherin in protection against symptomatic rotavirus infection. *Lancet.* 1998;351:1160.

Newman J. How breast milk protects newborns. *Scientific American.* December 1995:76–79.

Nommsen-Rivers L. The long-term effects of early nutrition: the role of breastfeeding on cholesterol levels. *J Hum Lact.* 2003;19:103–104.

Oddy WH et al. The relation of breastfeeding and body mass index to asthma and atopy in children: a prospective cohort study to age 6 years. *Am J Public Health.* 2004;94:1531–1537.

Oddy WH. Breastfeeding and asthma in children: findings from a West Australian study. *Breastfeeding Rev.* 2000;8:5–11.

Odze RD et al. Allergic colitis in infants. *J Pediatr.* 1995;126:163–170.

Okamoto Y, Ogra P. Antiviral factors in human milk: implications in respiratory syncytial virus infection. *Acta Paediatr Scand.* 1989;351(suppl):137–143.

Ostrea EM et al. Influence of breast-feeding on the restoration of the low serum concentration of vitamin E and beta-carotene in the newborn infant. *Am J Obstet Gyncecol.* 1986;154:1014–1017.

Owen CD et al. Infant feeding and blood cholesterol: a study in adolescents and a systematic review. *Pediatrics.* 2002;110:597–608.

Pabst HE et al. Differential modulation of the immune response to breast- or formula-feeding of infants. *Acta Paediatr.* 1997;86:1291–1297.

Paganelli R, Cavagni G, Pallone F. The role of antigenic absorption and circulating immune complexes in food allergy. *Ann Allergy.* 1986;57:330–336.

Palmer B. The influence of breastfeeding on the development of the oral cavity: a commentary. *J Hum Lact.* 1998;14:93–99.

Perera BJ et al. The impact of breastfeeding practices on respiratory and diarrhoeal disease in infants: a study from Sri Lanka. *J Trop Pediatr.* 1999;45:115–118.

Perez-Bravolt F et al. Genetic predisposition and environmental factors leading to the development of insulin-dependent diabetes mellitus in Chilean children. *J Mol Med.* 1996;74:105–109.

Petschow B et al. Influence of orally administered epidermal growth factor on normal and damaged intestinal mucosa in rats. *J Pediatr Gastroenterol Nutr.* 1993;17:49–57.

Picciano MF. Nutrient composition of human milk. In: Schanler RJ, ed. *Breastfeeding 2001, Part I. The evidence for breastfeeding. Ped Clin N Amer.* 2001;48:69–86.

Pickering LK, Kohl S. Human milk humoral immunity and infant defense mechanisms. In: Howell RR, Morriss FH, Pickering LK, eds. *Human Milk in Infant Nutrition and Health.* Springfield, Ill: Thomas; 1986:123–140.

Pisacane A et al. Breast feeding and urinary tract infection. *Lancet.* 1990;336:50.

Pisacane A et al. Breast feeding and multiple sclerosis. *Br Med J.* 1994;308:1411–1412.

Pisacane A et al. Breast-feeding and inguinal hernia. *J Pediatr.* 1995a;127:109–111.

Pisacane A et al. Breast feeding and acute appendicitis. *BMJ.* 1995b;310:836–837.

Popkin BM et al. Breast-feeding and diarrheal morbidity. *Pediatrics.* 1990;86:874–882.

Porro E et al. Early wheezing and breast feeeding. *Asthma.* 1993;30:23–28.

Prentice AM, Collinson AC. Does breastfeeding increase thymus size? *Acta Paediatr.* 2000;89:8–10.

Prentice AM et al. Breast-milk antimicrobial factors of rural Gambian mothers. *Acta Paediatr Scand.* 1984;73:796–812.

Prosser CG, Saint L, Hartmann PE. Mammary gland function during gradual weaning and early gestation in women. *Aust J Exp Biol Med Sci.* 1984;62:215–228.

Pullan CR et al. Breast-feeding and respiratory syncytial virus infection. *Br Med J.* 1980;281(6247):1034–1036.

Quigley MA, Kelly YJ, Sacker A. Breastfeeding and hospitalization for diarrheal and respiratory infection in the United Kingdom Millennium Cohort Study. *Pediatrics.* 2007;119:e837–e842.

Quinlan PT et al. The relationship between stool hardness and stool composition in breast- and formula-fed infants. *J Pediatr Gastroenterol Nutr.* 1995;20:81–90.

Rahman MM et al. Local production of rotavirus specific IgA in breast tissue and transfer to neonates. *Arch Dis Child.* 1987;62:401–405.

Raiha NCR. Nutritional proteins in milk and the protein requirement of normal infants. *Pediatrics.* 1985;75(suppl):136–141.

Raisler J, Alexander C, Campo P. Breastfeeding and infant illness: a dose-response relationship? *Am J Public Health.* 1999;89:25–30.

Ramsay DT et al. Anatomy of the lactating human breast redefined with ultrasound imaging. *J Anat.* 2005;206:525–534.

Ravelli A et al. Infant feeding and adult glucose tolerance, lipid profile, blood pressure, and obesity. *Arch Dis Child.* 2000;82:248–252.

Ravelomanana N et al. Risk factors for fatal diarrhoea among dehydrated malnourished children in a Madagascar hospital. *Eur J Clin Nutr.* 1995;49:91–97.

Read L et al. Changes in the growth-promoting activity of human milk during lactation. *Pediatr Res.* 1984;18:133–138.

Reid B, Smith H, Friedman Z. Prostaglandins in human milk. *Pediatrics.* 1980;66:870–872.

Rigas A et al. Breast-feeding and maternal smoking in the etiology of Crohn's disease and ulcerative colitis in childhood. *Ann Epidemiol.* 1993;3:387–392.

Rosenbauer J, Herzig P, Giani G. Early infant feeding and risk of type 1 diabetes mellitus—a nationwide population-based case-control study in pre-school children. *Diabetes Metab Res Rev.* 2008;24:211–222.

Rosenberg M. Breast-feeding and infant mortality in Norway 1860–1930. *J Biosoc Sci.* 1989;21:335–348.

Rovet JF. Does breast-feeding protect the hypothyroid infant whose condition is diagnosed by newborn screening? *Am J Dis Child.* 1990;144:319–323.

Rubaltelli FR et al. Intestinal flora in breast- and bottle-fed infants. *J Perinat Med.* 1998;26:186–191.

Rudloff EH et al. Interleukin-6 in human milk. *J Reprod Immunol.* 1993;23:13–20.

Ruiz-Palacios GM et al. Protection of breast-fed infants against *Campylobacter* diarrhea by antibodies in human milk. *J Pediatr.* 1990;116:707–713.

Ruuska R. Occurrence of acute diarrhea in atopic and nonatopic infant: the role of prolonged breast-feeding. *J Pediatr Gastroenterol Nutr.* 1992;14:27–33.

Saarela AT, Kokkonen J, Koivisto M. Macronutrient and energy contents of human milk fractions during the first six months of lactation. *Acta Paediatrica.* 2005;94:1176–1181.

Saarinen KM et al. Breast-feeding and the development of cow's milk protein allergy. *Adv Exp Med Biol.* 2000;478:121–130.

Saarinen UM, Kajosaari M. Breastfeeding as prophylaxis against atopic disease: prospective follow-up study until 17 years old. *Lancet.* 1995;346:1065–1069.

Saarinen UM et al. Prolonged breast feeding as prophylaxis for recurrent otitis media. *Acta Paediatr Scand.* 1982;71:567–571.

Sadeharju K et al. Maternal antibodies in breast milk protect the child from enterovirus infections. *Pediatrics.* 2007;119:941–996.

Saint L, Smith M, Hartmann PE. The yield and nutrient content of colostrum and milk of women giving birth to 1 month postpartum. *Br J Nutr.* 1984;52:87–95.

Salmenpera L et al. Folate nutrition is optimal in exclusively breast-fed infants but inadequate in some of their mothers and in formula-fed infants. *J Pediatr Gastroenterol Nutr.* 1986;5:283–289.

SanGiovanni JP et al. Meta-analysis of dietary essential acuity in healthy preterm infants. *Pediatrics.* 2000; 105:1292–1298.

Sassen ML, Brand R, Grote JJ. Breast-feeding and acute otitis media. *Amer J Otolaryngol.* 1994;15:351–357.

Schroten H et al. Secretory immunoglobulin A is a component of the human milk fat globule membrane. *Pediatr Res.* 1999;45:82–86.

Serdula MK, Seward J, Marks JS. Seasonal differences in breast-feeding in rural Egypt. *Am J Clin Nutr.* 1986;44: 405–409.

Shehadeh N et al. Importance of insulin content in infant diet: suggestion for a new infant formula. *Acta Paediatr.* 2001;90:93–95.

Shing YW, Klagsburn M. Human and bovine milk contain different sets of growth factors. *Endocrinology.* 1984;115:273.

Shu XO et al. Infant breastfeeding and the risk of childhood lymphoma and leukaemia. *Int J Epidemiol.* 1995;24:27–34.

Siigur U, Ormission A, Tamm A. Faecal short-chain fatty acids in breast-fed and bottle-fed infants. *Acta Paediatr.* 1993;82:536–538.

Siimes MA et al. Exclusive breast-feeding for nine months: risk of iron deficiency. *J Pediatr.* 1984;104: 196–199.

Smith AM, Picciano MF, Milner JA. Selenium intakes and status of human milk and formula fed infants. *Am J Clin Nutr.* 1982;35:521.

Smulevich et al. Parental occupation and other factors and cancer risk in children: 1. Study methodology and non-occupational factors. *Int J Cancer.* 1999; 83:712.

Sommerburg O et al. Carotenoid supply in breast-fed and formula-fed neonates. *Eur J Pediatr.* 2000; 159:86–90.

Specker BL et al. Sunshine exposure and serum 25-hydroxyvitamin D concentrations in exclusively breast-fed infant. *J Pediatr.* 1985;107:372–376.

Steichen JJ, Krug-Wispe SK, Tsang RC. Breastfeeding the low birth weight preterm infant. *Clin Perinatol.* 1987;14:131–171.

Steel MG, Leslie GA. Immunoglobulin D in rat serum, saliva and milk. *Immunology.* 1985;55:571–577.

Stuff JE, Nichols GL. Nutrient intake and growth performance of older infants fed human milk. *J Pediatr.* 1989;115:959–968.

Svanborg C et al. HAMLET fills tumor cells by an apoptosis-like mechanism—cellular, molecular, and therapeutic aspects. *Adv Cancer Res.* 2003;8:1–29.

Swartzbaum JA et al. An exploratory study of environmental and medical factors potentially related to childhood cancer. *Med Pediatr Oncol.* 1991;19: 115–121.

Takahata Y et al. Interleukin-18 in human milk. *Pediatr Res.* 2001;50:268–272.

Takala AK et al. Risk factors of invasive *Haemophilus influenzae* type b disease among children in Finland. *J Pediatr.* 1989;115:694–701.

Tran TT et al. Effects of neonatal dietary manganese exposure on brain dopamine levels and neurocognitive functions. *Neurotoxicology.* 2002;145:1–7.

Udall JN et al. Liver disease in a1-antitrypsin deficiency. *JAMA*. 1985;253:2679–2682.

US Department of Health and Human Services. *Healthy People 2010*. Washington, DC: USDHHS; 2000.

Uvnas-Moberg K, Marchini G, Windberg J. Plasma cholecystokinin concentrations after breastfeeding in healthy 4 day old infants. *Arch Dis Child*. 1993;68:46–48.

Van Derslice J, Popkin B, Briscoe J. Drinking-water quality, sanitation, and breast-feeding: their interactive effects on infant health. *Bull WHO*. 1994;72:589–601.

van der Westhuyzen, Chetty M, Atkinson PM. Fatty acid composition of human milk from South African black mother consuming a traditional maize diet. *Eur J Clin Nutr*. 1988;42:213–220.

Verge CF et al. Environmental factors in childhood IDDM: a population-based case-control study. *Diabetes Care*. 1994;17:1381.

Victora CG et al. Evidence for protection by breastfeeding against infant deaths from infectious diseases in Brazil. *Lancet*. 1987;2:319–321.

Virtanen SM, Rasanen L, Aro A et al. Childhood diabetes in Finland Study Group: feeding in infancy and the risk of type 1 diabetes mellitus in Finnish children. *Diabet Med*. 1992;9:815.

Wagner V, Stockhausen JG. The effect of feeding human milk and adapted milk formulae on serum lipid and lipoprotein levels in young infants. *Eur J Pediatr*. 1988;147:292–295.

Wahlberg J, Vaarala O, Ludvigsson J. Dietary risk factors of the emergence of type 1 diabetes-related autoantibodies in 2 1/2 year-old Swedish children. *Br J Nutr*. 2006;95:603–608.

Wallace JM et al. Cytokines in human milk. *Br J Biomed Sci*. 1997;54:85–87.

Wasmuth HE, Kolb H. Cow's milk and immune-mediated diabetes. *Proc Nutr Soc*. 2000;59:573–579.

Widdowson EM, Colombo VE, Artavanis CA. Changes in the organs of pigs in response to feeding for the first 24 hours after birth: II. The digestive tract. *Biol Neonate*. 1996;28:272.

Wight NE. Donor human milk for preterm infants. *J Perinatol*. 2001;21:249–254.

Wilson JV, Self TW, Hamburger R. Severe cow's milk-induced colitis in an exclusively breast-fed neonate. *Clin Pediatr*. 1990;29:77–80.

Wilson-Clay B, Hoover K. *The breastfeeding atlas*, 4th ed. Manchaca, TX: LactNews Press, 2008.

Wirt DP et al. Activated and memory T lymphocytes in human milk. *Cytometry*. 1992;13:282–290.

Woolridge MW, Fisher C. Colic, "overfeeding," and symptoms of lactose malabsorption in the breast-fed baby: a possible artifact of feed management? *Lancet*. 1988;2:382–384.

Woolridge MW, Ingram JC, Baum JD. Do changes in pattern of breast usage alter the baby's nutrient intake? *Lancet*. 1990;336:395–397.

Yamauchi Y, Yamanouchi I. Breast-feeding frequency during the first 24 hours after birth in full-term neonates. *Pediatrics*. 1990;86:171–175.

Yoneyama K, Nagata H, Asano H. Growth of Japanese breast-fed and bottle-fed infants from birth to 20 months. *Ann Hum Biol*. 1994;21:597–608.

Zaman K et al. Children's fluid intake during diarrhoea: a comparison of questionnaire responses with data from observations. *Acta Paediatr*. 2002;91:376–382.

Zanardo V et al. Beta endorphin concentrations in human milk. *J Pediatr Gastroenterol Nutr*. 2001;33:160–164.

Ziegler EE et al. The vitamin deficiency in breastfed infants in Iowa. *Pediatrics*. 2006;118:603–610.

Composition of Human Colostrum and Mature Breastmilk

Constituent (per 100 mL)	Colostrum 1–5 days	Mature Milk > 30 days	Constituent (per 100 mL)	Colostrum 1–5 days	Mature Milk > 30 days
Energy, kcal	58	70	**Vitamins (Water Soluble)**		
Lactose, g	5.3	7.3	Thiamine, µg	15	16
Total nitrogen, mg	360	171	Riboflavin, µg	25	35
Protein nitrogen, mg	313	129	Niacin, µg	75	200
Nonprotein nitrogen, mg	47	42	Folic acid, µg	—	5.2
Total protein, g	2.3	0.9	Vitamin B_6, µg	12	28
Casein, mg	140	187	Vitamin B_{12}, ng	200	26
α-lactalbumin, mg	218	161	Vitamin C, mg	4.4	4.0
Lactoferrin, mg	330	167	*Minerals and Trace Elements*		
IgA, mg	364	142			
Urea, mg	10	30	Calcium, mg	23	28
Creatine, mg	—	3.3	Sodium, mg	48	15
Total fat, g	2.9	4.2	Potassium, mg	74	58
Cholesterol, mg	27	16	Iron, µg	45	40
Vitamins (Fat Soluble)			Zinc, µg	540	166
Vitamin A, µg	89	47			
Beta-carotene, µg	112	23			
Vitamin D, µg	—	0.04			
Vitamin E, µg	1280	315			
Vitamin K, µg	0.2	0.21			

Source: Used with permission from Casey CE, Hambidge KM. Nutritional aspects of human lactation. In: Neville MC, Neifert MR, eds. *Lactation: physiology, nutrition and breastfeeding.* New York: Plenum, 1983:203–204.

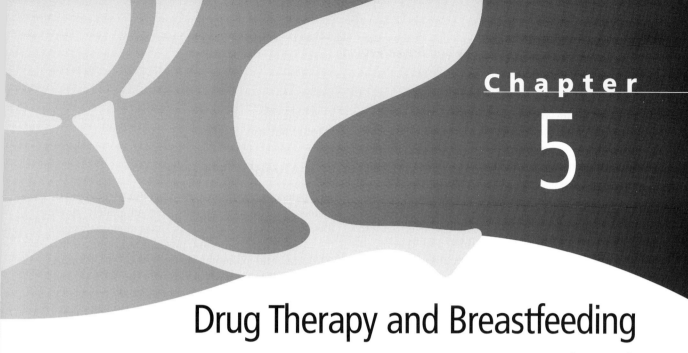

Drug Therapy and Breastfeeding

Thomas Hale

Introduction

HUMAN MILK PROVIDES the infant's first and best choice for protection against infectious disease during the first year of life. Not only is it perfectly suited for the infant's gastrointestinal (GI) tract, but its numerous growth factors enhance growth and maturation of a relatively permeable GI tract. The nutritional and immunologic benefits of human milk are exceptional, and many national and international health organizations now strongly recommend that all infants be breastfed (American Academy of Pediatrics, 2005). Key benefits to the infant include perfect nutrition, enhanced neurocognitive development, stronger immune function, and significant reductions in infectious disease, such as upper respiratory infections, otitis media, sudden infant death syndrome, and necrotizing enterocolitis (Cochi et al., 1986; Ford et al., 1993; Goldman, 1993; Goldman et al., 1994; Pisacane et al., 1992).

While recent studies suggest that the number of women who choose to breastfeed is rising, the number of women who discontinue breastfeeding to take a medication because of advice from their healthcare professional is high. Surveys in Western countries indicate that 90–99 percent of women who breastfeed will receive at least one medication during the first week postpartum (Bennett, 1996). Although it is not known how many women discontinue breastfeeding owing to concerns associated with using various medications, at least one Scandinavian study suggests that of mothers who discontinue breastfeeding prematurely, the use of medications is a major reason (Matheson et al., 1985).

Often clinicians recommend discontinuing breastfeeding while a mother is using a medication simply because they do not know if it is safe. Many manufacturers prescribing inserts often discourage breastfeeding to avoid risks of litigation. Some even suggest that no data are available when dozens of published works clearly show the safety of their product. However, sometimes the safety of a product is not absolutely clear. This is particularly true of new medications, which never have breastfeeding data.

We do know that certain pharmacokinetic parameters can be used to help distinguish between safe and unsafe medications. The most useful data available are studies that disclose the amount of drug that enters milk, but with new medications this information is seldom available. Therefore, the healthcare practitioner must sometimes use available kinetic tools to evaluate the overall risk to the infant.

The following review is designed to aid readers in their evaluation of medications in breastfeeding mothers and to provide current insight into this field. It is hoped that lactation consultants and other healthcare providers can use this data to evaluate the mother's situation and determine the true risk to the infant from the medication. Lactation risk categories (see Box 5–1), a tool for determining possible risks associated with taking a medication while breastfeeding, are used throughout this chapter.

The Alveolar Subunit

The parenchyma of the breast consists of approximately 8–12 ductal regions that ultimately drain toward the nipple (Figure 5–1). Ducts migrate through the mammary fat during pregnancy as progestins, estrogens, and placental lactogen rise. The forming ducts canalize themselves through the fat pad during the first and second trimesters of pregnancy,

---

BOX 5–1

Lactation Risk Category Descriptions

- **L1 Safest**: Drug that has been taken by a large number of breastfeeding mothers without any observed increase in adverse effects in the infant. Controlled studies in breastfeeding women fail to demonstrate a risk to the infant and the possibility of harm to the breastfeeding infant is remote; or the product is not orally bioavailable in an infant.
- **L2 Safer**: Drug that has been studied in a limited number of breastfeeding women without an increase in adverse effects in the infant. And/or, the evidence of a demonstrated risk that is likely to follow use of this medication in a breastfeeding woman is remote.
- **L3 Moderately Safe**: There are no controlled studies in breastfeeding women; however, the risk of untoward effects to a breastfed infant is possible; or, controlled studies show only minimal nonthreatening adverse effects. Drugs should be given only if the potential benefit justifies the potential risk to the infant.

- **L4 Possibly Hazardous**: There is positive evidence of risk to the breastfed infant or to breastmilk production but the benefits from use in breastfeeding mothers may be acceptable despite the risk to the infant (e.g., if the drug is needed in a life-threatening situation or for a serious disease for which safer drugs cannot be used or are ineffective).
- **L5 Contraindicated**: Studies in breastfeeding mothers have demonstrated that there is significant and documented risk to the infant based on human experience; or, it is a medication that has a high risk of causing significant damage to an infant. The risk of using the drug in breastfeeding women clearly outweighs any possible benefit from breastfeeding. The drug is contraindicated in women who are breastfeeding an infant.

Source: Adapted from Hale, 2008.

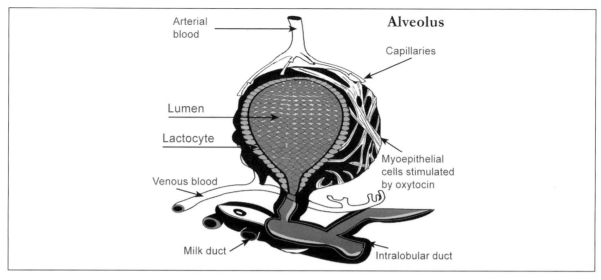

FIGURE 5–1 Structure of the alveolar subunit with blood supply and other structures.

ultimately ending in extensive lobulo-alveolar clusters, lined by the alveolar epithelium that actually creates milk (Neville et al., 1998).

The alveolar unit is lined with a specialized epithelial cell, presently called the lactocyte. The entire alveolar unit is thoroughly perfused with capillaries and lymphatics and is innervated with small nerves. Closely juxtapositioned to the basal membrane of the alveolus are numerous capillaries that are the primary source of immunoglobulins, fats, and many other components (including drugs) needed for the production of human milk (Figure 5–2). During pregnancy, the size and number of alveolar complexes increase significantly owing to the high level of maternal estrogen, progesterone, placental lactogen, prolactin, and oxytocin, all of which act directly on the mammary gland to bring about developmental changes (Neville et al., 2002). At this stage, milk production is largely suppressed by the high levels of progestins. With delivery of the placenta, progestins and estrogens rapidly disappear from the plasma of the mother and the lactocyte begins a rapid change from a quiescent state to a fully active secretory state (secretory lactogenesis).

During the early stages of lactation (colostral phase) when the lactocytes are small in size and the intercellular spaces are large, maternal substances, including drugs, lymphocytes, immunoglobulins, proteins, and other plasma substances, can easily transfer into human milk via these large intercellular

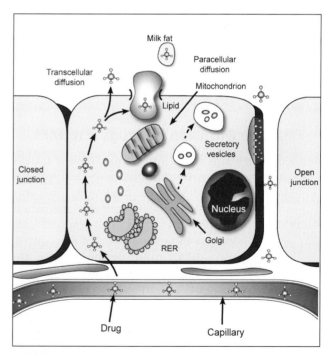

FIGURE 5–2 Transport of drugs and other substances through the alveolar epithelial cell.

Source: Adapted from Vorherr, 1974.

gaps. But with the drop in progestins, the lactocyte grows in size and subsequently narrows the intercellular gaps, eventually closing most of them.

As can be seen from the transition from colostrum to mature milk, these changes in milk occur due to rapid growth of the lactocyte, ending in closure of the tight junctions between the cells. At 36 hours following delivery, a major change in the components of milk occurs, which is complete by 5 days postpartum. With closure of the intercellular spaces, the transfer of maternal medications and other maternal proteins into the mother's milk is greatly reduced.

Drug Transfer into Human Milk

Drugs transfer into human milk largely as a function of their physicochemical characteristics, which include molecular weight, lipid solubility, protein binding, and alkalinity pKa (Atkinson & Begg, 1990; Hale et al., 2007b). Maternal factors include the relative oral absorption of the medication and the plasma levels of the medication. Of these many factors, the most influential are the following:

- Maternal plasma levels of the drug
- Molecular weight of the medication
- Oral bioavailability of the medication in mother and infant
- Protein binding of the medication

Passive Diffusion of Drugs into Milk

The transfer of drugs into human milk is usually facilitated by passive diffusion down a concentration gradient formed by the nonionized, free drug on each side of the semipermeable membrane (Miller et al., 1967). Normally, drugs transfer from areas of high concentration to areas of low concentration (passive diffusion). As described above, the overall rate and degree of transfer may be initially affected by the stage of alveolar development and the junctional condition of the lactocytes.

In the first 2–3 days with the production of small volumes of colostrum, the alveolar epithelial structure of the breast is quite open and porous, thus many maternal proteins, lipids, immunoglobulins, and medications easily transfer into the milk compartment. Often drug levels in milk

reach equilibrium with the plasma compartment (M/P ratio = 1). As the lactocyte begins to swell after several days, the intercellular junctions close. This subsequently leads to dramatically lower levels of drugs in the milk compartment after the first week postpartum. While it is true that the transfer of medications or any substance into milk may be higher during the initial stages of early lactation, the absolute amount of colostrum delivered is often quite low (50–60 mL/day on days 1 and 2); thus, the clinical dose of medication delivered to the infant during this time is actually very low.

Milk and maternal plasma should be viewed as distinct and separate compartments. For most drugs, their transfer in and out of the milk compartment is accomplished by passive diffusion. Although some active transport systems exist for immunoglobulins, electrolytes, and particularly iodides, facilitated transport systems are rather limited. We know of fewer than 10 drugs that are selectively transported into human milk. Transport systems for medications may be indicated by drugs that have high milk/plasma ratios, although many drugs are ion trapped in milk due to the lower pH of milk and higher pKa of the medication (see below). Regardless, in the case of higher milk/plasma ratios, it is apparent that either the drug is ion trapped in the milk or that it is pumped into milk at higher levels (e.g., iodides).

Drugs enter and exit the milk compartment largely as a function of their physiochemistry. The retrograde diffusion of drugs from the milk back into the plasma is well documented and is probably controlled by the same kinetic factors as entry (Schadewinkel-Scherkl et al., 1993). As the maternal plasma level of medication increases, so does the transfer into milk. Then, as the mother metabolizes or eliminates the medication and her plasma levels begin to drop, most drugs diffuse out of the milk compartment and back into the maternal plasma compartment to be eliminated by the mother (Figure 5–3). Following this reasoning, it is obvious that the diffusional forces that push medications into milk are highest at C_{max} (peak) in the mother and lowest during the trough period when the mother is eliminating the medication. Thus with shorter half-life medications, one can avoid higher exposure to medications by avoiding breastfeeding when the maternal plasma levels are highest, and

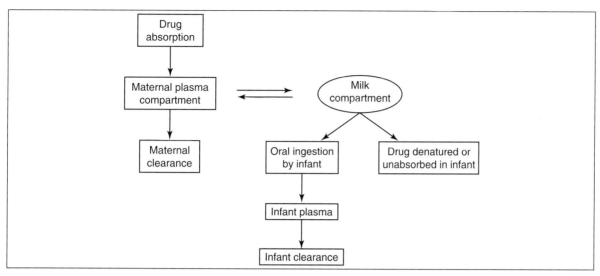

FIGURE 5–3 Compartment representation of drug transfer from plasma to the milk compartment.

instead, breastfeed when the maternal levels are much lower. While this works for some drugs, it will not work for medications with long half-lives, because the time period between C_{max} (peak) and the trough is prolonged.

Ion Trapping

Because the pH of milk is slightly more acidic than plasma (milk pH = 7.2; plasma pH = 7.4), certain weak bases (pKa > 8) may become more polarized and therefore fail to diffuse backward into the plasma once in milk. Thus, they are "trapped" in milk (ion trapping) and may produce higher milk/plasma ratios (Rasmussen, 1971). Ion trapping probably occurs with medications such as the barbiturates, ranitidine, and many others. Conversely, a weak acid is often trapped in the plasma compartment where it is more polar and enters milk relatively poorly due to its polarized state. Thus, it is unable to transfer through the lactocyte bilayer lipid membranes because of its high state of polarity.

Molecular Weight

With closure of the intercellular gaps, most medications must transfer via the "transcellular" pathway. To do so, they must enter the basal membrane of the lactocyte, diffuse gently through the cell, and exit via the luminal surface. The smaller the molecular weight of the medication (300 daltons or lower), the greater the diffusion across these bilayer lipid membranes. As the molecular weight of the medication exceeds 500–800 daltons, it becomes increasingly difficult to diffuse through bilayer membranes and enter milk. Thus, medications whose molecular weights exceed 1000 daltons seldom enter the milk compartment in clinically relevant amounts. Medications such as heparin, insulin, interferon (Kumar et al., 2000), and other large molecular weight drugs, simply do not pass into milk in clinically relevant amounts. A medication, such as lithium, with no protein binding and low molecular weight transfers into milk readily (Sykes et al., 1976). Many of the psychotropic drugs, such as the amphetamines, are low in molecular weight and highly lipid soluble, which accounts for their rapid entry into the central nervous system, as well as their higher milk/plasma ratios in human milk.

Lipophilicity

Although plasma contains lipid, it is relatively low compared to the 5–15 percent triglycerides found in human milk. As such, some medications that are lipid soluble may immerse themselves in the lipid fraction of milk and transfer to the infant. We actually know very little about the diffusion into and out of the lipid fraction of milk, but it is known that by selectively extracting the lipid fraction in milk, certain drugs are found in higher concentrations. Some medications during their transfer through the lactocyte dissolve themselves in the lipid droplets and are subsequently dumped into the alveolar lumen. Others may actually transfer completely through the cell and subsequently transfer into the lipid droplets within milk itself. For highly lipid-soluble drugs, such as many neuroleptic drugs (diazepam, chlorpromazine, etc.), a vast majority of the drug is found in the lipid fraction (Syversen & Ratkje, 1985). While scientifically interesting, the clinical use of this information is relatively small. The most important feature of lipid solubility is that the more lipid soluble the medication, the more likely it will transfer into human milk. A more practical feature of this is that most central nervous system (CNS) active drugs are both low in molecular weight and very lipid soluble, two kinetic parameters that permit them to transfer through the blood-brain barrier, as well as into human milk. Hence, greater concern for the infant should be taken with CNS active drugs.

Milk/Plasma Ratio

The ratio of the concentration of drug in the milk to that in the plasma is known as the milk/plasma ratio (M/P). The M/P ratio is quite useful in determining the relative transfer of medication into milk, but there are significant difficulties in accurately measuring it. Because of differences in the rate of drug transfer, the plasma and milk concentrations of medications don't always follow one another, and the time at which the samples are drawn becomes very important. The M/P ratio may be 1.14 at zero time and 0.31 at 3 hours following administration (Hale et al., 2002). As a result, the M/P ratio actually reflects the differential rate of entry of drug into plasma and milk and will often change from hour to hour (Sykes et al., 1976). Most importantly, the M/P ratio is of limited clinical use in assessing the likelihood that a clinically relevant dose will be transferred to the infant during breastfeeding. Even with some drugs that have high M/P ratios (e.g., ranitidine, cimetidine), the absolute dose transferred to the infant is still subclinical. Ultimately, it is the concentration of drug in the milk (relative infant dose) and the volume of milk ingested that

determine the clinical dose transferred to the infant. For this reason, low M/P ratios suggest that very little drug enters the milk. Conversely, high M/P ratios may or may not indicate high levels in milk because it ultimately depends on the maternal plasma level of medication.

Maternal Plasma Levels

Ultimately, one of the most important kinetic factors determining drug transfer to the infant is the maternal plasma level of the drug. Plasma concentrations of drugs vary according to the dose administered, the half-life of the medication, the volume of distribution, the oral bioavailability, and its protein binding. Drugs vary enormously in potency, some requiring only microgram doses, whereas others require huge doses (grams). Because of the enormous difference in potency, plasma levels of various drugs can vary from nanograms per mL to milligrams per mL. In general, as the molar concentrations of a drug in solution increases, the equilibrium gradient also increases to force the drug into other compartments. Thus, the more drug present, the higher the forces pushing it into the milk compartment. For this reason alone, the degree and rate of transfer of a drug into milk generally correlates with the plasma concentration curve. As the concentration in the plasma peaks (C_{max}), it is quite common that milk levels peak as well. While this is certainly not always true, such as with metformin (Hale et al., 2002), the majority of drugs exhibit this feature. Thus, it is important to understand that if a drug is not absorbed in the mother or is rapidly depleted from her plasma compartment to other compartments (rapid redistribution), the transfer to her milk compartment will be quite low. Drugs with brief half-lives will be eliminated so quickly that they seldom pose a major risk to the infant, unless the infant is feeding at C_{max}.

Bioavailability

The bioavailability of a medication generally refers to the amount of drug that reaches the systemic circulation after administration. Depending on the route of administration (oral, IV, IM, SC, topically), medications must ultimately pass into the systemic circulation prior to reaching their intended site of action or the milk compartment. Fortunately, many medications are unstable in the gastric milieu or are incompletely absorbed by infants. Most, but not all, topical medications are poorly absorbed transcutaneously, so they seldom attain significant plasma levels. If administered orally, the liver often sequesters or metabolizes many medications, preventing their entry into the plasma compartment. Thus, the poor bioavailability of many products reduces the exposure level in breastfed infants. Because infants receive drugs via the mother's milk, oral bioavailability is of major importance in evaluating potential risks to the infant. The absolute dose of a medication received via milk must be decreased by the percent of oral bioavailability. Obviously, poorly bioavailable drugs are ideal for breastfeeding mothers, as their absorption in the infant is likely poor. Box 5–2 includes medications that are virtually unabsorbed orally and are unlikely to cause problems in an infant. In some instances, however, the active medication may be concentrated in the GI tract of the infant causing problems. Diarrhea and thrush are common complications following the use of various antibiotics.

Drug Metabolites

Ordinarily, the primary function of drug metabolism is to make the drug more soluble so that it will be excreted by the kidneys. However, in many situations, the parent drug (prodrug) is actually metabolized to an active drug. This is true of valacyclovir, codeine, hydroxyzine, fluoxetine, and many others. Some of these metabolites actually have much longer half-lives than the parent drug, such as norfluoxetine (from Prozac), normeperidine (from Demerol), and cetirizine (from Atarax, hydroxyzine). So, in some cases, the metabolite and parent drug both must be evaluated for levels in milk and side effects. In the case of meperidine, it is the metabolite (normeperidine) that is believed to account for some of the toxicities of this drug.

Calculating Infant Exposure

Perhaps the most important clinical parameter is to calculate the actual dose (D_{inf}) received by the infant. To do so, you must know the actual concentration of medication in the milk and the volume of milk transferred. While this information is not always available, many drugs do have published studies providing the C_{max} concentrations or the average (C_{av}) concentrations for the drug. In many previous studies, the C_{max} was the most commonly reported value. Unfortunately, this frequently overestimates the amount of drug actually delivered to the infant. More recent studies now calculate the area under the curve (AUC) value for the medication (Hale et al., 2002). This methodology accurately estimates the average daily intake by the infant and is much more accurate than the C_{max} estimates.

BOX 5–2

Medications with Poor Oral Bioavailability and Low Risk

1. Heparin
2. Large molecular weight proteins
3. Insulin
4. Infliximab
5. Etanercept
6. Interferons
7. Aminoglycoside antibiotics
8. Third generation cephalosporins
9. Omeprazole
10. Lansoprazole
11. Inhaled steroids
12. Inhaled beta agonists

The volume of milk ingested is highly variable and depends on the age of the infant and the extent to which the infant is exclusively breastfed. Many clinicians use the 150 cc/kg/day value to estimate the amount of milk ingested by the infant. The formula below estimates the clinical dose to the infant:

$$D_{inf} = \text{drug concentration in milk (at } C_{max} \text{ or } C_{av}) \times \text{volume of milk ingested}$$

However, the most useful and accurate measure of exposure is to calculate the relative infant dose (RID):

$$\text{Relative infant dose} = \frac{D_{inf} \text{ (mg/kg/day)}}{\text{maternal dose (mg/kg/day)}}$$

This value is generally expressed as a percentage of the mother's dose. It provides a standardized method of relating the infant's dose to the maternal dose. In full-term infants, Bennett (1996) recommends that a relative infant dose of greater than 10 percent should be the theoretical "level of concern" for most medications. Nevertheless, the 10 percent level of concern is relative, and each situation should be individually evaluated according to the overall toxicity of the medication. In premature infants, this "level of concern" may require lowering appropriately, depending on the medication. In this regard, it should always be remembered that many neonates may have been exposed in utero to drugs taken by their mothers and that in utero exposure may be an order of magnitude greater than that received via breastmilk. Thus, the infants exposed in utero to methadone go through significant withdrawal upon delivery, even when breastfeeding.

Unique Infant Factors

A good clinical exam of the infant is mandatory to evaluate the relative risk of the medication to the infant. All infants should be categorized as low, moderate, or high risk for the medication of interest. Low-risk infants are generally older infants (6–18 months), who can metabolize and handle drugs relatively efficiently. Mothers in the terminal stage of lactation (> 1 year) often produce relatively lower quantities of milk. Thus, the absolute clinical dose transferred is often low to nil. Moderate-risk infants are those less than 6 months of age who suffer from various metabolic problems, such as complications of delivery, apnea, GI anomalies, or other metabolic problems. High-risk infants are premature infants, newborn, unstable infants, or infants with poor renal output.

Pediatric patients are often referred to as "therapeutic orphans" because of the lack of pharmacodynamic drug studies in neonates and infants. Fewer than 1 percent of all therapeutic agents used today have recommended dosing guidelines for the newborn or premature infant. The infant's GI tract is undergoing dynamic changes early postnatally. During the first week, a state of relative achlorhydria exists, and the pH continues to decrease slowly toward adult values in the next 2 years. Medications that are weak acids may have reduced absorption (phenobarbital), and drugs that are weak bases may have enhanced absorption. Because the infant's exposure is via the oral route, the oral bioavailability of the medication is of paramount importance. Drugs with high first-pass clearance (morphine) are rapidly cleared from the portal circulation and sequestered in the liver, even in infants. Drugs with poor stability in the gut (aminoglycosides, insulin, heparin) are rapidly degraded in the stomach or intestine and remain unabsorbed. Poor biliary function subsequently leads to poor lipid absorption and relative steatorrhea in newborn or premature infants. Therefore, lipid-soluble drugs, even if present in milk, would have poorer oral bioavailability in the infant. Gastric emptying time is much prolonged in premature infants and in some cases may alter the absorption kinetics altogether—the values for total body water are higher than in adults, protein binding is decreased in neonates, and the oxidative and conjugative capacity of the liver is greatly reduced in neonates (Besunder et al., 1988). Interestingly, while the metabolic capacity of the liver is reduced at first, it rapidly increases and actually approximates adult capacity by 9–12 months (Morselli et al., 1980). Ultimately, the evaluation of the safety of drugs in breastmilk depends on at least four major factors—the amount of medication present in milk, the oral bioavailability of the medication, the inherent toxicity of the drug, and the ability of the infant to clear the medication. Table 5–1 provides a list of medications of particular risk to newborn or premature infants. While we know milk levels for many hundreds of drugs and their approximate bioavailability, the ability of the infant to clear the medication is

TABLE 5–1	Drugs to Avoid in Breastfeeding Mothers of Premature or Newborn Infants

Drug	Possible Side Effect
Acebutolol	Has potential to cause hypotension in infant (Boutroy et al., 1986).
ACE inhibitors	May cause neonatal hypotension; wait several weeks postpartum (Hale & Berens, 2003).
Alcohol	May reduce milk production significantly (Mennella & Beauchamp, 1991).
Amphetamines	Potentially high milk levels reported; may cause stimulation of infant (Steiner et al., 1984).
Anticancer agents	Cytotoxicity, immune suppression reported (Hale & Berens, 2003).
Caffeine	Milk levels small, but neonatal half-life long; symptoms include jitteriness, stimulation (Stavchansky et al., 1988; Nehlig & Debry, 1994).
Cocaine	Potential high milk levels, intoxication, and stimulation of infant reported (Chasnoff, Lewis, & Squires, 1987).
Demerol	Neonatal sedation reported; neurobehavioral delay in neonates (Wittels, Scott, & Sinatra, 1990).
Dostinex	Reduces milk supply by inhibiting prolactin (Caballero-Gordo et al., 1991).
Ergotamine	Reduces milk supply by inhibiting prolactin (White & White, 1980).
Estrogens	May reduce milk supply (Booker & Pahl, 1967; Booker, Pahl, & Forbes, 1970; Gambrell, 1970).
Fluoxetine	Tremulousness, colic, crying, hypotonia reported (Lester et al., 1993).
Iodine	High levels in milk reported; may inhibit thyroid function in neonate (Postellon & Aronow, 1982).
Lithium	Levels high in milk, risk high to infant unless monitored closely (Llewellyn, Stowe, & Strader, 1998).
Marijuana	May suppress prolactin and/or milk supply; infant will be drug-screen positive for long periods (Hale & Berens, 2003; Perez-Reyes & Wall, 1982).
Parlodel	Reduces milk supply by inhibiting prolactin (Spalding, 1991; Canales et al., 1981).
Progestins	Early postnatal use may reduce milk supply (Hale, 2002).
Pseudoephedrine	May inhibit milk supply (Aljazaf et al., 2003).
Sulfonamides	Displaced bilirubin from binding site; hyperbilirubinemia possible; do not use in G6PD deficiency (Hale & Ilett, 2002).

highly variable and still requires individual evaluation by the clinician. Begg and colleagues (2000) estimated infant clearance to be 5, 10, 33, 50, 66, and 100 percent of adult maternal levels at 24–28, 28–34, 34–40, 40–44, 44–68, and more than 68 weeks postconceptual age, respectively.

Maternal Factors

The plasma compartment is the only source of medication for the milk compartment. If drugs are not absorbed by the mother and do not produce significant plasma levels, then they are of no risk to an infant. Medications that are not orally bioavailable in the mother (e.g., oral vancomycin, magnesium hydroxide, magnesium sulfate, and many others) do not normally attain significant plasma levels and are therefore not likely hazardous to a breastfed infant. This also includes most, but not all, topical preparations. Many topical steroids, antibiotics, and retinoids used over minimal surface areas are not well absorbed through the skin and are virtually undetectable in the plasma compartment. One-time injections of local anesthetics (such as for dental procedures) provide so little drug that plasma levels are minuscule. Hence, the acute use of many medications is not usually problematic as the overall dose transferred to the infant is low over time.

The amount of milk the mother produces is very important as well. Milk production the first or second day postpartum is so low that the overall dose of medication transferred is usually insignificant. Mothers who are 1–2 years postpartum generally have a significantly reduced milk supply, and their infants are much older. Thus, the clinical dose transferred in late-stage lactation is often reduced as well. Therefore, the risk of a medication in a mother with an 18-month old infant is relatively small unless the drug is extraordinarily toxic (radioactive or anticancer drugs).

Minimizing the Risk

The following factors may profoundly reduce exposure to medications and risk in the infant:

- Avoid feeding the infant or pumping the mother at C_{max}. Because milk levels are invariably a function of maternal plasma levels, collecting/breastfeeding at the peak (C_{max}) will always produce higher drug levels in milk. While useful for shorter half-life medications, it is of questionable use with long half-life medications.
- Temporarily withhold breastfeeding for brief exposures. If the mother can store sufficient milk for a brief exposure to medication, then the risk to the infant is eliminated. Milk produced during the exposure can be pumped and discarded.
- Choose medications that produce minimal levels in milk. For example, the antidepressants

sertraline (Zoloft) or paroxetine (Paxil) produce milk levels far less than fluoxetine (Prozac) (Bennett, 1996; Kristensen et al., 1998; Kristensen et al., 1999; Wisner et al., 1998).
- Choose medications that are commonly used in pediatric patients and are considered safe.
- Choose medications with high protein binding (warfarin) because tissue and milk levels will be lower.
- Choose medications with poor penetration into the CNS as they usually produce lower milk levels.
- Choose medications with higher molecular weights (heparin) as this factor greatly reduces transfer into milk.

Effect of Medications on Milk Production

Drugs That May Inhibit Milk Production

Some medications are well known to affect the rate of milk production. Because infant weight gain and development are directly associated with milk production, even modest changes in milk supply can produce major growth complications for the infant. Drugs that may potentially inhibit milk production include ergot alkaloids (bromocriptine, cabergoline (Dostinex), ergotamine), estrogens (Treffers, 1999; Sweezy, 1992), progestogens, pseudoephedrine (Aljazaf et al., 2003), and to a minor degree alcohol (Mennella & Beauchamp, 1991). Box 5–3 provides a list of drugs that are known to negatively affect milk production.

Estrogens have a long but poorly documented history of suppressing milk (Booker & Pahl, 1967; Booker et al., 1970; Gambrell, 1970). While they may have no effect whatsoever in some mothers, others may be exceedingly sensitive to them. The onset may be rapid or slow, and most mothers may not readily notice the change. Regardless, all mothers who take estrogen-containing birth control preparations should be forewarned of possible effects on milk production. When necessary, low-dose progestogen-only oral contraceptives should be used. However, even these can suppress milk production in some mothers if used too early

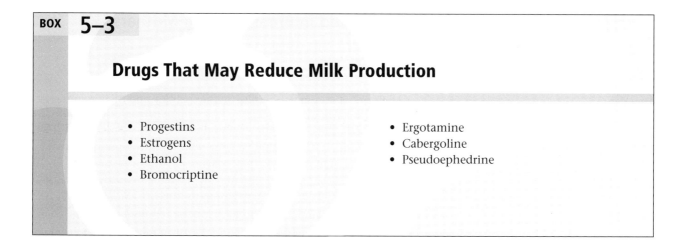

BOX **5–3**

Drugs That May Reduce Milk Production

- Progestins
- Estrogens
- Ethanol
- Bromocriptine

- Ergotamine
- Cabergoline
- Pseudoephedrine

postpartum. The most sensitive time for suppression is early postpartum before the mother's milk supply is established. Waiting as long as possible (weeks to months) prior to use is recommended. All mothers should be warned that in some cases reduced milk supply may result, and they should be observant for such changes.

Some members of the ergot family are well known to suppress prolactin levels. Bromocriptine has been used in the past to reduce engorgement and inhibit milk production, although it was associated with numerous cases of cardiac dysrhythmias, stroke, intracranial bleeding, cerebral edema, convulsions, and myocardial infarction (Dutt et al., 1998; Iffy et al., 1998; Pop et al., 1998; Webster, 1996). A newer analog, cabergoline, has proven much safer and is now recommended for both hyperprolactinemia and inhibition of lactation (Ferrari et al., 1995; Webster et al., 1992). Doses of 1 mg cabergoline administered early postpartum will completely inhibit lactation. For established lactation, 0.25 mg twice daily for 2 days has been found to completely inhibit lactation (Anonymous, 1991; Caballero-Gordo et al., 1991). In cases where mothers have received cabergoline inappropriately, immediate pumping and breastfeeding will probably return their milk supply to normal.

There are recent suggestions that the nasal decongestant pseudoephedrine may suppress milk production (Aljazaf et al., 2003). Studies are still under way, but mothers should be cautious using pseudoephedrine, particularly if they are late-stage lactation (> 8 months) or have a poor milk supply.

Table 5–2 lists other drugs that are usually contraindicated in breastfeeding mothers.

Drugs That May Stimulate Milk Production

The pituitary hormone prolactin is one of the major controllers of milk production. It is well known that while prolactin levels must be elevated for milk production to occur, higher levels of prolactin do not necessarily increase production (Chatterton et al., 2000). In essence, you have to have enough prolactin to maintain milk synthesis, but overwhelmingly high levels do not make more milk. Thus, prolactin levels and milk production are not necessarily related. Initially, antenatal prolactin levels are quite high (200 ng/mL or higher) and then over the next 6 months drop significantly, almost to slightly elevated levels in the 70 ng/mL range. Mothers whose prolactin levels fall to the nonpregnant, nonlactating range of < 20 ng/mL may suffer from poor milk synthesis.

In some mothers, particularly those with premature infants, prolactin levels may not be sufficient to support adequate lactation. In these patients, medications that inhibit dopamine receptors in the hypothalamus (metoclopramide, domperidone) may or may not stimulate milk production. Prolactin release from the pituitary is inhibited by dopamine from the hypothalamus. Any drug that inhibits dopamine will ultimately increase prolactin release.

Dopamine antagonists, such as domperidone, metoclopramide, risperidone, or the phenothiazine

TABLE 5–2	Drugs Generally Contraindicated in Breastfeeding Mothers

Drug	Possible Side Effect in Infant/Mother
Amiodarone	High risk of accumulation due to long half-life and high volume of distribution; cardiovascular risks are high; thyroid suppression risk is high (Brackbill, Kane, & Manniello, 1974a; Chatterton, 1978).
Antineoplastic agents	Some antineoplastic agents may be used following pumping and discarding of milk; others may not.
Chloramphenicol	Blood dyscrasias, aplastic anemia, etc. Possible in mother but not reported as a result of breastfeeding (Kuhnert et al., 1979b).
Doxepin	Dangerous sedation and respiratory arrest reported.
Ergotamine, Cabergoline, ergot alkaloids	Ergotism poisoning (vomiting and diarrhea) reported; may inhibit prolactin secretion; reduces milk production; Cabergoline in particular is a potent inhibitor of milk production.
Iodides	Iodides concentrate in milk; thyroid suppression has been noted; Betadine douches should be avoided.
Methotrexate and immunosuppressants	Potential for a range of symptoms associated with suppression of the immune system; cyclosporine appears to be low risk (Kuhnert et al., 1979a, 1980); methotrexate may concentrate in neonatal GI cells.
Lithium	RID high (18–23%); high potential for toxicity; monitor plasma levels and thyroid function routinely.
Radiopharmaceuticals	Brief to full interruption of breastfeeding recommended.
Ribavirin	No reported milk levels, but following chronic use may lead to hemolytic anemia; caution recommended.
Tetracycline (chronic)	Brief use ok (< 3 weeks); chronic use not recommended.
Pseudoephedrine	May reduce milk supply; caution recommended.

Source: Adapted from Hale & Ilett, 2002.

neuroleptics, are all well known to stimulate milk production in some patients. The two most commonly used dopamine antagonists are metoclopramide (Reglan) (Booker & Pahl, 1967; Booker et al., 1970; Budd et al., 1993; Ehrenkranz & Ackerman, 1986; Gambrell, 1970; Kauppila et al., 1981; Kauppila et al., 1983) and domperidone (Motilium) (Hofmeyr & Van Iddekinge, 1983; Hofmeyr et al., 1985; Petraglia et al., 1985). Metoclopramide is the most commonly used agent, and in some cases, profoundly stimulates milk production as much as 100%. Unfortunately, it may induce significant depression if therapy is continued over a month. The prolactin-stimulating effect of metoclopramide is dose related, with doses of 10–15 mg TID required for efficacy. The amount transferred into milk is small, ranging from 28 to 157 µg/L in the early puerperium (Kauppila et al., 1981), which is far less than the clinical dose administered directly to infants (800 µg/kg/d). The most significant side effect of metoclopramide is extrapyramidal symptoms, gastric cramping, and in some cases major depression.

Domperidone is apparently much safer as it does not penetrate the blood-brain barrier, thus causing no or few CNS side effects. However, it is unfortunately not available in the United States other than via compounding pharmacies. A recent study of domperidone suggests a mean milk volume increase of 44.5 percent over 7 days (da Silva et al., 2001). Milk levels of domperidone were only 1.2 ng/mL. These agents apparently do not always stimulate milk production in patients with prolactin levels already above normal or in those patients with inadequate breast tissue. But in many mothers with premature infants, these drugs may be quite efficacious. Because a mother's milk supply is dependent on an "elevated" prolactin level, the precipitous withdrawal of these agents may result in a significant loss of milk supply. A slow withdrawal is generally recommended over several weeks to a month to prevent loss of milk supply.

The dopamine agonists are often used inappropriately to stimulate milk production in mothers with moderate to low milk production. Before these agents are employed, mothers should be advised to breastfeed more often, pump after breastfeeding, and reduce the intervals between breastfeeding. In those cases where maternal prolactin levels are already elevated, the dopamine agonists often fail to work at all. Thus, measuring baseline prolactin levels just before breastfeeding or approximately 3 hours after breastfeeding will provide an accurate estimate of the mother's trough or baseline prolactin levels. These should be somewhere above 50–70 ng/mL.

The stimulation of milk production by the use of herbal medications is extraordinarily common therapy today. However, good supporting data suggesting that these agents stimulate milk production is minimal to nil. Fenugreek is the most commonly used herbal for this purpose. In a recent abstract of 10 women who ingested three capsules three times daily, the average milk production during the week increased significantly from 207 mL/day (range 57–1057 mL) to 464 mL/day (range 63–1140 mL) (Swafford & Berens, 2000). No untoward effects were reported; however, this was not a blinded or controlled study.

Review of Selected Drug Classes

Analgesics

Analgesics are the most commonly used medications in breastfeeding mothers. While the nonsteroidal anti-inflammatory drugs (NSAIDs) are most frequently used, opioids, such as morphine, codeine, and hydrocodone, are most commonly given during the early postpartum period for pain relief. Selected analgesics are reviewed in Table 5–3.

NSAIDs

Of the NSAID family, ibuprofen and ketorolac are perhaps ideal agents with low relative infant doses (< 0.6 percent). Not only is ibuprofen cleared for use in infants, its milk levels are generally subclinical. Naproxen is suitable for short-term use (a few days), but bleeding, hemorrhage, and acute anemia has been reported in a 7-day-old infant (Figalgo, 1989). Recent data from our laboratories on the newer COX2 inhibitors, such as celecoxib (Hale et al., 2004), suggest that milk levels are quite low, much less than 66 µg/L. While the use of this family is somewhat controversial, the coxibs family may yet prove to be useful and suitable alternatives to the older NSAIDs.

Aspirin, due to its causal association with Reye's syndrome, is not generally recommended in breastfeeding mothers. Given the very short half-life (31 min) of aspirin, the transfer of aspirin itself into milk is probably low to nil. The relative infant dose varies enormously and is reported to range from about 0.04 percent to as high as 10 percent of the maternal dose (Bailey et al., 1982). However, the amount of aspirin in milk is usually low, and it could be used in low maternal doses (82 mg/d) to inhibit platelet function. We do not know if the incidence of Reye's syndrome is dose related with aspirin. Would a single 82 mg/day dose increase the risk of Reye's syndrome? We do not know, but it would be extraordinarily remote. Most cases of Reye's syndrome were in children, 10–13 years old exposed to therapeutic doses of aspirin. It was rarely reported in infants.

Methadone

Methadone is widely used in the treatment of opiate addiction and is commonly used in pregnant patients. Methadone levels in milk are dependent on the dose, but generally range from 2.8 to 5.6 percent of the maternal dose (Begg et al., 2001; Wojnar-Horton et al., 1997). Because of these low levels in milk, neonatal abstinence syndrome may occur in a high percentage of breastfed newborns whose mothers took methadone during pregnancy (Ostrea et al., 1976; Strauss et al., 1974). In a recent study by McCarthy, methadone concentrations in milk ranged from 27 to 260 µg/L in patients receiving 25–180 mg/d (McCarthy & Posey, 2000). Assuming milk intake of 475 mL/d, the average infant would

TABLE 5–3	Relative Infant Dose and Clinical Significance of Selected Analgesics

Drug	Relative Infant Dose (%)	Clinical Significance	Lactation Risk Category
Fentanyl	< 3	Milk levels low; no untoward effects from exposure to milk.	L2
Indomethacin	0.4	Milk levels low; plasma levels low to undetectable in infants; caution with chronic administration.	L3
Ketorolac	0.16–0.4	Milk levels are very low; no untoward effects reported.	L2
Meperidine; pethidine	1	Neurobehavioral delay, sedation noted from long half-life metabolite; avoid.	L2 L3 postpartum
Methadone	2.6, 5.6, 2.4, 1.0	Milk levels low; approved for use in breastfeeding mothers; will not prevent neonatal abstinence syndrome.	L3
Morphine	5.8	Oral bioavailability poor; milk levels generally low; considered safe; observe for sedation.	L3
Naproxen	3.0	Long half-life; may accumulate in infant; bleeding, diarrhea reported in one infant; short-term use acceptable; avoid chronic use.	L3 L4 (chronic)

Source: Adapted from Hale & Ilett, 2002; Hale, 2008.

only receive 50 µg/d or 0.97 percent of the maternal dose in these studies.

Morphine and Congeners

The data on morphine is unfortunately somewhat varied. Older studies suggested the amount of morphine in milk was minimal to undetectable. In a study of epidural morphine, the concentration in milk following two 4 mg epidural doses was only 82 µg/L (Wittels et al., 1990). Other studies suggest higher levels (10–100 µg/L) (Robieux et al., 1990). Combined with its poor oral bioavailability (< 25%) and minimal milk levels, morphine does not appear to be significantly hazardous to most breastfeeding infants, so long as the maternal doses are low to moderate and the infant is stable. But all infants should be closely monitored for respiratory distress, sedation, or poor feeding.

Codeine and hydrocodone are without doubt the most commonly used opiate analgesics in breastfeeding mothers. Although some cases of neonatal sedation and apnea have been reported with codeine, the majority of infants are unaffected by these agents. While the studies on these drugs are poor, they suggest that after 48 hours of exposure to 12 doses of 60 mg codeine, the estimated dose of codeine in 2000 ml of milk was only 0.7 mg or 0.1 percent of the maternal dose. A recent fatal overdose in one infant has been reported, although this was in a mother who was a rapid metabolizer of codeine (Koren et al., 2006a). Bennett (1996) suggests the relative infant dose is 1.4 percent. Other than one fatality, few problems have been reported, although infant sedation can occur. Apparently, hydrocodone is not subject to genetic variations in its metabolism. Thus, it is probably a better choice than codeine in most mothers.

Meperidine

The use of meperidine in the perinatal period is increasingly controversial. Although the use of meperidine in obstetrics is common, it is gaining disfavor as more and more sedation and poor breastfeeding is reported in newborn infants. Meperidine administered to mothers has been found to produce neonatal respiratory depression, decreased Apgar scores, lower oxygen saturation, respiratory acidosis, and abnormal neurobehavioral scores (Brackbill et al., 1974a, 1974b; Hodgkinson et al., 1978, 1979). Meperidine is metabolized to normeperidine, which is both active and has a half-life of approximately 62–73 hours in newborns. Because of this prolonged half-life, neonatal depression after exposure to meperidine may be profound and prolonged (Brackbill et al., 1974a). Small but significant amounts of meperidine and normeperidine are secreted into human milk (Quinn et al., 1986) and have been found to produce changes in neurocognitive function in some infants (Wittels et al., 1990).

Fentanyl

The transfer of fentanyl into human milk is low. In women receiving doses varying from 50–400 µg intravenously during labor, the amount found in milk was exceedingly low, generally below the limit of detection (< 0.05 µg/L) (Leuschen et al., 1990).

Antibiotics

Aside from analgesics, the most commonly used class of medications in breastfeeding mothers are the antibiotics. Virtually all of the penicillins and cephalosporins have been studied and are known to produce only trace levels in milk (Blanco et al., 1983; Kafetzis et al., 1980, 1981; Matsuda, 1984; Shyu et al., 1992; Yoshioka et al., 1979; Bourget et al., 1993). Some changes in intestinal flora are to be expected (Table 5–4).

TABLE 5–4 **Relative Infant Dose and Clinical Significance of Antibiotics**

Drug	Relative Infant Dose (%)	Clinical Significance	Lactation Risk Category
Acyclovir	1.1, 1.5	Infant dose low; safe.	L2
Amoxicillin	1.3	Observe for change in intestinal flora; compatible.	L1
Ampicillin	0.24	Observe for change in intestinal flora; compatible.	L1
Azithromycin	5.8	Observe for change in intestinal flora; compatible.	L2
Cefazolin	0.8	Observe for change in intestinal flora; compatible.	L1
Cefepime	0.3	Observe for change in intestinal flora; compatible.	L2

(Continues)

TABLE 5–4	**Relative Infant Dose and Clinical Significance of Antibiotics (Continued)**		
Drug	**Relative Infant Dose (%)**	**Clinical Significance**	**Lactation Risk Category**
Cefoperazone	0.9	Observe for change in intestinal flora; compatible.	L2
Cefotaxime	0.3	Observe for change in intestinal flora; compatible.	L2
Cefoxitin	0.2	Observe for change in intestinal flora; compatible.	L1
Cefprozil	0.3	Observe for change in intestinal flora; compatible.	L1
Ceftazidime	0.9	Observe for change in intestinal flora; compatible.	L1
Ceftriaxone	0.9	Observe for change in intestinal flora; compatible.	L2
Cephalexin	0.5	Observe for change in intestinal flora; compatible.	L1
Ciprofloxacin	2.6, 2.0	Recently approved by AAP; one case of pseudomembranous colitis reported; observe for changes in gut flora.	L4
Clindamycin (oral)	1.6	Observe for changes in intestinal flora; pseudomembranous colitis reported in one infant; probably safe.	L3
Cloxacillin	0.8	Observe for change in intestinal flora; compatible.	L2
Dicloxacillin	1.2	Observe for change in intestinal flora; compatible.	L1
Doxycycline	4	Infant dose low; bioavailability poor; safe for acute use; do not use chronically.	L3 L4 chronic
Erythromycin	1.4	Observe for change in intestinal flora;	L1

(Continues)

TABLE 5–4	**Relative Infant Dose and Clinical Significance of Antibiotics (Continued)**		
Drug	**Relative Infant Dose (%)**	**Clinical Significance**	**Lactation Risk Category**
		compatible; hypertonic pyloric stenosis reported in one case.	
Fluconazole	12.6	Safe; no untoward effects have been reported.	L2
Gentamicin	2.1	Observe for change in intestinal flora; compatible.	L2
Isoniazid	13.5	Caution; monitoring of infant for liver toxicity and neuritis recommended.	L3
Metronidazole	13, 9.9, 12.6, 29	Milk levels moderately high, but significantly less than pediatric therapeutic dose (15 mg/kg/d); with high doses, discontinue breastfeeding for 12–24 hr after dose.	L2
Nitrofurantoin	0.7	Safe; no untoward effects reported; caution for infants with G6PD	L2
Ofloxacin	3.2	Probably safe but observe for changes in intestinal flora.	L3
Rifampicin	11	Probably safe; minimal data available.	L2
Streptomycin	0.6	Observe for change in intestinal flora; compatible.	L3
Tetracycline	1.35	Short-term use safe; bioavailability in milk is low to nil; caution with long-term use.	L2
Vancomycin	6.6	Safe; oral bioavailability low to nil; observe for changes in intestinal flora.	L1

Source: Adapted from Hale & Ilett, 2002; Hale, 2008.

The transfer of the older tetracyclines into human milk is very low. When mixed with calcium salts, the bioavailability of these tetracyclines is significantly reduced, and it is unlikely the infant would absorb the small levels present in milk. However, doxycycline absorption is delayed, not blocked, and its absorption may be significant. Short-term administration of these compounds for up to 3 weeks is permissible. Long-term use, such as for acne, is not recommended in breastfeeding mothers due to the possibility of dental staining in the infant and reduced growth rate in the epiphyseal growth plates.

The fluoroquinolones are somewhat controversial. Although the dose received via milk is low, pseudomembranous colitis has been reported, although this can occur with any antibiotic (Harmon et al., 1992).

Studies of the new fluoroquinolones suggest that ofloxacin (and its derivatives) concentrations in milk are probably lowest. Ciprofloxacin concentrations in human milk vary over a wide range, but are generally quite low (2.1–2.6 percent) (Cover & Mueller, 1990; Gardner et al., 1992; Giamarellou et al., 1989). Ciprofloxacin has recently been approved for use in breastfeeding mothers by the American Academy of Pediatrics (American Academy of Pediatrics, 2001). Ciprofloxacin ophthalmic products are poorly absorbed and the dose is low, so these products may be used in breastfeeding mothers.

Metronidazole is a commonly used antimicrobial in pediatric patients. Older studies in rodents suggesting that metronidazole may be mutagenic have never been duplicated in humans. Following an oral dose of 400 mg three times daily, the maximum concentration in milk averaged 15.5 mg/L (Passmore et al., 1988). Relative infant doses reported are moderate, approximating 10–13 percent of the maternal dose. Thus far, no untoward effects have been reported in a breastfed infant other than a metallic taste imparted to the milk. High maternal doses (PO), such as 2 g for treatment of trichomoniasis, may potentially produce high milk levels. In these patients, a brief interruption of breastfeeding is recommended for 12–24 hours.

Following the use of intravenous metronidazole, milk levels have not been reported. However, with a short withholding period of 2–3 hours to avoid the peak, maternal plasma levels rapidly fall to levels similar to those following oral administration. Intravaginal and topical applications do not produce significant plasma levels and do not require changes in breastfeeding recommendations.

Erythromycin and azithromycin levels in milk are quite low. Following a dose of 2 g erythromycin daily, milk levels varied from 1.6–3.2 mg/L of milk (Knowles, 1972). Azithromycin transfer to milk is minimal and produces a clinical dose of approximately 0.4 mg/kg/day (Kelsey et al., 1994). Erythromycin may not be a good choice in early postnatal mothers as it is known to increase the risk of hypertropic pyloric stenosis, even in breastfed infants (Sorensen et al., 2003).

Sulfonamides displace bilirubin from its albumin binding site, and therefore they should not be used in newborns. However, they can be used later, generally after 22 days of life in most infants when bilirubin levels drop to baseline. Sulfisoxazole milk levels are low, and only 1 percent of the maternal dose is transferred to the infant (Kauffman et al., 1980). The transfer of trimethoprim, which is commonly used in sulfonamide products, is minimal.

The use of antifungals in breastfeeding mothers is popular owing to suggestions of topical and intraductal candidiasis. However, recent evidence suggests that *Candida albicans* may not be present in the ductal system of breastfeeding women (Hale et al., 2007a), and others have suggested that this pain may be instead associated with *Staphylococcal aureus* infections. We do not know for certain that *C. albicans* is not present on the nipple of breastfeeding women. However, many clinicians remain resolute that *C. albicans* can indeed affect the ductal system in women. Until this is clarified, fluconazole will still be commonly used by clinicians.

The transfer of fluconazole has been studied and is reported to be less than 12 percent of the maternal dose. This is still considerably less than the clinical dose commonly used in neonates. While there is some risk of elevated liver enzymes, none have been reported following exposure to fluconazole in breast milk.

Topical antifungals, such as nystatin, clotrimazole, or miconazole are often used topically to treat candidiasis and are considered safe as long as minimal amounts are applied to limit oral absorption by the infant.

There are numerous other antibiotics in common use, and the reader is referred to other sources for a complete compilation of these drugs (Hale & Hartman, 2007; Hale, 2006).

Antihypertensives

Antihypertensives are commonly used early postnatally and sometimes much longer in breastfeeding mothers, but as a family, they require a higher degree of caution. Several beta blockers (atenolol, acebutolol) have been reported to produce dangerous cyanosis, bradycardia, and hypotension in some breastfed infants (Boutroy et al., 1986). Infants should be closely monitored for these symptoms following therapy. Certain beta blockers are safer than others, and the careful selection of an appropriate medication is highly recommended.

Early postpartum, some infants have difficulty controlling their blood pressure. ACE inhibitors should only be used cautiously in breastfeeding mothers until their infants can maintain adequate control of their blood pressure. It is therefore recommended that the ACE inhibitor family be avoided for at least several weeks postpartum in breastfeeding mothers, and they should not be used in premature infants. Afterward, captopril and enalapril are preferred due to lower milk levels.

Of the calcium channel blockers, nifedipine has been studied, and its concentration in milk is quite low. It has also been used extensively to control blood pressure in hypertensive breastfeeding patients and to treat Raynaud's phenomenon of the nipple. While the amount in milk varies depending on study, the clinical dose received by the infant is generally less than 8 µg/kg/day (Penny & Lewis, 1989). Four other studies of verapamil transfer into milk have reported relative infant doses of 0.1, 0.2, 0.3, and 1.0 percent, which is subclinical (Andersen, 1983; Anderson et al., 1987; Inoue et al., 1984; Miller et al., 1986).

Other antihypertensives, such as hydralazine and methyldopa, are commonly used in pregnant patients. Studies suggest that their breastmilk levels are quite low and do not produce clinical changes in breastfed infants (Jones & Cummings, 1978; Liedholm et al., 1982; White et al., 1985).

Psychotherapeutic Agents

Sedatives and Hypnotics

The most commonly used sedative medications are primarily benzodiazepines. Most of the benzodiazepine anxiolytics have been thoroughly studied in breastfeeding mothers. Levels of diazepam (Wesson et al., 1985), lorazepam (Whitelaw et al., 1981; Summerfield & Nielsen, 1985), and midazolam (Matheson et al., 1990) have been reported and are quite low (Table 5–5). However, some in this family have rather prolonged half-lives, and some medication does transfer to the infant as is evidenced by minor withdrawal symptoms.

TABLE 5–5	**Relative Infant Dose and Clinical Significance of Psychotropic Drugs**			
Drug	**Maternal Dose**	**Relative Infant Dose (%)**	**Clinical Significance**	**Lactation Risk Category**
Citalopram	20–60 mg/d	3.7	Infant levels extremely low; somnolence reported; most studies show no untoward effects.	L3
Diazepam	30 mg/d 30 mg/d	3.0 2.7	Sedation minimal; acute or occasional use acceptable; avoid prolonged exposure.	L3 L4 chronic

(Continues)

TABLE 5–5	Relative Infant Dose and Clinical Significance of Psychotropic Drugs (Continued)			
Drug	**Maternal Dose**	**Relative Infant Dose (%)**	**Clinical Significance**	**Lactation Risk Category**
Fluoxetine	20–80 mg/d (0.51 mg/kg/d) 7–65 mg/d (0.17–0.85 mg/kg/d)	3.4 4.4	Fluoxetine and norfluoxetine found in 55–77% of infants; not recommended in preterm or very young neonates, or in high maternal doses.	L2 in older infants L3 in neonates
Fluvoxamine	200 mg/d (2.86 mg/kg/d) 100 mg/d	0.5 0.52	No adverse effects in 2 infants; probably safe.	L2
Haloperidol	10 mg/d 29 mg/d	2.4 0.2	Infant dose minimal; no untoward effects noted; caution recommended.	L2
Lithium	15 mmol/d	56	Severe sedation in some infants; monitoring of milk and/or infant serum concentrations mandatory; plasma levels in infants vary from 30–40% of maternal levels 2 weeks postpartum.	L4
Lorazepam	5 mg/d 3.5 mg/d	2.5 2.8	Infant dose low; no untoward effects noted in breastfeeding infants; observe for sedation.	L3
Midazolam	15	0.6	Milk levels are low; no sedation noted in infants; use caution but probably safe.	L3
Olanzapine	15 mg/d	1.05	No adverse effects noted but data are preliminary; probably safe.	L3
Paroxetine	20–30 mg/d 10–50 mg/d	1.4 1.7–2.3	Minimally detected in several infants; no adverse effects; safe.	L2
Risperidone	6 mg/d	0.84	Single case; no infant data; use caution.	L3
Sertraline	50 mg/d 25–200 mg/d	0.9 0.3–1.9	Milk levels low; levels in some infants extremely low; no adverse effects; preferred; safe.	L2

(Continues)

TABLE 5–5	Relative Infant Dose and Clinical Significance of Psychotropic Drugs (Continued)			
Drug	**Maternal Dose**	**Relative Infant Dose (%)**	**Clinical Significance**	**Lactation Risk Category**
Temazepam	10–20 mg/d	No data	Milk concentrations in 9 mothers were extremely low; depending on dose, should be relatively safe.	L3
Venlafaxine	150–450 mg/d (6.1 mg/kg/d)	3.5	No adverse effects reported; use cautiously.	L3
	225–300 mg/d (2.9 mg/kg/d)	3.2		

Source: Adapted from Hale & Ilett, 2002; Hale, 2008.

The intermittent use of diazepam, midazolam, or lorazepam has not been associated with significant sedation in breastfed infants. In a prospective study of 42 women ingesting sedatives while breastfeeding, there were only three reports of slight sedation in their infants (Ito et al., 1993). Lorazepam has a shorter half-life than diazepam (12 hours) and when administered as premedication in 3.5 mg oral doses, milk concentrations were only 8–9 µg/L, which is far too low to be clinically relevant (Summerfield & Nielsen, 1985). Other studies suggest high levels (23–82 µg/L), but were not reported to produce neurobehavioral effects in breastfed infants (McBride et al., 1979).

In a mother who received alprazolam 0.5 mg 2–3 times daily (PO) during pregnancy, a neonatal withdrawal syndrome was reported in the breastfed infant the first week postpartum (Anderson & McGuire, 1989). These data suggest that the amount of alprazolam in breastmilk is insufficient to prevent a withdrawal syndrome following prenatal exposure. Further, in another case of infant exposure solely via breastmilk, the mother took alprazolam (dosage unspecified) for 9 months while breastfeeding and withdrew herself from the medication over a 3-week period (Anderson & McGuire, 1989). In this case, the mother reported withdrawal symptoms in the infant, including irritability, crying, and sleep disturbances. Thus, short-term use of certain benzodiazepines (i.e., diazepam, midazolam, or lorazepam) over a week or two is unlikely to produce problems, but long-term daily exposure could be problematic.

The use of phenothiazine sedatives, such as promethazine (Phenergan) or chlorpromazine (Thorazine), have been suggested to increase sleep apnea (Kahn et al., 1985) and the risk of SIDS (Cantu, 1989) and should probably be avoided in breastfeeding mothers if possible. The transfer of phenobarbital is moderate, averaging 2.74 mg/L following a dose of 30 mg four times daily (Nau et al., 1982). Maternal and infant plasma levels should be monitored occasionally and kept in the normal range to prevent high levels in the infant. Phenobarbital is not usually a major problem in neonates or premature infants, as the bioavailability of phenobarbital in premature infants is generally considered poor, but caution is recommended.

Antidepressants

The incidence of postpartum depression has either risen markedly or is being reported more often. At present, about 10–15 percent of postpartum women report clinical depression, although approximately 80 percent experience postpartum blues (O'Hara et al., 1990). In the past, the use of antidepressants in breastfeeding mothers has been discouraged. However, recent information suggests that depression itself has major negative implications for infants and that it may interfere with optimal parenting, producing significant neurobehavioral delay in infants (Lee & Gotlib, 1991; Sinclair & Murray, 1998; Zekoski et al., 1987). Many women presenting with depressive symptoms may not require pharmacotherapy. Early postpartum sleep deprivation and stress are clearly normal, and general support may be all that is required. But in some patients with severe depression, therapy is clearly indicated. For these reasons, it is important that major depression in breastfeeding women be closely monitored and, if necessary, treated.

In the past, the older tricyclic antidepressants were the mainstay of depressive therapy. Although they have been thoroughly studied in breastfeeding mothers and are generally considered safe, poor patient compliance and a high side effect profile generally preclude their use. Weight gain, sedation, anticholinergic symptoms, such as dry mouth, blurred vision, and constipation, are major drawbacks to their use as antidepressants. However, they still have a prominent use in prevention of migraine headaches and in chronic pain syndromes. Used in these conditions, lower doses at bedtime suffice and tend to reduce the untoward effects of this family. Thus, they are still commonly used for pain and migraine prevention.

With the introduction of the selective serotonin reuptake inhibitors (SSRIs), the use of antidepressants has increased enormously. In general, the SSRIs are well tolerated and highly effective, and we have an increasing number of studies showing they are quite safe in breastfeeding mothers. Clinical studies of sertraline (Zoloft) and paroxetine (Paxil) clearly suggest that transfer of these agents into milk is quite minimal, and virtually no side effects have been reported in numerous breastfed infants (Altshuler et al., 1995; Kristensen et al., 1998; Stowe et al., 1997, 2000). Withdrawal in newborns has been reported with sertraline, paroxetine, and other SSRIs (Sanz et al., 2005).

At least three case reports of colic, prolonged crying, vomiting, tremulousness, and other symptoms have been reported following the use of fluoxetine (Prozac) in breastfeeding women (Hale et al., 2001; Lester et al., 1993; Spencer & Escondido, 1993), although these numbers are probably quite small compared to the thousands of infants who have breastfed without side effect. In addition, there is some question as to whether these symptoms arose due to withdrawal from fluoxetine, rather than from serotonergic overload.

The mixed serotonin and norepinephrine reuptake inhibitor, venlafaxine, has been studied in nine breastfeeding women (Ilett et al., 1998, 2002). In the nine infants, the relative infants' doses for venlafaxine averaged 3.5 percent and for its active metabolite (o-desmethylvenlafaxine), 6.8 percent. Moreover, no adverse effects were noted in their infants despite milk concentrations of up to 8.2 mg/kg/d. Another report has suggested the infants born of mothers consuming venlafaxine may be at higher risk for a more severe withdrawal and that these symptoms may actually be reduced by breastfeeding (Koren et al., 2006b).

Citalopram is an SSRI antidepressant similar in effect to fluoxetine and sertraline, although more selective for the receptor site. In an excellent study of seven women receiving an average of 0.41 mg/kg/d citalopram, the average peak level (C_{max}) of citalopram was 154 µg/L and 50 µg/L for demethylcitalopram (Rampono et al., 2000). However, average milk concentrations (AUC) were lower and averaged 97 µg/L for citalopram and 36 µg/L for demethylcitalopram during the dosing interval. Low concentrations of citalopram (around 2–2.3 µg/L) were detected in only three of the seven infants' plasma. No adverse effects were found in any of the infants. The authors estimate the daily intake to be approximately 3.7 percent of the maternal dose.

The active metabolite of citalopram, escitalopram (Lexapro), has recently been studied. In a case report of a mother taking escitalopram (5 mg/day) while breastfeeding her newborn at 1 week of age, the reported milk level was 24.9 ng/mL. The infant daily dose was 3.74 µg/kg. At 7.5 weeks of age, the mother was taking 10 mg/day, and the milk concentration level was 76.1 ng/mL. The infant daily dose was 11.4 µg/kg. There were no adverse events reported in the infant (Castberg & Spigset, 2006). Another study of eight breastfeeding women taking an average of 10 mg/day showed the total relative infant dose of escitalopram and its metabolite to be 5.3 percent of the mothers. The drug and its metabolite were undetectable in most of the infants tested. No adverse events in the infants were reported (Rampono et al., 2006).

We have limited data on bupropion (Wellbutrin, Zyban), but milk levels have been reported to be low

(Briggs et al., 1993). However, the author has received three case reports suggesting that bupropion may reduce milk supply. Close monitoring of infant weight gain and the mother's milk supply is suggested.

Neonatal withdrawal symptoms characterized by poor adaptation, jitteriness, irritability, and poor gaze control after gestational exposure to selective SSRIs has been reported for fluoxetine (Chambers et al., 1996; Spencer & Escondido, 1993), sertraline, and paroxetine (Stiskal et al., 2001). However, long-term changes in psychomotor or neurodevelopment have not been noted (Nulman et al., 1997).

Antimanic Preparations

The treatment of bipolar syndrome in breastfeeding mothers is somewhat controversial. Lithium, valproate, and carbamazepine have relatively well-established efficacy in acute mania. However, due to the significant toxicity of lithium, some caution is recommended. Lithium is both small in molecular weight and unbound in the plasma compartment. As such, it produces relatively high levels in human milk and some reported toxicity (Llewellyn et al., 1998; Sykes et al., 1976; Tunnessen & Hertz, 1972). Research data suggest that lithium plasma levels in breastfed infants are moderate, approximately 30–40 percent of the maternal level (Fries, 1970; Sykes et al., 1976; Tunnessen & Hertz, 1972). However, lithium plasma levels can change dramatically with state of hydration, particularly in the infant with dehydration, and careful monitoring of plasma lithium levels in mother and infant is strongly recommended. Because lithium affects thyroid function, thyroid function tests should be routinely ordered as well.

Newer studies of valproic acid suggest that this medication is quite efficacious in treating acute mania. More rapid in onset, two placebo-controlled studies have reported clinically significant superiority of divalproex over placebo (Bowden et al., 1994; Pope et al., 1991). The transfer of valproic acid into milk is generally considered quite low. In a study of six women receiving 9.5 to 31 mg/kg/d valproic acid, milk levels averaged 1.4 mg/L while maternal serum levels averaged 45.1 mg/L (Nau et al., 1981). The average milk/serum ratio was 0.027. Most authors agree that the amount of valproic acid transferring to the infant via milk is low. Breastfeeding

would appear safe. However, the infant should be closely monitored for liver and platelet changes. Thus, in breastfeeding mothers with mania, valproic acid may be effective and safer than lithium.

Lamotrigine (Lamictal) has recently been approved for the treatment of mania. In numerous studies in breastfeeding mothers, relative infant doses ranged according to dose, but with doses of 200–400 mg/day, the RID ranged from 7.6 to 13 percent (Page-Sharp et al., 2006; Rambeck et al., 1997; Tomson et al., 1997; Ohman et al., 2000).

Antipsychotics

The published literature on the transfer of antipsychotics into milk is limited, but growing. However, older data seem to suggest that the phenothiazines and thioxanthenes transfer into milk in rather limited amounts.

In a number of small studies (Blacker, 1962; Wiles et al., 1978; Ohkubo et al., 1993; Uhlir & Ryznar, 1973; Citterio, 1964), the relative infant dose of chlorpromazine from breastmilk ranged from 0.25 percent and 0.14 percent after single doses of 1200 mg and 40 mg, respectively. In general, normal neurobehavioral development has been reported in infants exposed to chlorpromazine via milk (Ayd, 1973; Kris & Carmichael, 1957), although drowsiness and lethargy was reported in one infant who ingested milk containing 92 μg/L of chlorpromazine (Wiles et al., 1978). However, in another study, three infants exposed to both chlorpromazine and haloperidol via breastmilk showed developmental delay, and an infant exposed only to chlorpromazine was unaffected (Yoshida et al., 1998). However, chlorpromazine and other phenothiazines have been associated with neonatal apnea and SIDS and are poor choices for use in breastfeeding mothers (Boutroy, 1994; Kahn et al., 1985; Pollard & Rylance, 1994). For these reasons, the older phenothiazines and thiozanthines should probably be avoided in breastfeeding women.

Haloperidol transfers into breastmilk in moderately low concentrations, and reported relative infant doses range from 0.2–11.2 percent (Whalley et al., 1981; Stewart et al., 1980; Ohkubo et al., 1992; Sugawara et al., 1999). While adverse effects have been minimal in at least two cases (Whalley et al., 1981; Yoshida et al., 1998), in at least three other cases following exposure to both haloperidol and chlorpromazine via milk, neurobehavioral developmental milestones were not met (Yoshida et al., 1998).

The newer atypical antipsychotics may be the best choice of therapy for breastfeeding mothers. These include olanzapine, risperidone, and quetiapine.

Olanzapine transfer into milk has been studied in a total of 14 cases. Relative infant doses ranged from 0.9–1.6 percent, following maternal doses of 2.5–20 mg daily (Gardiner et al., 2003a; Croke et al., 2002; Ambresin et al., 2004; Kirchheiner et al., 2000). In seven of the infants, olanzapine was undetectable in the serum of the infants.

The transfer of quetiapine into human milk has only been studied in a total of eight cases. The relative infant dose ranges from 0.09–0.27 percent (Lee et al., 2004; Misri et al., 2006; Rampono et al., 2007). In none of the reported cases have side effects been noted in the breastfed infant.

The transfer of risperidone into human milk is also low and has been described in five women and four mother–baby pairs. Risperidone levels are reportedly quite low with an estimated relative infant dose of 4.3 percent (Hill et al., 2000). The metabolite was detected in infant plasma in one case (Aichhorn et al., 2005), and both risperidone and its metabolite were below the analytical limit of detection in another case (Ilett et al., 2004). No adverse effects have been detected in the four exposed infants studied (Ilett et al., 2004; Ratnayake & Libretto, 2002; Aichhorn et al., 2005).

Corticosteroids

The corticosteroids, in general, apparently do not transfer well into human milk. Following moderately high doses of prednisone (80 mg), the clinical dose transferred via milk is only 10 µg/kg, which is approximately 10 percent of the endogenous production (Ost et al., 1985). Prednisone and prednisolone transfer into milk has been found to be limited, even with larger doses (Berlin, 1979). Even following chronic doses of methylprednisolone (6–8 mg/d), no untoward side effects were noted in the infants (Coulam et al., 1982).

Steroids used via inhalation, such as fluticasone or budesonide, pose no problem for a breastfeeding mother or infant. Maternal plasma levels are low, and milk levels should be lower still, although no studies in breastfeeding mothers yet exist. These drugs were designed to have potent local effects, but minimal to nil oral absorption. Hence, milk levels will likely be minimal.

In the case of high intravenous doses (1–2 gm prednisone), such as for multiple sclerosis or acute immune reactions, plasma levels of these steroids fall rapidly due to redistribution. A brief interruption of up to 12 hours should suffice to limit exposure in the milk (Hale & Ilett, 2002).

With most lower potency topical steroids, the transcutaneous absorption is generally minimal. However, following the use of high-potency topical steroids over a large body surface, significant plasma levels are measurable. In these instances, a risk versus benefit assessment may be required concerning breastfeeding, particularly because these agents are extremely potent. In essence, use low- to moderate-potency topical steroids if possible.

Thyroid and Antithyroid Medications

The primary objective of treating patients with thyroid supplements is to increase their plasma thyroxine levels into the euthyroid range. Hence, it should be obvious that once accomplished, supplementation with thyroxine is no different than breastfeeding in a normal euthyroid mother. Regardless, the amount of thyroxine transferred into human milk is invariably low (Mizuta et al., 1983; Oberkotter, 1983). There are no contraindications to breastfeeding and using thyroid supplements as long as normal thyroxine levels in the maternal plasma are maintained.

In hyperthyroid states, both propylthiouracil (PTU) and methimazole have been thoroughly studied. PTU levels in milk are at least 10 fold lower than the maternal plasma level. Following a dose of 400 mg, the average amount of PTU transferred over 4 hours was only 99 ug (Kampmann et al., 1980). Using radiolabeled PTU, only 0.08 percent of the maternal dose transferred into milk over 24 hours (Low et al., 1979). Thus far, no changes in the infants' thyroid function have been reported.

Carbimazole is metabolized to the active metabolite, methimazole. Levels depend on maternal dose but appear too low to produce clinical effect. In one study of a patient receiving 2.5 mg methimazole every 12 hours, the dose to the infant was calculated at 16–39 µg/d (Tegler & Lindstrom, 1980). This was equivalent to 7–16 percent of the maternal dose. In a study of 35 lactating women receiving 5 to 20 mg/day of methimazole, no changes in the infant thyroid function were noted in any infant, even those at higher doses (Azizi, 1996).

Further, in a study of 11 women who were treated with the methimazole derivative, carbimazole (5–15 mg daily, equal to 3.3–10 mg methimazole), all 11 infants had normal thyroid function following maternal treatments (Lamberg et al., 1984). In a large study of over 139 thyrotoxic lactating mothers and their infants, even at methimazole doses of 20 mg/day, no changes in infant TSH, T4, or T3 were noted in over 12 months of study (Azizi et al., 2000).

Drugs of Abuse

It is all but impossible to determine if a drug-abusing mother will continue to do so while breastfeeding. Certain drugs of abuse are of major concern to a breastfeeding infant, and mothers need to be advised that the risk of the drug is simply too high to continue to breastfeed their infant. The risk versus benefit determination in women with a history of drug abuse and who want to breastfeed is enormously difficult. Each healthcare provider must evaluate the relative risk that the mother will return to the use of these various medications. While with some of these drugs the overall risk of the medication may be lower, some drugs of abuse are horribly detrimental to breastfeeding infants. In these cases, the risk assessment is extremely important. In mothers who appear unlikely to adhere to a drug-free environment while breastfeeding, they should probably be advised to feed formula.

Because most drugs of abuse are psychotropics, they readily pass into the brain and, in most instances, the breast milk compartment as well. The most dangerous compounds are the hallucinogens, such as LSD and phencyclidine. Mothers who are drug-screen positive for these substances should be strongly warned that these agents are the most dangerous of this group and pose significant hazard to their infants. Amphetamines and methylphenidate

do pass into milk, but the levels may not be high enough to pose a major hazard to most infants, although this is as yet unclear. Milk/plasma ratios with the amphetamines range from 3 to 7 (Steiner et al., 1984). Interestingly, cocaine levels in milk have never been reported. However, from kinetics we can be certain that cocaine undoubtedly enters milk avidly.

The effect of marijuana in breastfeeding mothers is rather unclear. Thus far, neurobehavioral effects on the infants have not been reported, even in heavy smokers (Perez-Reyes & Wall, 1982). Marijuana passes rapidly out of the plasma compartment and enters adipose tissue. Because of this rapid redistribution, milk levels are apparently low.

Marijuana is stored in fat tissues for long periods (weeks to months). Small to moderate secretion into breastmilk has been documented (Perez-Reyes & Wall, 1982). Analysis of breastmilk in a chronic heavy user revealed an eight-fold accumulation in breastmilk compared to plasma, although the dose received was insufficient to produce significant side effects in the infant. Studies have shown significant absorption and metabolism in infants, although long-term sequelae are conflicting. In one study of 27 women who smoked marijuana routinely during breastfeeding, no differences were noted in outcomes on growth, mental, and motor development (Tennes et al., 1985). In another study, marijuana in breastmilk was shown to be associated with a slight decrease in infant motor development at 1 year of age, especially when used during the first month of lactation (Astley & Little, 1990). This study's findings were confounded, however, by the use of marijuana during the first trimester of pregnancy. Interestingly, in this study, maternal use of marijuana during pregnancy and lactation had no detectable effect on infant mental development at 1 year of age.

The ingestion of heroin in breastfeeding mothers has not been well studied. Heroin is almost instantly deacetylated to its metabolite, morphine. While morphine is considered a good choice analgesic for breastfed infants, the major problem with heroin ingestion is the enormous dose sometimes used by addicts. Hence, levels of the metabolite (morphine) in milk could be potentially quite large and therefore hazardous to the infant.

Mothers should be advised that all of these psychotropic drugs of abuse readily enter milk and that their infants may be at high risk of sedation, apnea, or death if the dose is high enough. Further, all mothers should be advised that regardless of the clinical effect on the infant, their infants will be drug-screen positive for many days, perhaps weeks following their use. Suggested pumping and discarding periods are suggested in Table 5–6.

Radioisotopes

The use and transfer of radiolabeled substances are of major importance to breastfeeding mothers. Commonly used as diagnostic tools, the majority of these radioactive compounds have rather brief half-lives and don't pose a major problem for breastfeeding mothers. They can simply pump and discard their milk for 12–24 hours and continue to breastfeed. However, with the use of I-131, Gallium-67, or Thallium-201, longer pumping periods may be necessary and may preclude breastfeeding altogether.

A thorough summary of the most current literature concerning radioisotope transmission into human milk is available (Hale, 2006). Mothers who are required to take these medications are urged to follow guidelines set forth by Table 5–7.

TABLE 5–6	Suggested Duration for Interrupted Breastfeeding Following Use of Drugs of Abuse

Drug	Interrupt Feeding
Amphetamines, Ecstasy, MDMA	24–36 hours
Barbiturates	48 hours
Cocaine, crack	24 hours
Ethanol	1 hour per drink, or until sober
Heroin, morphine	24 hours
LSD	48 hours
Marijuana	24 hours
Phencyclidine, PCP	1–2 weeks

Source: Adapted from Hale & Ilett, 2002.

The most dangerous radioisotope is Iodine-131. It is concentrated in human milk (approximately 16–23 fold), may potentially destroy the infant's thyroid, and could ultimately increase the risk of thyroid carcinoma in the infant exposed to this isotope via milk. The NRC recommends discontinuing breastfeeding altogether. Because the levels of radioactive iodine in breast tissue is so high, women who require high doses of I-131 should probably discontinue breastfeeding for several weeks prior to use to avoid high radiation doses to their breast tissues.

Radiocontrast Agents

Radiocontrast agents or radio-opaque agents are used to enhance visualization of various tissue compartments. Two types are used: one group contains high concentrations of iodine, the other group contains the gadolinium ion. The iodinated groups are used for CAT scans, while the gadolinium products are used for magnetic resonance imaging (MRI scans).

In general, we recommend against the use of iodine-containing products in breastfeeding mothers. But in the case of the radiocontrast agents, the iodine molecule is covalently bound to the structure and is only minimally released. Thus, following the use of radiocontrast agents, the amount of free iodine is minimal, and they are not considered a risk to breastfed infants. In addition, the plasma half-life of these agents is quite short, less than 1 hour for most, and the oral bioavailability is virtually nil. Therefore, the absorption of clinically relevant amounts by breastfeeding infants is low. Table 5–8 provides the pharmacokinetic data and published milk levels on some of these agents. While most of the package inserts on these products suggest a 24-hour pumping and discarding of milk, this is obviously not necessary. The American College of Radiology has published a guideline on this subject and suggests that radiocontrast agents are not contraindicated in breastfeeding mothers (ACR Committee on Drugs and Contrast Media, 2001).

In MRI scans, gadolinium-containing compounds are used. Milk levels of gadopentetate are reported to be very low (Rofsky et al., 1993). Only 0.23 percent of the maternal dose was excreted over 24 hours of exposure. Further, the oral bioavailability of the gadolinium products is about 0.8 percent.

TABLE 5–7	**Nuclear Regulatory Guidelines on Radioisotopes and Breastfeeding**

| Radiopharmaceutical | Activity Above Which Instructions Are Required | | Examples of Recommended Duration of Interruption of Breastfeeding* |
	Mbq	mCi	
I-131 NaI	0.01	0.0004	Complete cessation (for this infant or child)
I-123 NaI	20	0.5	
I-123 OIH	100	4	
I-123 mIBG	70	2	24 hr for 370 MBq (10 mCi) 12 hr for 150 MBq (4 mCi)
I-125 OIH	3	0.08	
I-131 OIH	10	0.30	
Tc-99m DTPA	1000	30	
Tc-99m MAA	50	1.3	12.6 hr for 150 Mbq (4 mCi)
Tc-99m Pertechnetate	100	3	24 hr for 1,100 Mbq (30 mCi) 12 hr for 440 Mbq (12 mCi)
Tc-99m HAM	400	10	
Tc-99m MIBI	Tc-99m DISIDA	1000	
Tc-99m MDP	Tc-99m Glucoheptonate	1000	
Tc-99m PYP	900	25	
Tc-99m red blood cell in vivo labeling	400	10	6 hr for 740 Mbq (20 mCi)
Tc-99m red blood cell in vitro labeling	1000	30	
Tc-99m sulfur colloid	300	7	6 hr for 440 Mbq (12 mCi)
Tc-99m DTPA aerosol	1000	30	
Tc-99m MAG3	1000	30	
Tc-99m white blood cells	100	4	24 hr for 1,100 Mbq (5 mCi) 12 hr for 440 Mbq (2 mCi)
Ga-67 citrate	1	0.04	1 month for 150 Mbq (4 mCi) 2 weeks for 50 Mbq (1.3 mCi) 1 week for 7 Mbq (0.2 mCi)
In-111 white blood cells	10	0.2	1 week for 20 Mbq (0.5 mCi)
T1-201 chloride	40	1	2 weeks for 110 Mbq (3 mCi)

*The duration of interruption of breastfeeding is selected to reduce the maximum dose to a newborn infant to less than 1 millisievert (0.1 rem), although the regulatory limit is 5 millisieverts (0.5 rem). The actual doses that would be received by most infants would be far below 1 millisievert (0.1 rem). Of course, the physician may use discretion in the recommendation, increasing or decreasing the duration of the interruption.

Notes: Activities are rounded to one significant figure, except when it was considered appropriate to use two significant figures. Details of the calculations are shown in NUREG-1492, Regulatory Analysis on Criteria for the Release of Patients Administered Radioactive Material (Ref.2).

If there is no recommendation in Column 3 of this table, the maximum activity normally administered is below the activities that require instructions on interruption or discontinuation of breastfeeding.

Source: Adapted from Hale, 2008.

TABLE 5-8			

Radiocontrast Agents and Their Reported Milk Concentrations

Drug	Dose	Milk (C_{max})	Clinical Significance	Bioavailability	Lactation Risk Category
Gadopentetate	6.5 g	3.09 μmol/L	Only 0.023% of maternal dose; total dose = 0.013 μmol/24 hr; safe.	0.8%	L2
Iohexol	0.755 g/kg	35 mg/L	Mean milk level was only 11.4 mg/L; virtually unabsorbed; safe.	< 0.1%	L2
Iopanoic Acid	2.77 g	20.8 mg/ 19–29 hr	Only 0.08% of maternal dose; virtually unabsorbed; safe.	Nil	L2
Metrizamide	5.06 g	32.9 mg/L	Only 0.02% of maternal dose recovered over 44.3 hr; poor oral absorption; safe.	0.4%	L2
Metrizoate	580 mg	4 mg/L	Mean milk level 11.4 mg/24 hr; only 0.3% of maternal dose; safe.	Nil	L2

Source: Adapted from Hale & Ilett, 2002.

Summary

The data supporting the health benefits of breastfeeding is now significant, and it is strongly supported by numerous national academies and healthcare organizations. Far too often mothers are advised to discontinue breastfeeding so that they can be treated with a medication. In most cases, this advice is inaccurate and is simply given out of ignorance of this field. In most cases, drugs are quite safe for breastfeeding mothers to consume, and the healthcare practitioner is advised to seek accurate advice prior to disturbing breastfeeding.

It is true that all medications transfer into human milk. However, the vast majority do so in levels that are incredibly low, almost always subclinical, and pose no real risk for most infants. Nevertheless, all infants should be evaluated for risk prior to using medications in their mothers, and those infants deemed at high risk should only be exposed to medications that carry a minimal risk associated with their use. In reality, we do have a rather extensive database on drugs and their transfer into human milk.

By understanding the various mechanisms of transfer and those medications that pose the most risk, the clinician can usually develop strategies that can provide for the safe use of medications in mothers who breastfeed their infant. Such strategies involve using a safer medication or breastfeeding when the medication is low in the maternal plasma supply, or as a last resort, pumping and discarding the milk while the mother is treated.

Physicians and patients are advised to carefully choose those with lower relative infant doses (RID) and limited side effect profiles. But this might not always be possible, and each physician and mother must, as a team, determine the best choice for their individual case. Almost always, with the proper choice of medication, the mother can continue to breastfeed while undergoing drug therapy.

Key Concepts

- Avoid using medications when not absolutely necessary. This includes most herbal drugs.
- Choose drugs with shorter half-lives over those with longer half-lives.
- Choose drugs with less toxicity and those commonly used in infants.
- Choose drugs with poorer bioavailability to reduce oral absorption in infants.
- Choose drugs for which published milk studies exist.
- Evaluate the infant's medications. See if there are drug interactions.
- Evaluate the age, stability, and condition of the infant in order to determine if the infant can handle exposure to the medication.
- Preterm or unstable neonates may be more susceptible to adverse effects of medications because their clearance mechanisms have not matured.
- Understand that drugs that enter the CNS will also likely enter breastmilk. An increased level of concern is recommended.
- Always advise the mother to watch for changes in milk production with various drugs. Mothers forewarned are more observant of subtle changes.
- Most drugs can be safely used in breastfeeding mothers, but a risk versus benefit assessment is always required prior to use.
- Only a very few medications are unsafe under any circumstances.
- A relative infant dose of less than 10 percent is generally considered compatible with breastfeeding.

References

American Academy of Pediatrics. Transfer of drugs and other chemicals into human milk. *Peds.* 2001; 108(3):776–789.

American Academy of Pediatrics. Breastfeeding and use of human milk. *Peds.* 2005;115:496–506.

ACR Committee on Drugs and Contrast Media. Administration of contrast medium to breastfeeding mothers. *Am Coll Radiol.* 2001;57(10):13.

Aichhorn W, Stuppaeck C, Whitworth AB. Risperidone and breast-feeding. *J Psychopharmacol.* 2005;19(2): 211–213.

Aljazaf K et al. Pseudoephedrine: effects on milk production in women and estimation of infant exposure via breastmilk. *Br J Clin Pharmacol.* 2003; 56(1):18–24.

Altshuler LL et al. Breastfeeding and sertraline: a 24-hour analysis. *J Clin Psychiatry.* 1995;56(6):243–245.

Ambresin G et al. Olanzapine excretion into breast milk: a case report. *J Clin Psychopharmacol.* 2004; 24(1):93–95.

Andersen HJ. Excretion of verapamil in human milk. *Eur J Clin Pharmacol.* 1983;25(2):279–280.

Anderson P et al. Verapamil and norverapamil in plasma and breast milk during breast feeding. *Eur J Clin Pharmacol.* 1987;31(5):625–627.

Anderson PO, McGuire GG. Neonatal alprazolam withdrawal—possible effects of breast feeding. *DICP.* 1989;23(7–8):614.

Anonymous. Single dose cabergoline versus bromocriptine in inhibition of puerperal lactation: randomised, double blind, multicentre study. European Multicentre Study Group for Cabergoline in Lactation Inhibition [see comments]. *BMJ.* 1991; 302(6789):1367–1371.

Astley SJ, Little RE. Maternal marijuana use during lactation and infant development at one year. *Neurotoxicol Teratol.* 1990;12(2):161–168.

Atkinson HC, Begg EJ. Prediction of drug distribution into human milk from physicochemical characteristics. *Clin Pharmacokinet.* 1990;18(2):151–167.

Ayd F Jr. Excretion of psychotropic drugs in human breast milk. *Int Drug Ther News Bull.* 1973;8(9,10):33–40.

Azizi F. Effect of methimazole treatment of maternal thyrotoxicosis on thyroid function in breast-feeding infants. *J Pediatr.* 1996;128(6):855–858.

Azizi F et al. Thyroid function and intellectual development of infants nursed by mothers taking methimazole. *J Clin Endocrinol Metab.* 2000; 85(9):3233–3238.

Bailey DN et al. A study of salicylate and caffeine excretion in the breast milk of two nursing mothers. *J Anal Toxicol.* 1982;6(2):64–68.

Begg EJ. *Clinical Pharmacology Essentials. The Principles Behind the Prescribing Process.* Auckland, New Zealand: Adis International; 2000.

Begg EJ et al. Distribution of R- and S-methadone into human milk at steady state during ingestion of medium to high doses. *Br J Clin Pharmacol.* 2001;52(6):681–685.

Bennett PN. Use of the monographs on drugs. In: *Drugs and Human Lactation.* Amsterdam: Elsevier; 1996:67–74.

Berlin CM. Excretion of prednisone and prednisolone in human milk. *Pharmacologist.* 1979;21:264.

Besunder JB, Reed MD, Blumer JL. Principles of drug biodisposition in the neonate. A critical evaluation of the pharmacokinetic-pharmacodynamic interface (Part II). [Review]. *Clin Pharmacokinet.* 1988;14(5):261–286.

Blacker KH. Mothers milk and chlorpromazine. *Am J Psychiat.* 1962;114:178–179.

Blanco JD et al. Ceftazidime levels in human breast milk. *Antimicrob Agents Chemother.* 1983;23(3):479–480.

Booker DE, Pahl IR. Control of postpartum breast engorgement with oral contraceptives. *Am J Obstet Gynecol.* 1967;98(8):1099–1101.

Booker DE, Pahl IR, Forbes DA. Control of postpartum breast engorgement with oral contraceptives. II. *Am J Obstet Gynecol.* 1970;108(2):240–242.

Bourget P, Quinquis-Desmaris V, Fernandez H. Ceftriaxone distribution and protein binding between maternal blood and milk postpartum. *Ann Pharmacother.* 1993;27(3):294–297.

Boutroy MJ. Drug-induced apnea. *Biol Neonate.* 1994;65(3–4):252–257.

Boutroy MJ et al. To nurse when receiving acebutolol: is it dangerous for the neonate? *Eur J Clin Pharmacol.* 1986;30(6):737–739.

Bowden CL et al. Efficacy of divalproex vs lithium and placebo in the treatment of mania. The Depakote Mania Study Group. *JAMA.* 1994;271(12):918–924.

Brackbill Y et al. Obstetric meperidine usage and assessment of neonatal status. *Anesthesiology.* 1974a; 40(2):116–120.

Brackbill Y et al. Obstetric premedication and infant outcome. *Am J Obstet Gynecol.* 1974b;118(3):377–384.

Briggs GG et al. Excretion of bupropion in breast milk. *Annals Pharmacother.* 1993;27(4):431–433.

Budd SC et al. Improved lactation with metoclopramide. A case report. *Clin Pediatr (Phila).* 1993;32(1):53–57.

Caballero-Gordo A et al. Oral cabergoline. Single-dose inhibition of puerperal lactation. *J Reprod Med.* 1991;36(10):717–721.

Canales ES, Garcia IC, Ruiz JE, Zarate A. Bromocriptine as prophylactic therapy in prolactinoma during pregnancy. *Fertil Steril.* 1981;36:524–526.

Cantu TG. Phenothiazines and sudden infant death syndrome. *DICP.* 1989;23(10):795–796.

Castberg I, Spigset O. Excretion of escitalopram in breast milk. *J Clin Psychopharmacol.* 2006;26(5):536–538.

Chambers CD et al. Birth outcomes in pregnant women taking fluoxetine [comments]. *NEJM.* 1996; 335(14):1010–1015.

Chasnoff IJ, Lewis DE, Squires L. Cocaine intoxication in a breast-fed infant. *Pediatrics.* 1978;80:836–838.

Chatterton RT Jr. Mammary gland: development and secretion. *Obstet Gynecol Annu.* 1978;7:303–324.

Chatterton RT et al. Relation of plasma oxytocin and prolactin concentrations to milk production in mothers of preterm infants: influence of stress. *J Clin Endocrinol Metab.* 2000;85(10):3661–3668.

Citterio C. Riconoscimento e dosaggio di derivati fenotiazinici nella secrezione lattea. *Neuropsichiatria.* 1964;20141–146 (quoted by Toxnet/LactMed NLM Database).

Cochi SL et al. Primary invasive *Haemophilus influenzae* type b disease: a population-based assessment of risk factors. *J Pediatr.* 1986;108(6):887–896.

Coulam CB et al. Breast-feeding after renal transplantation. *Transplant Proc.* 1982;14(3):605–609.

Cover DL, Mueller BA. Ciprofloxacin penetration into human breast milk: a case report [comments]. *DICP.* 1990;24(7–8):703–704.

Croke S et al. Olanzapine excretion in human breast milk: estimation of infant exposure. *Int J Neuropsychopharmacol.* 2002;5(3):243–247.

da Silva OP et al. Effect of domperidone on milk production in mothers of premature newborns: a randomized, double-blind, placebo-controlled trial. *CMAJ.* 2001;164(1):17–21.

Dutt S, Wong F, Spurway JH. Fatal myocardial infarction associated with bromocriptine for postpartum lactation suppression. *Aust N Z J Obstet Gynaecol.* 1998;38(1):116–117.

Ehrenkranz RA, Ackerman BA. Metoclopramide effect on faltering milk production by mothers of premature infants. *Pediatrics.* 1986;78(4):614–620.

Ferrari C, Piscitelli G, Crosignani PG. Cabergoline: a new drug for the treatment of hyperprolactinaemia. *Hum Reprod.* 1995;10(7):1647–1652.

Figalgo I. Anemia aguda, rectaorragia y hematuria asociadas a la ingestion de naproxen. *Anales Espanoles de Pediatrica.* 1989;30:317–319.

Ford RP et al. Breastfeeding and the risk of sudden infant death syndrome. *Int J Epidemiol.* 1993; 22(5):885–890.

Fountain JR et al. Persistence of amethopterin in normal mouse tissues. *Proc Soc Exp Biol Med.* 1953;83(2):369–373.

Fries H. Lithium in pregnancy. *Lancet.* 1970;1(7658):1233.

Gambrell RDJ. Immediate postpartum oral contraception. *Obstet Gynecol.* 1970;36(1):101–106.

Gardiner SJ et al. Transfer of olanzapine into breast milk, calculation of infant drug dose, and effect on breast-fed infants. *Am J Psychiatry.* 2003;160(8):1428–1431.

Gardner DK, Gabbe SG, Harter C. Simultaneous concentrations of ciprofloxacin in breast milk and in serum in mother and breast-fed infant. *Clin Pharm.* 1992;11(4):352–354.

Giamarellou H et al. Pharmacokinetics of three newer quinolones in pregnant and lactating women. *Am J Med.* 1989;87(5A):49S–51S.

Goldman AS. The immune system of human milk: antimicrobial, antiinflammatory and immunomodulating properties. *Pediatr Infect Dis J.* 1993; 12(8):664–671.

Goldman AS et al. Immunologic protection of the premature newborn by human milk. *Semin Perinatol.* 1994;18(6):495–501.

Hale TW. *Medications and Mothers' Milk.* Amarillo, TX: Hale; 2008.

Hale TW, Berens PD. *Clinical Therapy in Breastfeeding Patients.* Amarillo, TX: Pharmasoft Publishing LP; 2003.

Hale TW, Hartman PE. *Textbook of Human Lactation.* Amarillo, TX: Hale; 2007.

Hale TW, Ilett KF. *Drug Therapy and Breastfeeding. From Theory to Clinical Practice.* London, UK: Parthenon Press; 2002.

Hale TW, Kristensen JH, Ilett KF. The transfer of medications into human milk. In: Hale TW, Hartmann PE (eds). *Textbook of Human Lactation.* Amarillo, TX: Hale; 2007b:465–478.

Hale TW, McDonald R, Boger J. Transfer of celecoxib into human milk. *J Hum Lact.* 2004;20(4):397–403.

Hale TW, Shum S, Grossberg M. Fluoxetine toxicity in a breastfed infant. *Clin Pediatr. (Phila).* 2001; 40(12):681–684.

Hale TW et al. Transfer of metformin into human milk. *Diabetologia.* 2002;45(11):1509–1514.

Hale TW et al. Presence of *Candida albicans* in symptomatic breastfeeding mothers [Abstract]. Academy of Breastfeeding Medicine; 2007. Abstract.

Harmon T, Burkhart G, Applebaum H. Perforated pseudomembranous colitis in the breast-fed infant. *J Pediatr Surg.* 1992;27(6):744–746.

Havelka J et al. Excretion of chloramphenicol in human milk. *Chemotherapy.* 1968;13(4):204–211.

Hill RC et al. Risperidone distribution and excretion into human milk: case report and estimated infant exposure during breast-feeding [letter]. *J Clin Psychopharmacol.* 2000;20(2):285–286.

Hodgkinson R et al. Neonatal neurobehavior in the first 48 hours of life: effect of the administration of meperidine with and without naloxone in the mother. *Pediatrics.* 1978;62(3):294–298.

Hodgkinson R et al. Double-blind comparison of maternal analgesia and neonatal neurobehaviour following intravenous butorphanol and meperidine. *J Int Med Res.* 1979;7(3):224–230.

Hofmeyr GJ, Van Iddekinge B. Domperidone and lactation [letter]. *Lancet.* 1983;1(8325):647.

Hofmeyr GJ, Van Iddekinge B, Blott JA. Domperidone: secretion in breast milk and effect on puerperal prolactin levels. *Br J Obstet Gynaecol.* 1985;92(2):141–144.

Iffy L et al. Severe cardiac dysrhythmia in patients using bromocriptine postpartum. *Am J Ther.* 1998; 5(2):111–115.

Ilett KF et al. Distribution and excretion of venlafaxine and O-desmethylvenlafaxine in human milk. *Br J Clin Pharmacol.* 1998;45(5):459–462.

Ilett KF et al. Distribution of venlafaxine and its O-desmethyl metabolite in human milk and their effects in breastfed infants. *Br J Clin Pharmacol.* 2002;53(1):17–22.

Ilett KF et al. Transfer of risperidone and 9-hydroxyrisperidone into human milk. *Ann Pharmacother.* 2004;38(2):273–276.

Inoue H et al. Level of verapamil in human milk [letter]. *Eur J Clin Pharmacol.* 1984;26(5):657–658.

Ito S et al. Prospective follow-up of adverse reactions in breast-fed infants exposed to maternal medication. *Am J Obstet Gynecol.* 1993;168(5):1393–1399.

Johns DG et al. Secretion of methotrexate into human milk. *Am J Obstet Gynecol.* 1972;112(7):978–980.

Jones HM, Cummings AJ. A study of the transfer of alpha-methyldopa to the human foetus and newborn infant. *Br J Clin Pharmacol.* 1978;6(5): 432–434.

Kafetzis DA et al. Transfer of cefotaxime in human milk and from mother to foetus. *J Antimicrob Chemother.* 1980;6(Suppl A):135–41135–141.

Kafetzis DA et al. Passage of cephalosporins and amoxicillin into the breast milk. *Acta Paediatr Scand.* 1981;70(3):285–288.

Kahn A, Hasaerts D, Blum D. Phenothiazine-induced sleep apneas in normal infants. *Pediatrics.* 1985;75(5):844–847.

Kampmann JP et al. Propylthiouracil in human milk. Revision of a dogma. *Lancet.* 1980;1(8171):736–737.

Kauffman RE, O'Brien C, Gilford P. Sulfisoxazole secretion into human milk. *J Pediatr.* 1980;97(5):839–841.

Kauppila A, Kivinen S, Ylikorkala O. A dose response relation between improved lactation and metoclopramide. *Lancet.* 1981;1(8231):1175–1177.

Kauppila A et al. Metoclopramide and breast feeding: transfer into milk and the newborn. *Eur J Clin Pharmacol.* 1983;25(6):819–823.

Kelsey JJ et al. Presence of azithromycin breast milk concentrations: a case report. *Am J Obstet Gynecol.* 1994;170(5 Pt 1):1375–1376.

Kirchheiner J, Berghöfer A, Bolk-Weischedel, D. Healthy outcome under olanzapine treatment in a pregnant woman. *Pharmacopsychiatry.* 2000;33:78–80.

Knowles JA. Drugs in milk. *Pediatr Currents.* 1972;21:28–32.

Koren G et al. Pharmacogenetics of morphine poisoning in a breastfed neonate of a codeine-prescribed mother. *Lancet.* 2006a;368(9536):704.

Koren G, Moretti M, Kapur B. Can venlafaxine in breast milk attenuate the norepinephrine and serotonin reuptake neonatal withdrawal syndrome? *J Obstet Gynaecol Can.* 2006b;28(4):299–302.

Kris EB, Carmichael DM. Chlorpromazine maintenance therapy during pregnancy and confinement. *Psychiatr Q.* 1957;31(4):690–695.

Kristensen JH et al. Distribution and excretion of sertraline and N-desmethylsertraline in human milk. *Br J Clin Pharmacol.* 1998;45(5):453–457.

Kristensen JH et al. Distribution and excretion of fluoxetine and norfluoxetine in human milk. *Br J Clin Pharmacol.* 1999;48(4):521–527.

Kuhnert BR et al. Meperidine and normeperidine levels following meperidine administration during labor. II. Fetus and neonate. *Am J Obstet Gynecol.* 1979a;133:909–914.

Kuhnert BR et al. Meperidine and normeperidine levels following meperidine administration during labor. I. Mother. *Am J Obstet Gynecol.* 1979b;133:904–908.

Kuhnert BR et al. Meperidine disposition in mother, neonate, and nonpregnant females. *Clin Pharmacol Ther.* 1980;27:486–491.

Kumar AR, Hale TW, Mock RE. Transfer of interferon alfa into human breast milk. *J Hum Lact.* 2000;16(3):226–228.

Lamberg BA et al. Antithyroid treatment of maternal hyperthyroidism during lactation. *Clin Endocrinol (Oxf).* 1984;21(1):81–87.

Lee A et al. Excretion of quetiapine in breast milk. *Am J Psychiatry.* 2004;161(9):1715–1716.

Lee CM, Gotlib IH. Adjustment of children of depressed mothers: a 10-month follow-up. *J Abnorm Psychol.* 1991;100(4):473–477.

Lester BM et al. Possible association between fluoxetine hydrochloride and colic in an infant. *J Am Acad Child Adolesc Psychiatry.* 1993;32(6):1253–1255.

Leuschen MP, Wolf LJ, Rayburn WF. Fentanyl excretion in breast milk [letter]. *Clin Pharm.* 1990;9(5):336–337.

Liedholm H et al. Transplacental passage and breast milk concentrations of hydralazine. *Eur J Clin Pharmacol.* 1982;21(5):417–419.

Llewellyn A, Stowe ZN, Strader JRJ. The use of lithium and management of women with bipolar disorder during pregnancy and lactation. *J Clin Psychiat.* 1998;59(Suppl 6):57–64; discussion 6557–6564.

Low LC, Lang J, Alexander WD. Excretion of carbimazole and propylthiouracil in breast milk [letter]. *Lancet.* 1979;2(8150):1011.

Matheson I. Drugs taken by mothers in the puerperium. *Br Med J (Clin Res Ed).* 1985;290(6481):1588–1589.

Matheson I, Lunde PK, Bredesen JE. Midazolam and nitrazepam in the maternity ward: milk concentrations and clinical effects. *Br J Clin Pharmacol.* 1990;30(6):787–793.

Matheson I, Pande H, Alertsen AR. Respiratory depression caused by N-desmethyldoxepin in breast milk. *Lancet.* 1985;2(8464):1124.

Matsuda S. Transfer of antibiotics into maternal milk. *Biol Res Pregnancy Perinatol.* 1984;5(2):57–60.

McBride RJ et al. A study of the plasma concentrations of lorazepam in mother and neonate. *Br J Anaesth.* 1979;51(10):971–978.

McCarthy JJ, Posey BL. Methadone levels in human milk. *J Hum Lact.* 2000;16(2):115–120.

McKenna WJ et al. Amiodarone therapy during pregnancy. *Am J Cardiol.* 1983;51(7):1231–1233.

Mennella JA, Beauchamp GK. The transfer of alcohol to human milk. Effects on flavor and the infant's behavior [comments]. *N Engl J Med.* 1991;325(14):981–985.

Miller GE, Banerjee NC, Stowe CM Jr. Diffusion of certain weak organic acids and bases across the bovine mammary gland membrane after systemic administration. *J Pharmacol Exp Ther.* 1967;157(1):245–253.

Miller MR et al. Verapamil and breast-feeding. *Eur J Clin Pharmacol.* 1986;30(1):125–126.

Misri S et al. Quetiapine augmentation in lactation: a series of case reports. *J Clin Psychopharmacol.* 2006;26(5):508–511.

Mizuta H et al. Thyroid hormones in human milk and their influence on thyroid function of breast-fed babies. *Pediatr Res.* 1983;17(6):468–471.

Morselli PL, Franco-Morselli R, Bossi L. Clinical pharmacokinetics in newborns and infants. Age-related differences and therapeutic implications. *Clin Pharmacokinet.* 1980;5(6):485–527.

Nau H et al. Valproic acid and its metabolites: placental transfer, neonatal pharmacokinetics, transfer via mother's milk and clinical status in neonates of epileptic mothers. *J Pharmacol Exp Ther.* 1981;219(3):768–777.

Nau H et al. Anticonvulsants during pregnancy and lactation. Transplacental, maternal and neonatal pharmacokinetics. *Clin Pharmacokinet.* 1982;7(6):508–543.

Nehlig A, Debry G. Consequences on the newborn of chronic maternal consumption of coffee during gestation and lactation: a review. *J Am Coll Nutr.* 1994;13:6–21.

Neville MC, McFadden TB, Forsyth I. Hormonal regulation of mammary differentiation and milk secretion. *J Mammary Gland Biol Neoplasia.* 2002;7(1):49–66.

Neville MC et al. The mammary fat pad. *J Mammary Gland Biol Neoplasia.* 1998;3(2):109–116.

Nulman I et al. Neurodevelopment of children exposed in utero to antidepressant drugs. *N Engl J Med.* 1997;336(4):258–262.

O'Hara MW et al. Controlled prospective study of postpartum mood disorders: comparison of childbearing and nonchildbearing women. *J Abnorm Psychol.* 1990;99(1):3–15.

Oberkotter LV. Thyroid function and human breast milk [letter]. *Am J Dis Child.* 1983;137(11):1131.

Ohkubo T, Shimoyama R, Sugawara K. Measurement of haloperidol in human breast milk by high-performance liquid chromatography. *J Pharm Sci.* 1992;81(9):947–949.

Ohkubo T, Shimoyama R, Sugawara K. Determination of chlorpromazine in human breast milk and serum by high-performance liquid chromatography. *J Chromatogr.* 1993;614(2):328–332.

Ohman I, Vitols S, Tomson T. Lamotrigine in pregnancy: pharmacokinetics during delivery, in the neonate, and during lactation. *Epilepsia.* 2000;41(6):709–713.

Ost L et al. Prednisolone excretion in human milk. *J Pediatr.* 1985;106(6):1008–1011.

Ostrea EM, Chavez CJ, Strauss ME. A study of factors that influence the severity of neonatal narcotic withdrawal. *J Pediat.* 1976;88(4 Pt. 1):642–645.

Page-Sharp M et al. Transfer of lamotrigine into breast milk. *Ann Pharmacother.* 2006;40(7–8):1470–1471.

Passmore CM et al. Metronidazole excretion in human milk and its effect on the suckling neonate. *Br J Clin Pharmacol.* 1988;26(1):45–51.

Penny WJ, Lewis MJ. Nifedipine is excreted in human milk. *Eur J Clin Pharmacol.* 1989;36(4):427–428.

Perez-Reyes M, Wall ME. Presence of delta9-tetrahydro-cannabinol in human milk [letter]. *N Engl J Med.* 1982;307(13):819–820.

Petraglia F et al. Domperidone in defective and insufficient lactation. *Eur J Obstet Gynecol Reprod Biol.* 1985;19(5):281–287.

Pisacane A et al. Breast-feeding and urinary tract infection. *J Pediatr.* 1992;120(1):87–89.

Plomp TA, Vulsma T, de Vijlder JJ. Use of amiodarone during pregnancy. *Eur J Obstet Gynecol Reprod Biol.* 1992;43(3):201–207.

Pollard AJ, Rylance G. Inappropriate prescribing of promethazine in infants [letter]. *Arch Dis Child.* 1994;70(4):357.

Pop C et al. Postpartum myocardial infarction induced by Parlodel. *Arch Mal Coeur Vaiss.* 1998;91(9):1171–1174.

Pope HG Jr et al. Valproate in the treatment of acute mania. A placebo-controlled study. *Arch Gen Psychiatry.* 1991;48(1):62–68.

Postellon DC, Aronow R. Iodine in mother's milk. *JAMA.* 1982;247:463.

Quinn PG et al. Measurement of meperidine and normeperidine in human breast milk by selected ion monitoring. *Biomed Environ Mass Spectrom.* 1986; 13(3):133–135.

Rambeck B et al. Concentrations of lamotrigine in a mother on lamotrigine treatment and her newborn child. *Eur J Clin Pharmacol.* 1997;51(6):481–484.

Rampono J et al. Citalopram and demethylcitalopram in human milk; distribution, excretion and effects in breast fed infants. *Br J Clin Pharmacol.* 2000; 50(10):263–268.

Rampono J et al. Transfer of escitalopram and its metabolite demethylescitalopram into breastmilk. *Br J Clin Pharmacol.* 2006;62(3):316–322.

Rampono J et al. Quetiapine and breastfeeding. *Ann Pharmacother.* 2007;41(4):711–714.

Rasmussen F. *Excretion of Drugs by Milk.* New York, NY: Springer-Verlag; 1971.

Ratnayake T, Libretto SE. No complications with risperidone treatment before and throughout pregnancy and during the nursing period. *J Clin Psychiatry.* 2002;63(1):76–77.

Robieux I et al. Morphine excretion in breast milk and resultant exposure of a nursing infant. *J Toxicol Clin Toxicol.* 1990;28(3):365–370.

Rofsky NM, Weinreb JC, Litt AW. Quantitative analysis of gadopentetate dimeglumine excreted in breast milk. *J Magn Reson Imaging.* 1993; 3(1):131–132.

Sanz EJ et al. Selective serotonin reuptake inhibitors in pregnant women and neonatal withdrawal syndrome: a database analysis. *Lancet.* 2005;365 (9458):482–487.

Schadewinkel-Scherkl AM et al. Active transport of benzylpenicillin across the blood-milk barrier. *Pharmacol Toxicol.* 1993;73(1):14–19.

Shyu WC et al. Excretion of cefprozil into human breast milk. *Antimicrob Agents Chemother.* 1992; 36(5):938–941.

Sinclair D, Murray L. Effects of postnatal depression on children's adjustment to school. Teacher's reports. *Br J Psychiatry.* 1998;172:58–63.

Sorensen HT et al. Risk of infantile hypertrophic pyloric stenosis after maternal postnatal use of macrolides. *Scand J Infect Dis.* 2003;35(2):104–106.

Spalding G. Bromocriptine (Parlodel) for suppression of lactation. *Aust NZ J Obstet Gynecol.* 1991;31:344–345.

Spencer MJ, Escondido CA. Fluoxetine hydrochloride (Prozac) toxicity in a neonate. *Pediatrics.* 1993; 92(5):721–722.

Stavchansky S, Combs A, Sagraves R, Delgado M, Joshi A. Pharmacokinetics of caffeine in breast milk and plasma after single oral administration of caffeine to lactating mothers. *Biopharm Drug Dispos.* 1999; 9:285–299.

Steiner E et al. Amphetamine secretion in breast milk. *Eur J Clin Pharmacol.* 1984;27(1):123–124.

Stewart RB, Karas B, Springer PK. Haloperidol excretion in human milk. *Am J Psychiat.* 1980;137(7):849–850.

Stiskal JA et al. Neonatal paroxetine withdrawal syndrome. *Arch Dis Child Fetal Neonatal Ed.* 2001; 84(2):F134–F135.

Stowe ZN et al. Sertraline and desmethylsertraline in human breast milk and nursing infants [comments]. *Am J Psychiatry.* 1997;154(9):1255–1260.

Stowe ZN et al. Paroxetine in human breast milk and nursing infants. *Am J Psychiatry.* 2000;157(2):185–189.

Strauss ME et al. Methadone maintenance during pregnancy: pregnancy, birth, and neonate characteristics. *Am J Obstet Gynecol.* 1974;120(7):895–900.

Sugawara K, Shimoyama R, Ohkubo T. Determinations of psychotropic drugs and antiepileptic drugs by high-performance liquid chromatogaphy and its monitoring in human breast milk. *Hirosaki Med J.* 1999;51(Suppl):S81–S86.

Summerfield RJ, Nielsen MS. Excretion of lorazepam into breast milk [letter]. *Br J Anaesth.* 1985;57(10):1042–1043.

Swafford S, Berens P. Effect of fenugreek on breast milk production. *BM News and Views.* 2000;6(3). Annual meeting abstracts. Sept 11–13.

Sweezy SR. Contraception for the postpartum woman. *NAACOGS Clin Issu Perinat Womens Health Nurs.* 1992;3(2):209–226.

Sykes PA, Quarrie J, Alexander FW. Lithium carbonate and breast-feeding. *Br Med J.* 1976;2(6047):1299.

Syversen GB, Ratkje SK. Drug distribution within human milk phases. *J Pharm Sci.* 1985;74(10):1071–1074.

Tegler L, Lindstrom B. Antithyroid drugs in milk. *Lancet.* 1980;2(8194):591.

Tennes K et al. Marijuana: prenatal and postnatal exposure in the human. *NIDA Res Monogr.* 1985;59:48–60.

Tomson T, Ohman I, Vitols S. Lamotrigine in pregnancy and lactation: a case report. *Epilepsia.* 1997;38(9):1039–1041.

Treffers PE. [Breastfeeding and contraception]. *Ned Tijdschr Geneeskd.* 1999;143(38):1900–1904.

Tunnessen WWJ, Hertz CG. Toxic effects of lithium in newborn infants: a commentary. *J Pediatr.* 1972;81(4):804–807.

Uhlir F, Ryznar J. Appearance of chlorpromazine in the mother's milk. *Act Nerv Super (Praha).* 1973;15(2):106.

Vorherr H. *The Breast: Morphology, Physiology and Lactation.* New York, NY: Academic Press; 1974.

Webster J. A comparative review of the tolerability profiles of dopamine agonists in the treatment of hyperprolactinaemia and inhibition of lactation [published erratum appears in *Drug Saf* 1996;14(5):342]. *Drug Saf.* 1996;14(4):228–238.

Webster J et al. Dose-dependent suppression of serum prolactin by cabergoline in hyperprolactinaemia: a placebo controlled, double blind, multicentre study. European Multicentre Cabergoline Dose-finding Study Group. *Clin Endocrinol (Oxf).* 1992;37(6):534–541.

Wesson DR et al. Diazepam and desmethyldiazepam in breast milk. *J Psychoactive Drugs.* 1985;17(1):55–56.

Whalley LJ, Blain PG, Prime JK. Haloperidol secreted in breast milk. *Br Med J (Clin Res Ed).* 1981;282(6278):1746–1747.

White GJ, White MK. Breast feeding and drugs in human milk. *Vet Human Toxicol.* 1980;22(1):18.

White WB, Andreoli JW, Cohn RD. Alpha-methyldopa disposition in mothers with hypertension and in their breast-fed infants. *Clin Pharmacol Ther.* 1985;37(4):387–390.

Whitelaw AG, Cummings AJ, McFadyen IR. Effect of maternal lorazepam on the neonate. *Br Med J (Clin Res Ed).* 1981;282(6270):1106–1108.

Wiles DH, Orr MW, Kolakowska T. Chlorpromazine levels in plasma and milk of nursing mothers. *Br J Clin Pharmacol.* 1978;5(3):272–273.

Wisner KL, Perel JM, Blumer J. Serum sertraline and N-desmethylsertraline levels in breast-feeding mother-infant pairs. *Am J Psychiat.* 1998;155(5):690–692.

Wittels B, Scott DT, Sinatra RS. Exogenous opioids in human breast milk and acute neonatal neurobehavior: a preliminary study. *Anesthesiology.* 1990;73(5):864–869.

Wojnar-Horton RE et al. Methadone distribution and excretion into breast milk of clients in a methadone maintenance programme. *Br J Clin Pharmacol.* 1997;44(6):543–547.

Yoshida K et al. Neuroleptic drugs in breast-milk: a study of pharmacokinetics and of possible adverse effects in breast-fed infants. *Psychol Med.* 1998;28(1):81–91.

Yoshioka H et al. Transfer of cefazolin into human milk. *J Pediatr.* 1979;94(1):151–152.

Zekoski EM, O'Hara MW, Wills KE. The effects of maternal mood on mother-infant interaction. *J Abnorm Child Psychol.* 1987;15(3):361–378.

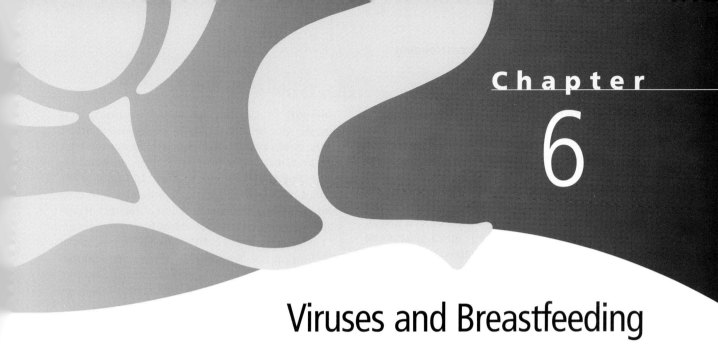

Viruses and Breastfeeding

Jan Riordan

Introduction

Mother-to-child transmission (MTCT) of a viral infection is a passage of infection that can occur during pregnancy, birthing, and the postpartum period. Specific concerns about infectious diseases and possible transmission through breastfeeding include the risks from mothers who acquire an infection while breastfeeding and the risks from mothers who acquired an infection during or before pregnancy. Questions abound:

- Which viruses are found in the milk of infected or seropositive women?
- What is the risk of transmission of such pathogens by breastfeeding?
- What effect does the infection have on the child?
- Do protective maternal antibodies in the milk limit transmission or reduce the severity of the viral infection in the child?
- Is there an effective treatment for the mother or the baby?

This chapter seeks to answer these questions, although we recognize that there are no simple answers to the complex puzzle of viral transmission from mother to infant.

Human milk, nature's most perfect vaccine model, plays a vital role in protecting the suckling young from viral infections. At the same time, a variety of animal and human viruses can be transmitted through mother's milk. Because breastmilk is a highly cellular fluid and viruses are intracellular (i.e., live within the cell), maternal–infant transmission by breastmilk is possible. HIV was isolated from breastmilk in 1985 and was found as cell-associated (DNA) and cell-free (RNA) (Thiry et al., 1985; Van de Perre et al., 1993). The transmission of cytomegalovirus (CMV) through breastmilk, for example, occurs frequently and provides a natural vaccine that confers active immunity to the infant against infection. CMV primary infection during pregnancy, on the other hand, can cause serious illness in a vulnerable infant, such as a preterm baby, especially if the viral load is high (van der Strate et al., 2001).

In contrast, hepatitis B virus and rubella virus appear in human milk, but breastfeeding does not appear to be a common mode of transmission for either. Human immunodeficiency virus (HIV) and human T-cell lymphotropic virus type I (HTLV-1) can be transmitted by breastmilk, with potentially adverse effects on the child.

HIV and Infant Feeding

The World Health Organization (WHO) and Joint United Nations Programme on HIV/AIDS (UNAIDS, 2007) have estimated that at the end of 2005 there were 40.3 million persons living with HIV/AIDS. Worldwide, approximately 300,000 children under 15 years of age are infected with HIV every year, most of them in sub-Saharan Africa and more recently an HIV epidemic in Papua New Guinea. MTCT of HIV accounts for most of these infections. In the United States estimates of the number of perinatal HIV infections peaked in 1991 and has declined since that time. The reduction is attributed to routine screening of pregnant women, use of antiretroviral (AVR) drugs for treatment and prevention, and by avoiding breastfeeding. With these interventions, rates of HIV transmission during pregnancy, labor, or delivery from mothers infected with HIV have been reduced to less than 2 percent compared with transmission rates of 25–30 percent with no interventions.

Since the last edition of this book, new research has cast a new light on prevention of breastfeeding and MTCT transmission. We now are recognizing that exclusive early breastfeeding dramatically lowers the risk of transmission through breast milk.

A breakthrough study (Coovadia, 2007) confirmed earlier studies (Coutsoudis et al., 1999) that when HIV-positive women breastfeed exclusively, their infants have a low risk of infection with HIV because the gut mucosa remains intact. On the other hand, mixed feedings with ingestion of contaminated fluids and food may lead to gastrointestinal injury and disruption of immune barriers. This risk is lower than that in infants who receive other food or liquids in addition to breast milk before 6 months. Mortality by age 3 months of breastfeeding babies who received food supplements is more than double that of those who were exclusively breastfed. Mixed feeding before or after 14 weeks nearly doubled transmission risk, and adding solids increased the risk 11-fold.

The possibility of breastfeeding while being HIV positive is promising because not being able to breastfeed can be deadly in a developing country. In a study (Brahmbhatt & Gray, 2003) of 14 developing countries, child mortality among the offspring of women who never breastfed was higher than among children who weaned. A finding from a Botswana perinatal trial documented a mortality rate at 7 months of age in formula-fed infants that is almost twice as high as that in breastfed babies (Thior et al., 2006). Of children in Botswana who were admitted to the hospital with severe diarrhea, 93 percent were not breastfeeding and were at the greatest risk of dying. Although replacement feeding does reduce HIV transmission, it is at the cost of substantial additional risks for infant mortality overall.

Eighty percent of US HIV-infected women are of childbearing age. Routine HIV testing and counseling to all pregnant women, and antiretroviral administration to those who are HIV positive, is now considered the standard of care in the United States. At the time of this writing, the CDC continues to recommend against breastfeeding by HIV-infected women living in developed areas. Breastfeeding by HIV-infected women in more developed countries has virtually ceased.

Antiretroviral therapy is profoundly effective in preventing perinatal transmission. Since the introduction of highly active antiretroviral therapy (HAART) in the mid-1990s the overall death rate of AIDS cases has decreased. Persons who are HIV positive can live for decades with what is now considered a chronic disease though they may suffer from complications of the disease and/or long-term use of medications.

Antiretroviral treatment to HIV-infected pregnant women and their newborns reduces the risk for perinatal transmission of HIV by approximately one half to two thirds (Connor et al., 1994; Karim, 2002).

Exclusive Breastfeeding

The first report that exclusive breastfeeding might reduce the risk of HIV infection was an influential prospective study of 549 HIV infected mothers in South Africa by Coutsoudis et al. (1999) who examined infant feeding practices as part of a vitamin A intervention trial. After adjusting for potential confounders, they found that infants who were exclusively breastfeeding had a significantly lower risk of HIV-1 transmission. Those infants receiving supplemental formula had the same risk as infants who were not breastfeeding. The probable reasons for this all or nothing phenomenon relates to maintaining the intestinal mucosal barrier. With mixed feedings bacteria and other contaminants may be introduced into the gut and cause inflammatory responses that damage the mucosa. HIV-1 is less likely to penetrate healthy gastrointestinal mucosa than damaged mucosa (Coutsoudis et al. 1999; Smith & Kuhn, 2000). Other investigators. most importantly the meticulous study by Coovadia and colleagues (2007) confirm this study's findings—a major breakthrough for areas of the world where replacement feedings are not easily available (Jackson et al., 2003).

At the same time, changing existing feeding practices to exclusive breastfeeding is an enormous challenge. Worldwide, few infants are exclusively breastfed in spite of a long duration of partial breastfeeding. Because of a wide range of cultural and traditional practices, other foods and liquids are given to infants early. In Tanzania, for example, almost half of the women in one study had introduced additional fluids to their babies after only a few days even though 85 percent started breastfeeding within the first 2 hours after birth (dePaoli et al., 2001). Moreover, formula marketing easily undermines exclusive breastfeeding.

Once feedings are no longer exclusive and supplements given, WHO recommends that HIV-infected women avoid breastfeeding completely. There is no evidence to support the exact timing for cessation. However early cessation reduces the risk of transmission by limiting the time the infant is exposed to HIV infection through breastmilk.

Treatment and Prevention

Before antiretroviral drugs were developed, perinatal transmission rates were 25–30 percent in the United States. Their use reduced perinatal transmission to about 8 percent or less. AZT and protease inhibitors block one step of the reproductive cycle of HIV and sharply reduce the risk of transmission from mother to infant. AZT, given in a combined regimen to the mother during pregnancy and labor, further reduces the transmission rate of HIV; however, AZT is expensive. Nevirapine, a new cheaper AIDS drug that can be taken by breastfeeding women, is now widely used around the world. A clinical trial in Uganda showed that the rate of new infections from breastfeeding at age 6 weeks to 12 months was not increased in infants of mothers receiving nevirapine (Owor et al., 2000).

Various interventions are now available for HIV-infected pregnant women in parts of Africa. Women receive short-course zidovudine during pregnancy and referral for highly active antiretroviral therapy. Women receiving a triple prophylaxis (zidovudine, lamivludine, and nevirapine) from 28 weeks gestation to 1 month postpartum significantly reduced HIV RNA levels and decreased the risk of breastfeeding-associated transmission (Giuliano et al., 2007). Resistance to antiretroviral medications, however, is a growing concern (WHO, 2007).

Risk factors that play a role in HIV transmission into human milk are listed in Box 6–1. General guidelines for avoiding perinatal transmission of HIV include the following:

- Screen for HIV—Knowing a mother's HIV status is critical for preventing transmission. Treatment with appropriate drugs can reduce the risk of perinatal transmission.
- Formula feeding if the mother is HIV-1 positive where safe, affordable alternatives are available—HIV can be transmitted from mother to infant through breastfeeding especially when supplements are given. The US Department of Health and Human Services states that HIV-infected women should not breastfeed or provide their breastmilk for the nutrition of their own or other infants, but these recommendations may change given new information.
- Exclusive breastfeeding if safe alternative supplements are not available—Where safe replacement feedings are not feasible, promotion of exclusive breastfeeding reduces risk of HIV-1 transmission to the baby. If replacement infant feedings are used, the risk of HIV transmission is exchanged for the risk of diarrhea and pneumonia if fuel to boil water for replacement-feeding preparation, sterilization, nutritional additives, and equipment are not available (Savage & Lhotska, 2000).
- After the cessation of exclusive breast feeding, HIV-infected women are recommended to avoid breastfeeding completely (WHO www.who.int, 2007).
- Deferring pregnancy—Women who are seropositive for HIV and areas not receiving ARV medications are advised to defer pregnancy. In countries where cesarean section delivery is available, surgical delivery can significantly reduce mother-to-baby HIV-1 transmission.

6–1

Risk Factors for HIV Transmission in Breastmilk

- Maternal viral load
- Duration of breastfeeding
- Type of breastfeeding (exclusive vs. mixed)

- Oral lesions in the infant
- Maternal breast lesions

In the case of vaginal birth, premature rupture of membranes and insertion of scalp electrodes should be avoided.

- Avoid practices that might increase exposure to HIV—Uninfected mothers who are breastfeeding should be especially careful to avoid high-risk practices (e.g., drug abuse or a sexual partner who is bisexual or has engaged in practices linked to HIV transmission) that might expose them to a primary HIV infection (Dunn et al., 1992; Van de Perre, 1991).

- Maintaining breast health by preventing entry of virus—Breast conditions such as mastitis, breast abscess, and nipple fissure may increase the risk of HIV transmission through breastfeeding. The extent of this association is not well documented (Smith & Kuhn, 2000).

Healthcare Practitioners

Practitioners who work with human milk or with breastfeeding women are concerned about their own protection. The Centers for Disease Control and Prevention (CDC) recommends precautions be used when handling blood and body fluids of all patients regardless of their infection status. These universal precautions apply to blood and other body fluids that contain visible blood (e.g., semen and vaginal secretions). Universal precautions *do not apply* to human milk unless it contains visible blood (CDC, 2008). Occupational exposure to human milk has not been implicated in the transmission of HIV. Gloves are not needed when touching the breasts

(e.g., in breast assessment), and they usually are not necessary when handling breastmilk either. However, if the healthcare worker comes in frequent contact with human milk (e.g., while working in human milk banking), he or she may choose to wear gloves. Also, if the mother has an open wound on her breast, glove wearing is warranted for the protection of both the mother and her care provider. Staff routinely wears gloves during delivery and for newborn care. Vigorous hand washing by the care provider—both before and after any physical contact with a client or with any body fluid—is standard practice for infection control and should be performed consistently to prevent transmission of *any* infection in the mother, the child, and the healthcare worker.

There is currently insufficient data that pasteurization of breastmilk is safe from risk of transmission (Giles & Mijch, 2005). Hartmann et al. (2006) have proposed a new approach for preventing MTCT that allows safe feeding of breastmilk of HIV positive mothers by treating their milk with a low concentration of sodium dodecyl sulfate, an alkyl sulfate microbicide.

Counseling

WHO technical guidelines emphasize that all HIV-infected mothers should receive feeding counseling that includes general information about the risks and benefits of various infant feeding options, and specific guidance in selecting the option most likely to be suitable for their situation (Coutsoudis, 2000). Results of the studies by Coutsoudis et al. (1999) and

Coovadia et al. (2007) that confirm the relative safety of exclusive breastfeeding for HIV MTCT necessitate a new public health mandate to teach mothers in resource-poor settings about the health benefits of practicing exclusive breastfeeding. Another mandate is teaching safer sex. HIV-infected women who do not practice safe sex risk acquiring drug-resistant HIV strains.

HIV-infected women come from all walks of life. Whatever the direct cause of their illness, their lives can be shattered by the knowledge that they are HIV positive. Few illnesses are associated with such high levels of stigma and social isolation. One woman complained that the healthcare workers at the local clinic acted "like they didn't want to talk to me or touch me. It's like I have AIDS written across my forehead, and they don't see anything else but that." Another noted, "I think I could be in a wreck and my arm would be hanging off and I'd be about to bleed to death, and all the doctors would see is someone with HIV" (Black & Miles, 2002).

In some areas where AIDS is rampant, white cream on a woman's face is visible evidence that she is breastfeeding. On a visit to South Africa I saw young women with white cream on their face as a signal to others that they were breastfeeding and thus HIV negative. Although HIV positive women desperately need help from family, friends, and other support groups, they may be isolated because HIV is a "secret" disease. Their counseling needs are necessarily complex, because these women must make difficult decisions while trying to cope with the implications of HIV for themselves and their families. In areas where antiretroviral drugs are available, the importance of adherence to the drug therapy is an essential topic.

Herpes Simplex Virus (HSV)

HSV-1, caused by *Herpesvirus hominus*, is a common viral infection in humans. HSV type 2 and HSV-1 genital infections are sexually transmitted diseases. HSV type 2 is associated more frequently with infection of the genital area and type I most often occurs in the face and mouth. Herpetic lesions can erupt anywhere in the body, including the breast or the genital area, usually as a result of direct contact. The infection may be either primary or recurrent.

Diagnosis is made either by culturing the lesion or by drawing serum-antibody titers.

The painful mucocutaneous blisterlike vesicles of herpes can appear within a few hours, or up to 20 days after exposure. After the lesions heal, the virus enters a dormant phase and resides in the nerve ganglia in the affected area. Usually the primary infection is the most severe. Neonatal HSV-1 infection is usually acquired when the newborn passes through an infected genital tract; congenital infection is responsible for the most serious illness in neonates. Vaginal delivery is safe in most women with a history of recurrent genital herpes unless active lesions are present at term. The American College of Obstetricians and Gynecologists (2002) officially recommends that a cesarean section be performed within 6 hours of rupture of membranes if active lesions are present. Cesarean delivery is not recommended when a woman with a history of recurrent infection has no obvious lesions and no symptoms of the infection.

The greatest threat of HSV-1 infection appears to be with neonates and when the mother experiences a first episode of genital herpes during pregnancy near term (Donahue, 2002). Primary infection means that the mother has insufficient antibodies that would help protect the infant from infection. Transmission rate to the newborn is 50 percent with a primary infection and only 1 to 3 percent if it is recurrent. Neonates may become seriously ill; beyond the first few weeks of the neonate's life, however, there are few adverse consequences. Despite the high prevalence of genital herpes in the general population, the incidence of neonatal herpes is low and ranges from 1 in 2,000 to about 1 in 10,000 births (Brown, 1995). It is doubtful that neonatal herpes is transmitted through human milk. Transmission during breastfeeding, if it occurs, is most likely from direct contact with a herpes vesicle on the breast.

Sealander and Kerr (1989) reported a case of a nursing toddler transmitting HSV to the mother through breastfeeding. In this case, the child's oral lesions (on the inner aspect of the lower lip) caused painful blisters on the mother's nipples. Culture of the child's oral lesions and the mother's nipple lesions were positive for HSV-1. After one week's cessation of breastfeeding, during which time the mother was given oral acyclovir—200 mg five times daily for five days—the mother resumed breastfeeding. The authors recommended that whenever a young child develops oral HSV lesions, the mother should be asked whether she is breastfeeding the child, so that the risk of contracting HSV from her child can be explained and appropriate intervention offered.

Sullivan-Bolyai et al. (1983) report a case of a mother with a maternal breast lesion identified as HSV-1. Although her infant experienced an uneventful nursery course and was discharged from the hospital at 2 days of age, the mother reported developing a "skin sore" on the areola of her left breast during her postpartum stay. On the fourth day of life, the baby appeared to have pustules in the corner of his mouth and on his chin. On day 6 and 7, HSV was also isolated from the mouth of the infant; on day 7, the virus was isolated from the mother's breast lesions. The infant died at 11 days of age. This case points out the need to avoid direct infant contact with an HSV-1 lesion. Although the mother's milk may be free of the virus, the lesion itself is not.

In another case, the milk from the mother of an infected infant was found to contain HSV; however, it appeared that the transmission had probably occurred at delivery, and it was unknown whether the infant became infected by the mother or the mother became infected by the infant (Duckle, Schmidt, & O'Connor, 1979).

Although HSV-1 can occasionally be cultured from breastmilk, this appears to be rare (Oxtoby, 1988). HSV-1 has not been isolated in any of the CMV studies that used culture techniques appropriate for HSV-1 (Pass, 1986), and no role in transmitting infection in the absence of a local HSV-1 lesion has been demonstrated. Breast lesions are seldom the first clinical evidence of herpes in the family (Sullivan-Bolyai et al., 1983). The primary herpetic lesion can be manifested in other family members who then pass it on (e.g., the father while making love with the mother, or a sibling who kisses a baby brother or sister). Therefore, transmission can be from mother to infant or from infant to mother; or some other family member can infect the infant, who then passes the virus on to the mother during feedings. HSV is an emotionally difficult topic and anxiety producing. There is no way to know when a reactivation will occur. In addition there are other issues such as disclosure of the disease to sexual partners and condom use.

Women with herpetic lesions on their breasts should refrain from breastfeeding; active lesions should be covered (AAP, 1997) to prevent contact by the suckling infant. In the absence of breast lesions, the newborn of a mother with HSV-1, if the baby is well, may breastfeed and be with the mother in her room; however, scrupulous hand washing, gowning, and covering of any lesions must be practiced to prevent possible cross-contamination. The mother does not need to wear rubber gloves while breastfeeding.

Treatment is usually directed toward symptomatic relief and prevention of a secondary infection. Acyclovir (Zovirax), valacyclovir, and famciclovir are antiviral medications used for HSV infections. Aggressive and early use of intravenous acyclovir results in apparent improvement for the mother and infant. Acyclovir can be given orally, applied topically, or given intravenously (usually when treating neonatal HSV). The routine administration of acyclovir to pregnant women with a history of recurrent infections is not recommended (Cline, Bailey-Dorton, & Cayelli, 2000). A new over-the-counter antiviral cream, docosanal (Abreva) is now available to treat cold sores and fever blisters. Cleaning affected areas with povidone-iodine (Betadine) solution is thought to help prevent a secondary infection, and applying Burrow's solution (aluminum acetate) may relieve some of the discomfort. Vitamin C or lysine and lysine supplements are frequently suggested to prevent recurrence, although their efficacy is unknown. A plan for care of a breastfeeding mother with HSV is described in Table 6–1.

Chickenpox / Varicella

Most people have immunity to chickenpox (varicella-zoster virus); therefore the issue of whether mothers with chickenpox can breastfeed is uncommon. Those who have not had chickenpox and are not immune (5–15 percent of adults) are potentially infectious for day 10 through day 21 after exposure. Lesions begin on the neck or trunk and spread to the face, scalp, mucous membranes, and extremities. Lesions first appear as small, flat, red blotches and progress to raised vesicles that form crusts over a period from 2 to 4 days. A vaccine (live attenuated virus) to prevent varicella was developed in 1995, and millions of doses of the vaccine have been administered since then. The CDC recommends vaccination of all susceptible healthcare workers.

TABLE 6–1	Clinical Care Plan for Breastfeeding Mother with Herpes Simplex (HSV) Infection	

Problem	Intervention	Rationale
Seropositive for HSV	Encourage continued breastfeeding unless breast lesions are present.	Provides protective antibodies to infant
Herpes	Instruct mother to wash hands thoroughly with soap before breastfeeding.	Helps prevent spreading infection
No breast lesion	Caution mother against touching baby or breast after touching lesion from any site.	Avoid risks of shedding
	Caution mother to avoid tub bath with infant; use universal precautions (hospital staff).	Avoid risks of shedding
Breast lesion present	Discourage breastfeeding from affected breast; encourage use of breast pump to maintain comfort and milk supply; after each use, sterilize pump part that comes in contact with breast.	Prevents infant's direct contact with lesion
Pain	Administer acetaminophen. Apply Burrow's solution topically. Employ imagery.	Analgesia Soothing effect Distraction by focusing
Feelings of shame	Reassure mother that HSV is not uncommon.	Mothers tend to blame themselves
Secondary infection	Cleanse lesion with Betadine.	Antibacterial

Because chickenpox can occur during the reproductive years, a woman may develop this infection while she is breastfeeding. If a mother contracts chickenpox while breastfeeding, she should continue to breastfeed because the antibodies in her milk confer immunity against chickenpox to her baby. This passive immunization may even spare the breastfed baby symptoms of chickenpox; if the disease is contracted, the course of the infant's disease is usually mild.

Congenital varicella syndrome can occur when chickenpox is contracted in the first half of pregnancy and cause serious problems for the fetus including low birth weight and neurological problems (McCarter-Spaulding, 2001). Fortunately, this condition is rare (one to six per 100,000 births).

A mother who develops chickenpox several days before she delivers her baby or has the virus within 48 hours after birth presents a special, complex medical case that can be potentially life threatening. Neonates of these women have a 17 to 30 percent likelihood of having a severe case of chickenpox because they do not have sufficient antibodies from their mother to lessen the severity of the infection (Cottrell & Carter, 1998). A woman with varicella who is admitted to the hospital for delivery is managed with airborne and contact infection control precautions using gowns, gloves, and masks. Following birth the mother and baby should be isolated from one another and others if the neonate does not develop lesions and discharged as soon as possible; however, this decision is usually made on an individual basis (McCarter-Spaulding, 2001). The mother can maintain her breastmilk supply by pumping and discarding the milk until she is no longer infectious. The mother should express breastmilk if the baby is

TABLE 6–2	**Viruses in Human Milk (Continued)**	

Virus	**Transmission**	**Recommendation**
Hepatitis C	Proven	Breastfeeding permitted if titers not high. No reported case of MTCT through breastmilk. Individual assessment if mother has acute HVC infection.
Herpes Simplex	Probably not transmitted through breastmilk	Breastfeeding permitted if no breast lesions. Handwashing and mask if oral or genital lesion present.
HIV	Proven	In developed countries, breastfeeding by HIV-infected mother should be avoided.
HTLV-1	Proven	HTLV-infected mother should not breastfeed.
Rubella	Proven	Neither postpartum immunization with rubella vaccine nor rubella should prevent a mother from breastfeeding her infant.
West Nile Virus	Probable	Breastfeeding permitted.

Source: Centers for Disease Control and Prevention, 2002; Pass, 1986; Stiehm & Keller, 2001.

The possibility of HIV transmission by human milk has had a negative effect on breastfeeding that is as yet unmeasured. In developing countries where replacement infant feeding is often lethal, this effect is a major concern (Coutsoudis, & Rollins, 2003). Even if antiretroviral treatment is available, such medications and artificial feeding are expensive. On the basis of realistic costs, decisions must be made as to whether individual families' incomes and countries' economic resources can support these high costs.

Key Concepts

- HIV-infected women should not breastfeed where safe, affordable alternatives are available. It is well established that HIV can be transmitted from mother to infant through breastfeeding.
- Where HIV-infected women have no other choice but to breastfeed, exclusive breastfeeding should be promoted. Exclusive breastfeeding includes teaching frequent emptying of the breast and breastfeeding management including effective attachment.
- HIV-infected pregnant women should receive feeding counseling that includes general information about the risks and benefits of infant feeding options, and specific guidance in selecting the option most likely to be suitable for their situation.
- Gloves are usually not necessary for handling breastmilk. If the healthcare worker comes in frequent contact with human milk, she may choose to wear gloves. If the mother has an open wound on her breast, glove wearing is warranted.
- In the absence of breast lesions, the newborn of a mother with HSV-1, if the baby is well,

may breastfeed and be with the mother in her room; however, scrupulous hand washing, gowning, and covering of any lesions must be practiced to prevent possible cross-contamination. Women with herpetic lesions on their breasts should refrain from breastfeeding.

- If a mother develops chickenpox several days before she delivers her baby or has the virus within 48 hours after birth, she should delay breastfeeding and pump her milk. Contact infection control precautions using gowns, gloves, and masks are indicated. Following birth the mother and baby should be isolated separately if the neonate does not develop lesions and discharged as soon as possible. The baby should be protected from direct contact with the mother's skin lesions. If the baby has lesions, the baby can be isolated with the mother, and breastfeeding may occur uninterrupted. Varicella-zoster immune globulin is given as soon as possible to modify and prevent further symptoms of the disease regardless of whether the mother has already received it during pregnancy.

- Cytomegalovirus, a prevalent infection, can be found in the human milk, genital tract, urine, and the pharynx and is transmitted by any close contact. Breastfeeding is an important means of conveying passive immunity to CMV. Although transmission through breastmilk has been documented, no serious illness or clinical symptoms in neonates secondary to breastfeeding have been reported. The danger of CMV infection lies in the potential transmission to the fetus or newborn of a woman who has a primary infection during pregnancy.

- Although the rubella virus can be passed through maternal milk lymphocytes to the infant, there is no evidence that the baby who acquires rubella in this manner becomes ill. Transmission of maternal antibodies against rubella, though at lower levels, is beneficial to the infant by serving as a natural vaccine. If the mother is immunized to rubella postpartum, the breastfeeding infant will develop antibodies to rubella but will not show symptoms of the disease.

- Infants born to an HBV-positive mother, already exposed to maternal blood during delivery, may breastfeed. The neonate should receive hepatitis B immunoglobulin (HBIG) within 12 hours after birth, followed by a series of injections of HBV vaccine. All infants should undergo pediatric follow-up including screening for HB_sAg.

- There is no evidence that breastfeeding confers risk of HCV infection. The overall rate of maternal–infant HCV transmission among breastfed infants is the same as that among formula-fed infants, and women who are infected should be allowed to breastfeed. The exception is the rare case of a mother with acute HCV infection acquired after delivery, a time when no neutralizing antibodies are present.

- Women who are HTLV-1 seropositive are usually advised not to breastfeed. In areas of the world where many mothers are HTLV-1 positive, restrictions against breastfeeding is equivocal. Children who are breastfed for a long period (> 6 or 7 months) are more likely to develop HTLV-1 infection than are those breastfed for a shorter period. Children born to seropositive carrier mothers passively acquire maternal antibodies prenatally that gradually disappear by 9 months of age.

- Mothers with West Nile virus can breastfeed.

Internet Resources

Position papers on HIV/AIDs and breastfeeding
http://global-breastfeeding.org

HIV/AIDS Surveillance Report. Statistics, teaching tools, PowerPoint presentations
http://www.cdc.gov/hiv/stats.htm

World Health Organization. Guidelines for antiretroviral drugs for treating pregnant women and preventing HIV infection in infants.
http://www.who.int/hiv/pub/guidelines/en

World Health Organization. HIV transmission through breastfeeding: a review of available evidence 2004.
http://www.who.int

West Nile virus and breastfeeding
http://www.cdc.gov/ncidod/dvbid/westnile/qa/breastfeeding.htm

References

Adu FD, Adeniji JA. Measles antibodies in the breast milk of nursing mothers. *Afr J Med Sci*. 1995;24: 385–388.

American Academy of Pediatrics. *1997 Red Book: Report of the Committee on Infectious Diseases*. 24th ed. Elk Grove Village, IL: American Academy of Pediatrics; 1997:73–79.

American College of Obstetricians and Gynecologists. *Management of herpes in pregnancy* [ACOG Practice Bulletin, No. 8]. Washington, DC: ACOG; 2002.

Bindo S et al. Transmission of cytomegalovirus. *Lancet*. 2001;357:1799.

Black BP, Miles MS. Calculating the risks and benefits of disclosure in African American women who have HIV. *JOGNN*. 2002;31:688–697.

Brahmbhatt H, Gray RH. Child mortality associated with reasons for non-breastfeeding and weaning: is breastfeeding best for HIV-positive mothers? *AIDS*. 2003;17:879–885.

Brown ZA. Preventing transmission of herpes simplex to newborns. *Contemp Nurse Pract*. 1995;Sept-Oct:29–35.

Buckhold KM. Who's afraid of hepatitis C? *Am J Nurs*. 2000;100:26–31.

Buimovici-Klein E et al. Isolation of rubella virus in milk after postpartum immunization. *J Pediatr*. 1977;6:939–941.

Centers for Disease Control and Prevention (CDC). West Nile virus infection and breastfeeding. http://www.cdc.gov/breastfeeding/disease/west_nile_virus.htm. Accessed August 12, 2008.

Centers for Disease Control and Prevention (CDC). Breastfeeding: diseases and conditions; hepatitis B and C infections. *MMWR*. 2007;12 June.

Cline MK, Bailey-Dorton C, Cayelli M. Update in maternity care: maternal infections diagnosis and management. *Primary Care*. 2000;27:13–33.

Connor EM, Sperling RS, Gelber R, et al. Reduction of maternal-infant transmission of human immunodeficiency virus type 1 with zidovudine treatment. *N Engl J Med*. 1994;331:1173–1180.

Cottrell BH, Carter C. Health care professionals: Have you had the chickenpox? *AWHONN Lifelines*. 1998;2:33–38.

Coovadia HM et al. Mother-to-child transmission of HIV-1 infection during exclusive breastfeeding in the first 6 months of life: an intervention cohort study. *Lancet*. 2007;369:1107–1116.

Coutsoudis A. Promotion of exclusive breastfeeding in the face of the HIV pandemic [commentary]. *Lancet*. 2000;356:1620–1621.

Coutsoudis A, Rollins N. Breast-feeding and HIV transmission: the jury is still out. *J Pediatr Gastroenterol*. 2003;36:434–442.

Coutsoudis A, Pillay K, Spooner E, et al. Influence of infant feeding patterns on early mother-to-child transmission of HIV-1 in Durban, South Africa: a prospective cohort study. *Lancet*. 1999;354:471–476.

Damato EG. Cytomegalovirus infection: perinatal complications. *JOGN Nurs*. 2002;31:86–92.

dePaoli M et al. Exclusive breastfeeding in the era of AIDS. *J Hum Lact*. 2001;17:313–320.

Donahue DB. Diagnosis and treatment of herpes simplex infection during pregnancy. *JOGNN*. 2002; 31:99–106.

Duckle LM, Schmidt R, O'Connor DM. Neonatal herpes simplex infection possibly acquired via maternal breast milk. *Pediatrics*. 1979;63:250–251.

Dunn DT et al. Risk of human immunodeficiency virus, type 1, transmission through breastfeeding. *Lancet*. 1992;340:585–588.

Fischler B et al. Vertical transmission of hepatitis C virus infection. *Scand J Infect Dis*. 1996;28:353–356.

Frederick IB, White RJ, Braddock SW. Excretion of varicella-herpes zoster virus in breast milk. *Am J Obstet Gynecol*. 1986;154:1116–1117.

Fujino T, Nagata Y. HTLV-1 transmission from mother to child. *J Reproduct Immunol*. 2000;47:197–206.

Furnia A et al. Estimating the time of HTLV-1 infection following mother-to-child transmission in a breast-feeding population in Jamaica. *J Med Virol*. 1999;59: 541–546.

Gibb DM et al. Mother-to-child transmission of hepatitis C virus: evidence for preventable peripartum transmission. *Lancet*. 2000;356(9233):904–907.

Giles M, Mijch A. Breast milk pasteurisation in developed countries to reduce HIV transmission. Do the benefits outweigh the risks? *Infect Dis Obstect Gynecol*. 2005;13:237–240.

Giuliano M et al. Triple antiretroviral prophylaxis administered during pregnancy and after delivery significantly reduces breast milk viral load: a study with the Drug Resource Enhancement Against AIDS and Malnutrition Program. *J Acquir Immune Defici Syndr*. 2007;44:286–291.

Hamprecht K et al. Epidemiology of transmission of cytomegalovirus from mother to preterm infant by breastfeeding. *Lancet*. 2001;357(9255):513–518.

Hardikar W. Advances in pediatric gastroenterology and hepatology. *J Gastroenterol Hepatol*. 2002;17: 476–481.

Hartmann SU et al. Biochemical analysis of human milk treated with sodium dodecyl sulfate, an alkyl sulfate microbicide that inactivates human immunodeficiency virus type 1. *J Hum Lact*. 2006;22:61–74.

Hill JB et al. Risk of hepatitis B transmission in breast-fed infants of chronic hepatitis B carriers. *Obstet and Gynecol*. 2002;6:1049–1052.

Hino S et al. Association between maternal antibodies to the external envelope glycoprotein and vertical transmission of human T-lymphotropic virus type 1. *J Clin Invest*. 1995;95:2920–2925.

Ho-Hsiung L et al. Absence of infection in breast-fed infants born to hepatitis C virus-infected mothers. *J Pediatr.* 1995;126:589–591.

Isaacs D. Neonatal chickenpox. *J Paediatr Child Health.* 2000;36:76–77.

Jackson DJ et al. HIV and infant feeding: issues in developed and developing countries. *JOGNN.* 2003;32:117–127.

Karim SA et al. Vertical transmission in South Africa: translating research into policy and practice. *Lancet.* 2002;359:92.

Kinoshita K et al. Milk-borne transmission of HTLV-1 from carrier mothers to their children. *Jpn J Cancer Res.* 1987;78:674–680.

Klein EB, Byrne T, Cooper LZ. Neonatal rubella in a breast-fed infant after postpartum maternal infection. *J Pediatr.* 1980;97:774–775.

Lal RB et al. Isotypic and IgG sub-class restriction of the humoral immune responses to human T-lymphotrophic virus type-1. *Clin Immuno Immunopathol.* 1993;67:40–49.

Lawrence RM. Cytomegalovirus in human breast milk: risk to the premature infant. *Breastfeeding Med.* 2006;1:99–107.

Losonsky GA, Fishaut JM, Strussenberg J et al. Effect of immunization against rubella on lactation products: I. Development and characterization of specific immunologic reactivity in breast milk. *J Infect Dis.* 1982;145:661–666.

McCarter-Spaulding DE. Varicella infection in pregnancy. *JOGN Nurs.* 2001;30:667–673.

Minamishima I et al. Role of breast milk in acquisition of cytomegalovirus. *Microbio Immunol.* 1994;38:549–552.

Nelson CT, Demmler GJ. Cytomegalovirus infection in the pregnant mother, fetus, and newborn infant. *Clin Perinatol.* 1997;24:151–160.

Oki T et al. A sero-epidemiological study on mother-to child transmission of HTLV-1 in Southern Kyushu, Japan. *Asia Oceania J Obstet Gynaecol.* 1992;44:371–377.

Oxtoby MJ. Human immunodeficiency virus and other viruses in human milk: placing the issues in broader perspective. *Pediatr Infect Dis.* 1988;7:825–835.

Owor M et al. The one year safety and efficacy data of the HIVNET 012 trial. *13th International AIDS conference.* Abstract, Durban, South Africa, 2000.

Pass RF. Viral contamination of milk. In: Goldman AS, Atkinson SA, Hanson A, eds. *Human Lactation 3: The Effects of Milk on Recipient Infant.* New York, NY: Plenum; 1986:279–287.

Polywka S et al. Low risk of vertical transmission of hepatitis C virus by breast milk. *Clin Infect Dis.* 1999;29:1327–1329.

Roberts EA, Yeung L. Maternal-infant transmission of hepatitis C virus. *Hepatology.* 2002;36:S106–S113.

Savage F, Lhotska L. Recommendations on feeding infants of HIV positive mothers. *Adv Exp Med Biol.* 2000;478:225–230.

Sealander JY, Kerr CP. Herpes simplex of the nipple: infant-to-mother transmission. *Am Family Pract.* 1989;39:111–113.

Smith MM, Kuhn L. Exclusive breast-feeding: does it have the potential to reduce breast-feeding transmission of HIV-1? *Nutr Rev.* 2000;58:333–340.

Stiehm RE, Keller MA. Breast milk transmission of viral disease. *Advances Nutr Res.* 2001;10:105–122.

Sullivan-Bolyai JS, Fife KH, Jacobs RF, et al. Disseminated neonatal herpes simplex virus type 1 from a maternal breast lesion. *Pediatrics.* 1983;71:455–457.

Tajiri H et al. Prospective study of mother-to-infant transmission of hepatitis C virus. *Pediatr Infect Dis J.* 2001;20:10–14.

Takahashi K et al. Inhibitory effect of maternal antibody on mother-to-child transmission of human T-lymphotrophic virus, type 1. *Int J Cancer.* 1991;49:673–677.

Thior I et al. Breastfeeding plus infant zidovudine prophylaxis for 1 month to reduce mother-to-child HIV transmission in Botswana: a randomized trial: the Mashi Study. *JAMA.* 2006;296:794–805.

Thiry L et al. Isolation of AIDS virus from cell-free breast milk of three healthy virus carriers. *Lancet.* 1985;326:891.

US Department of Health and Human Services. *HHS Blueprint for Action on Breastfeeding.* Washington, DC: US DHHS; 2000.

Van de Perre P. Postnatal transmission of human immunodeficiency virus type 1 from mother to infant: a prospective cohort study in Kigali, Rwanda. *N Engl J Med.* 1991;325:593–598.

Van de Perre P et al. Infective and antiinfective properties of breast milk from HIV-1 infected women. *Lancet.* 1993;34:914–918.

Van der Strate BW et al. Viral load in breast milk correlates with transmission of human cytomegalovirus to preterm infant, but lactoferrin concentrations do not. *Clin Diag Lab Immunol.* 2001;8:818–821.

World Health Organization. *Technical Consultation on behalf of the UNFPA/UNICEF/WHO/UNADIS Inter-Agency Task Team on Mother-to-Child Transmission of HIV.* Geneva, Switzerland: WHO; 2000:11–13.

World Health Organization. HIV transmission through breastfeeding: a review of available evidence 2004, http://www.who.int. Accessed July 27, 2007.

World Health Organization. Antiretroviral drugs for treating pregnant women and preventing HIV infection in infants in resource-limited settings: towards universal access. 2006. http://www.who.int/hiv/pub/guidelines/pmtctguidellines2006.pdf. Accessed July 13, 2007.

Yeung LT, King SM, Roberts EA. Mother-to-infant transmission of hepatitis C virus. *Hepatology.* 2001;34:223–229.

Section 3

Prenatal, Perinatal, and Postnatal Periods

A caring approach, knowledge, and clinical skills merge in lactation consultant services during pregnancy, the intrapartum, and the immediate postpartum. Problems that are most likely to be of concern in the early days of breastfeeding relate to method of birth, breast engorgement, sore nipples, and other problems that resolve quickly. Most breastfed infants are born at or near term and are healthy and thrive with only breastmilk. A few grow poorly when breastfed. Does this problem derive from the mother, the baby, or the hospital? How can the problem be resolved without compromising the breastfeeding relationship? Jaundice is an outcome of early extrauterine life, and how it is managed can influence the breastfeeding course. Those infants who are born early or at risk represent a small percentage of the total, yet they require extra care-giving by their mothers and the specialized technologies and care-taking available in neonatal inten-sive care units.

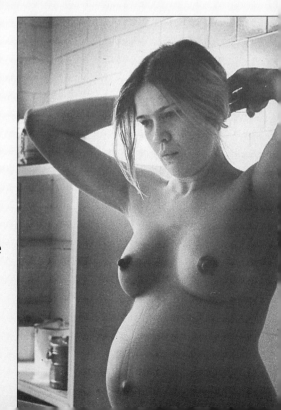

Donor milk banks represent a means of obtaining human milk for the occasional situation where it is needed to achieve exclusive breastfeeding. More and more hospitals keep human milk in their freezers for use when babies need supplement to their own mother's milk.

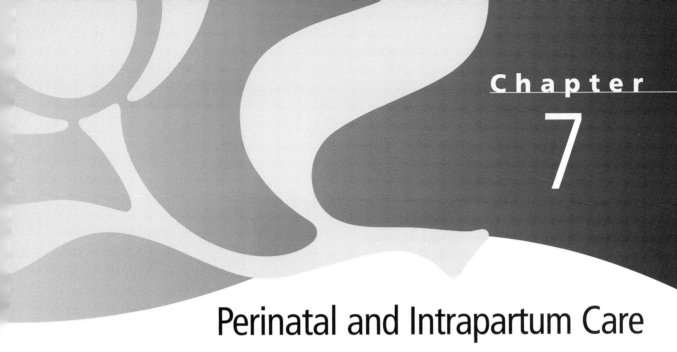

Perinatal and Intrapartum Care

Jan Riordan and Kay Hoover

HELPING WOMEN BREASTFEED is rewarding. With a basic understanding of the anatomy and physiology of the breast, infant behavior, infant suckling, and of the nutritional and immunological properties of breastmilk, the healthcare worker can contribute greatly to a woman's breastfeeding experience. However, the care provider must be prepared to offer practical assistance supported by relevant research findings and to meet the urgent needs of mothers with little or no breastfeeding experience. The provider must also be able to assist new mothers who, despite previous breastfeeding experience, are still anxious.

Mothering and breastfeeding are learned behaviors, and a mother's best "teacher" is her own baby. Lactation is automatic. It is a normal component of reproduction that begins during pregnancy and increases after birth. It is the baby's need, expressed through the behavior of breastfeeding that determines how much milk is made and how long milk continues to be produced. The baby breastfeeds within the caregiving environment that the mother provides, and everything that a woman has learned in her lifetime con-

tributes to her ability to accept the role of a breastfeeding mother. When reaffirmed as a person and supported in her early efforts to breastfeed, a mother will have most of what she needs to assume her new role and relish the unique joys it will provide her.

Breastfeeding Preparation

The best preparation for breastfeeding is for the woman to learn as much as possible before she embarks on her own childbearing adventure. Learning about breastfeeding can be accomplished in any number of ways. She can attend a community-based breastfeeding support group. Groups such as La Leche League and the Australian Breastfeeding Association hold regularly scheduled meetings to provide education and support for breastfeeding women. She may choose to take a prenatal breastfeeding class. Classes may be offered by healthcare facilities, such as hospitals or prenatal care providers' offices, public health or nutrition programs such as WIC, and independent lactation consultants.

Doulas and Childbirth Educators

Doulas are becoming accepted as a mother's coach to support her throughout labor and delivery (Trainor, 2002). Continuous support in labor by a trained doula reduces the need for analgesics, shortens the length of labor, decreases Cesarean deliveries, and improves breastfeeding outcomes (Campbell et al., 2006; Montgomery, Hale, Academy of Breastfeeding Medicine Protocol Committee, 2006). Doulas and childbirth educators encourage breastfeeding and integrate breastfeeding information into their prenatal teaching.

In addition to attending support group meetings or breastfeeding classes, mothers can prepare by reading books and watching videos or DVDs about breastfeeding, and by talking to women who have breastfed. Discussing breastfeeding with women who have had a positive experience is a good way to learn. The experienced breastfeeding mother acts as a mentor to the less knowledgeable woman. She can respond to the new mother's concerns and feelings and advise her on aspects of breastfeeding that are more difficult to address in written form or in a less personal setting.

Prenatal Preparation

Colostrum is produced throughout pregnancy. In some women, colostrum spontaneously leaks during sexual intercourse and late in pregnancy due to oxytocin. During pregnancy the breasts begin making milk and the nipples become more elastic, which may explain why some women characterize their nipples as "flat" or "inverted" at the beginning of pregnancy but not at the end. Prenatal preparation of nipple tissue is unnecessary and is not recommended.

How the nipple looks when the baby is not suckling bears little resemblance to its appearance in the baby's mouth, and it is not necessary for the nipple to be everted when not in the baby's mouth. Hoffmann's exercises for nipple inversion or flatness have no noticeable impact on the appearance of the nipple (Hoffmann, 1953) nor on the degree of inversion or protractility (MAIN Collaborative Group Preparing for Breast Feeding, 1994). If the nipples appear functional and are not inverted, the best preparation is to do nothing. If a couple enjoy involving the breasts and nipples in lovemaking,

such a practice would be sufficient to prepare the nipples for breastfeeding. Nipple stimulation during lovemaking is not recommended when the woman has a history of preterm labor.

Early Feedings

Following a vaginal birth, the baby should be dried and placed on the mother's abdomen or, in the case of a cesarean birth, on her chest (Figure 7–1). Mother and father have their first bonding experience with their new baby, which is almost always very emotional. If the perineum needs to be repaired, it can be done while the baby is skin to skin. The baby is placed on the mother's breast and gently encouraged to seek out and grasp his mother's nipple.

Early (in the first hour after birth) and frequent breastfeedings are encouraged for optimal functioning of both the infant and the mother for the following reasons:

- Suckling stimulates uterine contractions, aids in the expulsion of the placenta, and helps to control maternal blood loss.
- Breastfeeding and skin-to-skin contact colonizes harmless bacteria to protect the infant from pathogenic bacteria including methicillin-resistant *Staphylococcus aureus* (MRSA). The colonization rate of MRSA in the mouth of low birth weight infants could be lowered by spreading the mother's breastmilk over and

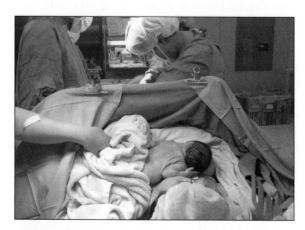

FIGURE 7–1 Newborn placed on mother's abdomen.

Source: Courtesy of Dr. Jack Newman.

into the mouth of such infant immediately upon entering the NICU (Kitajima, 2003).

- Mothers will breastfeed for a longer duration (Lawson & Tulloch, 1995; Lothian, 1995; Wright, Rice, & Wells, 1996; Ekström, 2003).
- The infant's suckling reflex is usually intense after birth. Gratification of this reflex "imprints" this biobehavior to facilitate learning to suckle (Anderson et al., 1982).
- The infant promptly receives the immunological components of the colostrum.
- The infant's digestive peristalsis is stimulated, thereby promoting elimination of the byproducts of hemoglobin breakdown. Jaundice is more likely to occur when feeding and peristalsis are delayed (see Chapter 11).
- Breast engorgement is minimized by the early and frequent removal of milk from the breast (Moon & Humenick, 1989).
- Lactation is accelerated, more milk is produced, and early and frequent intake of breastmilk lessens infant weight loss after birth (Chen et al., 1998; de Carvalho et al., 1982).
- Frequent removal of milk keeps the breast as empty as possible and stimulates the synthesis of breastmilk (Cregan & Hartmann, 1999).
- Attachment and bonding are enhanced at a time when both the mother and the infant are in a heightened state of readiness.
- Breastfeeding accelerates the baby's adaptation to extrauterine life, reduces crying, and increases the baby's blood glucose and temperature.

Epidurals and Other Birth Practices

Some neonates will take longer to learn how to latch onto the breast and feed effectively than others because of interventions during labor and birth and the postbirth care they receive. Most women in the United States and many who live in South American and European countries have epidurals during labor, and the number is rising, in certain places, to 90 percent. Epidurals are popular with women, some call it "the best thing since sliced bread." These women are unaware that such analgesia can delay and diminish neonatal suckling and be associated with shorter breastfeeding duration (Belin et al., 2005; Crowell, Hill, & Humenick, 1994; Riordan et al., 2000; Ransjo-Arvidson et al., 2001; Sepkoski et al., 1992; Jordan et al., 2005; Kroeger & Smith, 2004; Torvaldsen et al., 2006), especially if the amount of analgesia is high. Fortunately, anesthetists are using less analgesia in recent years.

Epidurals can have a "domino" effect—usually labor slows down after placement of the epidural—necessitating one intervention after another. For example, the body temperature of the mother and the baby may be elevated with epidurals (Lieberman et al., 1997; Ransjo-Arvidson et al., 2001; Viscomi, 2000), resulting in separation and septic workup to determine if an infection is present. Other research on the effect of epidurals on breastfeeding concluded that epidural use did not lead to breastfeeding problems or poor infant neurobehavior (Chang & Heaman, 2005). These more recent studies reflect the use of smaller analgesic dosages for epidurals.

Women who have a vacuum extraction during birthing abandon breastfeeding early (Hall et al., 2002), possibly due in part to a long, drawn out, and stressful labor and infant injury. If the birth was by cesarean, it takes longer for the mother's milk to come in.

Suctioning

Another disruption to early breastfeeding is suctioning the infant's mouth and nose after birth. The suction tends to cause the infant to have nasal edema and "stuffiness." Because the baby's airway is somewhat obstructed, the baby does not feed well until the swelling subsides. Oral suctioning can lead to breastfeeding difficulties because the baby's mouth or throat may be sore (Widström et al., 1987). In a randomized controlled pilot study newborns receiving bulb suctioning showed a statistically significant lower heart rate during the first 20 minutes after birth (Waltman et al., 2004). One pediatrician observed rough suctioning with a bulb syringe that resulted in perforation in the soft palate (Soppas, 2003).

Normal Patterns

Newborns spend 64 percent of their time sleeping (Sadeh, Dark, & Vohr, 1996). When skin-to-skin (kangaroo) care is practiced and access to the mother is not restricted after birth, the breastfeeding neonate exhibits a sleep pattern similar to that illustrated in Table 7–1. The initial alertness for the first 2 hours after birth and the eagerness of the

TABLE 7–1	First-day Sleep Patterns of Neonates	
Infant State		**Time Period**
Alert		Birth–2 hours
Light and deep sleep		2–20+ hours
Increasing wakefulness*		20–24 hours

*Often includes a cluster of 5 to 10 feeding episodes over 2 to 3 hours followed by deep sleep of 4 to 5 hours.

baby to breastfeed is followed by deeper sleep for several hours and then increased wakefulness and interest in breastfeeding. During this period of increased wakefulness, the baby will feed frequently, alternating between relatively short periods of light sleep and quiet wakefulness (Williams & Mueller, 1989). Mothers may interpret these "cluster feedings" as indicators that the baby is not getting any milk or is getting an insufficient amount. However, they actually constitute a series of mini-feedings, snacks, or courses in a larger banquet that is part of a single breastfeeding episode. A cluster of mini-feedings by the baby is usually followed by a period of deep sleep, during which time the mother should be encouraged to sleep.

The pattern of normal infant suckling was discussed in Chapter 3. Neonates who are kept in skin-to-skin contact with their mothers immediately after birth are more likely to learn how to suckle effectively and show increasing facility with each subsequent feeding than those who are separated. In general, full-term infants demonstrate a well-organized sequence of suckling behaviors, including bringing the hand to the mouth, rooting, and suckling within the first hour after birth (Widström et al., 1990).

The baby can be dried while skin-to-skin with his mother. Leaving the amniotic fluid on the baby's hands helps the baby find the breast (Varendi, Porter, & Winberg, 1996). Mother–infant body contact is as effective as supplemental heat in maintaining the healthy newborn's temperature (Johanson et al., 1992; Christensson et al., 1998). The placenta is normally expelled soon after birth, often before the infant latches on for the first time. If a delay occurs, breastfeeding may hasten detachment and expulsion of the placenta.

With the mother on her back and slightly inclined, or propped on her side with a pillow at her back for support, the baby may breastfeed in the delivery room/birthing suite. The ambience and homey comforts of a birthing suite encourage early breastfeeding. The father can share the enjoyment of these first moments together and can help position the mother and infant comfortably in the birthing bed.

Newborns usually lick or nuzzle the nipple at first. Given ample opportunity, the baby is able to crawl to the mother's breast, self-attach and suckle strongly within an hour (Righard & Alade, 1990; Righard, 1995). Those babies who have been affected by labor analgesia and anesthesia, and who may suckle only minimally at this time, should have an opportunity to lick or nuzzle the nipple. Regardless of the baby's initial suckling behavior, skin-to-skin holding by the mother is advantageous because it promotes colonization of harmless bacteria to protect the infant from pathogenic bacteria—a very pleasant method of infection control. Mothers whose infants have come in contact with their nipple/areolar complex choose to keep their babies with them for more time during the hospital stay (Widström et al., 1990). Explaining to the mother that "nuzzling" is normal behavior will help her to see this activity as a positive response rather than as disinterest in actual breastfeeding.

Sometimes the first breastfeeding takes place after the mother and her newborn are transferred from the delivery area to their room. Wherever it may be, if the mother is awake and oriented, it is best that she put her baby to breast as soon as possible (see Figures 7–2 and 7–3).

A positive, satisfying birthing experience gets breastfeeding off to a good start, and parents often recall this experience in great detail many years later. The caregiver's unhurried, nurturing approach helps to establish rapport with the mother. It is important to explain to the first-time mother that breastfeeding is not as automatic for her as the suckling and rooting reflexes are for her baby. Yet the experience is new to the baby too, and the first few times at breast offer opportunities for each to learn

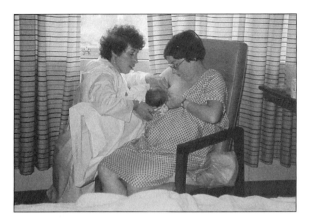

FIGURE **7–2**   Lactation consultant assisting mother at eye level during first breastfeeding.

from the other. Early breastfeeding is optimized in the following ways:

1. Wash your hands thoroughly. An alcohol-based hand rub may be used *in addition* to hand washing. Gloves (nonlatex) are worn as appropriate. Artificial fingernails should not be worn (Hedderwick et al., 2000; Winslow & Jacobson, 2000). Wearing these nails encourages growth of pathogens, and their sharp edges can hurt the mother and baby.

2. Arrange for privacy. Concentrating on learning a new skill is easier when it is private. Ask visitors to leave as appropriate. Sometimes mothers are too polite to ask visitors to leave in order to feed the baby (and/or rest!), and it is up to the nurse or lactation consultant to make this request. Shut the door of the mother's room or pull the curtains around her bed if she wishes.

3. Help the mother to find the most comfortable position and ensure that there are several pillows available. Full frontal contact of the baby's body with the mother's chest is a natural position. Women who have had a cesarean birth may prefer to sit in the hospital bed; others find it more comfortable to breastfeed while sitting in a comfortable chair with low arms. At the first feeding, to provide support, arrange pillows on her lap, behind her back, and under her arm and shoulder on the side on which the

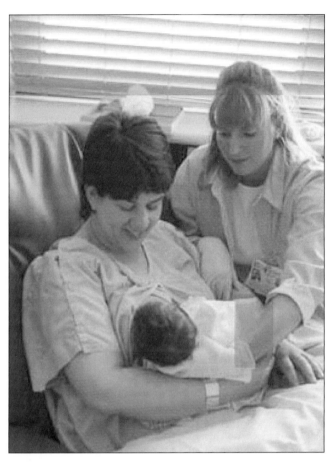

FIGURE **7–3**   Baby put to breast right after delivery.

baby is to feed. If the mother is in bed, raise the back of the bed to high Fowler's position with plenty of pillows for additional support. The mother who must remain flat may lie on her back or side with pillows at her back and between her knees. If wearing a hospital gown, open the snaps on the shoulders to pull down and expose the breast as needed.

4. Work with the mother at her eye level. If she is in a chair, kneel down; if she is in bed, pull up a chair; if the bed is electronically operated, raise the bed to bring her to your eye level. When an individual is engaging in a new activity, anyone standing higher than the learner provokes anxiety in the learner (Figure 7–2).

5. Help the mother to position the baby's head. The baby should be snuggled securely in the

mother's arms and facing toward her. This permits the mother to easily maintain eye contact with her baby. The baby's head should be free so he can bring it back in the event that his nostrils become blocked. By cradling the infant's thigh or the buttock of his lower leg with her hand, the mother can change the baby's position with ease. Be sure there is no pressure on the back of the baby's head. Other feeding positions are discussed later in this chapter.

6. Suggest that the mother support her breast with her hand if needed. Advise her to keep her thumb and fingers well behind the areola in a C-hold—a position in which the hand is shaped into a *C* (Figure 7–4). The mother can guide her breast to assist the baby in taking the breast into his mouth. Once latched, if the mother is concerned about the baby's ability to breathe, ask her to bring the baby's hips in close to her body, or lift her breast slightly so she can easily maintain the infant's airway.

7. Help the mother to position her baby so that his nose is at the level of the mother's nipple. Ask the mother to bring the baby's chin in contact with her breast. When the infant opens his mouth wide (rooting reflex) in response to this stimulus, he can self-attach or the mother can bring his shoulders to her breast in one quick movement of her hand or forearm, aiming the nipple toward the soft palate. The baby needs a wide gape to maximize the amount of breast tissue he grasps.

The baby's lips should be flanged outward and his nose slightly away from the surface of the breast so that he can easily breathe (Figure 7–5). Keep in mind that at the first feeding, the baby has never breastfed before and that the suckle/swallow/breathe pattern is a relatively complex series of actions that requires learning and practice.

8. Explain that an infant should be allowed to breastfeed as long and as often as he wants for these early feedings. This will stimulate the need-supply response. In some cases, the neonate will take only one breast before falling asleep, but most babies will take both breasts.

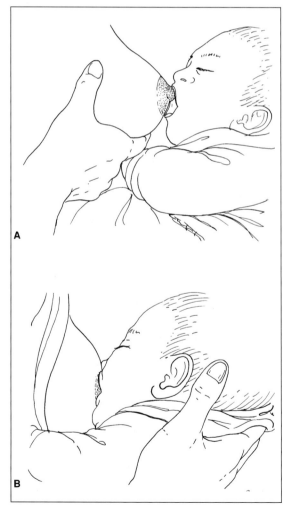

FIGURE 7–5 Latch-on. (A) Mouth gaped open. (B) Grasping breast.

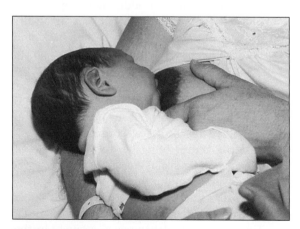

FIGURE 7–4 The C-hold.

As long as each breast is offered frequently (at least every 2 to 3 hours), single-breast feedings of whatever duration the baby wishes are an appropriate option (Woolridge, Ingram, & Baum, 1990). "Take turns with the breast you start on" and "Finish the first breast first" are easy suggestions if the mother is concerned about which breast to start on and when to move her baby from the first to the second breast.

9. Teach "baby watching." The recommendation is, "Watch the baby, not the clock." Feed the baby at the *earliest* sign of hunger. Crying is a *late* sign of hunger. A crying baby cannot latch on; the baby needs time to be consoled and to "settle down" emotionally and physiologically before he will become interested in feeding again. With crying, both the infant's blood pressure and intracranial pressure rises causing oxygen-depleted blood to flow back into the systemic circulation rather than into the lungs (Anderson, 1989). Box 7–1 describes the stages of the baby readying to feed.

10. Suggest that the mother feed until she notes cues from the infant suggesting satiety (suckling activity ceases, baby falls asleep and lets go on his own). The length of the feeding is up to the baby. If the baby lets go of the breast within 2 to 5 minutes, suggest to the mother that she burp the baby and return the baby to the same breast. Once the baby has fallen asleep and has come off the breast on his own, she can offer the other breast when the baby gives feeding cues again. If the mother is breastfeeding for the first time and feels more comfortable with knowing an approximate length of time to feed, suggest that she feed 20 to 30 minutes on the first side until satiety and that she then offer the other side. Toward the end of the feeding, the mother will probably become relaxed to the point of sleepiness—a delightful side effect of oxytocin secretion (Mulford, 1990).

Early feedings are a critical time for learning new information, especially the first-time mother who usually asks many questions. For example, noisy breathing during feedings indicating a "stuffy" nose worries some mothers who are concerned that the baby is having trouble getting enough oxygen. If the baby is feeding well, nasal stuffiness is usually not a problem and will resolve on its own. Neonates are obligate nose breathers. In a few instances a newborn's nares are congested to the point where the baby refuses to breastfeed because he cannot breathe and feed at the same time. In this case, saline drops

---

BOX 7–1

Cues in Baby Watching

Baby Cue	Stage of Readiness to Feed
Wiggling, moving arms or legs	Early
Rooting, fingers to mouth	Early
Fussing, squeaky noises	Mid
Restless, crying intermittently	Mid
Full cry, aversive screaming pitch, color turns red	Late

Source: Anderson, 1989.

or a hydrocortisone solution in the nose will help alleviate the problem. Mothers also worry if the baby gets the hiccups, another normal baby behavior.

If breastfeeding is painful after the first 30 seconds, the mother should be taught how to break the infant's suction on the breast by placing her finger in the corner of his mouth between his gums so she can take him off and start over again. If the mother and baby are having problems with latching, compress her breast to assist the baby in taking more breast tissue into his mouth.

Skin-to-Skin (Kangaroo) Care

Ideally, first breastfeedings take place in the first hour of life with the baby placed on the mother's abdomen skin-to-skin and close to her breasts. With skin-to-skin contact the infant is placed directly on the mother's bare chest and covered with a warmed blanket. When healthy infants are placed skin-to-skin on the mother's abdomen and chest shortly after birth, they are alert, and they can crawl, stimulated by the mother's touch, across her abdomen reaching her breast. Then baby smells, mouths, and licks the mother's nipple and finally attaches to the breasts and feeds (WABA, 2007).

Until recently skin-to-skin (kangaroo) care was used with premature infants (see Chapter 13) as seen in Figure 7–6. Now it is recommended for parents of all babies. A plethora of research and books published in the past few years uniformly support this practice. The following are risks of *not* using skin-to-skin care during the perinatal period:

- Unstable temperatures in the baby—Close physical contact helps regulate neonatal temperatures (Walters et al., 2007; Fransson, Karlsson, & Nilsson, 2005; Bergman, Linley, & Fawcus, 2004). With twins each breast responds individually to the infant's thermal needs (Ludington-Hoe et al., 2006).
- Shorter duration of exclusive breastfeeding (Vaidya, Sharma, & Dhungel, 2005)
- More maternal stress and less satisfaction with breastfeeding (Anderson, 2004)
- Greater "stress of being born" of the baby as demonstrated by higher vasoconstriction in the periphery, more crying
- Less desire by the mother to hold her infant (Anderson, 2004)

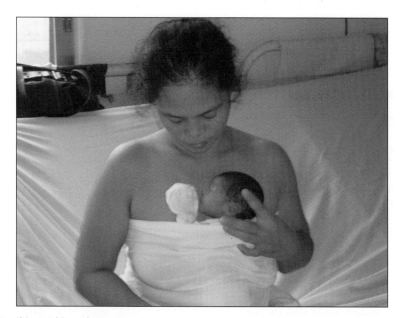

FIGURE 7–6   Skin-to-skin or kangaroo care.

Source: Courtesy of Shannon E. Perry.

- Less ability of the baby to smell the natural scent of his mother's milk (Marlier & Schaal, 2005) resulting in less milk ingestion in preterm babies and a longer hospital stay (Raimbault, Saliba, & Porter, 2007)
- Greater pain and more crying during painful procedures such as heel-lancing and blood collection (Johnston, 2003)

Pain Medications

A common question asked of lactation specialists in the perinatal period concerns the use of pain medications for nursing mother. Acetaminophen (Tylenol) and ibuprofen (Advil, Motrin) are commonly used for pain control postpartum. Both are safe and effective.

Meperidine (Demorol) should not be used as it can cause cyanosis, respiratory depression, and risk of apnea (see Chapter 5 on drug therapy). Morphine or fentanyl is preferred to meperidine for patient-controlled IV analgesia after a cesarean birth (Montgomery, Hale, ABM, 2006).

While oxycodone (Percocet, Percodan) is popular for post-cesarean births, it is not usually recommended for use in breastfeeding mothers because of limited information on its excretion into breastmilk. Breastfed infants may receive >10 percent of a therapeutic infant dose, which poses only minimal risk to the infant because of the low volume of breastmilk ingested in the first few days after delivery (Seaton, Reeves, & McLean, 2007).

Feeding Positions

The new mother needs to know ways to position her neonate at breast. The most frequently taught techniques are the cradle (Figure 7–7), the cross-cradle (across-the-lap, Figure 7–8A), the football (or clutch or under the arm) (Figure 7–8B), and the side-lying position (Figure 7–9). Although there is nothing magical about a particular position, the mother may feel uncomfortable experimenting with different positions prior to her discharge from the hospital. However, she needs to be encouraged to experiment and to use whatever position works best for her and her infant (Table 7–2). Mothers who had vaginal deliveries reported less fatigue if they breastfeed in

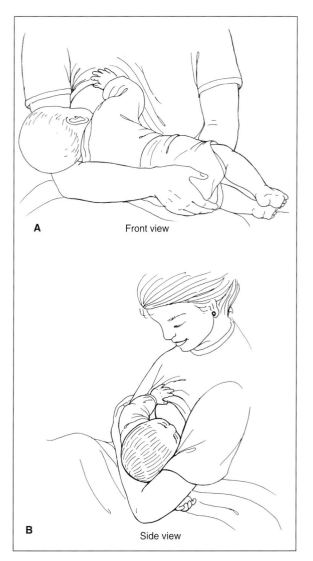

A Front view

B Side view

FIGURE 7–7 Madonna (cradle) position. (A) Front view. (B) Side view.

the side-lying position rather than the sitting position (Milligan, Flenniken, & Pugh, 1996).

Latch-On and Positioning Techniques

Methods for teaching new mothers how to latch on and position the baby on the breast are considered fundamental in lactation clinical practice. When problems arise, achieving optimal latch and positioning is often the first and often the only treatment needed to fix most breastfeeding problems.

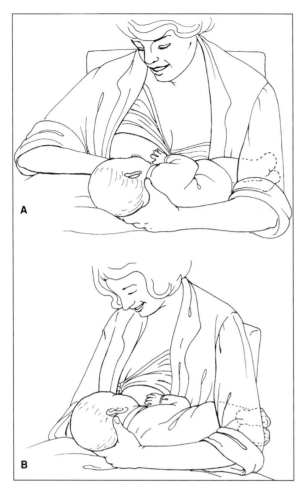

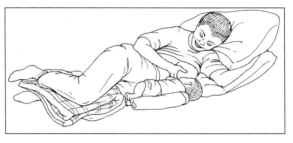

FIGURE **7–9**   Side-lying position.

FIGURE **7–8**   (A) Cross-cradle or modified clutch hold. (B) Football or clutch hold.

Different methods list techniques for achieving a "correct," "proper," or "good" latch and/or positioning. Some include the exact alignment that the baby's head must be with his body during a feeding. Another recommends that the baby's chin be buried in the breast, his nose not touching the breast (Newman, 2006). Rebecca Glover emphasizes the use of one finger to tilt the nipple toward the baby's nose. Suzanne Colson recommends the "post natal lie" with full frontal contact of the baby with the mother. Dr. Tina Smillie recommends the baby be angled across the mother's body and allowed to self-attach (personal communication, L. Smith, 2007). Marmet and Shell (2007) describe over 20 types of positioning at the breast. An example of another

technique is teaching the mother the mechanics of breastfeeding using the sandwich analogy:

> *Using the sandwich as a model, the breast must first be shaped into an oval and then it must be approached from below starting with the nose near the sandwich stuffing. The head tips back slightly and the mandible comes up and forward to fix itself well back on the sandwich. The maxilla is the last part to land on the sandwich, and it is then possible to take a large and satisfying bite (Weissinger, 1998).*

The many methods for latching the baby onto the breast reflect a growing interest in clinical techniques to help breastfeeding women by placing the baby on the breast a certain way. These techniques are useful because they emphasize to the mother (and father) that getting off to the right start by getting the baby to take the breast a certain way will optimize breastfeeding. Basically the mother needs to find a position that works for her and her baby.

Evidence should change and direct our practice, yet we have little evidence that positioning does make a difference. An Australian study (Henderson, Stamp, & Pincombe, 2001) examined teaching of correct latch-on and positioning by conducting a randomized trial on 160 first-time mothers. The mothers who received education on positioning breastfed their babies just as long as the group that did not. The mothers who had received education on positioning reported less nipple pain than the control group, but the study observers who collected the data noted no observable differences in nipple trauma between the two groups suggesting a halo

TABLE 7–2	Positive and Negative Elements of Infant Feeding Positions	
Positioning	**Positive Elements**	**Negative Elements**
Cradle	"Classic" position. Most frequently pictured and most often used.	Baby's head tends to wobble around on the mother's arm. Mother has minimal control over baby's head.
Football or clutch	Provides control of baby's head. Good for low birth weight or 36–39 weekers with minimum head control. Avoids incision of Cesarean birth. Best position to be able to see the baby's mouth.	Some teaching and coaching required on how to position baby. Baby's bottom needs to be against the back of mother's chair so his head can extend back and there is room between his chin and chest.
Cross-cradle	Provides good head control. Along with football hold, allows for ease with bringing the baby to the breast.	Least familiar to caregivers. Some mothers are not comfortable holding their babies in this manner.
Side-lying	Minimizes fatigue (Milligan, Flenniken, & Pugh, 1996). Enables mother to rest more completely than is possible if she is sitting up.	Not always taught in hospital. Mothers may fear smothering baby in this position. Difficult for the mother to see to assist the infant with attachment.

effect on mothers in the experimental group. Clearly, we need to be wary of assuming that "correct" latch-on is evidence based.

The Infant Who Has Not Latched On

Occasionally, an otherwise healthy newborn will not latch onto his mother's breast, even after several attempts. Birth is a strenuous event. Most nurses and lactation consultants have witnessed the frustrating situation in which a distraught mother repeatedly tries to breastfeed her neonate only to have the baby fall into a deep sleep. Most hospital protocols call for supplementation to be started if the baby has not latched on by *12 hours postpartum*; a few hospitals use *24 hours* as the cutoff time before supplementation when the baby has not latched on to the breast.

The appropriate action in this situation is to keep the baby skin-to-skin with his mother and teach her to watch for cues that the baby has cycled through the period of deep sleep and is beginning to awaken. Movement of head, arms, and legs; mouthing; and grimacing are all early cues that the baby is slowly awakening. This is the time to be alert to his interest in latching. Teaching parents these baby cues is a valuable element in early postpartum care. Poor

latch-on in this very early time is common (Dewey et al., 2003) and is not oral aversion or a breastfeeding "strike" discussed in other sections of this book. The baby's lack of interest may be due to labor-related or postbirth narcotics, or to the infant's neurological immaturity. Forcing the baby on the breast before the baby is rousable and shows active interest may result in an aversive reaction (Widström & Thingström-Paulsson, 1993).

In the unusual event of an infant who cannot attach to the breast after several attempts, a visual evaluation of the infant's mouth is appropriate. The roof of the mouth should be wide and gently domed. The tongue should be long enough to extend over the lower gum. The baby's response to a feather-light stroking of the center of the lower lip should be noted. In most cases, the alert infant will open his mouth wide and the tongue will come forward in response to such stimulation, as if seeking its source. The infant's frenulum (the small tissue tag under the tongue) should be far enough away from the tip of the tongue to prevent stricture during suckling. If the frenulum appears tight, a visual examination should be performed to determine whether the frenulum prevents the tongue from elevating or extending sufficiently to produce the wavelike motion necessary for effective suckling.

Digital Examination

Occasionally, a digital examination may be appropriate. The healthcare provider must use a clean, gloved finger with a short nail. A finger (pad side up, nail side down) is slid into the baby's mouth with baby's permission. The tongue should groove around the finger. When the pad of the finger lightly touches the palate, the baby usually initiates a suck response that includes massaging by the tongue on the underside of the finger from knuckle to the fingertip.

In a healthy newborn, the strength of oral negative pressure is such that the examiner will feel as if the nail bed is being pulled deeper into the baby's mouth. The nature of the suckling action should be rhythmic, although some neonates quickly realize that the finger does not reward suckling and so they cease doing so after several attempts. Because the finger is not a breast, with its soft areolar and nipple tissue, suckling at the breast should be the first experience for the infant. Thereafter, a finger assessment may be attempted, although it is not necessary in most cases and should be used judiciously.

Even if the baby is found to have an anatomical variation, such variation may not interfere with effective suckling. However, infants with a cleft palate, a high palatal arch, or a short tongue may require interventions provided by a therapist knowledgeable in treating these oral problems before the baby can breastfeed effectively.

Most maternal and infant problems resolve with time. The full-term infant is born with additional extracellular fluid (shed in the first few days after birth) that sustains him for a short time. Urine output usually exceeds fluid intake for the first 3–4 days after birth (Wight, 2003). However, after 24 hours without receiving fluid nutriment, the neonate is at risk for dehydration. If there is no protocol, it is a nurses' decision when to supplement. Some nurses are quick to give formula often with a bottle; others prefer to pump and give breastmilk via syringes and continue attempts at breastfeedings.

Figure 7–10 presents a flow chart that can be used as an algorithm indicating appropriate actions for early feedings or lack of feedings. We recommend the guidelines in Box 7–2 for intervention when the infant does not latch onto the breast 12 to 24 hours after birth.

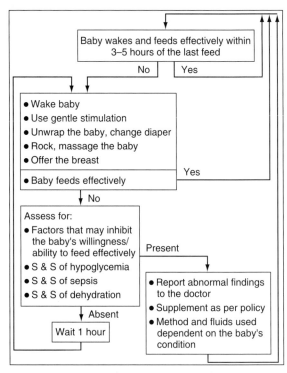

FIGURE 7–10 Breastfeeding flow chart.

Source: Reprinted with permission from Glover J. Supplementation of breastfeeding newborns: a flowchart for decision-making. *J Hum Lact.* 11:1995;127–131.

Plan for the Baby Who Has Not Latched On

The most important concern when a baby is not latching is to feed the baby. One easy technique is to teach the mother how to hand express her milk onto a spoon, and then feed her baby the drops of colostrum from the spoon. Often when staff members hear, "Feed the baby" they picture a bottle in the baby's mouth. If a baby is not latching, giving a bottle can lead to the discontinuation of breastfeeding (Howard et al., 2003). Supplementing in the first 24 hours can be done using a spoon with drops of colostrum or, once the volume of milk has increased to 10 ml or more, with finger-feeding or cup-feeding.

Women produce a small amount of milk during the first few days. These small amounts of colostrum give the baby an opportunity to practice suck-swallow-breathe. The baby should have lots of practice time before the milk increases in volume. After 1 week, the baby should be taking a full volume of

BOX 7–2

Guidelines for the Infant Who Does Not Latch-On (According to Hours Postpartum)

0–24 Hours

- For full-term healthy baby, no supplement is necessary providing that the baby has periods of awake and quiet, and vital signs and blood sugar are within normal limits.
- Attempt to breastfeed during quiet, alert times or at least every 3 hr.
- Have parents hold baby skin-to-skin.
- Encourage a quiet environment.
- If not latched-on by 18–24 hr, provide electric pump and instruct in use. Pump at least 8 times in 24 hr.
- Alternative: teach mother hand expression.

24–48 Hours

- In hospital (every 3 hr) attempt to breastfeed.
- If unsuccessful after 10 minutes, feed baby with expressed breastmilk + water to equal 10–15 cc. Use formula if no breastmilk available.
- Apply nipple shield if the baby is too weak to latch or mother has flat or inverted nipple(s).
- Continue to pump.
- After discharge attempt to breastfeed every 3 hr. If unsuccessful after 10 minutes, feed baby expressed breastmilk to equal 10 to 15 cc.
- Use alternative feeding methods as appropriate: finger feed, spoon, cup, slow flow nipple.
- Continue skin-to-skin contact and quiet environment.
- Continue to pump at least 8 times/24 hr.

> 48 Hours

- Attempt to breastfeed baby every 2–3 hr.
- If unsuccessful, feed baby with expressed breastmilk = 30–60 ml or expressed breastmilk + formula to equal 30–60 cc. Use formula if no breastmilk available.
- Consider nipple shield if the baby is too weak to latch or mother has flat or inverted nipple(s).
- Use alternative feeding method: cups, finger feed, slow flow nipple.
- Continue skin-to-skin contact and quiet environment.
- Continue to pump at least 8 times/24 hr.

Source: Adapted with permission from Memorial Hospital, Breastfeeding guidelines, 2003, Colorado Springs, Colorado.

milk. Table 7–3 lists expected breastmilk intake for the neonate's first 5 days after birth. The equation for milk intake based on infant weight is 2.5 times the baby's weight in pounds equals the number of ounces the baby needs in 24 hours. For example, an 8-pound baby needs 20 ounces (2.5×8) of milk in

TABLE 7–3	Neonatal Feeding Amounts for First Five Days Following Birth (Full-Term Infants)		

Day	Per Feeding	Total in 24 Hours
1	Few drops to 5 cc (< 1 tsp)	Few drops to 1 oz (2 tb)
2	5 to 15 cc (< 0.5 oz or < 1 tb)	1 to 4 oz (1/4 to 1/2 cup)
3	15 to 30 cc (0.5 to 1 oz or 1 to 2 tb)	4 to 8 oz (1/2 to 1 cup)
4	30 to 45 cc (1 to 1.5 oz or 2 to 3 tb)	8 to 12 oz (1.5 cups)
5	45 to 60 cc (1.5 to 2 oz or 3 to 4 tb)	12 to 18 oz (1.5 to 2 cups)

24 hours when he is 1 week old. This equation works for the first 10 weeks. After that, a baby needs less in proportion to his weight.

Establishing the Milk Supply

When a baby is not latching onto the breast, the mother needs to establish her milk supply mechanically. Before she leaves the hospital, a multiple-user, hospital-grade electric breast pump with a double pump kit should be made available to her. She should pump both her breasts at the same time for about 10 to 15 minutes, 8 to 10 times in 24 hours. While she is pumping, she can massage her breasts. The postpartum nurses can show the mother how to hold both pump kits to her breasts with one arm, so she has a hand free to massage her breasts while pumping. The hospital should provide a form for her to keep a record of the milk expressed each time.

When a baby has not latched on yet, it is important for the mother and baby to remain skin-to-skin for as many hours a day as possible (Meyer & Anderson, 1999). Skin-to-skin contact will help the baby learn to breastfeed. Part of the discharge teaching by the postpartum nurse or lactation consultant needs to include the importance of continuing skin-to-skin holding until the baby has learned to breastfeed well. It is important for the mother to remove as much milk as she possibly can, so once her milk supply increases in amount (usually on the third day) she needs to pump until the milk drips or spray subside, stop pumping,

massage her breasts, and begin pumping again. Repeat the above two times. She should be able to complete the pumping process within 30 minutes.

Mother's Nipples and Breast Problems

When a baby is having difficulty latching, it is usually a baby problem, but the mother's nipples may be a contributing factor. On occasion the woman's nipples may be too big for the baby to accommodate all of her nipple and enough of the breast tissue to extract milk. In such a case, she will need to bring in the milk supply herself, feed her milk to her baby, and wait for the baby to grow into her nipple size.

If the mother's nipple is flat, inverted, or retracts when the baby compresses the breast with his gums, it is difficult for the baby to attach. Many babies figure out how to make their mother's breasts work for them, but other babies need some help. Teaching the mother to compress and shape her breast tissue for the baby to feel in his mouth when the nipple retracts may be just enough of a signal for the baby to continue suckling. Other techniques that have been tried, but not researched, include the following:

- Push down on the breast gently as the baby latches on. It can assist the infant to pull more nipple and areola into his mouth.
- Pull back on the breast tissue so the nipples will protrude.

- Pump the breasts just before the feed to pull out the nipples.
- Use a nipple shield (must pump or express after feedings, monitor diaper output and weigh baby) twice weekly.
- Use a "nipple expanding" device to pull out flat or inverted nipples, such as the customized syringe (Kesaree et al., 1993) or a commercial expander (Evert it, Niplette).
- Wear shells between feedings to push areolar puffiness back into the breast (see section on breast edema later in this chapter) so the baby can latch.
- Express some milk to soften the breast for the baby if the woman is engorged.
- Reverse pressure softening if her breasts are swollen from IV fluids (uncommon).

Large-breasted women sometimes find breast-feeding challenging simply because they have difficulty dealing with their large breasts and the newborn at the same time. Finding a place for the baby to be secure, so the mother can use both hands to deal with her large breast, can be the answer for these women. Care should be taken to position the baby so the weight of the breast is not resting on the baby's chest. The baby may feel his airway is being threatened with pressure on his chest. It may be just as threatening as pressure to the back of the baby's head.

Women are creative in finding a position that will work for them. Positions women with large breasts have used successfully include the following:

- Sitting in a chair next to her hospital bed with the bed elevated to the level of her breast. The baby and her breast are supported by the bed.
- Using a side lying position to support both the baby and her breast.
- Using her dining room table at home to support her baby and her breast.

Baby Problems That May Cause Difficulty with Latch-On

The baby needs an intact palate, a tongue that can cup and extend over the lower lip, lips that flange and seal, and a mouth that does not hurt. If the baby is having any problems along these lines, he may not be able to attach well to the breast to breastfeed.

The baby needs to be able to breathe while feeding at the breast. A baby with laryngomalacia (floppy laryngeal structures pulled into the airway upon inspiration with audible stridor) or tracheomalacia (softening of the cartilaginous ring surrounding the trachea with stridor upon expiration) will need careful positioning to be able to breastfeed (McMillan et al., 1999). A side-lying or prone feeding position may work well for these babies. If the baby is having trouble breathing for any other reason (stuffy nose, swollen nares, obstructed nares, weight of the breast on his chest, etc.), he will not breastfeed.

The baby who is in pain resulting from birth trauma or surgical intervention may be temporarily unable to respond to internal hunger cues or external stimuli. Fractured clavicle, sore head, cranial suture out of line, hematoma, forceps marks, vacuum extraction trauma and circumcision may all contribute to an apparent disinterest in feeding for several hours.

Sometimes a baby will refuse one breast. This could be due to pain on one side of the body such as from a broken clavicle, an injury on one side of his head, or a painful shoulder. A few women have related stories of their children who were blind in one eye who resisted breastfeeding when the good eye was blocked. One woman reported the same response from her baby who was deaf in one ear and did not like to feed lying on the side that blocked his "hearing" ear.

Birth is a tiring process. Neonates may be drugged from the labor medications taken by their mothers. Some babies exhibit an exaggerated gag reflex. They may act as if they are backing away from the breast. Practicing sucking on a mother's clean finger may be an effective way to help these babies. If the baby has a tendency to hold his tongue in the wrong place, there are several strategies to assist the baby. If the baby is sucking the roof of his mouth, the baby may be working at stabilizing his jaw. By providing chin support, the baby may be able to lower his tongue.

If the baby holds his tongue behind the lower gum, the parents can play an imitation game with the baby and stick their tongues out at him. Babies tend to imitate their parents. Also, gently tapping a finger on the baby's lips should elicit interest on the baby's part to stick out his tongue in search of the finger.

When a baby is having difficulty latching, keep an eye, ear, and nose out for potential stimuli that could be potentially obnoxious to the baby. The smell of perfume, soaps, body lotions, room deodorizers, and so on may disturb him. Loud noises, such as barking dogs or a mother yelling at older children, can scare the newborn. If anything is touching the baby's cheeks—such as his undershirt or a baby blanket or the mother's fingers—the baby may turn toward them and ultimately away from the breast. Removing anything that could be in the way will help the baby. The most disturbing stimulus of all is pressure on the back of the baby's head. The baby becomes very worried that his nose will become blocked. Suggest that the mother support the baby's shoulders and hold the baby's ears with her index finger and thumb. The web between the finger and thumb make a second neck for the baby. In this way the baby knows he has control of his head and can lift his head back to free his airway if needed.

Previous negative experiences may cause aversion to the breast. If the baby's head has been pushed into the breast, the baby may start to cry when offered the breast. If the negative experience persists, the baby shuts down when offered the breast. The parents describe the baby as falling asleep when offered the breast. When the baby has breast aversion, feeding the baby another way is important (see Chapter 10). Have the mother hold the baby skin-to-skin against her chest at nonfeeding times. Gradually move the baby, over the course of several days, to the breastfeeding position. Once the baby can be placed in the mother's arms in a breastfeeding position without the aversive behavior, the baby can be offered the breast after having been fed half of his milk for that feeding. Attempts to latch should be kept to a short time. These attempts should stop before the baby gets upset. Babies who are hypertonic or hypotonic may need the additional help of a curled or flexed position for breastfeeding.

Late-Preterm Infants

The most frequent length of gestation in the United States is 39, not 40 weeks, largely because of the increase in births between 34 and 36 completed weeks of gestation. Births between 34 completed weeks and less than 37 completed weeks are now called *late-preterm infants* (NICHD, 2005). Late-preterm infants treated as full-term infants pose a special situation. They fall between the cracks—they are not considered preterm infants unless they have medical problems, but they do not behave as full-term infants. These vulnerable infants often are treated like full-term infants even though they have the same risks of complications as infants born prematurely (Simpson & Creehan, 2008). The unborn baby gains about one half pound per week, so babies born at 34 weeks may be one and a half pounds smaller than those born at 37 weeks.

In times past, these late-preterm babies were placed in a special nursery; now they are placed on the regular postpartum unit with their mothers. This is good for establishing breastfeeding, but as lactation consultants working in the postpartum area will testify, most late-preterm infants require considerable time and effort before they are able to breast-feed effectively.

Characteristics of the late-preterm infant may include the following (see Color Plate 40):

- Neurologic disorganization and poor state control—They can go from a highly alert state to deep sleep rapidly, and the environment should be kept quiet to avoid overstimulation.
- Poor muscle tone or floppiness requires careful positioning and extra support during feedings.
- Poor temperature control because of less body fat—Unnecessary suction or excessive handling can cause thermal and metabolic stress (Wight, 2003).
- Immature rooting and suckling. The suckle/swallow/breathe pattern may be uncoordinated.

Mothers of late-preterm babies are more likely to have a medical problem such as hypertension, diabetes, prolonged rupture of membranes, or cesarean delivery that may affect breastfeeding.

The baby will need good shoulder girdle support for head control, placed facing the mother with the baby's arms separated and hugging the breast, and the baby's hips should be well supported almost as high as the head (Tully, 2002). Figure 7–11 shows a 36-week-old premature baby at breast.

The usual pattern of these infants is to grasp the breast and suckle for a short time and then stop to rest (pacing the feed). Once a bolus of milk is in the baby's mouth and he drops his tongue to swallow,

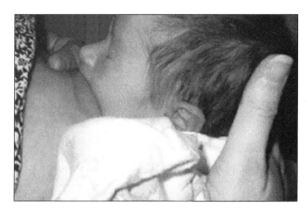

FIGURE **7–11** A 36-week-old premature baby at breast.

he may not have the maturity to bring his tongue into position to initiate the next suckle. The inability of these babies to maintain sustained periods of at least 10 suck/swallows/breathe patterns limits milk transfer and puts them at risk for high bilirubin levels, hypoglycemia, dehydration, and insufficient weight gain. Interventions for these infants must be individual; however, skin-to-skin (kangaroo) holding, keeping them warm, allowing longer periods of rest between feedings, and limiting stimulation are all important for optimizing the baby's ability to feed well when awake.

There are two basic principles involved with breastfeeding the late-preterm baby (Wight, 2003):

1. Feed the baby the mother's pumped milk.
2. Establish and maintain the mother's milk supply.
3. Provide support while she waits for her baby to mature.

Many of these babies feed best on approximately a 4-hour schedule until they are close to term age, at which time they go to the more usual 2- to 3-hour feeding pattern and begin to waken for feedings voluntarily. Trying to force a baby to waken before the fourth hour from the *beginning* of the last feeding may cause the baby to put a lot of energy into trying to maintain the sleep state he needs. However, at the fourth hour most of these babies wake willingly and feed vigorously taking a sufficient volume to justify six feedings in 24 hours. For some babies, short but frequent feedings work better.

The mother will need to pump after each breastfeeding to establish her milk production. This expressed milk can be given to the baby if the baby cannot obtain enough milk by breastfeeding. Because this small baby is learning to breastfeed, an alternative feeding method that does not provide sucking, such as cup or spoon, are options to consider. Nipple shields work well for these babies if they are having trouble maintaining latch-on and the mother has a good milk supply.

The mother–baby dyad will need extra care in such cases. Follow-up phone calls and early return for weight checks is mandatory. Mothers of 34 to 37 weekers who have breastfed a full-term baby previously need just as much help as first-time breastfeeders. They remember a vigorous baby who knows how to feed effectively. Her past experience does not prepare her for a sleepy baby who gives little feedback. Also, the mother who is engorged should be encouraged to pump or express sufficient milk to establish her milk supply.

Feeding Methods

Cup-Feeding

Babies can be fed by cup from birth, and many low birth weight infants are cup-fed around the world until they are mature enough to exclusively breastfeed (Gupta, Khanna, & Chattree, 1999). Many maternity units in the United Kingdom and elsewhere that are striving to attain baby-friendly status give supplements by cup in order to meet the award criteria of not using bottles.

Oro-motor skills used in sipping and lapping from a cup differ from those used while suckling at the breast or at the bottle because there is no object in the baby's mouth (Mizuno & Kani, 2005). Despite these differences, cup-feeding low birth weight infants was found to be at least as safe as bottle-feeding with no differences in physiological stability, choking, spitting, apnea, and bradycardia during feeds for both feeding methods (Malhotra et al., 1999; Marinelli, Burke, & Dodd, 2001; Mizuno & Kani, 2005). In a controlled trial (Howard, 2003) 700 healthy term infants were randomized to early or late introduction to a pacifier and within each group to cup or bottle for any supplement. The authors concluded that administration time, amounts ingested, and physiologic stability did not differ with cup- and bottle-feeding.

In another study, infants took less volume and required more time to feed as they were learning to cup-feed than when learning to bottle-feed. (Dowling et al., 2002). Freer (1999) found that a drop in oxygen saturation can occur in the preterm infant while cup-feeding. Other drawbacks are milk spillage and that the baby is deprived of sucking. In two early cup-feeding studies (Davis et al., 1948; Freeden, 1948), full-term babies cup-fed efficiently, taking milk faster by cup than by bottle or breast. In the 1940s, newborns were in the hospital for 10 days. Given more time, they became very proficient at cup-feeding.

The following are appropriate times to cup-feed:

- When baby is unable to latch on to the breast for whatever reason
- When the mother is not present on the neonatal unit
- When parents and staff wish to avoid the infant becoming addicted to the bottle
- When breastfeeding is not possible for any reason

The following are *not* appropriate times to cup-feed:

- Infant has been recently extubated with possible damage to the vocal cords
- Infant has a poor gag reflex.
- Infant is extremely lethargic.
- Infant has neurological deficits.
- Premie has respiratory unstable condition.

For cup-feeding, a small cup with a rounded edge is preferred. In India, a special cuplike device called a *paladai* is used for feeding premature babies in some neonatal intensive care units. The nurses in these units prefer the *paladai* to a regular cup (Malhotra et al., 1999). Medicine cups holding small quantities are readily available in hospitals. They are thus appropriate for early feedings when volume will rarely exceed 1 to 2 oz. Commercial feeding cups such as the Softfeeder, which resembles a spoon and has a control valve, are also available.

How to Cup-Feed

The following is how to cup-feed:

- Hold the baby in an upright position that is comfortable for both you and the infant.

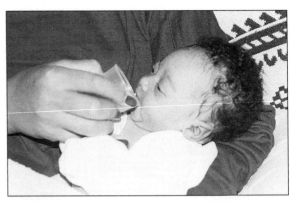

FIGURE 7–12   Baby cup-feeding.

Source: Courtesy of Kay Hoover, MEd, IBCLC.

- Secure the baby's arms and hands to prevent him from knocking the cup.
- Place a cloth diaper under the baby's chin to catch spillage (weigh before and after feed).
- Place and support the baby in an upright, sitting position (see Figure 7–12).
- Bring the cup to a position resting on his lower lip with the rim at the corners of his mouth. Avoid putting pressure on the lower lip.
- Tip the cup slightly to allow access to the fluid. Do *not* pour the milk into the baby's mouth.
- Let baby "pace" the feeding by watching his cues. Keep cup in position while the baby stops lapping.

Cup-feeding can be difficult for parents to learn. Teaching them the technique should include a "return demonstration" to make certain they are doing it safely (Hedberg-Nyqvist, 1999; Wilson-Clay & Hoover, 2005). As long as the caregiver does not attempt to pour too much milk into the baby's mouth, risk of aspiration is minimal and the feeding can be accomplished quickly (Lang, Lawrence, & Orme, 1994; Thorley, 1997). Some infants will "fight" the cup and refuse to lap the milk from the cup. Each infant must be treated individually.

Finger-Feeding

Finger-feeding with a feeding tube is an alternative feeding method for neonates (Figure 7–13). It is used by some lactation consultants when the baby is too sleepy to breastfeed, if the baby does not latch on well for any reason, if the mother and baby are

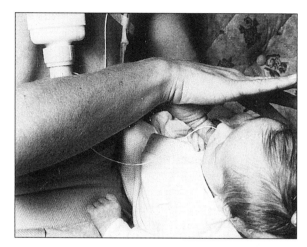

separated (Newman, 2002), or if the baby cannot bottle-feed. Proponents of finger-feeding believe that it facilitates proper use of the oral muscles, promotes optimal coordination of suck/swallow/breathe, and allows the baby to pace the feeding (Hazelbaker, 1997). Critics claim that the technique is invasive and addictive. Instructions for finger-feeding a neonate are presented in Box 7–3.

Nipple Shields

Nipple shields have a controversial history, largely due to the bad reputation of the old type of shields that were made of rubber or latex. Babies of mothers using these old type of shields were unable to ingest sufficient breastmilk often resulting in slow weight gain and failure to thrive. As a result, nipple shields came to be viewed as interfering with, rather than assisting the new mother in breastfeeding.

The newer ultrathin silicone nipple shields are especially helpful for a mother with flat or inverted nipples, for preterm babies who have trouble latching and maintaining suction, or for babies who have developed a preference for a bottle nipple and thus refuse the breast.

When a woman first uses a silicone nipple shield, she needs to use a multiuser electric pump (like the ones used in the hospitals) and pump her milk four to six times a day after breastfeeding to establish a milk supply. The baby needs to be weighed twice a week and diapers monitored for adequate stools and wetness. Once the baby is gaining well (about an ounce a day), the mother can gradually wean off pumping as long as the baby continues to gain appropriately.

In many cases, the short-term use of a nipple shield will preserve the breastfeeding relationship while the baby learns to breastfeed (Meier et al., 2000; Nicholson, 1993; Wilson-Clay, 1996). A La Leche League mother movingly described how a silicone nipple shield "saved her breastfeeding relationship" with her baby (Clemmit, 2003).

Placing a feeding tube (attached to a syringe with the milk supplement) inside of the nipple shield during a feed is particularly helpful (Figure 7–14). This technique gives the baby several advantages:

- An immediate reward for latching on and suckling
- An opportunity to stimulate the breast and remove breastmilk
- Control over the amount and flow of supplement ingested
- Nutriment (calories and fluids)

To apply a silicone nipple shield, smooth a thin layer of water inside the nipple shield brim, then flip up the brim of the shield (like that of a sombrero), and turn half of the teat of the shield in on itself. Center the shield directly over the nipple, and gently pat down the brim (Wilson-Clay, 2003). The silicone will reshape itself and pull the nipple partway into the shield teat. For additional discussion on nipple shields, see Chapter 12.

Hypoglycemia

Newborns experience a decrease in blood glucose after birth as they adapt to the extrauterine environment and then regain blood glucose rapidly (Eidelman, 2001). This transient hypoglycemia in the immediate postpartum period occurs in almost all mammalian species (Wight, 2006) and is an adaptive phenomenon as the newborn changes from the fetal state of continuous transplacental glucose feeding to that of intermittent feeding after birth. This dynamic process is self-limiting and is usually not pathologic.

Hypoglycemia is partially a matter of definition. Whether a baby is considered to have a low blood

BOX 7–3

Finger-Feeding a Neonate

- Ensure that your hands are clean and the nail on the finger or thumb you use is cut short before you begin. Wearing a latex-free glove or finger cott is preferable when the baby is finger-fed by someone other than the mother or father.
- Prop the baby, making sure his head is stable and slightly tilted back.
- If using a feeding-tube device (#5 French, 15 in. long), the tube can be held close to the end of the finger.
- Connect the feeding tube with a syringe or feeding bottle with expressed breastmilk or, if necessary, formula depending on the situation. If using a bottle, the feeding tube can be inserted through a cut made in the rubber nipple. If using a syringe, choose the size most appropriate for the circumstances (usually 10 to 30 cc).
- Select a large digit, since the breast fills the baby's mouth.
- Stroke the baby's lips gently until the baby opens his mouth. Slide your finger or allow the baby to suck the finger in

with the nail bed resting on his tongue and the pad side up. The tip of the finger needs to extend to the juncture of the hard and soft palates. The tube can be taped to the pad side of the parent's finger. In most instances, the baby will begin sucking as soon as he feels the finger pad on the hard palate.
- Push milk from the syringe into the baby's mouth ONLY if the baby is sucking.
- If the baby is sucking effectively, the person who is finger-feeding the baby will feel a pulling sensation along the nail bed with each exertion of negative pressure (suckle), as if the nail is being pulled deeper into the baby's mouth.
- Monitor color and vital signs, especially if the baby is low birth weight or has poor muscle tone or oral structural deficits.
- Record the amount of human milk (or formula) that the baby takes.
- Show the mother (and the father) how to finger-feed.

---

glucose level depends on the laboratory values used as criteria for hypoglycemia and the reliability of the methods used to measure blood glucose. Before deciding what is abnormal, one must first establish what is normal. What are normal blood sugar levels for newborns? Based on the author's experience with teaching an Internet course to graduate nurses across the United States and beyond, hypoglycemia protocols vary widely according to region, and routine glucose testing after birth is common even though it is not recommended by the Academy of Breastfeeding Medicine and other physician organizations.

On the whole, breastfed infants have lower blood sugar levels (58 mg/dL) compared with formula-fed infants (72 mg/dL), according to Hawdon, Ward-Platt, and Aynsley-Green (1992). In the same study, blood sugar levels were correlated with the intervals between the feeds—the more frequent the feeding, the higher the glucose concentration.

While there are still no universally accepted "cutoff" glucose levels for hypoglycemia, several guidelines have been recommended. The Academy of Breastfeeding Medicine published a table (Table 7–4) of recommended low thresholds for

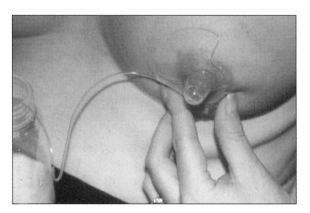

FIGURE 7–14A Feeding tube device under a silicone nipple shield.

(A) Feeding tube device placed under nipple shield. Baby would need to be able to suck well in order to pull the milk out of the bottle and through the tubing. This is a good technique to keep the baby feeding at the breast until he can latch on to the breast and get out enough milk directly. It could also be used for a baby who has become accustomed to a bottle nipple.

Source: Courtesy of Kay Hoover, MEd, IBCLC.

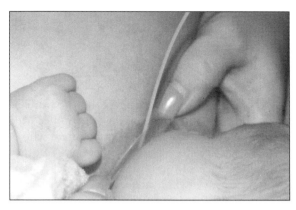

FIGURE 7–14B (B) Baby receives supplementation from feeding tube and breastfeeds at the same time. As soon as baby attaches, milk can be squeezed into the nipple shield to give the baby an immediate reward for any attempts made at the breast. Use with baby who has gotten used to bottle-feeding, has a weak suckle, or has difficulty latching onto the breast.

Source: Courtesy of Kay Hoover, MEd, IBCLC.

blood glucose based on hours after birth using data from a meta-analysis (Alkalay et al., 2006). On the basis of research findings from a large sample of well, full-term infants, Heck and Erenberg (1987) recommend that hypoglycemia in full-term infants be defined as serum glucose concentration of less than 30 mg/dL on the first day after birth or less than 40 mg/dL on the second day after birth. Srinivasan et al. (1986) recommended similar levels. If the higher level of 40 mg/dL were used for the first day postpartum, 20.6 percent of well, full-term infants would be considered hypoglycemic and would receive unnecessary supplements (Sexson, 1984). Brand (2005) evaluated the effects of transient hypoglycemia on the first day of life in 75 healthy term, large for gestational age infants, on their later neurodevelopment. There were no significant differences between children with normal glycemic levels and hypoglycemia at 4-year follow-up using standardized development scales. The Academy of Breastfeeding Medicine (2006) has published hypoglycemia guidelines that are available on the Internet (www.bfmed.org).

Severe neonatal hypoglycemia leads to potential brain damage and can result in serious sequelae such as seizures. Prolonged hypoglycemia can be avoided by close clinical observation of vulnerable infants while avoiding excessive invasive management (Moore & Perlman, 1999). Clinical symptoms that indicate possible hypoglycemia in neonates include the following:

- Jitteriness
- Exaggerated reflexes
- High-pitched cry

TABLE 7–4 Recommended Low Threshold: Plasma Glucose Level (PGL)

Hour After Birth	< 5th Percentile PGL (mg/dL)
1–2 (lowest point)	28 (1.6 mmol/L)*
3–47	40 (2.2 mmol/L)
48–72	48 (2.7 mmol/L)

* To convert mmol/L of glucose to mg/dL, multiply by 18. To convert mg/dL of glucose to mmol/L, divide by 18 or multiply by 0.055.

Source: Adapted from Alkalay, 2006.

- Seizures
- Lethargy
- Rapid breathing
- Hypothermia
- Poor suck and refusal to feed

Hypoglycemia is of particular concern with certain health conditions: the infant of a mother with diabetes, a postmature neonate, or an infant who is small for gestational age. The infant of a mother with diabetes is most apt to experience hypoglycemia shortly after birth, because he continues to produce a high level of insulin, which depletes the blood glucose within hours after birth. The degree of infant hypoglycemia is usually in proportion to the success achieved in controlling the mother's blood glucose during her pregnancy. Symptomatic neonates are given 10 to 15 percent glucose intravenously immediately after birth until they stabilize.

Postmature infants also need early, frequent breastfeedings to normalize their glucose levels. Lethargy and poor feeding in these babies may contribute to hypoglycemia; thus any interest shown in feeding should be followed by immediate, unrestricted access to the breast for as often and as long as the baby wishes. Most postmature neonates, after a first breastfeeding, show increased interest in subsequent breastfeeding, thus reducing the risk of continued hypoglycemia.

The newborn who is small for his gestational age is also at risk for hypoglycemia. A prompt first breastfeeding followed by very frequent breastfeeding thereafter is usually sufficient to bring the baby's blood glucose level to normal. In some cases, continued poor feeding may require a supplement. Start with the mother's own milk. If no milk can be obtained with hand expression, and there is no banked human milk, then formula may have to be used. This practice need not be repeated once the baby is breastfeeding well. The following conditions are associated with low blood sugar:

- Small for gestational age
- Postmature
- Discordant twin (smaller)
- Large for gestational age (LGA) > 90th percentile or weight
- Infants of diabetic mothers
- Low birth weight infants < 2500 gms
- Postasphyxia, cold stress, sepsis, and other stresses

Intrapartum management plays a role in the neonate's glucose level. Use of hypertonic glucose infusions during labor can lead to elevation in maternal blood glucose, which can in turn result in fetal hyperglycemia and hyperinsulinemia and eventually neonatal hypoglycemia.

The blood level is first measured at bedside using glucose testing strips. These strips are cheap and practical; however, they vary significantly from true blood glucose levels. Studies comparing different reagent strips have estimated that as many as 20 percent of truly normal glycemic infants are falsely labeled as hypoglycemic leading to unnecessary lab tests and treatments. Ho (2004) compared five glucometer devices and found *none* were satisfactory as the sole measuring device. Measuring blood glucose concentrations in asymptomatic babies in the first 2 postnatal hours is unnecessary and can cause parents to become anxious and worried for no reason. It also interferes with establishing breastfeeding and can result in serious disruption of the initiation and duration of breastfeeding (Haninger & Farley, 2001).

Placing the baby skin-to-skin with his mother helps stabilize his blood sugar. Christensson et al. (1998) report average blood glucose of 57.6 mg/dL in the skin-to-skin group and 46.6 mg/dL in the group cared for away from their mothers.

If the neonate is unable to suckle or feedings are not tolerated, begin IV therapy. If glucose remains low despite feedings, IV glucose should be started and the IV rate adjusted by monitoring changes in blood glucose. Infants with symptoms of hypoglycemia should have more aggressive therapy. Guidelines for documented hypoglycemia are seen in Boxes 7–4 and 7–5 (Wright, Marinelli, Academy of Breastfeeding Medicine Protocol Committee, 2006).

Cesarean Birth

Over 20 percent of births in the United States are by cesarean, and the rate is rising. Many European and South American countries have similar and even higher rates of surgical birth. Part of the rise is due to women themselves requesting to have a Cesarean delivery because they want to deliver early to avoid discomforts of the last few weeks (in fact, the average gestation period in the United States is now 8 months, instead of 9!), and because they can make definite plans for returning to work, getting child care, and so on. Moreover, delivering a baby by

BOX **7–4**

General Management Recommendations: ABM Protocol

Early and exclusive breastfeeding meets the nutritional and metabolic needs of a healthy, term newborn infant:

- Initiate breastfeeding within 30 to 60 minutes of life and continue on demand.
- Routine supplementation is unnecessary.
- Initiate skin-to-skin contact of mother and infant.
- Feedings should be frequent; 10–12 times per 24 hours in the first few days after birth.

Glucose screening is performed only on at-risk or symptomatic infants:

- Routine monitoring of blood glucose in all term infants is unnecessary and may be harmful.
- An at-risk infant should be screened for hypoglycemia with a frequency and duration related to the risk factor of the individual infant.
- Monitoring continues until normal, preprandial (prefeeding) levels are consistently obtained.
- Bedside glucose screening tests must be confirmed by formal laboratory testing.

Source: Adapted from Academy of Breastfeeding Medicine, June, 2006.

---

cesarean delivery is convenient for the physicians, too, who may subtly try to persuade their patients to deliver by cesarean.

The impact of cesarean delivery on breastfeeding has been extensively studied. Although its effects are difficult to disentangle from other interventions, generally, breastfeeding rates and the duration of mothers who deliver by cesarean birth are about the same as those who have vaginal births. The mother's commitment to breastfeeding plays a substantial role despite unexpected birth outcomes. A greater commitment to breastfeeding, regardless of the manner of birth, results in longer duration of breastfeeding (Janke, 1988).

Cesarean births are associated with delayed lactogenesis and a delay in initiating breastfeeding (Chen et al., 1998; Dewey et al., 2003; Evans et al., 2003; Grajeda & Perez-Escamilla, 2002; Leung, Lam, & Ho, 2002; Rowe-Murray & Fisher, 2002). Recovery from major surgery takes more time, is more painful and stressful, and represents additional risks compared to an uneventful vaginal birth, which explains why breastfeeding occurs later. In a recent study, one third of the women delivered by cesarean birth

believed that their ability to breastfeed was affected negatively to a large or very large extent by postoperative pain (Karlstrom et al., 2007).

Women's reactions to having a cesarean birth vary. Although some women may interpret an unexpected cesarean birth as a reflection on her adequacy, cesarean births are so frequent now that parents tend to view cesarean birth as a normal or alternative mode of delivery. Childbirth educators and others have effectively conveyed the message that cesarean birth does not have to be a threat and that they can be awake to experience the event and the baby's father can be present at the birth.

In working with a mother who has had a cesarean birth, the nurse or the lactation consultant needs to do the following:

- Assess the mother's degree of physical comfort and awareness. If she is not fully conscious, she is not ready to put her baby to breast. Once the mother is alert and able to hold her baby, however, she can begin breastfeeding.
- Relieve discomfort with pain medicine.

BOX **7–5**

Management of Documented Hypoglycemia

Asymptomatic infant:

- Continue breastfeeding (approximately every 1 to 2 hours) or feed 3 to 10 mL/kg of expressed breastmilk or substitute nutrition.
- Recheck blood glucose concentration before subsequent feedings until the value is acceptable and stable.
- Avoid forced feedings.
- If glucose remains low despite feedings, begin intravenous glucose therapy.
- Breastfeeding may continue during IV glucose therapy.
- Carefully document response to treatment.

Symptomatic infant or infants with plasma glucose levels < 20 to 25 mg/dL (< 1.1 to 1.4 mmol/L):

- Initiate intravenous 10 percent glucose solution.

- Do not rely on oral or intragastric feeding to correct extreme or symptomatic hypoglycemia.
- The glucose concentration in symptomatic infants should be maintained > 45 mg/dL (> 25 mmol/L).
- Adjust intravenous rate by blood glucose concentration.
- Encourage frequent breastfeeding.
- Monitor glucose concentration before feedings as the IV is weaned until values stabilize off intravenous fluids.
- Carefully document response to treatment.

Source: Adapted from ABM clinical protocol #1: Guidelines for glucose monitoring and treatment of hypoglycemia in breastfed neonates (Revision June, 2006). *Breastfeeding Medicine.* 1(3):178–184.

- Ask the mother how she wants to hold her infant. Some mothers, particularly those still receiving intravenous pain medication or those who have had an epidural narcotic, are quite comfortable holding their babies in the cradle position using pillows for support. Others are hesitant to hold the baby at all until they have been reassured that they can do so without touching or placing any pressure near their abdominal incision.
- Suggest that if the mother holds her baby in a clutch position (see again Figure 7–8B), she will avoid the sensitive incision area. As the pain of her incision decreases, the mother can be instructed and assisted in the use of positions other than the football hold, as discussed later in this chapter. By the second or third day postpartum, the side-lying position is generally comfortable, especially if the mother is adequately supported with pillows at her back and beneath her abdomen.
- Provide a breast pump if the baby cannot breastfeed. Assist the mother in pumping her breasts about every 4 hours during the day and skip a pumping at night. Although pumping the breasts in the immediate postpartum period neither hastens lactogenesis nor improves later milk transfer (Chapman et al., 2001), most hospitals routinely have mothers pump if breastfeeding is delayed.

The baby born by cesarean may be lethargic, particularly if the birth followed a long period of exposure to analgesia or anesthesia in labor. If so, explain to the mother that a delay in feeding will not deter breastfeeding; rather, her milk supply will be established slightly later than it would be following a vaginal birth.

Breast Engorgement

Breast engorgement is a major issue in the early postpartum period as the breast, under the influence of hormonal shifts, increases milk production rapidly from 36 to 96 hours postpartum. Although the gradual buildup of fluid in the breasts following parturition is a welcome sign of breastmilk, breast engorgement is a common problem in the early days after birth and a common reason for early weaning. Because women leave the hospital before their breasts become full or engorged, the situation is usually handled at home or in a postdischarge visit at a clinic or medical office.

For most women engorgement is at its height from 3 to 5 days after birth and slowly recedes but may last 2 weeks for some (Humenick, Hill, & Anderson, 1994). During normal engorgement, the mother's breast tissue usually remains compressible, thus enabling the infant to attach comfortably and efficiently, without risk of trauma to the breast or nipple tissue. Extreme breast fullness rarely lasts more than 24 hours, during which time breastfeeding can continue without discomfort. The mother with breast fullness should be encouraged to view this state as a transitory indication of milk production that will begin to regulate to meet the baby's needs as the infant breastfeeds.

Multiparous women are more likely to report more intense engorgement than primiparous women, and distinct patterns of breast engorgement can be identified (Humenick, Hill, & Anderson, 1994). Severe breast engorgement, a pathologic condition, and often the consequence of mismanagement, is painful. It can be caused by any situation that allows milk stasis to occur. There are several situations that lead to uncomfortable engorgement:

- Supplements (Wright, Rice, & Wells, 1996)
- Delayed initiation of feedings at the breast

- Infrequent feedings
- Time-limited feedings
- Removing the baby from the first breast to ensure feeding from both breasts at every feeding (Lawson & Tulloch, 1995)

Breast implants can also lead to severe engorgement. Sometimes the tissue around the nipple and areola becomes so taut that the infant is unable to grasp the nipple. When the baby is unable to latch onto the breast, the mother's discomfort mounts, and her breast and nipple tissue may be so tight that even leaking cannot occur. Under such conditions, further trauma to the tissue is apt to occur when a vigorous baby attempts unsuccessfully to grasp and draw the breast into his mouth.

Various treatments for engorgement have been suggested:

- Medications: Anti-inflammatory medications
- Heat treatments: Warm compresses, warm showers. Use warm treatments *before* breastfeeding.
- Cold treatments: Cold compresses, frozen vegetable bags (wrapped in a towel), cold gel packs. Use cold treatments *after* breastfeeding.
- Cabbage compresses: Fresh cabbages, cold or room temperature (Roberts, Reiter, & Schuster, 1995; Rosier, 1988)
- Breast massage and milk expression: Massaging the breast and expressing milk to relieve engorgement. This technique is commonly practiced worldwide, especially in Japan.
- Ultrasound: Ultrasound treatments are used for both plugged ducts and engorgement.
- Pumping: Pumping reduces build-up of milk.

Research on engorgement is unique in that the condition slowly and inevitably resolves itself no matter what treatment is used; thus a group of mothers (preferably randomized) receiving the treatment must be compared simultaneously with a group who do not receive the treatment. Snowden, Renfrew, and Woolridge (2002) analyzed eight randomized control trials involving 424 women receiving treatments for breast engorgement in an attempt to discover which treatments were effective (see Table 7–5). They concluded that cabbage leaves, cold packs, gel packs, oxytocin, and ultrasound treatments were all ineffective. Only pharmacological

TABLE 7–5 Meta-analysis of Studies on Postpartum Breast Engorgement

Treatment	Outcome
Anti-inflammatory drugs	Increase total improvement rating and reduce symptoms compared with placebo. Danzen (OR 3.6, 95%, CI 1.27–10.26); Kimotab (OR 8.02, 95%, CI 2.76–23.3).
Cabbage leaves	No difference between treatment and control groups.
Cold packs	No difference between treatment and control groups.
Gel packs	No difference between treatment and control groups.
Oxytocin	No difference when compared with saline injections.
Ultrasound treatments	No benefit. Decrease in pain due to the warmth of treatment rather than ultrasound waves themselves.

Source: Snowden, Renfrew, & Woolridge, 2002.

treatment using anti-inflammatory medications (Danzen and bromelain/trypsin complex) significantly improved symptoms of engorgement.

Whatever intervention is used, the mother should be encouraged to offer the breast frequently to avoid painful engorgement. Any method that reduces the sensation of tightness in the breast tissue is likely to help the mother. If the mother is breastfeeding, how often and how long her infant is suckling should be assessed. During the first 2 weeks, the average number of minutes a baby spends breastfeeding in 24 hours is about 2.7 hours (de Carvalho, 1982). If the baby is being offered the breast fewer than eight times in 24 hours, and for less than an average of 20 minutes per feeding, it may not be enough. If the mother is unable to increase the number of feedings, she may obtain relief with the judicious use of hand expression or a fully automatic intermittent electric breast pump.

A fever of unknown origin in a mother during the first week postpartum may be another sign of breast engorgement. Occasionally, fever from engorgement can be 101°F or higher. If the woman is not breastfeeding and her breasts are engorged, she can apply cold (causing vasoconstriction) to reduce fluid filtration into the interstitium. As in other areas of the body, tissue edema in the breast is reduced by cold and is increased by heat.

Breast Edema

Women who receive excessive intravenous fluids throughout labor may develop edema of their breast. This edema is different from the normal physiologic engorgement that precedes lactogenesis. The mother's breasts can be as "hard as rocks" and the nipples distended. As a result, the neonate may be unable to latch onto her breasts until the edema has subsided. Breast edema can be treated with areolar compression, a method to reduce nipple/areola edema manually by using gentle positive pressure (Miller & Riordan, 2004). The healthcare provider can perform the following intervention or the mother can do it herself:

1. Ask mother to wash her hands thoroughly. Explain what you plan to do to the mother and ask her permission. Nails should be short and preferably unpolished. No artificial nails.

2. Do a "press test" to determine areolar edema. Apply firm but gentle pressure with the index finger and thumb on either side of the areola behind the nipple. Hold it there until the edema can be felt to be giving way. Remove your fingers to see if there are finger impressions remaining in the tissue. If there are, then areolar edema is present.

3. Apply pressure again slightly behind the softened spot. Hold the pressure until the area under your fingers softens. Apply steady inward pressure toward the chest wall for 60 seconds or longer, concentrating on the areola where it joins the base of the nipple. Next, move the fingers behind the softened area to the firm tissue and apply pressure again.

4. Start behind the nipple, rotate the fingers clockwise, and move back along the areola holding the pressure until the tissue is soft before moving the fingers again. If fingernails are short, press with the curved fingertips of both hands simultaneously with the nail

nearly touching the sides of the nipple. The goal is to create a ring of small "dimples" or pits on the areola at the base of the nipple. (If performed by the healthcare provider, the flat part of two thumbs or two fingers can also be used. This will require another 60 seconds of pressure in opposite quadrants to soften the same general area.)

5. Rotate finger pressure, displacing the edema into the breast tissue until the areola is soft and the nipple is pliable.

6. Plan on the procedure taking anywhere from a few minutes to 30 minutes to move the edema out enough to latch the infant onto the breast. The length of time will depend on the severity of the edema.

The effect of areolar compression, also called reverse pressure softening (Cotterman, 2004), is fourfold: (1) it moves excess interstitial fluid inward in the direction of natural lymphatic drainage; (2) it relieves overdistension of the milk ducts and reduces latch discomfort; (3) it enables the infant to draw the breast deeply into his mouth so that the stripping action of the tongue can remove the milk; (4) it stimulates the nerves supplying the nipple and areolar complex, thus triggering the milk ejection reflex (Cotterman, 2003).

Areolar compression (Color Plate 20) should be done *before* pumping the breast. Pumping the breast first before areolar compression can cause further accumulation of edema in the areola, especially when maximum settings are used. The negative pressure of a pump tends to draw excess interstitial fluid *toward* the areola and nipple instead of moving it *away* from the area, thus worsening the problem. Once edema is displaced, the nipple will stretch outward making latching easier.

Hand Expression

Although many women in the United States think first of using a breast pump to obtain milk, expressing milk by hand is a skill that has been used by many mothers for millennia. The mother's own hands represent several advantages over breast pumps:

- They cost her nothing.
- They may trigger a more effective milk ejection reflex.

- They are always available.
- They compress the breast for milk removal.

After the mother has practiced this skill, she may find she can obtain more milk more quickly than women who use an electric device for the same purpose! Techniques vary across cultures and are most effective when the breasts are compressed well behind the nipple (Figure 7–15). Every postpartum nurse and every lactation consultant should be able to instruct a mother in hand expression. Pushing back toward the chest wall with her fingers and then rolling the fingers together is recommended rather than sliding the fingers down the breast, to avoid inadvertently bruising or abrading the skin. The mother should be cautioned that she might have greater difficulty with expression if she is attempting to relieve engorgement or her breasts are very tender. She should be encouraged to be patient, to shower or use warm compresses, and to stimulate

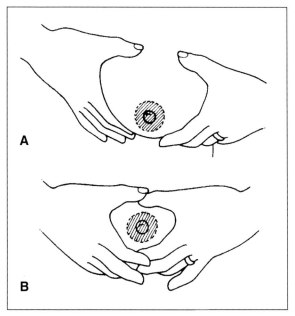

FIGURE 7–15 Hand expression. (A) Wash hands and any collection equipment to be used. Sit comfortably, and place the collection cup under the breast. Apply warm, moist towel to enhance milk flow. Massage breasts and nipples to stimulate milk ejection reflex. Use gentle pressure using a circular motion, moving around the breast. (B) Squeeze the breast gently, rolling the hands forward from the chest toward the nipple. *(Continues)*

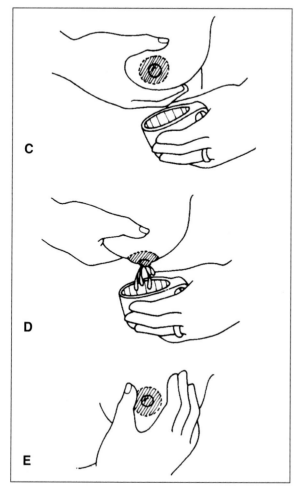

milk ejection with gentle breast massage in advance of attempting to express her milk.

If breast massage is practiced with each expression, encourage the mother to avoid creating a ritual that becomes so time consuming that it interferes with the process. This is particularly relevant if the mother is expressing her milk at work or some other site where she has only a limited time in which to accomplish it. An experienced mother who can demonstrate the technique to the novice can often provide the most effective teaching.

Clinical Implications

Assessment is a critical first step in working with a mother who has a newborn. For example, if the mother had maternal analgesia and her baby is sleepy and is breastfeeding infrequently, the hospital caregiver can do the following:

- Encourage and facilitate the mother to hold her baby skin-to-skin.
- Reassure the mother that the baby's sleepiness may be the result of the analgesia to which he was exposed prior to the birth.
- Encourage the mother to take every opportunity when the baby is awake to offer the breast.
- Suggest that the mother let the baby stay on the first breast until he has let go on his own before offering the second breast.
- Provide specific suggestions regarding home visitation and follow-up with a lactation consultant in private practice and a community-based breastfeeding support group. If the mother experienced difficulty in breastfeeding with an earlier baby, the caregiver may need to reassure the concerned or anxious mother that a similar condition need not recur, or if it does recur, what to do about it.

Breastfeeding Assessment

The infant's first few times breastfeeding should be assessed early in the neonatal period. Such assessment enables the healthcare worker to determine how well the infant roots, latches on, and suckles. Minor adjustments of maternal position or infant position can be made without interrupting or interfering with the mother and infant as they begin to

FIGURE 7–15 (C) Place thumb and forefingers approximately 2 to 3 cm (1 to 1 1/2 inches) behind the nipple and press into the breast. (D) Press inward toward the chest wall squeezing gently with a slight rolling action toward the nipple. Release pressure and repeat as needed to obtain milk. If pain results, something is wrong and the mother should be observed in order to identify what may be causing the mother discomfort. (E) Change position of the fingers around the areola to express milk from as many ducts as possible. Within 3 to 5 minutes, the milk flow may slow; this is a signal to express milk from the other breast. Both sides may be expressed as often as the mother wishes in a given session or until she tires. Particularly in the beginning, the mother should expect to spend 20 to 30 minutes expressing milk. As she becomes more adept at it, the time will decrease even as the amount of milk obtained increases.

learn how to breastfeed together. Several assessment tools specific to feedings at the breast are available and can be found in Chapter 20, Appendix A.

Assessment tools are useful for evaluating infant suckling over several feedings to show mothers that their babies are learning with each feeding and are becoming more efficient at obtaining milk. They can also be used to alert the caregiver to specific "red flags." If the mother–baby dyad is not feeding effectively, they may need special attention to prevent a problem with dehydration and weight loss. Breastfeeding assessment tools also remind the mother that what her baby does is both complex and predictable and that he needs lots of opportunities to practice, just as she needs many opportunities to learn how to hold and position him for optimal breastfeeding. The ease of using these tools means that the mother can evaluate for herself what occurs at each feeding. Despite the usefulness of these tools, reliability and validity testing indicate that they need further development (Riordan & Koehn, 1997). Newer investigations are leading us closer to more valid methods of clinical prediction of breastfeeding outcomes. Of the commonly used breastfeeding indicators, audible swallowing best predicts the actual intake of breastmilk (Riordan & Gill-Hopple, 2002; Riordan, Gill-Hopple, & Koehn, 2005). We also know that certain perinatal events predict that the mother will stop breastfeeding by 7 to 10 days postpartum (Hall et al., 2002), so these mothers need extra help (see Table 7–6).

Discharge Planning

Over the past 30 years the average length of a hospital stay in the United States has declined by nearly 60 percent, to 1.4 days. Mothers and infants often return home in the first 24 to 48 hours after a vaginal birth and 2 to 4 days after a cesarean birth. Early discharge from the hospital, a fact of life for most new mothers and their neonates, has had a major impact on postpartum care. It is the responsibility of the hospital caregiver to highlight critical points that the parents need to pay attention to when they are newly home with their baby. Foremost among these concerns is seeing to it that the baby feeds often and effectively.

Early discharge does not appear to negatively affect breastfeeding; in fact some studies indicate that mothers who leave the hospital early breastfeed longer (Edmonson, Stoddard, & Owen, 1997; Margolis & Schwartz, 2000). At the same time, early discharge may negatively influence the mother's feeling of competence in her mothering, particularly if she is unprepared or unsure of how to care for her newborn. Contact with mother-to-mother organizations can help the mother to place her experiences in the context of other women's comments about their breastfeeding course. In addition, more home health visits are being done to provide the care that used to be provided in longer-term hospitalization. Pediatricians and other physicians, cognizant of the postdischarge void in medical coverage, are routinely scheduling appointments with the family of a breastfed baby within 48 to 72 hours after discharge as recommended by the American Academy of Pediatrics.

The goal of discharge planning is twofold: to prevent common problems and to provide emotional support (Page-Goertz, 1989). With such a brief time in the hospital, the mother needs a caregiver who imparts as much basic information as

| TABLE 7–6 | Modifiable Perinatal Variables Predicting That a Mother Will Stop Breastfeeding by 7 to 10 Days Postpartum | |

Perinatal Events	P Value	Odds Ratio
Long breastfeeding intervals	0.0001	1.1–1.3
More than 2 bottles	0.001	1.7–4.8
Vacuum vaginal delivery	0.0017	1.7–9.3
Long duration of Pitocin	0.0492	1.00–1.11

Source: Adapted from Hall et al., 2002.

possible without overwhelming her. She also needs reinforcement of her self-confidence in her role as a new mother. These two goals are mutually reinforcing and, as the caregiver instructs the mother in the prevention of problems, she is in a position to simultaneously enhance the new mother's self-esteem and self-confidence; in short, the mother is able to "take control" of her experience (Hall & Carty, 1993). The mother's perceptions of her infant not only reflect how she and the baby will interact but can also influence how long she breastfeeds.

Weight Loss

Infants are routinely weighed before discharge to home. Exclusively breastfed neonates lose more weight than those completely or partially formula fed according to a study of 773 Canadian infants (Box 7–6) (Martens & Romphf, 2007).

If the parents are not aware that neonatal weight loss is normal in the first few days of life, they should be reassured that their baby will begin to gain weight in a few days. Review the following basic feeding techniques before the parents return home.

Basic Feeding Techniques

In teaching basic feeding techniques to a new mother, priority must be given to certain guidelines:

- Feed the baby frequently (8 or more feedings in a 24-hour period). Using a visual aid such as the size of the baby's fist to demonstrate the

size of the newborn's stomach is an excellent way to illustrate why the neonate needs frequent feedings: his stomach is simply too small to hold large quantities at a time! Additionally, the curds formed by human milk digest quickly. Artificial baby milk forms large curds that take longer to digest than human milk. The formula-fed infant feeds fewer times.

- Offer (and keep the baby on) the first breast until he has completed that side. If he wants more, offer the second breast for as long as the baby wants. Some babies will be satiated with one breast; others prefer two, and still others may have some early marathon feedings in which they move from one to the other several times!

- Avoid watching the clock. The best timer of the feeding is the baby. After breastfeeding is established, the mother may identify cues that the baby is happy with one breast at each feeding or wants both breasts at each feeding.

- Avoid the use of artificial teats, pacifiers (dummies), supplemental infant formula, water, or glucose water feeds for the first 2 to 4 weeks. The infant may substitute nonnutritive suckling for milk intake at the breast, resulting in poor weight gain. The pacifier can also become a source of nipple confusion (Powers & Slusser, 1997) and a possible marker for other difficulties that can result in shorter breastfeeding duration. Telling the mother why pacifiers can interfere with early, effective breastfeeding will give her the ammunition she may need to fend

---

BOX 7–6

Percentage of Infant Weight Loss at Hospital Discharge According to Type of Feeding

Exclusively breastfed	5.49	Completely formula-fed	2.43
Partially breastfed	5.52		

Source: Martens & Romphf, 2007.

off well-meaning but uninformed attempts to "assist" her with unnecessary, potentially interfering practices. The exception is preterm infants, who may benefit from nonnutritive suckling during the period that they are unable to take oral feedings (see Chapter 13).

- Identify various ways in which the mother can recognize that her infant is getting sufficient milk. These include the following:
  - Listening for and identifying the infant's swallows
  - Baby waking on his own for at least 8 feedings in 24 hours
  - Monitoring the diaper output

Signs That Intervention Is Needed

Slow infant weight gain is addressed in depth in Chapter 10. Briefly, the following signs indicate a need for healthcare intervention:

- Scant, concentrated urine, brick dust urine (from urate crystals) after day 2, or no urine at all
- Infrequent stools (fewer than four per day after day 3)
- Stools that have not turned yellow by day 5 or 6
- Lethargy (difficult or impossible to waken for feedings)
- Extreme fretfulness (never contented after any feeding)
- No swallowing is felt or heard during feedings; when a feeding is evaluated, the clinician does not observe an "open-pause-close" pattern of suckling (Newman, 1996)
- The mother is experiencing nipple soreness that is more intense if it existed earlier, or that suddenly develops if it was previously absent.
- The mother's breasts are clinically engorged and very painful, making it difficult or impossible for the baby to breastfeed.
- The baby is not latching onto the breast.
- The baby is not waking on his own to feed at least 8 times in 24 hours.

Discharge

At discharge, the parents need clear, simply written materials that provide step-by-step information and are individualized as much as possible. Materials with drawings or photographs of positioning and other techniques are helpful. The hospital caregiver should establish a definite plan for follow-up: making a phone call to the mother at a specific time postdischarge or providing her with the phone numbers of the hospital "warm line" and of lactation consultants or La Leche League leaders in the area. If the baby has breastfeeding problems, a referral to an LC prior to her discharge from the hospital is appropriate. Home health, nurse casemanager, or follow-ups at a breastfeeding clinic are other options.

Discharge packs (i.e., marketing packs) containing formula should be discouraged for the breastfeeding mother. It is logical that such a practice can undermine the mother's confidence and plant doubt about her ability to breastfeed, especially for the immigrant mother (see Chapter 24). Yet results of studies on the effects of discharge packs on breastfeeding duration are contradictory (Chezem et al., 1998; Howard & Howard, 1997; Janson & Rydberg, 1998; Rosenberg et al., 2008).

To settle the question, Snowden, Renfrew, and Woolridge (2000) conducted a systematic review of nine randomized controlled trials involving 3730 North American women. The meta-analysis showed that when comparing marketing discharge packs with any of the controls (no intervention, nonmarketing pack, and combinations of these), exclusive breastfeeding was reduced at all time points in the presence of commercial hospital discharge packs but mixed feeding (nonexclusive breastfeeding) was not affected. Discharge packs may not exert as large an influence on breastfeeding duration as some other determinants, but many of the other more powerful influences such as education, race, income, marital status, or return to work are not as readily amenable to change (Howard & Howard, 1997).

The intent of health maintenance organizations (HMO) and insurers in encouraging early postpartum discharge is corporate profits since earlier discharge means greater profit. With about 4 million births annually (United States) and maternity beds averaging $1000 per day, insurers save $4 billion annually for every day they shorten the hospital stay.

Early discharge does not appear to result in earlier weaning if postpartum follow-up is integrated into care (Quinn, Koepsell, & Haller, 1997). Several studies (Lee et al., 1995; Pascale et al., 1996; Soskolne et al., 1996) link early postpartum discharge with increased hospital readmission for both jaundice and dehydration when the breastfeeding mother and baby are not followed up. Others failed to demonstrate negative effects (Edmonson, Stoddard, & Owens, 1997).

In many countries other than the United States, midwives and home health visitors routinely visit new mothers. The optimal time for a follow-up visit or telephone call is no later than 2 to 4 days after discharge from the hospital. This is an especially crucial period because enough time has passed to make an accurate evaluation of the mother's milk supply and the infant's intake. Just as hospitals are becoming baby friendly, healthcare providers in the pediatric office or outpatient clinic should strive to be breastfeeding friendly by assisting breastfeeding mothers and babies after discharge.

S u m m a r y

Consumer advocacy, the expectations of parents, childbirth and breastfeeding education, early hospital discharge, frequent cesarean births, and new technologies all affect birthing and early breastfeeding. No longer do we view the mother and her infant as separate entities; rather we care for them as a natural, single unit. Many hospitals now boast a family-centered birthing unit or labor-delivery room providing postpartum care where the mother and infant are cared for together in one room. Birthing rooms today look much like a bedroom with a comfortable reclining chair for the mother's support person; hookups for medical equipment are concealed behind wall prints and other decorations. A major benefit of this kind of mother–baby care is that families receive more comprehensive, coordinated care, which facilitates breastfeeding.

At the same time that we are seeing improvements in mother–baby care, the use of medical interventions, particularly epidural analgesia, has skyrocketed. Two opposing forces appear to be battling each other for control of childbirth: on one side, childbirth education, midwifery, doula services, and free-standing birthing centers; on the other, hospitals with routine epidural injections, high rates of cesarean births, and other technologies that medicalize the intrapartum experience.

Too few mothers learn enough about breastfeeding in the hospital before being asked to assume full responsibility for themselves and their babies. Only sporadically are they informed of the red flags that indicate that they should seek expert help and when to do so. Thus what should be a natural function is perceived as complicated. New mothers need reassurance that they can enjoy an uncomplicated breastfeeding experience and that common concerns can be easily managed.

As public awareness grows that breastfeeding sustains the baby's health and government and insurance companies become more aware of cost savings, breastfeeding will be promoted as the feeding of choice. Insurance companies will provide household help and visiting nurses to assess breastfeeding mothers and infants, in addition to giving substantial rebates to mothers who breastfeed. Breastfeeding will be not only socially acceptable but socially responsible.

K e y   C o n c e p t s

- The best preparation for breastfeeding is to learn as much as possible about mothering before the birth of the baby and find a support system.
- Nipple rolling, "toughening," and other forms of nipple preparation during pregnancy are not necessary and should be avoided.
- Neonates are initially alert for about 2 hours after birth, followed by deep sleep until 20 hours, and then increased wakefulness and interest in frequent breastfeeding.
- If there are no complications, the first breastfeeding should take place during the first hour after the infant's birth. After the infant has been dried, the infant can be placed on the mother's body to breastfeed skin-to-skin.
- Privacy, comfortable positioning, and optimal latch-on are all basic skills necessary

to assist mothers and neonates in early breastfeeding.

- Techniques for latch-on and positioning vary according to the practitioner. "Correct" positioning is, as yet, not evidence based.

- When a baby is not latching onto the breast, it is important to encourage skin-to-skin holding, feed the baby, establish the mother's milk supply, and find hands-on help to correct the situation and encourage skin-to-skin holding.

- If cup-feeding is done carefully, it has been found to be as safe as bottle-feeding. However, infants who are cup-fed spill more milk than infants who are bottle-fed. Babies who are poor candidates for cup-feedings are those with a poor gag reflex, neurological deficits, and respiratory problems.

- During the first 2 days infants who are breastfed and infants who are cup-fed ingest less milk than infants who are bottle-fed.

- New parents should watch the baby, not the clock, to determine when the baby is ready to feed. Feed the baby at the *earliest* sign of hunger. Crying is a *late* sign of hunger.

- Late-preterm infants (born between 34 and 38 weeks) need special help and careful, frequent follow-up, as these babies tend to breastfeed poorly at first.

- Short-term use of a silicone nipple shield in certain situations (nipple inversion, low birth weight infants) can preserve the breastfeeding relationship while the baby learns to feed.

- Generally accepted guidelines for hypoglycemia in full-term infants is serum glucose concentration of less than 30 mg/dL in the first day after birth or less than 40 mg/dL after the second day. Invasive procedures for determining glucose levels can be avoided by early skin-to-skin contact between mother and baby, frequent breastfeeding, and close clinical observation.

- Generally speaking, women who deliver by cesarean birth breastfeed as frequently and for as long as those who have vaginal births. Special concerns related to breastfeeding are pain control, comfortable positioning, and early initiation of breastfeeding.

- Normal breast engorgement starts at 3 to 5 days after birth and then slowly recedes over the first 2 weeks. During normal engorgement the mother's breast tissue usually remains compressible, thus enabling the infant to suckle comfortably and efficiently. Early and frequent breastfeeding is thought to prevent severe engorgement.

- A meta-analysis of eight randomized control trials on treatments for breast engorgement concluded that only pharmacological treatment using anti-inflammatory medications significantly improved symptoms of engorgement.

- The full-term infant is born with additional extracellular fluid that sustains him for a short time. Urine output usually exceeds fluid intake for the first 3–4 days after birth.

- Excessive intravenous fluids during labor can lead to postpartum breast edema. The technique of areolar compression can help reshape the breast and nipple area so that the neonate is able to latch on to the breast.

- Hand expression is a time-honored skill that costs nothing, is easy to learn, and is always available.

- Early discharge does not appear to affect breastfeeding if there is postpartum care and support. If follow-up care is not provided, costly readmissions to the hospital result. The goal of discharge planning is to prevent common problems and to provide emotional support. With such a brief time in the hospital, the mother needs a caregiver who imparts as much basic information as possible without overwhelming her and is able to answer her questions with research-based information.

- At hospital discharge 2–3 days postpartum, the average weight loss of exclusively breastfed neonates is about twice that of those formula-fed.

- Basic and priority discharge teaching includes teaching the mother her baby's feeding cues, how to latch her baby onto the breast, how to know the baby is getting enough milk, and who to call for help with breastfeeding.

- Marketing or discharge packs reduce the length of exclusive breastfeeding; however, they do not exert as large an influence on breastfeeding duration as some other determinants.

Internet Resources

Academy of Breastfeeding Medicine. Clinical protocols for hypoglycemia
http://www.bfmed.org
Meta-analysis research on clinical aspects of breastfeeding:

http://www.breastfeedingonline.comwww.update-software.com/Cochrane/default.htm
Video of newborn crawling to mother's breast
http://www.breastcrawl.org

References

Alkalay AL et al. Population meta-analysis of low plasma glucose thresholds in full-term normal newborns. *Am J Perinatol.* 2006;23:115–119.

Anderson GC et al. Development of sucking in term infants from birth to four hours postbirth. *Res Nurs Health.* 1982;5(1):21–27.

Anderson GC. Risk in mother-infant separation postbirth. *Image: J Nurs Schol.* 1989;21(4):196–199.

Anderson GC et al. Skin-to-skin care for breastfeeding difficulties postbirth. In: Field T, ed. *Touch and Massage in Early Child Development.* New Brunswick, NJ: Johnson & Johnson; 2004:116–136.

Belin Y et al. Effect of labor epidural analgesia with and without fentanyl on infant breast-feeding: a prospective, randomized, double-blind study. *Anesthesiology.* 2005;103(6):1211–1217.

Bergman NJ, Linley LL, Fawcus SR. Randomized controlled trial of skin-to-skin contact from birth versus conventional incubator for physiological stabilization in 1200- to 2199-gram newborns. *Acta Paediatr.* 2004;93:79–85.

Brand PLP et al. Neurodevelopmental outcome of hypoglycemia in healthy, large for gestational age, term newborns. *Arch Dis Child.* 2005;90:78–81.

Campbell D, Scott KD, Klaus MH, et al. Female relatives or friends trained as labor doulas: outcomes at 6 to 8 weeks postpartum. *Birth.* 2006;34(3):220–227.

Chang ZM, Heaman MI. Epidural analgesia during labor and delivery: effects on the initiation and continuation of effective breastfeeding. *J Hum Lact.* 2005;21:305–309.

Chapman DJ, Young S, Ferris AM, Perez-Escamilla R. Impact of breast pumping on lactogenesis stage II after Cesarean delivery: a randomized clinical trial. *Pediatrics.* 2001;107(6):E94.

Chen DC, Nommsen-Rivers L, Dewey KG, Lonnerdal B. Stress during labor and delivery and early lactation performance. *Am J Clin Nutr.* 1998;68(2):334–344.

Chezem J et al. Lactation duration: influences of human milk replacements and formula samples of women planning postpartum employment. *JOGN Nurs.* 1998;27(6):646–651.

Christensson K et al. Randomised study of skin-to-skin versus incubator care for rewarming low-risk hypothermic neonates. *Lancet.* 1998;352(9134):1115.

Clemmit S. Nipple shield perspective. *New Beginnings.* 2003;20(2):58–59.

Cornblath M et al. Controversies regarding definition of neonatal hypoglycemia: suggested operational thresholds. *Pediatrics.* 2000;105(5):1141–1145.

Cotterman KJ. Too swollen to latch on? Try reverse pressure softening first. La Leche League. *Leaven.* 2003;39(2):38–40.

Cotterman K. Reverse pressure softening: a simple tool for easier latching during engorgement. *J Hum Lact.* 2004;20(2):227–237.

Cregan M, Hartmann PE. Computerized breast measurement from conception to weaning: clinical implications. *J Hum Lact.* 1999;15(2):89–96.

Crowell MK, Hill PD, Humenick SS. Relationship between obstetric analgesia and time of effective breastfeeding. *J Nurse Midwifery.* 1994;39(3):150–156.

Davis HV, Sears RR, Miller HC, Brodbeck AJ. Effects of cup, bottle and breastfeeding on oral activities of newborn infants. *Pediatrics.* 1948;2:549–558.

de Carvalho M et al. Milk intake and frequency of feeding in breastfed infants. *Early Hum Dev.* 1982;7(2):155–163.

Dewey LA et al. Risk factors for suboptimal infant breastfeeding behavior, delayed onset of lactation, and excess neonatal weight loss. *Pediatrics.* 2003;112:607–619.

Dowling DA et al. Cup-feeding for preterm infants: mechanics and safety. *J Hum Lact.* 2002;18(1):13–20.

Edmonson MB, Stoddard JJ, Owen LM. Hospital readmission with feeding-related problems after early postpartum discharge of normal newborns. *JAMA.* 1997;278(4):299–303.

Eidelman A. Hypoglycemia and the breastfed neonate. *Pediatr Clin No Amer.* 2001;48(2):377–387.

Ekström A, Widström AM, Nissen E. Duration of breastfeeding in Swedish primiparous and multiparous women. *J Hum Lact.* 2003;19(2):172–178.

Evans KC et al. Effect of caesarean section on breast milk transfer to the normal term newborn over the first week of life. *Arch Dis Child Fetal Neonatal Ed.* 2003;88(5):F380–F382.

Fransson AL, Karlsson H, Nilsson K. Temperature variation in newborn babies: importance of physical contact with the mother. *Arch Dis Child Neonatal Ed.* 2005;90:500–504.

Freeden RC. Cup-feeding of newborn infants. *Pediatrics*. 1948;2:544–548.

Freer Y. A comparison of breast and cup-feeding in preterm infants: effect on physiological parameters. *J Neonatal Nurs*. 1999;5:15–21.

Glover J. Supplementation of breastfeeding newborns: a flowchart for decision-making. *J Hum Lact*. 1995; 11:127–131.

Grajeda R, Perez-Escamilla R. Stress during labor and delivery is associated with delayed onset of lactation among urban Guatemalan women. *J Nutr*. 2002; 132(10):3055–3060.

Gupta A, Khanna K, Chattree S. Cup-feeding: an alternative to bottle feeding in a neonatal intensive unit. *J Trop Pediatrics*. 1999;45(2):108–110.

Hale TW. *Medications and Mothers' Milk*. 11th ed. Amarillo, TX: Pharmasoft Publishing; 2004:411.

Hall RT et al. A breastfeeding assessment score to evaluate the risk for cessation of breastfeeding by 7 to 10 days of age. *J Pediatr*. 2002;141(5):659–664.

Hall WA, Carty EM. Managing the early discharge experience: taking control. *J Adv Nurs*. 1993;18(4):574–582.

Haninger NC, Farley CL. Screening for hypoglycemia in healthy term neonates: effects on breastfeeding. *J Midwifery Women's Health*. 2001;46(5):292–301.

Hawdon JM, Ward-Platt MP, Aynsley-Green A. Patterns of metabolic adaptation for preterm and term infants in the first neonatal week. *Arch Dis Child*. 1992; 67(4 spec no):357–365.

Hazelbaker AK. In defense of finger-feeding. *Medela Rental Round-up*. 1997;14(2):10–11.

Hedberg-Nyqvist K. A cup feeding protocol for neonates: evaluation of nurses' and parents' use of two cups. *J Neonatal Nurs*. 1999;5:31–35.

Heck LJ, Erenberg A. Serum glucose levels in term neonates during the first 48 hours of life. *J Pediatr*. 1987;110(1):119–122.

Hedderwick SA et al. Pathogenic organisms associated with artificial fingernails worn by healthcare workers. *Infect Control Hosp Epidemiol*. 2000;21(8):505–509.

Henderson A, Stamp G, Pincombe J. Postpartum positioning and attachment education for increasing breastfeeding: a randomized trial. *Birth*. 2001;28(4):236–242.

Hoffmann JB. A suggested treatment for inverted nipples. *Am J Obstet Gynecol*. 1953;66:346.

Ho HT, Yeung WK, Young BW. Evaluation of "point of care" devices in the measurement of low blood glucose in neonatal practice. *Arch Dis Child Fetal Neonatal Ed*. 2004;89(4):F356–F359.

Howard C, Howard F. Discharge packs: how much do they matter? *Birth*. 1997;24(2):98–101.

Howard C et al. Randomized clinical trial of pacifier use and bottle-feeding or cupfeeding and their effect on breastfeeding. *Pediatrics*. 2003;111:511–518.

Humenick SS, Hill PD, Anderson MA. Breast engorgement: patterns and selected outcomes. *J Hum Lact*. 1994;10(2):87–93.

Janke JR. Breastfeeding duration following Cesarean and vaginal births. *J Nurs Midwifery*. 1988;33(4):159–164.

Janson S, Rydberg B. Early postpartum discharge and subsequent breastfeeding. *Birth*. 1998;25(4):222–225.

Johanson RB et al. Effect of post-delivery care on neonatal body temperature. *Acta Paediatr*. 1992; 81(11):859–862.

Johnston CC et al. Skin-to-skin (kangaroo) care is effective in diminishing pain response in preterm neonates. *Arch Pediatr Adolesc*. 2003;157:1084–1088.

Jordan S et al. The impact of intrapartum analgesia on infant feeding. *BJOG*. 2005;112(7):927–934.

Karlstrom A et al. Postoperative pain after cesarean birth affects breastfeeding and infant care. *JOGNN*. 2007;36:430–440.

Kesaree N et al. Treatment of inverted nipples using a disposable syringe. *J Hum Lact*. 1993;9(1):27–29.

Kitajima H. Prevention of methicillin-resistant *Staphylococcus aureus* infection in neonates. *Pediatrics International*. 2003;45:238–245.

Kroeger M, Smith L. *Impact of Birthing Practices on Breastfeeding: Protecting the Mother and Baby Continuum*. Sudbury, MA: Jones and Bartlett; 2004.

Lang S, Lawrence CJ, Orme RL. Cup-feeding: an alternative method of infant feeding. *Arch Dis Child*. 1994;71(4):365–369.

Lawson T, Tulloch MI. Breastfeeding duration: prenatal intentions and postnatal practices. *J Adv Nurs*. 1995; 22(5):841–849.

Lee KS et al. Association between duration of neonatal hospital stay and readmission rate. *J Pediatr*. 1995;127(5):758–766.

Leung GM, Lam TH, Ho LM. Breast-feeding and its relation to smoking and mode of delivery. *Obstet Gynecol*. 2002;99(5 pt 1):785–794.

Lieberman E et al. Epidural analgesia, intrapartum fever, and neonatal sepsis evaluation. *Pediatrics*. 1997;99(3):415–419.

Lothian JA. It takes two to breastfeed: the baby's role in successful breastfeeding. *J Nurs Midwifery*. 1995;40(4):328–334.

Ludington-Hoe S et al. Breast and infant temperatures with twins during shared skin-to-skin (kangaroo) care. *JOGNN*. 2006;35:223–231.

MAIN Collaborative Group Preparing for Breast Feeding. Treatment of inverted and nonprotractile nipples in pregnancy. *Midwife*. 1994;10:200–214.

Malhotra N et al. A controlled trial of alternative methods of oral feeding in neonates. *Early Hum Develop*. 1999;54(1):29–38.

Margolis L, Schwartz JB. The relationship between the timing of maternal postpartum hospital discharge and breastfeeding. *J Hum Lact*. 2000;16(2):121–128.

Marinelli K, Burke GS, Dodd VL. A comparison of the safety of cupfeedings and bottlefeedings in premature infants whose mothers intend to breastfeed. *J Perinatol.* 2001;21(6):350–355.

Marlier L, Schaal B. Human newborns prefer human milk: conspecific milk odor is attractive without postnatal exposure. *Child Develop.* 2005;76(1):155–168.

Marmet C, Shell E. Therapeutic positioning for breastfeeding. In: Genna CW, ed. *Supporting Sucking Skills in Breastfeeding Infants.* Sudbury, MA: Jones and Bartlett; 2007.

Martens P, Romphf L. Factors associated with newborn in-hospital weight loss: comparisons by feeding method, demographics, and birthing procedures. *J Hum Lact.* 2007;23(2):233–241.

McMillan JA et al. *Oski's Pediatrics.* Philadelphia, PA: Lippincott Williams & Wilkins; 1999.

Meier P et al. Nipple shields for preterm infants: effect on milk transfer and duration of breastfeeding. *J Hum Lact.* 2000;16(2):106–114.

Meyer K, Anderson GC. Using skin-to-skin (kangaroo) care in a clinical setting with full-term infants having breastfeeding difficulties. *MCN.* 1999;24(4):190–192.

Miller V, Riordan J. Treating postpartum breast edema with areolar compression. *J Hum Lact.* 2004;20(2):223–226.

Milligan RA, Flenniken PM, Pugh LC. Positioning intervention to minimize fatigue in breastfeeding women. *Appl Nurs Res.* 1996;9(2):67–70.

Mizuno K, Kani K. Sipping/lapping is a safe alternative feeding method for preterm infants. *Acta Paediatrica.* 2005;94:574–580.

Moon JL, Humenick SS. Breast engorgement: contributing variables and variables amenable to nursing intervention. *JOGN Nurs.* 1989;18(4):309–315.

Moore AM, Perlman M. Symptomatic hypoglycemia in otherwise healthy, breastfed, term newborns. *Pediatr.* 1999;103(4 Pt 1):837–839.

Mulford C. Subtle signs and symptoms of the milk ejection reflex. *J Hum Lact.* 1990;6(4):177–178.

Montgomery A, Hale TH, Academy of Breastfeeding Medicine. ABM clinical protocol #15. *Breastfeeding Medicine.* 2006;1(4):271–277.

National Institute of Child Health and Human Development Workshop (NICHD). Optimizing care and long-term outcome of near-term pregnancy and near-term newborn infant. Workshop held July 18–19, Bethesda, MD, 2005.

Newman J. Decision tree and postpartum management for preventing dehydration in the "breastfed" baby. *J Hum Lact.* 1996;12(2):129–135.

Newman J, Pitman T. *The Latch.* Amarillo, TX: Hale Publishing; 2006:28.

Nicholson WL. The use of nipple shields by breastfeeding women. *Aust Coll Midwives J.* 1993;6(2):18–24.

Page-Goertz S. Discharge planning for the breastfeeding dyad. *Pediatr Nurs.* 1989;15(5):543–544.

Pascale JA et al. Breastfeeding, dehydration, and shorter maternity stays. *Neonatal Network.* 1996;15(7):37–41.

Powers NG, Slusser W. Breastfeeding update 2: clinical lactation management. *Pediatr Rev.* 1997;18(5):147–161.

Quinn A, Koepsell D, Haller S. Breastfeeding incidence after early discharge and factors influencing breastfeeding cessation. *JOGN Nurs.* 1997;26(3):289–294.

Raimbault C, Saliba E, Porter RH. The effect of the odour of mother's milk on breastfeeding behaviours of premature neonates. *Acta Paediatr.* 2007;96:368–371.

Ransjo-Arvidson AB et al. Maternal analgesia during labor disturbs newborn behavior: effects on breastfeeding, temperature and crying. *Birth.* 2001;28(1):5–11.

Righard L. How do newborns find their mother's breast? *Birth.* 1995;22(3):174–175.

Righard L, Alade MO. Effect of delivery room routines on success of first breastfeed. *Lancet.* 1990;336(8723):1105–1107.

Riordan J, Gill-Hopple K. Testing relationships of breastmilk indicators with actual breastmilk intake. Presented at: National Institute of Nursing Research, State of the Science Nursing Congress; Washington, DC, September 26, 2002.

Riordan J, Gill-Hopple K, Angeron J. Indicators of effective breastfeeding and estimates of breast milk intake. *J Hum Lact.* 2005;21(4):406–412.

Riordan J, Koehn M. Reliability and validity testing of three breastfeeding assessment tools. *JOGN Nurs.* 1997;26(2):181–187.

Riordan J et al. The effect of labor pain relief medication on neonatal suckling and breastfeeding duration. *J Hum Lact.* 2000;16(1):7–12.

Roberts KL, Reiter M, Schuster D. A comparison of chilled and room temperature cabbage leaves in treating breast engorgement. *J Hum Lact.* 1995;11(3):191–194.

Rosenberg KD et al. Infant formula marketing through hospital: the impact of commercial hospital discharge packs on breastfeeding. *Am J Public Health.* 2008;98:1–6.

Rosier W. Cool cabbage compresses. *Breastfeed Rev.* 1988;12(1):28–31.

Rowe-Murray HJ, Fisher JR. Baby friendly hospital practices: cesarean section is a persistent barrier to early initiation of breastfeeding. *Birth.* 2002;29(2):124–131.

Sadeh A, Dark I, Vohr B. Newborns' sleep-wake patterns: the role of maternal, delivery, and infant factors. *Early Hum Develop.* 1996;44:113–126.

Seaton S, Reeves M, McLean S. Oxycodone as a component of multimodal analgesia for lactating mothers after Caesarean section: relationships between maternal plasma, breastmilk and neonatal plasma levels. *Aust NZJ Obtstet Gynaecol.* 2007;47:181–185.

Sepkoski CM et al. The effects of maternal epidural anesthesia on neonatal behavior during the first month. *Dev Med Child Neurol.* 1992;34(12): 1072–1080.

Sexson WR. Incidence of neonatal hypoglycemia: a matter of definition. *J Pediatr.* 1984;105(1):149–150.

Simpson KR, Creehan PA. *Perinatal Nursing.* 3rd ed. Philadelphia: Lippincott Williams & Wilkins, AWHONN; 2008:636.

Snowden HM, Renfrew MJ, Woolridge MW. Commercial hospital discharge packs for breastfeeding women (Cochrane Review). In: *The Cochrane Library.* Oxford: *Update Software,* Issue 2, 2000.

Snowden HM, Renfrew MJ, Woolridge MW. Treatments for breast engorgement during lactation (Cochrane Review). In: The Cochrane Library. Oxford: *Update Software.* Issue 3, 2002.

Soppas P. Personal Communication. June 2003.

Soskolne EI et al. The effect of early discharge and other factors on readmission rates of newborns. *Arch Pediatr Adolesc Med.* 1996;150(4):373–379.

Srinivasan G et al. Plasma glucose values in normal neonates: a new look. *J Pediatr.* 1986;109(1):114–117.

Thorley V. Cup-feeding: problems caused by incorrect use. *J Hum Lact.* 1997;13(1):54–55.

Trainor C. Valuing labor support. *AWHONN Lifelines.* 2002;6:387–389.

Torvaldsen S et al. Intrapartum epidural analgesia and breastfeeding: a prospective cohort study. *Inter Breastfeed J.* 2006;1:24.

Tully MR. Breastfeeding the 34 to 38 week infant: a challenge for the health team. International Lactation Consultant Annual Meeting. Boca Raton, Florida, July 27, 2002.

Vaidya K, Sharma A, Dhungel S. Effect of early mother-baby close contact over the duration of exclusive breastfeeding. *Nepal Med Coll J.* 2005;7(2):138–140.

Varendi H, Porter RH, Winberg I. Attractiveness of amniotic fluid odor: evidence of prenatal olfactory learning? *Acta Pediatr.* 1996;85(10):1223–1227.

Viscomi CM. Maternal fever, neonatal sepsis evaluation and epidural labor analgesia. *Reg Anesth Pain Med.* 2000;25(5):549–553.

Walters MW et al. Kangaroo care at birth of full term infants: A pilot study. *Amer J Maternal Child Nurs.* 2007;32:375–381.

Waltman PA et al. Building evidence for practice: a pilot study of newborn bulb suctioning at birth. *J Midwifery Womens Health.* 2004;49:32–38.

Widström AM, Thingström-Paulsson J. The position of the tongue during rooting reflexes elicited in newborn infant before the first suckle. *Acta Paediatr.* 1993;82:281–283.

Widström AM et al. Gastric suction in healthy newborn infants: effects on circulation and developing feeding behaviors. *Acta Paediatr Scand.* 1987;76(4):566–572.

Widström AM et al. Short-term effects of early suckling and touch of the nipple on maternal behavior. *Early Hum Develop.* 1990;21(3):153–163.

Wiessinger D. A breastfeeding teaching tool using a sandwich analogy for latch-on. *J Hum Lact.* 1998;14(1):51–56.

Wight N. Breastfeeding the borderline (near-term) preterm infant. *Pediatric Annals.* 2003;32(5):329–337.

Wight N. Hypoglycemia in breastfed neonates. *Breastfeed Med.* 2006;1:253–262.

Wight N, Marinelli KA, Academy of Breastfeeding Protocol Committee. ABM clinical protocol #1. Guidelines for glucose monitoring treatment of hypoglycemia in breastfed neonates. *Breastfeed Med.* 2006;1:178–184.

Williams J, Mueller S. A message to the nurse from the baby. *J Hum Lact.* 1989;5(1):19.

Wilson-Clay B. Clinical use of silicone nipple shields. *J Hum Lact.* 1996;12(4):279–285.

Wilson-Clay B. Nipple shields in clinical practice: a review [editorial]. *Breastfeed Abstracts.* 2003;22(2): 11–12.

Wilson-Clay B, Hoover K. *The Breastfeeding Atlas.* Austin, TX: LactNews Press; 2005.

Winslow EH, Jacobson AF. Can a fashion statement harm the patient? Long and artificial nails may cause nosocomial infections. *Am J Nurs.* 2000;100(9):63–65.

Woolridge MW, Ingram JC, Baum JD. Do changes in pattern of breast usage alter the baby's nutrient intake? *Lancet.* 1990;336(8712):395–397.

World Alliance for Breastfeeding Action (WABA). Breastfeeding: the 1st hour. Malaysia: Penang; 2007. http://www.WABA.org/my. Accessed August 11, 2007.

Wright A, Rice S, Wells S. Changing hospital practices to increase the duration of breastfeeding. *Pediatrics.* 1996;97(5):669–675.

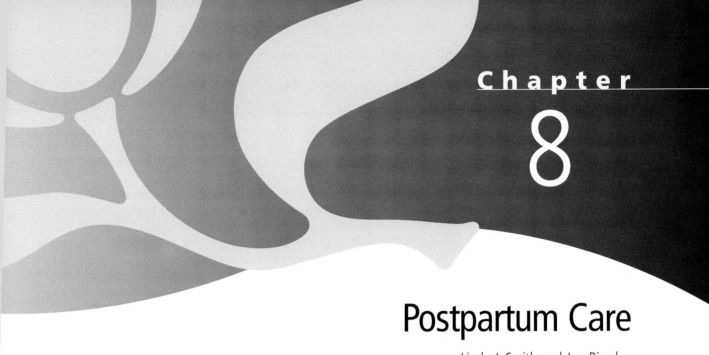

Chapter

8

Postpartum Care

Linda J. Smith and Jan Riordan

THIS CHAPTER FOLLOWS the mother–infant dyad after birth in the early postpartum period and will first address normal behavior and physiology and then cover common problems during the "fourth trimester" for the mother, the baby, and the family.

In a 2006 US nationwide survey, 61 percent of mothers intended to exclusively breastfeed, yet only 51 percent were exclusively breastfeeding at 1 week postpartum. One third of those surveyed reported that the hospital staff was neutral or negative about breastfeeding; 66 percent received formula samples, 44 percent of babies received a pacifier, and 37 percent were supplemented with formula. Sixty-two percent of mothers reported that they were exhausted, and 59 percent experienced breast or nipple pain (Declercq et al., 2006). If this is our report card for supporting and promoting breastfeeding in the postpartum period, we have considerable room for grade improvement.

Concerns about adequate milk supply and nipple pain are the top reasons that mothers stop breastfeeding early. Parents are also concerned about engorgement, leaking, jaundice, use of pacifiers, and

cosleeping with their baby during the first few weeks postpartum.

Immediate Postbirth Events

Normally, the mother–baby dyad have skin-to-skin contact immediately after birth. The baby is dried, both are kept warm, and the baby is immediately supported in skin-to-skin contact with mother's chest or abdomen. Within 5–70 minutes (Righard & Alade, 1990; Bullough, Msuku, & Karonde, 1989), the baby is able to use his inborn capabilities to crawl, wiggle, or scoot his way to one breast or the other, latch on comfortably, and receive a bolus of colostrum due to the powerful oxytocin responses following birth (Uvnas-Moberg et al.,1990). Simultaneously, mother and baby's central nervous systems are flooded with pleasurable, familiar experiences including smell, hearing, touch, and warmth. The mother's body is the baby's natural habitat, which provides all basic biological needs and determines behavior. The newborn both initiates and maintains breastfeeding; the mother responds with caring and maintains breastfeeding while continuing to transition into her new role as a mother.

First Weeks—Principles and Expectations

The early weeks of the mother–baby dyad's new relationship is characterized by symbiotic functions and rhythmicity. Sleeping rhythms of mother and baby are congruent when they are in close physical contact. Mothers need rest to recover physically and emotionally from even relatively uncomplicated births; babies need rest, food, and comfort to continue developing all body systems; both need nourishing food frequently to build tissue and strength; and both respond profoundly to multiple sensory messages of the other. Shared sleep is inextricably connected with and supportive of breastfeeding (McKenna, Mosko, & Richard, 1997), yet bed sharing or cosleeping has been the subject of much controversy and is addressed later in this chapter.

Feeding, Sleeping, and Behavior Patterns of the Neonate

After the first few weeks of life, the breastfed infant has a tendency for wakefulness with frequent feedings in the late afternoon and evening (Emde, Gaensbauer, & Harmon, 1976). These wakeful and sometimes fussy periods at the end of the day are often critical ones for the inexperienced breastfeeding mother who is unsure of her ability to breastfeed and unaware that wakefulness and frequent feeding at this time are normal. Lactation consultants (LCs) can expect that many of the distress calls from the mother during the second month after delivery stem from the mother's lack of knowledge of this common pattern.

The baby's gastric and metabolic functions closely parallel his circadian sleep cycle and the mother's lactation synthesis patterns. A baby's stomach empties of human milk in about 60–90 minutes. The capacity of a 1-week-old baby's stomach is about 30–35 ml (Zangen et al., 2001). The average volume of a single letdown reflex is about 35–40 ml (Ramsay et al., 2005). From days 2 through 6, babies have 5–10 daily breastfeeding sessions, with milk intake increasing rapidly to between 395 and 868 ml (Kent, 2007). By 1 month, babies take an average volume of 750–800 ml per day. (Kent et al., 2006). Given the baby's stomach capacity, the negative consequences of overfeeding (gastric distention, discomfort, vomiting/spitting, reflux), the rapid gastric emptying time of human milk, and the total daily calories needed for growth, we can expect that a baby will typically breastfeed many times per day.

Kent et al. (2006) published an analysis of 24-hour feeding patterns of healthy, exclusively breastfeeding babies age 1–6 months. Thirteen percent of the babies always took both breasts at a feed; 30 percent never took both breasts (i.e., they fed from only from one breast per feed); and most alternated between one and both breasts. Feeds ranged from 6 to 18 per day, and on average, the babies took 11 feeds per day, with between-feed intervals varying between 50 minutes to 6 hours. A large feed did not predict a long interval before the next feed; conversely, a small feed did not predict a short interval before the next meal. The time-tested concept of letting the baby "finish the first side first" was reinforced by this rigorous study. Expectations that reassure us that the baby is getting enough milk and is progressing normally are displayed in Table 8–1.

The newborn's rest–activity cycle is about 60–90 minutes (Ludington-Hoe et al., 2006). Breastfed babies sleep approximately 14 hours per day (less than previous recommendations for infant sleep), cycling with approximately 10 hours of wakefulness (Quillin & Glenn, 2004; Quillin, 1997). Mothers get more restful quiet sleep when breastfeeding exclusively (Doan et al., 2007) and safely bed sharing (Quillin & Glenn, 2004). For the infant, quiet sleep plays an important role in memory processing and neurodevelopment. The hormones released in both mother and baby's body enhance and facilitate bonding and calm, restorative sleep (Uvnas-Moberg & Eriksson, 1996). Therefore, *safe* bed-sharing facilitates breastfeeding, maternal rest and relaxation, and infant well-being.

Common Problems in the Early Days and Weeks

Preventing problems is always easier than fixing a problem later. Prenatal breastfeeding education (Dyson, McCormick, & Renfrew, 2005) and mother-friendly care during labor (Hodnett et al., 2007; Shealy et al., 2005) establish the foundation for a smooth postpartum course. Immediate and

TABLE 8–1 Reassuring Signs of Adequate Milk Intake and Normal Postpartum Progress in the First Week

Reassuring Signs	Rationale
Baby is skin to skin on mother's chest several times a day for at least 60–90 minutes or until self-wakening.	Skin-to-skin touch increases milk production; keeps baby close to mother's breast, and self-regulated sleep cycles support normal development.
Baby is in mother's arms most of the time, and sleeps calmly and safely within arm's reach (in proximity) when not being held.	Holding is comforting, increases oxytocin responses, which aid digestion and milk production and facilitate bonding and development.
Baby is alert ~ 10 hours a day, cues for feeds at least 8 or more times, and is obviously satiated after feeds.	An alert baby cues the mother to indicate that he is hungry and then that he is satisfied.
Baby rarely cries; mother responds quickly to early feeding cues before active crying begins.	Crying is a late sign of hunger, and raises stress hormones in both mother and baby.
Baby actively suckles at least 140 minutes per day, 5–16 times with audible swallowing; and releases the breast spontaneously.	At least that amount of time at breast is needed to obtain sufficient milk (de Carvalho, Robertson, Merkatz et al., 1982). Swallowing reflects milk intake (Riordan, Gill-Hopple, & Angeron, 2005).
After feeds, mother's nipple is comfortable, wet, and intact; breasts are softer after feeds than before; and both mother and baby are comfortable and possibly drowsy.	Nipple creasing, pain, damage, and/or milk stasis suggest poor milk transfer. Hormones foster relaxation and calmness in both.
Baby and mother are satisfied with feedings.	Mothers accurately report problems with feedings.
Baby's mucus membranes are wet and skin turgor is elastic and responsive. Gently pinched skin does not remain above the normal surface (tenting).	The absence of tenting after pinching indicates that infant is sufficiently hydrated.
By the end of the first week, baby passes five or more loose, yellow stools per day.	Frequent stool output is one indicator of adequate nutrient intake (Nommsen-Rivers, 2008).
By the end of the first week, six or more soaking wet diapers per day; urine is clear (not dark or concentrated).	Urine output is an indicator of adequate hydration after the first few days.
Mother reports that her milk "came in."	Mothers know their bodies.
Mother is confident in her ability to calm and feed her baby.	Confidence is an indicator of normal maternal role acquisition.

sustained skin-to-skin contact beginning moments after birth and for many hours every day is the most effective and evidence-based strategy to normalize mother–baby behavior; support normal lactogenesis; avoid breast and nipple pain; assure abundant milk production; assure adequate nutrition, hydration, and comfort for the newborn; and enhance the mother's confidence and ability to breastfeed and care for her baby (Anderson et al., 2003).

Baby Is Not Latching, Sucking or Feeding Effectively

A newborn's inability to latch and suck is intensely frustrating for the mother, health professionals, and especially the baby. Until recently, most professionals believed that "breast refusal" was primarily due to maternal factors, including flat or inverted nipples, overfull or engorged breasts, poor positioning, or "nipple confusion" resulting from the baby learning to suck on an artificial teat or pacifier. Certainly the mother's breast shape, size, and configuration play a role in the baby's ability to latch and feed comfortably. However, as knowledge and skills improve, lactation consultants have begun to look more closely at other events and conditions that can harm the infant's ability to latch on the breast and suckle.

Conditions that can lead to early latch and suck problems include:

- Immaturity or prematurity, illness, or birth injuries (Hughes et al., 1999)
- Facial or jaw asymmetry (Wall & Glass, 2006)
- Jaundice, and/or facial anomalies such as tongue-tie or cleft lip or palate (Genna, 2008).

Birth practices and medications administered to the mother during labor can be significant barriers to the infant's ability to latch and feed effectively:

- Epidural anesthesia or analgesia (Jordan et al., 2005; Riordan, Gill-Hopple, & Angeron, 2005; Beilin et al., 2005; Torvaldsen et al., 2006; Montgomery & Hale, 2006)
- Instrument delivery (Hall et al., 2002; Baumgarder et al., 2003)
- Long, difficult labor (Dewey et al., 2003; Smith, 2007)
- Cesarean surgery (Evans et al., 2003; Karlstrom et al., 2007)

If the baby cannot latch because of *prematurity, illness, or facial or oral structural anomalies,* collaboration with other professionals is necessary. While diagnosis and treatment plans are being developed, the lactation specialist should assist the mother to collect her milk frequently by hand-expression and/or pumping, and feed it to the baby using a carefully selected device. The lactation consultant's close monitoring of the baby's development of sucking abilities, the mother's milk production, and the mother's emotional status plays a central role in long-term breastfeeding (Genna, 2008).

If the baby is not latching because he is *"sleepy" or drugged from birth medications* (Ransjo-Arvidson et al., 2001), patience and sufficient calories (expressed colostrum or breastmilk) will buy time until the drugs are metabolized and the baby can smoothly coordinate sucking, swallowing, and breathing. Keep the mother and baby together, skin to skin, as close to continuously as possible. Be patient, because the age and maturity of the baby, dosage and combination of drugs, and other birth interventions can affect the baby's ability to recover and begin to breastfeed well. Some babies require several days to several weeks to recover fully.

If the baby *can only latch in one posture or position or on one breast*, help the mother to use that posture, position, or breast at frequent intervals. Express milk from the other breast to avoid problems related to milk stasis. With patience and sufficient calories, most babies will gradually improve in skill and be able to breastfeed in other postures, positions, and from both breasts within a fairly short time (Genna, 2008). Although research is scant, some professionals have reported that therapeutic modalities such as physical or occupational therapy (Wall & Glass, 2006), chiropractic treatment or cranial-sacral therapy, or osteopathic manipulative therapy (Fraval, 1998) may be helpful in resolving structural or postural asymmetries in collaboration with the baby's primary care provider.

If the baby cannot latch because of the *mother's breast or nipple size or structure*, then gentle mechanical strategies may alter the breast or nipple shape sufficiently to allow latching and sucking. These strategies include, but are not limited to, brief use of a breast pump or "nipple extender" device to draw out the nipple, massage to soften the breast, shaping the nipple and areola complex, breast support, and short-term use of a thin silicone nipple shield (Chertok, Schneider, & Blackburn, 2006). Follow the mother–baby dyad closely if any of these devices are being used, and discontinue their use when the baby can latch and suck effectively,

If the baby *latches or sucks in a way that causes pain or nipple damage, or insufficient milk intake,* the first strategy is to remove the baby from the breast and try again using a different technique or position. A persistently painful latch indicates an infant sucking problem that needs further investigation. Suboptimum latch and suck causes pain for the mother and leaves milk in her breast, which then compromises milk production and reduces infant milk intake. Normally, the nipple tip rests deeply in the baby's mouth, and may move an average of 4 mm anterior of the hard–soft palate juncture (Jacobs et al., 2007). Figure 8–1 shows a breastfeeding "seal" on the breast. The tongue cups around the

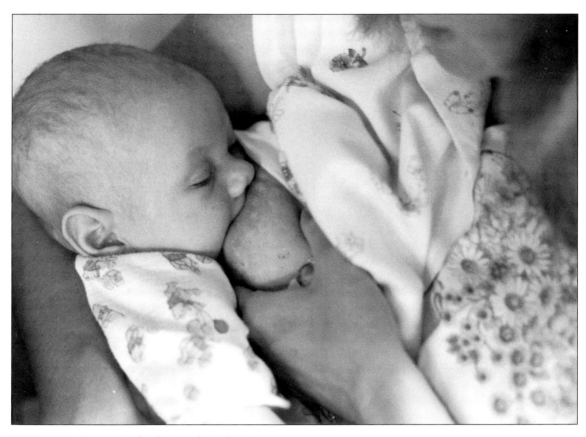

FIGURE 8-1   Breastfeeding "seal" on breast.

nipple, comfortably extending the nipple back into the baby's mouth.

If the baby takes only the nipple tip, the upward movement of the baby's tongue during sucking will compress the nipple tip against the hard palate, causing nipple pain and damage, and restrict flow through the milk ducts, resulting in milk retention in the breast and an underfed baby (Geddes, 2007). A repositioning of the baby further onto the breast, and/or facilitating the baby's self-directed attachment, may quickly result in an effective comfortable latch (Cadwell, 2007). If a comfortable, effective latch is not achieved in a few tries, it may be counterproductive to continue attempts to latch to the point of causing nipple damage. Fear of nipple pain and damage can quickly inhibit mother's motivation to continue (Thorley, 2005). At that point, further careful investigation of the cause(s) of poor latch will direct further strategies for resolution.

In any case, the lactation consultant should continue to help the mother support milk production, observe changes in the baby, and support the mother's motivation and confidence.

Some babies cannot latch and breastfeed comfortably because of *birth injuries*, including nerve injuries or damage such as brachial plexus injury/brachial palsy; fractures of the skull, clavicle, or other bones; wounds, bruises, or lacerations of the scalp, face, oropharynx or elsewhere; swellings including cephalhematoma and caput succedaneum; muscle abnormalities including torticollis; and/or major severe complications such as subgaleal hemorrhage or intracranial hemorrhage (Parker, 2005, 2006). The baby may have no outward signs or symptoms; moderate to severe pain with severe crying or crying unrelated to hunger; difficulty in some positions at breast; and/or difficulty feeding, regardless of the method used. The breastfeeding mother's instincts may serve her well in the case of hidden injuries, as she is acutely aware of even subtle aspects of her baby's behavior.

Torticollis

Torticollis is a positional deformity that is the result of a cramped intrauterine environment; as a result, the baby develops asymmetrical mandibles and/or tilted jaws that can make latching on to the mother's breast difficult. With torticollis, the baby consistently turns his head to one side (usually right) and tilts to the other side (usually left) because of a tight muscle. Other signs are a misalignment of the eyes and ears, one ear cupped forward and asymmetry of the jaws (see Color Plates 41, 42, 43). Assessing for torticollis is covered in Chapter 20. Typically the baby prefers to breastfeed on one side and may have other feeding difficulties (Wall & Glass, 2006). Popular use of seated baby carriers

exacerbates the condition because it confines the baby's head position.

Since the "Back to Sleep" campaign to prevent SIDS, the incidence of torticollis has increased. Before the campaign infants often slept prone and stretched the tight neck muscle over time by turning their head from one side to the other; thus, the condition resolved on its own. Parents can be taught to gently use these techniques to stretch the muscle on the affected side (Stellwagen, Hubbard, & Vaux, 2004):

- Turn the baby's head, chin to shoulder, while stabilizing the chest with one hand and hold for 10 seconds. Repeat three times on the other side.
- Tilt the head, ear to shoulder, while stabilizing the chest and hold for 10 seconds. Repeat three times on each side.

See Table 8–2 for general behaviors that assess breastfeeding. Other evidence-based breastfeeding tools that measure breastfeeding are in Chapter 20.

TABLE 8–2	**Assessing a Breastfeeding**	
Behavior to Assess	**Criteria**	**Rationale**
Rooting	Searches with mouth and face, turns face toward breast	Readiness to feed; intact nerve responses
Angle of gape	120–160 degree angle of jaw	Allows deep latch
Shape of cheeks	Full and rounded, no dimpling or puckering	Normal pressures in mouth
Tongue placement	Under the tongue, extends past lower gum ridge, may extend past lower lip	When tongue is down, milk flows comfortably and well
Audible swallows	Quiet "ta" sound every suck or every few sucks	No clicks, slurps, smacking that indicate loss of seal
Mouth "sealed" on breast (see Figure 8–1)	Tongue cupped around breast; lips flanged; can't easily pull off	Seal indicates adequate intraoral pressures for milk flow
Smooth rhythm of suckle/swallow/breathe	Long bursts of sucking with swallows and breathing; short pauses	Coordination needed for adequate intake
Comfortable nipple and breast	May feel nipple extend and stretch; no pain or pinching	Pain indicates poor latch or other problem
Nipple shape postfeed	Same shape as before feed; wet	Distortion indicates poor latch or suck
Breast fullness postfeed	Softer after feed than before; may not be "empty"	No change in fullness indicates lack of milk transfer

TABLE 8–3	**Clinical Care Plan for Sore Nipples**

Assessment	Interventions	Rationale
Nipples appear slightly red and chapped; appear shiny in dark-skinned mother.	Reassure mother that discomfort is temporary and will improve.	Breast is sensitive at start of breastfeeding. Some early nipple soreness may be caused by stretching of nipple/areola.
Mother complains of soreness at latch-on or at start of pumping. Soreness subsides when milk-ejection reflex occurs.	Discontinue if soap or antiseptic is used to cleanse breasts. Apply purified lanolin or hydrogel. Use all-cotton bra.	Skin becomes dry; maintains natural skin oils and moisture.
Mother winces as infant grasps breast (or draws nipples into mouth).	Massage breast to start milk-ejection reflex and to stimulate flow. Place crushed ice in plastic bag (or a bag of frozen vegetables covered with a washcloth) to nipples.	Massage softens nipple/breast before latch-on. Cold relieves discomfort.
Nipple sticks to bra or breast pad.	Moisten bra or breast pads before removing. Wear breast shell.	Protects keratin skin layer.
Mother is using breast cream.	Discontinue using cream and note any change.	Mother may be allergic to cream.
Crescent-shaped abrasions are seen above and/or below nipple. Nipple tip is blanched after suckling. Discomfort and pain occurs throughout feeding.	Review positioning, making sure infant's mouth is open wide before latching-on and baby is held high on mother's chest with entire body facing mother. Reposition as necessary. Gently press on baby's chin to pull it downward.	Infant is gumming and pinching nipple and/or sliding up and down because of poor positioning.
Mother has sore nipples that do not heal. Baby makes clicking sound while suckling or has frequent bursts of shallow suckles. Baby's tongue feels retracted behind lower gum.	Hold infant so that breast is positioned deep in baby's mouth. Bring tongue forward. Make sure baby's lips are flanged outward.	Baby is suckling tongue and not breast. Shallow latch promotes tongue retraction. Tongue retraction prevents normal perfusion to nipple.
A bright, pinkish-red color extends beyond nipple/areola. Mother complains of pain throughout feeding.	Apply antifungal medication to nipples. Treat family for candidiasis.	Prompt treatment alleviates problem. Candidiasis spreads with warm, moist contact among family members.
Mother has persistent, painful, reddish lesions on breast that do not appear to be candidiasis.	Refer to healthcare provider for possible treatment with antibiotic for bacterial infection.	Topical (or systemic in severe cases) antibiotics are effective in treating bacterial infection.

(range 24–102 hours) (Kulski & Hartmann, 1981; Arthur, Smith, & Hartmann, 1989) (see Chapters 3 and 7). *Edema*, an accumulation of abnormal quan-tities of fluid in the interstitial spaces, may be present already or occur simultaneously with the rapid rise in milk volume under certain conditions, and is usually short-lived. *Milk stasis* or breastmilk retention is an uncomfortable breast fullness that can occur at any time during lactation when too much milk remains in the breast, causing distention of the alveoli and distortion of the individual secretory cells. Milk stasis is caused by ineffective and/or infrequent removal of milk from the breast, or overfullness. Since milk storage capacity of the breasts is variable, some breasts will reach an overfull, distended state quicker than others. Milk storage capacities in mothers who are exclusively breastfeeding ranges from 81 to 606 mL per breast (Daly, Owens, & Hartmann, 1993; Kent et al., 2006), and capacities may change during the duration of breastfeeding (Ramsay et al., 2006).

Milk Stasis

Milk stasis is easier to prevent than correct later. The best prevention (and resolution) for *milk stasis* is early, frequent, and effective breastfeeding by a well-positioned baby with a normal, effective latch and suck response (Snowden, Renfrew, & Woolridge, 2001; Enkin et al., 2000). The causes of milk stasis can include poor suck, scheduled feeds, milk synthesis that exceeds the baby's ability to remove available milk, and factors that keep the baby away from the breast. Regardless of the causes, the result is the same: milk is retained in the breast. Depending on the storage capacity of each individual breast, at some point the breast's capacity to store milk is exceeded, and the process of involution begins. First, components of the milk itself exert a feedback inhibition on the mammary secretory epithelial cells (lactocytes) resulting in a slower rate of milk synthesis (Daly, Owens, & Hartmann, 1993). If milk is not removed, eventually the physical distension of the alveoli causes further disruption of milk synthesis (Cregan & Hartmann, 1999).

Removal of retained milk will reverse these processes as long as draining the breast is begun soon after stasis occurs. Unrelieved milk stasis triggers mammary involution. At some point in time involution becomes irreversible as the lactocytes, necessary for milk synthesis, are deactivated (or destroyed through apoptosis) for that particular lactation cycle (Neville & Neifert, 1983). It is unknown when the point of irreversibility is reached in women. Milk stasis can also lead to

plugged ducts and inflammatory reactions in the breast, then to infectious mastitis, and then, if not corrected, to breast abscess (Walker, 2006). Milk stasis is primarily a mechanical problem; therefore, a mechanical solution is needed. The core strategy in addressing all forms of milk stasis is frequent, thorough removal of milk from the breast, preferably by the baby, by hand-expression, and/or by pumping.

When milk stasis occurs for more than a few hours, for any reason and especially in the first few days after birth, it is crucial to assure frequent and adequate milk removal for both the baby's sake and to assure long-term lactation functional capacity of the breast. The rate of growth of mammary tissue necessary for ongoing milk synthesis slows after a few weeks. Milk production on day 6 is significantly associated with milk production at week 6 (Hill & Aldag, 2005). Therefore, the top priority is removing milk from the breast, which then can be provided to the baby.

Hand-expression is often more comfortable compared with pumping, especially during the colostral phase. Short expression or pumping periods may be more effective than long sessions. Pump or express until at least two milk ejection reflexes (letdown) are observed, then continue until drops of milk no longer flow for 2 minutes (Engstrom et al., 2007). Empty breasts may secrete milk rapidly (up to 2 ounces or 58 ml per hour per breast), so be prepared to repeat the process frequently, especially if the breasts have relatively small storage capacity. On average, breasts make milk at a rate of 1 ounce (30 ml) per breast per hour.

Edema

Breast edema is uncommon and generally short lived. Edema in the tissue surrounding the milk ducts (interstitial) appears to inhibit full dilation of the milk ducts during the milk ejection reflex, thus causing milk stasis in the breast. Lactation consultants have reported an apparent increase in breast and areolar edema following administration of IV fluids during labor, although research is lacking on this phenomenon. Ankle edema is commonly seen, however.

It is possible that overhydration during labor leads to dilution of plasma protein, resulting in increased interstitial fluid in the breast after birth

(Kroeger & Smith, 2004). First, try breastfeeding, hand-expression, or pumping to remove some milk. If the edema is severe enough to prevent adequate milk removal (by any means), then edema must be reduced before further attempts at milk removal. Application of cold packs for about 20 minutes (followed by removing the cold packs for at least the same length of time); gentle massage to mobilize lymph (Chikly, 2004); anti-inflammatory medications, reverse pressure softening using the flower hold (Cotterman, 2004) (see Figure 8–4), or areola compression (Miller & Riordan, 2004) (see Color plate 20 for instructions on areola compression) are suggested strategies to reduce edema and increase milk flow (International Lactation Consultants Association [ILCA], 2005). Applying heat to swollen breast tissue is *not* appropriate. Once milk is flowing freely, milk removal can be accomplished by any method, preferably the baby's direct breastfeeding.

Milk Supply

"Not enough milk" is a major worry during the first few weeks postpartum, and it is the most common reason given by mothers for early weaning and for supplementation; however, actual milk *production* insufficiency is quite rare. Mammalian survival has depended for millennia on sufficient breastmilk production to meet the needs of the young. If actual milk insufficiency occurred frequently, the species' survival would be in jeopardy.

Unrealistic expectations of infant behavior are major issues for mothers and professionals alike. Babies need frequent feeds because their small stomach capacity parallels lactation secretion patterns, as outlined earlier in this chapter. Expecting breasts or babies to go for long stretches between large meals is physiologically unrealistic, inappropriate, and counterproductive. Unethical marketing of infant formula continues to play a major role in fostering "milk supply" insecurities among families and even professionals.

Any event, behavior, custom, or practice that keeps the baby away from the breast or causes milk to remain in the breast for long periods (more than 4–6 hours) has the potential to inhibit milk production. These factors include, but are not limited to, scheduled feeds, use of bottles without corresponding expression of milk, use of pacifiers so that suckling time at the breast markedly decreases (see section on pacifiers), and/or maternal or infant illness. See Table 8–4.

Most mothers have sufficient lactation capacity to synthesize at least one third more milk than their

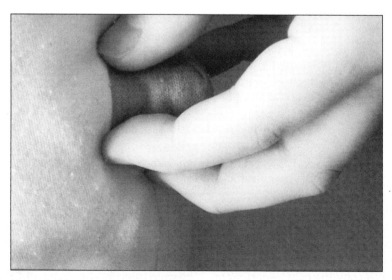

FIGURE 8-4 Flower hold reverse pressure softening.

Source: Courtesy of Rachel Myr.

| TABLE 8–4 | **Concerns or Worries About Milk Supply** |

Stated Concern or Worry	What Is Probably or Actually Happening	What to Do About This
Baby is fussy, irritable, cries or whimpers frequently	Probably hungry for milk, sucking, mother, and/or all of the above. If not hungry and being carried, then possibly sick or injured.	Breastfeed again. Increase carrying and skin-to-skin contact. Check for poor latch or poor suck or scheduled feeds.
Baby sucks fist or roots again soon after a feed	Probably hungry again, or low intake in previous feed	Breastfeed again. Increase carrying and skin-to-skin contact. Check for poor latch or poor suck or scheduled feeds.
Baby shakes head, can't stay latched, comes off nipple frequently	Breasts too full; suck problem and/or tongue-tie	Express milk and feed by cup and get baby's suck evaluated.
Baby has consistently long (> 30 minutes per side) or short (< 5 minutes per side) feeds; falls asleep but doesn't release breast	May be normal if baby is thriving and healthy. If baby is not thriving, or mother is exasperated, seek skilled help.	Express milk and feed by cup while baby is evaluated thoroughly.
Baby eagerly takes formula or pumped milk from a bottle right after a feeding	Normal if suck is poor; may be a very rapid-flow nipple, and baby can't control the flow of milk easily	Express milk and feed by cup while baby and mother are evaluated thoroughly.
Mother does not feel the let-down (milk-ejection) reflex	Multiple let-downs occur during feeds but mothers may not sense any, or only the first (Ramsay et al., 2006).	Reassure and encourage mother to watch and listen for infant swallowing or milk flowing during pumping.
Breasts still full and hard after feeds	Poor milk transfer; often because of poor latch, poor infant suck, and/or edema	Express or pump milk; investigate infant suck
Breasts are soft most of the time.	Normal	Reassure
Can't pump much milk	Some mothers do not release milk to any pump.	Breastfeed; hand-express or try a different pump
Baby wants to breastfeed "constantly"	Probably normal or unrealistic expectation of infant behavior	Observe; track length and duration of feeds and infant output; follow up.
Previous breast surgery	Surgery may affect lactation capacity	Follow closely especially in the first week postpartum.
Breasts too small (or large)	Probably a cultural myth; rarely is a true insufficiency	Evaluate and reassure; refer to mother-support groups.

baby typically takes (Daly et al., 1996). However, if the breasts are not drained of about 67 percent of the milk most of the time by the baby's suckling or expressing, the rate of milk synthesis slows down to match the lowered demand; therefore, total daily production falls. Breast storage capacity also matters. If a mother has small breasts and low milk storage capacity, her baby will need to feed more frequently to obtain all the milk he needs. Mothers with large breasts may have a large storage capacity and, as a result, may be able to provide larger feeds at longer intervals (if her baby is willing). If a baby cannot remove sufficient milk from the breast, milk synthesis will quickly diminish unless the mother begins pumping or expressing milk. Regular milk removal will maintain the mother's milk supply while the causes of her baby's poor suck are investigated and resolved.

Temporary Low Milk Production or Delayed Onset of Lactogenesis

The onset of lactogenesis II (the onset of copious milk secretion, or "milk coming in") occurs on average 30–40 hours after the delivery of the placenta, which causes a sharp drop in circulating progesterone. Retained placental fragments can inhibit the fall of progesterone, thereby delaying onset of lactogenesis II (Neifert, McDonough, & Neville, 1981). During lactogenesis II, lactose synthesis rapidly increases, drawing water into what has been colostrum and resulting in a sweeter and less viscous fluid referred to as "transitional milk." Mothers perceive this event on average about 50 to 60 hours postbirth (range 24–102 hours), after the increased rate of synthesis is well underway and as their breasts fill with milk.

Delayed onset of lactogenesis II is associated with cesarean birth and high levels of stress to the mother and fetus during birth (Scott, Binns, & Oddy, 2007; Chen et al., 1998; Chapman & Perez-Escamilla, 1999; Dewey, 2001). Premature delivery, insulin-dependent diabetes mellitus, obesity, and endocrine disturbances can delay lactogenesis II and impede the successful establishment of lactation. Whether delay is a maternal physiological response, due to delayed or ineffective suckling or a combination of factors, has not yet been clearly established. Early, frequent, and effective breastfeeding appears to be the most important factor in establishing normal lactation. Prolactin bursts associated with the infant suckling or breast pumping support the continued growth of secretory tissue for several weeks or months after birth (Cox et al., 1999).

Very few women are physically unable to make sufficient milk for one baby. Neville and Morton (2001) categorize failed lactogenesis as (1) preglandular, owing to retained placenta or lack of pituitary prolactin; (2) glandular, caused by surgical procedures or insufficient mammary tissue; or (3) postglandular, caused by ineffective or infrequent milk removal.

They observe that the latter category has received insufficient attention. Studies have reported breast hypoplasia as a marker of lactation insufficiency (Huggins, Petok, & Mireles, 2000). See Table 8–5.

TABLE 8–5	Strategies to Increase Milk Production
Strategy	**Rationale**
Breastfeed on cue; at least 8–16 sessions per day	This is how breastfeeding works.
Drain each breast thoroughly at least once a day.	Empty breasts make more milk rapidly.
Empty the breast(s) more often.	Milk is made rapidly when breast is emptiest and slower as the breast fills with milk. Milk stasis causes build-up of inhibiting factors; pressure of retained milk distorts cell function.
No long periods (> 5 hours) without milk removal	Five hours is longer than most babies go between feeds; overfull breasts cause slower milk production.
Change or add method(s) of milk removal.	Babies with effective suck are best; hand-expression, hospital-grade pumps, other pumps
Increase diameter of pump flange.	Larger diameter flanges allow duct expansion and more flow
Massage breasts gently.	Mechanically compresses alveoli (Jones, Dimmock, & Spencer, 2001)
Stop hormonal medications.	Estrogen suppresses lactation; progesterone may also.
Check endocrine levels.	Endocrine system affects lactation.
Check for pregnancy.	Pregnancy will reduce milk volume and change composition.
Use lactation-enhancing drugs as a last resort.	Drugs have side effects including psychological ones.

Too Much Milk (Oversupply)

A few women have too much milk, which can be just as big a problem as not having enough. The baby chokes, twists, and pulls back to escape the sudden flow of milk upon letdown. The mother's breasts leak to the point that it interferes with daily activities such as wet clothes and embarrassment in public places.

Usually oversupply problems disappear as the supply-and-demand mechanism adjusts itself, but not always. Babies may have a problem with suckle/swallow/breathe coordination—in other words, this may be a baby problem, not a maternal problem. There are two approaches to dealing with a baby who chokes or gags because of high breastmilk volume or rapid flow: deliberately reduce milk volume and/or carefully investigate suckle/swallow/breathe problems in the baby. Since "oversupply" can mask an infant problem, be sure to investigate the baby's ability to feed before attempting to alter milk production (Genna, 2008). The baby's suckling coordination almost always improves over time, and the mother's milk supply will almost always regulate itself to what the baby takes. If the baby consistently chokes when the mother's milk lets down or has difficulty handling fast-flowing milk, carefully evaluate the baby before deciding this is an oversupply issue. A baby with true gastroesophageal reflux may have some of the same symptoms (see Chapter 19).

Wilson-Clay and Hoover (2005) suggest that the mother try these methods to deal with oversupply:

- Use only one breast at each feeding. Over time her body will make less milk.
- Use the same breast for several feedings (remove a little milk in other breast for comfort).
- "Pace" the feeding, meaning remove the baby from the breast and let him rest before resuming the feed.
- Consider consulting with a physician about medications (Sudafed 60 mg, Benadryl). In severe cases, use low-dose birth control pills under close medical supervision.

If milk production greatly exceeds the baby's need for an extended period (more than a few weeks), carefully investigate the mother–baby dyad's feeding patterns looking for pacifier use, scheduled feeds (length and/or frequency), nighttime sleeping and feeding arrangements, hours regularly spent apart and milk expression during separations, and family health and social issues. Also refer the mother to a provider who can thoroughly evaluate her endocrine function and other health factors. Meanwhile, if the mother's milk production is so high that she is experiencing clogged milk ducts or mastitis, then reducing milk production may be necessary.

Effect of Pharmaceutical Agents on Milk Supply

The lactation consultant should always ask the mother if she is taking any prescription or over-the-counter drugs. Estrogen-containing contraceptives will quickly reduce milk supply. Some women will experience a reduction in supply from progestin-only preparations if they are used prior to 6 weeks postbirth (see Chapter 5 on drugs). Dopamine antagonist drugs used for treating gastroesophageal reflux are known to raise serum prolactin levels, although circulating prolactin plays more of a permissive than regulatory role in milk synthesis. Metoclopramide (Reglan) and

TABLE 8–6	**Strategies to Help Reduce or Lower Milk Production**
Strategy	**Rationale**
Allow up to two-thirds of the milk to remain in the breast unless doing so causes discomfort.	Feedback inhibition of lactation (properties of the milk itself) down-regulates the rate of milk synthesis.
Let the baby finish the first side first; don't press him to take the second side.	Infant appetite usually regulates milk production.
Express or pump the full breast, removing less than two thirds of the milk in the breast. Save the milk for future use.	Avoid overdistension and pain. Collected milk can be used later.
Use lactation-inhibiting drugs as a last resort.	Drugs have side effects; some permanently affect lactation.

domperidone (Motilium) are used to increase a mother's low milk supply, especially when she has given birth prematurely (da Silva et al., 2001). Both metoclopramide and domperidone pass into milk with no measurable effects on the infant. Unlike domperidone, metoclopramide affects the central nervous system and is associated with maternal depression in long-term (more than 4 weeks) use (see Table 8–6). (See Chapter 5 for a detailed discussion of these drugs.)

Breast Massage

Massage of the lactating breasts is not the same technique as manual expression of milk. Several techniques have been described or taught by various authors or sources. Jones et al. conducted a randomized controlled trial of methods of milk expression following preterm delivery and found that double-pumping with massage increased milk volume but not fat concentrations (Jones, Dimmock, & Spencer, 2001). Foda et al. studied Oketani massage and found higher levels of lipids after expression (Foda et al., 2004). Lymph drainage massage anecdotally shows promise when edema is present. Massage may be helpful as long as it is performed gently, preferably by the mother herself, and in combination with regular and frequent milk removal by any means, preferably the baby (see Table 8–7).

TABLE 8–7 Breast Massage Techniques

Description or Technique	Author, Source, Date
"Massage the milk producing cells and ducts. Start at the top of the breast. Press firmly into the chest wall. Move fingers in a circular motion on one spot on the skin. Stroke the breast area from the top of the breast to the nipple with a light tickle-like stroke. Shake the breast while leaning forward so that gravity will help the milk eject."	Marmet C. Lactation Institute, 1978–1998.
"The mother sits in a chair and someone standing behind her briskly rubs the knuckles of a fist from the base of the mother's neck to the bottom of her shoulder blades on both sides of her spine."	La Leche League, traditional.
"Gentle tactile stimulation of mammary and nipple tissue using a hand action that rolled the knuckles downward over the breast, beginning at the ribs and working towards the areola."	Spencer et al., 1998.
"When the baby is nibbling at the breast and no longer drinking with the "open mouth wide—*pause*—then close mouth" type of suck, compress the breast. *Do not roll your fingers along the breast toward the baby, just squeeze.* Not so hard that it hurts, and try not to change the shape of the areola (the part of the breast near the baby's mouth). With the compression, the baby should start drinking again with the "open mouth wide—*pause*—then close mouth" type of suck. *Use compression while the baby is sucking* but not drinking! Keep the pressure up until the baby no longer drinks even with the compression, and then release the pressure. Often the baby will stop sucking altogether when the pressure is released, but will start again shortly as milk starts to flow again. If the baby does not stop sucking with the release of pressure, wait a short time before compressing again. The reason for releasing the pressure is to allow your hand to rest, and to allow milk to start flowing to the baby again. The baby, if he stops sucking when you release the pressure, will start again when he starts to taste milk."	Newman, 2005.

(Continues)

TABLE 8-7	**Breast Massage Techniques (Continued)**

Description or Technique	Author, Source, Date
Oketani massage is *performed by midwives* with special training and technique. "Connective tissue massage developed by the midwife Sotomi Oketani involving manual separation of adhesions between the breast base and the major fascia of the pectoral muscles with the aim of helping to restore and maintain natural breast contour and normal breast function. The most salient characteristics of the Oketani method are the following: (1) the massage causes no discomfort or pain to the mother, (2) the mother will suddenly feel general relief and comfort, (3) lactation is enhanced regardless of the size or shape of the mother's breasts and nipples, (4) deformities such as inversion, flattening, or cracking of the nipples are rectified, and (5) nipple injuries and mastitis are prevented." Commentary by Hiroko Hongo, La Leche League International, *Leaven* 43(1), 2007.	Oketani, 1985; described by Foda et al., 2004.
Lymph drainage therapy is gentle massage of the lymphatic drainage channels in the breast, thought to move stagnated fluid, reduce edema, and improve cellular function. Dr. Chikly teaches this technique to *mothers* for self-care and to *physical therapists and other qualified therapists.*	Bruno Chikly, DO (Chikly, 2004).

Nausea During Milk Ejection Reflux

Maternal nausea while breastfeeding is uncommon but distressing. A mother known to the authors reported that she had been nauseated throughout her pregnancy. Although baby was thriving at 6 weeks, breastfeeding was not going well because she continued to suffer nausea and frequent vomiting when the milk ejection reflex occurred. She tried ginger as well as several homeopathic remedies to no avail. Both a pharmacologist and the LC recommended that the mother take Zofran, the drug that is used for nausea by people receiving chemotherapy. Eating before breastfeeding and wearing pressure bands for motion sickness was also suggested. The mother's nausea gradually abated over the next few weeks.

Clothing, Leaking, Bras, and Breast Pads

Breastfeeding mothers' clothing should allow frequent, easy access to her breasts. Beyond ease of access to the breasts, no special garments are needed. A well-fitting bra is not a therapeutic device, yet may increase the mother's comfort as long as the bra does not constrict or compress any part of the breast or shoulders.

Excessive leaking that requires the use of bra pads (breast pads) is often an artifact of scheduled feeds. In the early weeks, most women synthesize more milk than their baby requires. By around 6 weeks, daily milk supply has adjusted itself to the baby's needs, with sufficient residual milk volume to meet short-term increased needs. The letdown reflex is triggered by infant cues and other activities associated with breastfeeding. If worn, absorbent pads or milk-blocking devices should be comfortable, nonirritating, replaced when wet, and leave no residue that could be ingested by the baby. Direct pressure for a few seconds on a leaking breast, such as by crossed arms, is usually sufficient to temporarily inhibit leaking. Feeding the baby on cue and around the clock help prevent leaking.

Infant Concerns

Pacifiers

Pacifiers undermine exclusive breastfeeding for the first 6 months (Santo, de Oliveira, & Giugliani, 2007; Mitchell, Blair, & L'Hoir, 2006; Nelson, Yu, & Williams, 2005). The most common use of a pacifier is to deliberately postpone or stretch out the time between breastfeeds (Barros et al., 1995). Breastfed infants who use a pacifier frequently have approximately one fewer breastfeeding per 24 hours ($P = < .01$) than those who did not use a pacifier (Aarts et al., 1999). Since milk production is directly linked to frequent effective feeds, this reduction in the infants' total time at breast contributes to shorter and less exclusive breastfeeding among pacifier users (Howard et al., 1999b; Vogel, Hutchison, & Mitchell, 2001).

Routine and social use of pacifiers has been linked to the following:

- Dental and orthodontic problems (Peres et al., 2007)
- Accidents and injuries including fatal choking; increased oral thrush and other infections (Mattos-Graner et al., 2001)
- Delayed or altered speech development, behavior, and brain development (Lehtonen et al., 1998; Paul, Dittrichova, & Papousek, 1996)
- Deficits in attachment and maturation (Barros et al., 1997; Gale & Martyn, 1996).

Despite the risks, pacifiers are used by 50 to 80 percent of breastfeeding mothers (Howard et al., 1999b). Their use is more common in populations of lower socioeconomic status (Mathur, Mathur, & Khanduja, 1990) and in those experiencing breast-feeding problems (Righard & Alade, 1997; Santo, de Oliveira, & Giugliani, 2007). Step eight of the Baby-Friendly Hospital Initiative (UNICEF & WHO, 2006) (see Chapter 2) specifies "Give no pacifiers or artificial nipples to breastfeeding infants."

Pacifier use has been recommended as a strategy to reduce risk of SIDS (Hauck, Omojokun, & Siadaty, 2005; Hauck, 2006) on the basis of case-control studies that showed an association between lack of pacifier use on the infant's last night and an increased risk of SIDS. The AAP Task Force on Sudden Infant Death Syndrome recommended the following:

Consider offering a pacifier at nap time and bedtime: Although the mechanism is not known, the reduced risk of SIDS associated with pacifier use during sleep is compelling, and the evidence that pacifier use inhibits breastfeeding or causes later dental complications is not. Until evidence dictates otherwise, the task force recommends use of a pacifier throughout the first year of life according to the following procedures:

- *The pacifier should be used when placing the infant down for sleep and not be reinserted once the infant falls asleep. If the infant refuses the pacifier, he or she should not be forced to take it.*
- *Pacifiers should not be coated in any sweet solution.*
- *Pacifiers should be cleaned often and replaced regularly.*
- *For breastfed infants, delay pacifier introduction until 1 month of age to ensure that breastfeeding is firmly established (Task Force on Sudden Infant Death, 2005).*

The mechanism by which pacifiers might reduce the risk of SIDS, or by their absence increase the risk remains unknown. The quality of the research supporting the recommendation of universal use of pacifiers has been challenged by other researchers. Pacifiers generally fall out within 5–30 minutes of the infant's falling asleep (Franco et al., 2000; Weiss & Kerbl, 2001), leading to the speculation that other factors, including the frequent attention of a responsible adult who replaces the pacifier, may be the apparently protective mechanism.

Sucking, swallowing, and breathing are intimately related, each function affecting the others (Wolf & Glass, 1992). Sucking may affect respiratory centers in the brain; therefore, sucking may have a role in eliciting or maintaining breathing. Pollard studied night-time nonnutritive sucking in infants aged 1 to 5 months using infrared cameras. Babies who slept with their mothers sucked on their mother's breasts, their mothers' fingers, their own fingers, or pacifiers. If the babies were sleeping separately from mother, they sucked on their own fingers or pacifiers. The routine pacifier-users rarely sucked their digits. Digit sucking has state-modulating effects and may be suppressed by pacifier use (Pollard et al., 1999).

The 2005 AAP Breastfeeding Policy recommends "Pacifier use is best avoided during the initiation of breastfeeding and used only after breastfeeding is well established (Gartner et al., 2005). Given the lack of evidence of benefit and documented risks of pacifiers to the breastfed infant (Howard et al., 2003), breastfeeding mothers should be cautioned to avoid pacifiers except in limited situations.

Stooling Patterns

The stools of the breastfed newborn go through several predictable, observable changes and can be used as a partial indicator of milk intake (ILCA, 2005; Gartner et al., 2005). Black, tarry stools (meconium) are passed in the first days. With each subsequent milk feed, the stool gradually lightens in color, changing from dark to greenish to yellow (see Color Plate 53, Meconium) and becomes less sticky, softer, and more liquid (see Table 8–8). Stools may contain small curds, or have a mushy consistency. Color ranges from greenish-yellow to mustard-yellow, and the odor is a characteristic sweet, "yeasty," or cream cheese odor. By 2 weeks, breastfed babies' fecal flora is very different from formula-fed infants. Formula-fed children had fecal flora similar to that of the adult, in which coliforms and enterococci predominate, whereas the flora of the breastfed baby is dominated by lactobacilli and bifidobacteria (Penders et al., 2006).

In the early weeks of lactation, the whey–casein ratio of human milk is 90:10 (90 percent whey, 10 percent casein). Whey is the liquid portion of the milk, full of immune factors, and low in calcium and minerals. This early composition is perfect for the newborn's higher need for immune protection than minerals for long bone growth. By about 6 weeks, the stools may be firmer and may be passed slightly less often, reflecting the whey–casein ratio as it has evolved to approximately 80:20. The gradual increase in casein relative to whey results in slightly thicker, more formed stools (more like toothpaste or soft peanut butter) that may be passed less often. By the middle of the infant's first year, the whey–casein ratio has evolved to 60:40 or even 50:50—exactly paralleling the infant's increasing bone and muscle development and mobility (Kunz & Lonnerdal, 1992).

Shrago et al. studied stools of exclusively breastfed babies over the first 2 weeks and reported an average of 4 stools per day (range 0.8–7.2) in first 5 days; the first yellow stool appeared on day 4 (range day 3–15) (Shrago, Reifsnider, & Insel, 2006). Frequent feeds were correlated to appearance of yellow stool and more feeds per day, the sooner yellow stools appeared, and the faster babies gained weight. Nommsen-Rivers et al. (2008) reported a "significant relationship between diaper output and

TABLE 8–8	Stooling Patterns		
Time Period	**# per Day**	**Appearance/Color**	**Amount**
0–2 days	1+	Meconium (black, thick tarry)	Scant to copious
3–4 days	1–3	Black to green to yellow, looser	Increasing volume
4–7 days	1–4+	Yellow, seedy, runny to loose	Copious by day 6
1–6 weeks	3–5+	Yellow, seedy, runny to loose	Copious
6 weeks–6 months	3–5+; may skip days	Yellow; soft; may thicken over time because of milk compositional changes	Copious and may be passed less often
6 months and onward		Loose; color and aroma may change as family foods are added	

breastfeeding adequacy, but the relationship was not strong enough to be used as a screening tool. Less than 4 stools on day 4 in combination with milk onset delay may be screening tool."

If breastfeeding is not exclusive (for example, when the child begins eating family food, or if infant formula is given), stools become darker, with larger and firmer curds, and with more odor. The formula-fed infant tends to pass larger, more copious, more odorous, but less frequent stools (Quinlan et al., 1995). As the proportion of solid foods increases, stools will reflect the new foods with a change in odor, color, and consistency. Sometimes portions of undigested food may be visible in the stool.

In the first 4 to 6 weeks, newborns pass stool many times a day. If more than 24 hours passes without a stool, the child should be seen by a healthcare provider and adequate caloric intake assessed in other ways (Neifert, 2001). Lack of sufficient milk intake is the most common reason for lack of stooling; therefore, more attention to frequent effective breastfeeding and/or increasing milk intake should quickly increase infant output. A healthy, thriving exclusively breastfed child over 6 weeks old may stool only a few times a week or even less. As long as the stool is soft and profuse and the infant is otherwise thriving and content, that pattern is not unusual. If unusual stool patterns persist, the lactation consultant should collaborate with the baby's primary-care provider to investigate other diseases or conditions. Hirschsprung's disease, cystic fibrosis, infant botulism, cow's milk allergy (Vanderhoof et al., 2001; Daher et al., 2001), and other bowel disorders may be underlying unusual bowel patterns (see Chapter 19).

Hyperbilirubinemia Testing

Nurses and lactation consultants are a part of the management of infants on all levels of care, including monitoring bilirubin levels. AAP guidelines mandate that every baby be screened for bilirubin levels after 24 hours of life regardless of symptoms of jaundice and other symptoms. Normal and abnormal levels are determined by a nomogram, a graph that depicts risk zones based on the baby's age in hours and the bilirubin level (see Chapter 11). In the past few years, noninvasive handheld devices have

been used to measure bilirubin transcutaneously in neonates. The advantage is that the bilirubin level can be determined without a blood sample, a welcome advancement because they avoid the pain of a stick on the baby's heel to withdraw blood, especially since physicians tend to order more frequent bilirubin testing if the baby is breastfeeding. Readings are taken on the baby's forehead and sternum. Newer versions of these handheld devices are reasonably accurate regardless of skin color and show a close correlation between serum bilirubin and transcutaneous bilirubin (TcB) (Maisels et al., 2004).

A disadvantage is that when TcB devices are used, hospital protocols call for more frequent monitoring of bilirubin levels, usually every 12 hours. This close monitoring of bilirubin with TcB devices results in the likelihood that the baby will be given formula and put under "bili" lights even though the bilirubin level may not be abnormal but only rising. We now see babies placed under triple "bili" lights with a bilirubin of 8 at 24 hrs. Similar to the problem with using labor monitors, healthcare personnel tend to focus on the machine and not the individual. The nurse will depend on the nomogram protocol for bilirubin levels to decide when to intervene instead of using her judgment and looking at the "whole" picture, such as the baby's behavior, skin color, and amount of stool output (Gagnon et al., 2001).

If a serum (blood) bilirubin test must be done, it can be combined with serum testing routinely drawn for genetic screening (PKU, congenital hypothyroidism, etc.). Staff should try to time the procedure with a breastfeeding. Breastfeeding reduces pain levels during any painful procedure, and there is ample evidence that infants tolerate the discomfort of heelsticks or blood draws much better while they are nursing (Abdulkader et al., 2007; Phillips, Chantry, & Gallagher, 2005; Shah, Aliwalas, & Shah, 2006). According to one nurse/LC, "I try to do all my breastfeeding babies' heel sticks while they are at mom's breast. Even if they aren't latched on, they receive such comfort from mom that they cry less" (see Figure 8–5).

Prolonged, elevated bilirubin levels (greater than 5 mg/dL [85 umol/L]) in the otherwise healthy, thriving breastfed infant during the third week or even into the second month of life is common and requires no intervention beyond observation and assurance of adequate feeding (Gartner & Herschel,

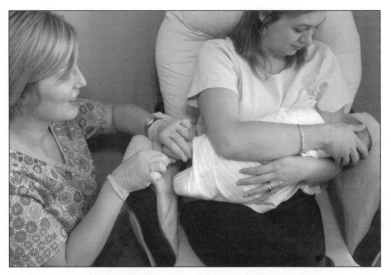

A mother breastfeeding a baby while the nurse does a heel stick.

2001). Home health nurses may be called upon to assess levels of jaundice and arrange appropriate treatment (Madlon-Kay, 2001).

If the baby is or becomes jaundiced after hospital discharge, review the information in Chapter 11. The lactation consultant should stay in close contact with the baby's primary care provider and carefully monitor and assist with breastfeeding. Keep the mother and baby close together; assure adequate milk transfer during direct breastfeeding with an electronic scale; monitor quality and quantity of direct breastfeeding; and help the mother express and feed her milk by alternate means if direct breastfeeding is not meeting the baby's caloric needs. Continue skin-to-skin contact and attempts at direct breastfeeding until the baby is effectively and comfortably obtaining milk and the jaundice has resolved.

Crying and Colic

Breastfed babies who are fed on cue and held and carried many hours a day rarely cry. An infant cries to signal a need, which may be for food, comfort, warmth, mother's presence (Christensson et al., 1995), pain, illness, and/or fear. Crying increases stress, increases blood pressure and potential for brain bleeds (Anderson, 1989), and releases potent chemicals that can alter and even damage the baby's brain (Schore, 2001; Christensson et al., 1992; Michelsson et al., 1996). It is never appropriate to "let a baby cry it out," make a baby cry to "teach him a lesson," or deliberately ignore a baby's cries. Prompt response reduces the baby's stress, enhances parental enjoyment of the baby, and increases parents' confidence in their new role. When parents and caregivers quickly respond to the baby's signals, a long, secure, and trusting relationship begins to develop and parents become more skilled in reading their baby's cues.

Before an assessment of colic is made, all other causes of crying should be investigated and ruled out, especially hunger, illness and injury, and lack of carrying and touch. Crying is a *late* sign of hunger (Gartner et al., 2005). Reinforcing the mother's prompt response to her baby's feeding cues is always appropriate and eliminates most cases of hunger-induced crying. Lack of knowledge about normal (frequent and sometimes clustered) feeding patterns of breastfed babies has led many mothers and even professionals to identify a baby's cries as "colic" when in fact the child was simply hungry or needed to be held or carried. Attempting to enforce a strict schedule for feeds is inappropriate and can result in serious underfeeding, dehydration, failure to thrive (Aney, 1998), reduction in milk supply, and undermining of the mother's confidence in caring for her baby. Breastfeeding should be the first strategy to soothe infant cries, because it instantly and automatically brings the infant his mother's presence, food, comfort, warmth, natural endorphins, and immune protection (Gray et al., 2002; Carbajal et al., 2003).

Wessel's (1954) 3-3-3 definition of colic (crying more than 3 hours a day, more than 3 days a week, and lasting more than 3 weeks) helps distinguish colic from hunger or other temporary illness or conditions. Unlike other cries, colic usually is characterized by a high-pitched wail or scream, as if the baby is in severe pain (St James-Roberts, 1999). Colic appears to be the result of sudden spasmodic abdominal cramping, with knees drawn up and sometimes a distended abdomen. Food protein hypersensitivity or allergy is the primary cause of true colic (Gupta, 2007). Disturbances in parental or maternal–child interactions may contribute to colic (Gupta, 2002) and parental expectations may play a role. Canivet et al. (2005) recommend providing closer attention, information and support to very young women, women who do not cohabit with the father, and women with high trait anxiety.

When investigating causes for persistent crying and colic (in collaboration with primary care providers), first carefully document everything consumed by the infant and mother for several days. Cow milk protein allergy or intolerance can also appear as gastroesophageal reflux related to cow's milk protein allergy (Cavataio, Carroccio, & Iacono, 2000; Salvatore & Vandenplas, 2002). If the child is sensitive to cow's milk protein, he is likely also sensitive to other foods or allergens (Iacono et al., 1998). Smoking, including maternal smoking during pregnancy (Sondergaard et al., 2003) may play a role in colic, and has other serious negative consequences for the infant (Fleming & Blair, 2007).

Cow's milk has been shown to be the single most commonly ingested allergen in infants (Greer, Sicherer, & Burks, 2008). Cow's milk is the major source of protein in most manufactured infant formula. Direct ingestion (from whole milk or infant formula) causes the worst symptoms; intake via mother's milk also occurs. Other less common allergens include legumes (including soy-based formula and peanuts), beef, chicken and eggs, grains such as corn and wheat, and high-acid fruits and vegetables. Babies who develop colic in response to foods in the breastfeeding mother's diet often exhibit allergic

symptoms when exposed to the same foods later in life. Dietary supplements taken by the baby or mother can also cause infant distress.

After ruling out hunger and illness, the lactation consultant may help the mother identify or rule out an allergic response to cow's milk or other allergens. For the breastfed baby under 6 months, the following steps are helpful:

1. Purify the baby's diet. Ensure that the baby gets nothing other than mother's milk by direct breastfeeding for at least 2 to 3 weeks. Avoid all bottles (even containing mother's expressed milk), teats and pacifiers, vitamins, and supplements. If the baby has already begun to take other supplements or table foods, those items are the most likely offenders. Make sure the baby is breastfed on cue around the clock during this time.

2. At the same time, ask the mother to begin keeping a detailed written diary of her food and beverage intake, any medications or supplements taken by her or the baby, the baby's breastfeeding patterns, and the baby's behavior. Include any unusual events affecting the family. Continue keeping this diary for several weeks.

3. Examine the food and behavior diary carefully for emerging patterns, including the mother's cravings, foods avoided or disliked, large quantities or regular ingestion of common allergens (especially cow's milk or dairy products), and maternal symptoms of allergies.

4. If no discernable pattern emerges in a few weeks, consult with a professional allergist, pediatric gastroenterologist, or other specialist for further evaluation.

If the baby is truly sensitive to cow's milk protein or another component of cow's milk, it may take several days to weeks for the offending substance to be cleared from the baby's body. Estep and Kulczycki (2000) report that bovine IgG antibody levels were markedly higher in the milk of mothers of colicky babies than in the milk of mothers whose babies were not colicky. Bovine IgG has a long half-life, and its presence in high levels may require an extended period of elimination. If the mother's avoidance of cow's milk clearly relieves baby's colic symptoms, she may need to continue to avoid all dairy products while consuming nondairy sources of calcium or nondairy calcium-containing supplements (Carroccio et al., 2000; Iacono et al., 1998). Soy protein is also a common allergen, is present in many formulas, and not recommended for babies with documented allergy to cow's milk (Greer, Sicherer, & Burks, 2008).

If the mother wants to resume eating dairy products, she should start with very small amounts such as a tablespoonful of hard cheeses (cheddar, Swiss) or yogurt during the first week. If the baby shows no reactions, she can expand the trial to include small amounts of soft cheeses such as cottage cheese or Gouda during the second week. If her baby is still asymptomatic, then butter, ice cream, and cooked milk can be tested, again in small quantities. The reintroduction of liquid milk should be attempted last, and in small quantities. She should continue keeping the written diary of symptoms and foods during the trial period. Some babies are so sensitive that the mother must eliminate most or all forms of dairy products for prolonged periods, even weeks or months. If the mother is also sensitive or allergic to dairy products, she may feel better as well.

Various remedies for colic, reflux, and/or persistent crying (after increasing physical contact, ruling out hunger and allergies as discussed above) have been proposed, including the following:

- Increased carrying on the back or chest (Barr et al., 1991, 1999)
- Carrying baby in the prone position on the parent's arm
- Swaddling (van Sleuwen et al., 2007)
- Giving oral sucrose (Barr et al., 1999)
- Spinal manipulation (chiropractic treatment) (Wiberg, Nordsteen, & Nilsson, 1999)

Mothering a baby who cries for hours a day can exhaust and undermine the confidence of any mother (Pauli-Pott et al., 2000) and shorten the duration of breastfeeding (Howard et al., 2006). Lactation consultants should stay in close contact with mothers of colicky breastfed babies as they investigate possible causes for the baby's distress, if for no other reason than to provide the mother with emotional support during these difficult times. Encourage and support the mother to provide more skin-to-skin contact, breastfeeding, and breastmilk that are comforting to the baby. Even unsuccessful attempts to comfort the baby are valuable, because abandoning the baby to its pain is worse. Weaning the baby to infant formula will almost certainly make the baby's distress even worse.

Regurgitation

Do neonates regurgitate less often if they are breastfed? Most regurgitations in the early newborn period are essentially benign and are related to neither food allergy nor anatomic or functional intestinal obstruction. But contrary to expectations, human milk feeding did not confer a protection from regurgitating compared with formula feedings according to one study (Barak et al., 2006).

Multiple Infants

An increase in the number of women delaying childbirth until after 30 and advances in techniques to treat infertility have contributed to a large increase in the number of multiple births in the last decade (Martin, 2007). Lactation consultants are likely to work with these families, as these women choose to breastfeed at about the same rate as women giving birth to single infants (Leonard, 2007; Bowers & Gromada, 2005).

Many expectant parents are uncertain whether breastfeeding is possible following a multiple birth, and their decisions regarding infant feeding are often influenced by information received from healthcare providers. Parents of multiples may be reassured that breastfeeding two or more infants generally is possible. Reports have even described mothers' experiences of breastfeeding conjoined twins (Bains, 2006; LaFleur & Niesen, 1996). Many mothers of twins, triplets, and quadruplets have breastfed for a year and longer. Research and case studies have demonstrated that most mothers of multiples are capable of producing most or all of the milk that two to four infants require (Berlin, 2007; Bleyl, 2001; Auer & Gromada, 1998; Mead et al., 1992; Saint, Maggiore, & Hartmann, 1986).

Breastfeeding is especially important for twins, triplets, and other higher-order multiples. In addition to offering optimal nutrition and immunological protection to these often preterm or otherwise compromised infants, breastfeeding helps ensure frequent mother–infant interaction with each baby. Although the frequency of feedings may be overwhelming for many new mothers, multiples' frequent feedings give a mother many daily opportunities to sit or lie down to rest while breastfeeding (Gromada, 2007). Figure 8–6 shows comfortable positions for nursing two infants simultaneously. Note that pillows support the mother's body and arms and help hold the babies in position. The pillows can be bed pillows strategically placed to help cradle the babies or special "nursing pillows" designed for nursing twins.

Full-Term Twins or Triplets

Full-term or late preterm (near-term) multiple infants have the same needs as any full-term singleton; the mother's role, however, is more complex since she must meet the needs of two or more newborns. In addition, the mother of multiples is more likely to have had complications of pregnancy and childbirth, and she may require more time to recover physically.

Mothers of multiples need help and support with early feedings, as they feel overwhelmed when first trying to figure out how to manage feedings with more than one infant. Some are anxious to initiate simultaneous feedings, as they have heard it saves time. However, it is important to first assess each infant at breast separately, as it is not unusual for one or more of the babies to breastfeed poorly even when the infants are born at term. Ongoing, individual assessment is particularly important for late preterm (near-term) multiples, even when they are basically stable and able to be with their mother, as feeding difficulties, hypoglycemia, and hyper-bilirubinemia are more common among these newborns (Jain, 2007).

Preterm or Ill Multiples

When multiple infants are born prematurely or have other medical complications, direct breastfeeding may be delayed for days or weeks. The LC should advise the mother to begin expressing milk for her infants within hours of giving birth (Bowers & Gromada, 2005). If a mother has had complications, she may need assistance when expressing milk (Gromada & Spangler, 1998).

Simultaneous pumping using a rental hospital-grade electric pump is the most effective way to obtain maximum amounts of milk and to maintain

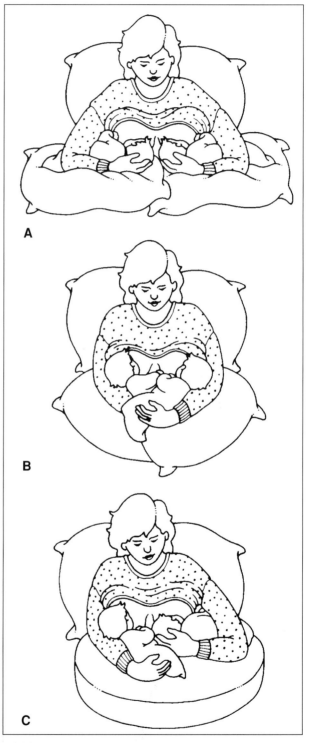

FIGURE 8–6   Positions for nursing twins.
(A) Double clutch. (B) Double cradle.
(C) Cradle-clutch.

lactation (see Chapter 12). Most hospitals with neonatal intensive care units have these pumps available for mothers to use. Anticipatory guidance for any expectant mother of multiples should include helping the mother to find a breast-pump rental location in her area.

When direct breastfeeding is initiated for two or more preterm or ill newborns following days or weeks of pumping, the LC is responsible for assisting the mother in developing an individualized, evidence-based plan for transitioning each multiple to the breast. For instance, Auer and Gromada (1998) described the approach of a mother of quadruplets who used interim bottle-feedings with each baby until she increased milk production. As with other aspects of breastfeeding, strategies for transitioning two or more infants to direct breastfeeding should look at each infant's signs, or cues, that the individual infant may be ready to progress. In addition, the process of transitioning multiple infants to direct breastfeeding may take time, and a mother may become discouraged. However, one study found preterm twins eventually progressed to full, direct breastfeeding at rates comparable to term infants (Liang, Gunn, & Gunn, 1997). Regular skin-to-skin contact sessions between a mother and one or more of her babies helps "normalize" the transition period, and skin contact with one baby at a time often facilitates the transition to direct breastfeeding due to baby-led latching.

Putting It All Together

Caring for and breastfeeding multiple newborns require a different kind of organization by the mother than caring for a single newborn or two infants of different ages (Bowers & Gromada, 2005). Encourage the mother to keep simple 24-hour charts for each infant's daily activities, especially those related to feeding and intake, until lactation is well-established and adequate weight gain for each infant indicates the multiples are able to breastfeed effectively. The charts should record the number of breastfeedings, any pumping sessions and/or alternative feedings, and the number of wet diapers and stools for each infant. Maintaining individual charts reassures the mother that all babies are receiving sufficient nutrients.

Whether a mother or her babies are ready for simultaneous feedings in the immediate postpartum period or not, a demonstration of the various single and simultaneous feeding positions will help a mother realize that she has many choices for comfortable breastfeeding. Simultaneous feedings can save time, and many mothers feed two babies at once during the first few weeks postpartum; however, some mothers and many multiples need more time to learn to work together for simultaneous feedings (Bowers & Gromada, 2005). Also, a mother may need someone to support each infant's head during individual latch-on until she and her infants become more comfortable with simultaneous feeding. Some mothers or infants indicate a preference for individual feedings, which give a mother the opportunity to enjoy some one-on-one time with each child. Perhaps the most common scenario is a combination of simultaneous and single feedings.

In addition to an interest in simultaneous feedings, many mothers also have questions about a feeding rotation and when to alternate breasts and babies. Almost any feeding rotation will work when all infants breastfeed on cue. Most mothers offer one breast per feeding. Then they may alternate breasts every feeding or they may alternate only every 24 hours, which often is easier to remember. Mothers of odd-number sets, such as triplets, may have to alternate babies and breasts more frequently than every 24 hours. Some mothers assign each of twins a particular breast, but alternating babies and breasts appears to have more advantages unless one baby consistently cues to feed from a particular breast. Also, assigning a breast, which allows each infant to self-regulate production in that particular breast, may be a useful strategy when a mother experiences an "overactive" milk-ejection reflex and/or milk overproduction with one or more infants exhibiting signs of lactose overload, or if one or more infants has frequent refluxes or has actual gastroesophageal reflux disorder (GERD).

The caregiver must remain sensitive to infant differences when a mother is forming an attachment, or bond, with each infant. Because humans are designed to form an attachment with one person at a time, the attachment process is more complex. It is also more likely to be disrupted with multiples, particularly if the twin or triplet birth was not discovered until shortly before the infants' birth or if one infant is sicker than the others (Gromada, 2007). Healthcare providers are in a position to help parents see and relate to each baby as an individual, rather than as part of a multiple unit. Promoting attachment behaviors, such as skin-to-skin contact during an infant's hospitalization and also once discharged home, is especially important with a multiple that has been less able to interact or establish eye contact with parents because of postnatal complications or illness. The healthcare provider can point out each infant's unique qualities as she helps the mother breastfeed and get to know her offspring.

Household help is not a luxury for mothers recuperating from a multiple pregnancy and birth who must feed and care for, and form attachments with, more than one neonate simultaneously. Another pair of hands and ongoing assistance with household chores allows a mother to spend more time and energy breastfeeding and meeting the other needs of her infants. Since taking care of babies is more fun than cleaning and cooking, the mother (and father) should make it clear that the helper is expected to assume household tasks, and that the mother feeds and takes care of the babies.

A lack of physical and emotional support, feelings of isolation, sleep deprivation, and other stressors associated with the care of multiple infants may contribute to the higher risk for postpartum mood or anxiety disorders in these mothers (Leonard, 1998). Because of the negative effects such a problem may exert on breastfeeding and attachment, healthcare providers should be aware of their increased likelihood and assess mothers of multiples for these disorders.

Needs, problems, and solutions vary with each multiple-birth situation. However, practical strategies to promote effective breastfeeding with multiple infants and maternal recovery may include the following ideas:

- Develop both short- and long-term breast-feeding goals with a mother to help her think of breastfeeding as a commitment and to get through the often overwhelming first few weeks or months of frequent feedings and/or pumping sessions.
- Link the mother with other women who have successfully breastfed multiples.

- Show the mother how to position and stabilize two infants for simultaneous feedings using pillows. Whether using pillows available at home or a special nursing pillow, each baby should be positioned so that the hips are significantly lower than the head. (This may be especially important for preterm or late preterm twins who are at greater risk for reflux or GERD.) The mother in Figure 8–6c is using a special pillow designed for feeding multiples. This pillow is longer and wider, which gives it a deeper "shelf," than some of the nursing pillows used for a single infant.
- Review the basics of breastfeeding, maintenance of milk production, and advantages of breastfeeding with the mother of multiples during the hectic early weeks and months of breastfeeding.
- Help the mother develop a plan to alternate infants and breasts as needed.
- Suggest that the mother create a "breastfeeding station" that she supplies with nutritious liquids and foods, breast pads, infant wipes, children's books (if she has older children), a cell or portable telephone, and a television remote.
- Emphasize the need for housekeeping help for at least several months. Recommend she advise any helper that she expects them to be supportive of breastfeeding.
- Encourage parents to ask well-wishers who want to "do something" for the family to help by delivering a meal or sending food. The care of multiples leaves little time to prepare food, and the caloric needs of a mother breastfeeding multiple infants are greater than for a mother breastfeeding a single infant. Suggestions for nutritious and convenient homemade foods may be helpful.

Partial Breastfeeding and Human Milk Feeding

Because mothers of multiple infants are more likely to be affected by complications or other factors that may interfere with effective early breastfeeding and milk production, they are more likely to supplement or complement breastfeeding with formula.

Complementing may take the form of "topping off" an occasional or daily breastfeeding, or it may involve replacing one or more breastfeedings with an alternative feeding.

With guidance from an LC who respects the overwhelming amount of infant care the mother faces daily and the lack of time to work on resolving problems, most mothers will be able to decrease the use of alternative feedings in favor of direct breastfeedings. Some mothers continue to offer an alternative feeding on a daily or weekly basis in order to have help with feedings or to sleep without interruption for a few hours. Many mothers prefer to express their own milk for feedings. Caution the mother that milk production might decrease if the total number of breastfeedings or pumping sessions dips below 8 to 10 in 24 hours.

Alternative feeding methods to provide expressed human milk is common with the increased availability of hospital-grade, electric breast pumps. Mothers of higher-order multiples find it helpful to pump, as it can be daunting to directly breastfeed three or more babies (Gromada, 2007). Mothers have maintained lactation and human milk feeding without the use of other supplements for several months. Pumping leaves the door open to later direct breastfeeding. Multiples wean as individuals; they may stop breastfeeding at about the same time or one may wean before the other(s).

Breastfeeding During Pregnancy and Tandem Nursing

The risk of a subsequent pregnancy occurring during the first 6 months of exclusive or full breastfeeding is extremely low (Van der Wijden, Kleijnen, & Van den Berk, 2003). The key points are "fully breastfeeding" and "in the first 6 months." Globally, over 50 percent of women will become pregnant while still breastfeeding their youngest child. When asked, many of these mothers report that the emotional needs of the child is their principal motivation to continue breastfeeding, followed by their belief in child-led weaning.

A mother who conceives while breastfeeding may experience any or all of the following:

- Nipple and/or breast tenderness: Hormonal changes may cause sudden onset of nipple or breast pain that appears to be hormonal in nature. The usual remedies for breast or nipple pain are often ineffectual.
- Maternal fatigue: The hormones of early pregnancy often impel women to want to sleep, although this is difficult for the mother of an active toddler to do. The fatigue is related to hormonal changes of pregnancy, not to continued breastfeeding, and it will diminish as the pregnancy progresses. Pregnant women with young children, whether breastfeeding or not, should be encouraged to nap when the child naps.
- Decline in milk supply and number of feedings: About 70 percent of mothers report a decrease in their milk production during a subsequent pregnancy. Most nursing children breastfeed less often than they did as infants. As the pregnancy progresses, the milk volume usually declines. Sometimes the child will wean during this period. If already talking, she or he may complain that the milk is "all gone," or that it takes "too long to get it."
- Change in taste of milk: As the hormones of pregnancy (especially estrogen) begin to affect the breast secretory tissue, lactose in the milk will decrease while sodium increases, changing the taste. The talking nursling may state quite clearly how the milk tastes or may simply indicate by his actions that it is not the same.
- Uterine contractions: Women experience uterine contractions during breastfeeding. There is no documented danger to the mother or fetus when mothers breastfeed through a healthy pregnancy uncomplicated by risk factors for preterm labor (Moscone & Moore, 1993). Little is known about the effect of breastfeeding during pregnancy in the presence of such risk factors.
- Weaning: Some nursing children wean before their sibling is born, presumably because of the decline in milk volume, the milk's change in taste, and/or their mother's urging to wean. As the mother's body changes shape, her lap will also disappear, which may bother the nursing child. The child may wean spontaneously if the mother responds to the child's request to breastfeed but does not offer breastfeeding first.

A maternal history of preterm labor and birth with a previous pregnancy, repeated spontaneous abortion, "incompetent" cervix, current multiple gestation, or other risks for preterm labor and birth should be taken into consideration when contemplating continued breastfeeding through the pregnancy. The mother who continues to breastfeed during a subsequent pregnancy will need to eat a nutritious diet; she may take supplemental vitamins as a precaution. In one study (Moscone & Moore, 1993), most mothers reported continued good general health throughout their pregnancy as well as healthy outcomes in the new baby.

Tandem nursing refers to the situation when a mother continues breastfeeding her child through a subsequent pregnancy including after the new baby is born. The well-referenced book on this topic is "Adventures in Tandem Nursing" by Hillary Flower (Flower, 2003). In La Leche League circles before this book was published, tandem nursing was called "nursing siblings who are not twins."

A mother who breastfeeds during pregnancy and/or continues into tandem nursing may face criticism from her family, friends, and healthcare providers. The lactation consultant may be asked for her opinion after the mother has been told by her physician that she must wean her child—even in the absence of indicators that continuing to breastfeed is a risk for the mother or her developing fetus. In developing countries, traditional beliefs about weaning when the mother's pregnancy is confirmed may also reduce the frequency of breastfeeding during a subsequent pregnancy. The lactation consultant or nurse who openly accepts individual decisions and behavior of breastfeeding women can be helpful in providing information and guidance that supports the mother's decisions.

Sleeping, SIDS, and Bed Sharing

Throughout history and around the world, mothers and babies usually sleep together, especially in the early months of exclusive breastfeeding. Anthropologic studies confirm that mother–infant bed sharing represents the most biologically appropriate sleeping arrangement for humans and is both ancient and ubiquitous because breastfeeding is not easily managed without it. Between 44 and 75 percent of breastfeeding mothers sleep with their babies all or part of the night in Western nations (McKenna & McDade, 2005). "For species such as primates, the mother *is* the environment" (Hrdy, 1999). Bed sharing results in more and longer breastfeeding episodes (McKenna, Mosko, & Richard, 1997; Blair & Ball, 2004), more frequent suckling (Ball et al., 2006), more maternal touching and looking, and faster and more frequent maternal responses (Baddock et al., 2006). Mothers get more sleep when they are bed sharing (Quillin & Glenn, 2004) and exclusively breastfeeding (Doan et al., 2007).

Despite the historical, biological, and cultural traditions of shared sleeping, concerns about infant deaths from suffocation or overlying and sudden infant death syndrome (SIDS) confuse parents, causing heated "where should the baby sleep" debates. The terms *bed sharing* and *cosleeping* are poorly defined in the research literature (Chantry et al., 2006). Delineating safe and unsafe conditions of shared sleep is critical to breastfeeding, because the majority of exclusively breastfeeding mothers will bring their babies into their bed for all or some sleeping sessions (Lahr, Rosenberg, & Lapidus, 2007). The chief concern about bed sharing is smothering or rollover deaths.

SIDS

SIDS is a diagnosis of exclusion, meaning other possible causes of death were ruled out during autopsy or investigation. Major risk factors for SIDS identified in 1991 were maternal smoking, prone position, and formula feeding (Mitchell et al., 1991). Further research has identified maternal smoking during pregnancy as a major risk factor in nearly every epidemiological study of SIDS, and may account for 50 to 80 percent of SIDS deaths, a fourfold risk (Fleming & Blair, 2007). Smokers in the household, daily exposure to secondhand smoke, and all-night bed sharing with a smoker increase risks to the infant (Lahr, Rosenberg, & Lapidus, 2005), even if the smoker is a breastfeeding mother or smokes outside the house. Prone position continues to be a risk factor for SIDS, and may be more accurately described as positional asphyxia (Moon, Horne, & Hauck, 2007). In earlier studies, formula-feeding was found to double the risks of SIDS (McVea, Turner, & Peppler, 2000). In a more rigorous systematic review, formula feeding was found to be associated with a 56 percent increase in SIDS deaths (Ip et al., 2007), possibly because of decreased arousability (Horne et al., 2004), more infections (Horne et al., 2002) and/or other factors. SIDS deaths, by definition, are *not* caused by smothering, overlying, entrapment, or suffocation.

Smothering

Smothering or other sudden unexplained infant death (SUID or SUDI) may be labeled "SIDS," even though other causes or risk or causative factors may be present. If a baby is found dead in a crib, the crib is usually not blamed for the death unless the crib was a clearly causative factor. However, if a baby is discovered dead in an adult bed next to a sleeping adult, the adult and/or the bed are often automatically blamed for the baby's death. "Overlying" (smothering) deaths usually involve alcohol or drug use by the bed partner (Blair et al., 1999; Gessner, Ives, & Perham-Hester, 2001), a bed partner other than the baby's parent (Hauck et al., 2003), and/or an unsafe surface such as a couch or sofa (Blair et al., 2006). *Unsafe sleep surfaces* can trap a baby in a dangerous position. Couches, some cribs, reclining chairs, and other surfaces that are not firm, flat, and clean are risky surfaces, especially if the infant is out of visual distance of a responsible adult (Carpenter et al., 2004). *Entrapment* deaths usually involve wedging of the infant between two objects or spaces between objects.

Breastfeeding mother–baby dyads sleep differently from formula-feeding mothers or other people. Breastfeeding mothers typically adopt a protective posture with the baby facing the mother, side-lying, with the baby's head at breast level ("cuddle-curl") (see Figure 8–7). The mother's arm above the baby's head prevents the baby from creeping up onto pillows, while the mother's bent lower leg prevents the baby scooting down to the foot of the bed (Richard et al., 1996; Baddock, Galland, Bolton, Williams, Taylor et al., 2006).

When bed sharing, mother and baby demonstrate more mutual arousals, more maternal touching and looking, increased breastfeeding, and faster and more frequent maternal responses (Baddock et al., 2007). Some argue that a mother should stay awake during feeds and return her baby to a crib for sleep; however, the hormones of breastfeeding induce relaxation and drowsiness in mother and baby, which is a major

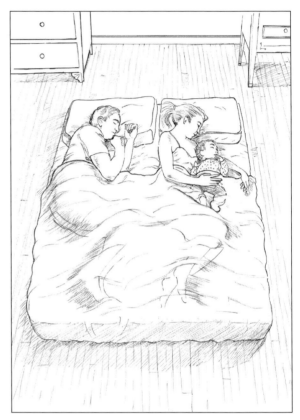

FIGURE 8–7   Protective posture: safe bedsharing supports breastfeeding.

Source: Sleeping With Your Baby: A Parent's Guide to Cosleeping, by James J. McKenna, PhD (Platypus Media, 2006). Reprinted with permission. All rights reserved.

advantage of breastfeeding (Levine et al., 2007). By 6 weeks of attempting to breastfeed without bed sharing, a majority of breastfeeding mothers manage night feeds by (1) supplementing with formula, which *reduces* maternal sleep (Doan et al., 2007); (2) try a sleep-training scheme such as feeding water in a darkened room, or (3) sleep next to their babies (Ball, 2003). The first two strategies undermine exclusive breastfeeding for 6 months. Safe bed sharing extends the duration of any breastfeeding and lengthens the period of exclusive breastfeeding (McKenna, Mosko, & Richard, 1997).

There is currently not enough evidence to support routine recommendations against "all bed sharing" to reduce risks of SIDS or smothering. If the mother does not bed share, then the baby should sleep supine in a safe crib within visual distance of a responsible adult (Task Force on Sudden Infant Death, 2005). Parents need factual, evidence-based information about specific risks of unsafe bed sharing conditions, unsafe cribs, and other practices that increase risk to the baby (McKenna, 2007). See Table 8–9.

Clinical Implications

Even when new mothers have adequate knowledge about breastfeeding and have social and clinical support, most still will benefit from a visit by a skillful breastfeeding advisor during the early postpartum period. Early and close follow-up by healthcare professionals skilled in breastfeeding should begin at birth and continue within 48 hours of release from hospital care or 3–5 days after birth and again within 2–3 weeks after birth (Gartner et al., 2005). An in-person evaluation at 72–96 hours is especially important (Dewey et al., 2003). Assessing and reinforcing expected milestones and screening for breastfeeding problems is an integral part of postpartum visits. According to adult education principles described in Chapter 23, this is a "teaching moment" in which the parents are highly receptive to information that helps them deal with practical life dilemmas.

Priority teaching for parents includes the following:

- Keep the baby close, and feed on cue around the clock.
- Be sure the baby is actually getting milk. Listen for audible swallowing. Finish the first breast before offering the second so that the baby will receive the creamier milk as the feeding progresses. Watch the baby for cues that he is finished with the feed. Do not limit the frequency or duration of feeds.
- Provide a phone number to call with questions or concerns, especially if the mother thinks the baby is not feeding well, or any nipple or breast pain occurs.
- Reinforce the mother's skill in breastfeeding with comments such as "You are making lots of good milk for your baby," "You are very responsive to your baby's need to be close and breastfed often," or "You look so comfortable and peaceful holding your baby skin to skin!"

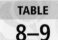

| TABLE 8–9 | **Safety Issues for Breastfeeding and Bed Sharing** |

Do **Practice Safety During Bed Sharing If**	*Do Not* **Bed Share All Night If**
Bed partners:	**Bed partners:**
Exclusively breastfeeding mother Conscious decision by both parents to bed share Nonsmoking (never smoke) Sober and drug free Parents of the baby No pets	Formula feeding or supplementing with formula Accidental bed sharing Any tobacco smoking, even outside Alcohol and/or drug use Nonparents; siblings Animals
Baby's position:	**Baby's position:**
Baby on his back (supine) Baby unwrapped, free to wiggle and move	Baby in prone or side-lying position Baby is swaddled or bundled in a blanket
Bedding/sleep surface:	**Bedding/sleep surface:**
Firm, flat, clean mattress No holes, spaces, or places that could trap baby Tightly fitting sheets under baby No pillows or blankets near baby's face No thick duvets or comforters Room comfortable temperature, not overheated	Couch or sofa; arm chair; soft or saggy mattress; waterbed Holes, spaces, or places that could trap baby Loose sheets or blankets under baby Pillows or blankets around baby Thick covers on or over baby Overheated room

Summary

The postpartum period is the time of transition from pregnancy to life with a child. Understanding normal patterns of breastfeeding helps lactation consultants identify problems and answer questions from parents and other professionals. Even when all is going well, mothers can benefit from additional support from peers, mother support groups, and lactation professionals.

Key Concepts

- The breastfeeding mother–baby dyad is a single psychobiological organism. The concept that "separation is harmful" replaces and supersedes the earlier understanding that "contact is advantageous."
- The number of feedings and the duration of feeding vary widely from mother to mother. However, reassuring signs of adequate infant intake include 8 to 12 or more effective feeds per day, profuse daily infant stools after day 4, and comfortable maternal breasts.
- The breastfed infant has a tendency to be wakeful, fussy, and want to breastfeed, frequently feeding in the late afternoon and evening. Parents should be reassured that this pattern is normal expected behavior.
- Abundant ongoing milk production depends on frequent, thorough removal of milk from the breast by the baby or by alternative means. Milk production calibrates to meet the infant's needs by about 6 weeks. About one-third of the milk available remains in the breasts over and above the baby's typical daily intake.
- Expecting breasts or babies to go for long stretches between large feeds is physiologically unrealistic, inappropriate, and counterproductive.
- Edema and milk stasis are two different phenomena and can occur simultaneously. The best prevention is immediate breastfeeding in the first hour after birth, and frequent effective breastfeeding thereafter.
- "Too much" or "too little" milk are often indicators of an underlying infant suckling problem. Before reducing milk volume, rule out infant factors.
- If a baby cannot latch and comfortably feed, keep the baby in nearly continuous skin-to-skin contact and help the mother express milk for the baby. Follow the family until the baby is feeding well.

- Early-onset nipple pain is often "mechanical" pain, related to improper infant latch or suck, nipple stretching and compression, or irritation from devices. Sudden-onset nipple pain after comfortable breastfeeding is often a sign of infection from bacteria, yeasts, or other organisms.
- Topical preparations do not prevent nipple pain nor speed healing. Gentle massage may increase milk flow during pumping or expressing milk.
- Pacifiers interfere, and should be avoided except in short-term, therapeutic situations.
- Infant stools change from black, tarry meconium to green and then to profuse, soft, yellow stools over the first week. In the first month or so, stools are passed every day. Over time, stools may become thicker and passed less often because of milk compositional changes.
- Jaundice is often a marker for poor feeding. Continued breastfeeding and/or feeding expressed milk is recommended for jaundiced infants.
- Breastfed babies who are fed on cue and held and carried many hours a day rarely cry. Crying is a late sign of distress and/or hunger. Crying is harmful for babies, and every effort should be made to immediately comfort and/or feed the baby.
- Sensitivity or allergy to cow's milk protein is a frequent cause of colic. Allergy to cow's milk protein or other foods calls for skilled and careful dietary management.
- Multiple infants have the same needs as any singleton. The mother's role is more complex because she must meet the needs of two or more newborns, and she is more likely to have had complications of pregnancy and childbirth, including requiring more time to recover physically.
- The risk of a subsequent pregnancy occurring during the first 6 months of exclusive or full breastfeeding is extremely low.

Internet Resources

Academy of Breastfeeding Medicine (ABM):
www.bfmed.org

American Academy of Pediatrics (AAP):
www.aap.org

Center for Evidence-Based Medicine:
www.cebm.net

Cochrane database/reviews of research on breast-feeding topics:
www.cochrane.org

International Lactation Consultant Association (ILCA):
www.ilca.org

La Leche League International (LLLI):
www.lalecheleague.org

Medline/PubMed:
www.ncbi.nlm.nih.gov/entrez/query.fcgi

US Centers for Disease Control and Prevention:
www.cdc.gov/breastfeeding

References

Aarts C et al. Breastfeeding patterns in relation to thumb sucking and pacifier use. *Pediatrics.* 1999;104(4):e50.

Abdulkader HM et al. Effect of suckling on the peripheral sensitivity of full-term newborn infants. *Arch Dis Fetal Neonatal Ed.* 2007;92:F130–F131.

Amir LH, James JP, Donath SM. Reliability of the Hazelbaker assessment tool for lingual frenulum function. *Int Breastfeed J.* 2006;1(1):3.

Anderson GC. Risk in mother-infant separation post-birth. *Image J Nurs Sch.* 1989;21:196–198.

Anderson GC et al. Early skin-to-skin contact for mothers and their healthy newborn infants. *Cochrane Database Syst Rev.* 2003(2):CD003519.

Anderson JE, Held N, Wright K. Raynaud's phenomenon of the nipple: a treatable cause of painful breast-feeding. *Pediatrics.* 2004;113(4):e360–e364.

Aney M. Babywise advice linked to dehydration, failure-to-thrive. *AAP News.* 1998;14(4):21.

Arthur PG, Smith M, Hartmann PE. Milk lactose, citrate, and glucose as markers of lactogenesis in normal and diabetic women. *J Pediatr Gastroenterol Nutr.* 1989;9(4):488–496.

Auer C, Gromada KK. A case report of breastfeeding quadruplets: factors perceived as affecting breast-feeding. *J Hum Lact.* 1998;14(2):135–141.

Baddock SA et al. Differences in infant and parent behaviors during routine bed sharing compared with cot sleeping in the home setting. *Pediatrics.* 2006; 117(5):1599–1607.

Baddock SA et al. Sleep arrangements and behavior of bed-sharing families in the home setting. *Pediatrics.* 2007;119(1):e200–e207.

Bains C. Breastfeeding a challenging dance: lots of patience required to help newborns nurse. *Winnipeg Free Press.* November 11, 2006:6.

Ball HL. Breastfeeding, bed-sharing, and infant sleep. *Birth.* 2003;30(3):181–188.

Ball HL et al. Randomised trial of infant sleep location on the postnatal ward. *Arch Dis Child.* 2006;91(12): 1005–1010.

Barak M et al. The prevalence of regurgitations in the first 2 days of life in human milk—and formula-fed infants. *Breastfeeding Med.* 2006;1(3):168–171.

Barr RG et al. Carrying as colic "therapy": a randomized controlled trial. *Pediatrics.* 1991;87(5):623–630.

Barr RG et al. Differential calming responses to sucrose taste in crying infants with and without colic. *Pediatrics.* 1999;103(5):e68.

Barros FC et al. Use of pacifiers is associated with decreased breast-feeding duration. *Pediatrics.* 1995; 95(4):497–499.

Barros FC et al. Breast feeding, pacifier use and infant development at 12 months of age: a birth cohort study in Brazil. *Paediatr Perinat Epidemiol.* 1997; 11(4):441–450.

Baumgarder DJ et al. Effect of labor epidural anesthesia on breast-feeding of healthy full-term newborns delivered vaginally. *J Am Board Fam Pract.* 2003; 16(1):7–13.

Beilin Y et al. Effect of labor epidural analgesia with and without fentanyl on infant breast-feeding: a prospective, randomized, double-blind study. *Anesthesiology.* 2005;103(6):1211–1217.

Berlin CM. "Exclusive" breastfeeding of quadruplets. *Breastfeed Med.* 2007;2(2):125–126.

Blair A et al. The relationship between positioning, the breastfeeding dynamic, the latching process and pain in breastfeeding mothers with sore nipples. *Breastfeed Rev.* 2003;11(2):5–10.

Blair AC, Smith LJ. Birth injuries and breastfeeding. Presented at: International Conference on the Theory and Practice of Human Lactation Management and Breastfeeding Research; 2007; Orlando, FL: Healthy Children/Center for Breastfeeding.

Blair PS, Ball HL. The prevalence and characteristics associated with parent-infant bed-sharing in England. *Arch Dis Child.* 2004;89(12):1106–1110.

Blair PS et al. Babies sleeping with parents: case-control study of factors influencing the risk of the sudden infant death syndrome. CESDI SUDI research group. *BMJ.* 1999;319(7223):1457–1461.

Blair PS et al. Major epidemiological changes in sudden infant death syndrome: a 20-year population-based study in the UK. *Lancet.* 2006;367(9507):314–319.

Bleyl J. Breastfeeding triplets: Personal reflections. In: Blickstein I, Keith L, eds. *Iatrogenic Multiple Pregnancy:*

Clinical Implications. New York, NY: Parthenon Publishing Group; 2001.

Bowers NA, Gromada KK. *Care of the Multiple-Birth Family: Pregnancy and Birth.* White Plains, NY: March of Dimes; 2005.

Bullough CH, Msuku RS, Karonde L. Early suckling and postpartum haemorrhage: controlled trial in deliveries by traditional birth attendants. *Lancet.* 1989;2(8662): 522–525.

Cadwell K. Latching-on and suckling of the healthy term neonate: breastfeeding assessment. *J Midwif Womens Health.* 2007;52(6):638–642.

Canivet CA et al. Infantile colic and the role of trait anxiety during pregnancy in relation to psychosocial and socioeconomic factors. *Scand J Public Health.* 2005;33(1):26–34.

Carbajal R et al. Analgesic effect of breast feeding in term neonates: randomised controlled trial. *BMJ.* 2003;326(7379):13.

Carpenter RG et al. Sudden unexplained infant death in 20 regions in Europe: case control study. *Lancet.* 2004;363(9404):185–191.

Carroccio A et al. Evidence of very delayed clinical reactions to cow's milk in cow's milk-intolerant patients. *Allergy.* 2000;55(6):574–579.

Cavataio F, Carroccio A, Iacono G. Milk-induced reflux in infants less than one year of age. *J Pediatr Gastroenterol Nutr.* 2000;30(Suppl):S36–S44.

Centuori S et al. Nipple care, sore nipples, and breast-feeding: a randomized trial. *J Hum Lact.* 1999; 15(2):125–130.

Chantry C et al. *ABM Protocol #6: Guideline on Cosleeping and Breastfeeding.* New Rochelle, NY: Academy of Breastfeeding Medicine; 2006.

Chapman DJ, Perez-Escamilla R. Identification of risk factors for delayed onset of lactation. *J Am Diet Assoc.* 1999;99(4):450–454; quiz 455–456.

Chen DC et al. Stress during labor and delivery and early lactation performance. *Am J Clin Nutr.* 1998; 68(2):335–344.

Chertok IR, Schneider J, Blackburn S. A pilot study of maternal and term infant outcomes associated with ultrathin nipple shield use. *J Obstet Gynecol Neonatal Nurs.* 2006;35(2):265–272.

Chikly B. *Silent Waves: Theory and Practice of Lymph Drainage Therapy.* 2nd ed. Scottsdale, AZ: IHH Publishing; 2004.

Christensson K et al. Temperature, metabolic adaptation and crying in healthy full-term newborns cared for skin-to-skin or in a cot. *Acta Paediatr.* 1992; 81(6-7):488–493.

Christensson K et al. Separation distress call in the human neonate in the absence of maternal body contact. *Acta Paediatr.* 1995;84(5):468–473.

Cotterman KJ. Reverse pressure softening: a simple tool to prepare areola for easier latching during engorgement. *J Hum Lact.* 2004;20(2):227–237.

Cox DB et al. Breast growth and the urinary excretion of lactose during human pregnancy and early lactation: endocrine relationships. *Exp Physiol.* 1999; 84(2):421–434.

Cregan MD, Hartmann PE. Computerized breast measurement from conception to weaning: clinical implications. *J Hum Lact.* 1999;15(2):89–96.

Daher S et al. Cow's milk protein intolerance and chronic constipation in children. *Pediatr Allergy Immunol.* 2001;12(6):339–342.

da Silva OP et al. Effect of domperidone on milk production in mothers of premature infants: a randomized, double-blind placebo controlled trial. *Can Med Assoc J.* 2001;164:17–21.

Daly SE, Owens RA, Hartmann PE. The short-term synthesis and infant-regulated removal of milk in lactating women. *Exp Physiol.* 1993;78(2):209–220.

Daly SE et al. Frequency and degree of milk removal and the short-term control of human milk synthesis. *Exp Physiol.* 1996;81(5):861–875.

de Carvalho M et al. Milk intake and frequency of feeding in breast fed infants. *Early Hum Dev.* 1982; 7(2):155–163.

Declercq E et al. *Listening to Mothers II: Report of the Second National US Survey of Women's Childbearing Experiences.* New York, NY: Childbirth Connection; 2006.

Dewey KG. Maternal and fetal stress are associated with impaired lactogenesis in humans. *J Nutr.* 2001; 131(11):3012S–3015S.

Dewey KG et al. Risk factors for suboptimal infant breastfeeding behavior, delayed onset of lactation, and excess neonatal weight loss. *Pediatrics.* 2003; 112(3 Pt 1):607–619.

Doan T et al. Breast-feeding increases sleep duration of new parents. *J Perinat Neonatal Nurs.* 2007;21(3): 200–206.

Dyson L, McCormick F, Renfrew MJ. Interventions for promoting the initiation of breastfeeding. *Cochrane Database Syst Rev.* 2005(2):CD001688.

Emde RN, Gaensbauer TJ, Harmon RJ. Emotional expression in infancy. Psychological issues. Monograph 37. New York, NY: International Universities Press; 1976.

Engstrom JL et al. Comparison of milk output from the right and left breasts during simultaneous pumping in mothers of very low birthweight infants. *Breastfeed Med.* 2007;2(2):83–91.

Enkin M et al. *A Guide to Effective Care in Pregnancy and Birth.* 3rd ed. New York, NY: Oxford University Press; 2000.

Estep DC, Kulczycki A Jr. Treatment of infant colic with amino acid-based infant formula: a preliminary study. *Acta Paediatr.* 2000;89(1):22–27.

Evans KC et al. Effect of caesarean section on breast milk transfer to the normal term newborn over the first week of life. *Arch Dis Child Fetal Neonatal Ed.* 2003;88(5):F380–F382.

Fleming P, Blair PS. Sudden Infant Death Syndrome and parental smoking. *Early Hum Dev.* 2007;83(11): 721–725.

Flower H. *Adventures in Tandem Nursing.* Schaumburg, IL: La Leche League International; 2003.

Foda MI et al. Composition of milk obtained from unmassaged versus massaged breasts of lactating mothers. *J Pediatr Gastroenterol Nutr.* 2004;38(5): 484–487.

Franco P et al. The influence of a pacifier on infants' arousals from sleep. *J Pediatr.* 2000;136(6):775–779.

Fraval MM. A pilot study: osteopathic treatment of infants with a sucking dysfunction. *J Am Acad Osteopath.* 1998;8(2):25–33.

Gagnon AJ et al. Indicators nurses employ in deciding to test for hyperbilirubinemia. *J Obstet Gynecol Neonatal Nurs.* 2001;30(6):626–633.

Gale CR, Martyn CN. Breastfeeding, dummy use, and adult intelligence. *Lancet.* 1996;347(9008):1072–1075.

Gartner LM, Herschel M. Jaundice and breastfeeding. *Pediatr Clin North Am.* 2001;48(2):389–399.

Gartner LM et al. Breastfeeding and the use of human milk. *Pediatrics.* 2005;115(2):496–506.

Geddes DT. Inside the lactating breast: the latest anatomy research. *J Midwif Womens Health.* 2007; 52(6):556–563.

Genna CW. *Supporting Sucking Skills in Breastfeeding Infants.* Sudbury, MA: Jones and Bartlett; 2008.

Gessner BD, Ives GC, Perham-Hester KA. Association between sudden infant death syndrome and prone sleep position, bed sharing, and sleeping outside an infant crib in Alaska. *Pediatrics.* 2001;108(4): 923–927.

Gray L et al. Breastfeeding is analgesic in healthy newborns. *Pediatrics.* 2002;109(4):590–593.

Greer FR, Sicherer SH, Burks AW. Effects of early nutritional interventions on the development of atopic disease in infants and children: the role of maternal dietary restriction, breastfeeding, timing of introduction of complementary foods, and hydrolyzed formulas. *Pediatrics.* 2008;121(1):183–191.

Griffiths DM. Do tongue ties affect breastfeeding? *J Hum Lact.* 2004;20(4):409–414.

Gromada KK. *Mothering Multiples.* 3rd Rev. ed. Schaumburg, IL: La Leche League International; 2007.

Gromada KK, Spangler AK. Breastfeeding twins and higher-order multiples. *J Obstet Gynecol Neonatal Nurs.* 1998;27(4):441–449.

Gupta SK. Is colic a gastrointestinal disorder? *Curr Opin Pediatr.* 2002;14(5):588–592.

Gupta SK. Update on infantile colic and management options. *Curr Opin Investig Drugs.* 2007;8(11):921–926.

Hall RT et al. A breast-feeding assessment score to evaluate the risk for cessation of breast-feeding by 7 to 10 days of age. *J Pediatr.* 2002;141(5):659–664.

Hauck FR. Pacifiers and sudden infant death syndrome: what should we recommend? *Pediatrics.* 2006; 117(5):1811–1812.

Hauck FR, Omojokun OO, Siadaty MS. Do pacifiers reduce the risk of sudden infant death syndrome? A meta-analysis. *Pediatrics.* 2005;116(5):e716–7e23.

Hauck FR et al. Sleep environment and the risk of sudden infant death syndrome in an urban population: the Chicago Infant Mortality Study. *Pediatrics.* 2003;111(5 Part 2):1207–1214.

Hill PD, Aldag JC. Milk volume on day 4 and income predictive of lactation adequacy at 6 weeks of mothers of nonnursing preterm infants. *J Perinat Neonatal Nurs.* 2005;19(3):273–282.

Hodnett E et al. Continuous support for women during childbirth. *Cochrane Database Syst Rev.* 2007(3): CD003766.

Horne RS et al. Arousal from sleep in infants is impaired following an infection. *Early Hum Dev.* 2002;66(2): 89–100.

Horne RS et al. Comparison of evoked arousability in breast and formula fed infants. *Arch Dis Child.* 2004;89(1):22–25.

Howard CR et al. The effects of early pacifier use on breastfeeding duration. *Pediatrics.* 1999b;103(3):E33.

Howard CR et al. Randomized clinical trial of pacifier use and bottle-feeding or cupfeeding and their effect on breastfeeding. *Pediatrics.* 2003;111(3): 511–518.

Howard CR et al. Parental responses to infant crying and colic: the effect on breastfeeding duration. 2006;1(3):146–155.

Hrdy SB. *Mother Nature: A History of Mothers, Infants, and Natural Selection.* New York, NY: Pantheon Books; 1999.

Huggins KE, Petok ES, Mireles O. Markers of lactation insufficiency: a study of 34 mothers. In: Auerbach KG, ed. *Current Issues In Clinical Lactation 2000.* Sudbury, MA: Jones and Bartlett Publishers; 2000.

Hughes CA et al. Birth trauma in the head and neck. *Arch Otolaryngol Head Neck Surg.* 1999;125(2):193–199.

Iacono G et al. Persistent cow's milk protein intolerance in infants: the changing faces of the same disease. *Clin Exp Allergy.* 1998;28(7):817–823.

ILCA. *Clinical Guidelines for the Establishment of Exclusive Breastfeeding.* Raleigh, NC: International Lactation Consultant Association; 2005.

Ip S et al. *Breastfeeding and Maternal and Infant Health Outcomes in Developed Countries.* Rockville, MD: Agency for Healthcare Research and Quality; 2007. AHRQ publication 07-E007.

Jacobs LA et al. Normal nipple position in term infants measured on breastfeeding ultrasound. *J Hum Lact.* 2007;23(1):52–59.

Jain L. Morbidity and mortality in late-preterm infants: more than just transient tachypnea! *J Pediatr.* 2007; 151(5):445–446.

Jensen RG. *Handbook of Milk Composition.* San Diego, CA: Academic Press; 1995.

Jones E, Dimmock PW, Spencer SA. A randomised controlled trial to compare methods of milk expression after preterm delivery. *Arch Dis Child Fetal Neonatal Ed.* 2001;85(2):F91–F95.

Jordan S et al. The impact of intrapartum analgesia on infant feeding. *BJOG.* 2005;112(7):927–934.

Karlstrom A et al. Postoperative pain after Cesarean birth affects breastfeeding and infant care. *JOGNN.* 2007;36:430–440.

Kent JC. How breastfeeding works. *J Midwif Womens Health.* 2007;52(6):564–570.

Kent JC et al. Volume and frequency of breastfeedings and fat content of breast milk throughout the day. *Pediatrics.* 2006;117(3):e387–e395.

Kroeger M, Smith LJ. *Impact of Birthing Practices on Breastfeeding: Protecting the Mother and Baby Continuum.* Sudbury, MA: Jones and Bartlett; 2004.

Kulski JK, Hartmann PE. Changes in human milk composition during the initiation of lactation. *Aust J Exp Biol Med Sci.* 1981;59(1):101–114.

Kunz C, Lonnerdal B. Re-evaluation of the whey protein/casein ratio of human milk. *Acta Paediatr.* 1992;81(2):107–112.

LaFleur EA, Niesen KM. Breastfeeding conjoined twins. *J Obstet Gynecol Neonatal Nurs.* 1996;25(3):241–244.

Lahr MB, Rosenberg KD, Lapidus JA. Bedsharing and maternal smoking in a population-based survey of new mothers. *Pediatrics.* 2005;116(4):e530–e542.

Lahr MB, Rosenberg KD, Lapidus JA. Maternal-infant bedsharing: risk factors for bedsharing in a population-based survey of new mothers and implications for SIDS risk reduction. *Matern Child Health J.* 2007;11(3):277–286.

Lavergne NA. Does application of tea bags to sore nipples while breastfeeding provide effective relief? *J Obstet Gynecol Neonatal Nurs.* 1997;26(1):53–58.

Lawrence RM, Lawrence R. *Breastfeeding—A Guide for the Medical Profession.* 6th ed. St. Louis, MO: CV Mosby; 2005. Appendix P.

Lehtonen J et al. The effect of nursing on the brain activity of the newborn. *J Pediatr.* 1998;132(4):646–651.

Leonard LG. Depression and anxiety disorders during multiple pregnancy and parenthood. *J Obstet Gynecol Neonatal Nurs.* 1998;27(3):329–337.

Leonard LG. *Breastfeeding Multiples.* Vancouver, BC: British Columbia Reproductive Care Program (BCRCP); 2007.

Levine A et al. Oxytocin during pregnancy and early postpartum: individual patterns and maternal–fetal attachment. *Peptides.* 2007;28(6):1162–1169.

Liang R, Gunn AJ, Gunn TR. Can preterm twins breast feed successfully? *N Z Med J.* 1997;110(1045):209–212.

Livingstone V, Stringer LJ. The treatment of *Staphyloccocus aureus* infected sore nipples: a randomized comparative study. *J Hum Lact.* 1999;15(3):241–246.

Ludington-Hoe SM et al. Neurophysiologic assessment of neonatal sleep organization: preliminary results of a randomized, controlled trial of skin contact with preterm infants. *Pediatrics.* 2006;117(5):e909–e923.

Madlon-Kay DJ. Home health nurse clinical assessment of neonatal jaundice: comparison of 3 methods. *Arch Pediatr Adolesc Med.* 2001;155(5):583–586.

Maisels MJ et al. Evaluation of a new transcutaneous bilirubinometer. *Pediatrics.* 2004;113(6):1628–1635.

Martin J. *Births: Final Data for 2005.* Hyattsville, MD: National Center for Health Statistics; 2007.

Mathur GP, Mathur S, Khanduja GS. Non-nutritive suckling and use of pacifiers. *Indian Pediatr.* 1990;27(11):1187–1189.

Mattos-Graner RO et al. Mutans streptococci oral colonization in 12–30-month-old Brazilian children over a one-year follow-up period. *J Public Health Dent.* 2001;61(3):161–167.

McKenna JJ. *Sleeping With Your Baby: A Parents's Guide to Cosleeping.* Washington, DC: Platypus Media; 2007.

McKenna JJ, McDade T. Why babies should never sleep alone: a review of the co-sleeping controversy in relation to SIDS, bedsharing and breast feeding. *Paediatr Respir Rev.* 2005;6(2):134–152.

McKenna JJ, Mosko SS, Richard CA. Bedsharing promotes breastfeeding. *Pediatrics.* 1997;100(2 Pt 1):214–219.

McVea KL, Turner PD, Peppler DK. The role of breastfeeding in sudden infant death syndrome. *J Hum Lact.* 2000;16(1):13–20.

Mead LJ et al. Breastfeeding success with preterm quadruplets. *J Obstet Gynecol Neonatal Nurs.* 1992;21(3):221–227.

Michelsson K et al. Crying in separated and non-separated newborns: sound spectrographic analysis. *Acta Paediatr.* 1996;85(4):471–475.

Miller V, Riordan J. Treating postpartum breast edema with areolar compression. *J Hum Lact.* 2004;20:223–226.

Mitchell EA, Blair PS, L'Hoir MP. Should pacifiers be recommended to prevent sudden infant death syndrome? *Pediatrics.* 2006;117(5):1755–1758.

Mitchell EA et al. Results from the first year of the New Zealand cot death study. *N Z Med J.* 1991;104(906):71–76.

Montgomery A, Hale TW. ABM clinical protocol #15: analgesia and anesthesia for the breastfeeding mother. *Breastfeed Med.* 2006;1(4):271–277.

Moon RY, Horne RS, Hauck FR. Sudden infant death syndrome. *Lancet.* 2007;370(9598):1578–1587.

Moscone SR, Moore MJ. Breastfeeding during pregnancy. *J Hum Lact.* 1993;9(2):83–88.

Neifert MR. Prevention of breastfeeding tragedies. *Pediatr Clin North Am.* 2001;48(2):273–297.

Neifert MR, McDonough SL, Neville MC. Failure of lactogenesis associated with placental retention. *Am J Obstet Gynecol.* 1981;140(4):477–478.

Nelson EA, Yu LM, Williams S. International Child Care Practices study: breastfeeding and pacifier use. *J Hum Lact.* 2005;21(3):289–295.

Neville MC, Morton J. Physiology and endocrine changes underlying human lactogenesis II. *J Nutr.* 2001;131(11):3005S–3008S.

Neville MC, Neifert M. *Lactation: Physiology, Nutrition and Breastfeeding.* New York, NY: Plenum Press; 1983.

Newman J. Handout #15: Breast Compression [Web page]. 2005. Available at: http://www.bflrc.com/newman/handouts/0501-HO15-Breast_Compression.htm. Accessed January 2, 2009.

Newton N. Nipple pain and nipple damage; problems in the management of breast feeding. *J Pediatr.* 1952;41(4):411–423.

Nommsen-Rivers LA et al. Newborn wet and soiled diaper counts and timing of onset of lactation as indicators of breastfeeding inadequacy. *J Hum Lact.* 2008;24:27–33.

Parker LA. Part 1: early recognition and treatment of birth trauma: injuries to the head and face. *Adv Neonatal Care.* 2005;5(6):288–297; quiz 298–300.

Parker LA. Part 2: Birth trauma: injuries to the intra-abdominal organs, peripheral nerves, and skeletal system. *Adv Neonatal Care.* 2006;6(1):7–14.

Paul K, Dittrichova J, Papousek H. Infant feeding behavior: development in patterns and motivation. *Dev Psychobiol.* 1996;29(7):563–576.

Pauli-Pott U et al. Infants with "Colic"-mothers' perspectives on the crying problem. *J Psychosom Res.* 2000;48(2):125–132.

Penders J et al. Factors influencing the composition of the intestinal microbiota in early infancy. *Pediatrics.* 2006;118(2):511–521.

Peres KG et al. Social and biological early life influences on the prevalence of open bite in Brazilian 6-year-olds. *Int J Paediatr Dent.* 2007;17(1):41–49.

Phillips RM, Chantry CJ, Gallagher MP. Analgesic effects of breast-feeding or pacifier use with maternal holding in term infants. *Ambul Pediatr.* 2005; 5(6):359–364.

Pollard K et al. Night-time non-nutritive sucking in infants aged 1 to 5 months: relationship with infant state, breastfeeding, and bed-sharing versus room-sharing. *Early Hum Dev.* 1999;56(2-3):185–204.

Quillin SI. Infant and mother sleep patterns during 4th postpartum week. *Issues Compr Pediatr Nurs.* 1997; 20(2):115–123.

Quillin SI, Glenn LL. Interaction between feeding method and co-sleeping on maternal-newborn sleep. *J Obstet Gynecol Neonatal Nurs.* 2004;33(5): 580–588.

Quinlan PT et al. The relationship between stool hardness and stool composition in breast- and formula-fed infants. *J Pediatr Gastroenterol Nutr.* 1995; 20(1):81–90.

Ramsay DT et al. Ultrasound imaging of milk ejection in the breast of lactating women. *Pediatrics.* 2004;113(2):361–367.

Ramsay DT et al. The use of ultrasound to characterize milk ejection in women using an electric breast pump. *J Hum Lact.* 2005;21(4):421–428.

Ramsay DT et al. Milk flow rates can be used to identify and investigate milk ejection in women expressing breast milk using an electric breast pump. *Breastfeed Med.* 2006;1(1):14–23.

Ransjo-Arvidson AB et al. Maternal analgesia during labor disturbs newborn behavior: effects on breast-feeding, temperature, and crying. *Birth.* 2001;28(1): 5–12.

Richard C et al. Sleeping position, orientation, and proximity in bedsharing infants and mothers. *Sleep.* 1996;19(9):685–690.

Ricke LA et al. Newborn tongue-tie: prevalence and effect on breast-feeding. *J Am Board Fam Pract.* 2005;18(1):1–7.

Righard L, Alade MO. Effect of delivery room routines on success of first breast-feed. *Lancet.* 1990; 336(8723):1105–1107.

Righard L, Alade MO. Breastfeeding and the use of pacifiers. *Birth.* 1997;24(2):116–120.

Riordan J, Gill-Hopple J, Angeron J. Indicators of effective breastfeeding and estimates of breast milk intake. *J Hum Lact.* 2005;21:406–412.

Saint L, Maggiore P, Hartmann PE. Yield and nutrient content of milk in eight women breast-feeding twins and one woman breast-feeding triplets. *Br J Nutr.* 1986;56(1):49–58.

Salvatore S, Vandenplas Y. Gastroesophageal reflux and cow milk allergy: is there a link? *Pediatrics.* 2002;110(5):972–984.

Santo LC, de Oliveira LD, Giugliani ER. Factors associated with low incidence of exclusive breastfeeding for the first 6 months. *Birth.* 2007;34(3):212–219.

Schore AN. Effects of a secure attachment relationship on right brain development, affect regulation, and infant mental health. *Infant Ment Health J.* 2001a; 22(1):7–66.

Scott JA, Binns CW, Oddy WH. Predictors of delayed onset of lactation. *Matern Child Nutr.* 2007;3(3): 186–193.

Shah PS, Aliwalas LI, Shah V. Breastfeeding or breast milk for procedural pain in neonates. *Cochrane Database Syst Rev.* 2006;3:CD004950.

Shealy K et al. *The CDC Guide to Breastfeeding Interventions.* Atlanta, GA: Centers for Disease Control and Prevention; 2005.

Shrago LC, Reifsnider E, Insel K. The Neonatal Bowel Output Study: indicators of adequate breast milk intake in neonates. *Pediatr Nurs.* 2006;32(3): 195–201.

Smillie CMM. Baby-Led Breastfeeding: The Mother-Baby Dance [DVD]. Geddes Production; 2007.

Smith LJ. Impact of birthing practices on the breastfeeding dyad. *J Midwif Womens Health.* 2007;52(6): 621–630.

Snowden HM, Renfrew MJ, Woolridge MW. Treatments for breast engorgement during lactation. *Cochrane Database Syst Rev.* 2001(2):CD000046.

Snyder JB. *Variation in Infant Palatal Structure and Breastfeeding.* Pasadena, CA: Pacific Oaks College; 1995.

Sondergaard C et al. Psychosocial distress during pregnancy and the risk of infantile colic: a follow-up study. *Acta Paediatr.* 2003;92(7):811–816.

Spencer SA, Jones E, Dobson J et al. *Breastfeeding: A Multimedia Learning Resource for Healthcare Professionals.* Bradford: Matrix Multimedia; 1998.

Srinivasan A et al. Ankyloglossia in breastfeeding infants: the effect of frenotomy on maternal nipple pain and latch. *Breastfeeding Med.* 2006;1(4):216–224.

St James-Roberts I. What is distinct about infants' "colic" cries? *Arch Dis Child.* 1999;80(1):56–61; discussion 62.

Stark Y. *Human Nipples: Function and Anatomical Variations in Relationship to Breastfeeding.* Pasadena, CA: Pacific Oaks College; 1993.

Stellwagen L, Hubbard E, Vaux K. Look for the "stuck baby" to identify congenital torticollis. *Contemp Pediatr.* 2004:21–55.

Task Force on Sudden Infant Death. The changing concept of sudden infant death syndrome: diagnostic coding shifts, controversies regarding the sleeping environment, and new variables to consider in reducing risk. *Pediatrics.* 2005;116(5):1245–1255.

Thorley V. Latch and the fear response: overcoming an obstacle to successful breastfeeding. *Breastfeed Rev.* 2005;13(1):9–11.

Torvaldsen S et al. Intrapartum epidural analgesia and breastfeeding: a prospective cohort study. *Int Breastfeed J.* 2006;1:24.

UNICEF, WHO. *BFHI: Revised and Updated Materials.* New York, NY: UNICEF; 2006.

Uvnas-Moberg K, Eriksson M. Breastfeeding: physiological, endocrine and behavioural adaptations caused by oxytocin and local neurogenic activity in the nipple and mammary gland. *Acta Paediatr.* 1996;85(5):525–530.

Uvnas-Moberg K et al. Oxytocin and prolactin levels in breast-feeding women. Correlation with milk yield and duration of breast-feeding. *Acta Obstet Gynecol Scand.* 1990;69(4):301–306.

Van der Wijden C, Kleijnen J, Van den Berk T. Lactational amenorrhea for family planning. *Cochrane Database Syst Rev.* 2003(4):CD001329.

van Sleuwen BE et al. Swaddling: a systematic review. *Pediatrics.* 2007;120(4):e1097–1106.

Vanderhoof JA et al. Allergic constipation: association with infantile milk allergy. *Clin Pediatr (Phila).* 2001;40(7):399–402.

Vogel AM, Hutchison BL, Mitchell EA. The impact of pacifier use on breastfeeding: a prospective cohort study. *J Paediatr Child Health.* 2001;37(1):58–63.

Walker M. *Breastfeeding Management for the Clinician: Using the Evidence.* Sudbury, MA: Jones and Bartlett; 2006.

Wall V, Glass R. Mandibular asymmetry and breastfeeding problems: experience from 11 cases. *J Hum Lact.* 2006;22(3):328–334.

Wambach K et al. Clinical lactation practice: 20 years of evidence. *J Hum Lact.* 2005;21(3):245–258.

Weber MW, Clinical Signs Study Group. Clinical signs that predict severe illness in children under age 2 months: a multicenter study. *Lancet.* 2008;371:135–142.

Weiss PP, Kerbl R. The relatively short duration that a child retains a pacifier in the mouth during sleep: implications for sudden infant death syndrome. *Eur J Pediatr.* 2001;160(1):60.

Wessel MA et al. Paroxysmal fussing in infancy, sometimes called colic. *Pediatrics.* 1954;14(5):421–435.

Wiberg JM, Nordsteen J, Nilsson N. The short-term effect of spinal manipulation in the treatment of infantile colic: a randomized controlled clinical trial with a blinded observer. *J Manipulative Physiol Ther.* 1999;22(8):517–522.

Widstrom AM, Thingstrom-Paulsson J. The position of the tongue during rooting reflexes elicited in newborn infants before the first suckle. *Acta Paediatr.* 1993;82(3):281–283.

Wilson-Clay B, Hoover K. The breastfeeding atlas. Austin, TX: LactNews Press; 2005.

Wolf LS, Glass RB. *Feeding and Swallowing Disorders in Infancy: Assessment and Management.* Tucson, AZ: Therapy Skill Builders; 1992.

Zangen S et al. Rapid maturation of gastric relaxation in newborn infants. *Pediatr Res.* 2001;50(5):629–632.

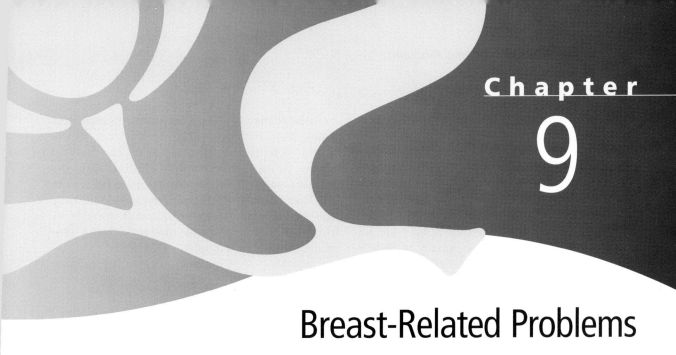

9

Breast-Related Problems

Jan Riordan and Karen Wambach

AN OUNCE OF PREVENTION is worth a pound of intervention. Many difficulties women encounter while breastfeeding can be prevented by the self-care measures and breastfeeding education discussed in preceding chapters. When a woman fully understands how her body works, she is at less risk for frustration and failure when she encounters a barrier to breastfeeding. This chapter deals with specific breast problems and identifies how health professionals can help.

Clinicians who work with breastfeeding women agree that breast and nipple problems can be common barriers to breastfeeding. During prenatal visits, women should be screened for unusual looking breasts, areolas, or nipples and lack of breast enlargement. Any of these, coupled with previous breastfeeding difficulties, are high-risk indicators for breastfeeding problems.

Before discussing the more clinical aspects of breast-related problems, including surgery, it is important to address the emotional significance of the female breasts. Breasts are part of a woman's internalized body image that she develops around adolescence and carries with her for the rest of her life. They represent a woman's deepest sense of womanhood. Any change in her breasts (e.g., breast surgery) threatens this feminine internal view of self

and creates disequilibrium. When a woman's breasts are altered by illness or infection, it can be a "double whammy": both her femininity and her ability to breastfeed can be threatened.

Nipple Variations

Inverted or Flat Nipples

There are two types of nipple inversion: (1) retractile/umbilicated where the nipple can be pulled out (everted), and (2) invaginated ("true" inversion) where the nipple cannot be everted. About 3 percent of Korean women have nipple inversion. Most of these are retractile (73–92 percent) and are bilateral (Park, Yoon, & Kim, 1999) (see Color Plates 47 and 48). Congenital inversion probably results from a failure of the underlying mesenchyme to proliferate and move the nipple out of its normally depressed position.

Retractile inversion sometimes resolves itself from the beginning to the end of pregnancy. In many cases, the degree of inversion is such that it does not affect the ability of the baby to grasp the areolar tissue and draw the nipple into the mouth, although this action might take longer. Lactation consultants have observed that women who have markedly inverted nipples early in their first pregnancy and who breastfeed have much less inversion with subsequent pregnancies. In some cases, these women have reported that their nipples, which initially inverted between feedings with the first baby, no longer do so with second and later infants.

The degree to which inverted nipples are an impediment to breastfeeding is partially caused by the belief that they prevent breastfeeding. How the nipple looks when it is not in the baby's mouth, however, does not always predict how well it functions. In most cases, as long as the mother positions the baby well back on the areola so that the entire nipple is placed well back in the baby's mouth, there is no reason why a mother with inverted nipples should forgo breastfeeding. During suckling, the nipple elongates to double its resting length (Smith, Erenberg, & Nowak, 1988). Such reactivity to infant suckling helps to explain by inference why the degree of inversion appears to lessen after weeks or months of repeated suckling by the infant.

When the clinician examines the mother's breasts and nipples in the third trimester of pregnancy, discussion about breastfeeding can continue. If the mother has flat or inverted nipples at that time, she can be taught that following birth, exercising the nipple just before latching on by a newborn appears to loosen the nipple tissue and helps to separate adhesions that cause retraction or inversion. Commercial "nipple enhancers" designed to evert flat or inverted nipples are available for purchase (Maternal Concepts, 2003). The infant also stretches the nipples during feedings.

Hoffman's exercises (exercises of the nipples during pregnancy) and breast shells, two traditional methods for treating inverted nipples, appear to be ineffective and are no longer recommended (Alexander, Grant, & Campbell, 1992).

The first intervention for treating a retractable inverted or flat nipple should be to stimulate and shape the nipple just before the feeding. For a flat nipple (not inverted), massage the nipple or apply a cold cloth to help the nipple to evert outward. For an inverted nipple, instruct the mother to shape her nipple by placing her thumb about 1.5 to 2 inches behind the nipple (with her fingers beneath) and pulling back into her chest. This works best in a side-lying position. Any pump can be used to help pull out the nipple immediately before the infant feeds. Placing a silicone nipple shield (described in Chapter 12) on the inverted nipple is another method of dealing with the problem of the baby not being able to latch onto the breast because of nipple inversion. The baby can usually ingest sufficient breastmilk through the thin shield, and at the same time his suckling stimulates the mother's nipples.

Absence of Nipple Pore Openings

Very rarely, duct pore openings on the mother's nipple are absent. Two cases have been reported. In one case, the mother's right breast enlarged abnormally starting her third month of pregnancy. Following delivery of her baby, the breast became extremely engorged and she was unable to express any milk from that breast. An ultrasound revealed that she had no nipple pores and no ducts leading from the nipple to the larger ducts, which caused extreme enlargement of the right breast. (Her left breast was normal.) Cosmetic surgery was offered to this mother, but because she was newly emigrated from India and had no insurance, she refused the surgery (V. Miller, personal communication, June 2003). The other reported was similar. Despite many attempts to breastfeed and then to pump, a Korean mother was unable to express even one drop of breastmilk.

Large or Elongated Nipples

Nipples come in assorted sizes and shapes and, like all anatomical structures, are genetically influenced. Clinicians report that Asian women are more likely to have unusually long nipples. Generally, nipples that are larger or longer than normal are less likely to cause problems in breastfeeding than are inverted or flat nipples. In fact, they are often viewed as an anatomical gift that will make breastfeeding easier. Although this is true in many cases, exceptionally long or large nipples (See Color Plate 45) may detract from breastfeeding, especially if the infant is small. Infants of mothers with extra-long nipples have been observed to gag after latch-on and to slide back toward the nipple tip (See Color Plate 46), which in some cases causes the mother to develop sore nipples.

Plugged Ducts

No one knows the specific cause of plugged ducts, but they are usually found in mothers who have an abundant milk supply and who do not adequately drain each breast. Pathological changes within the breast that cause the plug are vaguely referred to in the literature as a stasis, clogging of milk, or local accumulations of milk or dead cells that have been shed. A plugged duct is indicated by either of these two sets of symptoms: complaints of tenderness, heat, and possible redness in one area of the breast, or (if the plug is located in a duct close to the skin) a palpable lump of well-defined margins without a generalized fever. Sometimes, a tiny white milk plug can be seen at the opening of the duct on the nipple. One mother described it as "little bits of a hard white substance" that is just beneath the surface of milk duct outlets. Color Plate 11 shows a milk plug.

Clinicians are aware of a higher frequency of plugged ducts during the winter season. Although the reason for this is not clear, it may be related to the restricting effects of winter clothing or simply to the cold weather. There is also some evidence that, whereas some women are predisposed to developing plugged ducts, others never encounter it through multiple breastfeeding experiences. Plugged ducts can also lead to mastitis, especially if ignored or untreated. Box 9–1 presents self-care measures to recommend to a mother with a plugged duct.

In acute situations, briskly massaging the breast effectively dislodges the blocked milk. If a mother has chronically recurring plugged ducts, some physicians elect to open the duct with a sterile needlelike instrument. After this is done, the milk may forcibly shoot out from the duct, giving the mother relief, or strings of coalesced milk may be the "plug" that is released. It should be noted that this procedure can be followed by recurring pain in the affected area and should be done only in extreme cases.

Incomplete drainage caused by a skipped feeding or a constricting bra, poor nutrition, and stress have

---

BOX 9–1

Self-Care for Treating a Plugged Duct

- Continue to breastfeed often. Begin feeding on the affected breast to promote drainage.
- Depress the breast during the feed to prevent plugged ducts (Fetherston, 1998).
- Massage the affected breast before and during feeding to stimulate flow of milk. Support the breast with a cupped hand and use firm massage, starting at the periphery of the breast, using thumb to encourage flow of milk while baby suckles. (Another option is to massage the breast in a hot shower or bath.) Outside of the shower, try using an electric vibrator (on low setting).

- Soak the affected breast(s) by leaning over a basin of warm water, and gently massaging them.
- Change position of the infant during feedings to ensure drainage of all the sinuses and ductules in the breast. At least one position should result in the baby's nose being pointed toward the site of the plugged duct.
- Avoid any constricting clothing, such as an underwire bra or the straps on a baby carrier.
- Try taking lecithin, an oily substance, 1 tb/day (found in health food stores) (Lawrence & Lawrence, 1999, p. 273).

all been implicated in the development of plugged ducts, but a cause-and-effect relationship has never been substantiated. Assessment should include a review of these possibilities with the mother and a review of events leading up to the plugged duct, especially if the mother has a repeated problem. There is no need for an antibiotic to treat a plugged duct unless a fever and mastitis develop.

Mastitis

Lactation mastitis can develop during the early postpartum weeks after the mother leaves the hospital. Nurses and lactation consultants who practice in a clinic may be the first to speak with the mother whose symptoms suggest early indication of mastitis. The advice dispensed during this initial call can prevent the condition from advancing to an abscess, especially if the mother mistakenly thinks she should stop breastfeeding or has already done so.

Mastitis is usually a benign, self-limiting infection, with few consequences for the suckling infant. The initial symptoms of puerperal mastitis are fatigue, localized breast tenderness, headache, and flulike muscle aches (Wambach, 2003). If a breastfeeding mother complains that she has the "flu," the first consideration is to rule out infectious mastitis. Typically, fever, a rapid pulse, and the appearance of a hot, reddened, and tender area on the breast follow fatigue, headache, and muscular aching (see Color Plate 19). The infection is usually unilateral and located in one area (usually in the upper outer breast quadrant because most of the breast tissue is there), although it can occur in any area of the breast (Wambach, 2003). It can occasionally occur in both breasts simultaneously and may involve a large portion of the breast.

In worldwide studies published within the last 10 years, the incidence of lactation mastitis ranged from 4 to 27 percent depending on methods, especially subject selection, used in the study (Amir et al., 2007; Fetherston, 1995; Foxman et al., 2002; Vogel et al., 1999). Mastitis is most likely to occur in the first several weeks after delivery (Amir, 1999; Amir et al., 2007; Potter, 2005; Wambach, 2003). About one third of the cases in long-term breastfeeding mothers occur after the infant is 6 months old (Riordan & Nichols, 1990). The risk of mastitis is higher among women who have breastfed

previously, especially those with a history of mastitis (Foxman et al., 2002; Wambach, 2003)— thus removing an enduring myth that mastitis results from inexperience with breastfeeding. Symptoms last approximately 2 to 5 days. Breast pain and redness peak on days 2 and 3 and return to normal by day 5. Fatigue is the slowest symptom to dissipate. A number of risk factors predispose a woman to mastitis:

- Stress and fatigue (Fetherston, 1998; Riordan & Nichols, 1990): Mothers who had mastitis rate stress and fatigue as major factors leading to the infection; typically they describe themselves as exhausted as a result of circumstances above and beyond the normal stresses of taking care of the infant—for example, getting ready for holiday celebrations.
- Cracked or fissured nipples, and nipple pain (Amir et al., 2007; Fetherston, 1998; Foxman, Schwartz, & Looman, 1994; Vogel et al., 1999): A breakdown in the epidermis provides an avenue of entry into the breast tissue, although breakdown is not a prerequisite for a breast infection. Mastitis from sore, cracked nipples usually occurs in the first few weeks postpartum.
- Plugged or blocked ducts (Fetherston, 1998): Some women repeatedly develop plugged ducts, some of which lead to a full-blown infection. It is not uncommon to be able to see this plug as a white "head" and to feel pressure and tenderness around the plug. Gentle massage above the area of tenderness while the baby is breastfeeding from that breast may help, particularly if the plug is newly formed.
- Ample milk supply and/or decrease in number of feedings (Vogel et al., 1999): Women with an abundant milk supply experience more plugged ducts (and subsequent mastitis) than those with a normal supply.
- Engorgement and stasis: A decrease in the frequency of feedings presents the potential for engorgement or milk stasis. Infrequent feedings and milk stasis is frequently mentioned in the literature as being associated with mastitis. But there is little evidence that this is true. In fact, at least one researcher (Foxman et al., 2002) discovered that women without a history of mastitis who fed six or fewer times a

day had a rate of mastitis five times lower than those who fed 10 or more times a day. The daily use of a pacifier was associated with a *reduced* risk for mastitis in another study (Vogel et al., 1999)—just the opposite of conventional wisdom. Although it is logical to assume that the natural washing mechanism associated with breastmilk removal helps remove bacteria, bacteria can adhere to the epithelial cells lining the duct especially if there is trauma (Fetherston, 2001). Moreover, the presence of bacteria in milk is normal and breastmilk is not a good medium for bacterial growth.

Other conditions, such as breast trauma, constriction from tight bra or sleeping position (Fetherston, 1998), using a manual pump (Foxman et al., 2002), poor maternal nutrition, and vigorous exercise (particularly of the upper arms and chest) have been mentioned anecdotally as factors leading up to mastitis. These also should be noted in the assessment and history in the event that they predispose the mother to mastitis.

Treatment for Mastitis

The treatments for hastening recovery include continued breastfeeding, application of moist heat, increased fluids, bed rest, pain medication (acetaminophen, ibuprofen) and the judicious use of antibiotics (Table 9–1). It is well established in the medical literature that mastitis is most commonly associated with the presence of *Staphylococcus aureus*. However, if a culture is done, bacteria normally present on the skin (Coagulase-negative staphylococci, non-B-hemolytic streptococci) may be the only isolates in the milk culture. Osterman and Rahm (2000) compared mastitis symptoms according to bacteria found in a milk culture by dividing a sample of women with mastitis into two groups: Group A had only the bacteria normally present on the skin. Group B's culture contained potential pathogenic bacteria. The only differences in symptoms between the two groups were that women with pathogenic bacteria in their milk were more likely to have sore nipples before the mastitis and to develop the mastitis earlier postdelivery than those with normal bacteria. There were no differences in other symptoms such as fever and shivering.

Only rarely is a streptococcus involved; when it is, it may be present in breastmilk without causing clinical mastitis. Treatment with antibiotics can eradicate the organism from the milk (Oliver et al., 2000). Although untreated cases heal almost as quickly as treated ones, the standard antibiotic for lactation mastitis is a penicillinase-resistant penicillin or a cephalosporin that covers *S. aureus* for 6 to 10 days.

For chronic mastitis, erythromycin at low doses (regular 250–500 mg doses every 6 hours) or trimethoprim-sulfamethoxazole (Bactrim, Septra) over

TABLE 9–1	**Selected Antibiotics for Mastitis**	
Generic Name	**Trade Name**	**Adult Dosage Ranges**
Penicillinase-Resistant Penicillins		
Amoxicillin + clavulanate	Augmentin	875 mg 2× daily
Cloxacillin	Cloxapen, Tegopen	250–500 mg PO q6h
Dicloxacillin	Dynapen	125–250 mg PO or IM q6h
Flucloxacillin	Flucil	250–500 mg 4× daily
Oxacillin	Prostaphlin	500 mg–1 gm PO or IM q4–6h
Cephalosporins		
Cephalexin	Keflex	250–500 mg PO q6h
Cephradine	Velosef	250–500 mg PO q6h
Cefaclor	Ceclor	250–500 mg PO q8h

a longer period of time have been recommended (Cantlie, 1988). However, staphylococci rapidly develop resistance against erythromycin. Trimethoprim-sulfamethoxazole and erythromycin are also options when the mother is allergic to penicillin. In a case report, trimethoprim-sulfamethoxazole (2 tablets per day for 10 days) was effective in preventing recurrence of mastitis in a patient with multiple incidences of mastitis who was allergic to penicillin (Hoffman & Auerbach, 1986). These medications can be taken during breastfeeding without known untoward reactions in the infant.

Eglash and Proctor (2007) reported a case of bacterial lactiferous duct infection. Initial antibiotic choice was clindamycin 300 mg every 6 hours. Two weeks later the patient reported a lack of improvement and a painful right nipple crack that was worsening. The woman was treated with 14 days of fluconazole in addition to clindamycin. Two weeks later she reported feeling no better, and she was taken off clindamycin and fluconazole and treated with azithromycin 500 mg daily for 5 days. One week later the patient called to report that the nipple cracks were healing, and she had less breast pain. After 2 more weeks of azithromycin, the patient called to say that all of her pain was resolved, her nipple crack was almost healed and she was fully nursing her baby. The authors concluded that lactating women with chronic breast pain who have suspected bacterial lactiferous duct infection might need 4–8 weeks of an antibiotic that will cover *S. aureus*.

In the dairy industry, giving antioxidants such as vitamin E to cows is commonly recognized for preventing mastitis. Echinacea, one of the most popular herbal remedies, stimulates the immune system and may help to keep the infection in check (Binns, 2000). Mothers with mastitis reported taking vitamin C supplements (Wambach, 2003) to fight infection.

Another new alternative treatment for mastitis is the application of a solution of bacteriocin nisin to the nipple and areola. Nisin, a food-grade antimicrobial peptide, produced by strains of *Lactococcus lactis*, shows promise as an alternative to antibiotics for the treatment of staphylococcal mastitis (Fernandez et al., 2008).

Oxytocin nasal spray and acupuncture are used to treat mastitis in Sweden at the discretion of the midwife. Oxytocin nasal spray, used in the belief that drainage of the breast will be aided by the contractual effect of oxytocin on the lactiferous ducts, did hasten recovery from mastitis (Kvist et al., 2007). Acupuncture relieved the severity of symptoms in the same study) but did not reduce the number of contact days needed with healthcare services in order for inflammatory symptoms to subside (Kvist et al. 2007).

A mother with mastitis feels ill and is often emotional and discouraged (Amir & Lumley, 2006). She may ask, "Why does this have to happen to me?" and she may contemplate weaning. In addition, her supply of milk in the affected breast may be diminished for several weeks following the infection. She needs mothering herself, a role that the lactation specialist can assume as she reassures the mother that the infection will eventually resolve. To stop or limit breastfeeding will only increase the risk of infection or recurrence. Tender loving care goes a long way in helping her through this difficult time. She also needs specific advice and a plan for care (Table 9–2) as well as a long-term plan for self-care. A considerable number of mothers develop mastitis more than once during the course of lactation. Therefore, certain women may be prone to the condition, and prevention is important. Review with the mother all the possible factors that preceded and may have contributed to her bout(s) of mastitis. Then encourage the mother to seek medical help early if symptoms recur. Some mothers, especially if they are experienced long-term breastfeeders, do not consult their physicians, even though their mastitis warrants medical attention.

Types and Severity of Mastitis

Attempts have been made to classify types of mastitis. Generally, the distinctions are based on severity of symptoms and whether antibiotics should be started. Gibberd (1953), for instance, described two types of mastitis: cellulitis and adenitis. Cellulitis is thought to involve the interlobular connective tissue that has been infected by the introduction of bacteria through cracked nipples; it is treated with antibiotics. In adenitis, the breast ducts are presumably blocked, and the clinical symptoms are less severe. Treatment involves getting the milk flowing with heat, expression, and pumping. Antibiotics are used only if the infection is not resolving (Livingstone, 1990).

TABLE 9–2	**Mastitis Teaching Plan**	

Content-Goal	Teaching
Prevention	
Reduction of stress and fatigue related to childbearing responsibilities	Prioritize tasks from most important to least important. Encourage other family members to assist in routine household tasks. Hire household help if possible. Delay return to job as long as possible. Hold one informal open house for friends and relatives to see new baby. Use voicemail to filter calls. Turn down social invitations. Ignore e-mail. Take day naps when infant sleeps.
Plugged ducts	Breastfeed often (at least 8 to 12 times per day). Massage any reddened area of breast, especially while breastfeeding.
Change in number of feedings	Pump or express milk if a feeding is skipped.
Engorgement-stasis	Pump or express milk if breasts become overfull or distended. Wear bras without support underwires.
Care If Mastitis Occurs	
Self-care and relief of discomfort	Recognize early signs and symptoms: redness, fatigue, fever, chills. Rest with infant and fluids at bedside. Continue frequent breast-feedings.
Medical care	Monitor oral temperature. Place moist, warm packs at place of infection and over nipple. Expect slightly reduced milk supply in affected breast postinfection. Take antibiotics if needed. (They may not be necessary if fever is already subsiding.) Take antipyretic to reduce fever.

Subclinical lactation mastitis is a condition only recently described. While testing breastmilk of women in Bangladesh and Tanzania to determine vitamin A levels, Willumsen et al. (2000) found a quarter of the women tested had both a raised sodium–potassium ratio and elevated interleukin-8 (IL-8) indicating an infection without clinical symptoms. Fetherston (2001) challenged the idea of a subclinical infection by pointing out that a high sodium level in breastmilk without other symptoms is not a reliable indicator for an infection or a subclinical infection. There are known confounding factors where sodium is normally higher, such as initiation of lactation, involution, and pregnancy. Subclinical mastitis is presumably associated with an increase in the HIV load in breastmilk and could lead to higher rates of mother-to-child transmission of HIV (see Chapter 6).

Infectious versus noninfectious mastitis is another proposed classification. Noninfectious mastitis occurs when milk is not removed from the breast and milk production slows and infection results if milk stasis remains unresolved (i.e., the milk is not "washed" out of the breasts) (World Health Organization, 2000). Thomsen et al. (1985) proposed three classifications of mastitis—milk stasis, noninfectious inflammation, and infectious mastitis—based on leukocyte counts in milk from the infected breast. They recommended that antibiotic treatment be used only for infectious mastitis, the most severe classification. Although this taxonomy is helpful in theory, laboratory studies on mastitic milk are seldom done in practice. By the time the mother reports the problem to a healthcare provider, she usually has been ill for several hours, if not a day or two; the peak of the infectious process may have already passed, and she is getting well by the time she seeks medical treatment. There are other drawbacks: (1) leukocyte counts do not always correspond with bacterial counts (Fetherston, 2001), (2) the milk sample must be collected before any antibiotics are started, (3) laboratory studies take several days, and (4) the testing expense may not be covered by health insurance. Whatever the classification of mastitis, the mother suffering from symptoms clearly needs to be treated. If she has repeated mastitis, a culture of her milk and a review of risk factors are indicated.

Breastmilk composition changes during a breast infection (Table 9–3) (Fetherston, Lai, & Hartmann, 2006). Levels of some anti-inflammatory components, such as lactoferrin and sIgA rise to protect the baby from untoward effects from consuming mastitic milk (Buescher & Hair, 2001). Elevated levels of sodium and chloride caused by the temporary opening of the normally tight junctions between secretory cells in the paracellular pathways cause the breastmilk to taste salty. Sodium, chloride, and lactose are increased even when women have recovered from systemic symptoms. After the resolution of mastitis, the affected breast undergoes a temporary "resting" phase and usually produces less milk than it did before the infection.

In determining how a breast infection should be treated, it would be helpful to know the severity of the infection. With that in mind, investigators (Fetherston, Wells, & Hartmann, 2006) measured levels of serum C-reactive protein and compared them with mastitis symptoms since C-reactive protein is a marker of infection. They found that although an increasing severity of breast and systemic symptoms in mastitis was predictive of an increase of serum C-reactive protein in milk and blood, the presence of serum C-reactive protein in similar concentrations in both the mastitic and asymptomatic breast suggests it is of little use in making a differential diagnosis between infective versus noninfective forms of mastitis.

When a lactating woman has recurrent mastitis that does not respond to antibiotic therapy, inflammatory carcinoma must be ruled out. Inflammatory breast cancer can be mistaken for mastitis because the symptoms of an inflamed, edematous breast are similar. Breast cancer is different from mastitis because inflammatory carcinoma rarely produces fever, there is no palpable mass, and the symptoms

TABLE 9–3 **Breast Milk Components in Mastitis Compared with "Healthy" Asymptomatic Breasts**

Milk Component	Mastitis Breast (estimated mean)	"Healthy" Breast (estimated mean)
Sodium (mmol/L)	21.8	14
Chloride (mmol/L)	30	21
Lactose (mmol/L)	159	174
Glucose (mmol/L)	1.39	1.6
Lactoferrin (g/L)	3.45	3.2
sIgA (g/L)	1.22	1.25

Source: Adapted from Fetherston CM, Lai CT, Hartmann PE. Relationships between symptoms and changes in breast physiology during lactation mastitis. *Breastfeed Med.* 2006;3;136–145.

do not respond to antibiotic treatment. This woman should be referred to a surgeon experienced in this area who will perform a biopsy and other laboratory diagnostic tests to determine if inflammatory carcinoma is present (Merchant, 2002). If it is, lactation is a secondary consideration, as the mother will need intensive treatments that will preclude lactation.

Breast Abscess

A small percentage of breast infections develop into an abscess. The incidence is decreasing probably because we are more educated in prevention of abscess (Vogel et al., 1999). Amir et al. (2004) reported 3 percent of the women with mastitis in her sample developed an abscess, also noting the lower incidence than previously reported in the literature. An abscess, like a boil, is basically a collection of pus that must be drained (see Color Plates 13, 16, and 17). If the abscess is small, the pus may be aspirated with a fine needle under ultrasound guidance. According to Merchant (2002), ultrasound may be helpful but drainage is usually not performed after the ultrasound, even with symptoms of an abscess. Merchant contended "the erythema, tenderness, and induration can become worse and that breast necrosis may be considerable before adequate drainage is done." For a larger abscess, the physician makes an incision and drains the area. Love (2000) offers this advice:

> Surgeons never sew up a drained abscess; that would lock bacteria into the cavity, and almost ensure the infection's return. I'd tell my patients to go home and rest; then, after 24 hours, begin taking daily showers; let the water run over the breast and wash away the bacteria. Then put a dressing over it to absorb oozing fluids from the incision.

A drain is placed in the incision to promote drainage; in addition, manual expression helps to eliminate pus and milk. The incision heals from the inside out within a week or two. Treatment of abscesses varies across cultures. Efrem (1995) reported on 285 cases of breast abscess in lactating Nigerian women. Most (85 percent) grew *S. aureus*, 5 percent grew coliforms, and 10 percent grew no organism.

All of the cases responded well to treatment by incision and drainage followed by packing daily with ribbon gauze soaked in magnesium sulphate solution (135 cases), Euseol (100 cases), and honey (50 cases).

Breast and Nipple Rashes, Lesions, and Eczema

Breast rashes and lesions on the nipple or areolar area are unusual and often difficult to diagnose. They are particularly distressing if they are painful. In one case (Brackett, 1988), a mother described a periodic burning sensation in the breast not related to actual breastfeeding. Most of the mother's areola was itchy, flaky, and red. The family lived without air conditioning during hot, humid weather. In addition, the mother swam in a chlorinated pool each day, often wearing her bathing suit for some time after returning home. Thrush was ruled out as a possible cause of her problem. The mother stopped swimming and her rash resolved within 2 weeks.

Eczema is a painful, burning, itching dermatitis with redness, eruption of vesicles, and crusting and oozing papules. It also can be a chronic problem as a dry erythematous (red) and scaling dermatitis. About half of breastfeeding women who develop nipple and areola eczema have a history of eczema; the other half develop it as a contact dermatitis following introduction of solids to the baby. Topical corticosteroid ointments are the mainstay of treatment for eczema. They should be carefully wiped off the nipple area *before* the feeding and applied to the affected areas *after* the baby has fed. Topical antibiotics such as mupriocin, polysporin, and fusidic acid have been shown to reduce bacterial count and clinical severity. If the symptoms develop soon after the baby starts eating solid foods, the mother should identify and eliminate any infant foods that might have contributed to the onset of eczema. Rinsing the affected nipple and areola with the mother's own expressed milk or with water, then patting the area dry, is also helpful (Barankin & Gross, 2004).

Amir (1993) described a case in which a breastfeeding mother with celiac disease developed red, scaly, and cracked nipples. The mother appeared to have eczema, possibly infected, involving most of both breasts. A topical steroid ointment (betamethasone dipropionate 0.05% [Diprosone]) was applied four times daily and a topical antibiotic was used twice daily. Two weeks later, the eczema had resolved, and the mother was able to continue breastfeeding without pain. Box 9–2 presents interventions that will help prevent such disorders.

A more severe breast skin problem is redness and itching accompanied by tiny ulcers on the nipple and areola that resemble chickenpox. Breastfeeding is extremely painful. As the ulcers heal, they form scabs. The baby may or may not have similar perioral skin lesions. This condition requires referral to a physician, who should evaluate the mother for a possible staphylococcal or viral infection. Culture of the lesion should be taken during its early stages before the lesion begins to dry and heal over. Color Plate 8 and Color Plate 38 depict cracked nipples with a possible bacterial infection. In Color Plate 38 the mother's nipple had possible impetigo with raised red pimplelike bumps, cracking at the nipple base, and yellow crusting at the tips of the nipples.

Treatment will depend on laboratory results of a culture of the lesion and maternal serum antibody titers. If the lesion is herpes simplex it is advisable for the mother to wean the infant or to pump her milk until the lesions are healed. The mother will be treated with an antiviral medication.

The lactation consultant described the breast lesions from herpes (Color Plate 14) as looking like chickenpox. The healing lesions were scabbing, the active lesions were oozing ulcerations, and the new lesions were tiny, bright-red flat areas. The mother complained of extreme "razor blade–like" pain during feedings. Two physicians, who offered differing diagnoses, evaluated her. Her pediatrician suggested that it might be herpes virus, whereas her dermatologist thought the mother had a staphylococcal infection. Neither physician obtained a culture or serum antibody titers.

The woman was first treated for a staphylococcal infection, which worsened the problem, and then with an antiviral agent (Zovirax). The lesions began to resolve shortly after the mother applied Zovirax to her nipples and areola. The mother interrupted breastfeeding her 10-month-old baby for 2 weeks while the lesions healed. During this time, she pumped and hand-expressed her milk. She resumed full breastfeeding at the end of that time. The child had "fever blisters" every 3 or 4 months for some time after this episode, and the mother developed more breast lesions a few months after the first infection, which she again treated successfully with Zovirax. For more discussion on herpes simplex virus, see Chapter 6.

Candidiasis (Thrush)

When a mother has persistent sore nipples, candidiasis (also referred to as candidosis) is likely. The yeast, *Candida albicans* (also called *Monilia* or

---

BOX 9–2

Interventions for Breast and Nipple Rashes and Infections

- Discontinue irritant.
- Take frequent showers.
- Wear all-cotton bras.
- Expose breasts to sunlight (15 minutes) and to air.
- Apply a medicated cream on the affected area twice a day. (Bactroban, an antifungal, antibacterial, and hydro-cortisone combination, is available over the counter.) Remove cream with clean cotton swab if used on nipple-areola.
- Rinse nipple-areola area with warm water after each feeding. Pat dry, then air-dry with hair dryer on the low setting.

thrush) is the likely cause when it occurs orally. *Candida* thrives in the warm, moist areas of the infant's mouth and on the mother's nipples. The infant's mouth can become infected during vaginal birth and can then infect the mother's breast and nipple during breastfeeding. Candidiasis should be suspected if the mother has been breastfeeding without discomfort and then rapidly develops extremely sore nipples, burning or itching, and possibly, shooting pain deep in the breast. Staphylococcal infections can be mistaken for *Candida*, or the problem can be polymicrobial, meaning both bacteria and *Candida* are involved (C. M. Smillie, Treatment for nipple candidiasis, personal communication, December 2002).

Although *Candida* is naturally occurring yeast that lives in the mucous membranes of the gastrointestinal and genitourinary tract and on the skin, the use of antibiotics promotes overgrowth (candidiasis); consequently, infants and women who have received antibiotic therapy are more susceptible to candidiasis (Chetwynd et al., 2002). The increasing use of intrapartum antibiotic prophylaxis for group B streptococcus has been cited as contributing to the rising numbers of cases of breast *Candida* overgrowth (Tanguay, McBean, & Jain, 1994).

Mothers with vaginal candidiasis and nipple trauma are also predisposed to candidiasis of the breast. In checking for candidiasis, inspect the woman's breasts for inflammation of the nipples and areola. The inflammation is usually a striking deep pink, sometimes with tiny blisters (see Color Plate 12). The mother will complain of severe tenderness and discomfort, especially during and immediately after feedings.

The baby may have a diaper rash, with raised, red, sore-looking pustules or red, scalded-looking buttocks. Also examine the child's mouth carefully for white patches surrounded by diffuse redness. The absence of symptoms in the child's mouth, however, does not rule out thrush, because the infant may be asymptomatic. On the other hand, thrush symptoms in the baby (fussiness, refusing breast) can go unnoticed or can be attributed to something else. Whenever any woman has recurrent yeast infections, her sexual partner should be considered a potential reservoir of infection. Pacifiers and bottle nipples are another source of recurrent thrush infection; they may harbor persistent oral *Candida*

colonization and should be replaced or boiled after each exposure in the infant's mouth.

Candidiasis is a "family" disease; it spreads quickly among family members, especially with intimate contact involving warm, moist areas of the body, as is the case with breastfeeding and with sexual contact. Candidiasis that develops during breastfeeding can persist and recur unless all areas of possible infection in the baby, mother, and her sex partner are treated promptly and aggressively. The infant's mouth and anal area, and the mother's breasts (nipples and areola) and vagina are prime sites for *Candida* infection; all should be treated simultaneously if warranted.

Diagnosis

Candidiasis is most often diagnosed based on history, physical examination of the baby, and to a lesser degree, physical examination of the mother (Brent, 2001). According to Brent's survey of 312 members of the Academy for Breastfeeding Medicine, use of laboratory tests and cultures is infrequent (i.e., only 7 percent of providers used such methods), supposedly because cultures of the fungus may take days to grow and is difficult to differentiate from normal skin colonization.

To offset the well-recognized lack of evidence regarding accurate diagnosis of candidosis, Morrill and colleagues (2003, 2004, 2005) have conducted research on detection of *Candida* on the nipple and areolar skin and in breast milk, diagnosis of mammary candidosis, and risk factors for candidosis. First, a new culture technique for detecting *Candida* in breast milk was developed by Morrill et al. (2003) because the natural inhibition of *Candida* growth by lactoferrin in the milk samples can result in false negative cultures. By adding iron to the breast milk the ability to detect *Candida* growth was increased two- to three-fold and markedly reduced the likelihood of false negative culture results. Morrill and team (2004) also evaluated the sensitivity, specificity, and positive predictive value (PPV) of signs (shiny or flaky skin of nipple/areola) and symptoms (burning pain of nipple/areola, sore but not burning nipples, stabbing breast pain, and nonstabbing breast pain) of mammary candidosis reported by lactating women at 2 and 9 weeks postpartum, based on laboratory confirmation of the presence of

Candida on the nipple/areola or in breast milk at 2 weeks postpartum. Positive predictive value for colonization was highest when there were 3 or more signs and symptoms simultaneously or when flaky or shiny skin of the nipple/areola was reported together or in combination with breast pain.

Finally, in a prospective study of 100 lactating and 40 nonpregnant, nonlactating women (controls), the team of researchers led by Morrill (2005) sought to document risk factors for *Candida* colonization and the relationship between *Candida* colonization and breastfeeding at 9 weeks postpartum. None of the nonpregnant control subjects tested positive for *Candida*, somewhat contradictory to the assumption that *Candida* is normally present in many people. Risk factors for colonization of mother were bottle use in the first 2 weeks postpartum and pregnancy duration of longer than 40 weeks. Risk factors for the infant were bottle use in the first 2 weeks postpartum and presence of siblings. Among women who tested positive at 2 weeks, 43 percent were still breastfeeding at 9 weeks postpartum compared to 69 percent who did not test positive ($P < .05$). The authors concluded that use of signs and symptoms could be helpful to clinicians in determining the need for cultures and for immediate treatment while awaiting culture results. Their risk factor research suggests that avoidance of bottle use in the early postpartum may reduce mammary candidosis. Furthermore, such preventive practice may help to decrease early termination of breastfeeding due to infection and pain.

An Alternate View of Candidiasis

Hale (2008) questions the presumption that sore and inflamed nipples with pain radiating into the axilla are due to infection with *Candida albicans* since most studies have not actually found culturable *Candida* present in breastmilk. It was assumed that they were unable to grow *Candida albicans* from breastmilk because the fungus was destroyed or its growth inhibited by agents present in human milk such as lactoferrin. Because we presumed that we could not culture or grow *Candida* from breastmilk, studies of ductal *Candida* infection in breastfeeding women have been limited. It now appears that this original data is inaccurate. *Candida albicans* is a normal fungal organism found on all human skin. As many as 80 to 90 percent of infants have culturable *Candida* present in their mouths. According to Hale, many of the original studies did not sufficiently clean the mother's nipple and the source of the *Candida* may have actually been the saliva from the infant's mouth, and not growth on the mother's nipple.

Treatment

Despite the availability of antifungal medications, there are few clinical trials and little research on their effectiveness in treating candidiasis of the lactating dyad. Clinical trials with healthy versus immunocompromised infants are even more rare. A recent small (n = 34) randomized study in two US military clinics compared nystatin and fluconazole oral suspensions for treatment of oral candidiasis in otherwise healthy infants (Groins et al., 2002). Clinical cures for nystatin were 6 of 19 (32 percent) and for fluconazole 15 of 15 (100 percent). Microbiologic cures for nystatin at 10 days was 1 of 18 (5.6 percent) and for fluconazole at 7 days was 11 of 15 (73 percent) with 10 of these 11 cures (91 percent) by day 3. Breastfeeding mothers of the infants, regardless of study group, were prescribed nystatin cream for application to their nipples twice daily for duration of the infant's treatment. The authors did not report on the outcomes for mothers in this study. Thomassen et al. (1998) reported that treatment for mothers with mammary candidosis symptoms with 50 mg of fluconazole was ineffective, and Chetwynd et al. (2002) recommended higher dosing (100 mg) of fluconazole for a longer duration (several weeks) might be necessary for treatment.

Generally, treatment of candidiasis for the infant includes placing an antifungal medication (e.g., nystatin) in the infant's mouth with a medicine dropper after feedings and swabbing it over the mucosa, gums, and tongue. The mother applies an antifungal topical cream or lotion to her nipples and breast before and after each feeding and to the infant's entire diaper area if there is any redness. The mother may also have vaginal yeast infection and if indicated, should simultaneously use an antifungal intravaginal preparation. Clotrimazole (Gyne-Lotrimin) is an over-the-counter drug in the United States and is available as a vaginal suppository or as a cream but is not sold as a gel.

Other recommendations that can be made to the mother on a case-by-case basis include the following:

- "Air dry" the nipples and, if possible, expose them directly to the sun for a few minutes twice a day.
- Throw away disposable breast pads as soon as they become wet.
- Dry the external genitalia with a hair dryer on a warm setting.
- Wear 100 percent cotton underpants and bras that can be washed in very hot water and/or bleach to kill spores.
- Avoid baths with other members of the family.
- Restrict alcohol, cheese, bread, wheat products, sugar, and honey.
- Take 1 tablet acidophilus daily (40 million–1 billion viable units, found at health food stores) for 2 weeks beyond the disappearance of symptoms.
- Use condoms during coitus because cross-infection with a sexual partner is possible (Wilson-Clay & Hoover, 2002).

Nystatin is the most commonly used medication for candidiasis although its effectiveness is poor by some reports (Chetwynd et al., 2002; Groins et al., 2002), and occasionally it can cause gastrointestinal symptoms in the baby. Its use should be limited to never-treated cases of thrush. Nystatin oral suspension is painted on the baby's oral mucosa and tongue with a large cotton swab after every breastfeeding. In the case of frank thrush and persistent candidiasis, fluconazole is safe and effective, and should be prescribed for both the mother and infant. The amount of fluconazole that transfers through the mother's milk is not sufficient to treat the baby. One expert breastfeeding physician recommends that treatment of mother and infant be based on a holistic assessment of the case, as well as the assumption that *Candida* is a problem of host that causes overgrowth of the fungus (N. Powers, personal communication, 2007):

- If the mother has symptoms, and the baby never had obvious oral thrush, the baby is not considered particularly "susceptible," and thus do *not* treat the baby.
- If the baby has obvious thrush and the mother has symptoms, treat *both*.

- If the baby has obvious thrush and the mother has no symptoms, treat both or treat the baby, and have the mother call immediately if she develops symptoms.

Another treatment is painting ketoconazole suspension on the breast twice a day for 5 days, followed by prolonged nystatin application. If the mother has allergies, the healthcare provider must be aware that Seldane (terfenadine) should *not* be taken in conjunction with the antifungal drugs ketoconazole or itraconazole or the antibiotic erythromycin (see Chapter 5). Mixing these drugs can be life threatening.

Table 9–4 presents a list of recommended dosages for commonly used antifungal medications. Dr. Jack Newman's All Purpose Nipple Ointment (Newman & Pitman, 2000) is a combination nipple ointment of antifungal and cortisone agents.

After taking an antifungal medication, mothers need encouragement and follow-up; they may not get immediate relief from pain. In fact, after starting treatment the pain may become worse before it begins to fade. If nystatin does not clear the fungal infection, other antifungal medications, such as miconazole (Monistat), clotrimazole (Gyne-Lotrimin), naftifine (Naftin), or oxiconazole (Oxistat), should be tried. Johnstone and Marcinak (1990) reported a case in which nystatin oral suspension was applied to the infant's mouth lesions with a clean cotton swab four times daily for 2 weeks, and to the mother's nipples immediately after feedings. This treatment was ineffective. The mother then applied clotrimazole gel to her nipples and to the baby's oral lesions every 3 hours. After five applications, both mother and baby were symptom free. In another case of persistent candidiasis and thrush, fluconazole was the only effective treatment. For early cases, suggest that after feedings the mother try warm vinegar soaks (1 part vinegar, 4 parts water) followed by air drying and an antifungal preparation (La Leche League International, 2000).

Gentian violet, an old-fashioned antifungal drug, may be used as a second line of treatment following other antifungal treatment failure. A well-known drawback of this remedy is that gentian violet stains anything with which it comes into contact, although blotting with alcohol and then a detergent solution helps to remove the dye. The more significant and

TABLE 9–4	Selected Antifungal Preparations

Drug Name	Preparations	Usual Dosage
Clotrimazole (Lotrimin, Mycelex)	Creams, solutions, vaginal cream, and vaginal tablets.	Skin cream: apply twice daily. Vaginal cream or tablet: 100 mg/day for 7 days or 200 mg/day for 3 days.
Gentian violet	Dilute solution 0.25% or 0.5%.	Topical: infant: 2 to 3 times over several days. Do not repeat.
Fluconazole (Diflucan)	Oral.	Adult: 400 mg loading dose, then 100 mg twice daily for at least 2 weeks until pain-free for a week. Pediatric: loading dose of 6–12 mg/kg; then 3–6 mg/kg.
Ketoconazole (Nizoral)	Oral tablets.	Adult: 200–400 mg/day, given in single dose. Pediatric: children weighing less than 20 kg, 50 mg/day; children weighing 20–40 kg, 100 mg/day.
Miconazole (Monistat)	Skin cream or lotion: creams, lotions, vaginal cream, and vaginal suppositories.	Vaginal cream or suppository: 100 mg/day for 7 days. Skin cream or lotion: apply 3 to 4 times per day.
Nystatin (Mycostatin)	Suspensions, cream, powders, ointment, and vaginal suppositories; *Candida* resistance to nystatin is growing.	Oral: for adults: 1.5–2.4 million into units/day divided 3 to 4 doses; for infants: 400,000–800,000 units/day divided into 3 to 4 doses; Topical: 1 million units applied twice a day. Duration of therapy: at least 2 days after symptoms disappear; vaginal: 1–2 million units/day.
Newman's All Purpose Nipple Ointment	Ointment mixed by a pharmacist. Clotrimazole can be left out if 10% dosage is not available. Use until pain-free.	Mupirocin 2% ointment (15 gm); Nystatin 100,000 unit/ml ointment (15 gm); Clotrimazole 10% vaginal cream (15 gm); Betamethasone 0.1% ointment (15 gm).

dangerous side effect of gentian violet is irritation and ulceration of the infant's oral mucous membrane (Utter, 1990). A case study (Baca, Drexler, & Cullen, 2001) described a very serious case of obstructive laryngotracheitis secondary to gentian violet exposure necessitating endotracheal tube placement, several days of intensive care hospitalization, and feeding tube placement secondary to refusal of the infant to breastfeed. Given the availability of other antifungals with few side effects, the authors recommended extreme caution and consideration in prescribing gentian violet.

Another recommendation from Dr. Nancy Powers is to "treat" anything that comes into contact with the baby's mouth (pacifiers, nipples, teethers, or toys) or the mother's breasts (breast-pump parts, bras, breast pads) to destroy the heat-resistant spores. This treatment can be accomplished by soaking articles in a vinegar and water solution for 30 minutes, boiling the articles for 20 minutes, or sterilizing pump parts in microwaveable bags sold for pumps. Likewise, Dr. Christina Smillie, a pediatrician who treats only breastfeeding patients, views *Candida* as a normal flora that is everywhere, and its treatment should be focused on regaining healthy skin so the mother can resist infection.

It is not clear whether expressed milk of a mother with candidiasis should be saved and frozen for later use. Freezing deactivates yeast but does not kill it. Generally, it is advisable to tell mothers with candidiasis who are pumping not to freeze their milk until they have completed a course of medication treatment and are symptom free. In the situation where the mother has a large supply of stored milk, and both mother and infant are symptomatic, home pasteurization of the stored milk may be considered.

In one case of candidiasis infection of the breast (see Color Plate 12), the infant remained symptom-free for the entire 4-month period, whereas the mother had repeated episodes of candidiasis. Within 4 days after resolving the painful blistering and redness, she experienced a new flare-up. After four such episodes in 4 months, she obtained medication for both her infant and herself; after 5 days of treatments after *every* suckling episode, she was symptom-free and remained so (Johnstone & Marcinak, 1990).

According to conventional wisdom, when candidiasis infection is severe, it can involve the lower ducts and sinuses of the breast in addition to the outer skin of the nipples and breast. When the ducts are infected, the mother is very likely to feel a burning sensation deep in the breast, which is distinct from the burning sensation of the breast skin itself. Often the inner burning persists several minutes after the baby has come off the breast. When the mother is treated with oral antifungal medication, the pain

subsides (Chetwynd et al., 2002; Johnstone & Marcinak, 1990). It has been suggested that the more severe the candidiasis infection, the longer it takes for the treatment to work and for the pain to disappear.

Breast Pain

Breast pain that may derive from any number of sources can be both disconcerting and discouraging. Breast pain may be involved with the following conditions (Wilson-Clay & Hoover, 2002):

- Pinched nipple from poor latch-on
- Vasospasm or Raynaud's phenomenon
- Plugged duct
- Damaged nipples
- Nipple infection: bacterial, *Candida*, or both
- Engorgement
- Forceful milk ejection
- Rapid refilling of ducts
- Mastitis

In some cases, pressure on the brachial plexus can result in shooting pain in the breast. Identifying the cause of this pressure (e.g., a badly fitting bra or baby-carrier straps that are pulled too tightly across the mother's back) is a key to alleviating such pain.

Women have reported feeling shooting pain that coincided with powerful ejection of milk. Such episodes are most likely to occur in the first month of the breastfeeding course. When the milk-ejection reflex subsides, the pain often subsides as well. This temporary pain tends to occur more often in primiparous women; often the same mothers who have experienced it with a first breastfeeding baby do not experience a recurrence with later infants. This pain may reflect distension of the milk ducts, which is more obvious in the early first breastfeeding course than at later periods.

In cases in which the mother reports very intense pain coincidental with a vigorous milk-ejection response, the caregiver should encourage the mother to gently massage her breasts before putting the baby to breast to enhance the likelihood of some initial leaking of milk before the baby's active suckling stimulates milk ejection. When the milk begins to drip freely, sprays, and then subsides, subsequent suckling is less likely to result in such intense discomfort. By the end of the first month, such pain is usually no longer present when the milk-ejection reflex is activated.

Plagued by recurrent plugged ducts, mastitis, and sinus infection that were treated with antibiotics, one mother eventually developed episodes of deep pain in both breasts. Although her breasts were not red or hot to the touch, and she did not have any hardness over ducts, there was a burning and shooting pain inside. Finally, a pediatric nurse practitioner suggested she take high doses of acidophilus since she thought that the problem might be ductal yeast infection. After two months of this treatment the mother had no recurrence of either breast pain or a plugged duct (Buraglio, 2003).

Women who have nipple pain are highly anxious and distressed. However, once the pain resolves, their distress also resolves (Amir et al., 1996). Heads and Higgins (1995) looked at nipple trauma in relation to nipple pain between 3 and 5 days postpartum. Visible evidence of nipple damage and nipple trauma was observed in 38 (55 percent) of the 69 women in the study. Damage occurred most commonly in the form of minor grazes (61 percent) or blisters (23 percent). Women who had a strong personal commitment to breastfeed their babies reported less nipple pain than did those who were not so strongly committed.

Vasospasm

In breast vasospasm, the nipple appears blanched after the feeding, sometimes turning blue or red before returning to its normal color (see Color Plate 39). The mother feels extreme pain during the "spasm." This cluster of symptoms is often referred to as *Raynaud's phenomenon of the nipple*. Raynaud's phenomenon (an intermittent ischemia usually affecting fingers or toes) is more prevalent in women, and there usually is a family history.

Blanching of the nipple can occur not only during feedings but also between feedings according to one report (Lawlor-Smith & Lawlor-Smith, 1997). Exposure to cold precipitates nipple blanching and pain, and is relieved by warmth and covering the breast. Breast pain associated with Raynaud's is severe and throbbing and is often mistaken for *Candida albicans* infection. In a report of 12 mothers with Raynaud's, eight mothers and their infants received multiple courses of antifungal therapy without relief before

the diagnosis of Raynaud's was made (Anderson, Held, & Wright, 2004). Three of the mothers reported a history of breast surgery. Another report (Morino & Winn, 2007) of a breastfeeding mother with Raynaud's concluded that there was a definite association between the woman's symptoms and her emotional stress. To diagnose Raynaud's phenomenon accurately, symptoms of cold stimuli, classic triphasic color change of Raynaud's phenomenon (white, blue, and red) in their nipples, or biphasic color change (white and blue) must be present (Anderson, Held, & Wright, 2004).

Treatment with nifedipine (30 mg/day for 2 weeks) has been reported as effective for treating vasospasm without side effects (Anderson, Held, & Wright, 2004; Garrison, 2002; Page & McKenna, 2006). Nifedipine is a calcium channel blocker and vasodilator used to treat hypertension; its transfer through breastmilk to the baby is not significant (Penny & Lewis, 1989). Prompt treatment will allow mothers to continue to breastfeed pain free while avoiding unnecessary antifungal therapy. Taking ibuprofen and applying warmth to the breasts, either by taking a warm shower or by covering the breasts with a heating pad, help to alleviate discomfort.

Milk Blister

Infrequently, a milk blister—a whitish, tender area—develops on the upper areola. Nipple-pore milk that has been sealed over by the epidermis and has triggered an inflammatory response probably causes a milk blister. This obstruction then prevents the duct system from draining, so milk buildup behind the occlusion causes symptoms of a blocked duct (Noble, 1991). The spot may be white or yellow, depending on how long it has been present. The skin on and around the area may be reddened (see Color Plate 11).

Persistent and very painful during feeding, a milk blister can remain for several days or weeks and then spontaneously heal by a peeling away of the epithelium over the affected area. If it does not spontaneously heal, an optional treatment is to break the epithelial tissue using a sterile needle, sometimes along with sterile tweezers and small sharp scissors to entirely remove the excess skin. Aspiration may be necessary to draw out the fluid. Compressing around the areola to express out any stringy plugs may help to prevent future blisters from arising (Newman & Pitman, 2000). A mother who had a nipple probe for a chronically plugged duct and blister developed a lot of pain and insisted on weaning to get relief.

A less invasive treatment is rubbing the area with a damp cloth after softening the skin by immersion in warm water. With ice packs, an analgesic to relieve discomfort, and a topical antibiotic, breastfeeding can continue and healing is rapid.

In addition to the larger blister, tiny blisters that appear to have a whitish fluid, possibly milk, may appear on nipples. These blisters are sore and painful. Vitamin E ointment (applied sparingly and wiped off before feedings) and wearing breast shells (to relieve the pressure from clothing on the nipples) relieve discomfort and possibly aid healing.

Mammoplasty

Breast augmentation and reduction are increasingly common surgical procedures. Although augmentation is performed for cosmetic effect, reduction of very large breasts is often performed to reduce discomfort from neck and back pain and the need to "feel normal" (Grassley, 2002).

Sooner or later, the clinician will see a client who has had breast augmentation or reduction and who wants to know whether she will be able to breastfeed her baby. The ability to breastfeed after these surgeries depends on the type of surgery, the specific technique used, whether neural pathways were severed, and the amount of breast tissue removed. Generally speaking, full breastfeeding is possible with augmentation surgery but usually not after reduction surgery, unless feedings are supplemented; however, exceptions occur in both instances with any breast surgery. An explanation of the differences in the operative procedures is crucial to understanding the subsequent effect on lactation.

Gigantomastia

Gigantomastia of pregnancy is a rare, debilitating condition characterized by massive enlargement of breasts and result in tissue necrosis, ulceration, and infection. Because it appears in the early weeks of pregnancy, most believe there is a hormonal cause, although the exact mechanism is unknown.

A literature review shows that about one third of women with this problem eventually undergo breast reduction or a mastectomy (Swelstad et al., 2006). An inferior pedicle technique can be successfully performed in women with gigantomastia (Lacerna et al., 2005). A search of the MEDLINE and *Web of Science* database for the words *breastfeeding*, *lactation*, and *gigantomastia* revealed no reports.

Breast Reduction

The ability to breastfeed after breast reduction depends on whether the surgeon deliberately leaves nerve pathways and blood supply intact or the tissue is removed without regard for these structures (Soderstrom, 1993). Since adipose tissue of the breast is inseparably connected to glandular tissue, breast reduction cannot be done by simply removing the adipose tissue (Nickell & Skelton, 2005). Women with the least amount of glandular tissue removed have a greater opportunity to lactate (Marshall, Callan, & Nicholson, 1994), particularly if the fourth intercostal nerve that branches to the breast and areola is left intact (see Chapter 3).

The two techniques used for breast reduction are the *pedicle technique* and the *free-nipple technique*. The pedicle technique can be located laterally, medially, or inferiorly. Studies on pedicled breast reduction report breastfeeding success rates that vary from 19 to 72 percent. The inferior pedicle technique is common for women of childbearing age. The nipple and areola remain attached to the breast gland on a pedicle, and the tissue is "reduced." A wedge is removed from the sides of the underside of the breast (Figure 9–1). Because the breast, its ducts, its blood supply, and some nerves remain intact, breastfeeding has been possible after this operation but the success of breastfeeding cannot be predicted.

Half of the women reported having a small amount of milk, the other half a reasonable or large amount following the superior pedicle technique (Cherchel, Azzam, & De Mey, 2007). The free-nipple technique (auto transplantation of the nipple) involves removing the nipple and areola entirely from the breast and preserving it in saline (much like a graft) while the additional breast tissue (usually fatty tissue) is removed. Then the nipple and

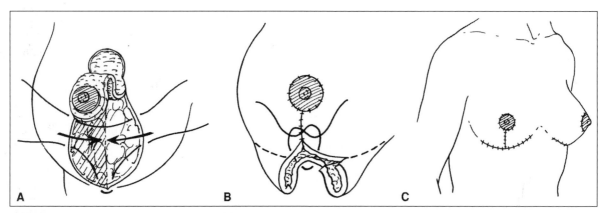

FIGURE 9-1   Breast reduction. (A) Wedge of breast tissue removed, areola pulled up, gap closed. (B) Excess tissue removed, skin closed with stitches. (C) Postoperative appearance.

areola is stitched back in place. This technique is used for women with extremely large breasts and is designed to reduce risks and complications and to position the nipple approximately on the substantially resculpted breast. Breastfeeding may be possible with the pedicle technique, but it is rarely possible with the free-nipple technique, because the blood supply of the nipple and areola is completely severed and damage to the nerves occurs.

Breast reduction usually interferes with the ability to breastfeed (Grassley, 2002; Souto et al., 2003). Brzozowski et al. (2000) studied 78 women who had undergone an inferior pedicle reduction mammoplasty and subsequently had children. For the first 2 weeks postpartum, 19 percent of these women breastfed exclusively, 10 percent breastfed with formula supplementation, and 18 percent were unsuccessful in breastfeeding. Half of the sample did not even attempt breastfeeding. Others (Marshall et al., 1994; Souto et al., 2003) found similar discouraging results. Even so, reports of successful breastfeeding after reduction surgery should encourage women to try breastfeeding and then supplement if it becomes necessary (Ashford, 2001; Kakagia, Tripsiannis, & Tsoutsos, 2005). Kakagia et al. reported breastfeeding success among those who attempted to breastfeed, defined as exclusive breastfeeding without formula supplementation for at least 3 weeks, following 3 different techniques of reduction mammoplasty: 71 percent for superior pedicle, 77 percent for inferior pedicle, and 63 percent for horizontal pedicle techniques. Twenty-two percent of the women had not made any attempt to breastfeed following the

reduction surgery. The authors concluded that reduction with pedicled transposition of the nipple–areola complex with preservation of adequate subareolar breast tissue did not adversely affect breastfeeding based on operative technique, but that lack of encouragement and support to women who had surgery was a detriment to choosing to attempt breastfeeding.

Breast scars after a reduction are illustrated in Color Plate 26. Several cases of spontaneous galactorrhea after reduction mammoplasty are reported in the literature; all of these women had not breastfed for several months before the surgery (Menendez-Graino et al., 1990; Song & Hunter, 1989).

The health professional should provide a forthright discussion about the likelihood of successful lactation and about options for supplemental feedings, especially in the later months. Plastic surgeons, though they may be sympathetic to breastfeeding, are most interested in the surgical technique and the cosmetic results; they are generally uninformed about breastfeeding. The women in one study (Souto et al., 2003) reported that almost 80 percent of their surgeons indicated that breast reduction would not affect lactation. Most of these women were young and desired to have children in the future. Only half of them worried about not being able to breastfeed.

The breast-reduced mother's reactions to her inability to breastfeed may vary according to culture. The US mother who has had breast reduction may accept whatever extent she can breastfeed without regretting that she had the surgery. Women with heavy, pendulous breasts report back, neck, and shoulder pain. They may feel depressed and stigmatized, and experience negative comments from both men and women about their breast size, including cruel jokes during their adolescence (Grassley, 2002; Guthrie et al., 1998). Mothers who have had breast reduction surgery may feel guilty or angry about not being able to breastfeed (Engstrom, 2000).

Mastopexy

Mastopexy, like a facelift, is a "breastlift"—cosmetic surgery where sagging breasts are uplifted and made firmer (Figure 9–2). The operation involves removing excess skin and breast tissue and elevating the nipple. It may be done either in the hospital or in the physician's office. Although there may be a slight loss of sensation in the nipple or areola, the operation "theoretically" should not affect the ability to breastfeed; however, the first author has worked with mothers who had this operation and had a very difficult time producing sufficient milk in order to maintain adequate growth for their infants.

Breast Augmentation

Because cosmetic surgery to "augment" or enlarge the breasts is increasingly popular, lactation consultants are likely to have clients who have had this procedure (Figure 9–3). The US Food and Drug Administration in 2006 lifted a 14-year ban on the use of silicone gel breast implants after decades of contentious debate and litigation following complaints and lawsuits in the 1970s and 1980s that the devices ruptured and became hard and painful and that some women developed cancer and autoimmune diseases. Before 2006, almost all women in the United States undergoing augmentation received saline-filled implants. But because implants of silicone gel are softer than saline implants, they are preferred.

Four techniques are used to enlarge the breasts:

- The infrasubmammary procedure calls for an incision to be made under the breast and for the implant to be placed under the breast tissue. One disadvantage is that the scar is very visible and is easily irritated by a bra.
- In the periareolar technique, an incision is made around the areola-nipple. Although the scar is less visible than in the infrasubmammary procedure, there is often a loss of sensation.
- The transareolar technique involves an incision made across the areola-nipple area. This procedure is rarely done now. Full lactation is almost always impossible after this procedure, because the glandular tissue, nerve, and blood supply are extensively disrupted. This should be made clear to any woman who contemplates having this procedure.
- An axillary enlargement is done by making an incision underneath the arm and placing the implant below the gland or muscle. Although there are few scars and no interference with

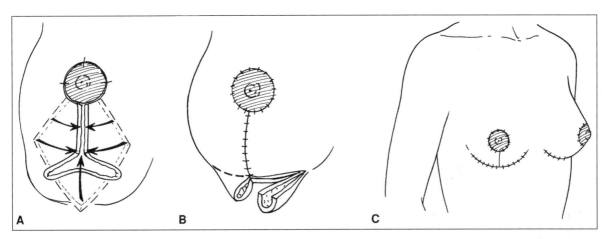

FIGURE 9–2 Breast "lift" or mastopexy. (A) Skin edges pulled together. (B) Excess tissue removed. (C) Postoperative appearance.

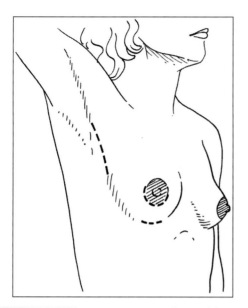

FIGURE 9–3 Breast augmentation. Incision is made through the armpit, underneath the breast, or under the areola.

breast tissue and lactation, this type of implantation makes breast cancer harder to detect, and there is a possibility of contractures. It is more common for surgeons to place saline implants under the muscle where it interferes less with mammograms (Figure 9–4).

Augmentation has minimal impact on initial breastmilk production, but because of the breast implants these women have greater problems with engorgement in the early days after birth. After initial engorgement, breastfeeding may go along well for days or weeks with the infant gaining weight until the rapidly growing baby's demand for milk may exceed the mother's ability to produce. The lactation consultant who works with these mothers needs to inform mothers of the possibility that supplementation may be necessary to ensure continued infant growth.

Women who had previous breast surgery have a greater than threefold risk of lactation insufficiency as compared with women who had not had surgery. Hughes and Owen (1993) interviewed 26 women with augmentation surgery and found that only one third were successful with breastfeeding. Neifert et al. (1990), Hurst (1996), and Hill et al. (2004) had similar findings. Women who had periareolar

and transareolar incision had greater incidence of lactation insufficiency. Neifert et al. (1990) studied 319 primiparous women who were breastfeeding healthy, full-term infants. The mothers with periareolar incisions were more than four times as likely to have insufficient milk than were those with no breast surgery. Women with breast incisions in other locations had no statistically significant increase in risk compared with those who never had breast surgery. In Hurst's study of 42 women who had augmentation surgery, 64 percent had insufficient lactation. Of the women who had periareolar surgery, none lactated sufficiently, compared with 50 percent who made sufficient milk if they had submaxillary or axillary augmentation (Hurst, 1996).

Why do some women with the "right" type of incision for augmentation still have difficulty lactating? In addition to the type of incision, the pressure of the implant must also be considered. Postpartum breast engorgement can occur despite ductal damage, but milk production continues only in part of the breast. Lobes that cannot empty because of severed ducts quickly undergo cellular-wall involution caused by intramammary pressure atrophy, suggesting that increased pressure, when prolonged and unrelieved, can cause an atrophy of the alveolar cellular wall and diminished milk production (Hurst, 1996; Neifert et al., 1990).

In addition to insufficient milk production issues, reports of galactorrhea, galactocele formation, and extreme engorgement have been reported in the literature, some occurring soon after surgery under the hormonal influence of birth control pills (i.e., without pregnancy) and some following pregnancy (Acarturk, Gencel, & Tuncer, 2005; Caputy & Flowers, 1994; Deloach, Lord, & Ruf, 1994). Thus, augmentation can lead to other lactation-related types of problems that women should be made aware of before having surgery. Furthermore, it is essential for the healthcare provider to discuss the potential impact of surgery on adequacy of breastmilk production. Some women who have had augmentation surgery become upset that their surgeons did not discuss with them the surgery's negative impact on breastfeeding. These women are also angry with themselves for proceeding with the surgery without having been completely informed. Because childbearing and lactation were not a priority at the time of breast surgery, many did not ask the surgeon

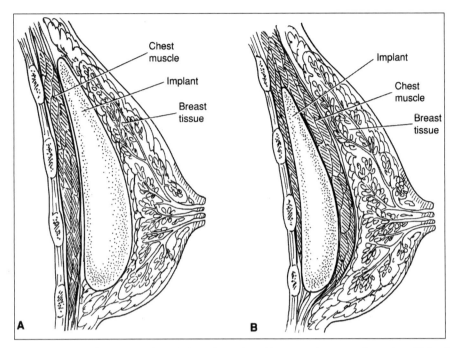

FIGURE **9–4** Location of breast implant. (A) Implant placed between breast and muscles. (B) Implant placed under muscles.

about their future ability to breastfeed (Hughes & Owen, 1993).

Nearly half of Breast Implant Surveillance Reports to the FDA on breast implants were about breastfeeding problems. There were concerns related to the health of the breastfeeding infant and the potential for silicone contamination of breast milk (Brown et al., 2006).

Breast Lumps and Surgery

What happens if a breastfeeding mother develops a lump or nodule in her breast? Warnings by the American Cancer Society have made American women keenly aware of breast lumps, and the woman discovering one is usually anxious and perhaps frightened. However, a breast lump in a lactating woman is most often a galactocele, a milk-filled lacteal cyst caused by plugged milk in the ducts (Stevens et al., 1997). A galactocele is usually tender and will atrophy rather rapidly and disappear in a matter of days. To aspirate a cyst, the physician first cleans and anesthetizes the skin, immobilizes the mass with his or her hand and inserts a 20- to 22-gauge needle to draw out fluid. This procedure

collapses the cyst and solves the problem. Cysts are almost never malignant. If the lump does not resolve or reduce in size, the mother should be examined and biopsied. The type of biopsy will depend on the size and palpability of the lump. If a biopsy is necessary, one of the following methods are used (Love, 2000). (In the two types of nonsurgical biopsies where needles are used, a single stitch may be needed to close the incision.)

- A fine-needle biopsy draws out a few cells.
- Larger-gauged hollow needles are used to remove a small piece of the lump (called a core or "tru-cut" biopsy).
- In surgical or "open" biopsies, the surgeon takes out a large piece of the lump or removes it entirely.

Stereotactic biopsy has become standard procedure to excise microcalcifications. In this procedure, the breast is suspended through an opening on the surgical table and a mammogram is performed to locate the exact position of calcifications, which are biopsied.

Most diagnostic procedures are performed on an outpatient basis either in a freestanding ambulatory clinic or in a minor operating room. Using the lowest dosage possible of local anesthetic (usually Lidocaine) and breastfeeding just before the biopsy minimizes the amount of anesthetic the infant might ingest. When the mother resumes breastfeeding depends on her comfort level and the type of procedure used, but she certainly should be able to resume within 12 hours. Although the area will be tender, resuming feeds needs to be weighed against the discomfort of engorgement and listening to the cries of an unhappy child. If breastfeeding is not resumed within 12 hours, the mother should pump her breasts to relieve the intramammary pressure. Too much milk pressure and stasis could lead to undue stress on the surgical site and infection.

Some surgeons prefer that the mother discontinue nursing either completely before the surgery or at least stop feedings from the affected breast. Milk can leak and mix with blood, which makes a "messy" surgery. Love (2000) suggests that if the mother is thinking of weaning anyway, it is probably a good time to do so. Otherwise, the mother should look for another surgeon. A graduate student of the first author decided to continue breastfeeding after stereotactic biopsy but waited until the evening of the surgery. She made sure that when her daughter latched-on, she was not near the incision site. Despite some leaking of blood-tinged milk from the incision site, the incision healed cleanly and quickly.

Day (1986) described a case in which a woman underwent biopsy of her right breast after suspicious calcifications were found by xeromammography. Biopsy was accomplished with a wedge-shaped resection at the nine o'clock position through a circumareolar skin incision with excellent cosmetic result. The pathology report indicated a benign "fibrocystic" condition. After the delivery of her next baby, the woman's breasts became engorged symmetrically. By the fourth postpartum day, she noted that her right breast remained engorged after breastfeeding, although her left breast seemed relieved of its milk supply. The client subsequently used warm packs, starting feedings on the right side only and using an electric breast pump in efforts to build up her milk supply in the treated breast. At no time was more than 2 ml of milk obtained from the right breast using the electric pump, despite the mother's having previously breastfed her first child on both breasts.

Many mothers have shared their breastfeeding experiences after breast surgery in La Leche League's publications, which are a rich source of clinical information. One mother (Hart, 1980) had a lump removed as an outpatient. The following day, her breast started swelling with stored milk because her baby had not nursed from that breast. After expressing by hand for 12 days, she began feeding her infant again on the affected breast. Her milk supply in the affected breast returned, though for 2 to 3 days nursing was uncomfortable.

Another woman (Paster, 1986) underwent a breast biopsy under general anesthesia for a lump that was deep within her breast. By 12 hours after the procedure, she was able to nurse on the affected side. Although painful at first, by the second or third day, breastfeeding was quite tolerable. The mother found that putting pressure (splinting) on the dressing helped to allay the feeling that the baby would pull the incision apart. At first, there was some lessening of milk production because about 25 percent of the ducts had been disturbed. Subsequently, the mother nursed another baby without noticing any difference in milk production in the affected breast.

In a third case (Resico, 1990), the nipple was cut during surgery from top to bottom and lifted to remove a golf ball-sized lump. The surgeon suggested that the mother not attempt to breastfeed when she became pregnant, because he thought he had severed milk ducts during surgery. Surprisingly, the mother was able to breastfeed from that breast. This suggests one of two possibilities: either some of the ducts were not actually severed, or it is possible for milk ducts to recanalize after having been severed.

Galactoceles

Galactoceles—milk-filled cysts in the lactating breast—are fairly uncommon. The etiology of galactoceles is thought to be an inflammation or infection-induced blockage of the mammary ducts. The condition can also occur in children infrequently (Welch, Babcock, & Ballard, 2004). Galactoceles can mimic other lesions of the breast, both benign and malignant. Ultrasound is generally used in the diagnosis along with needle aspiration of milk. Needle aspiration also is an effective treatment in most patients with galactoceles (Rampaul, 2005; Sawhney et al., 2002; Wang, Lee, & Kim, 2007).

Case studies in the literature provide descriptions from which clinicians can be informed about galactoceles. Bevin and Persok (1993) described a case in which a mother had a palpable chronic galactocele behind the left areola for 10 years, during which time she breastfed several children. The left breast was the site of many plugged ducts, breast infections (some requiring antibiotics), and a breast abscess. At various stages, 10 to 20 ml of milky fluid was aspirated, but the lump refilled quickly. No single treatment was helpful. However, on one occasion, antibiotic treatment caused the galactocele to disappear temporarily. Optimal management of a galactocele has yet to be determined.

A more recent case report from London was quite unusual (Rampaul, 2005) as it described multiple galactoceles in both axillae of a lactating woman. A 31-year-old woman presented with a 1-week history of bilateral swellings of the axillae, having been diagnosed with bilateral hidradenitis suppurativa (a chronic skin inflammation marked by the presence of blackheads and one or more red, tender bumps) 4 years earlier. She was 3 weeks postpartum, with engorged lactating breasts and both axillae were swollen with numerous discrete palpable lumps each measuring about 1.5 cm within each axilla. Ultrasonography revealed multiple thin-walled cysts. A cyst in the upper outer quadrant of the left breast was also present and on aspiration was shown to contain milk. The axillary cysts were not aspirated, as they were identical on imaging to the breast galactocele. This case also had an episode of milk secretion bilaterally in the axillae that spontaneously resolved, though there were no accessory nipples on examination. It was thought that the prior episodes of hidradenitis may have acted as a nidus (site of infection) in this case and the cause of the galactoceles.

Galactoceles have also been reported in the literature in women who have undergone breast augmentation (Acarturk, Gencel, & Tuncer, 2005). In the case described by Acarturk et al. massive engorgement started in the last month of pregnancy, caused major discomfort, and the woman did not attempt lactation. Although the authors attributed the engorgement to bilateral galactocele formation, there is no description of ultrasonic examination or needle aspiration of the breasts.

Fibrocystic Disease

Fibrocystic breast disease (benign breast disorder) is a general term that describes a number of benign breast conditions. It should not be assumed that fibrocystic disease actually refers only to a disorder in those breasts with cysts or nodules; the term is also used to include evidence of hyperplasia, metaplasia, and atypia, among other conditions (Brucker & Scharbo-DeHaan, 1991). The American Cancer Society recommends that clinicians use the term fibrocystic changes; nevertheless, healthcare insurers commonly use the diagnosis of fibrocystic disease because it guarantees reimbursement.

About half of all women of childbearing age will develop one of these conditions at some point. Years of menstrual cycling will eventually produce dense or fibrous breast tissue. Women usually develop cysts in their thirties. Because of its occurrence rate, the condition is sometimes referred to as a nondisease.

From 50 to 75 percent of all breast biopsies are done because of clinical diagnoses of fibrocystic disease (Norwood, 1989). About one fourth of women with fibrocystic disease develop gross evidence of a cyst or a fibroadenoma, a smooth, round lump that moves around easily when palpated. Fibroadenomas can vary from the size of a pea to the size of a lemon. A needle aspiration helps to confirm the diagnosis. If no fluid can be aspirated, a fibroadenoma is likely. Tissue is sent to the laboratory to confirm the diagnosis. Fibroadenomas are harmless in themselves and, if the woman is lactating, most surgeons choose to delay surgery at least until lactation ceases and the child is completely weaned. In middle-aged or older women, fibroadenomas are usually removed at the time they are diagnosed. A mother with persistent benign breast disease is commonly advised to reduce or eliminate caffeine (coffee, tea, cola, chocolate) and to take vitamin E supplements.

Bleeding from the Breast

Red-tinged, pink, or rusty breastmilk is relatively rare, but it does occur and causes concern because it signals the presence of blood. There are several possible antecedent factors that lead to bleeding in the milk ducts. For example, one mother with severely retracted nipples had painless bleeding from her breasts after wearing breast shells late in pregnancy. After she reduced the wearing time of the shells, the bleeding ceased.

In other cases, the etiology of the bleeding is not so clear. Chele Marmet (1990) has worked with mothers whose milk appears brown or rusty looking, like rusty water emitted from pipes that have not been used for a long while. Hence, she calls it the "rusty-pipe syndrome." This syndrome appears to occur more often in primiparous mothers during the early stages of lactogenesis and is not associated with any discomfort. O'Callaghan (1981) reported 37 cases of this syndrome in the Australian women they followed. Most of these women reported that their breast discharge was either red or brown. Its earliest appearance was during the fourth month of pregnancy and was associated with antenatal breast expression in a little over half of the mothers. Dairy farmers report similar rusty milk from cows calving for the first time and suggest that the reason is slight internal bleeding from edema during the cow's first engorgement.

Bright-red bleeding from the breast in the absence of nipple soreness or cracking indicates that the mother should be assessed for the possibility of an intraductal papilloma. This is a small, benign, wartlike growth on the lining of the duct that bleeds as it erodes. Usually no mass or tumor is palpable, and there may or may not be moderate pain and discomfort. Often the bleeding stops spontaneously without any treatment, but if bleeding continues, the woman should be medically evaluated. She can pump her breasts to maintain lactation (on low setting) until the cause of the bleeding is identified. Cytologic evaluation, mammography, and ultrasound can be useful diagnostic tools in these cases (Berens, 2001). The physician will probably remove it surgically to confirm that it is an intraductal papilloma and not something more serious such as intraductal cancer. In any case, the lactation consultant can reassure the mother that the infant is not harmed by the intake of small amounts of serosanguinous discharge. Larger amounts may lead to the infant regurgitating the blood.

Breast Cancer

Breast cancer is the most common malignancy among women (US Cancer Statistics Working Group, 2007). About one fourth of all women receiving diagnoses of breast cancer are premenopausal and potentially fertile. Breast cancer in lactating women is a clinical issue. New technology detects tiny precancerous calcifications that require further investigation. More women choose to breastfeed now, especially those who become pregnant later in life.

Breastfeeding is one of the few potentially modifiable factors that help to prevent breast cancer. Two recent large meta-analyses (review of many studies) on the effect of breastfeeding on the development of breast cancer concluded that breastfeeding provides a protective function against breast cancer (Bernier et al., 2000; Collaborative Group on Hormonal Factors in Breast Cancer, 2002). Studies suggest that the inverse association between breast cancer and breastfeeding exists mainly among premenopausal women (Yang et al., 1997; Katsouyanni et al., 1996; Newcomb et al., 1994) particularly among those who breastfed for a long time (Katsouyanni et al., 1996; Newcomb et al., 1994; Zheng et al., 2001; United Kingdom National Case-Control Study Group, 1993) and gave birth at an early age (Brinton et al., 1995; Yoo et al., 1992).

For a woman who is at risk for breast cancer, prolonged breastfeeding may at least delay its occurrence before menopause. On the estimates obtained from the Collaborative Group on Hormonal Factors in Breast Cancer (2002), if women in developed countries had 2.5 children on average, but breastfed each child for 6 months longer than current average, about 5 percent of breast cancers would be prevented each year, and about 11 percent of breast cancers might be prevented yearly if each child were breastfed for 12 additional months.

An older study on women in fishing villages near Hong Kong who customarily breastfeed only with the right breast is probably the most dramatic example of the protective effect of breast cancer. These women had a fourfold increased risk of cancer in the unsuckled breast (Ing, Ho, & Petrakis, 1977). More recently, Daniels et al. (2004) provided evidence of the association between lifestyle, religious value systems, and risk factors for breast cancer. Their group surveyed 848 non-Hispanic white females from Utah, the state with the lowest female malignant breast cancer incidence rate in the United States, partly due to low rates among women of the Church of Latter-day Saints (LDS or Mormon), to determine the association between selected breast cancer risk factors and religious preference and religiosity. Parity, prevalence of breastfeeding, and lifetime total duration of breastfeeding were highest among Latter-day Saints (LDS) women who attended church weekly. Average months of breastfeeding per child were greater among weekly church attendees, regardless of religious preference. Oral contraceptive use and total duration of hormone replacement therapy use were greatest for individuals of any religion attending church less than weekly and for those with no religious preference. These findings provided strong support for the role of breastfeeding and parity in the relatively low breast cancer incidence rates previously identified among LDS in Utah.

Breastfeeding's protective effect may be because it reduces the number of ovulations proportionally to breastfeeding duration and intensity and maintains lower estrogen levels than if the woman was menstruating. In addition, breastfeeding can reduce concentrations of endogenous and exogenous carcinogens present in the ductal and lobular epithelial cells (Helewa, Levesque, & Provencher, 2002).

Although lactation lowers the risk of developing breast cancer, it *does not prevent* the rare woman from having a cancerous lump in her breast while she is breastfeeding. Pregnancy-associated breast cancer, defined as breast cancer diagnosed during pregnancy or up to 1 year after delivery, occurs in about 1 in 3000 pregnancies (American Cancer Society, 2008), are often advanced at the time of diagnosis and estrogen-receptor negative, but carry a similar prognosis to other breast cancers when matched for stage and age (Woo, Yu, & Hurd, 2003). There is some thought that cancer diagnosed during lactation likely was present during pregnancy and a delay in detection and treatment up to 19 months could result (Yang et al., 2006). Difficulties in evaluating the breast during pregnancy and lactation due to increased density, glandularity, and water content of the lactating breast may delay the diagnosis, and the sensitivity of conventional mammography has been questioned in a review of past research (Woo, Yu, & Hurd, 2003); however, newer research has demonstrated improvement in tumor detection despite the density of the breast (Yang et al., 2006). Furthermore, recent research has also indicated that magnetic resonance imaging is useful in detecting breast carcinoma in lactating women (Espinosa et al., 2005).

These research findings are encouraging given the common projection of increases in breast cancer during pregnancy and lactation due to the increasing number of women postponing childbearing until their 30s and even early 40s, when odds of developing breast cancer are greater normally.

Descriptions of breast cancer during lactation that are useful to the clinician working with breastfeeding mothers are still not common in the literature. A dated but important description was given by Petok (1995) who described several cases of breast carcinoma seen in her consulting practice: lobular carcinoma, ductal carcinoma, and inflammatory breast cancer. Most of these women came for treatment of what they called a plugged duct and described a large lump in the breast that had persisted for 1 to 2 weeks. The lumps were 4 to 6 cm in diameter and were irregularly shaped. One mass felt like two firm lumps clustered together. The lumps did not change after feedings or after the usual treatments for a plugged duct (hot compresses, frequent feedings, breast massage, pumping, etc.). Only one woman reported feeling pain at the site of the lump. In one woman, slight redness showed on the side of the breast opposite the lump. The redness lasted only a few days and then disappeared, although the lump did not change. This woman later developed peau d'orange (dimples on the breast similar to those on an orange peel). All of the infants were breastfeeding and gaining weight. None of the infants rejected the cancerous breast, as has been described in the literature (Hadary, Zidan, & Oren, 1995; Saber, 1996), although one did show a preference for the noncancerous breast. After diagnosis of breast cancer, two of the three women weaned their infants before beginning chemotherapy. The third woman continued to breastfeed for four months, despite the objections of her physician, before initiating chemotherapy.

Petok (1995) recommended referring the lactating mother to a physician for evaluation for the following reasons:

- Any mass that shows no decrease in size after 72 hours of treatment
- Afebrile mastitis-like symptoms that are unresolved after a course of antibiotics
- Recurrent mastitis or plugged ducts that appear at the same location

The initial referral is usually to a primary physician, who then refers to a general surgeon. Hesitation to refer out of fear of causing unnecessary concern by mentioning referral to rule out a tumor in a breastfeeding mother is unwise.

One of the myths about breastfeeding and breast cancer is that a baby can receive cancer-causing viral particles in human milk. This is not true: there is no evidence that breastfeeding after treatment for breast cancer carries any health risk to the child (Helewa, Levesque, & Provencher, 2002). There is neither an increase nor a decrease in incidence of breast cancer in breastfed daughters of women who have had breast cancer (Michels et al., 2001).

Rejection of the breast without apparent reason may be an early warning sign of breast cancer (as noted above). Although it is true that most of the time an infant rejects the breast for another reason, close surveillance and perhaps also a search for an occult breast carcinoma in the involved breast may enable earlier diagnosis and improved prognosis.

Pregnant women diagnosed with breast cancer are treated surgically and/or medically, with the same goals as those for nonpregnant women: local control of disease and prevention of systemic metastasis. International recommendations for treatment of breast cancer during pregnancy were recently published and focused on cancer diagnosed and treated during pregnancy, and did not include recommendations for women diagnosed during lactation because such cancer "can be assessed and treated according to standard guidelines" (Loibl et al., 2006, p. 239). Treatment plans, based on time of diagnosis and staging of the cancer, and with careful consideration of potential risks to the fetus, can include a range of breast surgeries and chemotherapy with anthracycline-based chemotherapy in the second and third trimesters of pregnancy. Radiation therapy should be delayed until after delivery, and agents such as the taxanes, trastuzumab, and tamoxsifen are not recommended during pregnancy, given the limited data available.

Special consideration for women who develop breast cancer during lactation include the following:

- The same considerations for diagnosis during pregnancy using imaging (mammogram, MRI, or ultrasound) hold for the lactating woman owing to the increased breast density and water content of the lactating breast.
- A biopsy is the gold standard of diagnostic measures and must be done (needle, core needle, or fine needle). Optimally the breast should be emptied of milk to reduce the risk of milk fistula. Some recommend inhibiting lactation using ice packs, binding, and/or lactation suppression medication (Woo et al., 2003).
- If a positive diagnosis of breast carcinoma is made, breastfeeding should be interrupted and treatment begun.
- Women receiving chemotherapy for breast cancer or for any other cancer should not breastfeed. All chemotherapeutic drugs cross into the milk. Although levels are low in milk, these compounds are potent antimetabolites, and they are potentially toxic to the infant.

Lactation Following Breast Cancer

Approximately 7 percent of fertile women treated for mammary carcinoma subsequently become pregnant, usually within the first 5 years. Their survival rate is the same as for women who were never pregnant (Deemarsky & Semiglazov, 1987; Donegan & Spratt, 1988). According to a comprehensive review of studies of pregnancy-associated breast cancer by Woo et al. (2003), outcome and survival rates are similar for both pregnant and nonpregnant women who are of similar age and disease stage at time of diagnosis. In some studies a so-called healthy mother effect was observed in which former cancer patients who become pregnant had a better 10-year survival rate than their matched controls. Overall, future pregnancies seemed safe for these mothers unless the cancer was estrogen-receptor positive that was not cured.

As long as the woman with a history of breast carcinoma remains clinically free of cancer, there is no therapeutic benefit in interrupting the pregnancy. If advanced cancer is diagnosed in the first or second trimester, however, treatment choices will be limited due to risks to the fetus and termination may be considered.

Women who have undergone treatment (surgery, radiation, chemotherapy) for breast cancer and later became pregnant and gave birth report common experiences (David, 1985; Green, 1989; Higgins & Haffty, 1994; Tralins, 1995; Varsos & Yahalom, 1991):

- There is little or no enlargement of the treated breast during pregnancy.
- The ability to lactate and breastfeed from the untreated breast is normal, but there is less likelihood of having a full milk supply from the treated breast and possible absence of lactation.
- Difficulty with latch-on sometimes occurs because the nipple on the breast may not extend as completely as might be expected.
- There is less likelihood of an absence of lactation with a circumareolar incision; lactation from the treated breast is less likely to occur in centrally located lesions (Higgins & Haffty, 1994). The interval from the time of treatment to the time of delivery does not appear to adversely affect lactation from the treated breast.

Finally, women with estrogen- or progesterone-positive breast cancer are candidates for antiestrogen therapy such as tamoxifen, which stops estrogen from binding to estrogen receptors and stimulating cancer cell growth. Tamoxifen is not recommended during pregnancy. It inhibits milk production and has a long half-life (Helewa, Levesque, & Provencher, 2002). Significant risks to the infant from exposure to tamoxifen probably outweigh the benefits of breastfeeding.

Women who have experienced breast cancer obviously have many concerns including fears of reoccurrence of cancer. In addition, women of childbearing age have many psychosocial issues related to their fertility, contraceptive choices, pregnancy, and breastfeeding following breast cancer. Connell et al. (2006) conducted a qualitative study of 13 women with breast cancer in Australia, interviewing them multiple times over a period of 18 months. Concerns related to breastfeeding among women who became pregnant during the study included fears and anxiety of further breast cancer activation and difficulty in detecting breast cancer. These fears, understandable as they may be, conflicted with the women's desire to be a good mother (i.e., breastfeeding is best for the baby). Certainly the lactation consultant and other healthcare providers who counsel women with a history of breast cancer must be aware of the potential for such fears and anxiety and ready to provide information and support for the woman.

Breast Screening

Noninvasive screening of the breast is extensively used to detect breast abnormalities in nonlactating women especially breast cancer in order to diagnose and treat it at an early stage. Types of screening techniques are listed below.

Mammogram

A *screening mammogram* is used to look for breast disease in women who appear to have no breast problems; it is essentially an X-ray of the breast. Some discomfort is felt from flattening the breasts, but it is necessary for an accurate evaluation. A *diagnostic mammogram* is the same as a screening procedure except it may include additional views to magnify suspicious areas to obtain a better analysis of breast tissue. Women with implants will receive a diagnostic mammogram.

Breast Magnetic Resonance Imaging (MRI)

MRI uses a magnetic field and pulses of radio wave energy to see what is inside the breast without having to do surgery. MRI of the breast has no known health hazards and shows images of dense breasts and implant. The woman lies on her stomach with both breasts hanging freely into a cushioned recess containing a breast coil receiver and lies still for up to 15 minutes while images are obtained. MRI is expensive and is not recommended by itself for early detection of breast cancer although it may be used along with other techniques.

Breast Ultrasound

Also known as sonography, ultrasound is a method in which high-frequency sound waves are used to "look inside" the breast. A handheld instrument placed on the skin transmits the sound waves through the breast. Echoes from the sound waves are picked up and translated into a computer image. It is generally use to evaluate breast problems that are found during a physical exam and after viewing mammogram results. There is no exposure to radiation during this test. An objective, reliable, noninvasive technique, it is also used to study the breast's anatomical structures and patterns of breastmilk flow.

Thermography Imaging

Thermography imaging maps and measures the heat on the surface of the breast with the use of a heat-sensing camera. It is based on the premise that temperature rises in areas with increased blood flow and metabolism, which could be interpreted as a problem. It is not an effective screening tool for early detection of breast cancer especially in lactating women who have a much higher level of breast blood flow and temperature than those who are not lactating.

Clinical Implications

With abscess drainage, lump removal, or biopsy, there is usually no reason the mother should stop breastfeeding. In fact, irrigating a biopsy wound with the many antimicrobial and anti-inflammatory factors in human milk may in fact facilitate healing. Even when a breast abscess is surgically drained, the mother can breastfeed on the unaffected side and possibly on the affected side, if the incision is far enough from the nipple so that the baby's mouth does not touch it when he breastfeeds. Sometimes, the baby feeds only from the unaffected breast while waiting for the affected breast to heal, and the mother hand-expresses or pumps milk from the affected side.

If the wound is left open to drain, breastfeeding can be "messy," because milk and other body fluids may leak from the ducts for as long as 4 weeks or more. The mother should be prepared to replace soiled dressings with clean pads. Milk leaking from the wound may slow healing. As a result, the mother is at risk for a breast infection or a milk cyst; a low-dose prophylactic antibiotic is sometimes used to avoid infection. A silicone nipple shield with the teat cut off (leaving a doughnut ring of silicone over her nipple) will hold down the bandage and keep the baby's mouth off it. Wounds closer to the nipple–areola and in the lower part of the breast usually take longer to heal. If the problems persist, gradual weaning from the affected side might be necessary while the baby feeds from the unaffected side.

Usually the mother resumes breastfeeding on the affected breast when the drain or stitches are removed and when she can tolerate it. A child's reaction to being prevented from feeding from the affected breast (sometimes his "favorite" breast) varies. Some cooperate without a fuss; others are distraught and actively fight to breastfeed there.

Any woman contemplating breast surgery needs to be fully informed about the procedure and the different techniques that are available. A chart that shows the anatomy and lactation functions of the breast is indispensable for explaining the possible effects of surgery. If the patient is highly motivated to breastfeed, it is the clinician's responsibility to counsel her and suggest techniques that are less disruptive to breastfeeding than are others. If the surgery is very likely to disrupt breastfeeding, that likelihood should be made clear to the woman before the operation. At the same time, it is almost impossible to predict whether breastfeeding will be successful. If supplements become necessary, a feeding tube could be used, thereby allowing the infant to suckle at the breast while receiving a supplement and stimulating milk production.

Summary

Breast-related problems constitute a substantial proportion of clinical breastfeeding counseling. The overuse of antibiotics that leads to candidiasis, the surge in the popularity of cosmetic breast surgery, and digital mammography are human-made barriers to breastfeeding unique to affluent countries.

Most of what lactation consultants do for their clients is to give of themselves—the therapeutic self. Therefore, when a mother faces surgery or other procedures on her breasts that are painful and that might also potentially alter and/or scar her breasts, it is the lactation consultant's responsibility to encourage her to talk, to openly express her feelings, and to answer her questions—and perhaps anticipate her unspoken fears—as completely as possible.

Women have the right to be fully informed about any medical procedure, especially a surgical one, because the outcome is apt to be irreversible. Part of the health professional's responsibility is to act as a client advocate. The client should know all options available to her (including the right to refuse surgery) and all probable outcomes before consenting to a medical procedure.

Key Concepts

- Breastfeeding knowledge prevents problems that can be common barriers to breastfeeding.
- A woman's feminine identity is closely related to her breasts. Any changes or issues, including those due to illness, disease, or breastfeeding, hold an emotional significance to her.
- Inverted nipples need not impede breastfeeding provided a mother receives accurate information and assistance in learning effective intervention techniques. The degree of inversion typically lessens as breastfeeding continues.
- Typically, the size and length of nipples varies greatly among women and is genetically influenced. Unusually long nipples can make it difficult for a small infant to breastfeed.
- Recurrent plugged milk ducts plague some mothers while other mothers never experience one. There is no conclusive evidence that shows one particular cause, but it is commonly thought that a constricting bra, poor nutrition, stress, and an inadequately drained breast are contributing factors.
- A red, tender spot in the breast that is warm to the touch characterizes a plugged milk duct. It is a palpable lump of well-defined margins and occurs close to the surface of the skin or can be located deeper in the breast.
- A breast infection or mastitis may or may not be the result of a plugged duct. It is characterized by the symptoms of a plugged duct, but will include a flulike muscular aching and fever.
- Mastitis is usually treated with a penicillinase-resistant penicillin or a cephalosporin that covers *Staphylococcus aureus* (the bacteria usually present) for 6 to 10 days. Trimethoprim-sulfamethoxazole and erythromycin are used to treat chronic mastitis.
- Breastfeeding mothers can experience unexplained rashes, eczema, and herpes lesions on the breast that are painful and can hinder breastfeeding. Accurate diagnosis and/or use of medications help to resolve the problem.
- *Candida* is a yeast naturally found in the mucous membranes of the gastrointestinal and genitourinary tract. Use of antibiotics promotes an overgrowth that can result in symptoms that include pain in the mother's breast and vagina and symptoms in the baby's mouth and diaper area. Oral and topical antifungal medications are prescribed. Sometimes, the mother's sexual partner requires treatment too.
- A breast vasospasm causes extreme breast or nipple pain and is often referred to as a variation of Raynaud's phenomenon, which affects fingers and toes. Exposures to the cold triggers painful nipple blanching where the nipple can experience a color change from white to blue to red. Treatment includes a vasodilator, Nifedipine, and topical use of heat to relieve pain.
- A milk blister can cause extreme pain when the epidermis seals over the ductal opening and prevents milk from draining. If it does not resolve naturally, it is possible to manually remove the excess skin to promote healing.
- Breast augmentation is now commonplace in our society. Silicone gel is again being used for breast implants. Breast augmentation is less likely to impede breastfeeding than is breast reduction. Women who have had previous breast surgery have a greater than threefold risk of lactation insufficiency when compared with women who have not had surgery.
- A breast lump in a lactating woman is typically caused by a galactocele, a milk-filled lacteal cyst. Although seldom malignant, a lump that does not resolve itself should be biopsied. After the biopsy, breastfeeding can usually resume within 12 hours.
- In all women, fibrocystic disease accounts for 50 to 75 percent of all breast biopsies. About

one fourth of women with fibrocystic disease develop a cyst or a fibroadenoma, a smooth, round lump that moves easily when palpated and is harmless. A needle aspiration will confirm the diagnosis.

- Slight bleeding from the breast occurs in a small percentage of women, typically with their first pregnancy or upon the birth of their baby. The breast discharge can appear pink to dark red or brown. It is painless, and if it continues during lactogenesis, it is not harmful for the baby to ingest.
- Bleeding from the breast that appears bright red with no other explanation could be an indication of intraductal papilloma, a small, benign, wartlike growth on the lining of the duct. After medical evaluation, a physician may elect to surgically remove it, to confirm that it is not intraductal cancer.
- About 25 percent of all women who are diagnosed with breast cancer are in their childbearing years. Only 2 to 3 percent of breast cancer is diagnosed during pregnancy and lactation.
- Premenopausal women who breastfed have protective factors from breast cancer based on how many children they have, how long each child was nursed, and the age of the mother when she gave birth.
- Breastfeeding's protective effect may come from a reduction in the number of ovulations and lower estrogen levels. Breastfeeding also reduces the concentration of carcinogens present in the ductal and lobular epithelial cells in the breast.
- Although rare, lactating breasts can develop breast cancer. Although improved, diagnosis is often delayed due to difficulty in palpating a lump and/or lack of sensitivity of mammography due to the density, glandularity, and water content of the lactating breast.
- A breastfeeding mother who has a lump that does not show change during the normal course of breastfeeding over a 72-hour period should have it evaluated.
- Breastfeeding mothers who suffer from recurring bouts of mastitis or a plugged duct that occurs in the same location should be evaluated.
- A mother diagnosed with breast cancer will not harm her baby by continuing to breastfeed. Although, when chemotherapy begins, the infant must be weaned. All chemotherapeutic drugs cross into the milk and are potentially toxic to the infant.
- Women who have been treated for breast cancer go on to have normal, uneventful pregnancies though lactation in the treated breast may be abnormal.
- After breast surgery, breastfeeding can resume as soon as the mother becomes comfortable with it. Until then, a breast pump can be used to relieve discomfort and to stimulate the milk supply.
- Breast surgery has many implications for a breastfeeding mother and baby. Healthcare professionals must provide accurate and realistic information and support for the mother who must contemplate breast surgery. The lactation consultant, in particular, must act as an advocate for the breastfeeding mother and baby as the mother evaluates all possible options available to her.

Internet Resources

Breast cancer in pregnancy and lactation:
- Centers for Disease Control and Prevention—http://www.cdc.gov/cancer/breast
- National Cancer Institute—http://www.cancer.gov/cancerinfo/pdq/treatment/breast-cancer-and-pregnancy
- American Cancer Society—http://www.cancer.org/docroot/CRI/content/CRI_2_6x_Pregnancy_and_Breast_Cancer.asp?sitearea

Breast surgery information for healthcare providers and mothers:

- BFAR: Breastfeeding After Reduction—http://www.bfar.org
- American Society of Plastic Surgeons—http://www.plasticsurgery.org

Thrush and other breastfeeding information for mothers and parents:
- http://www.iparenting.com/channels/breastfeeding
- http://www.breastfeed.com/articles/3268/1
- http://breastfeeding.com

References

Acarturk S, Gencel E, Tuncer I. An uncommon complication of secondary augmentation mammoplasty: bilaterally massive engorgement of breast after pregnancy attributable to postinfection and blockage of mammary ducts. *Aesth Plast Surg.* 2005;29:274–279.

Alexander JM, Grant AM, Campbell MJ. Randomised controlled trial of breast shells and Hoffman's exercises for inverted and non-protractile nipples. *Br Med J.* 1992;304:1030–1032.

American Cancer Society. Pregnancy and Breast Cancer [Web page]. 2008. Available at: http://www.cancer.org/docroot/CRI/content/CRI_2_6x_Pregnancy_and_Breast_Cancer.asp. Accessed January 5, 2009.

Amir LH. Eczema of the nipple and breast: a case report. *J Hum Lact.* 1993;9:173–175.

Amir LH. An audit of mastitis in the emergency department. *J Hum Lact.* 1999;15:221–124.

Amir LH, Lumley J. Women's experiences of mastitis: I have never felt worse. *Aus Fam Phys.* 2006;35:745–747.

Amir LH et al. Psychological aspects of nipple pain in lactating women. *J Psychosom Obstet Gynecol.* 1996;17:53–58.

Amir LH et al. Incidence of breast abscess in lactating women: report from an Australian cohort. *BJOG: Int J Obstet Gyn.* 2004;111:1378–1381.

Amir LH et al. A descriptive study of mastitis in Australian breastfeeding women: incidence and determinants. *BMC Public Health.* 2007;7:62–71.

Anderson JE, Held N, Wright K. Raynaud's phenomenon of the nipple: a treatable cause of painful breastfeeding. *Pediatrics.* 2004;113:e360–e364.

Ashford T. Breastfeeding success after breast reduction. *La Leche League International: New Beginnings.* 2001;July/August:128–131.

Baca D, Drexler C, Cullen E. Obstructive laryngotracheitis secondary to gentian violet exposure. *Clin Pediatr.* 2001;40:233–236.

Barankin B, Gross MS. Nipple and areolar eczema in the breastfeeding women. *J Cutan Med Surg.* 2004;8(2)n:126–130.

Berens PD. Prenatal, intrapartum, and postpartum support of the lactating mother. In: Schanler RJ, ed. Breastfeeding, part II: the management of breastfeeding. *Pediatric Clin No America.* 2002;48:365–375.

Bernier MO et al. Breastfeeding and risk of breast cancer: a meta-analysis of published studies. *Human Reproduct Update.* 2000;6:374–386.

Bevin TH, Persok CK. Breastfeeding difficulties and a breast abscess associated with a galactocele: a case report. *J Hum Lact.* 1993;9:177–178.

Binns SE. Light-mediated antifungal activity of echinacea extracts. *Planta Med.* 2000;66(3):241–244.

Brackett VH. Eczema of the nipple/areola area. *J Hum Lact.* 1988;4:167–168.

Brent NB. Thrush in the breastfeeding dyad: results of a survey on diagnosis and treatment. *Clin Peds.* 2001;40:503–506.

Brinton LA et al. Breastfeeding and cancer risk. *Cancer Causes Control.* 1995;6:199–208.

Brown SL et al. Breast implant surveillance reports to the U.S. Food and Drug Administration: maternal-child health problems. *J Long-Term Effect Med Implants.* 2006;16(4):281–290.

Brucker MC, Scharbo-DeHaan M. Breast disease: the role of the nurse-midwife. *J Nurse Midwifery.* 1991;36:63–73.

Brzozowski D et al. Breast-feeding after inferior pedicle reduction mammaplasty. *Plast Reconstruct Surg.* 2000;105:530–534.

Buescher ES, Hair PS. Human milk anti-inflammatory component content during acute mastitis. *Cellular Immunol.* 2001;210:87–95.

Buraglio T. Stress and deep breast pain. *New Beginnings.* 2003;20(1):9–10.

Cantlie HB. Treatment of acute puerperal mastitis and breast abscess. *Can Fam Physician.* 1988;34:2221–2226.

Caputy CG, Flowers RS. Copious lactation following augmentation mammoplasty: an uncommon but not rare condition. *Aesth Plast Surg.* 1994;18:393–397.

Cherchel A, Azzam C, De Mey A. Breastfeeding after vertical reduction mammaplasty using a superior pedicle. *J Plastic Reconstruct Aesth Surg.* 2007;60:465–470.

Chetwynd EM et al. Fluconazole for postpartum *Candida* mastitis and infant thrush. *J Hum Lact.* 2002;18:168–171.

Collaborative Group on Hormonal Factors in Breast Cancer. Breast cancer and breastfeeding: collaborative reanalysis of individual data from 47 epidemiological studies in 30 countries, including 50,302 women with breast cancer and 96,973 women without the disease. *Lancet.* 2002;360:187–195.

Connell S, Patterson C, Newman B. A qualitative analysis of reproductive issues raised by young Australian women with breast cancer. *Health Care Women Inter.* 2006;27:94–110.

Daniels M et al. Associations between breast cancer risk factors and religious practices in Utah. *Prev Med.* 2004;38:28–38.

David FC. Lactation following primary radiation therapy for carcinoma of the breast [letter]. *Int J Radiat Oncol Biol Phys.* 1985;11:1425.

Day TW. Unilateral failure of lactation after breast biopsy. *J Fam Pract.* 1986;23:161–162.

Deemarsky LJ, Semiglazov VF. Cancer of the breast and pregnancy. In: Ariel IM, Cleary JB, eds. *Breast Cancer: Diagnosis and Treatment.* New York, NY: McGraw-Hill, 1987:475–488.

Deloach ED, Lord SA, Ruf LE. Unilateral galactocele following augmentation mammoplasty. *Ann Plast Surg.* 1994;33:68–71.

Donegan WL, Spratt JS. *Cancer of the Breast.* Philadelphia, PA: W. B. Saunders; 1988:685–687.

Efrem SEE. Breast abscesses in Nigeria: lactational versus non-lactational. *J R Coll Surg Edinb.* 1995;40:25–27.

Eglash A, Proctor R. A breastfeeding mother with chronic breast pain. *Breastfeed Med.* 2007;2(2):99–104.

Engstrom BL. Women's views of counseling received in connection with breastfeeding after reduction mammaplasty. *J Adv Nursing.* 2000;32:1143–1151.

Escott R. Vasospasm of the nipple: another case [letter]. *J Hum Lact.* 1994;10:6.

Espinosa LA, Daniel BL, Vidarsson L, Zakhour M, Ikeda DM, Herfkens RJ. The lactating breast: contrast-enhanced MR imaging of normal tissue and cancer. *Radiology.* 2005;237(2):429–436.

Fernandez L et al. The bacteriocin nisin, an effective agent for the treatment of Staphylococcal mastitis during lactation. *J Hum Lact.* 2008;24:311–316.

Fetherston C. Risk factors for lactation mastitis. *J Hum Lact.* 1998;14:101–109.

Fetherston C. Mastitis in lactating women: physiology or pathology? *Breastfeed Rev.* 2001;9(1):5–12.

Fetherston CM, Lai CT, Hartmann PE. Relationships between symptoms and changes in breast physiology during lactation mastitis. *Breastfeed Med.* 2006;3;136–145.

Fetherston C, Wells JI, Hartmann PE. Severity of mastitis symptoms as a predictor of C-Reactive protein in milk and blood during lactation. *Breastfeed Med.* 2006;1(3):127–135.

Fetherston C. Factors influencing the initiation and duration of breastfeeding in a private Western Australian maternity hospital. *Breastfeed Rev.* 1995;3:9–14.

Foxman B, Schwartz K, Looman SJ. Breastfeeding practices and lactation mastitis. *Soc Sci Med.* 1994;38:755–761.

Foxman B et al. Lactation mastitis: occurrence and medical management among 946 breastfeeding women in the United States. *Amer J Epidemiol.* 2002;155:103–114.

Garrison CP. Nipple vasospasm, Raynaud's syndrome and nifedipine. *J Hum Lact.* 2002;18:382–385.

Gibberd GF. Sporadic and epidemic puerperal breast infections. *Am J Obstet Gynecol.* 1953;65:1038–1041.

Goldsmith HS. Milk rejection sign of breast cancer. *Am J Surg.* 1974;127:280–281.

Grassley JS. Breast reduction surgery. *AWHONN Lifelines.* 2002;6:244–249.

Green JP. Post-irradiation lactation [letter]. *Int J Radiat Oncol Biol Phys.* 1989;17:244.

Groins RA et al. Comparison of fluconazole and nystatin oral suspensions for treatment of oral candidiasis in infants. *Ped Infec Dis J.* 2002;21:1165–1167.

Guthrie E et al. Psychosocial status of women requesting breast reduction surgery as compared with a control group of large-breasted women. *J Psychosom Res.* 1998;45(4):331–339.

Hadary A, Zidan J, Oren M. The milk-rejection sign and earlier detection of breast cancer. *Harefuah.* 1995;128:680–681.

Hale T. *Candida albicans*: Is it really in the breast? ILCA Conference and Annual Meeting. Las Vegas, Nevada, July 23–27, 2008.

Hart J. Nursing after breast surgery. *La Leche League News.* 1980;22:10.

Heads J, Higgins LC. Perceptions and correlates of nipple pain. *Breastfeed Rev.* 1995;3(2):59–64.

Helewa M, Levesque P, Provencher D. Breast cancer, pregnancy, and breastfeeding. *J Obstet Gynecol Canada.* 2002;111:164–171.

Higgins S, Haffty BG. Pregnancy and lactation after breast-conserving therapy for early stage breast cancer. *Cancer.* 1994;73:2175–2180.

Hill P et al. Breast augmentation and lactation outcome. *MCN.* 2004;29:238–242.

Hoffman KL, Auerbach KG. Long-term antibiotic prophylaxis for recurrent mastitis. *J Hum Lact.* 1986;1:72–75.

Hoover HC. Breast cancer during pregnancy and lactation. *Surg Clin North Am.* 1990;70:1151–1163.

Hughes V, Owen J. Is breast-feeding possible after breast surgery? *MCN.* 1993;18:213–217.

Hurst N. Lactation after augmentation mammoplasty. *Obstet Gynecol.* 1996;87:30–34.

Ing R, Ho JHC, Petrakis NL. Unilateral breast-feeding and breast cancer. *Lancet.* 1977;2:124–127.

Johnstone HA, Marcinak JF. Candidiasis in the breast-feeding mother and infant. *JOGNN.* 1990;19:171–173.

Kakagia D, Tripsiannis G, Tsoutsos D. Breastfeeding after reduction mammaplasty: A comparison of 3 techniques. *Ann Plast Surg.* 2005;55:343–345.

Katsouyanni K et al. A case-control study of lactation and cancer of the breast. *Br J Cancer.* 1996;73:814–818.

Kvist LJ et al. A randomized-controlled trial in Sweden of acupuncture and care interventions for the relief of inflammatory symptoms of the breast during lactation. *Midwifery.* 2007;23:184–195.

Lacerna M et al. Avoiding free nipple grafts during reduction mammaplasty in patients with gigantomastia. *Ann Plast Surg.* 2005;55:21–24.

La Leche League International. *Treating Thrush.* Schaumburg, IL: The League; 2000.

Lawlor-Smith L, Lawlor-Smith C. Vasospasm of the nipple–a manifestation of Raynaud's phenomenon: case reports. *Br Med J.* 1997;314:644–645.

Lawrence RA, Lawrence RM. *Breastfeeding: A Guide for the Medical Profession.* St. Louis, MO: Mosby; 1999:273.

Lethaby AE et al. Overall survival from breast cancer in women pregnant or lactating at or after diagnosis. Auckland Breast Cancer Study Group. *Int J Cancer.* 1966;67:751–755.

Livingstone V. Problem-solving formula for failure to thrive in breast-fed infants. *Can Fam Phys.* 1990;36:1541–1545.

Loibl S et al. Breast carcinoma during pregnancy: international recommendations from an expert meeting. *Cancer.* 2006;106:237–246.

Love SM. *Dr. Susan Love's Breast Book.* 3rd ed. Cambridge, MA: Perseus; 2000:95–100.

Marmet C. Breast assessment: a model for evaluating breast structure and function. Presented at: La Leche League International Annual Seminar for Physicians; July 1990; Boston, MA.

Marshall DR, Callan PP, Nicholson W. Breastfeeding after reduction mammaplasty. *Br J Plas Surg.* 1994;47:167–169.

Maternal Concepts. http://www.maternalconcepts.com. Accessed December 26, 2007.

Menendez-Graino F et al. Galactorrhea after reduction mammaplasty. *Plast Reconstr Surg.* 1990;85:645–646.

Merchant DJ. Inflammation of the breast. *Obstetrics Gynecol Clin No Amer.* 2002;29:89–102.

Michels K et al. Being breastfed in infancy and breast cancer incidence in adult life: results from the Two Nurses' Health Studies. *Am J Epidemiol.* 2001;153:275–283.

Morino C, Winn S. Raynaud's phenomenon of the nipples: an elusive diagnosis. *J Hum Lact.* 2007;23:191–193.

Morrill JF et al. Detecting *Candida albicans* in human milk. *J Clin Microb.* 2003;41:475–478.

Morrill JF et al. Diagnostic value of signs and symptoms of mammary candidosis among lactating women. *J Hum Lact.* 2004;20:288–295.

Morrill JF et al. Risk factors for mammary candidosis among lactating women. *JOGNN.* 2005;34:37–45.

Neifert M et al. The influence of breast surgery, breast appearance, and pregnancy-induced breast changes on lactation sufficiency as measured by infant weight gain. *Birth.* 1990;17:31–38.

Newcomb PA et al. Lactation and a reduced risk of premenopausal breast cancer. *N Engl J Med.* 1994;330:81–87.

Newman J, Pitman T. *The Ultimate Breastfeeding Book of Answers.* Roseville, CA: Prima; 2000.

Nickell WB, Skelton J. Breast fat and fallacies: more than 100 years of anatomical fantasy. *J Hum Lact.* 2005;21:126–130.

Noble R. Milk under the skin (milk blister)—a simple problem causing other breast conditions. *Breastfeed Rev.* 1991;2:118–119.

Norwood SL. Fibrocystic breast disease. *JOGNN Nursing.* 1989;19:116–119.

O'Callaghan MA. Atypical discharge from the breast during pregnancy and/or lactation. *Aust NZ J Obstet Gynaecol.* 1981;21:214–216.

Oliver WJ et al. Neonatal group B streptococcal disease associated with infected breast milk. *Arch Dis Child Fetal Neonatal Ed.* 2000;83:48–49.

Osterman KL, Rahm V. Lactation mastitis: bacterial cultivation of breast milk, symptoms, treatment and outcome. *J Hum Lact.* 2000;16:297–302.

Page SM, McKenna DS. Vasospasm of the nipple presenting as painful lactation. *Obstet Gynecol.* 2006;208:806–808.

Park HS, Yoon CH, Kim HJ. The prevalence of congenital inverted nipple. *Aesth Plast Surg.* 1999;23:1446.

Paster BA. Surgery on the nursing breast. *New Beginnings.* 1986;2:92.

Penny WJ, Lewis MJ. Nifedipine is excreted in human milk. *Eur J Clin Pharmacol.* 1989;36:427–428.

Petok ES. Breast cancer and breastfeeding: five cases. *J Hum Lact.* 1995;11:205–209.

Potter B. A multi-method approach to measuring mastitis incidence. *Comm Pract.* 2005;78:169–173.

Rampaul RS et al. A tale of two axillae. *Breast J.* 2005;11:160–161.

Resico S. Nursing after breast surgery. *New Beginnings.* 1990;6:118.

Ribeiro GG, Palmer MK. Breast carcinoma associated with pregnancy: a clinician's dilemma. *Br Med J.* 1977;2:1524–1527.

Riordan J, Nichols F. A descriptive study of lactation mastitis in long-term breastfeeding women. *J Hum Lact.* 1990;6:53–58.

Rodger A, Corbett PJ, Chetty U. Lactation after breast conserving therapy, including radiation therapy, for early breast cancer. *Radiother Oncol.* 1989;15:243–244.

Romieu I et al. Breast cancer and lactation history in Mexican women. *Am J Epidemiol.* 1996;143:54–52.

Saber A. The milk rejection sign: a natural tumor marker. *Am Surg.* 1996;62:998–999.

Sawhney S et al. Sonographic appearances of galactoceles. *J Clin Ultrasound.* 2002;30:18–22.

Smith WL, Erenberg A, Nowak A. Imaging evaluation of the human nipple during breastfeeding. *Am J Dis Child.* 1988;142:76–78.

Soderstrom B. Helping the woman who has had breast surgery: a literature review. *J Hum Lact.* 1993;9:169–171.

Song IC, Hunter JG. Galactorrhea after reduction mamma-plasty. *Plast Reconstr Surg.* 1989;84:857.

Souto GC et al. The impact of breast reduction surgery on breastfeeding performance. *J Hum Lact.* 2003;19:43–49.

Stevens K et al. The ultrasound appearances of galactoceles. *Br J Radiol.* 1997;70:239–241.

Swelstad MR et al. Management of gestational gigantomastia. *Plast Reconstr Surg.* 2006;118:840–848.

Tanguay KE, McBean MR, Jain E. Nipple candidiasis among breastfeeding mothers. *Can Fam Phys.* 1994;40:1407–1413.

Thomassen P et al. Breastfeeding, pain and infection. *Gynecol Obstet Invest.* 1998;46:73–74.

Thomsen AD et al. Course and treatment of milk stasis, noninfectious inflammation of the breast, and infectious mastitis in nursing women. *Am J Obstet Gynecol.* 1985;149:492–495.

Tralins AH. Lactation after conservative breast surgery combined with radiation therapy. *Am J Clin Oncol.* 1995;18:40–43.

United Kingdom National Case-Control Study Group. Breast feeding and risk of breast cancer in young women. *Br Med J.* 1993;307:17–20.

US Cancer Statistics Working Group. *United States Cancer Statistics: 2004 Incidence and Mortality.* Atlanta, GA: Department of Health and Human Services, Centers for Disease Control and Prevention, and National Cancer Institute; 2007.

Utter AR. Gentian violet treatment for thrush: can its use cause breastfeeding problems? *J Hum Lact.* 1990;6:178–180.

Varsos G, Yahalom J. Lactation following conservation surgery and radiotherapy for breast cancer. *J Surg Oncol.* 1991;46:141–144.

Vogel A et al. Mastitis in the first year postpartum. *Birth.* 1999;26:218–225.

Wambach KA. Lactation mastitis: a descriptive study. *J Hum Lact.* 2003;19:24–34.

Wang IY, Lee JH, Kim KT. Galactocele as a changing axillary lump in a pregnant woman. *Arch Gynecol Obstet.* 2007;276:379–382.

Welch ST, Babcock DS, Ballard ET. Sonography of pediatric male breast masses: gynecomastica and beyond. *Pediatr Radiol.* 2004;34:952–957.

Willumsen JF et al. Subclinical mastitis as a risk factor for mother-infant HIV transmission. *Adv Exp Med Biol.* 2000;478:211–223.

Wilson-Clay B, Hoover K. *The Breastfeeding Atlas.* Austin, TX: LactNews Press; 2008.

Woo JC, Yu T, Hurd TC. Breast cancer in pregnancy. *Arch Surg.* 2003;138:91–98.

World Health Organization. *Mastitis: Causes and Management.* Geneva, Switzerland: WHO; 2000.

Yang PS et al. A case-control study of breast cancer in Taiwan—a low-incidence area. *Br J Cancer.* 1997;75:752–756.

Yang WT et al. Imaging of breast cancer diagnosed and treated with chemotherapy during pregnancy. *Radiology.* 2006;239:52–60.

Yoo K-Y et al. Independent protective effect of lactation against breast cancer: a case-control study in Japan. *Am J Epidemiol.* 1992;135:726–733.

Zheng T et al. Lactation and breast cancer risk: a case-control study in Connecticut. *Br J Cancer.* 2001;84:1472–1476.

Chapter 1

Low Intake in the Breastfed Infant: Maternal and Infant Considerations

Nancy G. Powers

Introduction

Low intake of breastmilk relative to the infant's needs is the common denominator for a number of different clinical end points. There are numerous causes of low intake and in turn numerous outcomes. The complex interrelationship of factors is illustrated in Figures 10–1 and 10–2, which contrast the normal and abnormal situations. Table 10–1 lists various authors' methods of organizing and approaching a conceptual framework for low intake and poor growth in the breastfed infant; however, none of these frameworks are able to encompass the interactions of *all* potential factors.

Infant intake and maternal milk supply are often similar to "the chicken and the egg" problem—which comes first? "Perceived insufficient milk supply" is the erroneous belief that the mother is not producing enough milk for her infant—when in reality she is. However, delayed lactogenesis or perceived insufficient milk creates vulnerability for *actual* low milk supply if supplements are unnecessarily introduced (Chen et al., 1998). If the infant receives a low volume of intake from breastfeeding but receives supplementation, then the infant will gain weight normally, but the mother's milk supply will decline further. The mother will likely be

concerned about low supply, but health professionals may dismiss the concern because the infant is growing well.

If the infant does not receive supplementation, low intake will result in weight loss or abnormally slow weight gain *in addition to* low maternal milk supply. Slow weight gain in the breastfed infant is a major concern to both parents and health professionals. When the breastfed infant is not gaining normally, the infant is the "identified patient." However, in order to evaluate the situation, *both mother and infant must be assessed* for their contribution to the breastfeeding relationship. In most cases, by careful history taking and examination, along with breastfeeding observation, the astute clinician will be able to develop a differential diagnosis for the dyad, which then allows specific management for the individual case.

The groundwork for optimal feeding with sufficient milk intake is laid during the first days and weeks of breastfeeding and lactation. The critical importance of mother and baby staying together, the baby having unrestricted access to the breast, the "proper" latch to prevent most common problems, and the avoidance of other foods and liquids for the baby, are addressed in other chapters of this text. This discussion of low intake in the breastfed

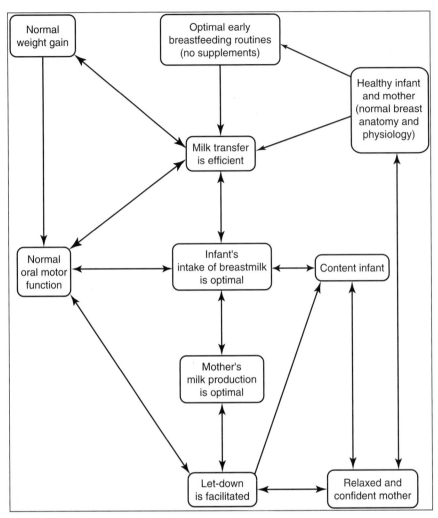

FIGURE 10–1 Positive cycle of milk intake and weight gain.

Source: Powers NG. Slow weight gain and low milk supply in the breastfeeding dyad. *Clin Perinatol.* 1999;26(2):399–430, with permission from Elsevier.

infant will begin with some general information regarding *normal* intake and growth patterns. Then we will move beyond the basics of early breastfeeding to examine more complex issues and interactions between mother and infant, as well as anatomic or physiologic variations, health status, medications, psychosocial, and medical factors.

Global Standards for Optimal Growth: The WHO Child Growth Standards

Since breastfeeding has become widely accepted as the optimal form of infant nutrition, many experts have advocated for *entirely new* growth standards based upon optimal breastfeeding practices. Routine measurements of weight, length (or height), and head circumference are a standard of care for infants and children. These measurements are typically plotted on a growth chart that reflects percentiles for the normal population at a given age. Since 1977, the World Health Organization (WHO) has used US-based National Center for Health Statistics (NCHS) reference data for height and weight to assess nutritional status of children worldwide. This reference data with corresponding growth charts was known as the NCHS/WHO reference; over the succeeding years, the limitations of the NCHS/WHO

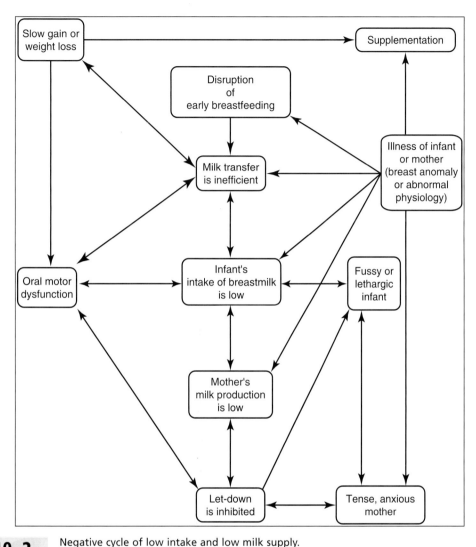

FIGURE 10–2 Negative cycle of low intake and low milk supply.

Source: Powers NG. Slow weight gain and low milk supply in the breastfeeding dyad. *Clin Perinatol.* 1999;26(2):399–430, with permission from Elsevier.

reference became well known (see previous editions of *Breastfeeding and Human Lactation*). In the United States, the Centers for Disease Control and Prevention (CDC) released a revised set of reference data referred to as the 2000 CDC Growth Charts. While the methodology was somewhat improved, the CDC 2000 reference—based on all US children and low rates of breastfeeding—was still inappropriate for much of the world's population.

In 2006, WHO released long-awaited, updated global growth standards, based upon optimal infant feeding practices. The Multicenter Growth Reference Study (MGRS) was nearly 15 years long—including

planning, data collection, and data analysis. All of the planning, methodology, and results are posted on the WHO Web site (http://www.who.int/child growth/en) and are published in *Acta Paediatrica* (2006). The new standards were developed from a large and detailed prospective study of infant growth and developmental milestones among breastfed infants (see study definition, to follow) in Brazil, Ghana, India, Norway, Oman, and the United States. The MGRS data were gathered on more than 8000 children between 1997 and 2003.

For purposes of the longitudinal study, the definition of *breastfeeding* required the following

TABLE 10–1	Assorted Schema for Poor Infant Growth During Breastfeeding	

Scheme	Concepts	Authors
Rate of gain:	Slow gain vs. impending failure to thrive vs. growth failure	Desmarais, 1990 Lawrence, 2005
Chronology:	Newborn vs. infant 6 weeks to 6 months vs. infant over 6 months	Lukefahr, 1990
Energy balance:	Decreased intake vs. increased losses vs. increased metabolic demands	Lawrence, 2005
Behavioral:	Content vs. fretful	Davies, 1978 Habbick, 1984
Etiology:	Maternal vs. infant	Lawrence, 2005 Neifert, 1983
Etiology:	Primary vs. secondary	Desmarais, 1990
Etiology:	Medical vs. psychosocial/cultural	Lawrence, 2005
Compartmental:	Milk synthesis vs. milk removal vs. milk intake Subcategories of each: preglandular, glandular, postglandular	Livingstone, 2002, 2005
Occurrence:	Common vs. rare	Powers, 1999
Appearance at presentation:	Apparently healthy vs. known illness	Powers, 1999

Source: Powers NG. Slow weight gain and low milk supply in the breastfeeding dyad. *Clin Perinatol.* 1999;26(2):399-430, with permission from Elsevier.

practices: exclusive or predominant breastfeeding for at least 4 months, introduction of appropriate complementary foods by 6 months, and continued partial breastfeeding for at least 12 months. Six gross motor milestones were included in order to correlate physical growth with developmental progress.

The study resulted in the following conclusions:

- Breastfeeding is the biological norm.
- Children all over the world grow and develop very similarly when optimally fed with human milk.
- Nutritional and environmental factors have greater influence than genetic factors on child growth.

The WHO standards for height, weight, and BMI are now "prescriptive" (demonstrating how children *should grow*) instead of "descriptive" (describing how children *actually have grown* in a given environment). The results are summarized in Box 10–1.

These standards apply to children from birth to age 5 years. The new growth charts are split into more age categories than were previously available, with a birth-to-6-month chart that details more frequent measurements than older charts. To quote the WHO MGRS study group (WHO, 2006) the differences between the previous NCHS/WHO growth standards and the MGRS will "vary—by anthropometric measure, sex, specific percentile or z-score curve, and age—in ways that are not easily summarized. Differences are particularly important in infancy." However, perhaps a few generalities can be stated: the new growth standards are likely to increase the prevalence of children labeled as underweight (in the 0- to 6-month age range), an increased prevalence of overweight in selected populations, and an overall increase in rates of stunting (low length/height for age) (see again Box 10–1).

At the time of writing of this chapter, implementation of the new standards has barely begun.

Results of the Multicenter Growth References Study (MGRS)

- Breastfeeding is the biological norm.
- Children all over the world grow and develop very similarly when optimally fed with human milk.
- Nutritional and environmental factors have greater influence than genetic factors on child growth.
- Global standards for height, weight, and BMI are now "prescriptive" (demonstrating how children *should grow*).
- Normal, optimally growing children are somewhat lower in weight and slightly taller than our previous standards have reflected.
- The new standards will generate higher rates of undernutrition from birth to 6 months of age.
- The new standards will generate lower rates of undernutrition after 6 months of age.
- The new standards will generate higher rates of overweight and obesity.

Source: Summarized from de Onis et al., 2007.

Implementation will require significant amounts of new training for health workers; the WHO goal is for the majority of countries to have adopted the new standards by the year 2010. Meanwhile in many locations, the NCHS/WHO reference or the 2000 CDC Growth Charts will remain in use. The WHO Child Growth Standards are depicted in Figures 10–3 to 10–5. In Figure 10–6 the 50th percentile of the 2000 CDC Growth Charts is superimposed on the WHO Child Growth Standards (birth to 2 years) for comparison.

US Growth Curves: Comparison to WHO Child Growth Standards

The growth charts now widely in use in the United States and also adopted in 99 other countries were published in the year 2000 by the CDC (www.cdc.gov/growthcharts). How do these charts compare to the WHO Child Growth Standards? The CDC curves are descriptive: they include a cross section of infants and children in five nutritional surveys conducted between 1963 and 1994. The CDC charts represent *only* infants from the United States. They include very few infants and children with optimal breastfeeding practices. In addition, there are no actual measurements taken between birth and 2 months of age. Finally, we must remember that with the use of *any* growth chart, the data have been gathered on a population basis. For any given child, we may see a pattern that does not exactly follow the lines on the charts—and these children must be evaluated individually according to health status, activity level, development, family traits, and other individual considerations—before jumping to conclusions based solely on numbers on a graph.

While the CDC curves represented an improvement from previous growth charts, the methodology is obviously quite different from that employed for the MGRS study. There has been a detailed analysis of the differences between the WHO Child Growth Standards and the 2000 CDC Growth Charts (de Onis et al., 2007). The CDC charts reflect a heavier and somewhat shorter sample than the WHO sample. The difference results in higher rates

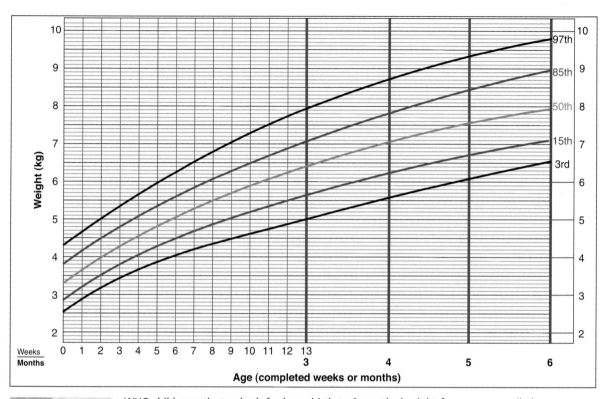

FIGURE 10–3   WHO child growth standards for boys, birth to 6 months (weight-for-age percentiles).

Source: World Health Organization. Child Growth Standards: Weight-for-Age: Birth to 6 Months, 2009. Available at: http://www.who.int/childgrowth/standards/chts_wfa_boys_p/en/index.html. Accessed January 6, 2009. Used with permission.

of undernutrition from birth to 6 months of age, lower rates of undernutrition after 6 months of age, and higher rates of overweight and obesity when using the WHO standards. See Table 10–2 for a summary of the comparisons.

We can compare the CDC and new WHO charts by looking at percentiles for *boys' weights* and *Z-scores* (a statistical method for comparing two items with different means and/or standard deviations). The publication by de Onis et al. uses Z-scores for boys, although they state that the same patterns are observed in girls. See Figure 10–6. We will compare *weight* charts because they show a greater magnitude of difference than do length/height charts.

Onset of Lactation and Newborn Weight Loss

The events of lactogenesis II are set in motion by the delivery of the placenta. There is wide individual variation in the rapidity of onset of copious milk secretion among women: some women take up to

2 weeks to produce the volume of milk that other women produce on the second or third day.

Meanwhile, in the first days after delivery, more than 95 percent of infants lose weight, primarily due to fluid loss as a natural consequence of declining maternal hormones. At the same time, their fluid intake is relatively low, due to the small (but normal) volumes of colostrum. A large comprehensive observational study by Dewey et al., 2003, studied primiparous and multiparous women (and their infants) who were breastfeeding. The study revealed that the average weight loss for breastfed infants (supplemented with less than 2 oz total) in the first three days of life was 5.5 ± 3.8 percent of their birth weight. Twelve percent of the infants lost 10 percent or more below birth weight. Only 5 percent of infants gained weight in the first 3 days. Onset of lactation (OL), as perceived by the mother, occurred in less than 72 hours postpartum in 59 percent of women. However, 33 percent of primiparas had OL later than 72 hours postpartum. Late OL (over 72 hours) was associated with seven times greater

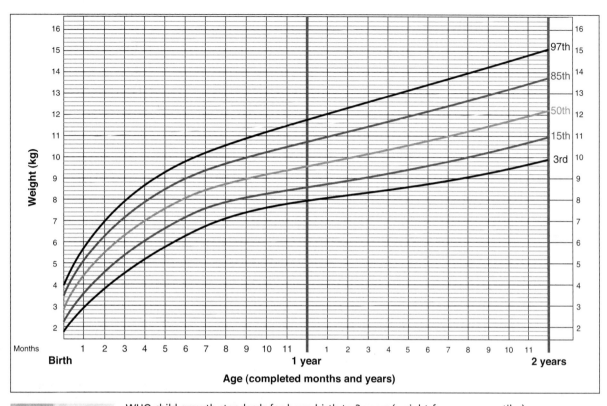

FIGURE 10-4 WHO child growth standards for boys, birth to 2 years (weight-for-age percentiles).

Source: World Health Organization. Child Growth Standards: Weight-for-Age: Birth to 2 Years. Available at: http://www.who.int/childgrowth/standards/chts_wfa_boys_p/en/index.html. Accessed January 6, 2009. Used with permission.

risk of excess infant weight loss than normal onset of lactation.

Dewey et al. (2003) also developed the concept of "SIBB" (suboptimal infant breastfeeding behavior) and found that 49 percent of infants had SIBB in the first 24 hours after birth. SIBB had some correlation to OL/infant weight loss. SIBB on day 0 and delayed OL were significant predictors of excess infant weight loss (10 percent or more below birth weight). Ninety-two percent of infant cases with excess weight loss could be predicted by combining SIBB on day 0 and delayed OL—one or the other, not necessarily both. Other risk factors identified for SIBB or excess infant weight loss were: primiparity, Cesarean section, flat or inverted nipples, long duration of stage II labor, total duration of labor over 14 hours, labor medications in multiparas and body mass index of over 37 kg/m². Heavier birth weight of infants born to primiparas was another risk factor for delayed OL. Risk factors for delayed lactogenesis, supplementation, and/or excess infant weight loss

(10 percent or more below birth weight) are summarized in Boxes 10–2 and 10–3.

The woman with slower onset of production will likely perceive more difficulties with supply in the early days (Chen et al., 1998; Segura-Millan, 1994). This causes anxiety, which interferes with letdown (limiting flow of colostrum) and further increases the tendency to provide supplements, which then further limits milk supply. This vicious negative cycle of events, labeled as "perceived insufficient milk," is correlated with shorter duration of breastfeeding. The cycle becomes difficult to reverse, and continues to spiral downward. In some cases, the milk supply is so low that "relactation" is required if the mother wants to continue breastfeeding (see Chapter 16 of this text regarding relactation).

Ongoing milk production is stimulated by milk removal, either by the infant or by some other means of expression, such as pumping (Peaker & Wilde, 1987). In the normal situation, larger birth weight

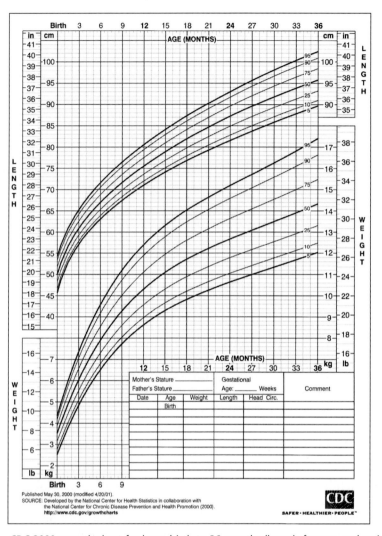

Published May 30, 2000 (modified 4/20/01).
SOURCE: Developed by the National Center for Health Statistics in collaboration with
the National Center for Chronic Disease Prevention and Health Promotion (2000).
http://www.cdc.gov/growthcharts

FIGURE 10–5   CDC 2000 growth chart for boys, birth to 36 months (length-for-age and weight-for-age percentiles).

Source: Centers for Disease Control and Prevention.

babies stimulate a larger volume of milk production than smaller babies, and the milk supply is primarily "infant driven" (Dewey & Lonnerdal, 1986; Dewey et al., 1991). In the abnormal situation, the milk supply is not appropriately stimulated, because the infant is not feeding frequently enough, is not staying at the breast for a sufficient length of time, the infant is ineffective at milk removal, or (rarely) the maternal physiology is unable to respond to the stimulation of the suckling infant. Underweight or poor quality nutrient intake in the mother has not been found to correlate with milk volumes in full lactation. Prepregnant overweight and obesity (based

on body mass index [BMI]) have consistently been found to be associated with slower onset of lactogenesis (Chen et al., 1998; Chapman & Perez-Escamilla, 1999; Hilson, 2004) and in a higher incidence of early cessation of breastfeeding (Hilson, Rasmussen, & Kjolhede, 1997). One possible mechanism for this finding is the diminished response to prolactin among overweight/obese women in the first week postpartum (Rasmussen, 2004). More recently, excessive pregnancy weight gain has been found to be associated with shorter durations of exclusive breastfeeding among *all* categories of prepregnant BMI that were studied (normal, overweight, obese)

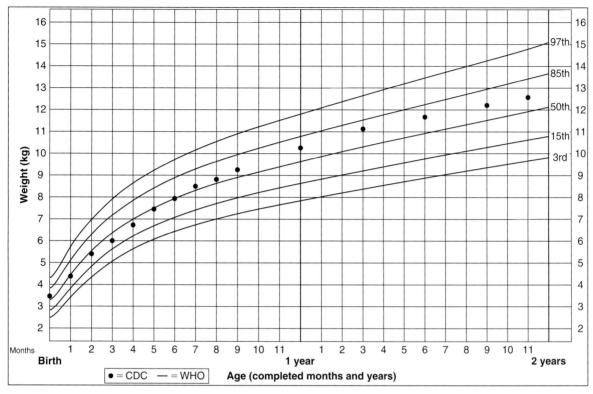

FIGURE 10–6 Comparison of the WHO and CDC weight-for-age percentiles for boys, birth to 2 years.

Source: Centers for Disease Control and Prevention. 2000 CDC Growth Charts. Available at:
http://www.cdc.gov/growthcharts. Accessed January 6, 2009. World Health Organization Child Growth Standards: Weight-for-Age: Birth to 2 Years.
Available at: http://www.who.int/childgrowth/standards/chts_wfa_boys_p/en/index.html. Accessed January 6, 2009.

(Hilson et al., 2006). This effect is additive in the woman who is obese prior to pregnancy.

Initial Newborn Weight Loss and Early Weight Gain

Infant weight loss of more than 7 percent from birth weight may be an indicator of breastfeeding difficulties and requires observation and evaluation of the breastfeeding process. Weight loss of more than 10 percent definitely requires intervention from the physician or lactation consultant (Academy of Breastfeeding Medicine, 2002; International Lactation Consultant Association, 2005). The American Academy of Pediatrics indicates the need for early follow-up of the breastfed infant. AAP guidelines (2005) state that an infant released from the hospital before 48 hours of age must be seen by a health professional at 3 to 5 days of age, when infant status and maternal milk production are at a critical juncture. Infants at risk for hyperbilirubinemia may need to be seen sooner. Thereafter, the infant should be seen as necessary to reevaluate breastfeeding and monitor weight gain. Return to birth weight is expected by 14 days of age. Once gaining, the average breastfed female infant gains 34 gm/day, while the male gains an average of 40 gm/day. For both genders, the minimum expected gain is 20 gm/day (Nelson et al., 1989) (see Table 10–3). Once above birth weight and gaining steadily, the baby is seen at routine health supervision intervals.

Low Intake and Low Milk Supply: Definitions and Incidence of Occurrence: Confusing Terminology, Limited Data, and Nonstandardized Research

Terminology surrounding abnormal growth can be confusing. Many texts have different definitions of the term *failure to thrive*. Most definitions of poor growth refer to deviations on growth charts, which,

TABLE 10–2	Comparison of 2006 WHO Child Growth Standards and 2000 CDC Growth Charts	
	WHO Child Growth Standards for Infants and Young Children	**2000 CDC Growth Charts**
Population—locations and dates	Global and diverse, from 1997 to 2003	United States only, primarily children of northern European descent from 1963 to 1994
Population—number of study subjects	• 882—longitudinal study (birth to 24 months) • 6669—cross-section study (2 to 5 years)	• Cross-sectional data • Data from 10 different data sets • Number of subjects varies for different ages of subjects
Population—nutrition	Optimal prescribed nutrition: • Exclusive or predominant breastfeeding for at least 4 months (longitudinal sample) or at least 3 months (cross-sectional sample) • Introduction of appropriate complementary foods by 6 months • Continued partial breastfeeding for at least 12 months	Observed nutrition in the United States: • Only 50% of children were *ever breastfed* • No information about exclusive breastfeeding • Very few infants were breastfed beyond 6 months of age
Population—environmental factors	• Strict criteria for site selection that would support optimal feeding routines • Other criteria that minimize environmental exposure to infectious diseases or environmental contaminants	• No environmental criteria
Population—health factors	Low-risk population • No maternal smoking (prenatal or postnatal) • Availability of energy-dense complementary foods • Socioeconomic conditions favorable to growth	Mixed population • No exclusion for smoking • Some data sets were collected from low-income populations
Data sampling (measurements)	Frequent sampling in the first 2 months	No sampling between birth and 2 months
Motor milestones	Included to assess association of physical growth and motor development	No measurement of developmental milestones

Source: Summarized from de Onis et al., 2007, and Dewey, 2001.

as discussed above, prior to the WHO Child Growth Standards, were not suitable for breastfed infants. Some authors refer to "slow gain" or "growth failure." In clinical practice, the term *failure to thrive* often carries negative connotations that imply poor parenting, neglect, or abuse. For these reasons, we will refer to the guidelines that are presented in Table 10–3 and the growth plots produced by the

BOX **10–2**

Maternal Risk Factors for Delayed Onset of Lactation (OL) (Later Than 72 Hours Postpartum)

Prenatal Factors

Excessive gestational weight gain (GWG) (Hilson, 2006)

Higher prepregnant BMI (Hilson, 2006)

Insulin-dependent diabetes mellitus (IDDM) with poor control (Neubauer, 1993)

Inverted or flat nipples (Dewey, 2003)

Obesity and excessive GWG are additive (Hilson, 2006)

Overweight and obesity (Chapman & Perez-Escamilla, 1999; Dewey, 2003; Hilson, 2006; Rasmussen, 2004)

Primiparity (Chen, 1998; Dewey et al., 2002, 2003; Grajeda & Perez-Escamilla, 2002; Hilson, 2006)

Intrapartum Factors

High cortisol levels (during labor) in multiparas (Chen, 1998; Grajeda & Perez-Escamilla, 2002)

Hospital delivery (vs. home delivery) (Chen, 1998)

Long duration of labor (Chen, 1998; Dewey, 2003)

Maternal exhaustion during labor and delivery (Chen, 1998)

Prolonged duration of stage II labor (Chapman & Perez-Escamilla, 1999; Dewey, 2003)

Unscheduled C-section (Chen, 1998; Dewey, 2003; Grajeda & Perez-Escamilla, 2002); C-section (Dewey, 2003)

Postpartum Factors

Exclusive formula feeding prior to onset of lactation (OL) (Chapman & Perez-Escamilla, 1999)

Heavier baby born to a primiparous mother (Dewey, 2003)

No rooming in (Perez-Escamilla & Chapman, 2001)

WHO Child Growth Standards (for examples see Figures 10–3 and 10–4), as opposed to any of the above jargon. If the infant falls into the category where concern is warranted, we must thoroughly evaluate the feeding process and intervene when necessary. Watchful waiting at this stage may be inappropriate, because unidentified problems often become more difficult to manage over time as the infant loses weight and the milk supply dwindles.

Much of the data regarding definitions of sufficient or insufficient weight gain in the breastfed infant is derived from the same studies that "define" sufficient and insufficient milk production. The infant's weight gain is often used as a proxy for maternal milk supply. This means that the definition of "adequate" infant weight gain will determine the "adequacy" of the milk supply. Unfortunately,

the studies have applied different definitions of adequate weight gain and used different time points to measure the babies' weights. Dewey et al. (2003) prospectively studied newborn weight loss in 280 infants. Twelve and a half percent lost 10 percent or more from birth weight by day 3. This initial excessive weight loss was correlated with delayed lactogenesis (see again Boxes 10–2 and 10–3). Neifert and colleagues (1990) found that 15 percent of infants gained less than 28.5 grams per day after the fifth day of life (Neifert, Seacat, DeMarzo, & Young, 1990). None of the infants in their study were identified as having any underlying medical problems. The cutoff point of 28.5 grams per day is probably too high, as the data from Nelson et al. (1989), discussed earlier, would have predicted 25 percent of normal infants gained less than 23 grams per day. Lukefahr (1990)

10–3

Risk Factors for Excessive Weight Loss in Infants (10 Percent or More Below Birth Weight in the First 3 Days of Life)

Maternal Factors

Delayed onset of maternal lactation (delayed OL) over 72 hours postpartum (Dewey, 2003)

Primiparity, if birth unmedicated (Dewey, 2003)

Labor pain medications, in multiparas (Dewey, 2003)

Infant Factors

Smaller infant size

Suboptimal infant breastfeeding behavior (SIBB) in the first 24 hours of life (Dewey, 2003)

Delayed onset of lactation over 72 hours postpartum (OL) (Dewey, 2003)

Infant stress (cord blood cortisol and glucose concentrations) (Chen, 1998)

Low-risk infant status at delivery (Dewey, 2003)*

Feeding-Related Factors

Lower mother–baby assessment (MBA) scores (Hilson, 2006)

*Curious result, paradoxical, hard to explain; this finding may be due to chance.

---

prospectively identified 38 breastfed infants with poor growth during a 4-year period in his private practice. When the infant presented with abnormal growth at over 1 month of age, organic causes were present in 50 percent of cases. It is difficult to draw conclusions because these three reports have different study designs, represent different patient selection biases, and have different definitions of "insufficient" weight gain.

Approaching the issue of low intake from the maternal side is equally confusing. The definition of insufficient milk is not standardized, and there are numerous confounding variables, biological as well as cultural and psychosocial. There is also the problem of determining a meaningful control group. Selection criteria, study design, and breastfeeding definition are different for each study.

As mentioned previously, in the study by Dewey et al. (2003) 12.5 percent of newborns lost more than 10 percent of birth weight—implying that there is also a 12.5 percent rate of insufficient milk supply at day 3 postpartum. In four addi-

tional studies of self-selected populations of US women who decided to breastfeed exclusively for at least 3 to 4 months, only a small percentage of women were unable to produce enough milk for their infants. Parity was mixed in these studies (Butte et al., 1984; Dewey et al., 1991; Neville et al., 1988; Stuff & Nichols, 1989). Neifert and colleagues' (1990) study—mentioned above in regards to the infant—used the same results to categorize 15 percent of US primiparas as unable to produce "sufficient milk." Table 10–4 summarizes the results of these six studies, but caution is urged in interpreting the findings; they serve to illustrate how little data we have, and how definitions can bias study results.

The definition of insufficient milk, for the purposes of this chapter, is as follows: insufficient breastmilk production to sustain normal infant weight gain despite appropriate feeding routines, maternal motivation to continue breastfeeding, and skilled assistance with breastfeeding problems.

| TABLE 10-3 | Variations of Growth in the Newborn and Young Infant | | |

Variations of Growth in the Newborn and Young Infant

Parameter	Normal: Follow Clinically	Possibly of Concern: Evaluate Breastfeeding	Abnormal: Evaluate Medical Condition and Breastfeeding
Initial weight loss (% below birth weight)	7% or less	8 to 10%	10% or more
Return to birth weight	By 2 weeks of age	Later than 2 weeks of age	Later than 2–3 weeks of age
Average daily weight gain (after return to birth weight)	Females 34 gm Males 40 gm	20–30 gm	Less than 20 gm
Weight loss after immediate newborn period	None		Any amount of unexplained weight loss
Growth curve—weight	Weight may cross percentiles downward *after* 3 months of age	Weight crossing percentiles downward in the first 3 months	Completely flat at any age
Growth curve—length	Length continues on a given percentile	Deceleration of rate of growth in length	Completely flat at any age
Growth curve—head circumference	Head size continues on a given percentile	Acceleration or deceleration of rate of growth of head	Crossing of percentiles for several consecutive measurements

Abnormal Patterns of Growth: The Baby Who Appears Healthy

Inadequate Weight Gain in the First Month

Once over birth weight, the neonate who gains less than 20 gm per day requires thorough medical and breastfeeding evaluation (see Box 10–4 and Tables 10–5 through 10–7). Poor feeding or poor weight gain can be subtle signs of illness in young infants. It is essential to keep illness (see again Box 10–2) as part of the differential diagnosis of feeding problems or poor weight gain. Yet, in the first month of life, problems with the feeding process are by far a more common cause of poor weight gain than are organic illnesses (Lukefahr, 1990; Neifert, Seacat, & Jobe, 1985). Detection and correction of the feeding problem should be addressed. Once feeding has improved, ongoing lack of weight gain may indicate underlying illness. Differential diagnosis and management are discussed later in this chapter.

The Late-Preterm Infant

Infants delivered at 35 to 37 weeks gestation (formerly called *near-term*) more closely resemble premature than term infants due to immaturity of most organ systems. Their immaturity predisposes them to the following complications: excessive sleepiness, feeding difficulties, low motor tone, dehydration, hyperbilirubinemia, apnea, hypothermia, hypoglycemia, and respiratory distress (Engle 2007). Overall, the late-preterm infant is two to three times more likely to be readmitted to the hospital; if not admitted to NICU and discharged before 48 hours of age, the risk may be as high as five to 10 times that of infants over 37 weeks gestation. Breastfeeding was found to be statistically significantly associated with readmission (Edmonson, Stoddard, & Owens, 1997; Engle, 2007; Soskolne et al., 1996). Neonatal

TABLE 10–4	**Frequency of Insufficient Milk in Selected Reports**		
Author	**Year**	**Number Insufficient of Total Number of Patients**	**Percent**
Dewey	2003	30 of 240	12.5
Dewey	1991	1 of 92	1
Neifert	1990	48 of 319	15
Stuff	1989	3 of 58	5
Neville	1988	0 of 13	0
Butte	1984	0 of 45	0

Source: Adapted from Powers NG. Slow weight gain and low milk supply in the breastfeeding dyad. *Clinic Perinatol.* 1999;26:399-430, with permission.

mortality (death at 0–27 days chronologic age) of late-preterm newborns is seven times that of term newborns. Infant mortality (death between 28 days to 1 year chronologic age) of late-preterm infants is three times higher (Engle, 2007).

Shapiro-Mendoza et al. (2008) reported that when maternal complications of antepartum hemorrhage or hypertensive disorders of pregnancy were present, the late-preterm infant has 11 times the morbidity of a term infant born to a mother with no maternal complications.

Oral–Motor Dysfunction (Ineffective Suckling)

When breastfed infants are put to breast frequently, yet fail to effectively remove milk, two problems may be responsible (separately or in combination). Either the infant is not attached properly or some form of suckling abnormality is present. The rate and pattern of suckling is flow dependent: higher suckling rates (nonnutritive) occur with decreased flow of milk (Bowen-Jones, Thomsen, & Drewett, 1982; Glass & Wolf, 1994). Thus ineffective suckling results in low milk supply and low flow, which further results in less efficient suckling (see again Figure 10–2).

Oral–motor dysfunction is a broad term encompassing abnormal motor tone and/or coordination of infant suck due to a variety of conditions. Oral–motor dysfunction may occur as an isolated and subtle finding in normal infants, often in conjunction with variations in motor tone and/or poor state regulation in the infant. Low-normal tone may result in weak suction and poor coordination, while high-normal tone results in clenching, biting, or vertical compression with the tongue. Infants with isolated oral–motor dysfunction can usually become proficient with at least one feeding method (bottle, cup, or finger-feeding). Oral–motor dysfunction will be an obvious concern when there are significant medical conditions such as neurological abnormality or cleft lip or palate. A variety of other sources (Lawrence & Lawrence, 2005; Glass & Wolf, 1994; Drane, 1996) provide in-depth discussion of suckling disorders. Unfortunately, much of the research on this topic is based upon observations of infants on artificial nipples, and their relevance to breastfeeding is uncertain. New research has begun using ultrasound along with intraoral pressure measurements to study suckling at the breast; in the near future we may have new data to inform us about suckling during breastfeeding.

Oral–motor dysfunction often presents with maternal nipple trauma and pain as well as with poor weight gain in the infant (see Figures 10–7 and 10–8). Clinically, these babies often remain calm or asleep only when at the breast. Although they appear to be asleep, when taken off the breast they cry hungrily. During active feeding, they will demonstrate a nutritive suck for only a few minutes after the initial letdown, before reverting to the nonnutritive suck (see case study in Box 10–5). In these cases it is frequently difficult to determine whether the initial problem was the infant's suck problem or the mother's milk supply, but odds favor the infant. In nearly all cases, maternal milk supply is determined

BOX 10–4

Infant and Maternal Conditions That May Contribute to Slow Weight Gain or Low Milk Supply

Infant

Allergy
Ankyloglossia (tongue-tie)
Biliary atresia
Cleft lip or palate
CNS abnormality
Congenital heart disease
Cystic fibrosis
Gastrointestinal infections
Gastrointestinal malformations
Gastroesophageal reflux
Hypocalcemia
Hypovitaminosis D
Inborn errors of metabolism
Increased caloric needs from chronic
disease, infection, malabsorption
Intestinal malabsorption syndrome
Neurological disorders
Oral–motor dysfunction (abnormal suck)
Prematurity
Renal disease
Rickets
Sepsis of the newborn
Thyroid disease
Urinary tract infection

Maternal

Autoimmune disease
Breast surgery
Chronic illness of any type
Connective tissue disease
Eating disorder
Hypopituitarism
Inverted nipples
Polycystic ovary syndrome
Postpartum hemorrhage
Pregnancy
Primary mammary glandular insufficiency
Psychiatric illness
Renal failure
Retained placenta
Stress
Theca lutein cyst
Thyroid disease

---

by the baby. An assessment of the infant's oral–motor behavior by a lactation consultant or an infant feeding specialist (e.g., an occupational, physical, or speech therapist) is required in this situation.

Gastroesophageal Reflux, Cow Milk Allergy, and Oversupply

The fussy breastfed baby may have gastroesophageal reflux disease or cow's milk allergy, or symptoms may be caused by maternal oversupply.

Primary care physicians encounter gastroesophageal reflux and/or milk allergy with sufficient frequency that these diagnoses are commonly made. Sometimes gastroenterologists or allergists have entered the picture. One review article states that about half of infants less than 1 year of age with GER have an associated cow's milk allergy. The diagnosis of cow's-milk-induced GER is made on the basis of an elimination diet and challenge (Salvador & Vandenplas, 2002). Even though breastfed infants are less likely than formula-fed infants

TABLE 10–5	History and Physical for Evaluation of the Breastfeeding Dyad		

Infant and Maternal History	Infant Examination	Maternal Examination	Laboratory Tests
• Prenatal risk factors • Previous feeding experiences • Prenatal care • Feeding plan and education • Perinatal history, especially labor, delivery, and first feeding		• Prenatal breast exam	
• Medical problems • Medications • Past medical history, especially breast surgery, postpartum hemorrhage, endocrine disorders	• Weight and growth parameters • Vital signs • General physical exam • Neurological exam, especially motor tone • Oral–motor exam (detailed)	• Vital signs • General physical exam • Thyroid exam	• General laboratory tests as indicated; consider thyroid function tests and/or endocrine consultation (prolactin levels are rarely helpful)
• Postnatal feeding and elimination history	• Breastfeeding observation	• Breast and nipple examination • Breastfeeding observation	• Test-weight, if indicated
• Infant temperament and sleep patterns • Maternal sleep, fatigue, appetite • Family history, especially atopy, diabetes, autoimmune diseases, cancer	• State transition, self-calming behaviors • General appearance, alertness, attentiveness • General exam	• General exam	
• Psychosocial history • Use of tobacco, alcohol, drugs	• Mother-infant interaction	• Mother-infant interaction • Signs of milk ejection reflex	• Depression screening or drug testing, if indicated

Source: Courtesy of Nancy G. Powers, MD.

to have reflux and/or allergy, there are occasional severe cases in the breastfed infant. Cow's milk allergy in the breastfed infant may require a strict elimination diet by the mother, as well as nutrition consultation for both diagnosis and management of this condition.

One variation of reflux in the breastfed infant is caused by oversupply of maternal milk, with delivery of high volumes of foremilk. The typical scenario for oversupply is a very chubby baby who is fussy or colicky, has very frequent watery or foamy stools (lactose overload—*not* lactose intolerance), and is fussy during feedings (see Chapters 8 and 19). Rarely, one may encounter failure to thrive in such an infant. Woolridge and Fisher (1988) reported a single case in which the dyad was

| TABLE 10–6 | Infant Factors: Problem-Oriented Management for Slow Gain or Insufficient Milk Supply |

Etiology	Management
Acute or chronic illness	• Medical management of specific entity
Ankyloglossia (short frenulum, tongue-tie)	• The presence of ankyloglossia associated with any feeding problem is usually an indication for frenotomy
Congenital anomalies	• Expression or pumping of milk to increase mother's production • Facilitate maternal let-down (relaxation techniques) • Patient attempts to latch baby at breast • Expanded definition of breastfeeding: the use of human milk by whatever feeding method is successful
Food allergy	• Maternal elimination diet; may take over 1 week for results • Maternal nutrition consultation • If severe or no response to elimination diet, refer to pediatric allergist and/or pediatric gastroenterologist
Gastroesophageal reflux	• Evaluate for maternal oversupply • Increase delivery of hindmilk (see special techniques for management) • Reduce maternal supply, if applicable • Position more upright during feeds • Frequent burping • Consider the possibility of overlapping cow's milk allergy • Medical management as indicated
Increased caloric demands	• Maximize volumes to 200 ml/kg/day if possible • Have the mother collect hindmilk • Add supplemental calories/nutrients to expressed breastmilk • See also "volume restriction" below.
Neurological conditions	• Expression or pumping of milk to increase mother's production • Chin/jaw support may be helpful • Feeding-tube device or alternative feeding method with expressed mother's milk or formula as needed for weight gain • Oral–motor therapy may be beneficial • Referral to lactation consultant • Referral to infant feeding specialist (e.g., pediatric occupational, physical, or speech therapist)
Oral–motor dysfunction	• Increased frequency of feeding • Expression or pumping of milk to increase mother's production • Feeding-tube device or alternative feeding method with expressed mother's milk or formula as needed for weight gain • Oral–motor exercises may be beneficial. • Referral to lactation consultant • Referral to infant feeding specialist
Prematurity, stable infant	• Promote skin-to-skin contact • Minimize heat loss • Feeding-tube device or alternative feeding method with expressed mother's milk, donor milk, or formula as indicated by weight loss/gain

(Continues)

TABLE 10–6 Infant Factors: Problem-Oriented Management for Slow Gain or Insufficient Milk Supply (Continued)

Volume restriction	• Additional caloric density may be indicated by supplemental means: commercial fortifier or carbohydrate or lipid • Have the mother collect hindmilk • Another alternative: skim the fat layer from stored expressed milk, then add this fat to additional expressed milk to achieve higher caloric density per given volume (approximately 8–10 calories per ml)

Source: Powers NG. Slow weight gain and low milk supply in the breastfeeding dyad. *Clinic Perinatol.* 1999;26:399-430. Adapted with permission.

successfully managed by measures that increased delivery of hindmilk, improved weight gain for the baby and gradually reduced maternal milk supply (Woolridge & Fisher, 1988).

Nonspecific Neurological Problems

Infant feeding problems with resultant poor weight gain may be the earliest indicator of various neurological problems. Developmental delays and neuromuscular disorders may not become apparent for many months, but subtle abnormalities in motor tone are usually present in infancy, and may present as oral–motor dysfunction (see previous section), with resultant growth problems. In the author's experience, neurologically based early breastfeeding problems are often characterized by inefficient feeding or disorganized feeding reflexes indicated by choking, brief apnea, or poor pacing of the suckle/swallow/breathe cycle. Inefficiency or disorganization typically causes very long feeding episodes during which the baby is not removing enough milk to gain weight and/or satiate his appetite. For the subtle neurological problems, these difficulties often occur across all feeding methods (breast, bottle, cup, finger-feeding) whereas in the infant with isolated oral–motor dysfunction, the baby can usually manage better on the bottle than on the breast.

Ankyloglossia (Tight Frenulum, Tongue-Tie)

A tight frenulum (Figure 10–9) may create breastfeeding problems such as low intake, low supply, sore nipples, blocked ducts or mastitis. Examination of the tongue may reveal a variety of findings: central depression of the tongue with bunching of the tongue laterally, retraction of the tongue (tongue may remain behind the lower gum line) with bunching of the tongue posteriorly, a "heart shaped" indentation or a cleft at the tip of the tongue that may prevent the upward mobility of the tip of the tongue. Reflexive biting, which would normally be inhibited by the presence of the infant's tongue over the lower gum, may cause a biting or chewing type of suck that is ineffective and painful (Genna, 2008).

Two randomized trials related to ankyloglossia were published in 2005 and 2006. The first study (Hogan, Westcott, & Griffiths, 2005), found an overall incidence of visible tongue-tie in 10.5 percent (201 of 1866) live births. The male to female ratio was 1.6 to 1. Of the 201, 44 percent had feeding problems, and the breastfeeding to bottle-feeding ratio was 5.8 to 1 among those with feeding problems. After accounting for dropout, 57 babies remained for randomization (40 were attempting breastfeeding and 17 were bottle feeding). Twenty breastfed and eight bottle-fed babies were randomized to receive "division" (i.e., release or frenotomy) of the tongue-tie. Twenty breastfeeding and nine bottle-fed babies were randomized to 48 hours of intensive assistance from a lactation consultant (controls). In the frenotomy group, 96 percent improved within 48 hours. One baby still did not breastfeed normally. In the control group, only one baby (3 percent) improved with 48 hours of intensive lactation support. Frenotomy versus control improved feeding significantly ($P < .001$). The results are summarized in Table 10–8. All of the control mothers subsequently requested division for their

TABLE 10–7	**Maternal Factors: Problem-Oriented Management for Slow Gain or Insufficient Milk Supply**

Etiology	Management
• Acute or chronic illness	• Medical management of specific entity
• Attachment difficulties	• Consistent skilled assistance with latch-on
• Nipple pain or trauma	• Expression (pumping) of milk 8 times/24 hr
• Inverted nipples	
• Breast abnormalities (breast surgery, breast trauma, insufficient glandular development)	• Follow infant weight gain closely the first month
	• Use feeding-tube device with formula as needed to maintain appropriate weight gain
	• Maximize production by proper positioning, frequent feedings, extra pumping
• Disruption of early breastfeeding	• Increase frequency of feedings
	• Nurse on both sides for sufficient lengths
	• Awaken baby at night for feedings
	• Household help and support for mother
	• Address sources of pain, anxiety, or stress
• Delayed milk ejection	• Relaxation techniques
	• Pain relief
	• Household help
	• Stress reduction techniques
	• Support groups or professional counseling
	• Intranasal oxytocin spray may be available via compounding pharmacy (expensive)
• Hormonal alterations (pregnancy, retained placenta, thyroid disorders, theca lutein cysts, hypopituitarism)	• Continue breastfeeding, tandem nursing is an option during pregnancy
	• Medical management of specific entity
• Ineffective milk removal (ineffective baby or pump)	• Review proper position and latch-on; check pump pressures
	• Chin support, if indicated
	• Express milk to increase supply; better pump if indicated
	• Evaluation by OT/PT/speech therapist
• Maternal medications	• Change to medications with similar therapeutic effect, but which will not affect milk supply
	• Feed baby more frequently to increase supply
	• Expression (pumping) of milk 8 times/24 hr
• Nipple shields	• Express or pump milk to increase or maintain supply
	• Wean from shield by removing it midfeed, or gradually cutting larger hole in tip
• Psychosocial problems	• Social work involvement
• Substance use/abuse	• Determine whether continued breastfeeding is appropriate

Source: Powers NG. Slow weight gain and low milk supply in the breastfeeding dyad. *Clinic Perinatol.* 1999;26:399-430. Adapted with permission.

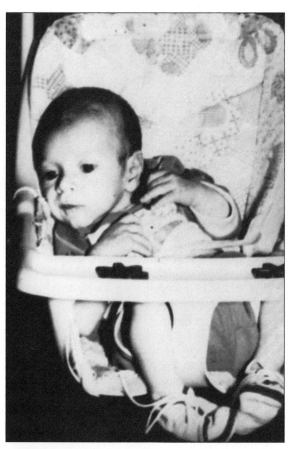

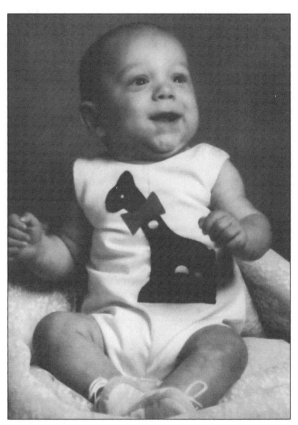

babies, and again, following frenotomy, 96 percent of the "control" group improved. Overall, feeding (breast or bottle) improvement occurred *immediately* in about 80 percent of the babies undergoing frenotomy; one baby took up to 7 days to improve. Considering the total study sample, 54 of 57 (95 percent) of babies improved feeding following frenotomy. The degree or extent of visible tongue-tie did not correlate with feeding difficulty or response to frenotomy.

The second study (Dollberg et al., 2006) included 25 term infant subjects who were randomized to either of two sequences utilizing either frenotomy or sham frenotomy. The groups were: (1) frenotomy, followed immediately by breastfeeding, then sham, followed immediately by breastfeeding (n = 14), or

(2) sham frenotomy followed by immediate breastfeeding, then frenotomy followed by immediate breastfeeding. The physicians performing the procedure/sham were blinded to the feeding evaluations done before and after each procedure. All other personnel and the mothers of the babies were also blinded to the procedure/sham. Care was taken to avoid vascular tissue and to limit bleeding. No baby had more than a few drops of blood loss. Breastfeeding assessment using the LATCH and nipple/breast pain scores was completed before and after each procedure/sham. The results indicated that immediately following frenotomy, pain score decreased significantly from 7.1 to 5.3 (*P* < .001). The LATCH score also increased (improved), though the results were not statistically significant.

These two studies, though small, provide strong evidence (randomized controlled trials, one that is

BOX	10–5

Low Intake and Low Milk Supply: A Case Study

Figure 10–7 shows a 6-week-old infant who looked and acted passive. When he went to breast, he immediately closed his eyes and appeared to be asleep; however, he could not be put down because he continually fussed and cried when not held at breast. Birth weight was 7 lb 11 oz (3.5 kg). At 2 weeks of age, the baby was 8% below birth weight, and the physician recommended formula supplementation by bottle. (Note: This is NOT the current recommendation!) The baby returned to birth weight within 1 week. The mother then made the decision to go off of supplementation, but at the 6-week visit the baby was only 6 oz (180 gm) above birth weight. The baby's physical examination did not suggest any physical problems other than weak suck. At this time, referral to a lactation consultant led to supplementation with a feeding-tube device. The baby started at 1 oz (30 ml) in the feeding-tube device (at breast) during seven daytime feedings, and breastfed two or three times at night. The infant's appetite quickly increased to 2 oz (60 ml) per feeding (or 14 oz/320 ml per day) for approximately 2 weeks. After catch-up growth, the amount of supplement in the feeding tube gradually declined over the next 2 months. By 4 months of age, the infant was fully breastfeeding without supplementaton, as seen in Figure 10–8. This case was delayed in diagnosis and management. If proper intervention had occurred at 2 weeks, the intervention would probably have been of much shorter duration.

double-blinded) that tongue-tie is associated with feeding difficulties, in breastfeeding infants more so than in bottle-feeding infants. Additionally, frenotomy is safe and is effective in improving a variety of feeding problems, and that the "degree" of visible tongue-tie does not correlate with the degree of feeding problem nor with the need for frenotomy. Screen for a family history of easy bleeding and check for extensive adhesions of the tongue to the floor of the mouth. If these conditions are not present, one may suggest consultation for frenotomy.

Abnormal Patterns of Growth: The Baby with Obvious Illness

The presence of a known medical complication, such as prematurity, infection, congenital heart disease, trisomy 21, congenital abnormalities, cystic fibrosis, and other health conditions (see again Box 10–4) puts the infant at risk for poor growth. These infants often have a combination of increased metabolic demands, low endurance for feeding, and lower growth rates despite close attention to feeding routines (Combs & Marino, 1993; Jones, 1988). Although these babies need increased caloric intake, volume restrictions may be necessary. Because such infants particularly benefit from human milk, special assistance must be provided to mothers regarding maintaining milk production while creative efforts are made to get adequate calories into the baby (see the section on special techniques for management at the end of this chapter). The goal is that with improved growth, the infant will eventually nurse completely at the breast. See Chapter 19 for detailed information regarding individual disorders and feeding implications.

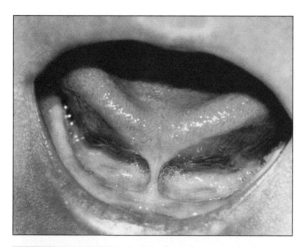

FIGURE **10–9**   A tight frenulum, attached at the tip of the tongue and at the alveolar ridge, limiting full motion of the tongue for suckling.

Source: Courtesy of Gregory E. Notestine; used with permission of Kathleen Auerbach.

Maternal Considerations: The Mother Who Appears Healthy

When there have been no previous known risk factors in the perinatal history, perhaps undiscovered risks are present, or some new disease process has arisen since delivery. What factors might be present and relatively asymptomatic other than the disruption of lactation? Box 10–4 lists maternal pathology associated with low milk production and low weight gain.

Delayed Lactogenesis

As mentioned earlier in this chapter, delayed lactogenesis may contribute to early supplementation, and subsequently, to a reduction in ultimate milk supply. (See again Box 10–2, which lists risk factors for delay of lactogenesis.)

Stress

Labor and delivery are stressful events. Chen and colleagues (1998) found that higher degrees of stress were associated with delayed onset of lactogenesis. New mothers also commonly experience a number of physical, social, and/or emotional stresses after

delivery, related to the life changing event of childbirth. These stresses are expected, and should not normally interfere with breastfeeding. Moderate to severe stress has been documented to inhibit oxytocin and subsequently interfere with milk production (see again Figure 10–2). Ruvalcaba (1987) reported some fascinating cases of sudden loss of milk and loss of milk flow in several women living in Mexico City during the 1985 earthquake. However, other mothers have been able to survive extreme circumstances while continuing to breastfeed their infants.

Inverted Nipples

Because inverted nipples can cause difficulty with proper latch-on, milk supply obviously may be adversely affected. Dewey and colleagues (2003) found that delayed onset of lactation was approximately twice as common among women with "flat or inverted nipples." Some experts have emphasized the importance of breast examination during the third trimester, with the intent to "treat" inverted nipples with various manual or mechanical methods. One prospective study found 6.7 percent of pregnant nulliparas ($n = 1926$) with at least one inverted or nonprotractile nipple (Alexander, Grant, & Campbell, 1992). This study is the only one performed to assess the efficacy of various treatments. There was no difference in breastfeeding outcomes between women who received treatment versus those who received none. Therefore, prenatal treatment is controversial, but knowledgeable and supportive care after delivery is essential.

Nipple Shields

Nipple shields are devices made of latex or silicone that cover the mother's nipple and areola, providing an artificial nipple for the infant while suckling at the breast. Nipple shields have been used to assist and maintain latch-on, to provide temporary relief from sore nipples, or to reduce rapid flow. Early studies indicated that use of shields impaired milk removal and subsequent milk production. More recent case reports and editorials (Bodley & Powers, 1996; Wilson-Clay, 1996; Pessl, 1996; Sealy, 1996) as well as research in preterm infants (Meier et al., 2002)

| TABLE 10–8 | Division of Tongue-Tie vs. Controls Improves Feeding Problems |

		Outcomes			
		Improvement	No Improvement	Total	*P* Value
All babies	Control	1	28	29	
	Division	27	1	28	.001
Breastfed	Control	1	19	20	
	Division	19	1	20	.001
Bottle-fed	Control	0	9	9	
	Division	8	0	8	.001

Source: Hogan M, Westcott C, Griffiths M. Randomized, controlled trial of division of tongue-tie in infants with feeding problems. *J Paediatr Child Health*. 2005;41:246-250. Reproduced with permission.

indicate that knowledgeable professionals may choose to use a silicone (not latex) shield in selected cases, after weighing the risks versus the benefits of this intervention (see Chapter 12). If a silicone nipple shield is used, the mother should express her milk at the end of or between nursing sessions to ensure an adequate milk supply. Eventually, the shield is removed and milk expression is discontinued. Close follow-up of weight gain and milk supply are imperative until the shield has been discontinued.

Hormonal Alterations

Milk production depends upon an array of primary and supporting hormones (see Chapter 3). Thus, it is not surprising to find that a variety of maternal conditions characterized by hormonal alterations will affect milk supply. Pregnancy superimposed on established lactation or retained placental fragments may decrease milk supply (Lawrence & Lawrence, 2005; Neifert, McDonough, & Neville, 1981). Hormonal characteristics of polycystic ovary syndrome and theca lutein cysts are suspected of inhibiting lactation, probably due to high circulating androgen levels (Hoover, Barbalinardo, & Platia, 2002). Although individual susceptibility varies, oral contraceptives containing estrogenic compounds will decrease milk production over several months (Hale, 2006).

Postpartum thyroiditis occurs in up to 5 percent of new mothers and may be associated with either hyper- or hypothyroidism (Wilson & Foster, 1992). Lactation experts generally agree that thyroid disorders in lactating women can affect milk supply.

Hypopituitarism (Sheehan's syndrome) following childbirth is a rare occurrence: postpartum hemorrhage with significant hypotension causes thrombotic infarction of the anterior pituitary and loss of those hormones. Thus prolactin is not secreted, resulting in failure of lactogenesis (Lawrence & Lawrence, 2005).

Medications and Substances

In rare situations, nonhormonal maternal medications will affect milk supply. Long-acting or high doses of short-acting thiazide diuretics may suppress lactation (Hale, 2006). One study of pseudoephedrine in eight lactating women demonstrated that milk production was decreased by 24% with a single 60 mg dose (Hale, 2006). Bromocriptine, which reduces prolactin levels, was once used for suppression of lactation but is no longer indicated for this purpose.

Several studies have demonstrated the detrimental effects of maternal smoking on milk ejection, milk volumes, infant weight gain, and total duration of breastfeeding (Hopkinson et al., 1992; Horta et al., 1997; Lawrence & Lawrence, 2005). Environmental (second-hand) smoke was shown in one study to be associated with shorter duration of breastfeeding (Horta et al., 1997).

Alcohol inhibits milk ejection in a dose-related fashion (Lawrence & Lawrence, 2005). In an experiment to analyze the effect of smell and taste upon breastmilk ingestion, Mennella (1997) found that infants ingested less breastmilk after their mothers drank an alcoholic beverage.

Breast Surgery

If a complete medical history has been obtained, the practitioner should have learned of prior breast surgery. However, some women hide this information from their spouse or partner. Others neglect to mention biopsy when asked about any previous surgery. Cosmetic breast surgery may be difficult to detect with routine physical examination. Neifert et al. (1990) published a report that implicated breast surgery as a major risk factor for decreased milk production. Periareolar incision was associated with a fivefold increase in risk of "insufficient milk" as determined by infant weight gain. A second study confirmed these results (Hurst, 1996). Recent surgical techniques for augmentation employ an axillary incision, and placement of implants underneath the pectoral muscle, which minimizes surgical damage to mammary structures and nerves. Many women with breast implants harbor anxiety about potential problems caused by previous breast surgery (especially those with silicone implants). At this time, silicone breast implants are not considered a contraindication to breastfeeding. Silicone is a ubiquitous substance, and levels are higher in cow's milk and infant formula than in human milk (Hale, 2006).

Another important consideration for patients who have undergone breast augmentation is to take a careful history regarding size, shape, symmetry, and development of the breasts prior to surgery. Unrecognized "insufficient glandular development of the breast" (see section below) may have been the reason for undergoing augmentation.

Breast reduction always involves disruption of mammary tissue, and breastfeeding outcomes are highly variable. In a 2003 controlled cohort study by Souto et al., 49 Brazilian women *status post* breast reduction surgery were matched with neighborhood controls. All subjects and controls in the study had initiated breastfeeding. The mean duration of exclusive breastfeeding for the reduction group was 4 days; for controls it was 3 months ($P < .001$). Women who had undergone breast reduction surgery had an 8.7 times higher risk of discontinuing exclusive breastfeeding at 1 month postpartum compared to controls; complete weaning at 4 months was 11.6 times higher. Individualized breastfeeding care plans are essential for women who have undergone breast reduction surgery, and close follow-up is required for their infants.

Insufficient Glandular Development of the Breast

In 1985, Neifert, Seacat, and Jobe reported "insufficient glandular development of the breasts" (sometimes alternatively referred to as "primary lactation failure") of three women. There were several strikingly similar features about these women. They had notable asymmetry of their breasts, and little or no breast changes during pregnancy. They were unable to nourish their infants despite maximum feeding frequency, effective milk removal, and professional breastfeeding assistance. They had normal prolactin levels. For their infants, increasing the frequency of feeding did not result in significant weight gain, and the infants required supplementation. The assumption, based on clinical findings, was that the syndrome is apparently analogous to arrested development of other organs or glands. Neifert et al. (1990) then published results of a prospective study initially designed to determine the frequency of this disorder. More than 400 women were recruited for the study, none of whom had the clinical characteristics of insufficient glandular development of the breast. The study did detect a significant number of women who had experienced breast surgery. Huggins, Petok, and Mireles (2000) published a descriptive report of 34 mothers with breast "hypoplasia." Lukefahr stated that one of the 38 mother/infant pairs in his report fit the clinical criteria for insufficient glandular development of the breast (J. L. Lukefahr, personal communication, 2002). Based upon Neifert et al.'s (1990) study and the experience of various lactation centers, it appears that approximately 1 out of 1000 (0.01 percent) lactating women may have this clinical syndrome. See Figure 10–10 and Color Plate 27. See Chapter 3 for further information on breast development and milk production.

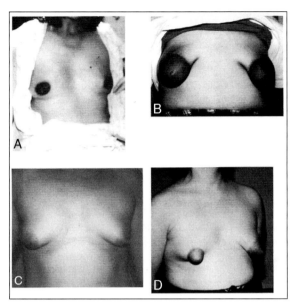

FIGURE **10–10** Women with variations of hypoplastic breasts. (A) Type 1 hypoplasia. (B) Type 2 hypoplasia. (C) Type 3 hypoplasia. (D) Type 4 hypoplasia.

Psychosocial Factors

Some women do not want to breastfeed but are being pressured to do so by a family member. Breastfeeding rarely goes well under these circumstances. Classic psychosocial failure to thrive (the result of emotional or physical neglect or abuse) is rarely seen in the breastfed infant, but it does occur. Parental drug or alcohol abuse or domestic violence may be a factor in some of these cases. Moderate to severe postpartum depression may result in excessive anxiety about the baby, alienation of the mother from her infant, and occasionally in overt abuse (Wisner, Parry, & Piontek, 2002). Two cases of Munchausen's syndrome by proxy have been reported in which the infant received ipecac in expressed maternal breast milk (Berkner, Kastner, & Skolnick, 1988; Sutphen & Saulsbury, 1988). Hypothyroidism must be considered in the differential diagnosis of maternal depression, and postpartum psychosis is often a manifestation of bipolar disorder (Wisner et al., 2002).

Maternal Nutrition

Several studies show no significant relationship between reduced maternal intake of calories or fluids and the volume of milk produced. Poor maternal nutrition will decrease birth weight of the infant, and smaller infants stimulate lower volumes of milk production (Institute of Medicine, 1991). The lactating woman needs to maintain good nutritional status for her own health as well as for future pregnancies. Rapid weight loss in well-nourished women requires further study to determine effects on milk volume. Much current research is focused on the effects of overweight and obesity upon lactation performance (see section of this chapter, "Onset of Lactation and Newborn Weight Loss" as well as Box 10–2) (Chapman & Perez-Escamilla, 1999; Dewey et al., 2003; Hilson et al., 1997; Hilson et al., 2006). Obviously, a woman with an eating disorder presents nutritional and psychosocial risks to the mother–infant relationship. See Chapter 15 for further information on maternal nutrition during lactation.

Anemia

One study (Henley et al., 1995) detected an association of anemia (postpartum hemoglobin of less than 10 g/dL) with "insufficient milk syndrome" (referred to earlier in this chapter as "perceived insufficient milk supply)." Even though this association was noted, the perceived insufficient milk supply was more closely correlated with early weaning than was anemia. More data is needed regarding anemia and effects on breastfeeding and milk supply.

Maternal Considerations: Obvious Illness

Acute illnesses may temporarily decrease milk supply, but production should rebound after the initial insult, especially in full lactation. Insulin-dependent diabetes mellitus was associated with delayed lactogenesis and lower volumes of milk production when diabetic control was poor (Neubauer et al., 1993; Perez-Escamilla & Chapman, 2001). Occasionally, mastitis will reduce milk secretion in the affected breast for the duration of lactation. The ability of women with other chronic illnesses to breastfeed depends upon their general condition (energy level, motor abilities, etc.) and the medications that they are required to take. There is currently no information regarding the effect of specific illnesses upon volume of milk production. Each case must be assessed and managed individually.

History, Physical Exam, and Differential Diagnosis

History

A complete history and physical exam for both mother and infant are critical to the evaluation of low intake or insufficient milk (see again Table 10–5; see also Chapter 20). Perinatal history includes prenatal risk factors, labor and delivery, medications, interventions, and any resuscitation efforts. A complete feeding history reviews a mother's previous feeding experiences, her feeding plan for this infant, the first feeding experience after delivery, and subsequent feeding difficulties or breast problems. Maternal past medical history and review of systems must include current routine medications, history of breast surgery, postpartum hemorrhage (risk for anemia or panhypopituitarism), or endocrine disorders. Family history and psychosocial history may also provide clues to slow weight gain due to familial conditions or family stress.

Physical Examination and Laboratory Tests

Physical examination (see again Table 10–5) for the mother is focused on areas of concern: vital signs, general skin condition, breasts, nipples, thyroid, and any other area suggested by careful history. A complete physical examination of the infant includes vital signs, weight, length, head circumference, and general examination with close attention to subtle neurological features and oral–motor exam (see also Chapter 20). Observation and evaluation of a breastfeeding session by a knowledgeable, experienced practitioner is an integral part of the objective assessment.

A multidisciplinary approach is recommended, with input from the primary care provider (family physician, obstetrician, pediatrician, midwife, nurse practitioner, or physician's assistant) and lactation consultant. In some programs with formal feeding teams, a pediatric developmental team (developmental pediatrician, speech pathologist, occupational and physical therapists), a pediatric gastroenterologist, or a pediatric allergist may conduct part of the feeding evaluation. Selective use of laboratory tests

may be helpful. Postpartum maternal thyroid disease is relatively common and may be asymptomatic aside from low milk production. Prolactin levels remain difficult to interpret, since they do not strictly correlate with milk volume. Prolactin levels are generally not very helpful in trying to evaluate or treat low milk supply.

Differential Diagnosis

After history and physical examinations have been completed, a differential diagnosis may be developed. Potential etiologies that can ultimately lead to a problem-oriented approach to management can be identified (see again Tables 10–6 and 10–7). Specific management suggestions are also included in the tables to assist with individualizing the treatment guidelines given below.

Clinical Management

Determining the Need for Supplementation

Many cases of slow weight gain in the breastfed infant will require a decision regarding *supplementation*—a term that is frequently used but rarely defined in relationship to breastfeeding. For the purposes of this chapter, and specifically for the management guidelines below, the term will be used to indicate the practice of giving the breastfed infant additional nutriment other than what he obtains directly from the breast. Supplementation may also include additional nutrients to increase the caloric density of human milk feedings (e.g., human milk fortifier). There are two important facets of supplementation to keep in mind: (1) the choice of type of supplement, and (2) the choice of method for supplementation.

Management guidelines in this chapter imply a hierarchy of preferences for type and method of supplementation. First choice for type of supplement is the mother's own expressed milk; pasteurized donor breastmilk (if indicated and if available) is the second choice; commercially prepared infant formula is the third choice. Choice for method of supplementation has not been well studied. Various experts (personal communications) have different preferences regarding various methods to supplement the breastfed baby. Some experts prefer to use the feeding-tube device and keep the baby at the breast (see Figures 10–11 and 10–12). Other experts prefer to have the baby bottle-feed to provide a rapid restoration of caloric intake, weight gain, and increase in energy for suckling once returned to the breast. Cup feeding has been well studied, is safe, hygienic, and practical for resource-poor settings (Howard et al., 1999; Howard, Howard, & Lamphear, 2003). Syringe or spoon feeding may provide other options, depending upon the specific circumstances of the case. Finger-feeding, though widely practiced, has no evidence base (see section "Oral–Motor Dysfunction" in this chapter).

Effective maternal milk expression (or pumping) is a mainstay for women who are supplementing their infants. This is best accomplished by professional electric pump or skilled hand expression (see Chapters 7 and 12 for information on breastmilk expression).

Intervention

The following management guidelines are suggested for a general approach to the slow-gaining baby. Figure 10–13 provides a flowchart of the general approach. Despite general recommendations, individualized management is required. (See again Tables 10–6 and 10–7, which give additional suggestions in this regard.)

1. Check the basics: Double-check proper positioning and latch-on. Increase the frequency, duration, and effectiveness of feedings at the breast, if these factors are not optimal, and if the infant is alert and hungry. Alternate breast massage and switch nursing may be used, if the infant is suckling actively during feedings. (See the section on special techniques for management of low intake or low supply later in this chapter.)

2. Have mother express breastmilk between feedings to increase her milk supply (see Box 10–6).

3. If the infant is clinically stable and exhibiting hunger cues, suggest optional supplementation with expressed breastmilk. If immediate supplementation is indicated by the criteria listed in Table 10–3 or by the clinical condition of the infant, use expressed breastmilk (or another alternative) to supplement the infant during or after breastfeeding.

4. Begin with ad lib supplemental feedings, following the baby's appetite. If the baby is not exhibiting hunger cues, aim for a *minimum* of 50 to 100 ml/kgm/24 hr, divided into 6 to 8

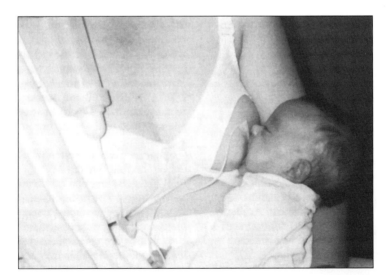

FIGURE 10–11 A mother and infant utilize a commercial feeding-tube device in order to deliver extra milk to the infant while the mother is able to feed the infant at breast and gradually increase her milk supply.

Source: Powers N, Slusser W. Breastfeeding update 2: clinical lactation management. *Pediatr Rev.* 1997;18(5):147-161. Reproduced by permission of *Pediatrics in Review.*

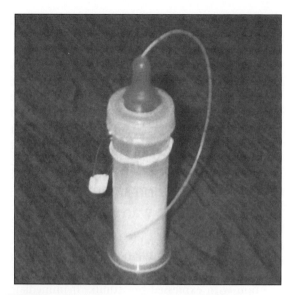

FIGURE 10–12 A homemade feeding-tube device can be made from supplies found in an office or hospital: a small bottle with slit nipple has a no. 5 French feeding tube threaded through the nipple with the hub resting in the milk. A rubber band and safety pin allow attachment of the device to the mother's clothing.

Source: Powers N, Slusser W. Breastfeeding update 2: clinical lactation management. *Pediatr Rev.* 1997;18(5):147-161. Reproduced by permission of *Pediatrics in Review.*

feedings (see Box 10–7). This minimum is suggested for infants who are not exhibiting hunger cues and whose stomachs are still small due to very low intake. Any infant may have more volume, as matched to appetite.

5. Increase the amount of supplement as indicated by infant appetite.
6. See other specific management suggestions in Tables 10–6 and 10–7.
7. Monitor and follow up infants under 3 months as follows:
   a. Monitor infant weight closely, every 2 to 4 days.
   b. Verify that weight stabilizes within 2 to 4 days.
   c. Verify that weight gain begins within 4–7 days.
   d. After 7 days, verify that the infant is gaining at least 20 gm/day (larger daily weight gain is preferable, some infants gaining 60 gm/day or more). Once weight gain

averages 20 gm/day or more, recheck every 1 to 2 weeks until infant establishes himself on a consistent growth curve.

8. If maternal milk supply has not increased within 1 week, do the following:
   a. Check the frequency of milk expression.
   b. Reevaluate maternal risk factors.
   c. Consider laboratory evaluation (especially maternal thyroid) as indicated.
   d. If maternal factors are involved, manage as indicated.
   e. Consider use of a galactogogue.
   f. If maternal evaluation is negative, reevaluate the infant.
9. If the infant does not gain weight as expected, consider the following:
   a. Verify that the infant is receiving the prescribed amount of supplemental feedings. Review specific amounts with the mother and ask her to keep written records.
   b. Determine whether the infant is willing to take the minimal amount of supplementation that is recommended. If not, strongly consider an organic illness or neurological problem.
   c. If the infant is actually ingesting the prescribed amount of supplement and still not gaining weight, evaluate the infant for illness or neurological problems.
   d. Arrange for lab tests as indicated.
   e. Treat infant illness as indicated.
   f. If the recommendations above are not effective and medical workup is underway, consider using special techniques that are discussed in the next section.

Reducing the Amount of Supplementation

As the mother's own milk production increases, the amount of other types of supplements (e.g., infant formula) will be reduced in favor of expressed breastmilk. Once maternal milk supply increases, the infant takes more milk directly from the breast and less milk by supplementary methods (infant appetite and satiety will determine this change). After the infant has attained a normal weight for age, the amount of supplementation may be reduced gradually to stimulate more milk production. This depends

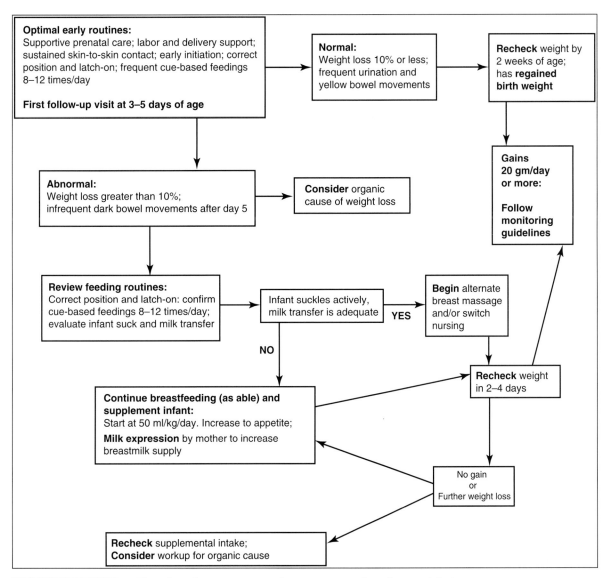

Flow chart for assessment and management of newborn weight loss.

Source: Courtesy of Nancy G. Powers, MD.

upon an increased frequency of breastfeeding as well as the infant being effective at milk removal. Continue to monitor weight gain while supplementation is reduced or withdrawn.

Family and Peer Support

Verbal, emotional, and physical supports are very important for a mother who is stressed by a significant feeding problem. In addition to support from family members, new mothers may find peer sup-

port in the community by checking with their physician, hospital of delivery, local breastfeeding support groups or the Internet.

When Maternal Milk Supply Does Not Increase

Most women who seek professional help with breastfeeding are highly motivated to breastfeed their infant. Sometimes, despite appropriate intervention and conscientious attempts by the mother

Measures That Encourage Increased Milk Production

- Apply moist heat to breasts a few minutes before feeding.
- Massage the breasts before and during feeding or pumping.
- Use relaxation techniques to reduce stress and enhance let-down.

- Feed your baby or express milk at least 8 times every 24 hours.
- Continue frequent milk removal, even if small amounts are obtained.

to follow the suggested treatment plan, her milk supply does not increase enough to fully meet the infant's needs. In some cases, her milk supply will remain at a minimal level or "dry up" completely. In these situations, the practitioner must acknowledge the emotional impact of this "failure" upon the maternal psyche: a grief reaction is common. It is often helpful for the mother to be able to talk openly with the healthcare provider or a close family member regarding her loss. If possible, they should reassure her that she did everything in her power to rectify the situation. As in any other grief situation, the passage of time will allow some degree of healing.

Special Techniques for Management of Low Intake or Low Supply

Breast Massage

Breast massage during feeding, discussed in Chapters 7 and 8, is a simple method of increasing volume and fat content of the breastmilk.

Switch Nursing

In normal breastfeeding, the baby is allowed to finish one breast before the mother switches to the other side. Infant-led feeding usually results in

optimal intake (Woolridge, Ingram, & Baum, 1990). However, for the infant who spends a large part of the feeding in a "nonnutritive" sucking pattern and is gaining weight slowly, the technique of switch nursing may be considered. Although there is no research regarding the technique, it is widely recommended. Switch nursing involves changing the baby frequently from breast to breast to facilitate more active swallowing and promote multiple letdowns during the feeding. The mother is taught to observe for a change from nutritive to nonnutritive suckling. At that point, she switches the infant to the other breast, and when nonnutritive sucking is again apparent, switches back. This pattern is repeated several times during a feeding. Switch nursing may not be useful if the baby has low endurance (due to prematurity, illness, or weight loss) or oral–motor dysfunction with an ineffective suck. If switch nursing is recommended, close follow-up of weight status is necessary.

Feeding-Tube Device

The infant can receive supplementation at the same time that he is suckling from the breast by use of a feeding-tube device that can be purchased commercially or constructed with syringes and feeding tubes (see again Figures 10–10 and 10–11). This technique provides extra volume of intake for the infant while continuing to stimulate the maternal milk supply and avoiding the potential risk of bottle preference.

BOX **10–7**

Amount of Supplement to Use in a Feeding-Tube Device

If a feeding-tube device is used to assist the baby in gaining weight, both the caregiver and the mother need to know how much supplement to give the infant. A general rule of thumb for *normal total intake* is 150 to 200 ml/kg/day of breastmilk or formula. Even if gaining slowly, most breastfed infants are getting *some* breastmilk from the breast, so we supplement with an amount that represents *partial* intake. Unless we use test weights, we will not know exactly how much the infant is receiving at the breast. A simple guideline is to begin with a minimum of 50 to 100 ml/kg/day divided into 6 to 8 feedings. The table below gives some approximate guidelines per feeding. Once supplementation has started, the amounts can be increased according to infant appetite and weight gain.

Infant Weight kg (lb)	Total Daily Intake: 150–200 ml/kg/day ml (oz per day)	Daily Supplement: 100 ml/kg/day ml (oz per day)	Approximate per Feeding Supplement: 6–8 times/day ml (oz per feeding)
2.5 kg (5 lb 8 oz)	375–500 ml (12.5–17 oz)	250 ml (8 oz)	30–40 ml (1 oz)
3.0 kg (6 lb 9 oz)	450–600 ml (15–20 oz)	300 ml (10 oz)	35–50 ml (1–2 oz)
3.5 kg (7 lb 11 oz)	525–700 ml (17.5–23 oz)	350 ml (12 oz)	40–60 ml (1.5 to 2 oz)
4.0 kg (8 lb 12 oz)	600–800 ml (20–27 oz)	400 ml (13 oz)	50–70 ml (2–2.5 oz)
5.0 kg (11 lb)	750–1000 ml (25–33 oz)	500 ml (17 oz)	60–80 ml (2–3 oz)

A feeding-tube device works well for young infants who have plenty of energy and good sucking ability but for whom the maternal milk supply has not been adequate. The mother must be carefully instructed regarding the use and cleaning of such a device (see Boxes 10–6 and 10–7).

Test Weighing

Infant test weighing has become widespread, though few practitioners understand its limitations (see Boxes 10–8 and 10–9). Test weighing involves the use of a sensitive scale (sensitivity of 2 gm or less) with digital readout and computerized integration to account for infant movement. The infant is weighed before and after feeding to determine the amount of breastmilk ingested. Weight gain in grams is approximately equal to the intake of the infant in milliliters (Woolridge et al., 1984). Test weighing on a regular office scale is not reliable and should not be done (Whitfield, Kay, & Stevens, 1981).

Test weighing should primarily be used as a research tool, because breastfed infants have large

BOX 10–8

Guidelines for Using a Feeding-Tube Device

1. Begin using the device when the mother and baby are most rested and when other household or family activities are unlikely to require the mother's attention. Use will become easier with practice.
2. Refer to Box 10–7 to estimate the amount of supplement to put into the feeding-tube device. Note that most babies will take less volume per feeding in the feeding-tube device than they would from a bottle feeding.
3. Prepare the feeding and begin the feeding process before the baby becomes overly hungry or fussy. Both mother and baby should be as relaxed as possible.
4. Fill the device and position the tubing so that it extends slightly past the end of the mother's nipple. Use any kind of hypoallergenic tape to hold the tubing in place. If the baby appears to be sucking only on the end of the tubing, pull it back so that it is flush with the end of the mother's nipple.
5. Look for the appearance of air bubbles in the reservoir. This indicates that the baby is actively swallowing.
6. Be aware that most babies will take most of the fluid in the device within the first 30 minutes. Different size tubes (to increase or decrease flow) are available with some commercial devices.
7. If the baby is actively suckling but the device is flowing very slowly or not at all, look for several potential problems:
   a. The tube may be kinked so as to block the flow. Check the tubing from bottle cap to baby's mouth.
   b. The tube may be blocked inside the baby's mouth by improper placement or kinking back on itself. Relatch the baby.
   c. The feeding-tube device may have developed a vacuum. Release the unused tube, or "prime" the device by pushing on the reservoir.
   d. The cap may be screwed on too tightly, blocking the flow. Loosen the cap and squeeze the container gently to activate the flow. If the device is working properly, there should be a steady drip from the end of the tubing.
   e. If *formula mixed from powder* is used in the device, small clumps of unmixed formula may block the tubing. Clean the tubing with hot soapy water pushed through with a syringe.
   f. The tubing was not properly cleaned and is blocked by old supplement. Try to clean the tubing again using hot soapy water pushed through with a syringe.
8. Clean the feeding-tube device soon after the feeding is finished (refer to manufacturers' instructions). The small diameter of the tubing is easily blocked.

Principles of Test Weighing an Infant

- The scale must be accurate to 2 gm or less, with computer integration for movement and a digital read-out.
- The infant must be weighed before and after every feeding for several days to get representative values.
- Infant intake in ml is approximately equal to infant weight gain in grams.
- The typical office scale is not accurate or reliable for test weighing.

- Test weighing may be used in complicated clinical situations to monitor intake and/or adjust volume of supplementation.

Source: Woolridge et al., 1984; Jensen & Neville, 1984; Whitfield, Kay, & Stevens, 1981.

feed-to-feed variability. Test weighing during one feeding does not offer an adequate representation of an "average" feeding or allow calculation of overall intake (Woolridge et al., 1984). In complicated situations where infant growth is of concern, test weighing may be used at each feeding to determine the need for supplementation (Meier et al., 1990). Alternatively, test weighing in the office may be used to "confirm" one's clinical impression of low intake or to "convince" the mother that the feedings are small. When test weighing is used for management of individual cases, it is crucial to have an electronic scale and to use the proper protocol with each weight, and for caretakers to keep detailed records of weights and feedings (see Box 10–10 for a sample procedure for performing infant test weights).

Galactogogues

Galactogogues are agents that promote milk production, such as drugs, herbs, or foods. Metoclopramide (Reglan) is indicated in selected cases, when all other aspects of milk production have been maximized. The recommended dose is 10 mg three times a day for 7 to 14 days (Ehrenkranz & Ackerman, 1986; Gupta & Gupta, 1985; Kauppila

et al., 1985). If there is a response to the drug, it is usually seen in 4–7 days after starting the prescription. Prescribing metoclopramide as a galactogogue is an "off label" use of the drug. Small amounts of the drug enter into the milk but have not been associated with clinical effects in the infant (Ehrenkranz & Ackerman, 1986; Gupta & Gupta, 1985; Kauppila et al., 1985). Maternal side effects of this drug include dizziness, nausea, sweating, and agitated depression. If depression occurs, the drug must be discontinued immediately, and symptoms typically resolve within 1 week. Some studies suggest that the increased milk production induced by metoclopramide will continue in the absence of the drug, while others indicate that milk production will drop off. The ultimate length of treatment will need to be individually based.

Domperidone, though not commercially available in the United States, is used as a galactogogue in other countries. The mechanism of action is similar to metoclopramide, but the advantage of domperidone is the lack of CNS side effects. In 2004, the FDA issued a statement that domperidone should not be used in lactating women due to concerns about arrhythmias seen with IV use of the drug. Oral use of domperidone has never been documented to cause

BOX 10–10

Procedure for Infant Test Weighing

Definition of test weighing: Weighing a baby before and after breastfeeding to determine intake.

Equipment: Digital scale with integration function that allows for movement of the infant, accurate to 2 gm (for example, Olympic Smart Scale or Medela Baby Weigh Scale).

Procedure:

- Before breastfeeding, place baby on the scale and weigh him. This is the "before" weight. It is fine to have clothing or a blanket but the final weighing must be done with exactly the same clothing and accessories as the initial weighing.
- Mother breastfeeds the infant. Do not change diaper yet.
- Reweigh the infant, with the exact same clothes, diaper, blanket, burp cloth, etc. This is the "after" weight. (It is possible to weigh before and after each breast, if the information is useful.)
- Subtract the first (before) weight from the second (after) weight. The difference in grams is considered the "intake" in milliliters. (Some scales automatically store the values and compute the difference for you. Refer to manufacturers' instructions.)
- If the "after" weight is smaller than the "before" weight, this means the baby has lost weight—which is possible. It also might mean that you forgot a blanket on the second weighing or that someone changed the diaper and removed weight.
- Burp cloth or clothing with any drool or emesis shall be included with the weight, to reflect original intake. (Record emesis in documentation of output.)
- If the infant receives a tube feeding at the same time as breastfeeding, subtract the amount given via tube to determine the amount of breastmilk ingested directly by breastfeeding.
- Record the intake of breastmilk and any supplement volumes.
- Parents can be taught to perform test-weights for the hospital or home setting. This allows them to start a feeding without waiting for a nurse to come and perform the test weights.

---

arrhythmias, so some physicians in the United States will arrange to have domperidone specially compounded for use as a galactogogue, though the cost may be prohibitive (Hale, 2006).

Though not strictly a galactogogue, oxytocin nasal spray (40 IU per ml) is used to stimulate milk ejection if mother's own letdown is inhibited by stress or pain. Oxytocin nasal spray is not commercially available, but like domperidone, may be specially compounded by selected pharmacies (Hale, 2006). Foods and herbs are used in many cultures to increase milk supply. Brewer's yeast and fenugreek have a long history as galactogogues, but only two abstracts are available for fenugreek (Swafford & Berens, 2000; Co, Hernandez, & Co, 2002), and no studies were found for brewer's yeast.

Hindmilk

Hindmilk refers to breastmilk that is obtained toward the end of the feeding episode as contrasted with the initial milk, called "foremilk." Fat content varies considerably from feed to feed, but within a given feeding, it rises steadily. There is no specific cutoff time for this definition, nor any specific fat percentage. The concept of foremilk and hindmilk imbalance is an artificial construct used for dyads when maternal production is significantly higher than infant intake. For example, a mother may be expressing 30 oz (900 ml) per day for a premature infant who is ingesting only 7 oz (210 ml) per day.

In cases where the mother is expressing milk for her infant, and has a generous supply (e.g., for a preterm or cardiac baby), she can fractionate her expressed milk by expressing milk for 2 to 3 minutes after letdown (foremilk), change containers to finish expressing (hindmilk) and use hindmilk to feed the baby (Valentine, Hurst, & Schanler, 1994). A sample of patient instructions is presented in Box 10–11. Very low birth weight infants who receive fortified breast milk must also receive fortification in hindmilk. If the infant is feeding at the breast, delivery of hindmilk may be increased by unlimited nursing on the first breast and/or by massage of the breast during feeding.

BOX 10–11

Patient Instructions: Hindmilk Collection

Hindmilk has been recommended for your baby in order to improve weight gain. When you start to breastfeed, there is a small amount of milk ready for your baby. Called "foremilk," this is the low-fat part of the feeding. As breastfeeding progresses, breastmilk contains more fat, and this later milk is called "hindmilk." Since hindmilk has more fat, it also has more calories than foremilk. Both foremilk and hindmilk are nutritious, so the use of hindmilk is a temporary measure. In order to obtain hindmilk, your current 24-hour milk production must be greater than the baby's 24-hour intake. To collect hindmilk for your baby, follow these guidelines:

- Review the general guidelines for breast pumping.
- Have containers ready, labeled "foremilk" and "hindmilk" (along with name and date).

- Pump for 2 to 3 minutes after the milk begins to flow.
- Stop pumping and save this milk, which should be labeled "foremilk."
- Continue pumping as usual.
- Put this milk into containers labeled "hindmilk."
- Use the containers of hindmilk for your baby until further notice.
- The foremilk may be stored in your home freezer for later use when the baby is older.

Summary

Low intake of breastmilk in the breastfed infant and low maternal milk supply are significant clinical problems. Early breastfeeding follow-up by a skilled provider at 3 to 5 days after delivery would allow early detection of many correctable problems that contribute to slow gain in the first month. By the time the baby's weight gain slows, the mother's milk supply has often already declined, so that both mother and infant must be evaluated and managed with a problem-oriented approach.

Infant or maternal illness, though unusual as a cause of slow weight gain, must always be considered a possibility so as not to overlook a condition that is potentially serious and/or treatable. If infant well-being requires supplementation, it is preferable to give him expressed breastmilk. Once the infant gains weight and the maternal milk supply improves, the amount of supplementation can gradually be decreased and the infant returned to full feedings at the breast. Rarely, maternal anatomy or physiology will preclude a full milk supply. In these cases, the mother is supported to provide as much breastmilk as possible while acknowledging the grieving process that comes with the loss of the desired breastfeeding experience.

Key Concepts

- Numerous factors, both maternal and infant, may affect infant intake and maternal milk supply; the interrelationships of these factors are complex.
- Proper positioning and latch-on are the foundation of efficient milk transfer and infant weight gain.
- Removal of milk by the infant determines the amount of milk production, and maternal limitations on milk supply are rare.
- If infant weight is low, then intake from breastfeeding is low, and the maternal milk supply is probably also low.
- During the first several weeks of breastfeeding, individual patterns of milk supply, infant intake, and infant growth patterns vary widely.
- Maternal undernutrition is not correlated with milk production.
- Maternal overweight, obesity, and excessive pregnancy weight gain are risk factors for delayed lactogenesis and early cessation of breastfeeding.
- Follow-up by a health professional must take place at 3 to 5 days postpartum, when breastfeeding progress is at a critical juncture: this may be an office visit or a home visit.
- Weight loss of more than 7 percent from birth weight warrants investigation of a potential feeding problem; weight loss of more than 10 percent from birth weight requires thorough assessment and intervention.
- Once gaining, the average newborn weight gain is 34 gm/day for females and 40 gm/day for males during the first 3 months.
- The *minimal* acceptable average weight gain is 20 gm/day during the first 3 months.
- If the infant is not gaining weight (not effectively removing milk), assume that the mother's milk supply has started to decline.
- In the first month of life, problems with the feeding process are more common than illness as a cause of poor weight gain.
- Infant illness should be suspected as a potential cause of poor feeding and poor weight gain, especially in the immediate postpartum period and after the first month of life.
- Now, with the release of the WHO Child Growth Standards, we have appropriate growth charts for optimally breastfed infants and young children. These standards are prescriptive and show how *all* babies should grow if optimally fed and nurtured.
- History and physical examination of both mother and infant, including breastfeeding observation, allows the clinician to develop a differential diagnosis for slow infant weight gain.
- Management of slow infant weight gain can be tailored to the suspected diagnosis.
- Two simple interventions for low intake—for an actively suckling infant—are breast massage during feeding and switch nursing.

- If supplementation is indicated, start with ad lib feedings. If the baby is not demonstrating hunger cues, start with 50 to 100 ml/kgm/day divided into 6 to 8 feedings. This should increase rapidly over the next few days.
- A mother's own expressed breastmilk is the preferred type of supplement.
- Supplementation can be given by feeding-tube device, cup, spoon, or bottle, depending on individual circumstances.
- As the maternal milk supply increases and the infant becomes more effective at the breast, the amount of supplementation may be decreased.
- Weighing the infant before and after feeding (test weighing) requires an electronic digital scale that is accurate to 2 gm or less.
- Test weighing is generally restricted to complicated clinical situations, to management of premature infants, or research projects.
- Medications and/or herbs may be an option for increasing milk production after other measures have been tried.
- Delivery of more hindmilk to the infant is one method of increasing caloric intake.
- A few women will be unable to resolve the problem of low intake and low supply; they are likely to undergo a grieving process.

Internet Resources

Academy of Breastfeeding Medicine:
  www.bfmed.org
American Academy of Pediatrics (AAP):
  www.aap.org
Centers for Disease Control and Prevention (CDC):
  www.cdc.gov/growthcharts
International Lactation Consultant Association:
  www.ilca.org

LactMed (drugs during breastfeeding)
  http://toxnet.nlm.nih.gov
La Leche League International:
  www.lalecheleague.org
World Health Organization:
  www.WHO.int

References

Academy of Breastfeeding Medicine. Protocol #3: Hospital guidelines for the use of supplementary feedings in the healthy term breastfed neonate, 2002. www.bfmed.org. Accessed October 31, 2008.

Alexander JM, Grant AM, Campbell MJ. Randomized controlled trial of breast shells and Hoffman's exercises for inverted and non-protractile nipples. *Br Med J*. 1992; 305:1030–1032.

American Academy of Pediatrics. Work group on breastfeeding: breastfeeding and use of human milk. *Pediatrics. 2005;*115:496–506.

Berkner P, Kastner T, Skolnick L. Chronic ipecac poisoning in infancy: a case report. *Pediatrics*. 1988;82:384–386.

Bodley V, Powers D. Long-term nipple shield use—a positive perspective. *J Hum Lact*. 1996;12:301–304.

Bowen-Jones A, Thomsen C, Drewett RF. Milk flow and sucking rates during breastfeeding. *Develop Med Child Neurol*. 1982;24:626–633.

Butte NF et al. Human milk intake and growth in exclusively breast-fed infants. *J Pediatr*. 1984;104(2):187–195.

Chapman DJ, Perez-Escamilla R. Identification of risk factors for delayed onset of lactation. *J Am Diet Assoc*. 1999;99:450–454.

Chen DC et al. Stress during labor and delivery and early lactation performance. *Am J Clin Nutr*. 1998;68(2):335–344.

Co MM, Hernandez EA, Co BG. A comparative study on the efficacy of the different galactogogues among mothers with lactational insufficiency. *Abstract, AAP Section on Breastfeeding*, 2002 NCE, October 21, 2002.

Combs VL, Marino BL. A comparison of growth patterns in breast and bottle-fed infants with congenital heart disease. *Pediatric Nursing*. 1993;19:175–178.

Davies DP, Evans T. The starved but contented breastfed baby. *Arch Dis Child*. 1978;53:763.

de Onis M et al. Comparison of the WHO child growth standards and the CDC 2000 growth charts. *J Nutr. 2007;*137:144–148.

Desmarais L, Browne S. Inadequate weight gain in breastfeeding infants: assessments and resolutions. In: Auerbach KG, ed. *Lactation Consultant Series*. Garden City Park, NY: Avery Publishing Group; 1990.

Dewey KG. Nutrition, growth and complementary feeding of the breastfed infant. *Ped Clin NA*. 2001;48:87–104.

Dewey KG et al. Maternal versus infant factors related to breast milk and residual milk volume: the DARLING study. *Pediatrics*. 1991;87(6):829–837.

Dewey KG, Lonnerdal B. Infant self-regulation of breast-milk intake. *Acta Paediatr Scand*. 1986;75:893–898.

Dewey KG et al. Risk factors for suboptimal infant breastfeeding behavior, delayed onset of lactation, and excess neonatal weight loss. *Pediatrics.* 2003; 112:607–619.

Dollberg D et al. Immediate nipple pain relief after frenotomy in breast-fed infants with ankyloglossia: a randomized, prospective study. *Jour Ped Surg.* 2006;41:1598–1600.

Drane D. The effect of use of dummies and teats on orofacial development. *Breastfeeding Review,* 1996:4:59–64.

Edmonson MB, Stoddard JJ, Owens LM. Hospital readmission with feeding-related problems after early postpartum discharge of normal newborns. *JAMA.* 1997;278:299–303.

Ehrenkranz RA, Ackerman BA. Metoclopramide effect on faltering milk production by mothers of premature infants. *Pediatrics.* 1986;78:614–620.

Engle WA et al. "Late-preterm" infants: a population at risk. *Pediatrics.* 2007;120:1390–1401.

Genna CW, ed. *Supporting Sucking Skills in Breastfeeding Infants.* Sudbury, MA: Jones and Bartlett Publishers, 2008:22–25.

Glass RP, Wolf LS. In coordination of sucking, swallowing, and breathing as an etiology for breastfeeding difficulty. *J Hum Lact.* 1994;10(3):185–189.

Grajeda R, Perez-Escamilla R. Stress during labor and delivery is associated with delayed onset of lactation among urban Guatemalan women. JNutr. 2002; 132:3055–3060.

Gupta AP, Gupta PK. Metoclopramide as a galactogogue. *Clin Pediatr.* 1985;24(5):269–272.

Habbick BF, Gerrard JW. Failure to thrive in the contented breastfed baby. *Can Med Assoc J.* 1984;131:765–768.

Hale T. *Medications and Mothers' Milk.* Amarillo, TX: Pharmasoft Publishing; 2006.

Henley SJ et al. Anemia and insufficient milk in first-time mothers. *Birth.* 1995;22:87–92.

Hilson JA, Rasmussen KM, Kjolhede CL. Excessive weight gain during pregnancy is associated with earlier termination of breastfeeding among white women. *J Nutr.* 2006;136(1):140–146.

Hilson JA, Rasmussen KM, Kjolhede CL. High prepregnant body mass index is associated with poor lactation outcomes among white, rural women independent of psychosocial and demographic correlates. *J Hum Lact.* 2004;20(1):18–29.

Hilson JA, Rasmussen KM, Kjolhede CL. Maternal obesity and breast-feeding success in a rural population of white women. *Am J Clin Nutr.* 1997;66:1371–1378.

Hogan M, Westcott C, Griffiths M. Randomized, controlled trial of division of tongue-tie in infants with feeding problems. *J Paediatr Child Health.* 2005;41: 246–250.

Hoover KL, Barbalinardo LH, Platia MP. Delayed lactogenesis II secondary to gestational ovarian theca lutein cysts in two normal singleton pregnancies. *J Hum Lact.* 2002;18(3):264–268.

Hopkinson JM et al. Milk production by mothers of premature infants: influence of cigarette smoking. *Pediatrics.* 1992;90(6):934–948.

Horta BL et al. Environmental tobacco smoke and the breastfeeding duration. *Am J Epidemiol.* 1997;146: 128–133.

Howard CR et al. Physiologic stability of newborns during cup and bottle-feeding. *Pediatrics.* 1999;104: 1204–1207.

Howard CR et al. Ramdomized clinical trial of pacifier use and bottle-feeding or cupfeeding and their effect on breastfeeding. *Pediatrics.* 2003;111:411–518.

Huggins KE, Petok ES, Mireles O. Markers of lactation insufficiency: a study of 34 mothers. In: Auerbach KG, ed. *Current Issues in Clinical Lactation, 2000.* Boston, MA: Jones and Bartlett; 2000.

Hurst NM. Lactation after augmentation mammaplasty. *Obstetr & Gyn.* 1996;87:30–34.

Institute of Medicine. *Nutrition During Lactation.* Washington, DC: National Academy Press; 1991.

International Lactation Consultant Association. *Clinical Guidelines for the Establishment of Exclusive Breastfeeding.* Raleigh, NC: ILCA Publications; 2005.

Jensen RG, Neville MC, eds. *Human Lactation: Milk Components Methodologies.* New York, NY: Plenum Press; 1984:5–21.

Jones WB. Weight gain and feeding in the neonate with cleft: a three-center study. *Cleft Palate J.* 1988;25: 379–384.

Kauppila A et al. Metoclopramide and breast feeding: efficacy and anterior pituitary responses of the mother and the child. *Eur J Obstetr Gynecol Reprod Biol.* 1985;19:19–22.

Lawrence RA, Lawrence R. *Breastfeeding—A Guide for the Medical Profession.* 6th ed. St. Louis, MO: CV Mosby; 2005.

Livingstone VH. Common lactation and breast-feeding problems. In: Ismail J, ed. *Manual of Breast Diseases.* Lippincott Williams & Wilkins; 2002:95–134.

Livingstone V. Neonatal insufficient milk syndrome (NIMS): a bio/psycho/social classification, (poster abstract). 10th Annual Conference of the Academy of Breastfeeding Medicine; October 21, 2005; Denver, CO.

Lukefahr JL. Underlying illness associated with failure to thrive in breastfed infants. *Clin Pediatr.* 1990;29(8): 468–470.

Martin MS, Schwartz RH. Tackling ankyloglossia in the office. *Contemp Ped.* 2008;25(1):59–64.

Meier PP et al. The accuracy of test weighing for preterm infants. *J Pediatr Gastroenterol Nutr.* 1990;10(1): 62–65.

Meier PP et al. Nipple shields for preterm infants: effect on milk transfer and duration of breastfeeding. *J Hum Lact.* 2002;16:106–114.

Mennella JA. The human infant's suckling responses to the flavor of alcohol in mother's milk. *Alcohol Clin Exp Res.* 1997;21:581–585.

Neifert MR. Failure to thrive. In: Neville MC, Neifert MR, eds. *Lactation: Physiology, Nutrition and Breastfeeding.* New York, NY: Plenum Press; 1983.

Neifert MR, McDonough SL, Neville MC. Failure of lactogenesis associated with placental retention. *Am J Obstet Gynecol.* 1981;140(4):477–478.

Neifert MR et al. The association between infant weight gain and breast milk intake measured by office test weights [abstract]. *Am J Dis Child.* 1990;144:420–421.

Neifert MR, Seacat JM, Jobe WE. Lactation failure due to insufficient glandular development of the breast. *Pediatrics.* 1985;76(5):823–828.

Neifert M et al. The influence of breast surgery, breast appearance, and pregnancy-induced breast changes on lactation sufficiency as measured by infant weight gain. *Birth.* 1990;17(1):31–38.

Nelson SE et al. Gain in weight and length during early infancy. *Early Hum Dev.* 1989;19:223–239.

Neubauer SH et al. Delayed lactogenesis in women with insulin-dependent diabetes mellitus. *Am J Clin Nutr.* 1993;58:54–60.

Neville MC et al. Studies in human lactation: milk volumes in lactating women during the onset of lactation and full lactation. *Am J Clin Nutr.* 1988;48:1375–1386.

Peaker M, Wilde CJ. Milk secretion: autocrine control. *News on Physiological Sciences.* 1987;2:124–126.

Perez-Escamilla R, Chapman DJ. Validity and public health implications of maternal perception of the onset of lactation: an international analytical overview. *J Nutr.* 2001;131:3021S–3024S.

Pessl MM. Are we creating our own breastfeeding mythology? *J Hum Lact.* 1996;12:271–272.

Powers NG. Slow weight gain and low milk supply in the breastfeeding dyad. *Clinics in Perinatology.* 1999;26:399–429.

Powers N, Slusser W. Breastfeeding update 2: clinical lactation management. *Pediatrics in Review.* 1997;18(5):147–161.

Ruvalcaba RHA. Stress-induced cessation of lactation. *West J Ed.* 1987;146:228–230.

Salvador S, Vandenplas Y. Gastroesophageal reflux and cow milk allergy: is there a link? *Pediatrics.* 2002;110:972–984.

Sealy CN. Rethinking the use of nipple shields. *J Hum Lact.* 1996;12(4):299–300.

Segura-Millan S, Dewey DG, Perez-Escamilla R. Factors associated with perceived insufficient milk in a low-income urban population from Mexico. *J Nutr.* 1994;124:202–212.

Shapiro-Mendoza CK et al. Effect of late-preterm birth and maternal medical conditions on newborn morbidity risk. *Pediatrics.* 2008;121:e223–e232.

Soskolne EI et al. The effect of early discharge and other factors on the readmission rates of newborns. *Arch Pediatr Adolesc Med.* 1996;150:373–379.

Stuff JE, Nichols BL. Nutrient intake and growth performance of older infants fed human milk. *J Pediatr.* 1989;115:959–968.

Sutphen JL, Saulsbury FT. Intentional ipecac poisoning: Munchausen syndrome by proxy. *Pediatrics.* 1988;82:453–456.

Swafford S, Berens P. Effect of fenugreek on breast milk volume [abstract]. *ABM News Views.* 2000;6(4):21.

Valentine CJ, Hurst NM, Schanler RJ. Hindmilk improves weight gain in low birth-weight infants fed human milk. *J Ped Gastr Nutr.* 1994;18:474–477.

Whitfield M, Kay R, Stevens S. Validity of routine clinical test weighing as a measure of intake of breast-fed infants. *Arch Dis Child.* 1981;56:919.

WHO Multicenter Growth Reference Study Group. WHO child growth standards based on length/height, weight and age. *Acta Paediatrica Suppl.* 2006;450:76–85.

Wilson JD, Foster DW, eds. *Williams Textbook of Endocrinology.* Philadelphia, PA: W. B. Saunders; 1992:441–442.

Wilson-Clay B. Clinical use of silicone nipple shields. *J Hum Lact.* 1996;12:279–285.

Wisner KL, Parry BL, Piontek CM. Postpartum depression. *N Engl J Med.* 2002;347:194–199.

Woolridge MW, Fisher C. Colic, "overfeeding" and symptoms of lactose malabsorption in the breast-fed baby: a possible artifact of feed management? *Lancet.* 1988;2(8607):382–384.

Woolridge MW, Ingram JC, Baum JD. Do changes in pattern of breast usage alter the baby's nutrient intake? *Lancet.* 1990;336:395–397.

Woolridge MW et al. Methods for the measurement of milk volume intake of the breast-fed infant. In: Jensen RG, Neville MC, eds. *Human Lactation: Milk Components and Methodologies.* New York: Plenum Press; 1984:5–21.

World Health Organization. Global strategy for infant and young child feeding: the optimal duration of exclusive breastfeeding. Presented at: 54th World Health Assembly (A54/INF.DOC./4); 2001.

Chapter 11

Jaundice and the Breastfed Baby

Lawrence M. Gartner

PHYSIOLOGIC JAUNDICE, caused by an elevation of serum unconjugated bilirubin, is a common clinical condition seen in approximately two thirds of newborn infants. In artificially fed infants the jaundice disappears within 1 week, and the serum bilirubin drops to adult normal levels by 10 to 14 days of life. In the great majority of breastfed infants, serum unconjugated bilirubin elevations persist for many weeks thereafter, falling to normal values by 1 to 2 months of age. Clinical jaundice also remains present in many breastfed infants until 3 to 6 weeks of life. This normal prolongation of physiologic jaundice in the healthy, thriving breastfed infant is known as *breastmilk jaundice*. Breastmilk jaundice, first recognized about 40 years ago (Newman & Gross, 1963; Stiehm & Ryan, 1965; Arias et al., 1964), results from the effect of an as yet unidentified factor in human milk that promotes an increase in intestinal absorption of bilirubin (Gartner, Lee, & Moscioni, 1983; Alonso et al., 1991). This factor is not found in colostrum, and only appears with the secretion of transitional and mature milk beginning on about the fifth day of life. This coincides with the observation that serum bilirubin concentrations of normal formula-fed and adequately breastfed infants are identical during the first 5 days of life; the higher bilirubin values in optimally breastfed

infants being seen after the fifth day of life. Although rarely necessary, discontinuation of breastfeeding for 24 to 48 hours in infants with breastmilk jaundice results in a prompt decline in serum bilirubin. Resumption of breastfeeding increases bilirubin levels although usually to lower levels than seen before discontinuation.

Because bilirubin is an effective antioxidant and newborns are deficient in naturally occurring antioxidants, it has been suggested that this mechanism for prolongation of physiologic jaundice (breastmilk jaundice) may be protective for the newborn (Stocker et al., 1987; Dore et al., 1999). To date, there is insufficient clinical evidence to confirm this intuitive and attractive concept, but recent animal studies strongly support the protective effect of hyperbilirubinemia in ischemic bowel injury (Hammerman et al., 2002). In addition, adults with life-long, low-grade unconjugated hyperbilirubinemia (Gilbert's syndrome) have been found to have significant reductions in heart disease and cancer, providing additional support for bilirubin acting as an effective antioxidant (Vitek, 2002; Schwertner, Jackson, & Tolan, 1994; Hunt et al., 1996; Temme et al., 2001).

Although most infants with breastmilk jaundice have low levels of unconjugated hyperbilirubinemia, generally below 10 mg/dl, occasional breastfed infants have more exaggerated bilirubin levels. These higher bilirubin levels are often caused by the presence of an independent acquired or inherited disorder that results in either increased bilirubin production or reduced clearance of bilirubin.

Inadequate breastfeeding, particularly in the early days of life, can also result in elevated levels of bilirubin (Gartner, 2001). This manifestation is known as *starvation jaundice of the newborn* (also known as *breast-nonfeeding jaundice)* and is the neonatal manifestation of the adult disorder, *starvation jaundice* (Whitmer & Gollan, 1983). In this condition, characterized by inadequate milk and caloric intake, but not necessarily by dehydration, there may be a delay in bilirubin clearance resulting from low stool output (de Carvalho, Robertson, & Klaus, 1985) with an increase in the intestinal absorption of unconjugated bilirubin. Exaggerated jaundice caused by poor breastfeeding should not be considered physiologic. It has been shown that in neonates who were adequately breastfed on demand, not according to a rigid time schedule, there was no difference in the percentage with an elevated level of bilirubin during the first days of life between those who were breastfed or those who were bottle-fed (Rubaltelli, 1993), nor was there a difference in the percentage of weight loss. After the fifth day of life, exaggerated hyperbilirubinemia and jaundice may be due to the combined effect of breastmilk jaundice and starvation jaundice of the newborn.

Despite the knowledge of an association between exaggerations of neonatal jaundice and breastfeeding, it would be a mistake to assume, without careful consideration, that because a neonate is breastfed and is jaundiced, breastfeeding is the sole, or main, cause of the jaundice. It would also be a mistake to believe that if the jaundice is associated with breastfeeding, it can never be harmful. This chapter will discuss neonatal jaundice, its physiologic and pathologic causes, its potential risks, and its evaluation and management.

Neonatal Jaundice

Jaundice, or icterus, is defined as a yellowish color of the sclerae and skin as a result of the deposition of bilirubin, a yellow molecule, in body tissues. Bilirubin is largely derived from red blood cell lysis and the breakdown of hemoglobin into globin and heme; subsequently, heme is degraded by the enzyme *heme oxygenase* to produce equimolar amounts of iron, biliverdin, and carbon monoxide. Biliverdin is reduced to bilirubin by biliverdin reductase (Dennery, Seidman, & Stevenson, 2001).

More than half of all newborns have some degree of visible jaundice. The intensity of jaundice is dependent on the balance of bilirubin production and bilirubin elimination. Serum bilirubin levels in newborns are higher than those in adults for several reasons (Gartner & Lee, 1992).

Increased Bilirubin Synthesis

The fetus in utero exists in a relatively low oxygen environment, stimulating increased erythropoieses and producing a large fetal red cell mass in order to assure adequate oxygen delivery to the tissues. The fetus also has a relatively large blood volume in addition to a high hemoglobin concentration compared to an adult or older child. The hematocrit of the newborn at birth increases further in proportion to the time between birth and clamping of the umbilical cord (Shurin, 1992). This increase in transfer of blood from the placenta to the newborn upon birth ensures an adequate volume of blood to fill the expanded vascular beds (e.g., lungs, intestine) and assures adequate iron for future metabolic needs, including new hemoglobin synthesis. Thus, within a few minutes, the newborn has a much greater volume of red cells relative to body weight than does an adult or older child. In addition, the life span of the red cells formed in utero (about 70 to 90 days) is shorter than that of the adult (100 to 120 days). This large volume of heme combined with a shorter life span of the red cells in the circulation results in synthesis of more bilirubin per unit of body weight than in the adult. In addition, the fetus produces red cells not only in the bone marrow but also in the liver and spleen. This very active erythropoiesis is driven by the hormone *erythropoietin*. Immediately after delivery of the infant into room air and the initiation of respiration, the blood oxygen level increases dramatically, resulting in a fall in erythropoietin production and complete cessation of erythropoiesis. These immature inactive red cells in the liver, spleen, and bone marrow are destroyed, producing additional bilirubin. All of the bilirubin formed in this process, *unconjugated bilirubin*, is insoluble in plasma, requiring that it be transported bound to serum albumin. In the fetus, the small amount of insoluble bilirubin formed was cleared from the circulation by passive diffusion across the placenta; but in the newborn, it must be eliminated by another pathway.

Bilirubin Metabolism

In the newborn, the insoluble bilirubin, also referred to as *unconjugated* or *indirect-reacting bilirubin*, must enter the liver cell (hepatocyte) by a process of facilitated diffusion, which, in the newborn, is less active than in an older child or adult, reducing the rate of clearance of bilirubin from the plasma. Once in the liver, bilirubin is conjugated with *glucuronic acid* via the enzyme *uridine diphosphate glucuronyl transferase* (UGT1A1) to become water-soluble *bilirubin glucuronide*, a requirement for transfer from the liver cell into bile and movement into the small intestine and ultimately into stool. Bilirubin glucuronide is also called *conjugated* or *direct-reacting bilirubin*. Compared to adults, newborns' conjugating system is relatively immature, as well as their uptake of bilirubin. The degree of imbalance between high bilirubin synthesis and limited liver cell uptake and conjugation of bilirubin causes the varying elevation of serum bilirubin concentration in blood and body tissues and the degree of severity of jaundice. This normal elevation of unconjugated bilirubin and the resulting visible jaundice is known as *physiologic jaundice of the newborn*.

Intestinal Metabolism of Bilirubin

For the conjugated bilirubin to be eliminated from the body, it must be passed in the neonatal stool. However, neonates, unlike adults, have a high level of an enzyme in the intestinal mucosa called *beta-glucuronidase*. This enzyme removes the glucuronide from the conjugated bilirubin, making the bilirubin once again water *insoluble* and thus available for transport back across the intestinal lumen into the neonate's circulation. This process, called the *enterohepatic circulation of bilirubin*, contributes to neonatal jaundice. The absence of intestinal bacteria in the neonate (which in the adult convert bilirubin into other metabolites), combined with the high level of beta glucuronidase in the intestine and high concen-

tration of unconjugated bilirubin leads to a marked increase of intestinal reabsorption of bilirubin in the neonate. This, in turn, increases the quantity of bilirubin in the circulation and the load of bilirubin presented to the liver for metabolism and excretion.

Assessment of Jaundice

Traditionally, clinicians have relied on visual inspection to determine the level of jaundice in newborns. As there is a craniocaudal progression in icterus of the skin with rising levels of bilirubin, the serum level of bilirubin has been inferred from the apparent level of demarcation of jaundice on the neonate's body. Newer information would suggest that the visual inspection for the estimation of bilirubin level is unreliable and inaccurate (Moyer, Ahn, & Sneed, 2000). This is particularly true in pigmented races. In this era of early hospital discharge of neonates, in which discharge commonly takes place at less than 48 hours of life, it is very hard to distinguish, simply by inspection, a pathological or abnormally high level of bilirubin from a normal level. For this reason, many experts now recommend that all neonates be screened by serum or transcutaneous level of bilirubin prior to hospital discharge and that this level be plotted on the nomogram of bilirubin level according to hours of age of the baby, as shown in Figure 11–1 (Bhutani, Johnson, & Sivieri, 1999). One can then readily determine into which risk category an infant falls. Significant hyperbilirubinemia, which is defined as bilirubin level greater than the 95th or 75th percentiles at any age strongly predicts that dangerously high serum bilirubin levels can be anticipated in the immediate future. This can be a guide as to what diagnostic testing may be indicated, whether or not the infant ought to be discharged to home, and when the early follow-up appointment should be scheduled.

Postnatal Pattern of Jaundice

Because of the physiological mechanisms described above, bilirubin levels rise in neonates after birth for a few days and then, typically, fall to the adult level. In the formula-fed healthy Caucasian term infant, bilirubin levels peak on day 2 to 3, which is often after hospital discharge has taken place. In preterm

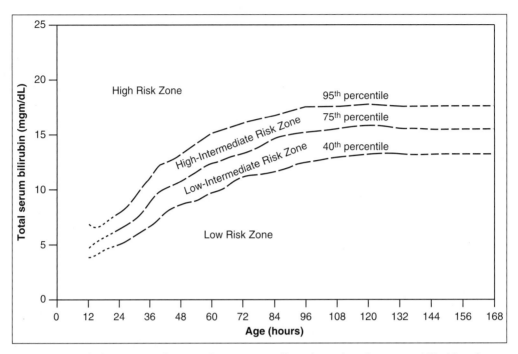

neonates and in infants of some racial groups—for example, in some full-term Asians—the peak may be later, days 4 and 5, and usually will be higher than in the Caucasian term newborn (Brown & Wong, 1965). Jaundice will have resolved in most infants by day 7 in the formula-fed normal term neonate, and by day 10 to 21 in the preterm neonate. The pattern of jaundice in the breastfed neonate, known as breastmilk jaundice, is more prolonged.

Breastmilk Jaundice

With its onset after the fifth day of life, in association with the appearance of transitional and mature milk, breastmilk jaundice is an extension of physiologic jaundice (Gartner & Herschel, 2001). The levels of jaundice rarely become dangerously high; if so, a careful evaluation for other causes of jaundice is essential (see below). Breastmilk jaundice is seen in healthy, thriving neonates who have good weight

gain; it may persist for many weeks. However, stools will be normal yellow in color, and the conjugated fraction of total bilirubin, which should be measured by 2 to 3 weeks of age in all infants who are still jaundiced, will be normal (less than 2 mg/dl and less than 10 percent of the total bilirubin).

Breastmilk jaundice is a normal physiologic phenomenon, not a disorder (Gartner & Herschel, 2001). Two thirds of all breastfed babies have an elevation in bilirubin, and half of those have visible jaundice during the second to fourth weeks of life. As bilirubin is a potent antioxidant, modest elevations of bilirubin may possibly be beneficial.

Breastmilk jaundice has been shown to result from an increase in the intestinal absorption of bilirubin, not to an inhibitor of the conjugating enzyme, UGT1A1 (Alonso et al., 1991). An as yet unidentified substance in the milk of the majority of breastfeeding mothers is responsible for this increase in intestinal reabsorption of bilirubin (Gartner, 2001).

Gilbert's syndrome, a benign inherited condition characterized by reduced activity of the bilirubin conjugating enzyme, has been associated with prolonged neonatal jaundice. Genetic studies of the promoter for the conjugating enzyme, UGT1A1, in a Scottish population (Monaghan et al., 1999) have revealed that there is a significant association between prolonged jaundice and breastfeeding in neonates who have an increase in the number of TATA box repeats. In Asians, a DNA sequence variant (Gly 71 Arg mutation) of the UGT1A1 gene has been shown to be associated with neonatal hyperbilirubinemia (Maruo et al., 1999). Fifteen of 17 Japanese infants with prolonged jaundice in association with breastfeeding had at least 1 UGT1A1 mutation (Maruo et al., 2000). Two different types of mutations of the gene for the UGT1A1 enzyme are major contributors to neonatal hyperbilirubinemia in European and Japanese populations. Thus, breastfeeding combined with this inherited defect in conjugation of bilirubin, may result in very high levels of bilirubin and in even greater prolongation of the hyperbilirubinemia and jaundice (Kaplan et al., 2003).

Although neonatal jaundice without other signs is almost never indicative of a bacterial infection, in 7.5 percent of afebrile, asymptomatic jaundiced newborns (predominantly formula-fed) younger than 8 weeks of age (mean age of 12 days) presenting to an emergency department, a urinary tract infection was diagnosed (Garcia & Nager, 2002). Bacterial infection in association with hyperbilirubinemia increases the risk of bilirubin toxicity and the development of kernicterus (Volpe, 2001). Diagnostic workup for bacterial infections is indicated in jaundiced infants who have signs of sepsis, including poor feeding, lethargy, hypotonia, respiratory distress and fever. It should be recognized, however, that these may also be early signs of bilirubin toxicity (kernicterus). In either situation, treatment to lower serum bilirubin concentrations is indicated (see below).

Starvation Jaundice

Breastmilk jaundice will usually be identified after the neonate has been discharged home, as it generally presents as a prolongation of the earlier physiologic jaundice. On the other hand, starvation jaundice (previously known as breastfeeding jaundice or breast-non-feeding jaundice), may be seen in the first few days after birth, but not before 24 hours (Gartner & Herschel, 2001). Again, other causes for jaundice must be considered and ruled out. Starvation jaundice is seen in neonates who have not established feedings because of maternal or neonatal factors or a combination of both. This is comparable to starvation jaundice seen in adults with inadequate caloric intake, in whom bilirubin levels rise above baseline (Whitmer & Gollan, 1983). A 24-hour period of complete caloric deprivation is sufficient in virtually all normal adults to double the serum bilirubin to approximately 2 to 3 mg/dl, a level that is *not* associated with visible jaundice. In those adults with Gilbert's syndrome, clinical jaundice may be evident when they go without eating for more than 24 hours because they double their bilirubin from an already elevated serum bilirubin concentration.

For infants who have not established effective breastfeeding, whether owing to sleepiness, prematurity, poor positioning and poor latch with inadequate milk transfer, or other conditions, it is unwise to send them home until the problem is resolved (Maisels & Newman, 1998; Neifert, 1998). Breastfeeding should be formally evaluated by a trained health professional at least twice each day in the hospital with attention to position, latch, and milk transfer. Failure to correct breastfeeding problems prior to hospital discharge may result in excessive weight loss (great than 7 to 10 percent), dehydration, hypernatremia, and excessive and dangerous levels of bilirubin, with a catastrophic outcome possible, such as kernicterus (bilirubin encephalopathy) (Johnson, Bhutani, & Brown, 2002), a permanent neurologic condition characterized by athetoid cerebral palsy and deafness. In addition to the risk of kernicterus, venous thrombosis has been reported in a few such instances (Gebara & Everett, 2001).

For neonates with jaundice and poor breastfeeding, the solution is not to stop the breastfeeding. The solution is to correct the breastfeeding problem and to restore fluid and caloric intake. In some instances, expressed milk, banked human milk, or artificial milk supplementation may be required for a time. The main point is that the baby must be fed and the mother must be supported. Regardless of the etiology of the jaundice, if breastfeeding is not going well, it must be improved, not abandoned.

Infants who develop elevated bilirubin levels in the early days of life due to starvation jaundice are also at increased risk of developing very high bilirubin levels when they enter the stage of breast-milk jaundice. If they have developed an exaggerated bilirubin pool early, that pool will multiply with mature human milk feeding due to enhanced intestinal bilirubin absorption. Conversely, good breastfeeding practices that keep early bilirubin at lower levels will prevent later excessive levels from developing.

Hyperbilirubinemia

Factors that have been associated with exaggerated hyperbilirubinemia may be categorized in the following way (Dennery, Seidman, & Stevenson, 2001), recognizing that there are often multiple reasons for hyperbilirubinemia in a given baby:

- Increased production of bilirubin (hemolysis)
  - Blood group incompatibility with isoimmunization (direct antibody [Coombs'] test DAT positive)
  - Inherited red blood cell abnormalities such as enzyme deficiencies (glucose-6-phosphate dehydrogenase deficiency) and red cell membrane defects (spherocytosis, elliptocytosis)
  - Birth "trauma" (ecchymoses, cephalhematoma, internal bleeding, subgaleal hemorrhage)
  - Genetic factors (Greek Island extraction, Asian race)
  - Prematurity (shortened erythrocyte lifespan)
  - Polycythemia
- Decreased elimination of bilirubin
  - Genetic variants/disorders of conjugation—Gilbert's syndrome, Crigler-Najjar syndrome, Asian race (Akaba et al., 1998)
  - Low oral intake of feedings (caloric deprivation)
  - Prematurity (immature hepatic metabolism)
  - Breastmilk feedings
- Multifactorial risks
  - Prematurity
  - Maternal diabetes
  - Urinary tract infection (Garcia & Nager, 2002)
  - Hypothyroidism

- G6PD deficiency with Gilbert's syndrome (Kaplan, 2001)
- Asian race (Young et al., 2001)

Bilirubin Encephalopathy

Bilirubin encephalopathy, also known as *kernicterus*, is a form of brain damage resulting from the entry of unconjugated bilirubin into the brain (Volpe, 2001; Shapiro, Bhutani, & Johnson, 2006). The damage to neurons occurs only in certain regions of the brain stem and cerebellum, particularly the basal ganglia. The initial presentation of bilirubin encephalopathy is characterized by lethargy, poor feeding, vomiting, and irregular respiration. This early stage may be reversible with prompt removal of bilirubin from the circulation and brain by exchange transfusion. If severe hyperbilirubinemia continues, the infant then manifests more severe neurologic signs characterized by opisthotonus (retrocollis), increased extensor tone of the extremities, high-pitched cry, fever, and seizures. While some infants may die in this stage, with modern intensive care most infants with bilirubin encephalopathy survive (Harris et al., 2001; Bhutani, Johnson, & Keren, 2005). Survivors of this more severe stage of bilirubin encephalopathy almost always have significant permanent neurologic damage, characterized by choreoathetoid cerebral palsy, deafness, and paralysis of upward gaze of the eyes. In the more severe forms of this disorder the child will not be able to sit, stand, walk, swallow, talk, or have any purposeful movements of the extremities. Despite the severity of the motor disability, these children often have normal intellectual function, probably because the cerebral cortex is not affected by bilirubin.

It was believed by many that this devastating outcome of hyperbilirubinemia was no longer of concern following the introduction of preventive treatment for severe hemolytic disease of the newborn secondary to Rh incompatibility, which was a common cause of severe hyperbilirubinemia in the past. Recent reports of infants with this condition have made it evident that bilirubin encephalopathy continues to occur (Centers for Disease Control, 2001), especially in (1) breastfed infants, (2) in infants who may weigh as much as full-term infants but yet their gestational age is less than 38 weeks, and (3) in those with large internal hemorrhage such as cephalhematomas.

The informal kernicterus registry at the University of Pennsylvania suggests that there is a rise in incidence of this devastating outcome (Johnson, Bhutani, & Brown, 2002). The cause of this rise is multifactorial. As a result of some articles in the pediatric literature, many pediatricians and others have adopted a more liberal and permissive approach to elevated bilirubin levels. Furthermore, it is suspected that early hospital discharge of newborns combined with an increase in the number who are breastfed, without timely follow-up within the first couple of days after discharge, is a contributing factor. Newborns are being sent home before feedings are established, without adequate assessment for the risk of significant jaundice and without appropriate and timely follow-up (Johnson, Bhutani, & Brown, 2002).

For a given neonate, it is not known at what level of bilirubin, and for what duration of exposure to that level, kernicterus may occur. Certain factors may increase the risk, in addition to the level of serum bilirubin. The form of bilirubin that crosses into the brain is unconjugated bilirubin that is not bound to plasma proteins, so-called free bilirubin. Low concentrations of serum albumin or the presence in sera of any substance that competes with bilirubin for albumin-binding sites may increase the risk of free bilirubin being available to enter the brain. This mechanism was recognized in the 1950s (Harris, Lucey, & Maclean, 1958) when an association was found between prophylactic sulfisoxazole antibiotic usage in preterm neonates and kernicterus. Sulfisoxazole competes with unconjugated bilirubin for albumin-binding sites and can displace bilirubin, which then may enter the brain. Benzyl alcohol, which at one time was used as a preservative in parenteral medications for newborns in intensive care nurseries, may have had the same effect. The potential for displacement of bilirubin from albumin-binding sites must be considered whenever a medication is prescribed for a newborn. Sulfisoxazole (Gantrisin) administered to infants was recognized as a major cause of kernicterus in infants with hyperbilirubinemia due to its competitive binding with bilirubin on albumin (Odell, Cohen, & Kelly, 1969). The commonly used antibiotic, ceftriaxone,

competes for bilirubin-binding sites on albumin (Martin et al., 1993), though no cases of kernicterus are known to have been attributed to this drug.

Hemolysis also appears to increase the risk of kernicterus; the mechanism of this effect remains undefined. In addition, factors affecting the integrity of the blood–brain barrier, such as asphyxia, acidosis, sepsis, or prematurity, may increase this risk. Although one must always consider the potential effect on the jaundiced neonate of drugs in breastmilk, all drugs commonly given to mothers antepartum or postpartum are safe with regard to neonatal jaundice, with the important exception of nalidixic acid, nitrofurantoin, sulfapyridine, and sulfisoxazole in mothers of infants with G6PD deficiency, because of the risk of hemolysis in the neonate (American Academy of Pediatrics, 2001). *Maternal* ingestion of fava beans is also dangerous to the breastfed neonate with G6PD deficiency because it is excreted in breastmilk and can cause hemolysis. Naphthalene mothballs and flakes should not be used in the home or in the clothes of any neonate because of the potential for vapors from these agents to produce hemolysis in infants with G6PD deficiency (Kaplan, Hammerman, & Feldman, 2000; Kaplan & Hammerman, 2004; Kaplan et al., 2004, 2005, 2006; Kaplan, Algur, & Hammerman, 2001).

Recent studies have suggested that G6PD deficiency in newborns only results in severe hyperbilirubinemia when there is severe hemolysis due to exposure to an inciting hemolytic agent with gross hemolysis or when the infant with G6PD deficiency also has a second inherited factor that reduces the capacity of the liver to conjugate bilirubin, such as abnormalities in the promoter region of the gene responsible for production of glucuronyl transferase, the hepatic conjugating enzyme (Gilbert's syndrome). In this latter group of infants, hemolysis may not be evident because it is relatively mild. Other investigators have also suggested that G6PD deficiency may in some way reduce the capacity of the liver to metabolize bilirubin. Although G6PD deficiency is relatively common worldwide, relatively few infants with it develop severe hyperbilirubinemia. Still, it has been recommended recently that newborn screening for G6PD deficiency be made a routine diagnostic procedure for all jaundiced neonates.

Evaluation of Jaundice

As noted above, it is currently recommended by experts that *all* neonates be screened for their level of bilirubin prior to hospital discharge (Johnson, Bhutani, & Brown, 2002). The serum bilirubin concentration combined with evaluation for various risk factors will provide guidance for future management (Newman, 2005; American Academy of Pediatrics, 2004).

With the availability of new transcutaneous devices for the noninvasive measurement of serum bilirubin that have been shown to be as accurate as routine laboratory methods for bilirubin screening (Rubaltelli et al., 2001; Felc, 2005), this can now be performed rapidly at the bedside. If the transcutaneous reading is 15 mg/dL or higher, confirmation with a serum bilirubin level is recommended (Bhutani et al., 2000). If the bilirubin level plotted on the nomogram is at or above the 75th percentile, the neonate is at risk for significant hyperbilirubinemia and will need careful assessment; delay of hospital discharge may be appropriate.

Every hospital using transcutaneous bilirubin devices should calibrate the instrument against their standard laboratory measurement of serum bilirubin in a series of babies before relying upon the device. Variations in accuracy may occur with different providers and with infants of different ages, skin color, and physical condition. The transcutaneous bilirubin device should be used as a screening tool, and elevated levels should always be confirmed with a serum bilirubin determination.

Diagnostic Assessment

Having established that the neonate has, or is at risk for, significant hyperbilirubinemia according to the nomogram of bilirubin level for hours of age, consideration must be given to the cause of the jaundice. Therapy will be guided, to some extent, by the cause. Most cases of hyperbilirubinemia are caused, at least in part, by increased bilirubin production from hemoglobin degradation (hemolysis) (Stevenson, Dennery, & Hinz, 2001). It is important to identify hemolysis because it may lead to very high levels of bilirubin, and/or to significant anemia. Hemolysis is also associated with an increased risk for bilirubin encephalopathy at all elevated serum bilirubin levels.

Traditional hematological tests (hematocrit, reticulocyte count, blood smear, direct antiglobulin [DAT; Coombs'] test) are generally not very helpful in making a diagnosis of hemolysis in the neonate (Newman & Easterling, 1994; Herschel et al., 2002). A clinical technique that is noninvasive and simple for estimating the rate of bilirubin production (hemolysis) is measurement of exhaled end-tidal carbon monoxide (CO), corrected for ambient CO (ETCOc) (Vreman et al., 1996). When red blood cells break down, hemoglobin is released. The heme moiety is degraded by the enzyme, heme oxygenase, to release iron, CO, and biliverdin in equimolar amounts. Biliverdin, a water-soluble nontoxic compound, is reduced to unconjugated bilirubin, a fat soluble compound. CO is excreted as a component of expired breath. Since CO and bilirubin are produced in equimolar quantities, measurement of expired CO provides an indication of the rate of bilirubin production. A device has been developed that can be used to measure ETCOc in newborns at the bedside, quickly and noninvasively. The result obtained with this CO detector is immediately available on a data strip printout and can be plotted on a nomogram of ETCOc levels for hours of age to identify infants with excessive hemolysis.

The advantage of ETCOc over the Coombs' test is that ETCOc will identify infants with hemolysis due to causes in addition to isoimmunization (Rh, ABO), such as G6PD enzyme deficiency or red cell membrane defects. Furthermore, a positive Coombs' test may be misleading as to the risk for hemolysis because many neonates with a positive test do not have significant hemolysis (Herschel et al., 2002). Other tests that may be diagnostic of hemolysis in adults are not usually helpful in neonates. The expired carbon monoxide measuring device is, unfortunately, no longer available for purchase at the time of publication of this book. At some time in the future, it may again be commercially produced.

Since the level of bilirubin is a result of the balance between production and elimination, one must also consider deficiencies in the elimination of bilirubin in the neonate with hyperbilirubinemia. A common underlying cause of increased hyperbilirubinemia in the newborn is a variation in the promoter region of the gene for the conjugating enzyme (glucuronyl transferase) UGT1A1, resulting in decreased activity of the conjugating enzyme. By itself, people with this disorder are asymptomatic although they may have mild unconjugated hyperbilirubinemia (Gilbert's syndrome); but in combination with even mild hemolysis or with starvation, bilirubin becomes significantly elevated. It has been shown that neonatal hyperbilirubinemia due to G6PD deficiency occurs in those neonates who also have Gilbert's syndrome (Kaplan, 2001).

Another reason for decreased elimination of bilirubin is an increase in the enterohepatic circulation of bilirubin (intestinal absorption), due to insufficient caloric intake (starvation jaundice) or, normally, due to ingestion of mature human milk (breastmilk jaundice).

Management of Jaundice

The reader is referred to the recent American Academy of Pediatrics *Clinical Practice Guideline on Management of Hyperbilirubinemia in the Newborn Infant 35 or More Weeks of Gestation* (American Academy of Pediatrics,

2004) and to the technical report that accompanies the clinical practice guideline (Ip S et al., 2004) for a detailed discussion of the management of neonatal jaundice.

The management of hyperbilirubinemia will depend to some extent on the cause, but ultimately on the level of bilirubin and the condition of the neonate. If the neonate is less than 38 weeks' gestation, or has hemolysis or other medical problems, the bilirubin level for initiating phototherapy may be somewhat lower than if the neonate is full-term, healthy, and does not have any type of hemolytic disease (Figure 11–2) (American Academy of Pediatrics, 1994). Very high or rapidly rising bilirubin levels may need to be controlled with an exchange transfusion (Figure 11–3), in which case feedings would be temporarily interrupted for the procedure. Neonates who are treated only with phototherapy should continue to be breastfed or receive other milk feedings since good caloric intake improves the effectiveness of phototherapy.

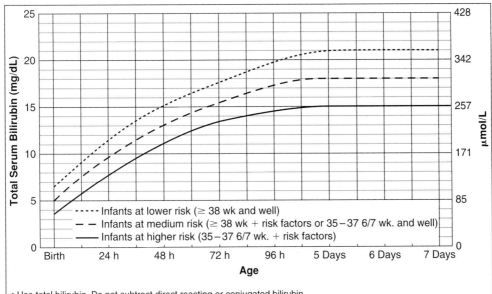

• Use total bilirubin. Do not subtract direct reacting or conjugated bilirubin.
• Risk factors = isoimmune hemolytic disease, G6PD deficiency, asphyxia, significant lethargy, temperature instability, sepsis, acidosis, or albumin < 3.0g/dL (if measured)
• For well infants 35–37 6/7 wk can adjust TSB levels for intervention around the medium risk line. It is an option to intervene at lower TSB levels for infants closer to 35 wks and at higher TSB levels for those closer to 37 6/7 wk.
• It is an option to provide conventional phototherapy in hospital or at home at TSB levels 2–3 mg/dL (35–50 μmol/L) below those shown but home phototherapy should not be used in any infant with risk factors.

FIGURE 11–2 Guidelines for phototherapy.

Source: American Academy of Pediatrics. Clinical practice guideline on management of hyperbilirubinemia in the newborn infant 35 or more weeks of gestation. *Pediatrics.* 2004;114:297-316. Reprinted with permission of the American Academy of Pediatrics.

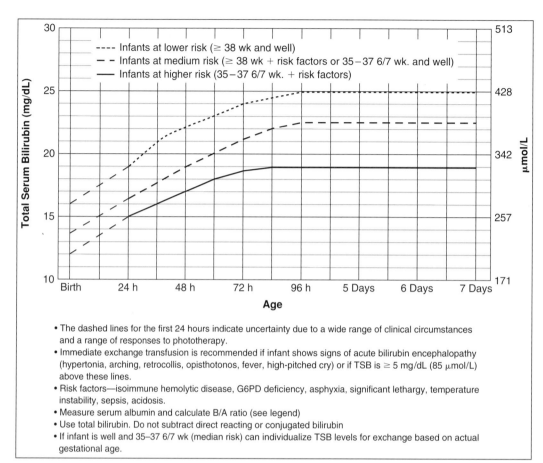

Source: American Academy of Pediatrics. Clinical practice guideline on management of hyperbilirubinemia in the newborn infant 35 or more weeks of gestation. *Pediatrics.* 2004;114:297-316. Reprinted with permission of the American Academy of Pediatrics.

FIGURE 11–3 Guidelines for exchange transfusion.

Phototherapy of hyperbilirubinemia is based on the knowledge that light wavelength in the blue spectrum (450–500 nanometers) is absorbed by bilirubin and results in a change in the structure of the bilirubin molecule such that the fat-soluble, unconjugated bilirubin becomes water soluble without having to be conjugated in the liver. This stereoisomer of bilirubin, a product of light therapy, can be excreted in the stool and urine without conjugation with glucuronic acid. Phototherapy treatment of jaundice should be reserved for those infants who meet the AAP criteria for intervention (American Academy of Pediatrics, 2004). When phototherapy is indicated, it should be performed intensively so that it is as effective as possible (Maisels, 1996). Home phototherapy does not have a role in treating neonates with significant hyperbilirubinemia who need close and thus frequent monitoring of bilirubin levels and who would otherwise be at risk for exchange transfusion if not properly and effectively managed with light therapy. Infants under phototherapy should be fed orally and do not need intravenous fluids unless they have signs of dehydration (Boo & Lee, 2002). Breastfeeding need not be interrupted; feeding with breastmilk may still continue while a baby is in the hospital under light therapy, though the more time the infant spends under the light, the faster the bilirubin will decline. In some instances, the newborn may need to be fed while under phototherapy if the level of bilirubin is high enough that exchange transfusion might become necessary if the hyperbilirubinemia cannot be lowered. In that case, the mother could pump and feed breastmilk. For most infants under phototherapy, interruptions of light treatment for up to 30 minutes every 2 to 3 hours will not significantly reduce the effectiveness of the phototherapy.

Acknowledgment

Marguerite Herschel, MD, was the original first author of this chapter in the previous edition of this book. Sadly, Dr. Herschel died shortly after publication of the book. Dr. Herschel was a marvelous and dedicated teacher and clinical researcher. Her research on neonatal jaundice is noted in this chapter.

S u m m a r y

The diagnosis, assessment, and management of neonatal jaundice should take place in the context of the breastfeeding. While it is known that there is an association between jaundice and breastfeeding, one must be very careful not to convey the wrong message to the mother and her family that breast-feeding is potentially dangerous or harmful to her baby. Mothers commonly feel guilty, believing they have caused the baby to be jaundiced (Hannon, Willis, & Scrimshaw, 2001).

As emphasized in this chapter, a careful evaluation for the etiology of the hyperbilirubinemia must be made, with jaundice associated with breast-feeding being considered as a diagnosis of exclusion. In any case, regardless of the cause, the breast-feeding must be optimized and supported. This often requires that the hospital staff be educated not to make remarks to mothers to the effect that they should supplement their babies with formula if they do not want the baby to have to remain in the hospital for treatment for jaundice. The staff on all shifts must be knowledgeable in helping babies and their mothers to have a proper latch and to feed frequently. They should also encourage mothers to speak up to get help. The staff must know the right questions to ask mothers to assess the adequacy of the breastfeeding. Staff must be able to make careful direct observations of feedings, the patterns of stools, and weight loss or gain. At least twice a day, a formal evaluation of breastfeeding for position, latch, and milk transfer should be made by a health-care provider who is trained in this methodology. The results of this assessment must be recorded in the infant's medical record.

Neonates with jaundice, who are breastfed, just as newborns with jaundice who are artificially fed, should be approached in a global manner in the diagnostic evaluation and management of the jaundice. This will ensure the optimal outcome for the neonate and family.

K e y   C o n c e p t s

- Jaundice, a yellow discoloration of the sclerae and skin, is caused by the deposition of bilirubin in those tissues. Bilirubin is a product of red blood cell—specifically hemoglobin—breakdown.
- Physiologic jaundice is a common clinical condition in the majority of newborn infants that generally resolves within the first week of life in the term artificial-milk fed neonate. Approximately 60 percent of all newborns will have some jaundice in the first week of life. Nearly all newborns will have some elevation of serum bilirubin concentration compared with adult normal values.
- Breastmilk jaundice, characterized by prolongation of physiologic jaundice, is a normal manifestation in at least one third of breastfed infants. Approximately two thirds of all breastfed infants will have an elevation of serum bilirubin concentration.
- Inadequate breastfeeding may lead to jaundice, particularly in the first few days of life, but not on day 1. This is the neonatal manifestation of the adult disorder, starvation jaundice.
- Despite the known association of jaundice and breastfeeding, other causes for jaundice must be ruled out before attributing jaundice solely to breastfeeding.
- The level of bilirubin in a neonate resulting in neonatal jaundice is determined by the balance between production and elimination of bilirubin.

- Increased production of bilirubin, owing to increased red cell breakdown (hemolysis), may lead to very high levels of bilirubin.
- Extreme hyperbilirubinemia may result in permanent brain damage, known as bilirubin encephalopathy (kernicterus).
- Kernicterus has become a public health problem. To prevent this tragic outcome, all neonates should be screened for bilirubin level prior to hospital discharge. Adequate breastfeeding must be documented prior to discharge. Follow-up with a healthcare provider must take place at 3 to 5 days of age or 1 to 3 days after discharge. At that visit, jaundice and breastfeeding must be assessed.

Internet Resources

American Academy of Pediatrics Practice Guideline. Management of Hyperbilirubinemia in the

Healthy Term Newborn: http://www.aap.org (Keyword: jaundice)

References

Akaba K et al. Neonatal hyperbilirubinemia and mutation of the bilirubin uridine diphosphate-glucuronosyltransferase gene: a common missense mutation among Japanese, Koreans and Chinese. *Biochem Mol Biol Int.* 1998;46:21–26.

Alonso EM et al. Enterohepatic circulation of nonconjugated bilirubin in rats fed with human milk. *J Pediatr.* 1991;118:425–430.

American Academy of Pediatrics. Clinical practice guideline on management of hyperbilirubinemia in the newborn infant 35 or more weeks of gestation. *Pediatrics.* 2004;114:297–316.

American Academy of Pediatrics, Committee on Drugs. The transfer of drugs and other chemicals into human milk. *Pediatrics.* 2001;108:776–789.

Arias IM et al. Prolonged neonatal unconjugated hyperbilirubinemia associated with breast feeding and a steroid, pregnane-3(alpha), 20(beta)-diol, in maternal milk that inhibits glucuronide formation in vitro. *J Clin Invest.* 1964;43:2037–2047.

Bhutani YK et al. End-tidal carbon monoxide (ETCOc) hours-specific nomogram: for early and pre-discharge identification of babies with increased bilirubin production. *J Perinatol.* 2001;21:S01.

Bhutani VK, Johnson LH, Keren R. Treating acute bilirubin encephalopathy before it's too late. *Contemp Pediatr.* 2005;22(5):57–74.

Bhutani VK, Johnson L, Sivieri EM. Predictive ability of a predischarge hour-specific serum bilirubin for subsequent significant hyperbilirubinemia in healthy term and near-term newborns. *Pediatrics.* 1999; 103:6–14.

Bhutani VK et al. Noninvasive measurement of total serum bilirubin in a multiracial predischarge newborn population to assess the risk of severe hyperbilirubinemia. *Pediatrics.* 2000;106:e17.

Boo NY, Lee HT. Randomized controlled trial of oral versus intravenous fluid supplementation on serum bilirubin level during phototherapy of term infants with severe hyperbilirubinemia. *J Paediatr Child Health.* 2002;38:151–155.

Brown WR, Wong HB. Ethnic group differences in plasma bilirubin levels of full-term, healthy Singapore newborns. *Pediatrics.* 1965;336:745–751.

Centers for Disease Control and Prevention. Kernicterus in full-term infants, United States, 1994–1998. *MMWR.* 2001;50:491–494.

de Carvalho M, Robertson S, Klaus M. Fecal bilirubin excretion and serum bilirubin concentrations in breast-fed and bottle-fed infants. *J Pediatr.* 1985;107: 786–790.

Dennery PA, Seidman DS, Stevenson DK. Neonatal hyperbilirubinemia. *N Engl J Med.* 2001;344: 581–590.

Dore S et al. Bilirubin, formed by activation of heme oxygenase-2, protects neurons against oxidative stress injury. *Proc Natl Acad Sci USA.* 1999;96: 2445–2450.

Felc Z. Improvement of conventional transcutaneous bilirubinometry results in term newborn infants. *Am J Perinatol.* 2005;22:173–179.

Garcia FJ, Nager AL. Jaundice as an early diagnostic sign of urinary tract infection in infancy. *Pediatrics.* 2002;109:846–851.

Gartner LM. Breastfeeding and jaundice. *J Perinatol.* 2001;21:S25-S29.

Gartner LM, Herschel M. Jaundice and breastfeeding. *Pediatr Clin North Am.* 2001;48:389–399.

Gartner LM, Lee KS. Jaundice and liver disease. In: Fanaroff AA, Martin RJ, eds. *Neonatal-Perinatal Medicine: Diseases of the Fetus and Infant.* St. Louis, MO: Mosby–Year Book, 1992:1075–1104.

Gartner LM, Lee KS, Moscioni AD. Effect of milk feeding on intestinal bilirubin absorption in the rat. *J Pediatr.* 1983;103:464–471.

Gebara BM, Everett KO. Dural sinus thrombosis complicating hypernatremic dehydration in a breastfed neonate. *Clin Pediatr.* 2001;40:45–48.

Hammerman C et al. Protective effect of bilirubin in ischemia-reperfusion injury in the rat intestine. *J Ped Gastro Nutr.* 2002;35:344–349.

Hannon PR, Willis SK, Scrimshaw SC. Persistence of maternal concerns surrounding neonatal jaundice. *Arch Pediatr Adolesc Med.* 2001;155:1357–1363.

Harris RC, Lucey JF, Maclean JR. Kernicterus in premature infants associated with low concentrations of bilirubin in the plasma. *Pediatrics.* 1958;21:875–884.

Harris MC et al. Developmental follow-up of breastfed term and near-term infants with marked hyperbilirubinemia. *Pediatrics.* 2001;107:1075–1080.

Herschel M et al. Evaluation of the direct antiglobulin (Coombs') test for identifying newborns at-risk for hemolysis as determined by end-tidal carbon monoxide concentration (ETCOc) and comparison of the Coombs' test with ETCOc for detecting significant jaundice. *J Perinatol.* 2002;22:341–347.

Hunt SC et al. Evidence for a major gene elevating serum bilirubin concentration in Utah pedigrees. *Arterioscler Thromb Vasc Biol.* 1996;16:912–917.

Ip S et al. An evidence-based review of important issues concerning neonatal hyperbilirubinemia. *Pediatrics.* 2004;114:e130–e153.

Johnson LH, Bhutani VK, Brown AK. System-based approached to management of neonatal jaundice and prevention of kernicterus. *J Pediatr.* 2002;40:396–403.

Kaplan M. Genetic interactions in the pathogenesis of neonatal hyperbilirubinemia: Gilbert's syndrome and Glucose-6-phosphate dehydrogenase deficiency. *J Perinatol.* 2001;21:S30–S34.

Kaplan M, Algur N, Hammerman C. Onset of jaundice in glucose-6-phosphate dehydrogenase-deficient neonates. *Pediatrics.* 2001;108:956–959.

Kaplan M, Hammerman C. Glucose-6-phosphate dehydrogenase deficiency: a hidden risk for kernicterus. *Semin Perinatol.* 2004;28:356–364.

Kaplan M et al. Predischarge bilirubin screening in glucose-6-phosphate dehydrogenase-deficient neonates. *Pediatrics.* 2000;105:533–537.

Kaplan M, Hammerman C, Maisels MJ. Bilirubin genetics for the nongeneticist: hereditary defects of neonatal bilirubin conjugation. *Pediatrics.* 2003;111:886–891.

Maisels MJ. Why use homeopathic doses of phototherapy? *Pediatrics.* 1996;98:283–287.

Kaplan M et al. Hyperbilirubinemia among African American, glucose-6-phosphate dehydrogenase-deficient neonates. *Pediatrics.* 2004;114:e213–e219.

Kaplan M et al. Neonatal hyperbilirubinemia in African American males: the importance of glucose-6-phosphate dehydrogenase deficiency. *J Pediatr.* 2006;149:83–88.

Kaplan M et al. Glucose-6-phosphate dehydrogenase activity in term and near-term male African American neonates. *Clinica Chimica Acta.* 2005;355:113–117.

Maisels MJ, Newman TB. Jaundice in full-term and near-term babies who leave the hospital within 36 hours. The pediatrician's nemesis. *Clin Perinatol.* 1998;25:295–302.

Martin E et al. Ceftriaxone-bilirubin-albumin interactions in the neonate: an in vivo study. *Eur J Pediatr.* 1993;152:530–534.

Maruo Y et al. Association of neonatal hyperbilirubinemia with bilirubin UDP-glucuronosyltransferase polymorphism. *Pediatrics.* 1999;103:1224–1227.

Maruo Y et al. Prolonged unconjugated hyperbilirubinemia associated with breast milk and mutations of the bilirubin uridine diphosphate-glucuronosyltransferase gene. *Pediatrics.* 2000;106:e59.

Monaghan G et al. Gilbert's syndrome is a contributory factor in prolonged unconjugated hyperbilirubinemia of the newborn. *J Pediatr.* 1999;134:441–446.

Moyer VA, Ahn C, Sneed S. Accuracy of clinical judgment in neonatal jaundice. *Arch Pediatr Adolesc Med.* 2000;154:391–394.

Neifert MR. The optimization of breast-feeding in the perinatal period. *Clin Perinatol.* 1998;25:303–326.

Newman AJ, Gross S. Hyperbilirubinemia in breast-fed infants. *Pediatrics.* 1963;32:995–1001.

Newman TB, Easterling MJ. Yield of reticulocyte counts and blood smears in term neonates. *Clin Pediatr.* 1994;33:71–76.

Newman TB, Liljestrand P, Escobar GJ. Combining risk factors with serum bilirubin levels to predict hyperbilirubinemia in newborns. *Arch Pediatr Adolesc Med.* 2005;159:113–119.

Odell GB, Cohen SN, Kelly PC. Studies in kernicterus. II. The determination of the saturation of serum albumin with bilirubin. *J Pediatr.* 1969;74:214–230.

Rubaltelli FF. Unconjugated and conjugated bilirubin pigments during perinatal development. IV. The influence of breast-feeding on neonatal hyperbilirubinemia. *Biol Neonate.* 1993;64:104–109.

Rubaltelli FF et al. Transcutaneous bilirubin measurement: a multicenter evaluation of a new device. *Pediatrics.* 2001;107:1264–1271.

Schwertner HA, Jackson WG, Tolan G. Association of low serum concentration of bilirubin with increased risk of coronary artery disease. *Clin Chem.* 1994;40:18–23.

Shapiro SM, Bhutani VK, Johnson L. Hyperbilirubinemia and kernicterus. *Clin Perinatol.* 2006;33:387–410.

Shurin SB. The blood and hematopoietic system. In: Fanaroff AA, Martin RJ, eds. *Neonatal-Perinatal Medicine: Diseases of the Fetus and Infant.* St. Louis, MO: Mosby–Year Book; 1992:941–989.

Stevenson DK, Dennery PA, Hinz SR. Understanding newborn jaundice. *J Perinatol.* 2001;21:S21–S24.

Stiehm ER, Ryan J. Breast-milk jaundice. *Amer J Dis Child.* 1965;109:212–216.

Stocker R et al. Bilirubin is an antioxidant of possible physiological importance. *Science.* 1987;235:1043–1046.

Temme EH, Zhang J, Schouten EG, Kesteloot H. Serum bilirubin and 10-year mortality risk in a Belgian population. *Cancer Causes Control.* 2001;12:887–894.

Vítek L et al. Gilbert syndrome and ischemic heart disease: a protective effect of elevated bilirubin levels. *Atherosclerosis*. 2002;160:449–456.

Volpe JJ. *Neurology of the Newborn*. 4th ed. Philadelphia, PA: WB Saunders; 2001:521–546.

Vreman HJ et al. Evaluation of a fully automated end-tidal carbon monoxide instrument for breath analysis. *Clin Chem*. 1996;42:50–56.

Whitmer DI, Gollan JL. Mechanism and significance of fasting and dietary hyperbilirubinemia. *Semin Liver Dis*. 1983;3:42–51.

Young BWY et al. Predicting pathologic jaundice: the Chinese perspective. *J Perinatol*. 2001;21:S73–S75.

Chapter

12

Breast Pumps and Other Technologies

Marsha Walker

SPECIAL DEVICES HAVE BEEN USED for hundreds of years to help breastfeeding mothers overcome various problems. Examples of someone, or something, other than a baby removing milk from the breasts are cited in medical literature as early as the mid-1500s (Fildes, 1986). Before breast pumps or other instruments were used to withdraw milk from the breasts, children, young puppies, or birth attendants were enlisted to do the job. By the 1500s the medical literature included discussions of "sucking glasses." These devices allowed women to remove milk themselves and were recommended for relieving engorgement or expressing milk when the nipples were damaged or when mastitis was present. Sucking glasses were also thought to help evert flat and inverted nipples. For the most part, vacuum was generated by mouth, and the devices were made of glass (Figure 12–1). Women could use a glass, glass vial, or glass bottle heated with very hot water and applied to the breast in order to draw out milk. French breast pumps in the 1700s resembled smoking pipes.

As technology advanced, so did breast pump materials and design. Combinations of materials such as brass, wood, glass, pewter, and rubber were used to make pumps like the syringe pump (Figure 12–2), the long-handled lever pump (Figure 12–3), and the

syringe pump with pewter flanges (Figure 12–4). Women pump their breasts for short periods of time to solve acute problems or to donate to a human milk bank, and for extended periods in order to provide human milk for their babies under such circumstances as employment, induced lactation, relactation, compromised milk supply, maternal or infant illness, or following a preterm birth. Win et al. (2006) reported that in a study of 587 mothers, those who

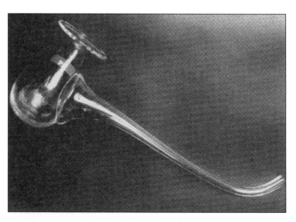

FIGURE 12–1 An American sucking glass, circa 1870.

Source: Courtesy of Canon Babysafe Ltd., Suffolk, England/Courtesy of Hollister/Ameda-Egnell.

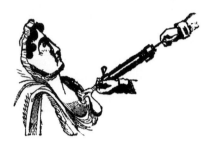

DRAWING THE BREASTS.

Where the breast is hard, swollen and painful, from inflammation, or the nipple sore from excoriation, the application of this instrument is attended with more ease to the patient than any other means, and she may without difficulty use it herself, by which she can regulate its action agreeably to her own sensations. The flat surface of the glass should be smeared with oil before it is put on, and the bulb preserved in a dependant position to receive the fluid. During the operation the small aperture in the brass socket must be closely covered with the finger, which being removed, admits air into the glass and causes it to be detached from the breast whenever it may be desired.

FIGURE 12–2 Expressing the breasts with a syringe pump, circa 1830.

Source: Courtesy of Canon Babysafe Ltd., Suffolk, England/Courtesy of Hollister/Ameda-Egnell.

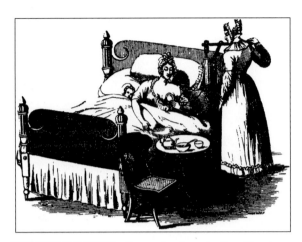

FIGURE 12–3 Expressing breastmilk with a long-handled lever pump, circa 1830.

expressed breast milk at one or more time periods were less likely to discontinue breastfeeding before 6 months. Binns et al. (2006) calculated that the proportion of mothers who had expressed breast milk almost doubled in the decade between 1993 and 2003. They attributed this to the increased encouragement of exclusive breastfeeding, a possible change in how clinicians managed early breastfeeding problems, and the availability of more efficient breast pumps.

Concerns of Mothers

Most mothers want a pump that works efficiently and comfortably at a reasonable cost. They want pumps that are easy to find, easy to use, and easy to clean. The amount of milk expressed and the time it takes to obtain it are the two issues most frequently mentioned by mothers when they are choosing or using a breast pump.

Satisfaction with breast pumps, however, is highly individual. In an informal survey conducted with more than 200 mothers (Walker, 1992), a pump was rated highly if it (1) worked quickly—

(less than 20 minutes total), (2) obtained two or more ounces of milk from each breast, and (3) did not cause pain. The mothers in this survey suggested pumping techniques to speed the process and to increase the volume of milk per pumping session. Many mothers expressed the most milk before or after the first morning feeding when the breasts were reported to be fullest (and intramammary pressure was the highest); later volumes steadily decreased throughout the day. Many mothers mentioned that if they were not relaxed, or if they were uncomfortable or felt rushed, their output dropped by one third to one half the usual amount.

The majority of mothers used one or more techniques to increase pumping efficiency. The two most frequently mentioned techniques were eliciting the milk-ejection reflex before starting to pump and massaging the breast while pumping. Both techniques increased pumping speed and milk output. Some mothers were able to double the amount pumped by using both of these techniques at each pumping session.

Stimulating the Milk-Ejection Reflex

Research conducted by the dairy industry supports the importance of eliciting the milk-ejection reflex before starting to express milk. In the dairy cow, premilking stimulation of the udder increases serum oxytocin levels (Merrill et al., 1987) and results in shorter time on the machine and a higher average rate of milk flow

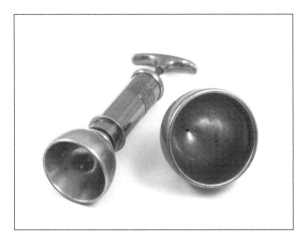

FIGURE **12–4** Pewter breast pump (Weedon), c.1830–1856.

Source: Courtesy of Phisick (www.phisick.com).

(Dodd & Griffin, 1977; Goodman & Grosvenor, 1983; Gorewit et al., 1983; Sagi, Gorewit, & Zinn, 1980). In the second edition of *Dairy Science,* Petersen (1950) cited several factors that contribute to poor milking: undue excitement at milking time, improper stimulation for the let-down of milk, too long an interval between stimulation of let-down and the beginning of milking, too slow milking, and incomplete withdrawal of milk. His observations regarding proper milking techniques parallel many recommendations of professionals and the expression techniques human mothers have discovered on their own. Animal models of lactation can serve as a frame of reference from which recommendations can be drawn and applied.

Avoid Undue Excitement at Milking Time

Many women use specific relaxation techniques and visual imagery before and during pumping. Feher et al. (1989) reported using a guided relaxation audiotape to increase milk output during breast pumping among mothers of preterm infants. Newton and Newton (1948) described the adverse effect of a painful or distracting stimulus during nursing on the milk-ejection reflex. Pain and psychologic stress can inhibit the milk-ejection reflex by reducing the number of oxytocin pulses during suckling episodes (Ueda et al., 1994). Opiate and B-endorphin release during stress can block stimulus-related oxytocin secretion (Lawrence & Lawrence, 2005).

Elicit the Milk-Ejection Reflex First

For 1 to 2 minutes before pumping begins, massaging with a hot, wet cloth is the most effective stimulus for let-down. Mothers have reported using hot compresses, showers, and breast massage before expressing to obtain the best results. Some report that they are most successful if they pump one side while the baby feeds on the other breast (as with pumping in dairy cattle when all teats are milked simultaneously), if the baby elicits the milk-ejection reflex first and they then pump, or if they hand express first or massage the breast first and then pump. Upon nipple stimulation, oxytocin is released in a pulsatile nature consisting of brief 3 to 4 second bursts of oxytocin into the bloodstream every 5 to 15 minutes. This shortens and widens the lactiferous ducts, increasing the pressure inside the breast and is essential for maximum removal of milk from the breast (Neville, 2001). Correlations between oxytocin pulsatility on day 2 and the duration of exclusive breastfeeding suggest that the development of an early pulsatile oxytocin pattern is of importance for sustained exclusive breastfeeding (Nissen et al., 1996). Oxytocin can also be released prior to the baby being placed at breast and is not dependent solely on tactile stimulation for release. It takes the baby between 54 and 60 seconds to elicit the milk-ejection reflex on the first side and 47 seconds on the second side, on average. Some pumps can take up to 4 minutes to elicit the milk-ejection reflex (mean 103.2 sec ± 89.2 sec) (Kent et al., 2003; Mitoulas, Lai, & Gurrin, 2002a). Studies done using a Medela Symphony pump show that the time the pump takes to stimulate the first milk ejection as detected by breast ultrasound is approximately 90 seconds (Ramsay et al., 2006). Some pumps are electronically programmed to "stimulate" milk ejection by initially providing low vacuum and rapid cycling then switching to a higher vacuum and lower cycling.

Massage Each Quarter of the Udder During Mechanical Milking

Massaging during breast pumping can markedly increase milk yield. Breast massage may increase fat content and milk yield when a baby is at breast. Bowles, Stutte, and Hensley (1988) and Stutte, Bowles, and Morman (1988) found that infants gained greater amounts of weight and mothers experienced little nipple pain or painful engorgement when the breasts were massaged by quadrant in an alternating pattern with the baby's suckling bursts. Breast massage represents a form of positive pressure, which adds to the pressure created within the milk ducts during let-down as it significantly increases the plasma oxytocin level (Yokoyama et al., 1994). The diameter of the milk ducts increases by approximately 79 percent after let-down, (Hartmann, 2000) with duct diameters drifting down after a 1- to 2-minute period following let-down (Hartmann, 2002). A pump needs to remove milk quickly before the volume of milk in the ducts decreases and another let-down is necessary to reestablish the pressure gradient between breast and pump. Adding external compression probably acts as an "artificial" let-down, increasing the positive pressure within the breast and helping milk flow toward the negative pressure created in the pump. The establishment of an effective pressure gradient that can be sustained over a long enough period of time will contribute to the optimal drainage of each breast.

When Hand-Milking, Avoid Point Compression and Digging In with the Fingertips

Point compression and digging in with the fingertips is likely to cause injury. The Marmet method of hand expression (Marmet & Shell, 1980) cautioned against this technique when a mother is hand-expressing her milk.

Remove the Milking Machine as Soon as the Milk Stops Flowing

Stopping the pump when the milk stops flowing reduces tissue injury. Many mothers switch to the other breast when the milk flow slows in the breast being pumped. Some mothers mention that pain is the cue for this switch, indicating a change in the pressure gradient. Auerbach (1990b) found that protracted pumping times did not significantly increase milk yield beyond a certain point. Those who pumped (sequentially or simultaneously) for longer than 16 minutes averaged total milk volumes of 55 cc or less. Mitoulas, Lai, and Gurrin (2002a) found that the rate of milk expression changed over the course of a 5-minute expression period, remaining constant the first 2.5 minutes but decreasing by

5 minutes. The variation among mothers was large, with some mothers delivering almost 2 oz in the first 30 seconds to others delivering no milk by the end of 5 minutes. If it takes a particular mother 4 minutes to elicit the milk-ejection reflex, she may need a much longer time to pump than another mother delivering 99 percent of the milk in her breasts into the pump within 5 minutes.

The dairy literature includes many recommendations that are applicable to human breast pumping. Even some of the modern electric breast pumps designed for mothers have similarities to the agricultural milking units. The Whittlestone pump incorporated the design of the double-chambered teat cups. The suction and rest phases of a commercial milking unit are either 60/40 or 70/30 (percentage of suction to percentage of rest per cycle). There are usually 60 cycles generated per minute (a calf generates about 120 cycles), and negative pressure is around 375 mm Hg (similar to the higher pressures seen in a few breast pumps, including hand pumps).

Breast pumps must also be easy to clean, affordable, and accessible. When recommending a pump, the caregiver should give a specific name and several places to find it to avoid acquisition of a pump that may be inappropriate or ineffective (Figure 12–5). Hospital or medical supply houses may have pumps originally designed as chest aspirators that are not as suitable for milk expression as those specifically designed for that purpose. Instructions for use may be inadequate, causing some mothers to forgo pumping and breastfeeding altogether. Many mothers have complained of the extra expense incurred if their pump broke (common with the battery pumps) and required replacement (Walker, 1992). Of 97 battery pumps used in the survey, 24 broke or stopped generating suction and had to be replaced (a 25 percent breakage rate). The life of a battery-operated pump is considered to be about 16 weeks (4 months) by some companies, a much shorter period than many employed mothers require. Batteries are a major expense for mothers who pump regularly; many purchase an A/C adapter to economize. The cost of the accessory kit and daily rental charges for an electric pump can be expensive, even with a long-term rental contract. Some insurance carriers and health maintenance organizations cover the cost of pump rentals only while a baby is hospitalized or for only a limited period of time.

Several mothers in the survey (Walker, 1992) purchased a hand pump solely to cut cost. Some were dissatisfied and purchased a second, more expensive pump that worked better. Pump prices vary considerably depending upon the type of store or organization that sells them. Some breastfeeding programs provide breast pumps at cost to their clients. Many hospitals give breastfeeding mothers a high-quality hand pump upon discharge rather than formula packs. Box 12–1 summarizes recommendations for mothers using a breast pump.

Hormonal Considerations

When milk expression using a pump is necessary, the device used must be efficient enough to activate prolactin and oxytocin release and to efficiently remove milk from the breasts.

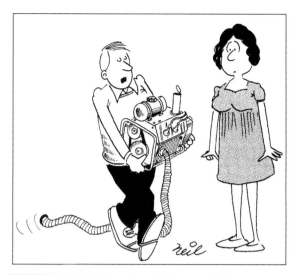

FIGURE 12–5 "They didn't actually have a breast pump…"

Source: Courtesy of Neil Matteson, © 1984.

BOX 12–1

Recommendations for the Nursing Mother Who Uses a Pump

General Pumping Recommendations

1. Read the instructions on the use and cleaning of a pump before expressing milk with any product.
2. Wash hands before each pumping session.
3. Frequency: For occasional pumping, pump during, after, or between feedings, whichever gives the best results. Most mothers tend to express more milk in the morning. For mothers employed outside the home, pumping should occur on a regular basis for the number of nursings that are missed. For premature or ill babies who are not at breast, the number of pumpings should total 8–10 or more each 24 hours for the 1st 14 days. Initiation of pumping should be delayed no longer than 6 hours following birth unless medically indicated. This ensures appropriate development and sensitivity of prolactin receptors. More frequent pumping will avoid the build-up of excessive backpressure of milk during engorgement.

(Continues)

BOX **12–1** (Continued)

4. Duration: With single-sided pumping, duration ranges from 10 to 15 minutes with an electric pump and 10 to 20 minutes with a manual pump. If double pumping with an electric or two battery-operated pumps, 7 to 15 minutes is optimal. Encourage mothers to tailor these times to their own situation.

5. Technique:
   - Elicit the milk-ejection reflex before using the pump.
   - Use only as much vacuum as is needed to maintain milk flow and remain comfortable.
   - Massage the breast in quadrants before and during pumping to increase intramammary pressure.
   - Allow enough time for pumping to avoid anxiety.
   - Use inserts or different sized flanges if needed to obtain the best fit between pump and breast.
   - Avoid long periods of uninterrupted vacuum.
   - Stop pumping when the milk flow is minimal or has ceased.

Recommendations for Specific Types of Pumps

1. Avoid pumps that use rubber bulbs to generate a vacuum.
2. Cylinder pumps:
   - When O rings are used, they must be in place for proper suction.
   - Gaskets must be removed after each use for cleaning to avoid harboring bacteria in the pump.
   - The gasket on the inner cylinder may be rolled back and forth to restore it to its original shape.
   - The pump stroke may need to be shortened as the outer cylinder fills with milk.
   - The mother may need to empty the outer cylinder once or twice during pumping.
   - Hand position should be palm up with the elbow held close to the body.
   - Hand position should be palm up with the elbow held close to the body.

3. Battery-operated pumps:
   - Use alkaline batteries, not rechargable batteries.
   - Replace batteries when cycles per minute decrease.
   - Interrupt vacuum frequently to avoid nipple pain and damage if the pump does not autocycle.
   - Use an AC adapter when possible, especially if the pump generates fewer than 6 cycles per minute.
   - Consider purchasing or renting an electric pump for pumping that will continue for longer than 1 or 2 months.
   - Use two pumps simultaneously if pumping time is limited or to increase the quantity of milk obtained.
   - Choose a pump in which the vacuum can be regulated.
   - Massage the breast by quadrants during pumping.

4. Semiautomatic pumps:
   - Vacuum may be easier to control if the mother does not lift her fingercompletely off the hole but rolls it back and forth rhythmically so that the vacuum is efficient but not painful.

(Continues)

> **BOX** **12–1** (Continued)
>
> 5. Automatic electric pumps:
>   - Use the lowest pressure setting that is efficient. Mothers may find that changing the vacuum and/or the cycling characteristics of the pump during each expressing session may increase milk volume.
>   - Use a double setup (simultaneous pumping) when time is limited in order to increase a milk supply, as well as for prematurity, maternal or infant illness, or other special situations.

Prolactin

A steady rise in prolactin during pregnancy prepares the breasts for lactation (Neville, 1983). Prolactin levels rise during pregnancy from about 10 ng/ml in the nonpregnant state to approximately 200 ng/ml at term. Baseline levels do not drop to normal in a lactating woman, but average about 100 ng/ml at 3 months and 50 ng/ml at 6 months. Prolactin levels can double with the stimulus of suckling. After about 6 months of breastfeeding, the prolactin rise with suckling amounts to only about 5 to 10 ng/ml. This is accounted for by the increased prolactin-binding capacity or sensitivity of the mammary tissue that allows full lactation in the face of falling prolactin levels over time. The high levels of prolactin during pregnancy and early lactation may also serve to increase the number of prolactin receptors and is dependent on tactile input for stimulation and release. In spite of the importance of prolactin to lactation itself, prolactin does not directly regulate the short-term or long-term rate of milk synthesis (Cox, Owens, & Hartmann, 1996). Once lactation is well established, prolactin is still required for milk synthesis to occur, but its role is permissive rather than regulatory (Cregan & Hartmann, 1999).

Prolactin concentration in the plasma is highest during sleep and lowest during the waking hours and operates as a true circadian rhythm (Stern & Reichlin, 1990). The prolactin response is superimposed on the circadian rhythm of prolactin secretion, thus the same intensity of suckling stimulus can elevate prolactin levels more effectively at certain times of the day when the circadian input enhances the effect of the sucking stimulus (Freeman et al., 2000). Prolactin levels only remain elevated after the first weeks postpartum if the baby is put to breast, or in the absence of breast stimulation by an infant, if a pump is used to mechanically maintain prolactin cycling. Small studies with wide variations in methodology have demonstrated the ability of various pumps to elevate prolactin levels (Howie et al., 1980; Neifert & Seacat, 1985; Noel, Suh, & Frantz, 1974; de Sanctis et al., 1981; Weichert, 1980; Whitworth et al., 1984; Zinaman et al., 1992).

Clinical Implications

1. The function of infant suckling (or mechanical milk removal) varies between lactogenesis II, the onset of copious milk production, and galactopoiesis (lactogenesis III), the maintenance of abundant milk production. Lactogenesis II occurs in the absence of milk removal over the first 3 days postpartum, but milk composition and volume will not proceed along the continuum to maximum milk production and mature milk composition in the absence of frequent milk removal after that time. While suckling (or mechanical milk

removal) may not be a prerequisite for lactogenesis II, it is critical for galactopoiesis. Delayed suckling by the infant, whether owing to premature delivery (Cregan, de Mello, & Hartmann, 2000), cesarean delivery (Sozmen, 1992), or other factors that necessitate mechanical milk removal, may affect the timing or delay the onset of lactogenesis II. Additional breast pumping after a couple of breastfeeds before the onset of lactogenesis II has not been shown to hasten the event or result in increased milk transfer to the baby at 72 hours (Chapman et al., 2001). In the absence of a baby at breast, the breasts need to be stimulated eight or more times every 24 hours. Pumping only once or twice during the day and never at night, when prolactin levels are at their peak, may contribute to delayed lactogenesis II. A faltering milk supply in the following weeks may be attributed to the lack of sufficient prolactin receptors and infrequent breast stimulation while lactation is being established.

2. Painful overdistension of the breasts (secondary engorgement) must be prevented. As alveolar pressure rises, lactation suppression begins. Painful engorgement lasting longer than 48 hours can potentially decrease the milk supply. Therefore, if a baby cannot keep up with a suddenly increased milk supply, the mother should express her milk. When milk production begins in the absence of a baby, pumping frequency may need to be temporarily increased to prevent involution of the alveoli caused by the back pressure of milk and the buildup of suppressor peptides that down-regulate milk volume. Wilde, Prentice, and Peaker (1995) have identified this peptide and named it the feedback inhibitor of lactation (FIL).

3. Early breastfeeding has a critical period during which frequent nipple stimulation and milk removal are necessary for a plentiful milk supply in later weeks. The clinician should offer management guidelines with this in mind, especially if mother and baby are separated. Woolridge (1995) provided a practical identification of six separate stages in the lactation process:

- Priming (changes of pregnancy)
- Initiation (birth and the management of early breastfeeding)
- Calibration (the concept that milk production gets underway without the breasts actually "knowing" how much milk to make in the beginning). Over the first 3 to 5 weeks, milk output is progressively calibrated to the baby's needs, usually building up (up-regulation) but occasionally down-regulating to meet the baby's needs.
- Maintenance (the period of exclusive breastfeeding)
- Decline (the period after complementary foods or supplements are added)
- Involution (weaning)

It is the second, third, and fourth time periods that are crucial to ensuring abundant milk production. Close attention must be given to alterations that could impact the breasts' ability to calibrate their milk output to the needs of the baby.

Daly et al. (1992, 1993) have shown that the degree of breast emptying is inversely proportional to the amount of milk made to replace it; that is, the more thoroughly that a breast is drained, the more milk is made. Daly and Hartmann (1995a,b) noted that breasts with smaller storage capacities may need to be expressed more frequently than breasts with larger storage capacities, even though both types of breasts are capable of synthesizing similar amounts of milk in 24 hours. Mothers with larger storage capacities are able to express a higher volume of milk with each pumping session but not necessarily more milk in a 24-hour period than mothers with smaller storage capacities. The volume of milk expressed is also related to the degree of fullness of the breast, with a fuller breast yielding more milk volume when pumped (Mitoulas, Lai, & Gurrin, 2002a). Full breasts tend to take less time to achieve the milk-ejection reflex, with a less full breast taking up to 120 seconds (Hartmann, 2002). Expressed milk volume tends to be higher from the right breast than the left with these differences sometimes being quite large but stable over time (Engstrom et al., 2007). Primiparous mothers and first time breastfeeders demonstrated the greatest differences. A possible explanation could be that the right breast preferentially receives more blood flow than the left which was demonstrated in a Doppler ultrasound study in women with established lactation (Aljazaf, 2004).

Oxytocin

Oxytocin is responsible for the milk-ejection reflex. By acting on the myoepithelial processes, oxytocin causes shortening of the ducts without constricting them, thus increasing the milk pressure. Cobo et al. (1967) measured milk-ejection by recording intraductal mammary pressure using a catheter placed in a mammary duct. Values were measured at 0.19 plus or minus 0.04 in/min and from 0 to 25 mm Hg on recording paper. Ductal contractions lasted about 1 minute and occurred at about 4 to 10 contractions every 10 minutes. Caldeyro-Barcia (1969) reported that intramammary pressure rose 10 mm Hg after 5 days postpartum with oxytocin release. Drewett, Bowen-Jones, and Dogterom (1982) and McNeilly et al. (1983) have shown by minute-to-minute blood sampling that oxytocin occurs in impulses at about 1-minute intervals. Thus oxytocin release is pulsatile and variable with intermittent bursts. These pressure changes cease when suckling stimulation ends. Oxytocin also responds in the same way to prenursing stimuli and mechanical nipple stimulation by a breast pump. The milk-ejection reflex, initiated by oxytocin release, serves to increase the intraductal mammary pressure and maintain it at sufficient levels to overcome the resistance of the breast to the outflow of milk. There is approximately 30 to 35 ml of milk ingested by the infant per milk-ejection (Hartmann, 2002). Milk ducts stay dilated approximately 1.5 to 3.5 minutes following let-down (Hartmann, 2002) making it beneficial to elicit multiple let-downs during the course of a pumping session. Ramsay et al. (2006) observed that the first milk ejection of the expression period released significantly more milk than subsequent milk ejections regardless of vacuum level. There is a significant decline in the rate at which milk is removed after the initial milk ejection (Ramsay et al., 2005). Women with the highest increase in ductal diameter and with more and longer milk ejections expressed more milk. This

may provide a partial explanation of why some mothers are able to express large amounts of milk in short periods of time and others whose anatomy may preclude to small ducts that do not dilate to a great extent and who do not experience as many let-downs during pumping may express lesser amounts of milk.

Pumps

Mechanical Milk Removal

A pump does not pump, suck, or pull milk out of the breast. It reduces resistance to milk outflow from the alveoli, allowing the internal pressure of the breast to push out the milk. The milk-ejection reflex produces an initial rise in the intramammary pressure; because of the pulsatile nature of oxytocin release and its short half-life, periodic rises in ductal pressure maintain the pressure gradient over time.

The classic work on breast pumps conducted by Einar Egnell (1956) was based on research in dairy cattle and Egnell's own experiments with a pump that created periodic and limited phases of negative pressure. Egnell assumed that the milk-secreting alveoli of the breast and the cow udder were similar, even though the two organs are anatomically different and do not drain in the same way. He postulated that the quantity of milk secreted is regulated by the counterpressure it exerts. This counterpressure rises as milk fills the available space; secretion ceases when the pressure reaches 28 mm Hg. Egnell's pump created a maximum negative pressure of 200 mm Hg below atmospheric pressure (760 mm Hg). He based this setting on previous research done with an Abt pump (on human mothers), which produced 30 periods of negative pressure per minute and was reported to rupture the nipple skin in every third breast. Placing his settings well below this level to avoid damaging the human nipple, Egnell calculated the difference between the pressure-filled alveoli and his pump's negative pressure as 760 + 28 − 560 = 228 mm Hg. He maintained that it was the pressure within the breast that activated milk outflow.

Egnell's original pump operated in four phases per cycle, with one cycle lasting from one initiation of suction to the next initiation of suction: (1) a period of increasing suction that is relatively short, (2) a decreasing phase of suction, (3) a resting phase, and (4) a slight amount of positive pressure when the decreased suction phase is finished. Egnell contended that mechanical pumping was safer than manual expression because he feared that the "high" positive pressure generated by "squeezing" the breast could damage the alveoli and ducts. He also speculated that manual expression would leave too much milk in the breast, a common concern in the dairy industry. However, in countries where manual expression is used to obtain mothers' milk when the baby is unavailable, increased breast damage has not been reported. The volume of expressed milk though, tends to be higher when using a breast pump compared to manual expression. Paul et al. (1996) showed that use of a cylinder pump resulted in significantly higher volumes of milk expressed per session compared to hand expression. Slusher et al. (2007) compared milk volumes expressed by hand, double-collection pedal pump, and double-collection electric pump. Both pumps resulted in higher expressed milk volumes compared to hand-expression, with the double-collection electric pump expressing the highest volume of milk. Many pump manufacturers still use Egnell's pressure settings as a guide. However, various pumps are still capable of generating more suction than stated in his calculations.

The vacuum applied to the breast by an infant during suckling is not constant. The vacuum is initiated, it rises, it is released, and it is maintained with a basal resting pressure to keep the nipple in the mouth. The vacuum stretches the teat to approximately twice its resting length, with a 70 percent reduction of the teat's original diameter (Smith, Erenberg, & Nowak, 1988; Weber, Woolridge, & Baum, 1986). Speculation on the function of vacuum ranges from thoughts that (1) vacuum facilitates the refilling with milk of the ducts within the teat following each swallow, or that (2) milk is released from the teat by vacuum caused when the jaw lowers and enlarges the oral cavity (Smith, Erenberg, & Nowak, 1988). In a breastfeeding ultrasound study, Jacobs et al. (2007) showed that the tongue in its uppermost position (securing the nipple in contact with the palate) did not compress any milk into the oral cavity. Tongue movement downward was followed by milk exiting the nipple.

An infant feeding at breast achieves a range of 42 to 126 suck cycles per minute with a mean of 74 sucks per minute (Bowen-Jones, Thompson, & Drewett, 1982). Suction is applied over approximately half of the suck cycle (Halverson, 1944). However, vacuum or suction is not the only force that an infant employs to extract milk from the breast. A compressive force from the tongue and jaw is also applied during the suction cycle to more effectively create milk transfer from the breast to the baby.

Computer modeling that compares breastfeeding and breast pumps has shown that there is an optimal time during the suction cycle when an infant applies the compressive peristaltic force of the tongue. This results in an asymmetric compression of the teat between the tongue and hard palate. Using a model that applied symmetric peristaltic compression of the teat during a suction cycle, Zoppou, Barry, and Mercer (1997a) found that the compressive force applied at the optimal time and speed during the suck cycle could significantly increase the mean fluid flow through the teat, while a compressive force applied at the wrong time in the pressure cycle restricted the flow of fluid. A compressive force applied by a breast pump approximately a quarter of the way through the suction cycle increased the milk volume over one suction cycle by 15 percent, while a compressive force that compressed the teat early in the suction cycle restricted milk flow into the teat and reduced milk volume (Zoppou, Barry, & Mercer, 1997b).

Compression

Whittlestone (1978) described a breast pump that not only accommodated the simultaneous pumping of both breasts but further adopted principles from the commercial dairy milking machines of providing a compressive force to the breast from a liner inside the pump flange that rhythmically contracted around the teat. He called this a physiologic breastmilker. Alekseev et al. (1998) found that adding the compressive stimulus changed the dynamics of milk expression. Using an experimental pump where the compressive stimulus could be switched on and off, it was found that in a 3- to 5-minute period of pumping, 50 percent of the milk could be removed from the breast, but when the compressive stimulus was turned off it took 1.5 to 2.0 times longer to express this volume of milk. Currently, the Whittlestone Breast Expresser (Figure 12–6) employs a compressive liner in its flanges.

The Whisper Wear breast pump (Figure 12–7) is worn under the bra and utilizes a flexible massaging cup. Other pumps have a soft flange that collapses over the teat when vacuum is applied.

The Evolution of Pumps

As breastfeeding rates increased and reasons for pumping changed, mothers and professionals have demanded products that are safe, efficient, and effective in both initiating and maintaining a good milk supply. The breast pump market offers a bewildering array of devices from which to choose. Three broad classifications of breast pumps will be discussed in this chapter: (1) hand pumps that generate suction manually, (2) battery-operated pumps with small motors that generate suction from power supplied by batteries, and (3) electric pumps in which suction is created by various types of electric motors. There is no intent to recommend any one

pump. A listing of companies that sell breast pumps can be found in Appendix 12-A. More extensive descriptions and pictures of pumps can be found at the company Web sites.

A Comparison of Pumps

The efficiency of pumps and how well they work for mothers have not received much discussion in the research literature. Many mothers and clinicians have turned to Internet sites that report mothers' evaluations of the various pumps they have used. These Web sites—www.breastpumpsdirect.com/breast-pump-reviews.asp, www.epinions.com, and www.amazon.com—list pump reviews. While not very scientific, the reviews run the gamut of pros and cons from a mother's perspective with some helpful hints about pump use, troubleshooting problems, and pumping situations.

Hand pumps are popular, relatively inexpensive, and readily available. Much information on the efficiency of hand pumps is anecdotal; some pumps work quite well, whereas others suffer from poor suction, excessive suction, cylinders that pull apart during pumping, and user fatigue from the repeated

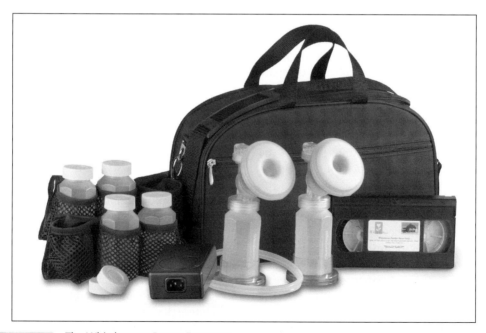

FIGURE 12–6   The Whittlestone Breast Expresser.

Source: Courtesy of Whittlestone, Inc., Benicia, CA.

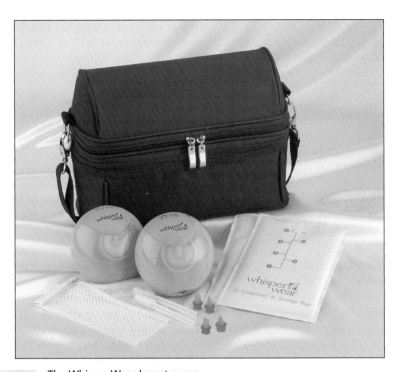

FIGURE 12–7   The Whisper Wear breast pump.

Source: Courtesy of Whisper Wear, Marietta, GA.

motions necessary to work the pumps. A few studies have examined the efficiency of hand pumps, as well as their ability to influence prolactin levels, the volume of milk expressed, and its fat and energy content. These studies are difficult to compare because study design and methodology vary widely. The results may depend on single or random milk samples, and on measurement of milk components obtained at different postpartum times.

Zinaman et al. (1992) studied differences in the volume of milk obtained and prolactin stimulation by various types of breast pumps, as well as by the mother's baby, in 23 women who were 28 to 42 days postpartum. Their results showed that a double setup (in which both breasts are pumped simultaneously) electric pump did better in stimulating prolactin levels than did battery or manual pumps, or hand expression, when only one breast was stimulated at a time. The White River electric pump was reported to stimulate the highest prolactin levels, cycling at 40 times per minute. Milk volumes were highest with this pump. Lowest milk volume was with hand expression and the Gentle Expressions battery pump, which produced 6 to 10 cycles per minute. When mothers rated their satisfaction with the pumps, the White River electric rated as one of the more uncomfortable to use. A singular problem with this study was its comparison of double pumping to breastfeeding a single baby or sequential pumping of one breast at a time. A more reliable test of pump efficacy would be to control for breast stimulation by using mothers of twins when comparing double pumping—or using other double-pump setups or two pumps simultaneously. Neifert and Seacat (1985) have shown the greater prolactin rise when both breasts are expressed simultaneously.

Fewtrell, Lucas, and Collier (2001) compared the efficacy of the Avent Isis manual pump and the Egnell electric pump in mothers who delivered preterm infants less than 35 weeks gestation. At 7 to 10 days, the mothers evaluated "consumer" characteristics of their assigned pump (ease of use, amount of suction, comfort, pleasant to use, and overall opinion of the pump). Mothers did not use or compare both pumps to each other. While mothers rated the Avent Isis as a more comfortable pump, mothers in both groups pumped a mean of three times per day with a mean volume of less than 7 ounces a day (199 ml/day, range 57 to 323 ml with the Avent Isis and 218 ml/day, range 126 to 341 ml with the electric pump). It is difficult to concur with the authors' conclusions that the manual pump reflected a significant advance in pumping milk for preterm infants when milk output was so low for the amount of time spent pumping. The study did not address the ability of the pumps to initiate a milk supply or maintain milk production over a long period of time.

Fewtrell et al. (2001) compared the efficacy of the Avent Isis manual pump and the Medela Mini electric pump in term 8-week-old babies. Each pump was tested on a single occasion with the second pump tested 2 to 3 days after the first, and the mothers rated the pumps on the same "consumer" scale as above. The rating factor for the mothers was only if the pump was pleasant to use, not the volume of milk expressed. These data also showed that irrespective of which pump was tested as the second pump, milk volumes were increased. However, when the second pump was the mini electric, milk volume was 164 ml ± 673 compared to 149 ml ± 671 with the manual pump. The value of this study remains unknown, as neither of the study pumps was used over time or validated as being capable of sustaining milk production in a mother who is dependent on a pump for this purpose.

Manual Hand Pumps

The various types of hand pumps rely on differing mechanisms to generate suction.

Rubber Bulb Models

Rubber bulb pumps are seldom seen in current clinical practice. Squeezing and releasing a rubber bulb generates a vacuum in these pumps. In most "bicycle horn" pumps, the rubber bulb is attached directly to the collection container. Some manufacturers separated the bulb from the collection container by modifying the angle at which it is attached to the pump or by adding a length of tubing. These modifications were thought to reduce the high potential for bacterial contamination of

the bulb caused by the easy backflow of milk. Backflow risk is reduced when the bulb is separated from the collection container. Vacuum control on these pumps is extremely difficult, thus increasing the likelihood of nipple pain and damage. Even with the use of a blood pressure-type bulb, vacuum control is left to chance. The "bicycle horn" pumps are inexpensive, but collect only about one half ounce of milk at a time and must be emptied frequently. The other pumps collect milk in a bottle. Mothers often complain of nipple pain during pumping and low milk yields, especially if they have used these pumps for more than a few weeks. Most mothers no longer see these pumps in stores, but some models may still be available and are a poor choice in any circumstance.

Squeeze-Handle Models

Squeeze-handle models (Figures 12–8 and 12–9), such as Avent Isis, Ameda One-Hand, Gerber Massaging Manual, First Years Easy Comfort, Medela Harmony, Dr. Brown Natural Flow, and Evenflo ComfortEase Manual, involve squeezing and releasing a handle that creates suction in the pump. They are typically used for occasional pumping and are a type that can be used when no electricity is available. These pumps are easily cleaned but their operation may present difficulties for women with hand or arm problems, such as arthritis or carpal tunnel syndrome. The hand and wrist can tire easily with repeated use.

Cylinder Pumps

Cylinder pumps consist of two cylinders. The outer cylinder generates vacuum as it is pulled away from the body. The inner cylinder with the flange is placed against the breast; a gasket at the other end helps form a seal with the edge of the outer cylinder. Gaskets may need to be replaced occasionally if they dry out, shrink, or lose their ability to form a seal. Gaskets can harbor bacteria and must be removed during cleaning, contrary to some user instructions. When placing the gasket back on the cylinder, roll it back and forth over the cylinder to help restore the shape. Some pumps come with extra gaskets.

Small plastic or silicone inserts can be placed in the inner opening to custom fit the pump to the breast. Silicone liners are available for some pumps; these are designed to collapse against the breast during the

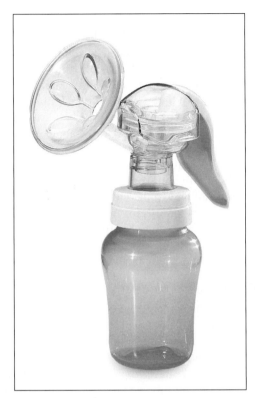

FIGURE 12–8 The Avent Isis squeeze handle manual pump.

Source: Courtesy of Canon Babysafe Ltd., Suffolk, England.

suction phase to provide external positive pressure. These pumps are lightweight, not too expensive, and easily cleaned.

Before recommending any of these pumps, the clinician should check if the pump automatically interrupts vacuum at a preset level, if there are adjustable vacuum settings, and if the pump has a collection bottle rather than an outer cylinder where milk accumulates during pumping. Some pumps also provide an extra cylinder for milk storage or have an angled rather than a straight flange. Some mothers report that the angled flange does not work as well as the straight pumps. As the outer cylinder fills with milk, the gasket is repeatedly dunked in the milk. Mothers who express more than 3 oz of milk at a time may have to empty these pumps more than once in a single pumping episode.

Efficiency of use varies from brand to brand. Some can also be adapted for use on the larger electric pumps. Higher vacuum is generated as the outer cylinder fills with milk. Mothers may need to shorten the outward stroke after collecting more than 1 oz.

Battery-Operated Pumps

These pumps use a small motor with usually either size AA 1.5-volt batteries or size C batteries. Most have a vacuum adjustment mechanism. Vacuum in some pumps can take up to 30 seconds to reach maximum level and is regulated by how frequently the vacuum is interrupted. The Whisper Wear pump is battery operated but is worn under the bra like breast shells and operates hands-free once secured in place.

Some of these pumps have a button to press in order to release the vacuum periodically and to simulate the rhythm of a nursing baby. All take varying periods of time for the recovery of suction following each release. This limits the number of suction/release cycles per minute to as few as six and may require relatively long periods of vacuum application to the nipple. To compensate for this, some mothers leave the suction on for much longer than the pump instructions recommend. Mothers in one survey mentioned 30 to 60 seconds. Four women never interrupted the suction during the entire pumping session because they could not get the milk flow restarted following vacuum interruption. Some pumps have preset automatic cycling.

Most pumps have AC adapters to decrease battery use. A major complaint about these pumps is their short battery life. This affects pumping efficiency because fewer cycles are generated as the batteries wear down. Batteries may have to be replaced as frequently as every second or third use. Rechargeable batteries are an option, but they usually require charging each night and may not produce as many cycles per minute as alkaline batteries. AC adapters usually allow the maximum number of cycles per minute that the motor can produce. Maximum suction after each vacuum release will often continue decreasing in amount throughout the pumping session. In contrast, the Medela battery pump automatically produces 32 cycles per minute with alkaline batteries, 30 cycles per minute with rechargeable batteries, and 42 cycles per minute with the A/C adapter.

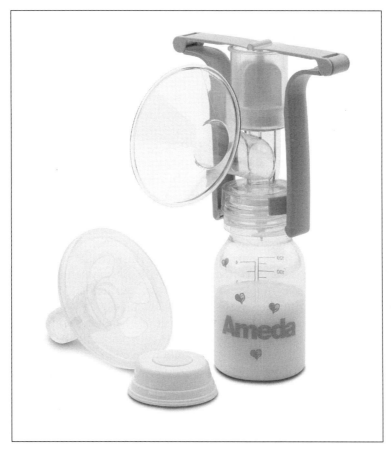

FIGURE **12–9** The Ameda One-Hand pump.

Source: Courtesy of Ameda, Inc.

Battery pumps require only one hand to operate, are lightweight, and are popular with mothers employed outside the home. Some mothers use two battery-operated pumps simultaneously to decrease pumping time when they are on a tight schedule. Mothers who plan to pump for several months while at work may consider a larger personal use pump or a long-term rental contract for an electric pump, because battery replacement can be very expensive—as can artificial formula if it must be used to substitute for breastmilk. Some of the pumps operate with a quiet hum while others are very noisy.

The Whisper Wear pump is worn under the bra and automatically cycles 35 to 60 times per minute. It has three cycling phases, an initial strong 1-minute latch phase that draws the nipple and areola into the cup, a second rapid cycling let-down phase at 60 cycles per minute, and a third phase with three adjustable pumping speeds (fast 50–58 cycles per min, medium 48 cycles per minute, and slow 35 cycles per minute). The flange or cup is soft silicone with some give for accommodating different size nipples as well as a massaging action that adds an element of positive pressure. The settings can be independently controlled for each breast. Battery life is up to 50 hours.

Electric Pumps

Electric breast pumps fall into one of three categories:

- Small semiautomatic pumps
- Personal use pumps (Figure 12–10) (lightweight portable pumps often used by employed mothers)
- Institutionally used pumps, such as those commonly rented and/or used in the hospital

Various types of electric motors are used in this group of pumps to generate suction. Semiautomatic pumps (Figure 12–11) require the mother to cycle suction by covering and uncovering a hole in the flange base, a process that creates a pumping rhythm designed to simulate the pattern of a suckling baby. These pumps maintain a constant negative pressure. Some lack a dial or mechanism to adjust the amount of suction. The actual amount of vacuum delivered to the nipple is determined by the degree of closure of the hole in the flange base. Many mothers learn to roll their finger three fourths of the way off the hole rather than to lift the finger completely, to generate vacuum faster for the subsequent cycle by preventing complete interruption of vacuum. However, too much negative pressure, or negative pressure applied for too long a period, increases the risk of damage to the nipple and underlying vascular structures. The initiation of suction places the greatest pressure on the nipple; thus it is most desirable that a pump generate suction quickly.

Automatic electric pumps are designed to cycle pressure rather than to maintain it. Because Egnell (1956) observed nipple damage when cycles were 2 seconds long (30 per minute), manufacturers increased the number of cycles so that they more closely simulate that of a nursing baby. Pressure setting parameters on these large pumps also attempt to mimic that of an infant. Mean sucking pressures of most full-term infants range from –50 to –155 with a maximum of –220 mm Hg (Caldeyro-Barcia, 1969). In pumps that have a preset pulsed suction (automatic pumps), there is typically a 60/40 ratio. Negative pressure is applied for 60 percent of the cycle; 40 percent of the cycle is the resting phase. The Medela Classic/Lactina pattern has a fixed number of cycles per minute (48) with relax times becoming longer in lower vacuum ranges. The Medela Symphony (Figure 12–12) operates with a "stimulation" phase at the start of the pumping session at 120 cycles per minute with variable adjustable vacuum of 50 to 200 mm Hg. This causes a change in the "expression" phase to cycle between 54 to 78 cycles per minute with vacuum from 50 to 250 mm Hg. The number of cycles per minute varies in this pump according to the set vacuum with higher vacuum levels resulting in

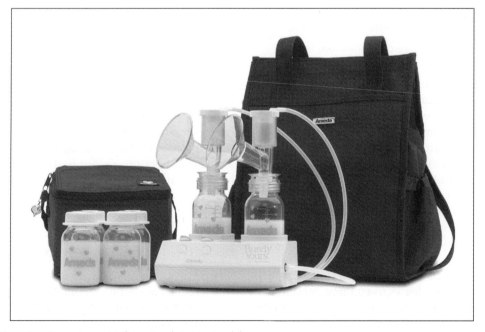

FIGURE 12–10   A personal use Purely Yours model.

Source: Courtesy of Ameda, Inc.

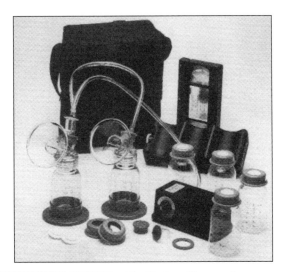

FIGURE **12–11** The Nurture III, a small semiautomatic pump.

Source: Courtesy of Bailey Medical Engineering, Los Osos, CA.

lower cycles per minute. At a minimum vacuum of 50 mm Hg the Symphony applies 78 cycles per minute, and at the maximum vacuum of 250 mm Hg, 54 cycles per minute are applied. The maximum pressure that these pumps will generate at their normal (high) setting is approximately 220 to 250 mm Hg. By comparison, the Nurture III semiautomatic pump produces 220 mm Hg after about 2.5 seconds using a single collecting kit (approximately 24 cycles per minute). With the double collecting kit, this same pump takes about 3.25 seconds to achieve this level, generating about 18 cycles per minute.

Negative pressure—a function of the volume of air in the accessory kit—increases as the bottle fills with milk. The pressure generated varies with different sized bottles (collecting containers) and from one manufacturer to another. When double-pump setups are used (with two collecting containers being filled simultaneously), the potential for very low negative pressure exists when the containers are empty; negative pressure increases as the bottles fill. Most accessory kits compensate for this by separating the collection containers from the power source so that the amount of air in the system remains constant regardless of the amount of fluid in the collection container. If a mother is using an accessory kit or pump without a similar feature, she can compensate by using a smaller collection bottle (Vol-u-feeders fit on some pumps), turning down the vacuum as the bottle fills, emptying the bottle more frequently, or cycling the suction more frequently on the hand, battery-operated, or semiautomatic pumps.

The Whittlestone Breast Expresser does not use alternating vacuum pulses but generates about 147 mm Hg on a constant basis with the inner flange liners rhythmically compressing the breast 45 times per minute.

Simultaneous and/or Sequential Pumping

All of the automatic electric pumps and a few of the battery-operated pumps have collection kits that allow pumping both breasts at the same time. Neifert and Seacat (1985) reported the experiences of 10 mothers who were 2 to 7 months postpartum. The women alternated between sequentially pumping each breast for 20 minutes and then pumping both breasts simultaneously for 10 minutes. Milk yield was about the same with both techniques but was obtained in one half the time with lower pump suction (260 mm Hg versus 320 mm Hg) when pumping was simultaneous. They also found a significantly higher prolactin rise with double pumping. This is similar to Tyson's report (1977) of a doubling in prolactin rise when two infants were put to breast simultaneously and echoes the findings of Saint, Maggiore, and Hartmann (1986), who reported larger milk volumes in mothers of twins (up to double that of singleton mothers).

Auerbach (1990b) studied 25 mothers with babies between 5 and 35 weeks of age. She investigated the amount of milk obtained with single and double pumping, whether it takes longer to pump with a single setup compared to a double setup, and whether the milk fat varies between the two methods of pumping. Results showed that highest milk yields with single pumping occurred over 10 to 15 minutes. With double pumping, maximum milk volumes were seen in 7 to 12 minutes. The maximum yield overall occurred with double pumping. Milk fat concentrations were only slightly higher for double pumping sessions with no time limits. However, the mothers preferred double pumping three to one. Mothers' preferences regarding pumping regimens

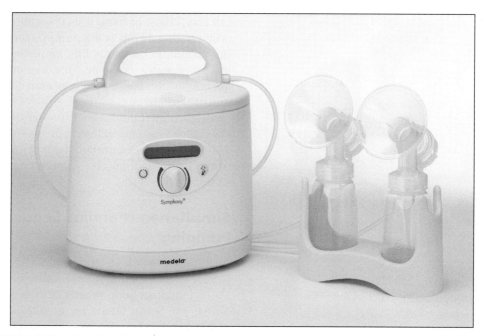

The Medela Symphony pump.

Source: Courtesy of Medela, Inc., McHenry, IL.

usually predicted how they obtained the highest yields. Groh-Wargo et al. (1995) studied 32 preterm mothers, half of whom pumped each breast in sequence; the other half pumped both breasts simultaneously. Daily frequency of pumping in both groups ranged from three to nearly five times. The single pumping group averaged 24 minutes for each pumping session; the bilateral pumping group expressed milk for an average of 16 minutes per session. Other aspects of simultaneous (SIM) versus sequential (SEQ) pumping have been studied, helping the clinician to construct pumping guidelines tailored to maximizing milk output for mothers encountering a variety of problems or situations (Table 12–1).

A number of factors combine to result in optimum milk expression: vacuum generated by the pump, cycling patterns of the vacuum, compressive forces from the pump flange, compressive forces external to the pump, oxytocin pulses, sequential or simultaneous pumping, number of times per day and per week of pumping sessions, time postpartum when pumping was initiated, type of flange, proper fit of the flange, comfort, and so on (Table 12–2).

Flanges

Most pumps have hard plastic shields called flanges. Some may have softer plastic or silicone flanges, soft inner liners, soft inserts, projections on the flange that compress the breast when vacuum is applied, or inserts that change the diameter of the nipple opening.

The Whittlestone Breastmilker Pump, developed in New Zealand, is a double-pumping flange design based on milking techniques used by the dairy industry. The Whittlestone design was an answer to early mechanical milking devices used on domestic animals, which consisted of a single-chambered teat cup attached to a vacuum source that withdrew milk by simple suction (Woolford & Phillips, 1978). This design was inefficient, and the cows objected to the discomfort. The teat cup that is now used consists of a metal case lined with soft rubber. The milking apparatus produces a regular collapsing of the rubber liner against the teat to cause stimulation. The Whittlestone breast cups consist of a solid casing attached to a pulsating vacuum source. A foam pad in the cup case is held in place by a liner. When negative pressure occurs in the cup

TABLE **12–1**	**Methods of Milk Expression: Selected Studies**

Study	Findings
Neifert & Seacat, 1985 *n* = 10 term infants	Milk yield similar, volume obtained in half the time with SIM with lower vacuum levels; increased prolactin rise with SIM.
Auerbach, 1990b *n* = 25 5–35 weeks postpartum term infants	SIM = highest milk yields in 7–12 minutes; higher milk volume SEQ = 10–15 minutes to reach maximum milk yield
Groh-Wargo et al., 1995 *n* = 32 Preterm infants Pumped 3–5 times/day	SIM = 16 minutes/session; 7.6 ± 3 hours/week SEQ = 24 minutes/session; 11.1 ± 3.1 hours/week Average 28 pumping sessions/week = 400 ml/day of milk did not see increased prolactin.
Hill, Aldag, & Chatterton, 1996 *n* = 9 Preterm infants Pumped 5 times/day during hospital stay Pumped 8 times/day at home through day 42	SEQ 5×5×5×5 20 minutes total; milk volumes decreased after 25 days; proportion of prolactin at day 42 was 52% of level at day 21. Milk yield ranges 158.4 g day 3–505.8 g day 20; SIM milk volumes continued to rise over entire study time; prolactin at day 42 was 85% of level at day 21. Milk volume ranges 41.4 g day 3 to 741 g on day 41.

Hill, Aldag, & Chatterton, 1999
n = 39
Preterm infants
Pumped 8 times/day
	SIM 10 minutes; milk weights higher each week of the study in SIM; pumping frequency = 31 + 11.93 times/to 45 + 10.88 times.
	SEQ 5×5×5×5 for 20 minutes; pumping frequency = 28 ± 8.9 times/week to 41 ± 9.05 times/week.
	Hours from birth to initiation of pumping:
	  SEQ—9.7 hours to 101 hours (4.2 days)
	  SIM—28.28 hours to 84.3 hours (3.5 days)
	Milk weights inversely correlated to number of hours from birth to initiation of pumping. Milk weights positively correlated with weekly frequency of pumping and kangaroo care.

Hill, Aldag, & Chatterton, 2001 *n* = 39 Preterm infants 2–5 weeks postpartum	Studied median number of hours from birth to initiation of pumping and median frequency of pumping over weeks 2–5 to categorize subjects into high and low pumping frequency and early and late pumping initiation. Early initiation = 30.9 ± 11.4 hours post delivery. Late initiation = 82.0 ± 37.9 hours post delivery. Low pumping frequency group = 4.9 times/day; range = 2.6–6.14 times/day. High pumping frequency = 7.0; range 6.25–8.10 times/day.

(Continues)

| TABLE 12–1 | Methods of Milk Expression: Selected Studies (Continued) |

Study	Findings
	Mothers with both late initiation and low frequency had lowest milk weights. Frequency of pumping was primary influence on milk weights.

Jones, Dimmock, & Spencer, 2001
   n = 36
Preterm infants
4 days total study time
	Compared simultaneous and sequential pumping on milk volume and energy yield.
	Secondary aim: measure the effect of breast massage on milk volume and fat content.
	Milk yield per expression:
	  SEQ with no massage = 51.32 ml
	  SEQ with massage = 78.71 ml
	  SIM with no massage = 87.69 ml
	  SIM with massage = 125.08 ml
	Fat concentrations were not affected.

Key: SIM = simultaneous pumping; SEQ = sequential pumping.

case, the liner moves against the pad, and the nipple and areola are drawn down into the conical portion of the liner (Whittlestone, 1978). Mothers reported that this pump is comfortable and efficient with a full milk supply. The current Whittlestone Breast Expresser uses a silicone liner and a lower vacuum level. The Whisper Wear pump utilizes a flexible massaging cup.

Johnson (1983) measured several aspects of flanges, including the diameters of the outer opening (flare), the inner opening, the depth of flare, and the length of the shank. She measured negative pressure at the inner opening of the flange and reported that the smaller the nipple cup the greater the pressure exerted on the tip of the nipple. The larger and deeper flanges may provide greater stimulation of the areolar region of the breast. Zinaman (1988) repeated the same measurements on 11 manual pumps, 4 battery pumps, and 7 electric pumps. Comparing these measurements among pumps highly rated in the other studies showed that the diameter of the flange ranged from 60 to 69 mm, depth ranged from 25 to 30 mm, and the inner opening was between 21 and 26 mm for the manual pumps. A woman with a large or wide nipple may have difficulty with a flange that has a small opening or a narrow slope.

Because one size of flange does not fit all breasts, some manufacturers provide a choice of different sized flanges (Table 12–3), silicone flange liners, or small plastic inserts that are placed at the level of the inner opening to change the diameter of the shank and inner opening. Silicone or soft plastic flange liners are supposed to cushion the pumping forces and are purported to "massage" the breast or mimic external compressive forces. Inserts placed in the flanges are designed to provide a better fit between pump and breast.

When vacuum is applied, the nipple and part of the areola elongate and are drawn past the inner opening and down into the shank or nipple tunnel (Biancuzzo, 1999). In general, the pump is more likely to be effective when the flange accommodates the anatomic configuration of the particular breast. However, mothers have various sized nipples. Ziemer and Pidgeon (1993), Stark (1994), and Wilson-Clay and Hoover (2005) measured nipple diameters that ranged from less than 12 mm at base to greater than 23 mm at base. Wilson-Clay and Hoover (2005) also observed that nipples swell during pumping. Thus a mother with large nipples may find that a standard size flange is too small to accommodate both the large nipple and subsequent swelling. Meier et al. (2004) observed a sample of

TABLE 12–2 **Comparison of Pressure, Hormonal Responses, and Mechanics Among Various Methods of Breastmilk Removal**

Negative Pressure Ranges

Baby	Hand Expression		Hand Pump	Battery Pump	Electric Pump
50–241 mm Hg 50–155 mm Hg average basal resting pressure to keep nipple in mouth 70–200 mm Hg	None		0–400 mm Hg	50–305 mm Hg	10–500 mm Hg

Positive Pressure Ranges

Baby	Breast and Milk-Ejection Reflex	Hand Expression	Hand Pump	Battery Pump	Electric Pump
Tongue .73–3.6 mm Hg	28 mm Hg when breast is full	Theoretically could exert > 760 mm Hg, which is atmospheric pressure	None to minimal	None to minimal	Without compression stimulus, none to minimal
Jaw 200–300 mm Hg	10–20 mm Hg with milk-ejection reflex				With compression stimulus

Hormonal Response Ranges

	Baby	Hand Expression	Hand Pump	Battery Pump	Electric Pump
Prolactin basal levels up to 200 ng/ml first 10 days, 10–90 days 60–110 ng/ml, 90–180 days 50 ng/ml, 180 days to 1 year 30–40 ng/ml	55–550 ng/ml	67 ng/ml 28–42 days postpartum	67 ng/ml 28–42 days postpartum	59.7 ng/ml 28–42 days postpartum	46–405 ng/ml Single pumping 92.1 ± 29.2 ng/ml Double pumping 136 ± 31.6 ng/ml
Oxytocin	5–15 units/ml 100 mU released during 10 minutes				

Mechanics

	Baby	Hand Expression	Hand Pump	Battery Pump	Electric Pump
Cycles per minute	36–126 cycles	Variable	Variable	5–60 cycles	2–84 cycles

(Continues)

| TABLE 12–2 | Comparison of Pressure, Hormonal Responses, and Mechanics Among Various Methods of Breastmilk Removal (Continued) | | | | |

Mechanics

	Baby	Hand Expression	Hand Pump	Battery Pump	Electric Pump
Duration of vacuum	.7 seconds	None	Variable	1–50 seconds	1–3 seconds
Duration of rest	.7 seconds	Variable	Variable		
Volume of milk per suck	.14 ml/suckle at the beginning of a feeding .01 ml/suckle at end of feeding				

mothers expressing milk for their preterm infants, with about half requiring a 27–30 mm flange (rather than a standard 23–24 mm flange) and as lactation progressed, 77 percent of the mothers found they needed a larger flange. Clinicians have observed damage on the areola presenting as suction rings or cracks at the junction of the nipple and areola from flanges that are too small. Such a misfit between flange and breast could endanger milk production if the teat were strangulated to the point where little to no milk could be expressed. Wilson-Clay and Hoover (2005) speculate that if a mother has a nipple size of approximately 20.5 mm (or the size of a US nickel) or larger she may benefit from using a larger than standard size pump flange. Lacking a clinical algorithm for nipple size and flange selection that would provide a path for decision making, some health professionals who have access to autoclaving or similar sterilizing facilities offer mothers the opportunity to try several different brands of breast pumps and flange sizes in order to ascertain optimal fit before they purchase or rent a pump. Some mothers find that they can achieve a good fit between a nipple that changes size during the pumping session and the use of an angled flange (Pumpin Pal).

Pedal Pumps

Medela, Inc. and BreastPump.Com, Inc. manufacture breast pump pedals that generate vacuum by pressing a foot down on a pedal. The leg muscles tend to be stronger than hand and arm muscles; thus this type of a pump may be useful for women with a compromised upper body, arms, or hands. The pumps run without electricity and may accommodate a number of different flange and tubing sets.

Clinical Implications Regarding Breast Pumps

The concerns of health professionals may vary considerably from those of mothers (Human Milk Banking Association of North America, 2005) and typically center around safe collection techniques and the maintenance of low bacteria counts in the expressed milk. Of equal importance are choosing the right pump for each individual situation, providing appropriate pumping instructions, and tempering all this with a consideration of the emotional toll that pumping can sometimes exact.

The professional literature includes reports of bacterial contamination of breastmilk and breast pumps. Factors related to nipple cleansing, hand washing, collection technique, type of pump, feeding method of preterm infants, pump-cleaning routines, and gestational age of the baby have all been identified as contributing to concern over high bacteria counts in expressed milk. Expressed breast milk is not sterile (el-Mohandes et al., 1993b). There is considerable disagreement over what constitutes an acceptable bacteria count, especially if the recipient

TABLE 12–3	Flange Sizes		
Company		**Flange**	**Tunnel Diameter**
Avent		One standard	22.2 mm flange with projections
Whisper Wear		One size	22.0 mm
Ameda		Custom flange	30.5 mm
		Custom flange	28.5 mm with insert
		Standard flange	25.0 mm
		Standard flange	23.0 mm with reducing insert
		Standard flange	21.0 mm with Flexishield
Medela		Personal Fit	21.0 mm small
		Personal Fit	24.0 mm standard
		Personal Fit	27.0 mm large
		Personal Fit	30.0 mm extra large
		Personal Fit	36.0 mm extra large
		Blown glass	40.0 mm

of the milk is a preterm infant (el-Mohandes et al., 1993a). Caution must be exercised in reviewing the literature because certain institutional practices may actually increase the likelihood of contamination problems with expressed milk.

With the increased use of both hand and electric pumps in the 1970s, many reports described contaminated milk as one source of bacteremia, but the reports lacked conclusive epidemiology. Hand-expression of breastmilk showed lower bacteria counts than breastmilk obtained by manual or electric pumps when pumps first began to be commonly used. Donowitz et al. (1981) reported an outbreak of *Klebsiella*-caused bacteremia in a neonatal intensive care unit (NICU). The electric breast pump was grossly contaminated and lacked proper bacterial surveillance. Once gas sterilization of pump parts was required between each mother's use of the equipment, the problem disappeared. However, all five affected babies in the report were fed milk by the nasoduodenal route, which delivers the milk directly to the small bowel, thus bypassing the protective action of gastric acid in the stomach. Four of the five infants had received broad-spectrum antibiotic therapy prior to the contaminated feedings, and therefore received contaminated milk in a bowel with altered protective gastrointestinal flora. Such a practice predisposes an infant to infection given even small challenges of bacteria.

Gransden et al. (1986) reported an outbreak of *Serratia marcescens* in a NICU via inadequately disinfected breast pumps (Kaneson manual and Egnell electric models). Kaneson pump parts (after being washed) were soaked in a solution of hypochlorite. Egnell pump parts were washed with the metal parts soaked in a solution of 0.5 percent chlorhexidine in 70 percent ethyl alcohol. The pumps were soaked for 1.5 hours in a 1 percent hypochlorite solution, and the solution was changed every 24 hours. Bacteria were isolated from the soaked pump parts as well as from the hypochlorite solution itself. When the Egnell pump parts were autoclaved and the Kaneson pumps were washed at 80°C, the problem was resolved. Often, the available chlorine in these chemical solutions is readily inactivated by small amounts of organic matter. The original disinfection technique in this study had several faults, including failure to completely dismantle the hand pump completely, failure to remove the rubber gasket, and failure to totally immerse the pump components.

Moloney et al. (1987) reported isolation of *Serratia marcescens, Staphylococcus aureus,* and *Streptococcus faecalis* from hand-operated and electric breast pumps. The pumps were disinfected in a hypochlorite solution as in the previous study. It is well known that there are infection risks from electrically operated breast pumps. With proper surveillance and sterilizing by autoclaving, gas (ethylene oxide), or high-temperature washing—rather than chemical sterilization—the risk of overgrowth and transmission of pathogenic bacteria can be substantially reduced. If pumps or pump parts are heat sensitive, consideration should be given to using pumps that do not depend on chemical sterilization.

Asquith, Sharp, and Stevenson (1985) compared Medela hand and electric pumps to manual expression in order to measure the amount of bacterial contamination. Boiling the personal use kits for 10 minutes worked well. The disposable kits were washed in hot soapy water and used for only 1 day. In some hospitals a fresh sterile kit is used for each pumping session, but this has not been shown to be a requirement for bacteriologically safe breastmilk.

Other approaches to reducing the bacterial count in expressed breastmilk have included expressing techniques and various breast-nipple cleansing routines. Asquith et al. (1984) noted that the bacterial content of milk is high when expression is first begun, regardless of collection technique. Asquith and Harod's earlier work (1979) recommended that stripping and discarding the first 10 ml of expressed milk would decrease total bacteria counts. They observed that bacterial contamination was high within the first 24 hours after birth or after initiation of pumping, whether or not the first 10 ml were discarded. Asquith and colleagues (1984) suggest that delayed expression of breastmilk is associated with high bacterial counts of nonnursing mothers of NICU infants: "Milk stasis and breast engorgement may provide an opportunity for bacteria, including 'normal flora' or pathogenic species, to incubate in the breast." Their recommendations for mothers of hospitalized newborns include initiation of expression as soon as possible on a frequent and regular basis, thereby avoiding excessive engorgement, and the discarding of the first 10 ml of milk with each pumping. Some mothers may get only 10 ml of colostrum or milk at first, so care should be taken to determine the necessity of discarding this early milk. Most NICU milk expression instructions no longer carry this recommendation.

Pittard et al. (1991) found no difference in the number of heavily contaminated (> 10,000 colony-forming units/ml [cfu/ml]) milk cultures when a clean versus a sterile collection container was used, or when manual versus mechanical collection techniques were employed. They did not observe increased levels of bacteria in the initial milk removed from the breast.

According to Meier and Wilks (1987), acceptable bacteria levels in expressed breastmilk are difficult to define and vary between healthy full-term infants and preterm, high-risk babies. Healthy term infants can tolerate some pathogens and relatively high levels of nonpathogenic bacteria (> 104 cfu/ml of milk). Preterm or high-risk infants with immature immune systems who are not nursing directly from the breast may be at greater risk from the same level of bacterial growth. The investigators' criteria for acceptable bacteria levels for preterm infants are the absence of any pathogens and a maximum concentration of 104 cfu/ml. Mothers in their study were instructed in hand washing, especially under and around the fingernails. The nipples and areolae were cleaned with pHisoDerm soap before each pumping session. Increased nipple soreness was not noticed in this study, but the number of weeks of pumping was not specified. Using these guidelines, 74 out of 84 expressed milk specimens had concentrations of less than 104 cfu/ml. It is not known whether this type of cleansing increases the risk for problems other than topical soreness, such as dry areolar skin that is susceptible to breakdown and infection, or a change in the pH of the skin, which affects the secretions of the glands of Montgomery.

Costa (1989) showed significantly lower bacterial counts when preterm mothers washed their nipples and areolae with pHisoDerm soap prior to each pumping session. Although Costa noticed no skin breakdown with this routine, it is unknown what adverse affects would be encountered from using this soap six to eight times a day over an extended period of time.

Thompson et al. (1997) demonstrated that preexpression breast cleaning with pHisoDerm and tap water were no more effective than plain tap water in producing expressed milk that was free from bacterial contamination. No control group that refrained from breast cleaning preparations provided a basis for comparison. Because breastmilk is not sterile, some bacteria will always be present, even if it is nonpathologic. In a larger study by Law et al. (1989), no cases of infant sepsis could be linked to the particular bacteria present in expressed breastmilk feedings received by an infant who was either colonized or septic.

Wilks and Meier (1988) describe guidelines for care of hospital breast pump equipment that include scrubbing collection kits and tubing with instrument cleaning solution after each use and autoclaving each item. The exterior of the pump should be cleaned with antiseptic solution each day and the pump cultured monthly. They also described other factors that may influence the amount of nonpathogens that a preterm baby can tolerate. These include the baby's clinical condition; the use of bolus feedings every 2 hours rather than continuous feedings; the use of refrigerated rather than frozen milk to retain active antiinfective properties; and feeding the baby directly from the breast as much as possible to receive unaltered antiinfective properties, thereby further decreasing the risk of infection.

Cultures were performed by D'Amico et al. (2003) in the NICU on breast pump kit attachments for the Medela Classic or Lactina that included three sites— the tubing, the small white barrier membrane, and the bottom of the collection bottle. Positive cultures were obtained from the bottom of a bottle and from the membrane area. The membrane was probably contaminated when mothers inadvertently touched it or tried to remove it for cleaning which they had been instructed not to do. A positive culture from the bottom of the bottle suggests that collection bottles should be inverted to dry or wiped dry with a paper towel so that remaining droplets do not provide a medium for bacterial growth.

Each year many pumps change or add features that reduce the chance of milk backflow and contamination. Some models now have in-line air filters in the pump; some use overflow bottles, and others have filters and/or protection against overflow in the accessory kit. Some have a completely closed collection system (Ameda), deemed the optimal manner in which to prevent contamination (Human Milk Banking Association of North America, 2005; Slusser & Frantz, 2001). When choosing a pump for milk collection for term or preterm babies, the professional should know whether and how the pump or accessory kit guards against contamination. This is especially important if the pump is operated by more than one user.

Cleaning Pumps

Mothers should generally follow the cleaning instructions provided with the pump. For most

purposes, hot soapy water, thorough rinsing, avoidance of abrasives, and air drying is sufficient to clean pump parts that come in contact with the milk. If tubing for electric pumps develops condensation, the tubing can be spun like a lasso to move out water droplets. Many mothers find it easier to remove the flanges and collection bottles from the tubing and run the pump for a few minutes which pulls in air and air dries the tubing. Alcohol can also be injected down the disconnected tubing to dry it and reduce the likelihood of contamination. Tubing can be boiled but may cause it to become opaque, making it more difficult to see condensation or milk droplets if present. Collection bottles should be inverted to dry or wiped dry with a clean paper towel. Sterilizing or disinfecting pump parts can be accomplished by boiling the parts, use of an electric sterilizer, placing the parts in a sterilizer bag made for the microwave, or using a dishwasher with a high temperature sanitizing cycle. Cloth towels should be avoided to either dry or store pump parts. Harsh chemicals and abrasive scrubbing should not be used so that small scratches are not created that could harbor bacteria or mold. Mothers sharing an electric pump (such as in a NICU or workplace) may wish to wipe the outside of the pump with a germicidal solution prior to use.

Maternal Concerns and Education Needs

Morse and Bottorff (1988) observed 61 nursing mothers and their emotional experiences related to expressing milk. Many were surprised that the ability to express their milk was not automatic. They often found that verbal and written instructions were unclear and confusing; many learned by trial and error. Mothers in this study emphasized that "instructions for one mother did not necessarily work for all." Some were embarrassed and others were frustrated when they obtained only small amounts of milk. Although success with expression increased a mother's self-confidence, women who perceived expression to be an important aspect of breastfeeding, but who were unable to express milk, displayed heightened feelings of inadequacy. The authors suggest modifying how expression is taught to include not only explicit how-to's but the encouragement of private exploratory practice and the use of humor by the instructor (when appropriate) to reduce embarrassment.

Many mothers receive only the instructions that come with the pump to use as a guide in learning milk expression and handling. These instructions vary widely in their recommendations on pumping techniques and even on the cleaning of the pump. Further confusion is possible if a mother uses more than one type of pump, especially if she fails to read all of the instructions carefully or if the instructions from one manufacturer conflict with those from another.

The concerns of mothers are rarely addressed in the professional literature on breast pumps and milk expression. Clinicians must remember that the best pump will do little for a mother whose emotional needs are not met and who lacks the guidelines necessary to use the equipment properly for optimal results.

When Pumps Cause Problems

In the United States, breast pumps are class II medical devices regulated by the US Food and Drug Administration (FDA) within the FDA's Center for Devices and Radiological Health. The FDA maintains a medical product reporting program, called Med-Watch, that enables consumers and healthcare providers to report problems with these devices. Problems with breast pumps could include defective parts, poor labeling, a malfunction of the pump, nipple damage or pain, or being ineffective at removing milk, and should always be reported to the manufacturer. It may be difficult to separate a pump that is ineffective or painful from how the pump is being used or simply if the flanges are too small for the mother. Few adverse events are reported to the FDA. More reports of injuries and malfunctions are reported on Internet Web sites than to the FDA (Brown et al., 2005). In addition, problems can be reported to the FDA online at the FDA's Web site, www.fda.gov. Clinicians can also access reports of problem devices through two databases:

1. Manufacturer and User Facility Device Experience (MAUDE) (www.accessdata.fda.gov/scripts/cdrh/cfdocs/cfMAUDE/Search.cfm), which represents reports of adverse events involving medical devices. The data consist of all voluntary reports since June 1993, user facility reports since 1991, distributor reports since 1993, and manufacturer reports since August 1996.

2. The Medical Device Reporting database (www.accessdata.fda.gov/scripts/cdrh/cfdocs/cfmdr/search.CFM) allows you to search the Center for Devices and Radiological Health's database information on medical devices that may have malfunctioned or caused a death or serious injury during the years 1992 through 1996. It is no longer being updated.

Some mothers give their used pumps to other mothers, borrow used pumps, or purchase previously used breast pumps to save money. This practice has the potential for improper functioning and cross-contamination (Box 12–2). Multiple use of single-user devices also typically invalidates the manufacturer's warranty. Most single-user pumps are open systems and may not have any protective barrier to prevent cross-contamination to multiple users. A borrowed pump can be ineffective or break, necessitating the purchase of a replacement pump. Because pumps have a limited lifetime, some mothers who borrow or purchase previously used pumps may put their milk supply at risk because the device cannot operate at its optimum.

Sample Guidelines for Pumping

The healthcare professional needs to base pumping recommendations on many factors and to take into account each mother's situation. For example, a mother whose premature infant is younger than 30 weeks of gestation and is not taking oral feedings needs instructions very different from those of a mother who is pumping during her hours of employment, or one who is only occasionally expressing milk. The mother of the premature infant needs a pump that has the following characteristics:

- Removes milk quickly
- Pumps both breasts simultaneously
- Promotes physiologic prolactin cycling
- Obtains milk with a high energy content
- Has an easily controlled vacuum
- Permits the vacuum to be applied for short periods of time to avoid tissue damage
- Produces high milk yield

BOX 12–2

FDA Policy on Used Breast Pumps

Should I Buy a Used Breast Pump or Share a Breast Pump?

You should never buy a used breast pump or share a breast pump.

Only FDA-cleared, hospital-grade pumps should be used by more than one person. With the exception of hospital-grade pumps, the FDA considers breast pumps single-use devices. That means that a breast pump should only be used by one woman because there is no way to guarantee the pump can be cleaned and disinfected between uses by different women.

The money you may save by buying a used pump is not worth the health risks to you or your baby. Breast pumps that are reused by different mothers can carry infectious diseases, such as HIV or hepatitis.

Buying a used breast pump or sharing a breast pump may be a violation of the manufacturer's warranty, and you may not be able to get help from the manufacturer if you have a problem with the pump.

Source: US Food and Drug Administration, 2007.

- Is easy to use
- Is heat resistant for sterilization
- Has a collection kit that is easily assembled and cleaned
- Is durable (will not stop working or break easily)
- Is economical
- Is accessible

A reasonable option for long-term pumping is an electric pump with a double collecting kit that is leased on a long-term basis. The mother should begin pumping as soon after the birth as possible and do so at least eight times each 24 hours (Hill, Aldag, & Chatterton, 1996).

The mother who has a healthy 2- to-3-month-old infant and is returning to full-time employment outside the home may have different needs. Although battery pumps are popular, using an AC adapter will help increase efficiency and decrease the cost of replacement batteries. This mother might also consider a long-term lease on an electric pump or the purchase of a personal-use pump. If this mother chooses to use a manually operated cylinder pump,

instructions should include proper hand positioning in order to avoid developing lateral epicondylitis, (i.e., tennis elbow) (Williams, Auerbach, & Jacobi, 1989). These instructions emphasize shoulder adduction, with the elbow lying against the body, the forearm in supination (turned up), and the wrist slightly flexed. A mother with carpal tunnel syndrome; arthritis; or other hand, wrist, arm, or shoulder problems may need to use an electric pump rather than a manual or battery-operated pump to avoid exacerbation of her symptoms.

A mother who expresses only small amounts of milk or who has a low milk supply should be advised to elicit the milk-ejection reflex by baby suckling, looking at a picture of her baby, listening to guided relaxation tapes, or practicing slow chest breathing before applying the pump, and to massage the breast by quadrants throughout the pumping session. She may need to sit in a quiet area that permits relaxation with a minimum of interruptions. Pumping early in the morning or on the opposite breast while the baby is nursing may also prove helpful. Flange size should be checked to

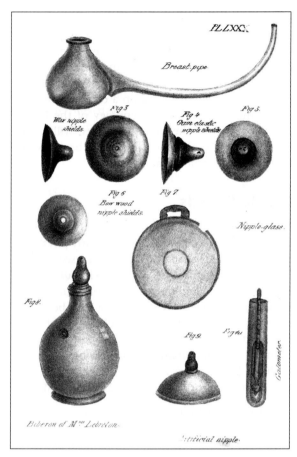

FIGURE **12–13**   Early nipple shields, circa 1833.

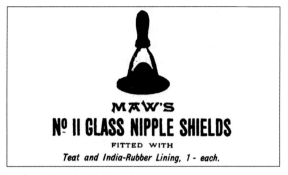

FIGURE **12–14**   Nipple shield and breast glass, circa 1864.

Review of Literature

Woolridge, Baum, and Drewett (1980) studied the effect of the all-rubber shield (Macarthy-Mexican Hat) and a thin latex shield on the suckling patterns and milk intake of 5- to 8-day-old babies of mothers with problem-free lactation experiences. The Macarthy-Mexican Hat reduced milk transfer by 58 percent and changed infant suckling patterns by increasing the suckling rate and the time spent pausing. This is a pattern typically seen when milk flow decreases. The thin latex shield reduced milk intake by 22 percent and had no significant effect on suckling patterns. This thin shield was being tested as part of an apparatus in a new system for measuring milk flow and composition during breastfeeding. The babies observed in this study had no difficulty latching onto mothers' nipples, and no nipple soreness was reported by the mothers in the study. Theoretically, if these problems existed, milk transfer and suckling patterns could be further compromised with the continued use of a thick shield. Using the same thin latex shield, Jackson et al. (1987) showed a 29 percent decrease in milk transfer during their study of nutrient intake in healthy, full-term newborns.

Amatayakul et al. (1987) measured plasma prolactin and cortisol levels in mothers, with and without a thin latex nipple shield in place. They found that prolactin and cortisol levels were unaffected by the shield but that milk transfer was decreased by 42 percent when the shield was in place during feedings. They postulate that this effect on milk volume is attributable to an interference with oxytocin release.

lining the inside to help "stimulate" the breast. This design was reported to be very painful to use. The rubber shields gradually became thinner (Evenflo) and were replaced with thin latex (Lewin Woolf, Griptight, Ltd.) and ultrathin silicone (Canon Babysafe, Medela, Ameda, Avent) seen today (Figure 12–15).

Early nipple shield use generated poor outcomes in many babies due to misuse, misunderstanding, the very thick nature of the device that prevented mothers from feeling the baby at breast (which probably reduced prolactin levels), and overall poor milk transfer. The barrier that the thick shield created between the baby's mouth and teat exceeded the limits of the mechanical requirements for milk removal. They became destructive to the course of lactation and risky to the health of the baby (Desmarais & Browne, 1990).

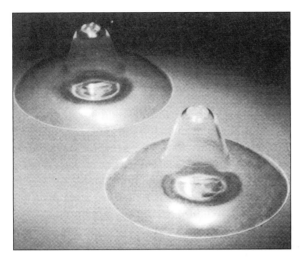

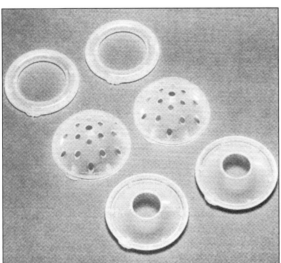

FIGURE **12–15**   Modern silicone nipple shields (above) and breast shells (below).

Source: Courtesy of Medela, Inc., McHenry, IL.

Auerbach (1990a) studied changes in pumped milk volume with and without the use of a thin silicone shield (Cannon Babysafe). Twenty-five mothers used a breast pump (Medela electric model) to provide milk samples, which prevented any change in infant suckling patterns from affecting milk volume amounts. Milk volume was significantly reduced when a shield was in place. Seventy-one percent of the total milk obtained was recorded when no shield was used. Pumping without a shield resulted in mean volumes five to seven times greater than when a shield was in place.

Nipple shield use has yielded more beneficial outcomes. Key to such outcomes is the use of ultrathin silicone shields, critical assessment by a skilled lactation consultant, and continuous follow-up. Babies who otherwise may have been unable to breastfeed have benefited from the judicious use of this device. However, there still remain drawbacks to much of the published research due to lack of prospective, randomized controlled trials of shield use; references to old studies conducted with thick rubber shields; using samples of babies with no feeding problems; using small samples; and often measuring only a single feeding (Table 12–4).

Types of Shields

Rubber Shields

Rubber shields are seldom seen today and should not be used.

Standard Bottle Nipples or Bottle Nipples Attached to a Glass or Plastic Base

These types of shields place the baby and his mouth one to two inches away from the mother's nipple, significantly altering positioning at breast. This does not permit compression of the milk sinuses or skin-to-skin stimulation of the nipple–areolar complex and may alter prolactin cycling. Milk may pool in the base, which holds the artificial nipple, and never reach the baby, or simply leak out the sides. These too are seldom seen and should not be used, nor should an artificial nipple itself be placed over a mother's nipple.

Latex and Silicone Shields

These are extremely thin, flexible shields with the nipple portion being firmer. Because the silicone is so thin, more stimulation reaches the areola, and milk volume is not as seriously depleted as with the other designs (Auerbach, 1990a). Because of the increasing reports of latex allergy in the general population, latex-containing shields should be avoided. Silicone shields are available in a number of sizes (Table 12–5).

Shield Selection and Instructions

There is little in the literature regarding shield selection and instructions for use. If the height of the

TABLE 12–4	Nipple Shield Research

Study	Description
Brigham, 1996	Reviewed 51 mothers, with 81% reporting positive outcomes in resolving breastfeeding problems.
Bodley & Powers, 1996	In 10 cases weight gain was appropriate during and following the period of nipple shield use.
Woodworth & Frank, 1996	Shield used for breast refusal.
Wilson-Clay, 1996	Experiences of 32 mothers using shields to resolve breastfeeding problems.
Clum & Primomo, 1996	9 of 15 preterm infants consumed 50% more milk at breast with an ultrathin shield than without a shield.
Meier, Brown, & Hurst, 2000	34 preterm infants showed increased milk transfer with a shield; 3.9 ml without the shield and 18.4 ml with the shield.
Chertok, Schneider, & Blackburn, 2006	32 mothers demonstrated no significant difference in hormonal levels and infant milk intake with and without ultrathin nipple shield use.

teat of a shield is greater than the length from the junction of the hard and soft palate to the lips, then the infant's jaw closure and tongue compression will fall on the shaft of the teat, and not over the breast. Wilson-Clay and Hoover (2005) also recommend that the base diameter should fit the mother's nipple and that better results occur with the shortest teat height and smallest base diameter. A summary of instructions includes the following:

- Apply the shield by turning it almost inside out.
- Moisten the edges to help it adhere better or warm the shield with hot water.
- Drip expressed milk onto the outside of the teat to encourage the baby.
- Hand express a little milk into the teat if necessary.

- Use alternate massage to help drain breast.
- Run tubing inside or outside of shield for supplementation.
- The baby's mouth must not close on the shaft of the teat.
- The latch should be checked to see that the baby is not just suckling on the tip of the teat.
- The shield should be washed in hot soapy water after each use and rinsed well.
- If yeast is present on the areola, the shield should be boiled.
- Some mothers may need more than one shield.
- Weight check about every 3 days until milk supply is stable and baby is gaining well.
- Check breasts for plugged ducts and areas that are not draining well.

TABLE 12–5	Silicone Shields

Product	Diameter (in.)	Height of Nipple (in.)	Width of Nipple (in.)	Number of Holes
Avent	2 6/8	7/8	5/8 at tip, 1 at base	3
Medela Standard	2 6/8	7/8	5/8 at tip, 1 at base	4
Medela Extra Small	2 6/8	6/8	3/8 at tip, 5/8 at base	3
Ameda	2 5/8	7/8	4/8 at tip, 7/8 at base	5

Weaning from the Shield

Recommendations regarding weaning from the nipple shield include:

- No set time; extended use of the ultrathin silicone shield has not been shown to be detrimental.
- Mothers start by just skin-to-skin next to nipple, starting the feed with the shield and removing it, and gradually trying feeds without the shield.
- The shield should not be cut.

Responsibilities

The healthcare professional has the following responsibilities regarding breastfeeding women and nipple shields:

- Document all of your encounters and instructions and communicate these to the primary healthcare provider.
- Understand the risks and advantages of using such a device (Box 12–3).
- Assess the situation before recommending a shield (Auerbach, 1989). Shields used as a quick fix to ensure infant feedings before early discharge act as "band-aid therapy." They cover up the problem without addressing the cause. Identify and take steps to correct the problem rather than issuing a shield as the initial therapy.
- Consider written informed consent. The mother and the provider who is recommending the shield sign the consent form. This ensures that everyone knows the risks of using a shield, as well as how to use it so that its dangers are minimized. It also serves as a teaching aid to professionals who are unaware of potential long-range problems. A copy should be given to the mother, another copy is retained in the medical record, and a third copy is sent to the pediatrician (Kutner, 1986).
- Ensure that the mother will receive close follow-up during the time the shield is in use.
- Realize that the risks of nipple shield use have legal implications for the hospital and/or professional who recommend them (Bornmann, 1986).

- Provide proper instructions and referrals if a shield is used as an interim recommendation to assist with breastfeeding. If a mother is discharged from the hospital using a shield, a community referral must be made to a lactation consultant or the nurse practitioner at the pediatrician's office for daily follow-up. Weight checks may need to be obtained twice a week. The pediatrician should be alerted to the problem that required use of the shield in the first place and should be aware of suggestions for discontinuing its use.

Breast Shells

Breast shells are two-piece plastic devices worn over the nipple and areola to evert flat or retracted nipples. Historically, these shells were called nipple glasses (center device in Figure 12–13) and were used to protect the mother's clothing from leaking milk, or applied if the mother had "too much" milk. Some brands are still marketed as a device for catching leaked milk between feedings. Currently, shells are not recommended for this use, although many mothers find them helpful for collecting drip milk from one breast while nursing or pumping on the opposite side. Some clinicians also recommend their use for engorgement, as their gentle pressure encourages milk to leak and for areolar edema to create a circular pit which exposes the nipple. The milk collected between feedings must be discarded because of potential high bacteria counts. If drip milk is collected during a feeding or pumping session, it can be stored as usual.

Inverted nipples are identified when the areola is compressed behind the base of the nipple and the nipple retreats into the surrounding skin. This is caused by the presence of the original invagination of the mammary dimple. Prenatally, breast shells were worn for increasingly longer periods of time throughout the day and removed at night. The constant gentle pressure around the base of the nipple was thought to release the adhesions anchoring the nipple, thus allowing it to protrude when the baby latches onto the breast. Shells can be worn between feedings, after the baby is born, if nipple flattening or retraction is identified postpartum or if the nipples still need correction. Current information shows that little correction of the nipple actually

12–3

Quick Guide to Nipple Shield Use

What Shields Do

- Therapeutically supply oral stimulation not provided by mother's nipples
- Create a nipple shape in infant's mouth
- Allow extraction of milk by expression with minimal suction and negative pressure
- Help compensate for weak infant suction
- Present a stable nipple shape that remains during pauses in suckling bursts
- Maintain the nipple in a protruded position
- Raise the rate of milk flow

What Shields Will Not Do

- Correct milk transfer problems or weight gain if the mother has inadequate milk volume
- Fix damaged nipples if the cause is not discovered and remedied
- Replace skilled intervention and close follow-up

Advantages of Nipple Shields

- Permit learning to feed at breast
- Allow supplementation at breast (i.e., thread tubing under or alongside of the shield)
- Encourage nipple protractility
- Will not overwhelm mother with gadgets
- Prevent baby fighting the breast

Disadvantages of Nipple Shields

- Used as a substitute for skilled care
- Used as a quick fix

- May exacerbate original problem
- May lead to insufficient milk volume, inadequate weight gain, weaning
- Prevent proper extension of the nipple back into the baby's mouth (Minchin, 1985)
- May pinch the nipple and areola, causing abrasion, pain, skin breakdown, and internal trauma to the breast if not applied properly
- Create nipple shield addiction (DeNicola, 1986), after which the baby will not feed at breast without the shield in place
- Predispose the nipple to damage when the baby is put to breast without the shield, as he may chew rather than suckle
- Discarded as a useful intervention in selected situations

Possible Indications for Nipple Shield Use

Latch Difficulty

- Nipple anomalies (flat, retracted, fibrous, inelastic)
- Mismatch between small baby mouth and large nipple
- Baby from heavily medicated mother
- Birth trauma (vacuum extraction, forceps)
- Oral aversion (vigorous suctioning)
- Artificial nipple preference (pacifiers, bottles)
- Transition baby from bottle to breast

(Continues)

BOX **12-3** (Continued)

- Baby with weak or disorganized suckle (slips off nipple, preterm, neurological problems)
- Baby with high or low tone
- Delay in putting baby to breast

Oral Cavity Problems

- Cleft palate
- Channel palate (Turner's syndrome, formerly intubated)
- Bubble palate
- Lack of fat pads (preterm, SGA)

- Low threshold mouth
- Poor central grooving of the tongue
- Micrognathia (recessed jaw)

Upper Airway Problems

- Tracheomalacia
- Laryngomalacia

Damaged Nipples

- When all else fails and mother states she is going to quit breastfeeding

takes place prenatally and that some women do not like using these devices (Alexander et al., 1992). Most clinicians no longer recommend prenatal use of this product.

Several brands of shells are available, all of which have a dome that is placed over a base through which the nipple protrudes when worn under a bra. Depending on the brand, the dome may have one or many ventilation holes. The domes with only one or two holes may not provide adequate air circulation to the nipple and areola. The retained moisture and heat (especially in hot weather) can create a miniature greenhouse effect that promotes soreness and skin breakdown. Extra holes can be drilled in the top of the dome. Some brands have many holes in the dome to help with this problem. Another form of breast shell with a wider base has been used for sore nipples to keep air circulating around them and to prevent them from adhering to a bra. Currently, most clinicians seldom recommend these devices.

Feeding-Tube Devices

Judicious use of feeding-tube devices enables many mothers and babies to breastfeed who otherwise would have lost this unique opportunity. Such devices consist of a container to hold breastmilk or formula and a length of thin tubing that runs from

the container to the mother's nipple. The tube is secured in place by nonallergenic tape or run under the nursing bra or nipple shield, and as the baby suckles at breast, supplement is simultaneously delivered. Providing milk in this manner may be a novel idea to the mother. Careful explanations should include how the feeding-tube device is used and the expected outcomes. Some mothers are put off by the thought of feeding their babies in what they consider a "nonnatural" way that at first appears complicated. Explaining that the device is a temporary aid in establishing the baby at breast while ensuring adequate nutrition helps the mother to accept tube feeding. Several commercial devices are on the market; in addition, noncommercial devices can be constructed from bottles or syringes and tubing.

Lact-Aid (USA)

Developed in 1971 for nursing the adopted baby, the Lact-Aid device created a breastfeeding experience for those mothers and babies who previously had no choice in terms of feeding methods. It is a closed system consisting of a presterilized, disposable four-ounce bag to hold milk—with a cap through which a length of fine tubing extends to the nipple. The bag hangs around the mother's neck on a cord. Air is squeezed out of the bag to facilitate milk flow. Powdered formulas will not flow readily through the device.

Supplemental Nutrition System (USA) Medela, Inc

The SNS device consists of a 5-oz plastic bottle with a cap through which a length of tubing is secured to each breast. This two-tube unit allows the tubing to be set up on both breasts at the same time and comes with three different sizes of tubing. It is a vented system with a cap that has notches for pinching off both tubes while setting up the unit and securing one tube while the baby is feeding from the other side. Flow rates are influenced by the size of the tubing used (small, medium, large), the height of the bottle, and whether or not the opposite tube is pinched off during the feeding. A smaller version is also available with only one tube.

Situations for Use

Feeding-tube devices can be recommended and used in many situations where other measures have failed or in order to prevent further complications.

Infant Suckling Problems

Babies with weak, disorganized, or dysfunctional suckling are candidates for feeding-tube devices.

Maternal Situations

Mothers can benefit from the use of feeding-tube devices in the following situations:

- Adoptive nursing (induced lactation) mothers (Auerbach & Avery, 1981; Sutherland & Auerbach, 1985)
- Relactation—meaning inducing a milk supply after a separation or interruption of breastfeeding (Auerbach & Avery, 1980; Bose et al., 1981)
- Breast surgery, especially breast reduction mammaplasty that involved moving the nipple
- Primary lactation insufficiency—Not enough functional breast tissue to support a full milk supply (Neifert & Seacat, 1985)

- Severe nipple trauma
- Illness, surgery, or hospitalization

Generally, a feeding-tube device is used to maintain a mother's milk supply, to deliver sufficient or extra nutrients to the baby, and to create a behavior-modification situation that shapes the baby's suckling pattern to one suitable for obtaining milk from the breast (or prevents the suckling pattern from changing). These devices allow feedings to be done at breast when formerly, in certain situations, bottles with artificial nipples were used. Because these devices are used only in special situations, it is imperative that the professional who recommends their use follow-up closely (daily if necessary) to ensure adequate milk intake by the baby, to validate correct use by the mother, and to wean from the device when it is appropriate to do so.

A baby using a feeding tube at breast must be able to latch-on and execute some form of suckling. For babies who are unable at first to do this because of complete nipple confusion, strong extensor positioning, hypotonia, or lethargy, finger-feeding with the device can be used as an interim measure (Bull & Barger, 1987), followed by attempts to feed at breast. The mother can place a tube on the pad of her index finger or whichever finger is closest in size to her nipple. She allows the baby to draw the finger into his mouth. Correct suckling will cause the milk to flow and will reward the desired behavior; no milk is removed if the baby bites the finger like an artificial nipple. While this also allows the father or other caregiver to feed the baby, some babies become unable to feed at breast because of the strong stimulus that the firm finger provides. Finger-feeding in this manner may prevent improper suckling patterns from being reinforced and move the baby to breast faster than if artificial nipples are used to feed the baby, but care must be taken that babies do not become so accustomed to this form of feeding that they are unwilling to suckle at breast.

When considering feeding-tube devices, the clinician should note the following guidelines:

- They can be used to temporarily assist the baby at breast but are generally not necessary if the baby is gaining weight adequately.
- In situations of adoptive nursing; breast reduction surgery; primary lactation insufficiency; and certain genetic, anatomic, or

neurologic problems in an infant, these feeding devices may require long-term use with or without breast pumping.

- Close follow-up is mandatory with short- or long-term use.
- Because the baby controls the flow, he will not aspirate or be overwhelmed by the fluid he receives. When he swallows or releases the vacuum, the milk flows backward and the baby must initiate another suckle to start the flow. If he cannot initially do this, the bottle or bag of supplement can be squeezed or the plunger of the syringe can be pushed slightly. The milk will not continuously drip or flow as with a bottle and artificial nipple.
- Risks of use include "addiction" to the device by the clinician, mother, and/or baby. The mother and baby should be weaned from the device as quickly as is appropriate. Some mothers may have difficulty believing that they can support a milk supply without the device and not trust themselves to provide for the baby. The clinician should avoid routine use of tube-feeding devices except where necessary. Some clever babies learn to suckle only on the tube, in which case it should be placed so it does not extend beyond the end of the mother's nipple. If the baby has become accustomed to the feel of the tubing, it can be moved to the corner of his mouth and gradually removed. One mother finally taped a one inch length of the tube to her areola and withdrew it after her baby latched-on.
- One or both tubes can be secured on either side of the areola or the top or bottom, whichever gives the best results.
- The clutch position may be easier to use at first because the mother has greater control of the infant's head.
- A gavage setup with a No. 5 feeding-tube can also be used as a feeding device.
- Tubing from a butterfly needle can also be used as it is smaller and softer than gavage tubing (Edgehouse & Radzyminski, 1990).
- A baby can also be fed by dropper, spoon, cup, or bowl if tubing is not available.
- Powdered formulas and special formulas may clog the smaller tubes if the formula is not mixed well. Larger sizes of tubing may be necessary to prevent clogging.
- The device should be rinsed in cold water after each use and then filled with warm soapy water that is squeezed through the tubing and rinsed well. Sterilization can be done once a day, usually by placing it in boiling water for 20 minutes. In the hospital some of the devices can be steamed or autoclaved (Rental Roundup, 1986).
- Feeding in public may be more difficult or obvious. The mother may prefer to use alternatives to tube feeding when she is away from home.

Summary

Just as the healthcare professional must base recommendations for use of breast pumps on various factors, the same holds true for the temporary use of other breastfeeding technologies. Too often a breastfeeding mother may see a device advertised as an aid to breastfeeding and assume that she needs to use it. If she then attempts to do so without thoroughly understanding its risks and benefits, actual and presumed, she could unwittingly interfere with the lactation course and the baby's ability to breastfeed. This is particularly true if she obtains the device from a person or institution that lacks a specialist in lactation management.

Nipple shields are most apt to be used when they are not necessary—in part because of their wide availability and in part because of their attractiveness in busy hospitals or practices, where healthcare workers offer the devices because they appear to "make the baby nurse." Thus, when a healthcare provider considers offering the device to a mother, careful instructions and emphasis on the temporary nature of the use of the device must be offered.

Feeding-tube devices are more complex and therefore potentially more off-putting than either breast shells or nipple shields. Mothers who insist upon using the device because they are convinced that their own milk supplies are inadequate to support appropriate infant growth need careful follow-up. Too often, the mother misinterprets the instructions or reads only enough to know how to put the device together and to clean it. The manner in which the device should be used is rarely completely understood from a single reading of the instructions that accompany the device. Healthcare providers or counselors who recommend the inappropriate use of feeding-tube devices can potentially interrupt the breastfeeding relationship or cause further problems. In addition, observation and assessment of the mother and infant as they breastfeed both with and without the device is a necessity if the healthcare provider is to make appropriate recommendations for an optimal outcome. In most cases, the nature of the problem that requires assistance of a feeding-tube device is such that the mother's anxiety level is high and the need to provide additional nutrition for the baby is critical. The lactation consultant, nurse, or other healthcare worker can expect that working with such a mother and baby will be time consuming and will require many more hours of follow-up time than is the case for other situations.

In all cases where any breastfeeding device or pump is used, the benefits of such technology must be weighed against the risks of interfering in the breastfeeding relationship. Anticipating the emotional response of mothers to devices and discussing them in a straightforward manner will assist the healthcare provider in determining whether and when to suggest a particular technology, as well as how to help the mother stop using it when it is no longer necessary. As with all other care, the use of a breastfeeding device of any kind must first be found to "do no harm."

Key Concepts

- Examples of mothers using a device to remove milk from the breasts are cited in medical literature as early as the mid-1500s. The various devices were typically used to relieve engorgement or to express milk because of damaged nipples or mastitis.

- Today women express breastmilk on a short-term basis to solve acute problems, but they also pump on a long-term basis to provide human milk for their babies following a preterm birth or during periods of employment, illness, induced lactation, or relactation.

- Mothers list the following criteria as important when choosing a breast pump: (1) quick and effective in removing milk, (2) comfortable to use, (3) reasonably priced, and (4) easy to find, use, and clean.

- To increase pumping efficiency, mothers use two techniques: (1) elicitation of the milk-ejection reflex before pumping, and (2) massage of the breasts while pumping. Research and literature from the dairy industry support both techniques.

- Other factors that contribute to pumping efficiency include using relaxation techniques and visual imagery and applying warm, moist heat to the breasts before and during pumping. To avoid breast or nipple injury, it is recommended that the pump be removed as soon as the milk stops flowing. When hand-expressing, fingertip compressions deep in the breast tissue should be avoided.

- Considering the bewildering array of breast pumps in the marketplace today, a caregiver recommending one should give a specific name and several places to find it. Prices vary considerably depending upon where it is purchased.

- When expressing milk, the device used must be efficient enough to activate prolactin and oxytocin release. The volume of milk expressed is also related to the degree of fullness of the breast, with a fuller breast yielding more milk volume when pumped. Full breasts tend to take less time to achieve the milk-ejection reflex, with a less full breast taking up to 120 seconds.

- Stage III of lactogenesis is dependent upon early and regular stimulation of the nipple and regular removal of milk from the breasts. Lactogenesis II occurs in the absence of milk removal, but lactogenesis III can be inhibited without regular milk removal. The amount of milk produced is dependent upon the rate the breast is emptied.

- A breast pump does not pump, suck, or pull milk out of the breast. It reduces resistance to milk outflow from the alveoli, allowing the internal pressure of the breast to push out the milk.

- Einar Egnell was the pioneer in breast pump design and based his design on research from the dairy industry. He designed a pump that created periodic and limited phases of negative pressure. It operated in four phases per cycle. Many pump manufacturers still use Egnell's pressure settings as a guide in current breast pump design.
- W. G. Whittlestone found that by providing a compressive force to the breast from a liner inside the pump flange, it enhanced the dynamics of milk expression. The compression is analogous to a baby's tongue and jaw compress the teat between the tongue and hard palate during the suction cycle. Some pumps currently offer a soft flange that collapses over the teat when suction is applied while others with a hard plastic flange offer an insert or liner that is intended to serve the same purpose.
- Breast pumps are divided into three broad classifications: (1) manual hand pumps, (2) battery-operated pumps, and (3) electric pumps.
- Manual hand pumps are easy to find, easy to use, and inexpensive. Some are more effective than others in expressing milk. These pumps are typically used in the short-term or occasionally. The hand and wrist can tire easily with repeated use. Because of nipple pain and low milk yields, the old-fashioned "bicycle horn" pump is not recommended.
- Battery-operated pumps use a small motor to create a vacuum that is usually adjustable. Most have a button the mother presses to release the vacuum in a rhythmic pattern to simulate the rhythm of a nursing baby. They are lightweight, easy to find and use, and are relatively inexpensive. One disadvantage of these pumps is the short battery life. Some have AC adapters. The time each pump takes to achieve optimal suction varies, and those that require up to 30 seconds can cause nipple pain.
- Electric pumps include some that are small and semiautomatic and use a small motor to create a vacuum that is adjustable. Most have an open hole in the flange that the mother covers and uncovers with her fingertip to create a rhythmic pattern to simulate the rhythm of a nursing baby. These pumps are moderately priced and most can do double pumping.
- Automatic electric pumps are designed to cycle pressure rather than maintain it. Pressure setting parameters are set to mimic a nursing infant. Pumps are now designed with adjustable cycling rates up to 120 cycles per minute. Vacuum pressure adjusts up to 250 mm Hg. These pumps are considered the most effective of all pumps and use the double collection kits. They cost more and are heavier than their handheld counterparts.
- All automatic electric pumps and some of the smaller semiautomatic pumps offer double collection kits that allow both breasts to be pumped simultaneously. When researched, prolactin levels were significantly higher and maximum milk yield occurred with double pumping.
- Product manufacturers offer flanges in different sizes to accommodate the anatomic configuration of a particular breast. If a nipple swells during pumping, the mother with a larger nipple may find that a standard size flange is too small to accommodate both the large nipple and subsequent swelling. Those mothers whose nipples are larger than 20.5 mm (the size of a US nickel) may benefit from a larger sized flange.
- Expressed breastmilk is not sterile, and there is considerable disagreement over what constitutes acceptable bacteria count, especially when pumping for a preterm infant. Many factors play a part in the bacteria level, including nipple cleaning, hand washing, collection techniques, type of pump, feeding method of preterm infant, pump-cleaning routines, and gestational age of infant. Some bacteria will always be present and are nonpathogenic. Healthy term infants can tolerate some pathogens and relatively high levels of nonpathogenic bacteria. Yet, preterm or high-risk infants may be at greater risk from the same levels of bacterial presence.
- There are infection risks from electric breast pumps with multiple users, and healthcare facilities must take the necessary precautions to prevent contamination.
- Colostrum and breastmilk inhibits bacterial growth at different rates in both full-term and preterm milk. Milk storage guidelines and practices differ depending on the health of the infant.

- Mothers who chose to discontinue pumping for their hospitalized infants cited insufficient milk collection as the first reason and complained that pumping was too time consuming.

- Mothers pumping for a hospitalized infant need much clinical encouragement and emotional support to ease embarrassment and frustration and gain understanding of the significance of collecting breastmilk for their hospitalized infant.

- Breast pumps are considered to be medical devices by the US Food and Drug Administration and as such are regulated within the FDA's Center for Devices and Radiological Health. They maintain a medical product reporting program to record problems with breast pumps as encountered by consumers and clinicians.

- The issue of mothers selling and buying used breast pumps remains pertinent. The FDA advises that there are certain risks presented by breast pumps that are reused by different mothers if they are not properly cleaned and sterilized. It is not recommended that a pump that is labeled as a single-user pump be reused or resold.

- Common pumping problems include sore nipples, low milk yield, erratic or delayed milk-ejection reflex, and dwindling milk supply over a long-term course of pumping.

- An erratic or delayed milk-ejection reflex can have an overwhelming impact on effective milk expression. A mother's feeling about pumping such as embarrassment, tension, fear of failure, pain, fatigue, and anxiety can inhibit the neurochemical pathways required for milk ejection. When a clinician knows a mother's feelings and attitudes about pumping, guidelines can be individually created for her specific situation.

- Early use of nipple shields generated poor outcomes. The thickness of material created a barrier that prevented a mother from feeling her baby at the breast and inhibited milk transfer.

- Nipple shields fell into disfavor when the ramifications of use became destructive to the course of lactation and risky to the health of the baby.

- Recent research and discussions of nipple shields have yielded more beneficial outcomes with the use of ultrathin silicone shields. Use of all other shields, including latex, is not recommended. Critical assessment and continuous follow-up by a skilled lactation consultant is essential. Babies who otherwise may have been unable to breastfeed have benefited from the judicious use of this tool.

- Nipple shields can therapeutically supply oral stimulation not provided by mother's nipples, create a nipple shape in an infant's mouth, and allow extraction of milk by expression with minimal suction. With negative pressure inside the shield tip keeping milk available, the shield may compensate for weak infant suck, present a stable nipple shape that remains during pauses in sucking bursts, maintain the nipple in protruded position, and impact the rate of milk transfer.

- The disadvantages of nipple shields include use as a substitute for skilled care or a quick fix. Their use may lead to insufficient milk volume, inadequate weight gain or weaning, and a nipple shield addiction after which the baby will not feed without the shield in place. They may also predispose the nipple to damage when the baby is put to breast without the shield, as he may chew rather than suckle.

- The proper size of nipple shield must be used. The teat height should not exceed the length of the infant's mouth from the juncture of the hard and soft palates to lip closure. The base diameter should fit the mother's nipple and better results occur with the shortest teat height and smallest base diameter.

- Breast shells are two-piece plastic devices worn over the nipple and areola to evert flat or inverted nipples. Historically, these shells were called nipple glasses and were used to protect the mother's clothes from leaking milk, or used if the mother had "too much milk." Milk collected in the shells must be discarded due to potential bacterial growth.

- When worn prenatally, breast shells were designed to create a constant gentle pressure around the base of the inverted nipple and were thought to release the adhesions anchoring the nipple. Current information shows little correction of the nipple actually happens prenatally.

- Although breast shells have been used to provide air circulation around sore nipples and to keep a bra from adhering to the nipple, most clinicians today seldom recommend these devices.
- Designed to supplement feedings at the breast, feeding-tube devices can enable many mothers and babies to breastfeed when they would otherwise have to use an alternate feeding method without the baby at the breast.
- Feeding-tube devices consist of a container to hold breastmilk or formula and a length of thin tubing that runs from the container to the mother's nipple. The tube is secured in place with nonallergenic tape.
- The use of a feeding-tube device is indicated for babies with weak, disorganized, or dysfunctional sucking. A partial list includes those babies who are preterm, hypertonic, or hypotonic; babies who have Down syndrome, cardiac problems, nipple preference, neurological impairment, or cleft lip or palate; infants who have experienced perinatal asphyxia, low, slow, or no weight gain, or weight loss due to ineffective suckling.
- The feeding-tube device is useful in maternal situations such as adoptive nursing and for mothers who are relactating, have had breast surgery, suffer from primary lactation insufficiency, have severe nipple trauma, are suffering from an illness, or are undergoing surgery or hospitalization.
- With finger-feeding, a mother places the tube on the pad of her index finger or whichever finger is closest in size to her nipple. The baby draws the finger into his mouth and with correct suckling, causes the milk to flow. This method also allows the father or other caregiver to feed the baby.
- Finger-feeding can also be used to take the edge off the baby's hunger before putting him to the breast and to help transition a baby to nursing at the breast.
- With the use of a feeding-tube device, the clinician must closely follow the progress in short- or long-term use. Risks of use include "addiction" to the device by the clinician, mother, and/or baby. The mother and baby should be weaned from the device as quickly as is appropriate.
- Healthcare professionals must employ judicious use of devices and other technology that are designed to aid in breastfeeding. As with all care, the use of a breastfeeding device of any kind must be found to "do no harm;" thereafter its benefits must outweigh the risks it represents in order for the breastfeeding relationship to be truly supported.

Resources for Mothers

Berggren K. Working Without Weaning. Amarillo, TX: Hale Publishing; 2006.

Casemore S. *Exclusively Pumping Breast Milk: A Guide to Providing Expressed Breast Milk for Your Baby.* Bath, Ontario: Gray Lion Publishing; 2004.

Colburn-Smith C, Serrette A. *The Milk Memos: How Real Moms Learned to Mix Business with Babies— And How You Can, Too.* New York: Tarcher; 2007.

Freeman P, Mannel R. ILCA's inside track: milk expression and pumping. *J Hum Lact.* 2007;23(3):281–282.

Pryor G, Huggins K. *Nursing Mother, Working Mother.* Rev. ed. Boston, MA: Harvard Common Press; 2007.

Pumpin' Pal's Pocket Guide to Breast Pumping: A How-To Breast Pumping Guide for New Moms and Working Moms. Pumpin' Pal; 2006.

Stafford S. *Pumping Breast Milk Successfully.* Lincoln, NE: iUniverse; 2003.

Internet Resources

http://groups.yahoo.com/group/epers
http://messageboards.ivillage.com/iv-ppexcluspump

http://www.mother-2-mother.com/ ExclusivePumping.htm

References

Alekseev NP et al. Compression stimuli increase the efficacy of breast pump function. *Eur J Obstet Gynecol Reproduct Biol.* 1998;77:131–139.

Alexander JM et al. Randomized controlled trial of breast shells and Hoffman's exercises for inverted and non-protractile nipples. *Br Med J.* 1992; 304(6833):1030–1032.

Aljazaf KMNH. *Ultrasound Imaging in the Analysis of the Blood Supply and Blood Flow in the Human Lactating Breast.* [Dissertation]. Medical Imaging Science, Curtin University of Technology, Perth, Australia; 2004.

Amatayakul K et al. Serum prolactin and cortisol levels after suckling for varying periods of time and the effect of a nipple shield. *Acta Obstet Gynecol Scand.* 1987;66:47–51.

Asquith M, Harod J. Reduction of bacterial contamination in banked human milk. *J Pediatr.* 1997;95: 993–994.

Asquith M, Sharp R, Stevenson D. Decreased bacterial contamination of human milk expressed with an electric breast pump. *J Calif Perin Assoc.* 1985; 4:45–47.

Asquith M et al. The bacterial content of breast milk after early initiation of expression using a standard technique. *J Pediatr Gastroenterol Nutr.* 1984;3: 104–107.

Auerbach KG. Using nipple shields appropriately. *Rental Roundup.* 1989;6:4–5.

Auerbach KG. The effect of nipple shields on maternal milk volume. *JOGNN.* 1990a;19:419–427.

Auerbach KG. Sequential and simultaneous breast pumping: a comparison. *Int J Nurs Stud.* 1990b;27: 257–265.

Auerbach KG, Avery JL. Relactation: a study of 366 cases. *Pediatrics.* 1980;65:236–242.

Auerbach KG, Avery JL. Induced lactation: a study of adoptive nursing by 240 women. *Am J Dis Child.* 1981;135:340–343.

Auerbach KG, Guss E. Maternal employment and breastfeeding: a study of 567 women's experiences. *Am J Dis Child.* 1984;138:958–960.

Auerbach KG, Walker M. When the mother of a premature infant uses a breast pump: what every NICU nurse needs to know. *Neonatal Network.* 1994; 13:23–29.

Bennion E. *Antique Medical Instruments.* Berkeley, CA: University of California; 1979:271.

Biancuzzo M. Selecting pumps for breastfeeding mothers. *JOGNN.* 1999;28:417–426.

Binns CW et al. Trends in the expression of breastmilk 1993–2003. *Breastfeed Rev.* 2006;14:5–9.

Bodley V, Powers D. Long-term nipple shield use—a positive perspective. *J Hum Lact.* 1996;12:301–304.

Bornmann P. Legal considerations and the lactation consultant—USA, Unit 3 (Lactation Consultant Series). Garden City Park, NY: Avery Publishing Group; 1986.

Bose C et al. Relactation by mothers of sick and premature infants. *Pediatrics.* 1981;67:565–568.

Bowen-Jones A, Thompson C, Drewett RF. Milk flow and sucking rates during breast-feeding. *Dev Med Child Neurol.* 1982;24:626–633.

Bowles B, Stutte P, Hensley J. Alternate massage in breastfeeding. *Genesis.* 1988;9:5–9.

Brigham M. Mothers' reports of the outcome of nipple shield use. *J Hum Lact.* 1996;12:291–297.

Brown SL et al. Breast pump adverse events: reports to the Food and Drug Administration. *J Hum Lact.* 2005;21:169–174.

Bull P, Barger J. Fingerfeeding with the SNS. *Rental Roundup.* 1987;4:2–3.

Caldeyro-Barcia R. Milk-ejection in women. In: Reynolds M, Folley S, eds. *Lactogenesis, the Initiation of Milk Secretion at Parturition.* Philadelphia, PA: University of Pennsylvania Press; 1969.

Chapman et al. Impact of breast pumping on lactogenesis stage II after cesarean delivery: a randomized clinical trial. *Pediatrics.* 2001;107(6):e94.http://www.pediatrics.org/cgi/content/full/107/6/e94. Accessed October 30, 2007.

Chertok IR, Schneider J, Blackburn S. A pilot study of maternal and term infant outcomes associated with ultrathin nipple shield use. *J Obstet Gynecol Neonatal Nurs.* 2006;35:265–272.

Clavey S. The use of acupuncture for the treatment of insufficient lactation (Que Ru). *Am J Acupuncture.* 1996;24:35–46.

Clum D, Primomo J. Use of a silicone nipple shield with premature infants. *J Hum Lact.* 1996;12:287–290.

Cobo E et al. Neurohypophyseal hormone release in the human: II. Experimental study during lactation. *Am J Obstet Gynecol.* 1967;97:519–529.

Costa K. A comparison of colony counts of breast milk using two methods of breast cleansing. *JOGNN.* 1989;18:231–236.

Cox DB, Owens RA, Hartmann PE. Blood and milk prolactin and the rate of milk synthesis in women. *Exp Physiol.* 1996;81:1007–1020.

Cregan MD, de Mello TR, Hartmann PE. Preterm delivery and breast expression: consequences for initiating lactation. *Adv Exp Med Biol.* 2000;478:427–428.

Cregan MD, Hartmann PE. Computerized breast measurement from conception to weaning: clinical implications. *J Hum Lact.* 1999;15:89–96.

da Silva OP et al. Effect of domperidone on milk production in mothers of premature newborns: a randomized double-blind, placebo-controlled trial. *Can Med Assoc J.* 2001;164:17–21.

Daly SEJ, Hartmann PE. Infant demand and milk supply. Part 1: infant demand and milk production in lactating women. *J Hum Lact.* 1995a;11:21–26.

Daly SEJ, Hartmann PE. Infant demand and milk supply. Part 2: the short-term control of milk synthesis in lactating women. *J Hum Lact.* 1995b;11:27–37.

Daly SEJ et al. The determination of short-term breast volume changes and the rate of synthesis of human milk using computerized breast measurement. *Exp Phys.* 1992;77:79–87.

Daly SEJ et al. The short-term synthesis and infant regulated removal of milk in lactating women. *Exp Phys.* 1993;78:209–220.

D'Amico CJ, DiNardo CA, Krystofiak S. Preventing contamination of breast pump kit attachments in the NICU. *J Perinatal Neonatal Nurs.* 2003;17: 150–157.

de Sanctis V et al. Comparison of prolactin response to suckling and breast pump aspiration in lactating mothers. *La Ric Clin Lab.* 1981;11:81–85.

DeNicola M. One case of nipple shield addiction. *J Hum Lact.* 1986;2:28–29.

Desmarais L, Browne S. Inadequate weight gain in breastfeeding infants: assessments and resolutions, Unit 8 (Lactation Consultant Series). Garden City Park, NY: Avery Publishing Group; 1990.

Dodd F, Griffin T. Milking routines, machine milking. Reading, England: National Institute of Research on Dairying, Shinfield, England; 1977:179–200.

Donowitz L et al. Contaminated breast milk: a source of *Klebsiella* bacteremia in a newborn intensive care unit. *Rev Infec Dis.* 1981;3:716–720.

Drewett R, Bowen-Jones A, Dogterom J. Oxytocin levels during breastfeeding in established lactation. *Horm Behav.* 1982;16:245–248.

Edgehouse L, Radzyminski S. A device for supplementing breast-feeding. *MCN.* 1990;15:34–35.

Egnell E. The mechanics of different methods of emptying the female breast. *J Swe Med Assoc.* 1956;40:1–8.

Ehrenkranz RA, Ackerman BA. Metoclopramide effect on faltering milk production by mothers of premature infants. *Pediatrics.* 1986;78:614–620.

el-Mohandes AE et al. Aerobes isolated in fecal microflora of infants in the intensive care nursery: relationship to human milk use and systemic sepsis. *Am J Infect Control.* 1993a;21:231–234.

el-Mohandes AE et al. Bacterial contaminants of collected and frozen human milk used in an intensive care nursery. *Am J Infect Control.* 1993b; 21:226–230.

Engstrom JL et al. Comparison of milk output from the right and left breasts during simultaneous pumping in mothers of very low birthweight infants. *Breastfeeding Medicine.* 2007;2:83–91.

Eteng MU et al. Storage beyond three hours at ambient temperature alters the biochemical and nutritional qualities of breast milk. *Afr J Reprod Health.* 2001;5:130–134.

Feher S et al. Increased breastmilk production for premature infants with a relaxation/imagery audiotape. *Pediatrics.* 1989;83:57–60.

Fewtrell MS et al. Randomised, double blind trial of oxytocin nasal spray in mothers expressing breast milk for preterm infants. *Arch Dis Child Fetal Neonatal Ed.* 2006;91:F169–F174.

Fewtrell MS, Lucas P, Collier S. Randomized trial comparing the efficacy of a novel manual breast pump with a standard electric breast pump in mothers who delivered preterm infants. *Pediatrics.* 2001;107:1291–1297.

Fewtrell M et al. Randomized study comparing the efficacy of a novel manual breast pump with a mini-electric breast pump in mothers of term infants. *J Hum Lact.* 2001;17:126–131.

Fildes V. *Breasts, Bottles, and Babies.* Edinburgh: Edinburgh University; 1986:141–143.

Freeman ME et al. Prolactin structure, function, and regulation of secretion. *Physiological Rev.* 2000;80: 1523–1631.

Gabay MP. Galactogogues: medications that induce lactation. *J Hum Lact.* 2002;18:274–279.

Goodman G, Grosvenor C. Neuroendocrine control of the milk-ejection reflex. *J Dairy Sci.* 1983;66: 2226–2235.

Gorewit R et al. Current concepts on the role of oxytocin in milk-ejection. *J Dairy Sci.* 1983;66: 2236–2250.

Gransden W et al. An outbreak of *Serratia marcescens* transmitted by contaminated breast pumps in a special care baby unit. *J Hosp Infec.* 1986;7: 149–154.

Groh-Wargo S et al. The utility of a bilateral breast pumping system for mothers of premature infants. *Neonat Network.* 1995;14:31–36.

Gross MS. Letter. *ILCA Globe.* 1995;3:5.

Gunn AJ et al. Growth hormone increases breast milk volumes in mothers of preterm infants. *Pediatrics.* 1996;98:279–282.

Halverson HM. Mechanisms of early infant feeding. *J Gen Psych.* 1944;64:185–223.

Hamosh M et al. Breastfeeding and the working mother: effect of time and temperature of short-term storage on proteolysis, lipolysis, and bacterial growth in milk. *Pediatrics.* 1996;97:492–498.

Hartmann P. Human lactation: current research and clinical implications. Presented at: Australian Lactation Consultants' Association Conference; October 12–15, 2000; Melbourne, Australia.

Hartmann P. New insights into breast physiology and breast expression and development of the Symphony breast pump. In: *Human Lactation—The Science of the Art Series*, CD. Baar, Switzerland: Medela AG, Medical Technology; 2002.

Hill PD, Aldag JC, Chatterton RT. The effect of sequential and simultaneous breast pumping on milk volume and prolactin levels: a pilot study. *J Hum Lact.* 1996; 12:193–239.

Hill PD, Aldag JC, Chatterton RT. Effects of pumping style on milk production in mothers of non-nursing preterm infants. *J Hum Lact.* 1999;15:209–216.

Hill PD, Aldag JC, Chatterton RT. Initiation and frequency of pumping and milk production in mothers of non-nursing preterm infants. *J Hum Lact.* 2001;17:9–13.

Howie P et al. The relationship between suckling-induced prolactin response and lactogenesis. *J Clin Endocrinol Metab.* 1980;50:670–673.

Human Milk Banking Association of North America. Best practice for expressing, storing and handling human milk in hospitals, homes and child care settings. Raleigh, NC: Human Milk Banking Association of North America; 2005.

Jackson D et al. The automatic sampling shield: a device for sampling suckled breast milk. *Early Hum Dev.* 1987;15:295–306.

Jacobs LA et al. Normal nipple position in term infants measured on breastfeeding ultrasound. *J Hum Lact.* 2007;23:52–59.

Johnson CA. An evaluation of breast pumps currently available on the American market. *Clin Pediatr.* 1983;22:40–45.

Jones E, Dimmock PW, Spencer SA. A randomized controlled trial to compare methods of milk expression after preterm delivery. *Arch Dis Child Fetal Neonatal Ed.* 2001;85:F91–F95.

Kent JC et al. Response of breasts to different stimulation patterns of an electric pump. *J Hum Lact.* 2003;19:179–186.

Kutner L. Nipple shield consent form: a teaching aid. *J Hum Lact.* 1986;2:25–27.

Law BJ et al. Is ingestion of milk-associated bacteria by premature infants fed raw human milk controlled by routine bacteriologic screening? *J Clin Microbiol.* 1989;27:1560–1566.

Lawrence RA, Lawrence RM. *Breastfeeding: A Guide for the Medical Profession.* 6th ed. St. Louis, MO: Mosby; 2005.

Marmet C, Shell E. Marmet technique of manual expression of breastmilk. Encino, CA: The Lactation Institute; 1980.

Maygrier J. *Midwifery Illustrated.* Philadelphia, PA: Carey & Hart; 1833:173.

McNeilly AS et al. Release of oxytocin and prolactin response to suckling. *Br Med J.* 1983;286:646–647.

Meier PP, Brown LP, Hurst NM. Nipple shields for preterm infants: effect on milk transfer and duration of breastfeeding. *J Hum Lact.* 2000;16:106–114.

Meier P, Motyhowski J, Zuleger J. Choosing a correctly-fitted breast shield for milk expression. *Medela Messenger.* 2004;21:8–9.

Meier P, Wilks S. The bacteria in expressed mothers' milk. *MCN.* 1987;12:420–423.

Merrill W et al. Effects of premilking stimulation on complete lactation, milk yield and milking performance. *J Dairy Sci.* 1987;70:1676–1684.

Minchin M. *Breastfeeding Matters.* Victoria, Australia: Alma Publications; 1985:142–145.

Mitoulas LR, Lai CT, Gurrin LC. Efficacy of breast milk expression using an electric breast pump. *J Hum Lact.* 2002a;18:344–352.

Moloney A et al. A bacteriological examination of breast pumps. *J Hosp Infect.* 1987;9:169–174.

Morse J, Bottorff J. The emotional experience of breast expression. *J Nurse Midwifery.* 1988;33:165–170.

Neifert M, Seacat J. Milk yield and prolactin rise with simultaneous breast pumping. Presented at: Ambulatory Pediatric Association Meeting, May 7–10, 1985; Washington, DC.

Neville M. Regulation of mammary development and lactation. In: Neville M, Neifert M, eds. *Lactation: Physiology, Nutrition and Breast-Feeding.* New York, NY: Plenum; 1983:118.

Neville MC. Anatomy and physiology of lactation. *Pediatr Clin North Am.* 2001;48(1):13–34.

Newton M, Newton N. The let-down reflex in human lactation. *J Pediatr.* 1948;33:698–704.

Nissen E et al. Different patterns of oxytocin, prolactin, but not cortisol release during breastfeeding in women delivered by cesarean section or by the vaginal route. *Early Hum Dev.* 1996;45:103–118.

Noel G, Suh H, Frantz A. Prolactin release during nursing and breast stimulation in postpartum and nonpostpartum subjects. *J Clin Endocrinol Metab.* 1974;38:413–423.

Paul VK et al. Manual and pump methods of expression of breast milk. *Indian J Pediatr.* 1996; 63:87–92.

Petersen W. Dairy science: principles and practice. Philadelphia, PA: Lippincott; 1950:373–387.

Pittard W et al. Bacterial contamination of human milk: container type and method of expression. *Am J Perinatol.* 1991;8:25–27.

Ramsay DT et al. Milk flow rates can be used to identify and investigate milk ejection in women expressing breast milk using an electric breast pump. *Breastfeeding Med.* 2006;1:14–23.

Ramsay DT et al. The use of ultrasound to characterize milk ejection on women using an electric breast pump. *J Hum Lact.* 2005;21:421–428.

Rental Roundup. New product. *SNS.* 1986;3:1–3.

Ruis H et al. Oxytocin enhances onset of lactation among mothers delivering prematurely. *Br Med J.* 1981;283:340–342.

Sagi R, Gorewit R, Zinn S. Milk-ejection in cows mechanically stimulated during late lactation. *J Dairy Sci.* 1980;63:1957–1960.

Saint L, Maggiore P, Hartmann P. Yield and nutrient content of milk in eight women breast-feeding twins and one woman breast-feeding triplets. *Br J Nutr.* 1986;56:49–58.

Slusher T et al. Electric breast pump use increases maternal milk volume in African nurseries. *J Trop Pediatr.* 2007;53:125–130.

Slusser W, Frantz K. High-technology breastfeeding. Part II: the management of breastfeeding. *Ped Clin North Am.* 2001;48:505–516.

Smith W, Erenberg A, Nowak A. Imaging evaluation of the human nipple during breastfeeding. *Am J Dis Child.* 1988;142:76–78.

Sozmen M. Effects of early suckling of cesarean-born babies on lactation. *Biol Neonate.* 1992;62:67–68.

Stark Y. *Human Nipples: Function and Anatomical Variations in Relationship to Breastfeeding* [master's thesis]. Pasadena, CA: Pacific Oaks College; 1994.

Stern JM, Reichlin S. Prolactin circadian rhythm persists throughout lactation in women. *Neuroendocrinology.* 1990;51:31–37.

Stutte P, Bowles B, Morman G: The effects of breast massage on volume and fat content of human milk. *Genesis.* 1988;10:22–25.

Sutherland A, Auerbach KG. *Relactation and induced lactation, Unit 1 (Lactation Consultant Series).* Garden City Park, NY: Avery Publishing Group; 1985.

Thompson N et al. Contamination in expressed breast milk following breast cleansing. *J Hum Lact.* 1997;13:127–130.

Toppare MF et al. Metoclopramide for breast milk production. *Nutr Res.* 1994;14:1019–1029.

Tyson J. Nursing and prolactin secretion: principal determinants in the mediation of puerperal infertility. In: Crosignani P, Robyn C, eds. *Prolactin and Human Reproduction.* New York, NY: Academic; 1977:97–108.

Ueda T et al. Influence of psychological stress on suckling-induced pulsatile oxytocin release. *Obstet Gynecol.* 1994;84:259–262.

US Food and Drug Administration, Center for Devices and Radiological Health. Breast Pumps—Choosing a Breast Pump. 2007. Available at: http://www.fda.gov/cdrh/breastpumps/choosing.html#4. Accessed January 7, 2009.

Walker M. How to evaluate breast pumps. *MCN.* 1987; 12:270–276.

Walker M. Breast pump survey. Unpublished manuscript; 1992.

Weber F, Woolridge MW, Baum JD. An ultrasonographic study of the organization of sucking and swallowing by newborn infants. *Dev Med Child Neurol.* 1986;28:19–24.

Weichert C. Prolactin cycling and the management of breastfeeding failure. *Adv Pediatr.* 1980;27:391–407.

Whittlestone W. The physiologic breastmilker. *NZ Fam Phy.* 1978;5:1–3.

Whitworth N et al. The effect of fetal genotype on the human maternal PRL response to labor, delivery and breast stimulation. *Abst Proc Int Cong Prolactin.* 1984;4:60.

Wilde CJ, Prentice A, Peaker M. Breast-feeding: matching supply with demand in human lactation. *Proc Nutr Soc.* 1995;54:401–406.

Wilks S, Meier P. Helping mothers express milk suitable for preterm and high-risk infant feeding. *MCN.* 1988;13:121–123.

Williams J, Auerbach K, Jacobi A. Lateral epicondylitis (tennis elbow) in breastfeeding mothers. *Clin Pediatr.* 1989;28:42–43.

Williams-Arnold LD. Human milk storage for healthy infants and children. Sandwich, MA: Health Education Associates; 2000.

Wilson-Clay B. Clinical use of silicone nipple shields. *J Hum Lact.* 1996;12:279–285.

Wilson-Clay B, Hoover K. *The Breastfeeding Atlas.* 3rd ed. Austin, TX: LactNews Press; 2005.

Win NN et al. Breastfeeding duration in mothers who express breast milk: a cohort study. *Int Breastfeed J.* 2006;1:28.

Woodworth M, Frank E. Transitioning to the breast at six weeks: use of a nipple shield. *J Hum Lact.* 1996;12:305–307.

Woolford M, Phillips D. Evaluation studies of a milking system using an alternating vacuum level in a single chambered teatcup. Proceedings of the International Symposium on Machine Milking. National Mastitis Council; 1978:125–149.

Woolridge MW. Breastfeeding: physiology into practice. In: Davies DP, ed. *Nutrition in Child Health.* Proceedings of conference jointly organized by the Royal College of Physicians of London and the British Paediatric Association. RCPL Press; 1995:13–31.

Woolridge M, Baum J, Drewett R. Effect of a traditional and of a new nipple shield on sucking patterns and milk flow. *Early Hum Dev.* 1980;4:357–364.

Yokoyama Y et al. Releases of oxytocin and prolactin during breast massage and suckling in puerperal women. *Eur J Obstet Gynecol Reprod Biol.* 1994; 53:17–20.

Ziemer M, Pidgeon J. Skin changes and pain in the nipple during the first week of lactation. *JOGNN.* 1993;22:247–256.

Zinaman M. Breast pumps: ensuring mothers' success. *Contemp Obstet Gynecol.* 1988;32:55–62.

Zinaman M et al. Acute prolactin, oxytocin response and milk yield to infant suckling and artificial methods of expression in lactating women. *Pediatrics.* 1992;89:437–440.

Zoppou C, Barry SI, Mercer GN. Dynamics of human milk extraction: a comparative study of breast feeding and breast pumping. *Bull Math Biol.* 1997a;59:953–973.

Zoppou C, Barry SI, Mercer GN. Comparing breast-feeding and breast pumps using a computer model. *J Hum Lact.* 1997b13:195–202.

Appendix 12-A

Manufacturers and Distributors of Breast Pumps and Feeding Equipment

Ameda Breastfeeding Products
(www.ameda.com)

Avent America, Inc., 475 Supreme Drive, Bensenville, IL 60106
(www.aventamerican.com)

Bailey Medical Engineering, 2216 Sunset Dr., Los Osos, CA 93402
Nurture III small semiautomatic breast pump
(www.baileymed.com)

BreastPump.com, Inc., P.O. Box 18475, Tucson, AZ 85731
VersaPed pedal pump
(www.BreastPump.com)

Evenflo Company, Inc., 1801 Commerce Drive, Piqua, Ohio 45356
(www.evenflo.com)

The First Years, 2021 9th Street East, Dyersville, IA 52040-2316
(www.learningcurve.com)

Gerber Products Co., 445 State Street, Fremont, MI 49412
(www.gerber.com)

Handi-Craft Company, 4433 Fyler Avenue, St. Louis, Missouri 63116

Dr. Brown's breast pump
(www.handi-craft.com)

Lact-Aid International, Inc., P.O. Box 1066, Athens, TN 37371
Feeding-tube device
(www.lact-aid.com)

Limerick, Inc., 2150 N. Glenoaks Blvd., Burbank, CA 91504-4327
PJ's Comfort electric pump
(www.limerickinc.com)

Lumiscope Company, Inc., 1035 Centennial Ave., Piscataway, NJ 08854
Gentle Expressions pump
(lumiscope.net)

Medela, Inc., P.O. Box 660, McHenry, IL 60051
(www.medela.com)

Playtex Products, Inc., P.O. Box 701, Allendale, NJ 07401
(playtexproductsinc.com)

Whisper Wear
(www.whisperwear.com)

Whittlestone, P.O. Box 2237, Antioch, CA 94531
(www.whittlestone.com)

Frontal view of lactating breast. (Based on an illustration by Ka Botzis.)

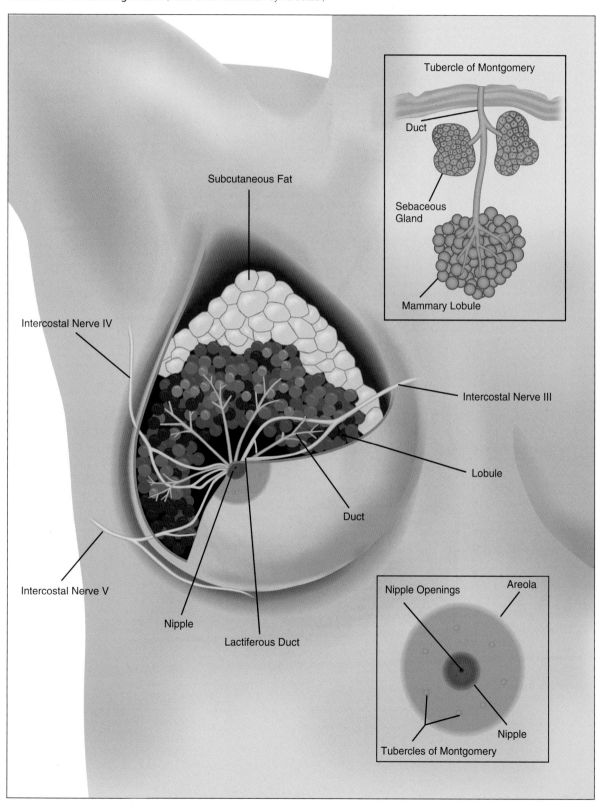

Tubercle of Montgomery

Duct

Sebaceous
Gland

Mammary Lobule

Subcutaneous Fat

Intercostal Nerve IV

Intercostal Nerve III

Lobule

Duct

Intercostal Nerve V

Nipple

Lactiferous Duct

Nipple Openings

Areola

Nipple

Tubercles of Montgomery

Side view of lactating breast. (Illustration by Ka Botzis.)

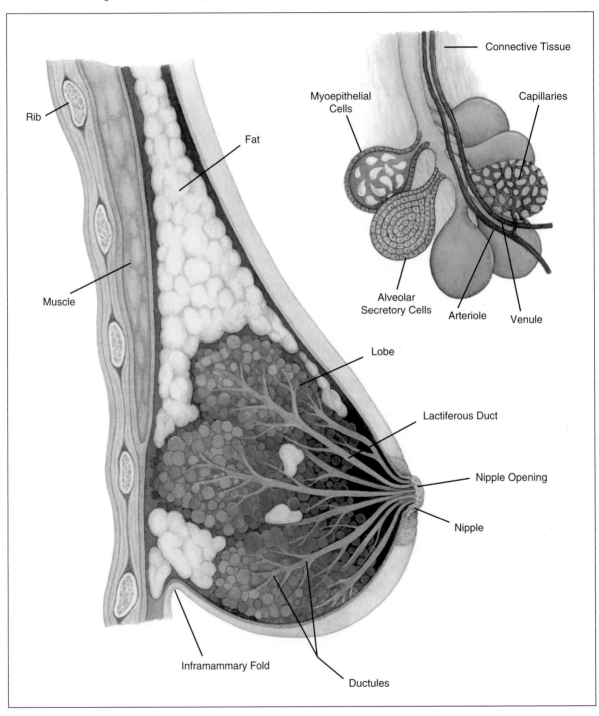

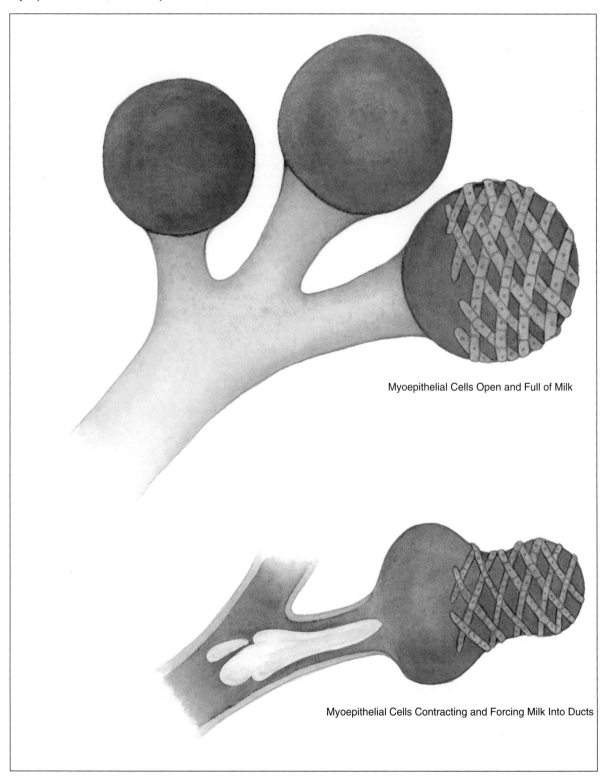

Myoepithelial Cells Open and Full of Milk

Myoepithelial Cells Contracting and Forcing Milk Into Ducts

BALT and GALT migration. B cells originate in the epithelium of the mother's intestinal tract or respiratory tract. These B-cell lymphocytes are sensitized by microbial antigens from bacteria in the mother's intestines and activated by a chemical from T-cell lymphocytes. The sensitized B cells migrate to the mother's breast by a special "homing" system (GALT or BALT) described in the text. Once there, they can secrete IgA that enters into breastmilk. When the infant consumes the milk, it coats his intestinal walls, providing protection. The B-cell lymphocytes can also travel in milk to the baby and secrete IgA antibodies in the infant's own intestinal tract. Either way, the infant has secretory IgA antibodies against the specific bacteria he will most likely encounter in his environment. (Based on an illustration by Ka Botzis.)

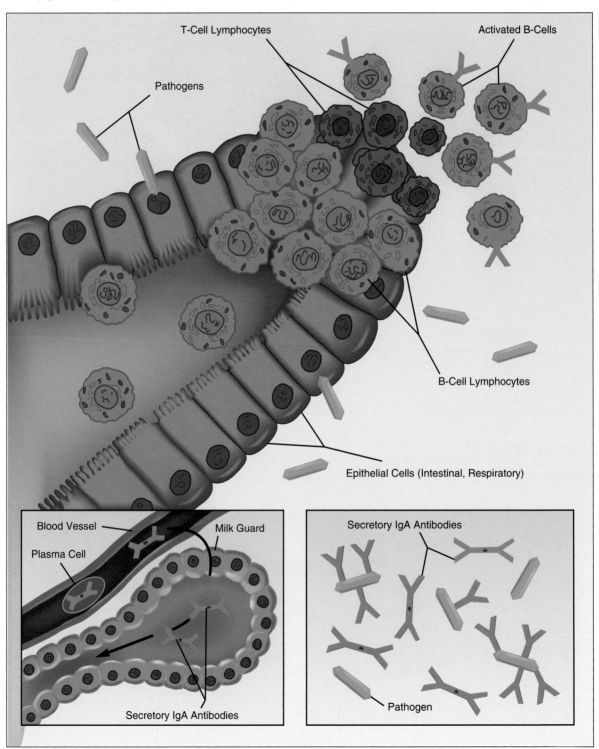

COLOR PLATE 5

Nipple bruised and cracked from poor positioning. This trauma occurred on postpartum day 1. It was corrected by lifting the baby out of the mother's lap and into her arms and turning the baby so that his entire body faced the mother.

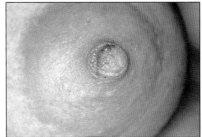

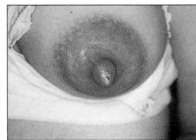

COLOR PLATE 6

Sore nipple with trauma from poor positioning. The white streak across the face of the nipple is a sign that the baby's lower jaw was too close to the tip of the nipple. Positioning the baby centrally across the mother's torso resulted in the baby driving his chin in closer to the breast rather than to the nipple. (Photo with permission from Barbara Wilson-Clay.)

COLOR PLATE 7

Nipple fissure that resulted from use of a poorly designed breast pump for three days. Even short-term use of a poorly designed pump can cause significant nipple damage. (Photo with permission of Catherine Watson Genna.)

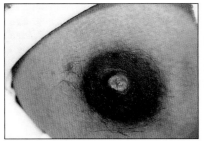

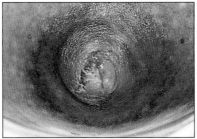

COLOR PLATE 8

Badly cracked nipple with possible bacterial infection. Such trauma can become an entry point for bacterial invasion and subsequent inflammation or infection. (Photo with permission of Kay Hoover.)

COLOR PLATE 9

Extreme engorgement. Engorgement occurred 30 to 36 hours postpartum, secondary to ineffective and infrequent breastfeeding and no expression or pumping when the infant did not obtain milk. (With permission from Chele Marmet/ Lactation Institute.)

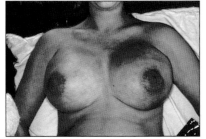

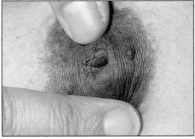

COLOR PLATE 10

Abraded folded nipple. The abrasion occurred when the nipple tissue remained wet between feedings; air-drying after each breastfeeding resolved the problem.

COLOR PLATE 11

Milk plugs at nipple pores, often characterized by acute pain. When milk is released from the duct, relief is immediate.

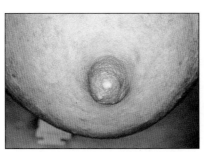

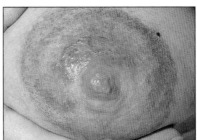

COLOR PLATE 12

Candidiasis **(thrush) of the breast.** This mother experienced four separate episodes in which her breasts, but not the baby's mouth, were treated. Within one week of simultaneous treatment of mother and baby, neither the baby's mouth nor the mother's breasts were infected.

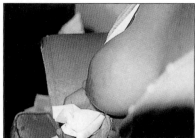

COLOR PLATE 13

Breast abscess prior to excision. A breast abscess will often present with generalized redness. When the affected area is palpated, it is hot and hard to the touch. (Photo with permission from Barbara Wilson-Clay.)

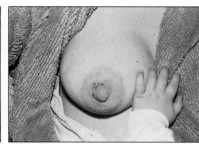

COLOR PLATE 14

Herpes on the areola. A thirteen-month-old nursing toddler contracted oral herpes by using a playmate's contaminated rattle; the mother was then infected. The breast lesion appeared soon after the baby's infection was identified. (With permission from Chele Marmet/Lactation Institute.)

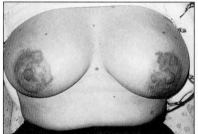

COLOR PLATE 15

Psoriasis of the nipples. Although previous lesions had occurred on her breasts (but never on her nipples or areolae), this mother developed psoriasis on her nipples within a week of her baby's birth. When the baby latched on at the beginning of each breastfeeding session, she felt pain, which gradually subsided as the feeding progressed. (Photo with permission of Karen Foard.)

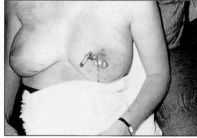

COLOR PLATE 16

Breast abscess with iodoform gauze drain in place; the safety pin is not holding the drain in place. (Photo with permission of Donna Corrieri.)

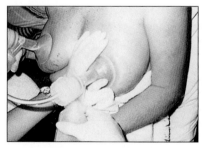

COLOR PLATE 17

Pumping the breast following abscess drainage. When a mother cannot put a baby to breast following treatment for a breast abscess, pumping may be necessary. The LC's gloved hand is placing gentle, even pressure over the area of the abscess drain to create a seal, in order to pump both breasts simultaneously and comfortably. (Photo with permission from Donna Corrieri.)

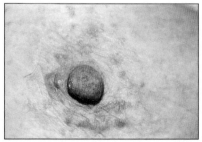

COLOR PLATE 18

Poison ivy on the areola. (Photo with permission of Kay Hoover.)

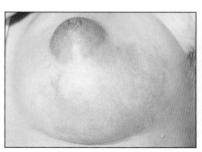

COLOR PLATE 19

Mastitis involving the lower outer quadrant of the breast. The mother was placed on intravenous antibiotics in the hospital, and lactation continued throughout the IV therapy. Her baby was housed with her during her hospitalization.

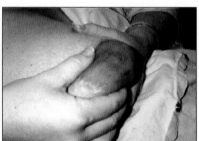

COLOR PLATE 20

This mother is displacing breast edema (different from engorgement) by applying pressure from the areola backwards toward the chest wall, rotating the fingers around the "clock" and moving back, holding the pressure until the tissue becomes soft. The procedure can take a few minutes to 30 minutes depending on the severity of the edema.

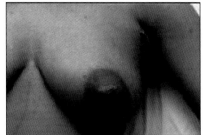

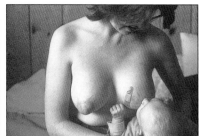

COLOR PLATE 22

Breastfeeding following biopsy for a benign tumor. The mother, with a totally breastfed infant, is shown four months postpartum. The tumor was discovered during lactation two weeks prior to biopsy. The baby is breastfeeding four hours after biopsy, the mother keeping the baby's hand away from the biopsy incision area. (With permission from Chele Marmet/Lactation Institute.)

COLOR PLATE 23

Nipple inversion. The mother had successfully breastfed her previous baby using both breasts.

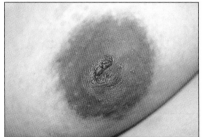

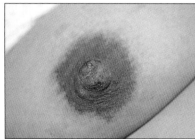

COLOR PLATE 24

Nipple eversion. Following gentle suction with a hand breast pump, the nipple completely everted.

COLOR PLATE 25

Burn scars on breast. This mother sustained third-degree burns as a child and experienced numerous subsequent reconstructive surgeries, including one to reconstruct her nipples. Although the breast tissue was difficult to compress because of extensive scar tissue, the baby was able to breastfeed.

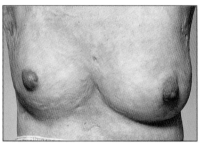

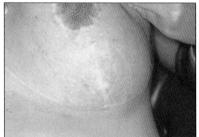

COLOR PLATE 26

Breast-reduction scars. This mother had breast surgery at age 28, two years before her first pregnancy; her bra size changed from a 32HH to a 36B prior to her first pregnancy. The nipples were not entirely detached, but both areolae were reduced in size and repositioned on the breast. Following surgery, the left breast had heightened sensation; the right nipple had no sensation at all. Some milk was obtained from each breast. (With permission from Chele Marmet/Lactation Institute.)

COLOR PLATE 27

Significantly different breast size and shape, suggestive of primary breast insufficiency; this mother was referred for a lactation consultation for her inadequate milk supply. (Photo with permission from Kay Hoover.)

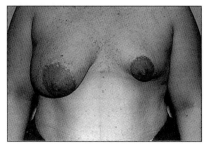

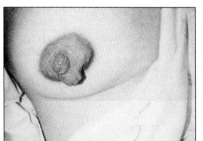

COLOR PLATE 28

Double nipple on the same breast. This mother's baby needed to gape widely enough to take both nipples into his mouth. (Photo with permission of Linda Stewart.)

Staph infection (impetigo). Raised red pimple-like "bumps," cracking at nipple base with yellow crusting at nipple tips. (Photo with permission from Vonie Miller.)

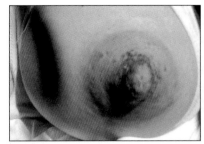

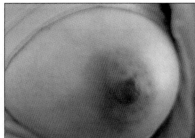

Vasospasm and skin tag. This nipple demonstrates the purple phase of color change associated with nipple vasospasm. An incidental finding is the small skin tag seen between 12 to 1 o'clock. (Photo with permission from Nancy Powers.)

Late preterm infant. Late preterm infants are placed on the regular postpartum unit with their mothers. Most late preterm infants require more time and effort to help them breastfeed because they are smaller and less mature neurologically.

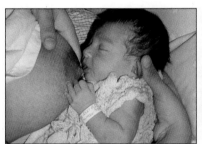

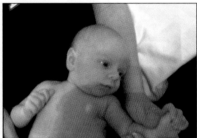

Torticollis, head turned to left. This infant with congenital muscular torticollis shows several classic findings shown in plates 41 through 43. The shortened and tightened sternocleidomastoid muscle causes the infant routinely to assume a "position of comfort" with his head tilted and turned to the left. Often there will be secondary changes to the shape of the skull, positional plaigiocephaly. (Photo with permission from Nancy Powers.)

Torticollis, jaw to side. In this photo, the same infant demonstrates obvious jaw asymmetry, with the left side slanting more acutely toward the ear while the right side is rounder and fuller. This is caused by the pressure of the baby's face and jaw against the left shoulder in utero. It will usually be accompanied by asymmetry of the gums as well.

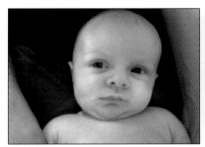

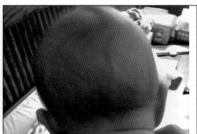

Torticollis, left ear out. The same infant as in the previous two photos demonstrates the left ear protruding further from the skull than the right side. It is also slightly larger. Compression of the ear against the shoulder in utero is responsible for overgrowth of the ear. This finding is most easily appreciated from the posterior view.

Nipple healing. (A) Day 1. Nipple skin condition the day of delivery before breastfeeding had commenced. Note the white flecks on the skin. (B) Day 3. Two small areas that appear to be blisters can be noted at the 7 o'clock position. (C) Day 5. A fissure on the nipple skin and eschar formation can be seen. (D) Day 7. Eschar remains adhered to the surface of the nipple. Nipple condition improved. (Magnification factor of 22.) (Used with permission from Ziemer M, Pidgeon J. Skin changes and pain in the nipple during the first week of lactation. *JOGNN*. 1993; 22:247–256.)

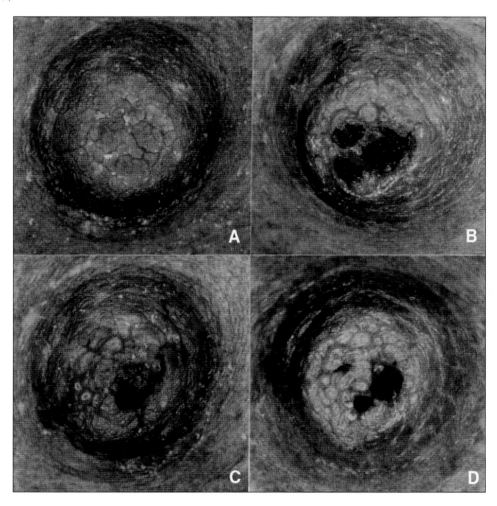

Large nipples. Unusually large nipples can cause latch on problems at first but tend to resolve as the baby grows. (Photo with permission of Barbara Wilson-Clay and Kay Hoover.)

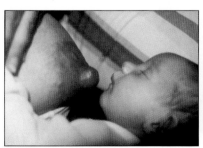

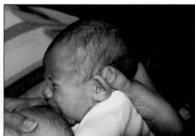

Gagging due to large nipple. Large nipples can cause gagging in early breastfeeds until the baby matures.

COLOR PLATE 47

Inverted nipple. This patient has bilateral significantly inverted nipples that evert during milk expression with a breast pump, but immediately return to the inverted state. In this photo, the right nipple/areolar complex is erythematous from pumping her breastmilk postpartum. (Photo with permission of Nancy Powers.)

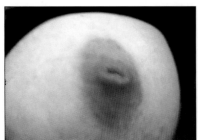

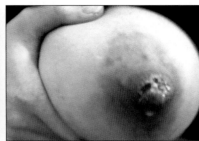

COLOR PLATE 48

Deep crack in inverted nipple. The same patient as previous photo show a deep crack on the left nipple that would not heal because the inversion kept the tissue "buried" without air or light. The nipple everted only immediately after applying the breast pump. (Photo with permission of Nancy Powers.)

COLOR PLATE 49

A large pigmented lesion appears on the areola to the left of the nipple. The referring clinician was uncertain what to recommend.

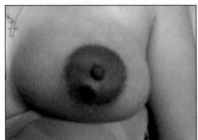

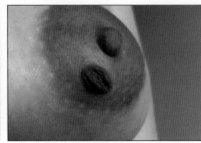

COLOR PLATE 50

Upon closer inspection, the lesion appears soft and deflated, but will erect with tactile stimulation. This lesion was surgically removed during pregnancy to help avoid interference with breastfeeding. It is a large supernumerary nipple.

COLOR PLATE 51

Tongue-tie. (Photo with permission from Linda Smith.)

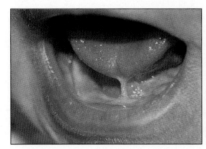

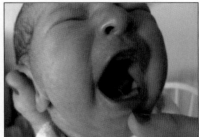

COLOR PLATE 52

Side view of tongue-tie. Exists in many variations. Accordingly, tongue movement and suckling ability can present with a variety of different clinical effects for mother and/or baby. (Photo with permission of Nancy Powers.)

COLOR PLATE 53

Normal yellow, frothy stool of exclusively breastfed baby at two months old.

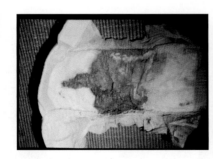

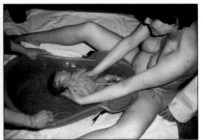

COLOR PLATE 54

Natural birth.

Breastfeeding the Preterm Infant

Nancy M. Hurst and Paula P. Meier

BREASTFEEDING AND BREAST MILK are the standard to which all other forms of infant nutrition are compared. Advances in neonatal care have resulted in the survival of very preterm (less than 32 weeks gestation) infants, presenting a challenging context for the establishment of breastfeeding. The importance of human milk in the management of preterm infants is well recognized (Gartner et al., 2005) and has been reported to improve host defenses, digestion and absorption of nutrients, gastrointestinal function, neurodevelopmental outcomes, and enhanced maternal psychological well-being (Schanler, 2001). Yet mothers of preterm infants encounter numerous, well-documented barriers to breastfeeding that are not experienced by mothers of healthy term infants (Callen et al., 2005; Meier, 2001).

To improve these breastfeeding outcomes, clinicians must use research-based strategies that target specific barriers to breastfeeding initiation and duration for mothers and their preterm infants. Numerous scientific reports have focused on delineating and studying these barriers in order to develop strategies to optimize breastfeeding outcomes (Baker & Rasmussen, 1997; Blaymore Bier et al., 1997; Cregan et al., 2002; Hedberg Nyqvist, & Ewald, 1999; Hurst, Myatt, & Schanler, 1998; Jaeger,

Lawson, & Filteau, 1997; Jones & Spencer, 2007; Killerstreiter et al., 2001; Nyqvist, Sjoden, & Ewald, 1999; Ortenstrand et al., 2001; Pietschnig et al., 2000; Pinelli, Atkinson, & Saigal, 2001; Lau et al., 2003; Wheeler et al., 1999). Compared to term infants, preterm infants have maturity-dependent physiologic and metabolic differences that require integration. Similarly, mothers of preterm infants experience unique physiologic and emotional challenges, such as maintaining lactation for several weeks, and coping with extreme vulnerability about infant intake during breastfeeding.

Suitability of Human Milk for Preterm Infants

Evidence for the benefits of human milk feeding for preterm infants continues to accumulate (Table 13–1). Specific bioactive factors, such as secretory IgA, lactoferrin, lysozyme, oligosaccharides, nucleotides, cytokines, growth factors, enzymes, antioxidants, and cellular components present in human milk have been implicated in reports of decreased rates of infections in premature infants fed human milk compared with those fed commercial formula (Akisu et al., 1998; Bernt & Walker, 1999; Hamosh, 2001; Hylander, Strobino, &

Dhanireddy, 1998; Newburg, Ruiz-Palacios, & Morrow, 2005; Newburg & Walker, 2007; Paramasivam et al., 2006; Schanler, Shulman, & Lau, 1999) Gastrointestinal effects of feeding human milk include enhanced intestinal lactase activity (Shulman et al., 1998b), more rapid gastric emptying (Ewer et al., 1994), and a decrease in intestinal permeability early in life (Shulman et al., 1998a), compared with preterm formula. The feeding of human milk has been associated with improved cognitive and motor development at 3, 7, 12, 18, and 30 months (Bier et al., 2002; Vohr et al., 2006, 2007; Wang et al., 2003), greater intellectual performance scores at 7.5 to 8.0 years of age (Lucas, Morley, & Cole, 1998), and faster brainstem maturation (Amin et al., 2000) compared with formula-feeding in former preterm infants. Human milk-fed infants have been found to have enhanced visual acuity (Birch

et al., 1993; Birch et al., 1992; Jorgensen et al., 1996; Uauy & Hoffman, 2000) and less incidence and severity of retinopathy of prematurity (Hylander et al., 2001) compared to preterm formula-fed infants—possibly due to the presence of very long-chain polyunsaturated fatty acids and antioxidant activity in human milk (Koletzko et al., 2001). Finally, the provision of the mother's own milk to her infant allows the mother a distinct role in the care of her infant, at a time when many of the infant's needs are met by the nursing and medical neonatal intensive care unit (NICU) staff.

Studies comparing human milk composition of mothers delivering prematurely compared to those delivering at term have shown specific differences, at least during the first few weeks, following delivery (Gross et al., 1980). The higher concentrations in preterm compared to term milk of several

 TABLE 13–1 **Benefits of Human Milk Feeding for Preterm Infants**

Host Defense

- Cellular functions (Blumer, Pfefferle, & Renz, 2007; Garofalo & Goldman, 1998; Hanson, 1999)
- Bioactive factors (Akisu et al., 1998; Bernt & Walker, 1999; Henderson et al., 2001; Newburg, Ruiz-Palacios, & Morrow, 2005; Newburg & Walker, 2007)
  - Secretory IgA (Eibl et al., 1988; Paramasivam et al., 2006)
  - Cytokines (Fituch et al., 2001; Ustundag et al., 2005)
  - Lactoferrin (Fituch et al., 2004; Goldblum et al., 1989; Hutchens, Henry, & Yip, 1991; van der Strate et al., 2001; Ward, Paz, & Conneely, 2005)
- Enzymes (Henderson et al., 2001)
- Reduced risk and severity of morbidities (Contreras-Lemus et al., 1992; Furman et al., 2003; Hylander, Strobino, & Dhanireddy, 1998; Hylander et al., 2001; Kosloske, 2001; Lucas & Cole, 1990; Schanler, Shulman, & Lau, 1999)

Gastrointestinal

- Hormones (Armand et al., 1996; Elmlinger et al., 2007)
- Lactase activity (Kunz & Rudloff, 1993; Shulman et al., 1998b)
- Growth factors (Diaz-Gomez, Domenech, & Barroso, 1997; Sangild et al., 2002)
  - Epidermal growth factor (Xiao et al., 2002)
  - Insulin-like growth factors (Elmlinger et al., 2007)
- Improved feeding tolerance (Aggett et al., 2006; Moody et al., 2000; Schanler et al., 1999; Schmolzer et al., 2006; Shulman et al., 1998b)

(Continues)

TABLE 13–1	Benefits of Human Milk Feeding for Preterm Infants (Continued)

Nutrition

- Amino acids (Moro et al., 1989; van den Berg et al., 2005)
- Lipid profile (Charpak & Ruiz, 2007; Genzel-Boroviczeny, Wahle, & Koletzko, 1997; Heird, 2001; Peterson et al., 1998; Saarela, Kokkonen, & Koivisto, 2005)
- Antioxidants (Korchazhkina et al., 2006; Shoji & Koletzko, 2007)
- Glutamine, taurine (Bernt & Walker, 1999; Rassin et al., 1983; van den Berg et al., 2005)

Neurodevelopment

- Omega-3 fatty acids (Farquharson et al., 1995; Heird, 2001; Lauritzen et al., 2005; Luukkainen et al., 1995)
- Cholesterol (Boehm et al., 1995; Singhal et al., 2004; Woltil et al., 1995)
- Improved visual acuity (Birch et al., 1993; Birch et al., 1992; Jorgensen et al., 1996; Uauy et al., 1992; Uauy & Hoffman, 2000)
- Enhanced neurocognitive outcomes (Amin et al., 2000; Bier et al., 2002; Lucas, Morley, & Cole, 1998; Lucas et al., 1994; Vohr et al., 2006, 2007; Wang et al., 2003)
- Maternal/infant bonding (Aguayo, 2001; Flacking, Ewald, & Starrin, 2007a; Hildebrandt & Gundert-Remy, 1983; Wheeler et al., 1999)

components, including sIgA and other anti-infective properties (Ballabio et al., 2007; Britton, 1986; de Ferrer et al., 2000); oligosaccharides (Miller et al., 1994); protein (Butte et al., 1984); fat (Luukkainen, Salo, & Nikkari, 1994); sodium, chloride, and iron (Lemons et al., 1982; Torres et al., 2006), has led some to speculate that the mother adapts to the higher needs of her preterm infant. Yet more recent studies examining the influence of gestational age at delivery and duration of lactation on the changing macronutrient composition of preterm milk theorize that these compositional differences are a result of the interruption of the gestational developmental processes occurring in the mammary gland (Maas et al., 1998). Whatever the etiology of these compositional differences, the clinical significance of these gestationally dependent differences in milk composition is apparent when short- and long-term health outcomes are compared for preterm infants receiving either human milk or formula-feedings. These outcomes, summarized in Table 13–1, suggest that human milk may provide optimal "nutritional programming" for preterm infants and may be protective against several prematurity-related health conditions

(Dvorak et al., 2003; Furman et al., 2003; Schanler & Atkinson, 1999; Schmolzer et al., 2006).

Yet despite these profound benefits, studies have shown the rate of linear growth and bone mineralization is negatively affected in preterm infants fed unfortified human milk (Nicholl & Gamsu, 1999; Schanler, Shulman, & Lau, 1999). Commercial fortifiers providing mineral supplementation of mother's own milk have shown a normalization of these indices (Kuschel & Harding, 2000; Schanler, 1998). Given these findings, current recommendations include the provision of fortified mother's own milk as the preferred feeding for preterm infants (Arslanoglu, Moro, & Ziegler, 2006; Canadian Pediatric Society (CPS), 1995; Schanler, 2001).

Mothers of Preterm Infants

A focus on the experiences of mothers of preterm infants reveals a time-dependent process involving varying degrees of alienation and separation from her infant (Jackson, Ternestedt, & Schollin, 2003), powerlessness related to her infant's daily care needs (Bialoskurski, Cox, & Wiggins, 2002), and a delay in her transition to motherhood (Flacking, Ewald, &

Starrin, 2007b; Shin & White-Traut, 2007). The ability to provide her breastmilk and breastfeed has been described as a contribution to infant care that only the mother can make and as one aspect of care that does not have to be forfeited in the event of preterm birth. These clinical impressions are confirmed in several qualitative studies of mothers of preterm infants interviewed during their infant's hospitalization (Bernaix et al., 2006; Sweet, 2006) and following (Flacking, Ewald, & Starrin, 2007b; Kavanaugh et al., 1997). These women, who received research-based in-hospital breastfeeding services (Meier et al., 1993), reported that "the rewards outweigh the efforts" in describing their breastfeeding experiences during the first month that their infants were home.

The mothers from Kavanaugh's study (1997) delineated and exemplified five rewards of breastfeeding their preterm infants. Most frequently reported was "knowing that they had given their infants a good start in life," with references to the health benefits of breastfeeding for premature babies followed by the mothers' enjoyment of the physical closeness and intimacy of breastfeeding, and their perception that their infants "preferred" the breast to bottle-feedings of expressed milk. A fourth reward was "making a unique contribution to infant care," but mothers circumscribed this reward to the NICU stay, when other caretaking opportunities were limited. Finally, the mothers felt that, even with the extra effort of feeding and continued milk expression in the home, breastfeeding was "convenient" for them.

Mothers of very preterm infants in various geographic and cultural environments reveal an incongruity related to their breastfeeding expectations and the realities they faced within the context of the NICU experience. Australian mothers viewed their expressed breast milk as an object, more easily scrutinized and examined by herself and others (Sweet, 2006). Swedish mothers described emotional swings from exhaustion to relief, secure to insecure, and viewing breastfeeding as reciprocal as well as nonreciprocal (Flacking, Ewald, & Starrin, 2007b). These altered expectations were validated in a cohort of women in a Midwestern United States NICU (Bernaix et al., 2006). Yet the process of breastfeeding and providing breast milk for their infants was universally described as an experience that strengthened the bonds between mother and preterm infant.

Thus, the literature suggests that breastfeeding and the provision of breast milk affords unique advantages for this vulnerable population that are in addition to the health benefits of breastfeeding for mothers of term healthy infants. These important findings provide scientific justification for the allocation of resources to improve breastfeeding outcomes for this vulnerable population.

Rates of Breastfeeding Initiation and Duration

Although breastfeeding statistics vary for individual countries, worldwide data suggest that mothers of preterm infants initiate and sustain breastfeeding at rates lower than the general population (Furman, Minich, & Hack, 1998; Jaeger, Lawson, & Filteau, 1997). Several conclusions and practice priorities can be drawn from this body of research.

First, breastfeeding initiation rates appear to be increasing for this population (Adams et al., 2001; Wagner et al., 2002), presumably because promotion efforts have made mothers aware of the health benefits of human milk. Second, the duration of breastfeeding for mothers and preterm infants is typically shorter than the mothers' initial goals. Third, rates for breastfeeding initiation and duration can be improved if mothers are provided with research-based, comprehensive breastfeeding services. Thus, a prerequisite for research and practice is to address the documented barriers to breastfeeding for mothers of preterm infants through the use of evidence-based strategies.

Research-Based Lactation Support Services

Research demonstrates that counseling mothers of preterm infants (regardless of their initial feeding intentions) increased the incidence of lactation initiation and breastmilk feeding without increasing maternal stress and anxiety (Miracle, Meier, & Bennett, 2004; Sisk et al., 2006). Several publications have provided models for provision of breastfeeding services in the NICU (Hurst, Myatt, & Schanler, 1998; Jones, 1995; Meier et al., 1993, 2004; Spatz, 2005), and included specific interventions within a four-phase temporal model: expression and collection of mothers' milk; gavage feeding of mothers' milk; in-hospital breastfeeding; and postdischarge breastfeeding management. A central feature of this model is that breastfeeding services are directed or coordinated by a nurse and/or physician with expertise in both lactation and intensive preterm infant care.

Making an Informed Decision

All mothers who are hospitalized for preterm labor should be approached by a health professional to provide specific infant feeding information. Emphasizing the importance of sharing research-based health benefits of breastfeeding with parents allows for an informed decision about feeding method (Meier, 2001; Meier & Brown, 1997; Rodriguez, Miracle, & Meier, 2005). If the mother has already given birth, breastfeeding should be discussed as soon after delivery as the mother is able to converse. The clinician should use specific information about the baby—such as maturity or health condition—and share with the mother research-based information that is relevant to her baby's situation.

Alternatives to Exclusive, Long-Term Breastfeeding

Many mothers, especially those who had not intended to breastfeed, remain indecisive or reluctant to begin milk expression if they feel they must make a commitment to exclusive breastfeeding for several months. Additionally, healthcare providers or family members may have advised them that breastfeeding is "too much" for them at a time when they are consumed with discomfort, anxiety, stress, and fatigue. These women should be encouraged to begin milk expression immediately after birth when the hormonal milieu is optimal so their infants can receive colostrum. Mothers should be told that they can cease milk expression at any time if they desire, and that professional help is available to help them discontinue pumping.

When women are indecisive and their initial plans include a day-by-day commitment to breastfeeding, several issues can help women make these important choices. For example, mothers who are unenthusiastic about pumping often ask how long they must provide milk for their infants. The practitioner can use infant milestones to place these

recommendations in a more pragmatic timeframe for the mother. For example, a mother can be told that the most important time for the preterm infant is the introduction and advancement of early feedings, and that her colostrum is ideal for this purpose. This translates into milk expression for approximately 1 week. The clinician can add that providing milk until term-corrected age for the infant is especially beneficial because of the unique nature of the lipids in preterm milk. Most mothers are willing to consider short-term "contracts" of this nature when they understand the day-by-day importance of their milk for their infant.

Some mothers will express milk with a breast pump, but do not want to feed their infants at the breast. The practitioner can introduce this option by stating: "Some women decide that they will use a breast pump to express milk and then feed it to their babies by bottle. Is this something that you would consider?" This approach informs mothers and reassures them that other women have chosen this option.

When the mother of a preterm infant selects an alternative to exclusive, long-term breastfeeding, the breastfeeding specialist and NICU staff must not imply that her choice is "second best." Instead, the previously indecisive mother should be praised for her commitment and respected for her choice. The mother should be made aware of resources to help her if she changes her breastfeeding goals in the future.

Models for Hospital-Based Lactation Support Services

A variety of hospital-based breastfeeding support services have been developed in recent years and serve as models for clinical areas choosing to improve their services. The Lactation Support Program and Mother's Own Milk Bank at Texas Children's Hospital in Houston was established in 1984 to provide support to mothers of hospitalized infants and improved quality control in the handling of expressed breast milk (Hurst, Myatt, & Schanler, 1998). Registered nurses with additional certification in lactation management provide mothers and their infants with instruction and support in milk volume maintenance and breastfeeding. The Mother's Milk Club at Rush-Presbyterian

Hospital in Chicago utilizes a peer-support group model in providing breastfeeding support to mothers of hospitalized, preterm infants (Meier, 2001). Mothers meet once a week to discuss issues related to breast pumping, expressed breast milk feeding, and initiation and progression of breastfeeding in the hospital and postdischarge. This support extends into the neonatal unit where mothers assist each other in their breastfeeding efforts. Similar mother-to-mother support groups have reported effective results in reducing maternal stress and greater perceived social support (Preyde & Ardal, 2003). Trained peer counselors utilized in the NICU and posthospitalization have also been shown to improve breastfeeding outcomes (Agrasada et al., 2005; Merewood et al., 2006).

Regardless of the model or combination of approaches used in a specific clinical environment, without the provision of evidence-based rationale for specific lactation management and breastfeeding policies and procedures to all staff involved, compliance will be less than optimal. Specifically, this information should include factual verbal and written materials and alternatives to exclusive, long-term breastfeeding for women who do not want to make these commitments. Establishing early in the neonatal period the mother's feeding plans and goals will allow for individualized strategies to ensure that these goals are realized and to allow for timely modifications when warranted.

Finally, a primary source of support for breastfeeding can be provided from other family members. A qualitative study examined the management styles observed in breastfeeding families of preterm infants (Krouse, 2002). Families were described as facilitating (positive and proactive), maintaining (passive and adaptive), or obstructing (negative and feeling out of control) in their management styles related to breastfeeding. Although this small sample of families received intensive breastfeeding support services, the diversity in management styles observed highlights the complexity in providing effective interventions to assist mothers in meeting their breastfeeding goals.

Initiation of Mechanical Milk Expression

Mothers of preterm infants must initiate and maintain lactation with a breast pump until their infants are able to regulate intake from the breast.

The pump-dependent state experienced by these mothers adds to their burdensome schedule and may last several weeks to several months. Mothers need research-based instruction and emotional support to persevere with their breastfeeding goals during this time.

Principles of Milk Expression

Little is known about the differences, if any, in the physiologic responses of maternal lactation following preterm compared to term gestation, or the effects of the NICU environment. Few studies have focused on the mother's physiologic response to exclusive, long-term breast pump use (Chatterton et al., 2000; Cregan et al., 2002; Hartmann & Cregan, 2001). Thus, the principles of lactation that have been studied for the healthy population are commonly applied to the mother who initiates and maintains lactation with a breast pump. Although giving birth prematurely does not appear to limit milk production, several factors surrounding the birth experience—prolonged bed rest, maternal complications, fatigue, stress, and irregular breast emptying—are documented prolactin inhibitors and can adversely affect milk volume. In high-risk pregnancies, a variety of conditions may exist that alter the normal progression and hormonal responses characteristic to pregnancy. A shortened gestation may prevent specific hormones to reach their maximum levels and therefore alter, delay, or prevent the normal onset of lactogenesis. Speculatively, a shortened gestation may result in a blunted or minimized response in the oxytocin, prolactin, and opiate effects on the maternal brain. Additionally, the immediate and prolonged separation of the mother from her preterm infant limits the close, physical contact associated with the stimulation of these lactogenic hormones (Carter & Altemus, 1997; Uvnas-Moberg, 1998).

The available research supports the practice of beginning milk expression with a hospital-grade electric breast pump as early as possible after delivery (Hill, 1999; Hopkinson, 1988). Factors shown to optimize milk yield include frequent milk expression of adequate duration to promote complete breast emptying (Hill, Aldag, & Chatterton, 2001). Clinically, advising mothers to express milk more frequently (e.g., 8–10 times daily) during the first week to 10 days postbirth may result in a milk volume approximating 750–1000 ml per day. Theoretically this practice may stimulate mammary alveolar growth during a time when circulating lactogenic hormones are elevated (Bialoskurski, Cox, & Wiggins, 2002). Some (Groh-Wargo et al., 1995) but not all studies (Fewtrell et al., 2001; Hill, Aldag, & Chatterton, 1999) have shown an advantage to simultaneous compared to sequential breast pumping. The predictors for risk of insufficient milk production at week 12 postpartum among mothers of preterm infants include multiple birth, week 6 inadequate milk supply, maternal age younger than 29 years, and intended length of lactation less than 34 weeks (Hill et al., 2007).

Selecting a Breast Pump

Studies by Hartmann and colleagues have provided objective determination of major parameters of breast pump efficacy, namely time to milk ejection, amount of milk removed, and rate of milk removal (Aljazaf et al., 2003; Daly et al., 1993; Daly et al., 1996). Mothers who initiate long-term milk expression need a hospital-grade electric breast pump and, as some studies have demonstrated (Hill et al., 1999; Slusher et al., 2007), may benefit from a double-collection kit.

The clinical challenge is ensuring that these breast pumps are available to mothers who need them. These pumps may be rented through pharmacies, lactation consultants, and home health agencies, but low-income mothers may be unable to incur the rental expense. A letter, such as the one in Figure 13–1, should be prepared on hospital letterhead, signed by a neonatologist and/or the NICU lactation specialist, and given to mothers for reimbursement purposes. Even with such a letter, the rental expense may be rejected by third-party payers, with an explanation that the mother can use a less expensive battery-operated model or that breastfeeding is "elective," and formula-feeding is cheaper.

It is helpful to have a packet of research-based materials, such as the following documents, that parents can use to challenge these decisions:

- An official letter on institutional letterhead that is specific to the infant's condition and the mother's breastfeeding needs
- Research reports that demonstrate the superiority of electric breast pumps (Becker, McCormick, Renfrew, 2008)

- Official statements and/or data that endorse the importance and health outcomes of human milk feeding for preterm infants (such as the American Academy of Pediatrics)

Milk Expression Technique

The mother's milk expression technique can influence the composition and bacterial content of her milk. Lipids provide at least 50% of the calories in human milk, and lipid concentration increases over a single milk expression (Daly et al., 1993; Woodward, Rees, & Boon, 1989). The last few drops of milk are very high in lipid, and can contribute a substantial proportion of the calories in the entire milk sample. Mothers should be advised of this relationship and encouraged to continue pumping until milk ceases to flow. Generally, 10–15 minutes of pumping per session is sufficient, but this may vary from woman to woman, and once lactation is established, some mothers may find that less time is required to achieve breast emptying.

The distribution of lipid in expressed milk is uneven in not only changing fat content as the breast is emptied, but also because milk fat (cream) rises to the top on the storage container after expression. Mothers should be advised to mix the milk thoroughly but gently before distributing into sterile storage containers. If the milk is not mixed, the infant can receive feedings with markedly different fat and caloric values, affecting metabolic processes and overall weight gain (Valentine, Hurst, & Schanler, 1994). An exception to this principle is the intentional feeding of hindmilk only, which is discussed later in this chapter.

Milk Expression Schedule

The actual number of daily milk expressions will depend upon each mother's breastfeeding goals. Mothers who need to produce maximal volumes of milk to achieve their goals should plan to express milk eight times per day. Included in this group are women who want to breastfeed exclusively at the time of infant discharge, provide hindmilk for infant feedings, and/or have given birth to multiples. Mothers who plan to provide milk for a limited time, such as until an infant's expected birth date, or those who plan to combine formula and

RUSH-PRESBYTERIAN-ST. LUKE'S MEDICAL CENTER   1653 WEST CONGRESS PARKWAY, CHICAGO, ILLINOIS 60612-3833 • 312.942.6640
RUSH UNIVERSITY   RUSH MEDICAL COLLEGE

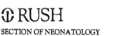

SECTION OF NEONATOLOGY
DEPARTMENT OF PEDIATRICS

Date

Insured:

Policy Number:

Re: Electric Breast Pump Rental

To Whom It May Concern:

Dr. _____, a neonatologist in the Special Care Nursery at
Rush-Presbyterian-St. Luke's Medical Center has prescribed human milk feedings for
_____, who was born on _____,and whose parents are
_____. Because this infant is too small and/or ill to feed
at the breast, the mother must remove her milk with an electric breast pump, store it, and
transport it to the Special Care Nursery so that it can be fed to her infant using a gavage tube.

A hospital grade electric breast pump with a double collection kit is necessary for extracting
milk under these circumstances. Randomized controlled trials have shown that manual and/or
battery-operated pumps, intended for occasional use by mothers of healthy infants, are
inadequate for mothers who must initiate and maintain lactation in the absence of a nursing
infant. Although hospital grade electric pumps can be purchased (approximately $900), they are
more economical to rent on a short-term basis. We estimate that this mother will require use
of the pump for approximately _____.

I trust that this information will expedite insurance coverage of the electric pump rental for this
mother and infant. Should there be additional questions, please contact me at the above
address/telephone.

Sincerely,

Paula P. Meier, RN, DNSc, FAAN
NICU Lactation Program Director

FIGURE 13–1   Sample letter to request third-party payment for breast pump.

breastfeeding, can pump less frequently. Instructing "short-term" breastfeeding mothers to express milk more than five or six times daily is unnecessary, and may discourage them from pumping at all.

The NICU staff can modify the nursery environment to enhance the probability that mothers will pump more frequently and consistently. Enabling mothers to remain at their infants' bedside while expressing milk with the electric breast pump (Meier, 2001) promotes frequent stimulation and sends a strong message to the mother regarding the importance placed (by the staff) on providing her milk to her infant. This arrangement also provides an opportunity for the mother to see, touch, or hold her infant while expressing milk. Bedside pumping incorporates the scientific literature on the use of relaxation and imagery in enhancing milk volume (Feher et al., 1989), and is convenient for the mother and staff. Additionally, the expectation that mothers will provide milk while in the NICU highlights their indispensable role in infant care. Anecdotally, mothers have reported that they express more milk at their babies' bedsides, and combined with skin-to-skin care and nonnutritive sucking at the breast, that bedside pumping gives them a purpose for frequent and lengthy NICU visits.

Written Pumping Records

Keeping a written log of pumping frequency and milk volumes expressed allows the mother to monitor her progress. Documenting the time, duration, and amount of milk expressed (Figure 13–2) provides useful information to the mother that can be shared with the NICU staff for assessment of milk volume maintenance. Evaluation of pumping

frequency and milk volumes obtained allows the NICU staff to assist the mother in modifying her pumping schedule (to be explained later) based on her individual milk synthesis rate.

Maintaining Maternal Milk Volume

Expressed Milk Volume Guidelines

An arbitrary guideline categorizing levels of 24-hour milk volume is useful in order to determine the need for appropriate intervention (Box 13–1). Most preterm infants will require at least 500 ml/24 hrs at the time of discharge. Providing specific guidelines

---

PUMPING RECORDS

Your name: _____
Your infant's medical record #_____

Use the table below and on the back of this form to keep track of the date, time, and volume of milk expressed from each breast for every pumping session. Once you complete this record please give it to one of the lactation consultants to make a copy. She can provide you feedback about your milk volume.

Tips for Increasing Your Milk Supply
Pump frequently—at least 6 to 8 times a day.
Massage your breasts before and during pumping.
Rest and sleep whenever you can.
Use relaxation techniques while pumping.
Hold your baby skin to skin whenever possible.

If you have any questions, please contact one of the lactation consultants.

Today's Date: _____

Time of day	Volume from left breast	Volume from right breast	Circle where you pumped
1.			Hospital / Home / Work / Other
2.			Hospital / Home / Work / Other
3.			Hospital / Home / Work / Other
4.			Hospital / Home / Work / Other
5.			Hospital / Home / Work / Other
6.			Hospital / Home / Work / Other
7.			Hospital / Home / Work / Other
8.			Hospital / Home / Work / Other
9.			Hospital / Home / Work / Other

♥ **Only you can provide the wonderful gift of breast milk for your baby** ♥

Texas Children's Hospital

Lactation Support Program, 2003

FIGURE 13–2   Sample of Pumping Records.

will help each mother assess her individual breastfeeding goals and need for more (or less) frequent pumping. As previously mentioned, encouraging mothers to maintain a written pumping record will allow an accurate accounting of each mother's individual milk expression pattern and need for appropriate interventions. In the event that a mother does not achieve a minimum milk volume of 350 ml/24 hrs by 10 to 14 days following delivery, strategies to stimulate milk synthesis should be initiated immediately. Maternal hormonal milieu is believed to confer maximum reponsivity to stimulate lactation during the first few weeks after delivery. Later attempts to increase milk production may be less successful.

Based on research demonstrating the variability from mother to mother regarding the rate of milk synthesis (Daly & Hartmann, 1995b), mothers can be advised that extending the nonpumping interval at night is appropriate or not. Calculating the volume attained at a pumping and dividing that volume by the interval (in hours) between milk expressions provides an estimate of the rate of milk synthesis. Calculating milk synthesis rates over a 24-hour period provides a picture of the mother's overall milk synthesis rate. Milk synthesis rates are calculated by taking the volume obtained divided by the number of hours since the last milk expression (e.g., 90 cc divided by 3 hours = 30 cc/hr). Studies have found that mothers with large milk storage capacities are able to maintain fairly consistent milk synthesis rates despite longer intervals between breast emptying (Kent et al., 1999). This is an invaluable benefit for mothers who must maintain their milk volumes over a long period of time.

Preventing Low Milk Volume

Milk expression guidelines as previously described are based on observational studies demonstrating that mothers who pump early and often following delivery experience higher milk yields (Hill et al., 1999). Yet despite the best efforts of some mothers, persistent low milk volumes occur—or milk production decreases over the many weeks following preterm delivery. Due to the lack of available research little is known about the physiology of long-term milk expression for mothers who are separated from their infants for extended periods following delivery. Therefore, strategies to manage low milk volume for mothers of preterm infants have focused on pharmacologic and nonpharmacologic enhancement of prolactin secretion (Budd et al., 1993; Emery, 1996; Milsom et al., 1998; Novak et al., 2000). Obtaining a thorough history from the mother is vital in order to provide appropriate interventions to manage low milk volume. Information regarding maternal medication use, history of breast surgery, infertility, thyroid conditions, polycystic ovarian syndrome, extended bed rest prior to delivery, and previous breastfeeding experience will provide a clearer picture of potential risk factors and

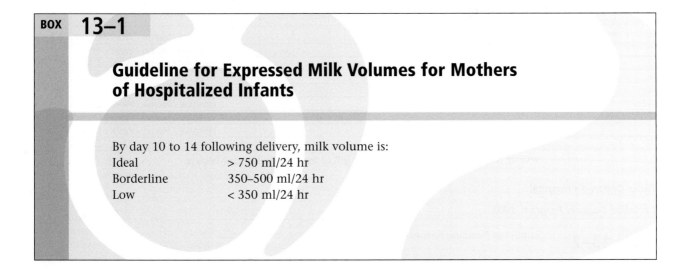

BOX **13–1**

Guideline for Expressed Milk Volumes for Mothers of Hospitalized Infants

By day 10 to 14 following delivery, milk volume is:
Ideal   > 750 ml/24 hr
Borderline   350–500 ml/24 hr
Low   < 350 ml/24 hr

possible effective interventions. Box 13–2 outlines the assessment and strategies to increase low maternal milk volume.

The use of certain maternal medications, including oral contraceptives, may diminish milk volume in mothers of preterm infants who are expressing milk with a breast pump. Although the obstetrician usually advises women that progestin-only contraceptives will not interfere with lactation, the mothers' experiences indicate that this may not be true for a less-established "vulnerable" milk supply. Anecdotally, mothers report that milk volume diminishes markedly within days of starting oral contraceptives, and returns to baseline shortly after they are discontinued. This phenomenon needs to be explored in controlled studies. But in the interim, clinicians should ask about oral contraceptive use if mothers report a rapid decline in a previously adequate volume. Some nonprescription medications,

such as pseudoephedrine (Aljazaf et al., 2003), have been associated with a 30% decrease in maternal milk volume. Since some mothers do not consider oral contraceptives and over-the-counter medications of concern when breastfeeding, it is best to ask about these groups of medications specifically. See Chapter 5 for additional information on medication/contraceptive use in breastfeeding mothers.

Most mothers of preterm infants experience a decrease in milk volume during the second month of milk expression (Hill, Brown, & Harker, 1995; Hurst, Myatt, & Schanler, 1998). Although no published studies have examined the physiology of this phenomenon, data from studies of term infants may offer some insight. Studies (Daly & Hartmann, 1995a,b) have documented that maternal milk volume is limited primarily by infant demand, rather than a finite capacity of the mother to produce milk. These findings suggest that, over days or weeks, the

---

BOX 13–2

Assessment of and Strategies to Increase/Prevent Low Milk Volume

- Obtain lactation risk history (e.g., breast surgery, endocrine disease, previous insufficient lactation).
- Review recent milk expression patterns:
  - Ensure frequent milk expression (> six times per day).
  - Encourage periodic breast massage concurrent with pumping to facilitate breast emptying.
  - Minimize nonpumping intervals of > 6 hours in a 24-hour period.
- Check efficiency/comfort of pump and fit of pump flange.
- Determine maternal medication use (including OTC drugs, birth control pills).

- Consider maternal stress, depression, and sleep deprivation:
  - Recommend 5–6 hours uninterrupted sleep.
  - Strategize ways to minimize steps in pumping routine and activities of daily living.
- Maximize maternal/infant contact:
  - Suggest pumping at the infant's bedside.
  - Encourage frequent and extended skin-to-skin holding of infant.
- Consider initiation of pharmacologic (e.g., metoclopramide, domperidone) or herbal galactogogues (e.g., fenugreek).

milk expression procedure may be ineffective in stimulating an optimal milk supply for mothers of preterm infants. In particular, a breast pump does not mimic the infant's physical closeness and responsiveness that may be essential for optimal hormonal regulation of milk volume. Thus, encouraging infant contact during and after milk expression in the NICU may represent a promising intervention in preventing and improving low milk volume.

Skin-to-Skin Care

Worldwide, studies have documented many benefits of skin-to-skin, or kangaroo, care: promoting physiologic stability in preterm and high-risk infants (Bauer et al., 1997; Bier et al., 1996; Bohnhorst et al., 2001; Browne, 2004; Cattaneo et al., 1998; Charpak et al., 2005; Dodd, 2005; Gazzolo, Masetti, & Meli, 2000; Tornhage et al., 1998; Whitelaw & Liestol, 1994), analgesia during heel sticks (Ludington-Hoe, Hosseini, & Torowicz, 2005), strengthening maternal-infant interaction (Korja et al., 2007), accelerating autonomic and neurobehavioral maturation in the infant (Feldman & Eidelman, 2003), and improving sleep patterns (Ludington-Hoe et al., 2006). Although the relationship between STS care and lactation has been studied less systematically, the duration of breastfeeding appears to be higher for STS infants than for incubator controls (Charpak et al., 2001; Ludington-Hoe et al., 1994). In one study mothers who participated in STS care had a significantly greater increase in milk volume between 2 and 4 weeks than mothers who did not practice STS care (Hurst et al., 1997). Furthermore, Hurst et al. speculated that STS holding may trigger the production of maternal milk antibodies to specific pathogens in the infant's environment through mechanisms in the enteromammary pathway. Additionally, STS holding has been positively correlated with improved maintenance of milk expression as evidenced by continued pumping frequency (Lau et al., 2007).

Mothers whose infants are in STS care have reported observing their infants' rooting and mouthing movements, and moving toward the nipple during STS sessions (Hurst et al., 1997). Mothers frequently note feelings of milk ejection, leaking, and expressing higher milk volumes immediately following STS care. Interestingly, the administration of exogenous oxytocin nasal spray prior to pumping does not result in significant improvement of milk production (Fewtrell et al., 2006). The apparent effects from the release of endogenous oxytocin are validated in studies of positive social interactions during the developing maternal-infant relationship (Uvnas-Moberg, 1997). During social interactions, oxytocin can be released by sensory stimuli perceived as positive, including touch, warmth, and odors (Uvnas-Moberg, 1998). Because the release of oxytocin can become conditioned to emotional states and mental images, the actions of this peptide may provide an additional explanation for the long-term benefits of positive experiences. However the conditioning of this response for the mother of a preterm infant, at least initially, is related to experiences far removed from her infant, such as entering the neonatal intensive care unit (NICU), turning on an electric breast pump, or walking into the entry of the hospital. How best to "normalize" this conditioning to its proper maternal-infant orientation is one of the challenges clinicians are faced with when working with this vulnerable population—and STS holding may provide an early antidote (Feldman et al., 2002).

Although a complete review of procedures for STS holding is beyond the scope of this chapter, several principles can be summarized:

- Infants can be safely placed in STS care while very small and mechanically ventilated (Gale, Franck, & Lund, 1993; Legault & Goulet, 1995; Tornhage et al., 1999).
- There is no scientific reason to restrict the duration of STS care, unless an infant becomes physiologically unstable while on the mother's chest. Typically, a STS care session is ended based upon the mother's availability, rather than infant criteria.
- The position of the infant in STS care is important in maintaining physiologic stability, and recliners are ideal in achieving this position. The infant should be placed upright between the mothers' breasts, with the side of the face against the internal surface of one breast (Figure 13–3). The recliner is angled back to allow the infant's body to remain at a 45- to 60-degree angle from the floor. A mirror

positioned to allow the mother to observe her infant's face is helpful during these sessions.

- STS sessions of 2 or more hours are ideal, and it is not uncommon for infants to display behaviors that suggest autonomic instability when returned to the incubator following STS care (Kirsten, Bergman, & Hann, 2001).

Evidence-Based Guidelines for Milk Collection, Storage, and Feeding

Guidelines for Collection and Storage of Expressed Mother's Milk (EMM)

The collection and storage of expressed mother's milk (EMM) for later use by the mother's own infant has an impact on milk composition and various constituents. Several factors should be considered, including the type of collection container and storage conditions. Even with meticulous technique, no mothers' milk is sterile (el-Mohandes et al., 1993; Thompson et al., 1997). Mothers' attention to hand washing and cleansing of milk expression equipment is extremely important in reducing colonization by pathogens other than normal skin flora (Tully, 2000). Milk collection and storage guidelines are summarized in Box 13–3 and place special emphasis on ensuring anything coming in contact with the milk or the breast be thoroughly cleaned prior to each pumping session. Special attention should be placed on disassembling all pump parts following each collection for washing to avoid harboring of bacterial growth. Glass (Pyrex) and rigid plastic (polypropylene) containers are preferable to use for storage of human milk, as both

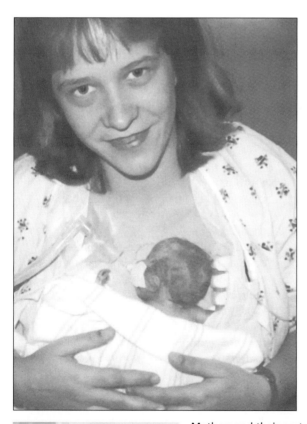
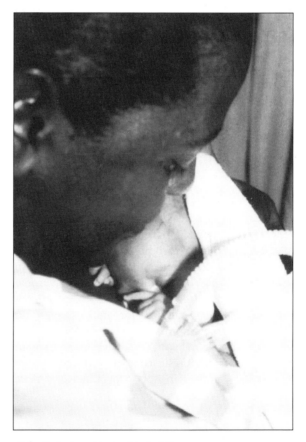

FIGURE **13–3A and B** Mothers and their preterm infants during skin-to-skin holding.

Source: Used with permission from the Lactation Support Program and Mothers' Own Milk Bank, Texas Children's Hospital, Houston, TX.

provide stability of water-soluble constituents and immunoglobulin A and are easy to handle (Goldblum et al., 1981; Williamson & Murti, 1996). Flexible, polyethylene bags are not recommended for milk collection and storage owing to significantly greater loss of cells (Goldblum et al., 1981) and chance of leakage during storage and handling. The temperature at which milk is stored is based on the duration of time until the infant receives the milk for feeding. Box 13–4 summarizes the criteria to determine the proper storage temperature to be used for human milk. The impact of various temperatures on milk constituents is included.

Preparing Expressed Mother's Milk for Infant Feeding

In most countries, preterm infants receive their mothers' milk by gavage until they are able to consume feedings directly from the breast. At this time,

infants are small and vulnerable to problems that can occur when EMM is handled unnecessarily. Proper procedures should be developed and adhered to in order to minimize bacterial growth and possible changes in milk constituents during storage and feeding. Box 13–4 describes the situational and environmental opportunities for bacterial contamination and guidelines for minimizing and preventing bacterial growth. Published guidelines for preparation of breast milk for the hospitalized infant can be useful in developing institutional NICU policies and procedures (HMBANA, 2006; Robbins & Beker, 2004).

NICU Area Used for Milk Preparation

Attention to the environment designated in the NICU for milk storage and preparation is important in ensuring optimal quality control in the provision of EMM for infant feeding. Use of similar procedures for storage of perishable food items should be adhered to, such as monitoring of refrigerator or

---

BOX 13–3

Guidelines for Collection and Storage of Mother's Own Milk for Preterm Infant Feeding

1. Wash hands and scrub under fingernails prior to each milk expression. Wipe the nipple area with water only (no soap) prior to each pumping.
2. Collect and store expressed milk in glass (Pyrex) or hard plastic (polypropylene) containers. Plastic bags are not recommended for milk storage for preterm infants.
3. Wash all milk collection equipment coming in contact with the breast milk with hot soapy water and rinse thoroughly following each use. Disassemble all parts prior to cleaning. Use a bottle brush to clean small crevices.
4. Sterilize milk collection equipment once a day by either boiling parts in water for 15–20 minutes or using a microwave sterilizing bag.
5. Label each bottle with infant's name, medical record number, date, and time of pumping. List any current maternal medications on the label.

BOX **13–4**

Guidelines to Minimize/Prevent Bacterial Growth of Mother's Own Milk for Infant Feeding

Milk Collection

- Instruct mother on proper collection technique including hand washing and maintenance of pumping equipment (see Box 13–3).

Milk Storage

- Use fresh, unrefrigerated milk within 1 hour of milk expression.
- Refrigerate milk immediately following expression when the infant will be fed within 24–48 hours.
- Freeze milk when infant is not being fed or the mother is unable to deliver the milk to the hospital within 24 hours of expression.
- Store each collection in a separate bottle. When pumping both breasts at the same time, two bottles can be combined into one.
- Ensure fresh/frozen milk is transported to the hospital on ice, in an insulated cooler to avoid thawing or warming.
- Thawed milk should not be refrozen.

Thawing

- Milk should be thawed gradually in a warm water bath not to exceed 20 minutes; alternately, frozen milk can be placed in the refrigerator to thaw.
- When using warm water bath method, do not submerge bottles in water.

- Label frozen milk with date and time when thawing in the refrigerator.

Milk Preparation

- Designate optimal physical space in the NICU for milk preparation.
- Gloves should be worn by staff when preparing or handling milk.
- When preparing feedings for more than one infant at a time, wash hands or change gloves, and wipe down counter between preparations.

Fortification

- Add fortification per physician's order ensuring complete mixing.
- Avoid vigorous shaking of milk to prevent disruption of milk fat membrane integrity (can result in adherence of milk fat to feeding tubes, bottles, etc.).
- Feed milk within 24 hours of addition of fortifier to EMM.

Warming

- EMM should be warmed to room temperature (27°C) prior to feeding in electric warming units or warm running water.
- Milk containers can be placed in the infant's incubator 30 minutes prior to feeding to warm.

(Continues)

BOX **13–4** **(Continued)**

- Use of unattended warm water baths for warming purposes should be discouraged as milk could be warmed to high temperatures resulting in changes in milk constituents.

Feeding

- For continuous milk infusions, limit infusion time to 4 hours.
- Avoid use of additional extension tubing for gavage feeding of EMM.

---

freezer temperatures and routine cleaning and maintenance of storage units and milk preparation spaces. Input from the hospital infection control department can be useful in developing appropriate guidelines for establishing an optimal environment for the storage and preparation of EMM.

Quality Control Issues

Mothers of hospitalized infants play a vital role in this process by ensuring correct labeling of each milk container with the infant's name, medical record number, date and time of collection, and use of any maternal medications. If the milk is to be transferred to another container by the nurse or other designated NICU staff prior to feeding, each individual syringe/bottle should be labeled appropriately. Human milk is a living fluid, not unlike blood, and should be handled as such. Proper hand washing and/or wearing gloves during handling should be practiced to avoid potential bacterial contamination of the EMM. Countertops and surfaces used for milk preparation should be wiped down with an appropriate antibacterial cleaner prior to preparation activities.

All milk that is to be used for infant feeding should be stored in the hospital under controlled conditions. All too often, mothers are told to store their expressed milk at home because of insufficient storage space in the NICU freezer. However, this approach would not be recommended for medications or blood; expressed milk should be no exception. When milk is out of sight of the NICU staff, there is no assurance that it has remained completely frozen and/or unopened before it is

subsequently fed to small preterm infants. A final consideration is ensuring that EMM in the NICU is not subject to tampering. There are no clear guidelines as to whether refrigerators and freezers should be locked or have restricted access, but this is a very important issue. Anecdotally, NICU staff and parents have expressed concern that suggests that EMM should be kept in an environment that eliminates the potential for tampering.

Every effort should be made to provide stringent quality control standards to minimize potential errors in which infants receive another mother's milk. Considering the risk of possible transmission of viruses (e.g., cytomegalovirus, hepatitis C, human immunodeficiency virus) via unpasteurized donor breast milk, administering another mother's milk to an infant is a serious error. Proper labeling of milk collection/preparation containers with the infant's name and medical record number and verification of this information (checked with another nurse) against infant's name band before feeding is an effective procedure to avoid potential errors.

Warming EMM for Feeding

Rapid heating, especially microwaving, has been demonstrated to adversely affect both the immunologic and nutritional properties of EMM (Hamosh et al., 1996; Quan et al., 1992). Refrigerated EMM should be gradually warmed (over 30 minutes) to approximately body temperature before being fed to small preterm infants (Newman et al., 2000). For the smallest infants, the feeding volume can be withdrawn into a syringe that is placed in the infant's incubator for gradual warming.

Special Issues Regarding the Feeding of EMM

The scientific literature supports feeding of fresh (unfrozen) milk when possible, because the anti-infective properties are maximally preserved (Hamosh, 2001; Hamosh et al., 1996). Ideally, preterm infants should receive at least one daily feeding of milk that has been pumped at the bedside, and fed without refrigeration. This milk retains all of the anti-infective properties and has been subjected to minimal handling and temperature changes. Many mothers will ensure that their infants have fresh milk available for feedings if they understand the rationale behind this practice. The staff can support this plan by developing a sequence of feeding the milk so it can be used within 48 hours of expression, and/or alternated with frozen milk when necessary. Additionally, it is important to emphasize to the mother that frozen milk still retains most of the anti-infective properties and is nutritionally superior to formula.

Volume Restriction Status

Special considerations regarding the feeding of EMM to preterm infants are based on the infant's fluid restrictive status at a time of greatest nutritional need. Although full feeding volume status for preterm infants are routinely considered to be a daily volume of 150 cc/kg/d, human milk-fed infants usually tolerate volumes much higher—up to 200 cc/kg/d (Schanler, 2001). The ability to handle a greater volume has been attributed to the faster gastric emptying rates observed with human milk (Moody et al., 2000). However, to achieve optimal bone mineralization at a vulnerable time in the preterm infant's development, human milk fortifiers are routinely mixed with the milk to provide greater intake of specific minerals, such as calcium and phosphorus (Sankaran et al., 1996; Wauben et al., 1998).

Commercial Nutritional Additives

Unfortified EMM is deficient in protein and selected minerals to support optimal growth and bone mineralization for small preterm infants (Schanler, 1998; Schanler, Hurst, & Lau, 1999; Schanler, Shulman, & Lau, 1999; Simmer, Metcalf, & Daniels, 1997). Thus,

for most preterm infants, these additional nutrients are provided in the form of commercial milk fortifiers. However, recent studies have raised concern that these commercial liquids and powders may affect the bioavailability and function of human milk components (Ewer & Yu, 1996; Jocson, Mason, & Schanler, 1997; Lucas et al., 1996; Quan et al., 1994; Schanler, 1998). Studies evaluating the effects of nutrient fortification on some of the general host defense properties of human milk have shown no effect on the concentrations of IgA (Jocson, Mason, & Schanler, 1997; Quan et al., 1994), and bacterial growth was not affected during 4 (Jocson et al., 1997) and 6 hours (Telang et al., 2005) at room temperature and decreased over 24 (Jocson et al., 1997) and 72 hours (Santiago et al., 2005) at refrigerator temperature. The results of these studies under simulated nursery conditions suggests that current practice should include limiting storage to 4 hours at room temperature and 24 hours in the refrigerator once fortification is added to the milk.

Hindmilk Feeding

The feeding of the hindmilk-only fraction of EMM has received considerable interest among clinicians (Griffin et al., 2000; Ogechi, William, & Fidelia, 2007; Valentine, Hurst, & Schanler, 1994). The lipid and caloric content of hindmilk is greater than that of foremilk or composite milk (e.g., a full pumping that includes fore- and hindmilk). By fractionating the hindmilk portion of a milk expression, mothers can provide high-lipid, high-calorie milk that promotes accelerated infant growth (Ogechi et al., 2007; Slusher et al., 2003; Valentine, Hurst, & Schanler, 1994). Although hindmilk feeding holds remarkable potential for preterm infant nutrition, the technique has not yet been subjected to randomized controlled trials.

There is tremendous within and between mother variation in breastmilk lipid content. Thus, a standard procedure for collection of hindmilk does not ensure a standard outcome. Clinically, the lipid and caloric content of milk can be estimated with the creamatocrit, a technique that involves centrifuging a milk specimen that has been drawn into a capillary tube (Lucas et al., 1978; Polberger & Lonnerdal, 1993). The creamatocrit, or the percent of total volume in the capillary tube that is equivalent to lipid, can be converted to an estimate of lipid and caloric content using one of the published regression graphs (Table 13–2). However, creamatocrits performed in this manner represent only a relative estimate of lipid and calories. A more accurate quantification of lipid and caloric content requires that the creamatocrit be standardized with one of the direct measures of total milk lipid, such as the Folch technique (Jensen, 1989).

Hindmilk and commercial fortifiers and additives are not interchangable, a point that is often misunderstood. Although commercial fortifiers provide small amounts of calories in the form of carbohydrates, their primary purpose is to supplement essential minerals, such as calcium and phosphorus, which are needed in higher concentrations than are present in human milk. In contrast, hindmilk does not "concentrate" these nutrients (Valentine, Hurst, & Schanler, 1994), but does provide an extremely efficient energy source by concentrating the endogenous milk lipids. Thus, the use of hindmilk does not replace the need for mineral supplementation, and commercial fortifiers are a relatively inefficient means of supplying extra calories.

Finally, the needs of the mother must be considered whenever her composite milk is not used exclusively. It is easy for mothers to infer that their milk is not "adequate" for their infants when it must be fortified or fractionated for hindmilk feedings. Mothers should be informed that their milk is ideal with respect to immunologic and nutritional properties—but the rapid growth of their very small infants requires temporary supplementation with commercial fortifiers and/or hindmilk.

Lactoengineering of own mothers' milk (OMM) through a combination of hindmilk and creamatocrit measures can be empowering for mothers of preterm infants (Griffin et al., 2000; Jennings,

Meier, & Meier, 1997). Specifically, mothers are assisted in expressing milk with a creamatocrit value that meets their individual infant's growth needs. When their infants demonstrate the desired weight gain pattern, mothers recognize that their milk modifications supported the desired growth.

Methods of Milk Delivery

A series of studies provides strong scientific support for the administration of EMM by intermittent rather than slow-infusion continuous gavage (Brennan-Behm et al., 1994; Schanler, Shulman, & Lau, 1999). In particular, milk lipids that comprise 50 to 60 percent of the calories in EMM adhere to the lumen of infusion tubings, and their loss results in a relatively dilute, low-calorie feeding (Brennan-Behm et al., 1994). The greatest lipid loss occurs during the slowest infusion rates (Greer, McCormick, & Loker, 1984; Stocks et al., 1985). Clinically, this means that the smallest babies, for whom caloric requirements are the highest, will receive EMM by the slowest infusion rates, resulting in a low-calorie milk. For this reason, EMM should be administered by slow intermittent bolus, rather than by continuous gavage infusion.

Maternal Medication Use

When small preterm infants receive their OMM by gavage, extra care must be taken to ascertain that maternal medications in the milk can be tolerated safely. Preterm infants, especially those who are extremely low birth weight, have immature metabolic and excretory pathways. As a result, drugs that may be safely given to mothers of term healthy infants may have adverse consequences for more vulnerable infants (Hale, 2003). Although a detailed

TABLE 13–2	Creamatocrit Readings and Associated Fat/Caloric Content of Human Milk								
Creamatocrit	3	4	5	6	7	8	9	10	11
Cal/oz	15.7	17.8	20	22.1	24.3	26.4	28.5	30.7	32.8
% of calories–fat	22	37	44	48.2	52.1	56	58.2	60.4	62.6

Source: Adapted from Lucas et al., 1978.

description of these issues is beyond the scope of this chapter, several principles should be considered when a mother of a preterm infant must take medications:

- The medication should be considered "safe" for healthy term infants (AAP, 2001; Hale, 2006; Premji & Chessell, 2001); if this is not the case, the medication should not be considered safe for the small preterm infant.
- If the medication or its metabolites has been shown to accumulate in newborn body tissues, its accumulation may be even more exaggerated for the preterm infant.
- Many mothers of preterm infants will have had complicated births and/or health conditions that necessitate a combination of medications.
- The infant may be receiving medications and/or other therapies that could interact with the maternal medications. The safety of these combinations—rather than the individual medications—must be considered.
- Extra caution is needed when lipid-rich hindmilk is being fed; medications that are lipophilic may cross readily into the milk.

Only healthcare professionals who have expertise in lactation, pharmacology, and neonatal care should provide advice concerning the safety of medications for small preterm infants. When in doubt about a specific medication, or a combination of medications, a national expert should be consulted. In all instances any information about maternal medications should be reviewed with the neonatologist who is responsible for the infant's care, and mothers should record any medications consumed on the individual milk container.

Transmission of Viruses and Other Pathogens Via EMM

Transmission of viruses (Jim et al., 2004; Omarsdottir et al., 2007; Yasuda et al., 2003) and other pathogens (Arias-Camison, 2003; Byrne, Miller, & Justus, 2006; Kotiw et al., 2003) in breast milk have been described. Several studies have reported cytomegalovirus (CMV) seropositive rates between 52 and 97 percent in mothers of preterm infants (Doctor et al., 2005; Hamprecht et al., 2001; Jim et al., 2004), with CMV positive breast milk as high

as 38 to 70 percent. Yet despite these high rates, postnatal asymptomatic and symptomatic CMV infections in preterm infants are low, at 25 percent and 1 to 5 percent, respectively (Miron et al., 2005; Mussi-Pinhata et al., 2004; Schanler, 2005). However, given the vulnerability of the very preterm immune compromised infant, consideration of exposure to high viral loads is of concern. One goal is the elimination of CMV from a mother's breast milk without damaging protective constituents. Freezing techniques to eliminate CMV virus are inconclusive (Curtis et al., 2005; Hamprecht et al., 2004; Sharland, Khare, & Bedford-Russell, 2002) and have not shown complete viral inactivation. As no recommendations related to CMV and breast milk feeding in very preterm infants exist, some clinicians have suggested using freeze-thawed milk combined with at least some fresh milk feeding each day for the most vulnerable infants to minimize possible exposure. Additionally, it is speculated that the *exclusivity* of EMM feeding may be protective against CMV infection given the "enveloping" characteristic of the virus. As it happens, this same characteristic exists with HIV and may be a factor in the protection provided by exclusive human milk feedings of infants of HIV+ women compared to mixed feedings.

Group B streptococcus (GBS) is the most common cause of sepsis in newborns, and preterm infants are more susceptible to infection than term infants. Breast milk feeding has been implicated as a source of several reports of infant GBS infection (Arias-Camison, 2003; Byrne, Miller, & Justus, 2006; Kotiw et al., 2003; Olver et al., 2000). Additionally, Methicillin-resistant *Staphylococcus aureus* (MRSA) has been isolated from EMM (Behari et al., 2004; Gastelum et al., 2005; Novak et al., 2000). Several explanations of etiology were put forth including a more virulent strain of GBS following the use of prophylactic antibiotics in labor; early introduction of mixed feedings/human milk fortifier; and high bacterial load during mastitis episode. Recommendations for management included infant blood and EMM cultures to document transmission and the withholding of EMM until adequate therapy is achieved (Byrne, Miller, & Justus, 2006; Kotiw et al., 2003). Interestingly, in a study of 161 mothers of infants born less than 30 weeks gestation, weekly milk cultures (from 1 to 11 weeks) were not predictive of infection (Schanler et al., 2005).

Feeding at Breast in the NICU

Early oral experiences may influence later oral feeding development. Many clinicians specializing in feeding disorders report a high percentage of their patients as former preterm infants. This is not surprising given the amount of negative oral insults experienced by these infants, such as intubation, suctioning, and insertion of feeding tubes. Thus the provision of positive oral experiences early in their development may counteract some of the negative effects by these negative, but necessary, procedures. Nonnutritive suckling and suckling at the emptied maternal breast provides a positive experience for preterm infants.

Suckling at the Emptied Breast

There are no universally established criteria for the initiation of breastfeeding (or bottle-feeding for that matter) for preterm infants. Although a minimum body weight or gestational age (commonly 34 weeks) has been used, more recent practice has been to consider each infant's individual abilities when determining the initiation of oral feeding, be that breast or bottle (Lau & Hurst, 1999; McGrath & Braescu, 2004; Medoff-Cooper, 2000; Simpson, Schanler, & Lau, 2002). Whereas judging the ability to breastfeed on the infant's achievement of consuming a prescribed milk volume by bottle, evidence-based research as previously described prove this practice inappropriate. In neonatal units whereby infants are allowed nonnutritive sucking at the emptied breast (Meier, 2001; Narayanan et al., 1991), the idea of "when to initiate" breastfeeding has been reconceptualized.

Controlled clinical trials have demonstrated many benefits of nonnutritive sucking (NNS) with a pacifier for preterm infants (Pinelli & Symington, 2007). Theoretically, these same benefits should extend to the preterm infant's suckling at the mother's recently pumped breast, an experience that may also maximize the mother's milk production. Initiating NNS at the emptied breast provides a maternal stimulus that is different from routine breast pump use, and as such, may increase milk yield. Additionally, mothers receive instant reinforcement from infants' behaviors that reflect enjoyment and physiologic stability while at the breast. For the infant, the ability to "taste" the milk allows

for optimal oral stimulation during a time when the oral cavity is bypassed via oral-gastric tube feedings. Another sensory experience—smell—may also condition the infant for breastfeeding as evidenced in a randomized study of preterm infants (30–33 weeks) exposed to their mother's own milk odor immediately following early breastfeeding attempts (Raimbault, Saliba, & Porter, 2007). During each breastfeeding session, infants exposed to the milk odor displayed longer sucking bouts and bursts, and also consumed more milk than the control (exposed to water) infants.

For small (< 1000 g) infants, the mother completely expresses milk from the breast just prior to the infant being placed in STS care at the breast. The infant should be supported in the football hold or across the chest, so that the infant's entire ventral surface is in direct contact with the lateral aspect of the mother's breast. The infant's temperature can be monitored noninvasively if this is a concern—however the same criteria and outcomes utilized for STS holding should apply during suckling at the emptied breast (Dodd, 2005). Although the infant should be held in proximity with the breast, no attempt should be made to "position" the infant's mouth and gums over the nipple and areola. Instead, licking and suckling on the nipple tip is all that is expected of very small preterm infants. In one NICU, NNS is begun as soon as small infants are extubated (Meier, 2001). Infants on NCPAP can participate in NNS; positioning across the lap with NCPAP tubings directed upward and over the breast is most effective (Figure 13–4). For larger infants, the mother can combine NNS at the emptied breast with administering her freshly expressed milk by gavage (Figure 13–5).

These early opportunities for the infant to suckle at the emptied breast allows the mother to observe the infant's behavior and developing signs for readiness to oral feeding. In this way the mother can provide invaluable input into the plan of care as it relates to advancement of oral feeding. For this reason, a specific postnatal/gestational age or body weight is not used as the criteria for advancing oral feedings (Nyqvist, Sjoden, & Ewald, 1999; Sidell & Froman, 1994). Observations made by the mother and nursing staff during early STS holding and suckling sessions allows for the development of an individualized plan of care regarding initiation and progression of oral feeding (Nyqvist et al., 1996;

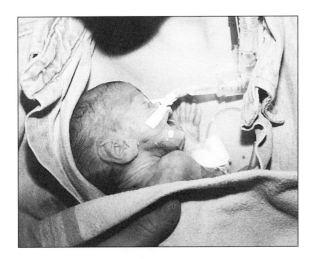

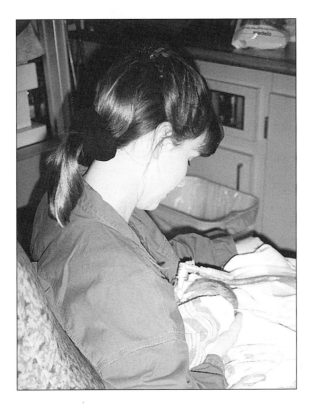

FIGURE **13–4A and B** Infants with NCPAP tubes positioned across mother's lap.

Source: Used with permission from the Lactation Support Program and Mothers' Own Milk Bank, Texas Children's Hospital, Houston, TX.

Shaker & Woida, 2007). As feeding at breast advances in the NICU, two principal topics should be discussed: the science and practice of initiating and advancing direct breastfeedings; and the measurement and facilitation of milk transfer.

The Science of Early Breastfeeding

Studies have demonstrated that preterm infants serving as their own controls had more stable measures of transcutaneous oxygen pressure and body temperature during breastfeeding compared to bottle-feeding (Blaymore Bier et al., 1997; Meier, 1988; Meier & Anderson, 1987), but less milk was transferred during breastfeeding than measured during bottle-feeding (Blaymore Bier et al., 1997; Furman & Minich, 2004; Martell et al., 1993; Meier & Brown, 1996). Table 13–3 represents the body of work present in the literature to date regarding breastfeeding behavior in preterm infants. These data suggest that the more stable patterns of oxygenation for breastfeeding than for bottle-feeding are a result of less interruption of breathing during breastfeeding—possibly as a result of a slower rate of milk flow during breastfeeding. To safely project a bolus of milk through the pharynx, an infant must coordinate sucking, swallowing, and breathing. Infant oral motor skills must not only be adequate for sucking, but sucking must be intricately coordinated with both swallowing and breathing (Gewolb et al., 2001). Considering the preterm infant's novice skills, the restricted milk flow experienced during breastfeeding may be a more optimal environment for development of oral motor skills.

To test this theory, Meier and Brown (1996) studied a cohort of clinically stable preterm infants who served as their own controls for serial breastfeeding and bottle-feedings from the time of oral feeding initiation until NICU discharge. The following variables were monitored and recorded continuously on an 8-channel polygraph: sucking event, respiratory event, body temperature, and oxygen saturation during each feeding session. Volume of milk intake was measured by test-weighing. Previous research in Meier's lab had validated the instruments that were used for the measurement of sucking (deMonterice et al., 1992) and milk intake (Kavanaugh, Meier, & Engstrom, 1989; Meier et al., 1990) in this research. Results revealed that during bottle-feedings preterm infants frequently did not breathe during sucking bursts; instead they alternated short bursts of sucking with pauses during which they breathed rapidly. Oxygen saturation measures in response to this

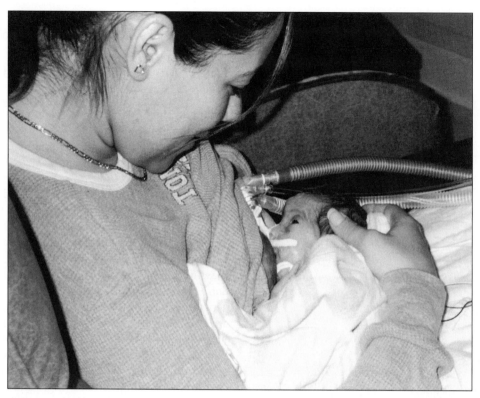

FIGURE **13–5**   Suckling at the emptied breast.

Source: Used with permission from Rush Mothers' Milk Club, Rush-Presbyterian St. Luke's Medical Center, Chicago, IL.

suck-breathe patterning varied. For most, but not all, infants who maintained short sucking bursts (e.g., minimal durations of not breathing), oxygen saturation remained relatively stable. For infants who attempted longer sucking bursts, or for those who demonstrated long durations of suspended breathing followed by short sucking bursts, oxygen saturation declined significantly. Examples of these patterns of suck-breathe coordination are depicted in Figure 13–6. During breastfeeding episodes these same infants integrated breathing within sucking bursts (Figure 13–7). A maturational trend was seen, in which less mature infants demonstrated brief episodes of suspended breathing within long sucking bursts. As the infants approached 34–35 weeks of gestation, the suck-breathe patterning approximated a ratio of 1:1.

These findings are consistent with those of previous researchers who described more stable patterns of oxygenation during breastfeedings than during bottle-feedings for preterm infants.

However, these findings explain the mechanism for this stability: less interruption in breathing during breastfeeding. Meier concluded that differences in suck-breathe patterning for bottle and breastfeeding may be due to the infant's ability to control the flow of milk during breastfeeding by subtle alterations in the suck mechanism. These alterations consisting of the infant's manipulation of intra- and intersuck intervals to accommodate breathing, may not be clinically apparent, but were detected during this research (Figure 13–7). Infants did not demonstrate similar suck-breathe patterning during bottle-feedings until they were several weeks older.

In a large cohort (n = 71) of Swedish preterm infants, breastfeeding was studied prospectively from initiation until discharge (Hedberg et al., 1999). In this Swedish hospital setting where early maternal contact was encouraged, infants demonstrated rooting, areolar grasp, and latching on as early as 28 weeks; nutritive sucking (as defined

TABLE 13–3	**Studies Related to Physiologic Effects of Breastfeeding in Preterm Infants**			
Reference	**Design/Sample (N)**	**Measures**	**Findings**	**Limitations**
Meier, 1988	Crossover; healthy preterm (5)	Respiratory rate PaO$_2$ Heart rate Temperature	tcPO$_2$ patterns were more stable and body temperature increased during Bfing compared to Bot	Small sample size Milk intake was not measured
Martell et al., 1993	Crossover; preterm infants Breastfed (16) Bottle-fed (46)	Milk intake measured: Bf—test weights @ 3 min. intervals Bot—ingested vol. during each SU period	Shorter feeding duration w/Bot compared to Bf	Only six infants were studied at all time periods—no explanation given—one possibility, infants were unable to sustain attachment to the breast for the initial attempts
Bier et al., 1993	Crossover; preterm (20); 9 infants ≥ 1 morbidities associated w/prematurity	Respiratory rate PaO$_2$ Heart rate Temperature Test weights NOMAS scores	No diff. in PaO$_2$ during Bf; 21% vs. 38% in Bf vs. Bot in O$_2$ desaturation (< 90%); Milk intake during Bf < during Bot; No diff. in temp, feeding duration, NOMAS scores	
Nyqvist, Sjoden, & Ewald, 1999	Observational; healthy preterm infants (71)	Describe the development of feeding behavior; Time to full oral feeds	1st experience Bf @ median 33.7 wks PMA; 51% of infants observed on 1st day of Bf intro; all but 2 infants showed rooting behavior	Total duration of latch and SU during each session and vigor of sucking behavior were not assessed; focus of study on infant behavior, not milk intake
Dowling, 1999	Crossover; healthy preterm (8)	Sucking parameters Respiratory rate PaO$_2$ Heart rate Test weight	SU bursts longer for Bot than Bf; no difference in SU rate between Bot and Bf; 10 Bf & 1 Bot feeding were not included due to no milk intake	Only one type of Bot nipple was tested; effect of orthodontic nipple on the time to full Bf/duration of Bf not reported

(Continues)

TABLE 13–3	Studies Related to Physiologic Effects of Breastfeeding in Preterm Infants (Continued)			
Reference	**Design/Sample (N)**	**Measures**	**Findings**	**Limitations**
Meier et al., 2000	Crossover, healthy preterm (34)	Milk transfer as measured by test weights w/ and w/o nipple shield (NS); duration of NS use; duration of Bfing	Mean milk transfer significantly greater for feedings w/NS (18.4 vs. 3.9 ml), with all infants consuming more milk w/NS in place; mean duration NS use 32.5 d. Mean duration of Bfing 169.4 days; No significant association between % of time NS used and Bfing duration	Maternal nipple characteristics were not reported
Chen et al., 2000	Crossover, healthy preterm (25)	PaO_2 Heart rate Respiratory rate Body temperature	PaO_2 and body temp significantly higher during Bfing; 2 episodes of apnea and 20 episodes of $PaO_2 < 90\%$ during Bot, none during Bf	Milk intake was not measured
Nyqvist et al., 2001	Observational; preterm (26)	SU and SW behavior as measured by electromyography (EMG)	Agreement between direct observations of SU and EMG data were high. Considerable variation between infants in extent of mouthing. No association with maturational level for any oral behavioral components.	Milk intake was not measured
Furman & Minich, 2004	Observational; preterm Breastfed (35) Bottle-fed (70)	A modified version PIBBS (Nyqvist, Sjoden, & Ewald, 1999)	At 35 wks corrected age, Bfing compared to Bot took in smaller volumes (6.5 vs. 30.5 ml, $P < .001$), fed less efficiently	Only 1 feeding session was observed for each infant; no subjective/object-ive measure of maternal milk ejection noted.

Key: Bf = breastfeeding; Bot = bottle feeding; PMA = postmenstrual age; SU = suck; SW = swallow.

by ≥5 ml intake) from 30.6 weeks; and repeated swallowing at 31 weeks. In a smaller cohort (n = 26) Nyqvist and colleagues (Nyqvist et al., 2001) used surface electrodes to record the oral behavior during breastfeeding of preterm infants. The preterm infants (mean gestational age 32.5 ± 2.1, range 26.7 to 36) showed a wide variation in sucking behavior, both in duration and intensity. Analyses of possible factors influencing the infants' oral feeding behavior revealed only one significant association, that is infants with a higher postnatal age had a higher mean duration of sucks (r = 0.39, $P < .05$).

The results of these studies demonstrate the infant's sucking ability at the breast and physiologic stability during breastfeeding. Thus, waiting to initiate breastfeeding until the infant demonstrates the

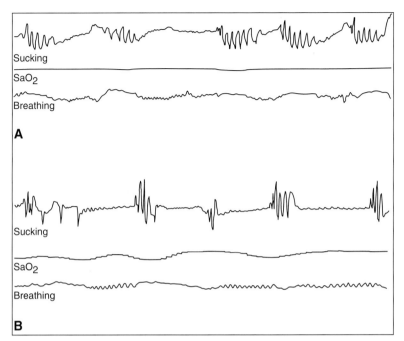

FIGURE 13–6 (A) Polygraphic recording demonstrating suck/breathe patterning and oxygenation during bottle-feeding for a preterm infant. In this recording, the infant alternates short sucking bursts with breathing but does not breathe within sucking burst. Oxygen saturation remains stable. (B) Polygraphic recording demonstsrating suck/breathe patterning and oxygenation during bottle-feeding for a preterm infant. Oxygen saturation fluctuates, with values as low as 78 percent during short sucking bursts.

Source: Reproduced by permission of Royal Society of Medicine Press, London.

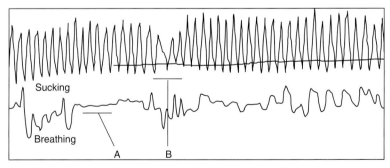

FIGURE 13–7 Polygraphic recording demonstrating suck/breathe patterning and oxygenation during breastfeeding for an infant of 33 weeks' gestational age. The infant breathes within this long (104 sucks) suckling burst until phase A, when breathing is interrupted for several sucks. In phase B, the infant alters the duration and amplitude of individual sucks, apparently to reinstitute a more regular breathing pattern, which continues through the remainder of the burst.

Source: Reproduced by permission of Royal Society of Medicine Press, London.

ability to consume entire bottle feedings is not a research-based criterion of readiness to breastfeed. Additionally, there may be benefit from these early "practice" sessions as evidenced in a small cohort of preterm bottle-feeding infants whereby a regimen of oral stimulation for 10 days prior to the initiation of oral feedings resulted in some, but not all, oral motor functions (Fucile, Gisel, & Lau, 2005). For clinical purposes, all infants should be monitored for physiologic stability during early oral feedings, regardless of method.

Progression of In-Hospital Breastfeeding

When infants are placed at the breast for daily nonnutritive sucking opportunities, the transition to "nutritive feedings" can be a natural progression appropriate to the infant's individual abilities. When it is determined that the infant should consume some "low-flow" milk, the mother can express some, but not all, of the milk from the breast. In this way, the preterm infant is introduced to small droplets of milk that do not necessitate prolonged closure of the airway for swallowing. As the infant matures, the mother can regulate the milk flow by pumping the amount of milk necessary to reduce the postmilk ejection flow. When the infant demonstrates the ability to coordinate sucking and breathing, the mother no longer needs to express milk prior to the feeding. This progressive increase in the rate of flow during breastfeeding is consistent with observations from studies in which suction and expression pressures were measured during low-flow bottle feedings for low birth weight infants (Lau et al., 1997; Scheel, Schanler, & Lau, 2005). Data from these studies suggest that less mature preterm infants can initiate feedings safely, provided that milk flow is restricted.

The preterm infant should be breastfed in a position that affords support to the head and neck, such as the football or the across-the-lap hold. The head of the preterm infant is heavy in relation to the weak musculature of the neck, and undirected head movements can easily collapse the airway, with resultant apnea and bradycardia. Use of these positions will also compensate for the preterm infant's disadvantage

in extracting milk from the breast. Specifically, the data from nonnutritive sucking and bottle-feeding studies reveal that suction pressures are maturationally dependent (Hafstrom & Kjellmer, 2000; Lau et al., 2000). With this limitation, the small preterm infant needs to be "placed" and "kept" on the nipple, because the limited suction pressures do not permit the infant to draw the nipple into the intraoral cavity to achieve milk extraction (Figure 13–8).

Milk Transfer During Breastfeeding

Factors Influencing Milk Transfer During Breastfeeding

Milk transfer during breastfeeding is dependent upon sufficient maternal milk secretion and ejection

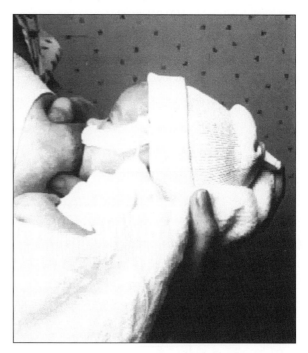

FIGURE 13–8 Providing support of the infant's head and support of the breast during breastfeeding.

Source: Used with permission from the Lactation Support Program and Mothers' Own Milk Bank, Texas Children's Hospital, Houston, TX.

concurrent with proficient infant oral motor skills. Table 13–4 provides an algorithm of the various components essential to achieve milk transfer during breastfeeding and the possible outcomes in the absence of each of these components. In examining this diagram it is apparent that the mother contributes important elements (milk synthesis/ejection and maternal nipple/areolar attributes) and the infant equally vital components (effective suck/swallow). Mothers and their preterm infants may experience problems with any or all of these components. Conversely, because these components are interactive, a problem with one, such as ineffective suckling, can be compensated for by adequacy in the other components. Application of this framework to intake-related

questions and problems is essential in determining the appropriate clinical intervention.

For example, most but not all preterm infants have ineffective and/or marginally effective suckling during early breastfeeding experiences. Typically, these infants suckle in short bursts and fall asleep quickly at the breast (Kavanaugh et al., 1995; Nyqvist, Ewald, & Sjoden, 1996; Nyqvist et al., 1996). Recently, feeding efficiency was compared in 35 breastfeeding and 70 bottle-feeding very low birth weight (< 1500 g) infants (Furman & Minich, 2004). A *single* feeding observation at a mean corrected age of 35 ± 1 weeks was performed for each study infant. Breastfeeding as compared with bottle-feeding infants transferred smaller milk

TABLE 13–4 Algorithm of Essential Components of Milk Transfer During Breastfeeding

	Essential Components									Outcome
	Maternal Components						**Infant Components**			
	MS*	+	ME	+	MA	→	SU	+	SW	=	MT
Clinical States										
1.	+		+		+		+		+	=	Adequate
2.	–		+		+		+		+	=	Insufficient*
3.	+		–		+		+		+	=	Insufficient
4.	+		+		–		+		+	=	Insufficient**
5.	+		+		+		–		+	=	Insufficient†
6.	+		+		+		+		–	=	Insufficient†

Clinical Interventions

No intervention required (1)

Interventions to increase MS required (2)

Strategies to elicit ME are required to facilitate milk flow (3)

Interventions to facilitate attachment to the maternal nipple (i.e., nipple shield) (4)

Strategies to improve infant SU response (5)

Strategies to improve infant SW ability (6)

Key: MA = maternal nipple/areolar attributes; ME = milk ejection; MS = milk synthesis; MT = milk transfer; SU = infant expression or suction or combination of both; SW = infant swallow.

* May be sufficient for the preterm infant considering lower milk volume needs.

** May be sufficient if infant can achieve sustained attachment despite MA.

† May be sufficient if attachment to breast and MS + ME are adequate.

volumes (median 6.5 vs. 30.5 ml, $P < .001$), fed less efficiently (median 0.6 vs. 2.2 ml/min, $P < .001$), and spent less time with sucking bursts (mean 33 vs. 55 percent, $P < .001$). One limitation to this study was a lack of objective and/or subjective evidence of maternal milk ejection during breastfeeding sessions. Maternal milk volume and ejection can compensate for marginally effective infant sucking. Anecdotally, it is not uncommon for some mothers, whose milk-ejection response has become conditioned to the higher suction pressures experienced with the mechanical breast pump, to have difficulty eliciting milk ejection during early breastfeeding attempts.

To document the progression of breastfeeding behavior observed for each individual mother–infant dyad, several tools have been used varying from simple approximation based on the observer's assessment (Jenson, Wallace, & Kelsay, 1994; Mulford, 1992) to detailed observations using checklists or coding forms (Nyqvist et al., 1996). The Preterm Infant Breastfeeding Behavior Scale (PIBBS) is a tool developed specifically for mothers of preterm infants (Nyqvist, Ewald, & Sjoden, 1996). The PIBBS was developed from observations of preterm behavior in collaboration between observers and mothers. By observing her infant in a more systematic way using the PIBBS, the mother develops greater sensitivity to her infant's behavioral pattern at the breast and is able to develop his capacity for nutritive suckling without restrictions of breastfeeding frequency or duration of breastfeeding sessions, irrespective of maturational level or age (see Appendix 13–A).

Several years ago Hurst at Texas Children's Hospital developed a checklist to document specific behaviors and observations made by the nurse or lactation consultant during a breastfeeding session in the NICU (Figure 13–9). This form was developed because existing breastfeeding tools lacked key components necessary to effectively evaluate the infant and maternal contributions to the dyad in the preterm population. Inclusion of this documentation in the infant's medical record provides pertinent information regarding the preterm infant's progress with breastfeeding that is then conveyed to the entire healthcare team. This checklist of key components provides an evaluation of the infant's sucking behavior and activity, as well as

the mother's milk ejection response and average pumped milk volume. However this tool is not used to place a "score" on the feeding session but merely to provide information as to relevant aspects of the contributions made by each member of the breastfeeding dyad allowing for appropriate interventions to be utilized.

Methods to Estimate Milk Transfer

Along with these key components observed during feeding, it is important to evaluate milk transfer once the preterm infant has been introduced to unrestricted milk flow during breastfeeding. Mothers and healthcare professionals are unable to use clinical indices to accurately estimate milk intake for preterm infants (Kavanaugh et al., 1995; Meier et al., 1996). However, clinicians are concerned that more accurate measures of milk intake are either too stressful for mothers or unnecessary for preterm infants (Meier, 1995; Walker, 1995). Similarly, many care providers are unaware that accurate measurement of milk intake for preterm infants is possible.

Test-weighing procedures, whereby the clothed infant is weighed pre- and postfeed (the difference in weight equals the volume consumed) provides an accurate measure of milk intake for clinical and research settings (Meier et al., 1994, 1996; Scanlon et al., 2002). Using test-weights, 1 g of weight gain approximates 1 ml of milk intake. When performed correctly, test-weighing is accepted as the technique of choice in clinical situations whereby milk intake needs to be measured accurately (Scanlon et al., 2002).

Test-weighing should be introduced in the NICU when it appears that milk transfer has occurred and/or discharge is imminent. For smaller preterm infants, the test-weight estimate permits individualized complementation of breastfeedings, so that 24-hour fluid and caloric requirements can be met. For larger infants awaiting NICU discharge, test-weights can be used to diagnose milk-transfer problems. For example, the infant may suckle marginally, but the mother's milk volume is adequate. It is impossible to know whether the mother's milk flow can compensate for the infant's suck unless volume of intake is measured.

PREMIE Breastfeeding Assessment

Recent Oral Feeding

Number of PO feeding attempts/d during previous 24 hours (circle one): None   1   3–5   8
Type of PO feeding attempt: Breast (#)_____   Bottle (#)_____
If bottle-fed, % of prescribed volume taken_____
If breastfed, was additional milk given via bottle or gavage pc: Yes___ No___

Maternal Nipple Attributes (Prior to Feeding)
(Check appropriate items.)
  ☐ Prominent
  ☐ Flat
  ☐ Inverted
  ☐ Other, describe:_____

Assessment of Breastfeeding Session:
(Check appropriate items.)

Predominant infant behavior	☐ Quiet/active alert ☐ Drowsy ☐ Deep sleep/crying
Rooting	☐ Obvious rooting w/ minimal stimulation ☐ Some rooting w/ stimulation ☐ No rooting
Effective latch-on	☐ Maintains effective latch ☐ Attempts latch, slips off or holds nipple in mouth ☐ No latch achieved
Milk ejection	☐ Obvious objective or subjective signs ☐ Possible signs, uncertain or not noticed ☐ No objective or subjective signs
Infant suck	☐ Rhythmic sucking ☐ Arrhythmic sucking ☐ No sucking
Evident swallowing	☐ Smooth swallowing ☐ Strained swallowing ☐ No swallowing

Nipple shield used? If so, which size: ☐ Small   ☐ Newborn

Maternal Milk Volume

Average pumped volume nearest to the time of the current feeding session_____(ml)

Milk Transfer

Infant weight prior to feeding_____(gm)   Following feeding_____(gm)
Total milk transfer during feeding (postfeed weight – prefeed weight)_____(gm)

FIGURE 13–9   PREMIE breastfeeding assessment.

Source: Used with permission from the Lactation Support Program, Texas Children's Hospital, Houston, TX.

Strategies to Facilitate Milk Transfer

Seldom does significant milk transfer occur during the first few breastfeeding sessions for preterm infants (Furman & Minich, 2004). However, as NICU discharge approaches, consistently small volumes of intake become a concern that must be evaluated. Selected problems of milk transfer are particularly common among preterm infants.

The single most important factor for mothers who will be breastfeeding a preterm infant at home is maintaining a milk supply that exceeds the baby's requirements at hospital discharge (Hill, Ledbetter, & Kavanaugh, 1997; Lawrence, 2001; Meier, 2001). With an adequate milk supply, the infant's immature sucking pattern may be less problematic. Mothers can plan for this by expressing their milk an extra time or two in the week before their baby's discharge. For mothers who have a borderline milk supply as NICU discharge approaches, the clinician should consider a regimen of metoclopramide (Emery, 1996) or domperidone (Novak et al., 2000) to augment the milk yield. Theoretically, the prolactin stimulus from the medication will be maintained by the infant's direct breastfeeding in the home.

Mothers should be reminded to express milk with the electric breast pump after each breastfeeding in the hospital. NICU staff and mothers seldom appreciate that a preterm infant cannot substitute for the breast stimulation provided by the electric breast pump, especially if the infant consumes only small milk volumes. Mothers frequently question how to coordinate milk expression with demand feedings because they are concerned their breasts will be empty when their infants awake to feed. An appropriate strategy in this situation is to emphasize the priority of maintaining milk yield by maintaining complete breast emptying during their transition of exclusive breastfeeding.

Many mothers of preterm infants deny feeling the sensations of milk ejection both when using the electric pump and when feeding their infants at breast. Thus, it is often difficult to evaluate the synchronization of milk ejection and infant sucking. One strategy that may be useful in evaluating milk ejection response is to instruct the mother to uncover the opposite breast during a breastfeeding session in order to observe the spontaneous dripping of milk during milk ejection. Typically, mothers experience a delay in milk ejection when infants are placed at the breast because the women are conditioned to the sensations of the breast pump. It is not uncommon for milk flow to begin just as the preterm infant falls asleep at the breast. If this situation persists for more than a few feedings, the mother can use the electric breast pump to initiate the milk flow. This can be done by placing the infant at one breast and the pump at the other, or by first initiating the milk flow with the breast pump and then placing the infant at breast.

Sustaining Attachment to the Maternal Breast

The sucking pattern of the healthy term infant is characterized by the rhythmic alternation of two types of pressure, negative (suction) and positive (compression) pressure (Dubignon & Campbell, 1969; Sameroff, 1968). Suction defines the negative intraoral pressure generated as the infant draws milk into the mouth and compression as the positive pressure resulting from the compression and/or stripping of the nipple between the tongue and the hard palate as milk is ejected into the mouth (Ardran, Kemp, & Lind, 1958; Nowak, Smith, & Erenberg, 1994, 1995; Waterland et al., 1998). The majority of milk transfer problems for preterm infants can be related to immaturity and inconsistency in suckling (Kavanaugh et al., 1995; Meier & Brown, 1996). The relatively low suction pressures and the infants' inconsistent, irregular sucking bursts do not sustain the milk flow needed for effective milk transfer or in many cases allow for sustained attachment to the maternal breast. These phenomena appear to be maturationally dependent. Until the infant achieves term-corrected age, strategies to increase the effectiveness of sucking to achieve sustained attachment to the breast are often necessary.

Weak sucking pressures (–2.5 to –15 mm Hg) measured in preterm infants may result in difficulties maintaining attachment to the maternal breast (Lau et al., 1997). Bottle-feeding studies by Lau and colleagues (Lau et al., 1997, 2000) concluded that sucking ability does not need to be at a mature level before preterm infants are introduced to oral feeding. These preterm infants were able to transfer milk during bottle feeding via compression only, using little or no suction pressure. Therefore the provision of a rigid nipple may allow the infant the ability to transfer milk without the need to generate suction pressure, utilizing instead the compression component of infant feeding. Interestingly, preterm infants have been shown to modify their sucking skills in order to maintain a rate of transfer that is compatible with the level of suck/swallow/breathe coordination they have attained at a particular time (Scheel et al., 2005).

It is this theoretical basis that may explain reports of improved milk transfer during breastfeeding in preterm infants using a thin, silicone nipple shield placed over the mother's nipple to facilitate sustained attachment (Clum & Primomo, 1996; Meier et al., 2000). A study of 34 preterm infants (Meier et al., 2000) revealed a significantly greater increase in milk transfer with the shield than for the previous breastfeeding without the shield (18.4 ml vs. 3.9 ml, $P = .0001$). In a retrospective study of 15 preterm infants, the nipple shield was introduced following at least five failed attempts to achieve breast attachment or milk transfer without the nipple shield (Clum & Primomo, 1996). Nine of the 15 infants consumed at least half or greater of the prescribed feeding amount with the nipple shield. Clinical indications for nipple shield use among this group included the inability of the infant to sustain attachment to the breast, holding the nipple in the mouth while falling asleep, and maternal nipple characteristics.

The results of these studies (Clum & Primomo, 1996; Meier et al., 2000) raise further questions as to the underlying etiology of the nipple shield's effect on infant and maternal breastfeeding responses. One possible explanation could be the nipple shield provides a uniform rigid structure that extends deeper into the infant's oral cavity thus allowing greater tactile stimulation (Figure 13–10). As a result of this stimulation the infant responds by compression and or compression/suction and sustained breast attachment. Consequently, a sustained attachment and compression of the shield results in stimulation of the underlying nipple/areolar tissue providing a stimulus for activation of the maternal milk-ejection reflex and improved milk flow and transfer. However these responses are only speculative as maternal nipple/areolar attributes and/or infant suction pressures were not measured in these studies. Although an ideal nipple shield for preterm infants has yet to be designed, the smallest, thinnest shield available is indicated for these babies.

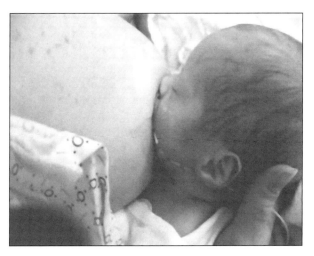

FIGURE **13–10** Preterm infant at breast with nipple shield in place.

Source: Used with permission from Rush Mothers' Milk Club, Rush-Presbyterian St. Luke's Medical Center, Chicago, IL.

The nipple shield is extremely well accepted by mothers, because it often represents the first breastfeeding experience in which the infant remains awake, sucks eagerly, and consumes measurable volumes of milk. However, mothers are concerned about providing the gentle pressure necessary to keep the infants correctly positioned over the areola, because of the plastic nature of shield. Thus, mothers need to be shown how to support the breast with the shield in place so that the infant can achieve an effective sucking position while keeping the shield away from the nose.

Clinicians often assume that preterm infants do not take as much milk with the shield in place as they would without its use. This concern seems to be based on the Auerbach 1990 data that demonstrated reduced milk transfer when mothers of term infants expressed milk with a breast pump with a nipple shield in place (as cited in Auerbach, 1992). Although this study addressed an important concept, the findings cannot be applied indiscriminately to infants as milk transfer was measured for milk expression with a breast pump—not infant feeding. Preterm infants, who are unable to transfer milk during breastfeeding prior to nipple shield use, actually increase milk intake when the shield is in place. Similarly, concern that use of the shield will reduce the milk yield over time is not applicable in this situation. Preterm infants who feed longer and more eagerly with the shield in place provide considerably more breast stimulation than breastfeeding without the shield.

Second, clinicians suggest that other feeding techniques, such as cup- or finger-feedings, be used as an alternative to the nipple shield. This approach appears to reflect an unscientific bias against the nipple shield, and is especially problematic because use of the shield means that the infant can feed at the breast. Mothers of preterm infants, who have spent weeks or months expressing milk, prefer to feed their babies at the breast, even if it entails temporary nipple shield use. And use of the shield saves time for mothers, because they do not need to offer a complement after breastfeeding, as is the case with a cup- or finger-feeding.

Finally, the duration of nipple shield use is a common concern, in that clinicians frequently ask how to "wean" babies from the shield. Data indicate that for a sample of preterm, low-birthweight infants who received the same research-based breastfeeding services, duration of breastfeeding was twice as long for the group of infants who were breastfed with the shield (Meier et al., 2000). Thus, common concerns that use of the nipple shield decreases the milk supply and shortens the duration of breastfeeding are not supported by the available research for preterm infants.

If the nipple shield is effective in correcting milk transfer problems in the hospital, its use should be continued after NICU discharge. Additionally, there is no scientific reason for recommending that infants be "weaned" from the shield as soon as possible. Typically, the infant will require the shield for adequate milk transfer until approximately term-corrected age. For most mothers, this coincides with 2 to 3 weeks of nipple shield use, over which time the infant's intake and weight gain can be monitored regularly. Mothers have described their individual approaches to discontinuing the shield, but in no case should they be advised to cut back or tamper with the integrity of the shield. Serial test-weights are helpful to most mothers as they transfer from the shield to feeding at the breast without the shield.

In addition to the nipple shield, other breastfeeding devices are frequently recommended to measure and facilitate milk transfer. A supplemental nurser can be helpful for the mother who has a limited milk supply and the infant is able to achieve sustained attachment and sucking mechanism at the breast. This device is especially helpful for borderline preterm infants (> 34 weeks gestation) who are still premature with respect to the ability to extract adequate volumes of milk. Providing they are able to sustain attachment, these infants can receive the extra milk they need with a supplemental nurser while feeding at the breast.

Discharge Planning for Postdischarge Breastfeeding

Unlike term healthy infants, preterm infants do not demonstrate predictable, easily detectible hunger cues until close to term-corrected age (Kavanaugh et al., 1995; Nyqvist et al., 1999; Ross & Browne, 2002), and mothers report difficulty in recognizing these behaviors (Reyna, Pickler, & Thompson, 2006). Thus, infants may consume minimal volumes at a breastfeeding and still sleep for several hours, if undisturbed. The use of test-weights permits the emergence of demand feeding behaviors, while retaining a safeguard against slow weight gain and dehydration in the days before NICU discharge.

When the infant has demonstrated the ability to consume all feedings orally, the neonatologist or neonatal nurse practitioner can prescribe a 24-hour minimal milk intake for the infant. The 24-hour volume can then be subdivided into 6- or 8-hour volumes to permit a modified demand-feeding schedule. For example, if an infant weighing 1700 grams needs a minimum of 300 ml per day, the mother and nurse can plan to feed 100 ml every 8 hours. Then, the infant is allowed to "demand," but must receive the prescribed 100 ml volume within an 8-hour period. Test-weights are measured with each breastfeeding, and the volume of complements and/or supplements is recorded. Thus, if the infant consumes 15 ml, 12 ml, and 18 ml within a period of 2 hours, the infant has been given the opportunity to self-regulate sleep and feeding. However, the infant still must consume the remaining 55 ml over the next 6 hours. NICU nurses can help mothers implement this plan in the days before infant discharge, so that mothers develop an understanding of how the infant coordinates sleep and feeding.

Many mothers of preterm infants, both borderline babies and those who are smaller, find it reassuring to measure milk intake and/or serial weight gain in the first days after infant discharge (Hurst et al., 2004). A portable, battery-operated scale that mothers can rent and perform test-weights and/or daily weights in the home is ideal for this purpose. The scale, which weighs to the nearest 2 g and automatically calculates milk intake from the pre- and postfeed weights, has been demonstrated to measure milk intake accurately for term and preterm infants (Meier et al., 1994). This scale can be a useful adjunct to breastfeeding management for mothers and preterm infants during the first week or two after discharge. However, mothers should be introduced to the proper use of the scale during the days prior to NICU discharge.

The United States is different from most developed countries in that preterm infants are typically discharged from the NICU before their expected birth dates, whether or not breastfeeding has been well established. In contrast, in some European countries, preterm infants are discharged only when weight gain on exclusive breastfeeding has been documented, which may be several weeks later than the United States (Akerstrom, Asplund, & Norman, 2007; Flacking et al., 2003; Nyqvist et al., 1999). In developing countries, preterm infants are frequently discharged at lower weights, but many of these infants are small for gestational age (Ramasethu, Jeyaseelan, & Kirubakaran, 1993) and/or maintained in skin-to-skin care in the home (Bergman & Jurisoo, 1994; Cattaneo et al., 1998; Charpak, Ruiz-Pelaez, & Charpak, 1994; Whitelaw & Liestol, 1994).

When these data are considered in combination, it appears that preterm infants remain at risk for underconsumption of milk by exclusive at-breast feeding until approximately term-corrected age (Meier & Brown, 1996). This is suggested by the low incidence of exclusive at-breast feeding in the early weeks after NICU discharge in the United States (Furman, Minich, & Hack, 1998; Hill, Ledbetter, & Kavanaugh, 1997); the longer hospitalization in European countries so that exclusive at-breast feeding is established (Nyqvist et al., 1999); and the slow weight gain on exclusive breastfeedings in the first 2–4 weeks after hospital discharge in developing countries. This commonality probably reflects a problem with the maturationally dependent "infant suckling" component of milk transfer, often expressed by mothers as "getting enough."

Getting Enough: Determining Need for Extra Milk Feedings

Studies from the United States have examined the phenomenon of "getting enough" for mothers and preterm infants (Hill, Ledbetter, & Kavanaugh, 1997; Kavanaugh et al., 1995). However, clinicians who work primarily with term, healthy infants do not always comprehend the difference between "getting enough" and "insufficient milk supply." As a result, mothers of preterm infants are frequently told to breastfeed their babies and/or pump more frequently, interventions that are focused upon the milk volume component of milk transfer. These recommendations are inappropriate for most mothers of preterm infants who describe problems with "getting enough." These women report that they can express adequate volumes of milk with the breast pump, but perceive that their infants do not take all of the milk available to them. Thus, effective interventions must focus on the infant suckling component of milk transfer. This distinction has important research and practice implications.

The most fundamental research issue is that accepted nomenclature for describing and classifying amount of breastfeeding does not fit the breastfeeding patterns for this population (Meier & Brown, 1997). For example, most mothers of preterm infants complement at-breast feedings with their own expressed milk during the early weeks at home (Hurst et al., 2004; Wooldridge & Hall, 2003), but the Labbok and Krasovec schema does not accurately capture this pattern. If this pattern is categorized as "exclusive breastfeeding," it overestimates mothers' successes and misrepresents data on duration of breastfeeding. Thus, research-based criteria to categorize the amount of breastfeeding for these mothers must be developed and standardized.

Research addressing the early postdischarge period must also include methods that accurately and reliably distinguish between insufficient maternal milk supply and the infant's ability to consume adequate milk volumes (Hill et al., 1997; Meier & Brown, 1997). These studies must incorporate available technology to measure milk volume and infant intake during breastfeeding, rather than relying on checklists or clinical indices that have been demonstrated to be inaccurate and/or unreliable. Similarly, other studies in which milk intake during breastfeeding was not measured have related slow weight gain and/or the need for continued milk fortification postdischarge to address deficiencies in the mothers' milk (Chan, Borschel, & Jacobs, 1994; Hall, Wheeler, & Rippetoe, 1993; Wauben et al., 1998). Thus, future postdischarge studies for preterm infants must include accurate instrumentation to differentiate among milk supply, milk "quality," and infant intake.

Methods to Deliver Extra Milk Feedings Away from the Breast

In most NICUs in the United States, the most common method of oral feeding when the mother is not available is by bottle. Several investigators have suggested that the differences in sucking patterns required during breastfeeding compared to bottle-feeding contribute to difficulties transitioning to exclusive breastfeeding. Alternative feeding devices are frequently recommended by clinicians to avoid "nipple confusion" (Cronenwett et al., 1992; Lang, Lawrence, & Orme, 1994; Neifert, Lawrence, & Seacat, 1995). Reports suggest that one such alternative feeding method—cup feeding—is safe when performed by experts (Lang et al., 1994; Rocha, Martinez, & Jorge, 2002), but few controlled clinical trials have established increased breastfeeding prevalence for these devices (Dowling et al., 2002; Rocha et al., 2002). An interesting finding revealed in one study showed the oral mechanisms used by preterm infants during cup-feeding as "sipping" rather than "lapping" in the majority of the 15 cup feeding sessions for eight preterm (mean gestational age at birth 30.6 wks) infants (Dowling, 2002). Additionally, a significant amount (38.5 percent) of milk spillage during cupfeeding was reported by Dowling et al. (2002) and others (Aloysius & Hickson, 2007).

Postdischarge Breastfeeding Management

Preterm infants are vulnerable to underconsumption of milk during the first weeks after discharge. Clinicians who are accustomed to helping mothers of term healthy infants, must acknowledge this phenomenon. Several key principles must be understood and incorporated into postdischarge breastfeeding plans for preterm infants:

- The practitioner must recognize that the clinical indices of intake used for healthy term infants, such as breastfeeding behaviors, wet diapers, frequency of stools, and sleep patterns, are not accurate or reliable for preterm infants. For example, a preterm infant may remain "hydrated," but still not consume enough milk to grow.
- Preterm infants may not consistently "demand," so mothers must not be told "You'll know when your baby is hungry."
- These infants should not be awakened more frequently than every 3 hours to breastfeed because sleep interruption interferes with growth hormone release, retarding weight gain.
- Mothers of preterm infants are not reassured with nonspecific comments such as "Trust your body." It is important to accept that mothers' concerns about intake are real, and not just a reflection of their NICU experience.

In summary, mothers of preterm infants need a safety net during the first weeks at home until their infants have demonstrated the ability to gain weight on exclusive breastfeedings. Milk transfer must be monitored regularly, such as every 48–72 hours, and accurately at this time, either through frequent visits to the primary care provider for serial growth measures, or by in-home test-weighing.

Care must be taken to listen to these women and their feelings of vulnerability with respect to infant intake. They must not be hurried through these processes, or told that they are not breastfeeding "correctly." For example, if a mother feels that she needs to give bottle supplements of her expressed milk in the first few days, she should not be warned about "nipple confusion," or told that alternative feedings should be used. Instead, her ability to determine and advocate what she feels is best for her infant must be interpreted as a sign of strength. It is important to remember that breastfeeding is only one activity that these women must deal with; their babies are vulnerable to many conditions, and mothers need time to sort out care priorities.

Similarly, mothers should be encouraged to continue the breastfeeding strategies that worked in the hospital until their infants have demonstrated an acceptable pattern of growth for at least a week or two. For many women, these devices will include a nipple shield and/or in-home weighing, and there are no data to support withdrawing these aids before the mother is ready. Finally, the mother needs access to both consumer support groups and a professional who is experienced with breastfeeding for preterm infants when discharge approaches.

Summary

In summary, breastfeeding for preterm infants and mothers is different from breastfeeding for healthy populations in many important ways. The vast body of research in this area suggests that these differences are physiologic, biologic, metabolic, and emotional, and that they are common across a variety of national boundaries and cultures. The challenge to researchers and clinicians who work with mothers and preterm infants is to continue to generate new studies and practices that incorporate findings from these scientific publications. Only research-based practices can address the many barriers to breastfeeding initiation and duration for this at-risk population.

Key Concepts

- Studies indicate that preterm infants are not just "small term infants" with respect to breastfeeding management, therefore research-based strategies that target specific barriers for this vulnerable population should be used.
- Human milk may provide optimal "nutritional programming" for preterm infants, and may be protective against several prematurity-related conditions.
- Based on current research related to the superiority of human milk for preterm infants parents should be provided accurate information in order to make an informed choice in providing mother's own milk for their preterm infant.
- Mothers providing breast milk for their preterm infants should be praised for their efforts regardless of the length of time of their commitments.
- Although giving birth prematurely does not appear to limit milk production, several factors surrounding the birth experience are documented prolactin-inhibitors and can adversely affect milk volume.
- The mother's milk expression technique can influence the composition and the bacterial count of the milk to be fed to her infant.
- Documenting the time, duration, and amount of milk expressed provides useful information to the mother that can be shared with the NICU staff for assessment of milk volume maintenance.
- It has been speculated that skin-to-skin holding may trigger the production of maternal milk antibodies to specific pathogens in the preterm infants' environment through mechanisms in the enteromammary pathway.
- Proper NICU procedures should be developed and adhered to in order to minimize bacterial growth and possible changes in milk constituents during storage and feeding.
- Special consideration regarding the feeding of expressed mothers' milk to preterm infants is based on the infant's fluid restrictive status at a time of greatest nutritional need.
- Unfortified expressed mothers' milk is deficient in protein and selected minerals to support optimal growth and bone mineralization for small preterm infants.
- Lactoengineering of expressed mother's milk through a combination of hindmilk and creamatocrit measures can impact the caloric density of the milk provided to preterm infants, as well as empowering their mothers.
- Early oral feeding experiences may influence later oral feeding development in preterm infants.
- There are no universally established criteria for the initiation of breastfeeding (or bottlefeeding for that matter) for preterm infants.
- In NICUs where infants are allowed nonnutritive suckling at the emptied breast, the mother is afforded valuable observation of her infant's

behavior and developing signs for readiness to oral feeding.

- Delayed initiation of breastfeeding until the infant demonstrates the ability to consume entire bottle feedings is not a research-based criterion of readiness to breastfeed.
- Milk transfer during breastfeeding is dependent upon sufficient maternal milk secretion and ejection concurrent with proficient infant oral motor skills.
- Test-weighing procedures provide the most accurate measure of milk intake for clinical and research settings.
- The single most important factor for mothers who will be breastfeeding a preterm infant at home is maintaining a milk supply that exceeds the infant's requirements at hospital discharge.
- The majority of milk transfer problems for preterm infants can be related to immaturity and inconsistency in suckling.
- For preterm infants who are unable to sustain attachment to the maternal breast and/or transfer milk, the nipple shield has proven an effective strategy as a milk transfer device.
- It appears that preterm infants remain at risk for underconsumption of milk by exclusive at-breast feeding until term-corrected age.
- Mothers' concerns regarding their preterm infants ability to "get enough" milk during breastfeeding are real and should not be dismissed.

Internet Resources

American Association for Premature Infants (AAPI), founded in 1992, is an organization dedicated to improving the quality of health, developmental, and educational services for premature infants, children, and their families: www.aapi-online.org.

Congenital Heart Information Network (CHIN), is an international organization that provides reliable information, support services, and resources to families of children with congenital heart defects and acquired heart disease: www.tchin.org.

iVillage Web site, a unique discussion board designated for mothers who are exclusively pumping their breastmilk for their infants: http://parenting.ivillage.com/newborn/nbreast feed/topics/0,,4rnn,00.html.

La Leche League International, parent and professional materials on breastfeeding a preterm infant: www.lalecheleague.org.

National Organization of Mothers of Twins Clubs, Inc. (NOMOTC), founded in 1960, is a group providing support, education, and information for mothers of twins: www.nomotc.org.

Parents of Premature Babies, Inc. (Preemie-L), is a Web site offering support to families of premature infants while the babies are hospitalized and following discharge: www.preemie-l.org.

Preemie Place is an online resource providing answers to questions, or information for a specific topic regarding prematurity: www.thepreemieplace.org.

Premature Baby Premature Child is a volunteer Web site providing parents with information to care for premature infants: www.prematurity.org.

Texas Children's Hospital provides a newsletter for parents of preterms and professionals: www.texaschildrens.org/lactation.

References

Adams C et al. Breastfeeding trends at a Community Breastfeeding Center: an evaluative survey. *J Obstet Gynecol Neonatal Nurs.* 2001;30(4):392–400.

Aggett PJ et al. Feeding preterm infants after hospital discharge: a commentary by the ESPGHAN Committee on Nutrition. *J Pediatr Gastroenterol Nutr.* 2006;42(5):596–603.

Agrasada GV et al. Postnatal peer counselling on exclusive breastfeeding of low-birthweight infants: a randomized, controlled trial. *Acta Paediatr.* 2005;94(8):1109–1115.

Aguayo J. Maternal lactation for preterm newborn infants. *Early Hum Dev.* 2001;65(suppl):S19–S29.

Akerstrom S, Asplund I, Norman M. Successful breastfeeding after discharge of preterm and sick newborn infants. *Acta Paediatr.* 2007;96(10): 1450–1454.

Akisu M et al. Platelet-activating factor levels in term and preterm human milk. *Biol Neonate.* 1998;74(4): 289–293.

Aljazaf K et al. Pseudoephedrine: effects on milk production in women and estimation of infant exposure via breastmilk. *Br J Clin Pharmacol.* 2003;56(1):18–24.

Aloysius A, Hickson M. Evaluation of paladai cup feeding in breast-fed preterm infants compared with bottle feeding. *Early Hum Dev.* 2007;83(9):619–621.

AAP. Transfer of drugs and other chemicals into human milk. *Pediatrics.* 2001;108(3):776–789.

Amin SB et al. Brainstem maturation in premature infants as a function of enteral feeding type. *Pediatrics.* 2000;106(2 pt1):318–322.

Ardran GM, Kemp FH, Lind J. A cineradiographic study of breastfeeding. *Br J Radiol.* 1958;31:156–162.

Arias-Camison JM. Late onset group B streptococcal infection from maternal expressed breast milk in a very low birth weight infant. *J Perinatol.* 2003; 23(8):691–692.

Armand M et al. Effect of human milk or formula on gastric function and fat digestion in the premature infant. *Pediatr Res.* 1996;40(3):429–437.

Arslanoglu S, Moro GE, Ziegler EE. Adjustable fortification of human milk fed to preterm infants: does it make a difference? *J Perinatol.* 2006;26(10):614–621.

Auerbach KG. Re: 'Changes in nutritive sucking patterns with increasing gestational age'. *Nurs Res.* 1992;41(2):126–127.

Baker BJ, Rasmussen TW. Organizing and documenting lactation support of NICU families. *J Obstet Gynecol Neonatal Nurs.* 1997;26(5):515–521.

Ballabio C et al. Immunoglobulin-A profile in breast milk from mothers delivering full term and preterm infants. *Int J Immunopathol Pharmacol.* 2007;20(1):119–128.

Bauer K et al. Body temperatures and oxygen consumption during skin-to-skin (kangaroo) care in stable preterm infants weighing less than 1500 grams. *J Pediatr.* 1997;130:240–244.

Becker, GE, McCormick FM, Renfrew MJ. Methods of milk expression for lactating women. *Cochrane Database Syst Rev.* 2008;(4): CD006170.

Behari P et al. Transmission of methicillin-resistant *Staphylococcus aureus* to preterm infants through breast milk. *Infect Control Hosp Epidemiol.* 2004; 25(9):778–780.

Bergman NJ, Jurisoo LA. The 'kangaroo-method' for treating low birth weight babies in a developing country. *Trop Doct.* 1994;24(2):57–60.

Bernaix LW et al. The NICU experience of lactation and its relationship to family management style. *MCN Am J Matern Child Nurs.* 2006;31(2):95–100.

Bernt KM, Walker WA. Human milk as a carrier of biochemical messages. *Acta Paediatr Suppl.* 1999; 88(430):27–41.

Bialoskurski MM, Cox CL, Wiggins RD. The relationship between maternal needs and priorities in a neonatal intensive care environment. *J Adv Nurs.* 2002;37(1):62–69.

Bier JA et al. Comparison of skin-to-skin contact with standard contact in low-birth-weight infants who are breast-fed. *Arch Pediatr Adolesc Med.* 1996;150(12): 1265–1269.

Bier JA et al. Human milk improves cognitive and motor development of premature infants during infancy. *J Hum Lact.* 2002;18(4):361–367.

Bier JB et al. Breast-feeding of very low birth weight infants. *J Pediatr.* 1993;123(5):773–778.

Birch E et al. Dietary essential fatty acid supply and visual acuity development. *Invest Ophthalmol Vis Sci.* 1992;33(11):3242–3253.

Birch E et al. Breast-feeding and optimal visual development. *J Pediatr Ophthalmol Strabismus.* 1993; 30(1):33–38.

Blaymore Bier JA et al. Breastfeeding infants who were extremely low birth weight. *Pediatrics.* 1997; 100(6):E3.

Blumer N, Pfefferle PI, Renz H. Development of mucosal immune function in the intrauterine and early postnatal environment. *Curr Opin Gastroenterol.* 2007;23(6):655–660.

Boehm G et al. Fecal cholesterol excretion in preterm infants fed breast milk or formula with different cholesterol contents. *Acta Paediatr.* 1995;84(3):240–244.

Bohnhorst B et al. Skin-to-skin (kangaroo) care, respiratory control, and thermoregulation. *J Pediatr.* 2001; 138(2):193–197.

Brennan-Behm M et al. Caloric loss from expressed mother's milk during continuous gavage infusion. *Neonatal Netw.* 1994;13(2):27–32.

Britton JR. Milk protein quality in mothers delivering prematurely: implications for infants in the intensive care unit nursery setting. *J Pediatr Gastroenterol Nutr.* 1986;5(1):116–121.

Browne JV. Early relationship environments: physiology of skin-to-skin contact for parents and their preterm infants. *Clin Perinatol.* 2004;31(2):287–298.

Budd SC et al. Improved lactation with metoclopramide. A case report. *Clin Pediatr (Phila).* 1993; 32(1):53–57.

Butte NF et al. Longitudinal changes in milk composition of mothers delivering preterm and term infants. *Early Hum Dev.* 1984;9:153–162.

Byrne B, Hull D. Breast milk for preterm infants. *Prof Care Mother Child.* 1996;6(2):39, 42–35.

Byrne PA, Miller C, Justus K. Neonatal group B streptococcal infection related to breast milk. *Breastfeeding Medicine.* 2006;1(4):263–270.

Callen J et al. Qualitative analysis of barriers to breastfeeding in very-low-birthweight infants in the hospital and postdischarge. *Advances in Neonatal Care.* 2005;5(2):93–103.

CPS. Nutrient needs and feeding of premature infants. Nutrition Committee, Canadian Paediatric Society. *CMAJ.* 1995;152(11):1765–1785.

Carter CS, Altemus M. Integrative functions of lactational hormones in social behavior and stress management. *Ann N Y Acad Sci.* 1997;807:164–174.

Cattaneo A et al. Kangaroo mother care for low birthweight infants: a randomized controlled trial in different settings. *Acta Paediatr.* 1998; 87(9):976–985.

Chan GM, Borschel MW, Jacobs JR. Effects of human milk or formula feeding on the growth, behavior, and protein status of preterm infants discharged from the newborn intensive care unit. *Am J Clin Nutr.* 1994;60(5):710–716.

Charpak N, Ruiz-Pelaez JG, Charpak Y. Rey-Martinez Kangaroo Mother Program: an alternative way of caring for low birth weight infants? One year mortality in a two cohort study. *Pediatrics.* 1994; 94(6 pt1):804–810.

Charpak N et al. A randomized, controlled trial of kangaroo mother care: results of follow-up at 1 year of corrected age. *Pediatrics.* 2001;108(5):1072–1079.

Charpak N et al. Kangaroo Mother Care: 25 years after. *Acta Paediatr.* 2005;94(5):514–522.

Charpak N, Ruiz J. Breast milk composition in a cohort of pre-term infants' mothers followed in an ambulatory programme in Colombia. *Acta Paediatr.* 2007; 96(12):1755–1759.

Chatterton RT, Jr. et al. Relation of plasma oxytocin and prolactin concentrations to milk production in mothers of preterm infants: influence of stress. *J Clin Endocrinol Metab.* 2000;85(10):3661–3668.

Chen CH et al. The effect of breast- and bottle-feeding on oxygen saturation and body temperature in preterm infants. *J Hum Lact.* 2000;16(1):21–27.

Clum D, Primomo J. Use of a silicone nipple shield with premature infants. *J Hum Lact.* 1996;12(4):287–290.

Contreras-Lemus J et al. Morbidity reduction in preterm newborns fed with milk of their own mothers. *Bol Med Hosp Infant Mex.* 1992;49(10):671–677.

Cregan MD et al. Initiation of lactation in women after preterm delivery. *Acta Obstet Gynecol Scand.* 2002; 81(9):870–877.

Cronenwett L et al. Single daily bottle use in the early weeks postpartum and breast-feeding outcomes. *Pediatrics.* 1992;90(5):760–766.

Curtis N et al. Cytomegalovirus remains viable in naturally infected breast milk despite being frozen for 10 days. *Arch Dis Child Fetal Neonatal Ed.* 2005; 90(6):F529–F530.

Daly SE et al. Degree of breast emptying explains changes in the fat content, but not fatty acid composition, of human milk. *Exp Physiol.* 1993;78(6):741–755.

Daly SE, Hartmann PE. Infant demand and milk supply. part 1: Infant demand and milk production in lactating women. *J Hum Lact.* 1995;11(1):21–26.

Daly SE, Hartmann PE. Infant demand and milk supply. part 2: The short-term control of milk synthesis in lactating women. *J Hum Lact.* 1995;11(1):27–37.

Daly SE et al. Frequency and degree of milk removal and the short-term control of human milk synthesis. *Exp Physiol.* 1996;81(5):861–875.

deMonterice D et al. Concurrent validity of a new instrument for measuring nutritive sucking in preterm infants. *Nurs Res.* 1992;41(6):342–346.

Diaz-Gomez NM, Domenech E, Barroso F. Breast-feeding and growth factors in preterm newborn infants. *J Pediatr Gastroenterol Nutr.* 1997;24(3):322–327.

Doctor S et al. Cytomegalovirus transmission to extremely low-birthweight infants through breast milk. *Acta Paediatr.* 2005;94(1):53–58.

Dodd V. Implications of kangaroo care for growth and development in preterm infants. *J Obstet Gynecol Neonatal Nurs.* 2005;34(2):218–232.

Dowling DA. Physiological responses of preterm infants to breast-feeding and bottle-feeding with the orthodontic nipple. *Nurs Res.* 1999;48(2):78–85.

Dvorak B et al. Increased epidermal growth factor levels in human milk of mothers with extremely premature infants. *Pediatr Res.* 2003;54(1):15–19.

Edelbauer M et al. Maternally delivered nutritive allergens in cord blood and in placental tissue of term and preterm neonates. *Clin Exp Allergy.* 2004;34(2):189–193.

Eibl MM et al. Prevention of necrotizing enterocolitis in low-birth-weight infants by IgA-IgG feeding. *N Engl J Med.* 1988;319(1):1–7.

Elmlinger MW et al. Insulin-like growth factors and binding proteins in early milk from mothers of preterm and term infants. *Horm Res.* 2007;68(3):124–131.

el-Mohandes AE et al. Bacterial contaminants of collected and frozen human milk used in an intensive care nursery. *Am J Infect Control.* 1993;21(5):226–230.

Emery MM. Galactogogues: drugs to induce lactation. *J Hum Lact.* 1996;12:55–57.

Ewer AK et al. Gastric emptying in preterm infants. *Arch Dis Child Fetal Neonatal Ed.* 1994;71(1):F24–F27.

Ewer AK, Yu VY. Gastric emptying in pre-term infants: the effect of breast milk fortifier. *Acta Paediatr.* 1996;85(9):1112–1115.

Farquharson J et al. Effect of diet on the fatty acid composition of the major phospholipids of infant cerebral cortex. *Arch Dis Child.* 1995;72(3):198–203.

Feher SD et al. Increasing breast milk production for premature infants with a relaxation/imagery audiotape. *Pediatrics.* 1989;83(1):57–60.

Feldman R et al. Comparison of skin-to-skin (kangaroo) and traditional care: parenting outcomes and preterm infant development. *Pediatrics.* 2002;110(1 pt1):16–26.

Feldman R, Eidelman AI. Skin-to-skin contact (Kangaroo Care) accelerates autonomic and neurobehavioural maturation in preterm infants. *Dev Med Child Neurol.* 2003;45(4):274–281.

Fewtrell M et al. Randomized study comparing the efficacy of a novel manual breast pump with a mini-electric breast pump in mothers of term infants. *J Hum Lact.* 2001;17(2):126–131.

Fewtrell MS et al. Randomised, double blind trial of oxytocin nasal spray in mothers expressing breast milk for preterm infants. *Arch Dis Child Fetal Neonatal Ed.* 2006;91(3):F169–F174.

Fidler N et al. Fat content and fatty acid composition of fresh, pasteurized, or sterilized human milk. *Adv Exp Med Biol.* 2001;501:485–495.

Fituch CC et al. Interlukin-10 concentration in milk of mothers delivering extremely low birth weight infants. *Pediatr Res.* 2001;49(4):398A.

Flacking R et al. Long-term duration of breastfeeding in Swedish low birth weight infants. *J Hum Lact.* 2003;19(2):157–165.

Flacking R, Ewald U, Starrin B. "I wanted to do a good job": Experiences of 'becoming a mother' and breastfeeding in mothers of very preterm infants after discharge from a neonatal unit. *Social Science & Medicine.* 2007;64:2405–2416.

Friedman S et al. The effect of prenatal consultation with a neonatologist on human milk feeding in preterm infants. *Acta Paediatr.* 2004;93(6):775–778.

Fucile S, Gisel EG, Lau C. Effect of an oral stimulation program on sucking skill maturation of preterm infants. *Dev Med Child Neurol.* 2005;47(3):158–162.

Furman L, Minich NM, Hack M. Breastfeeding of very low birth weight infants. *J Hum Lact.* 1998;14(1): 29–34.

Furman L et al. The effect of maternal milk on neonatal morbidity of very low-birth-weight infants. *Arch Pediatr Adolesc Med.* 2003;157(1):66–71.

Furman L, Minich N. Efficiency of breastfeeding as compared to bottle-feeding in very low birth weight (VLBW, <1.5 kg) infants. *J Perinatol.* 2004;24(11): 706–713.

Gale G, Franck L, Lund C. Skin-to-skin (kangaroo) holding of the intubated premature infant. *Neonatal Netw.* 1993;12(6):49–57.

Garofalo RP, Goldman AS. Cytokines, chemokines, and colony-stimulating factors in human milk: the 1997 update. *Biol Neonate.* 1998;74(2):134–142.

Gartner LM et al. Breastfeeding and the use of human milk. *Pediatrics.* 2005;115(2):496–506.

Garza C et al. Special properties of human milk. *Clin Perinatol.* 1987;14(1):11–32.

Gastelum DT, Dassey D, Mascola L, et al. Transmission of community-associated methicillin-resistant Staphylococcus aureus from breast milk in the neonatal intensive care unit. *Pediatr Infect Dis J.* 2005;24(12):1122–1124.

Gazzolo D, Masetti P, Meli M. Kangaroo care improves post-extubation cardiorespiratory parameters in infants after open heart surgery. *Acta Paediatr.* 2000;89(6):728–729.

Genzel-Boroviczeny O, Wahle J, Koletzko B. Fatty acid composition of human milk during the 1st month after term and preterm delivery. *Eur J Pediatr.* 1997;156(2):142–147.

Goldblum RM et al. Human Milk Banking I: Effects of Container Upon Immunologic Factors in Mature Milk. *Nutrition Research.* 1981;1:449–459.

Goldblum RM et al. Human milk feeding enhances the urinary excretion of immunologic factors in low birth weight infants. *Pediatr Res.* 1989; 25(2):184–188.

Goldman AS et al. Molecular forms of lactoferrin in stool and urine from infants fed human milk. *Pediatr Res.* 1990;27(3):252–255.

Greer FR, McCormick A, Loker J. Changes in fat concentration of human milk during delivery by intermittent bolus and continuous mechanical pump infusion. *J Pediatr.* 1984;105(5):745–749.

Griffin IJ, Abrams SA. Zinc absorption by infants. *Minerva Pediatr.* Jun 2003;55(3):231–242.

Groh-Wargo S et al. The utility of a bilateral breast pumping system for mothers of premature infants. *Neonatal Netw.* 1995;14(8):31–36.

Gross SJ et al. Nutritional composition of milk produced by mothers delivering preterm. *J Pediatr.* 1980;96(4):641–644.

Gunn TR et al. Does early hospital discharge with home support of families with preterm infants affect breastfeeding success? A randomized trial. *Acta Paediatr.* 2000;89(11):1358–1363.

Hale TW. Medications in breastfeeding mothers of preterm infants. *Pediatr Ann.* 2003;32(5):337–347.

Hale TW. *Medications and Mother's Milk.* Amarillo, TX: Pharmasoft Publishing; 2006.

Hall RT, Wheeler RE, Rippetoe LE. Calcium and phosphorus supplementation after initial hospital discharge in breast-fed infants of less than 1800 grams birth weight. *J Perinatol.* 1993;13(4):272–278.

Hamosh M. Bioactive factors in human milk. *Pediatr Clin North Am.* 2001;48(1):69–86.

Hamprecht K et al. Epidemiology of transmission of cytomegalovirus from mother to preterm infant by breastfeeding. *Lancet.* 2001;357(9255):513–518.

Hamprecht K et al. Cytomegalovirus (CMV) inactivation in breast milk: reassessment of pasteurization and freeze-thawing. *Pediatr Res.* 2004;56(4):529–535.

Hanson LA. Human milk and host defence: immediate and long-term effects. *Acta Paediatr Suppl.* 1999; 88(430):42–46.

Hartmann P, Cregan M. Lactogenesis and the effects of insulin-dependent diabetes mellitus and prematurity. *J Nutr.* 2001;131(11):3016S–3020S.

Hartmann PE et al. Physiology of lactation in preterm mothers: initiation and maintenance. *Pediatr Ann.* 2003;32(5):351–355.

Hedberg Nyqvist K, Ewald U. Infant and maternal factors in the development of breastfeeding behaviour and breastfeeding outcome in preterm infants. *Acta Paediatr.* 1999;88(11):1194–1203.

Heird WC. The role of polyunsaturated fatty acids in term and preterm infants and breastfeeding mothers. *Pediatr Clin North Am.* 2001;48(1):173–188.

Henderson TR et al. Gastric proteolysis in preterm infants fed mother's milk or formula. *Adv Exp Med Biol.* 2001;501:403–408.

Hildebrandt R, Gundert-Remy U. Lack of pharmacological active saliva levels of caffeine in breast-fed infants. *Pediatr Pharmacol (New York)*. 1983;3(3-4): 237–244.

Hill PD, Andersen JL, Ledbetter RJ. Delayed initiation of breast-feeding the preterm infant. *J Perinat Neonatal Nurs.* 1995;9(2):10–20.

Hill PD, Ledbetter RJ, Kavanaugh KL. Breastfeeding patterns of low-birth-weight infants after hospital discharge. *J Obstet Gynecol Neonatal Nurs.* 1997; 26(2):189–197.

Hill PD, Aldag JC, Chatterton RT. Effects of pumping style on milk production in mothers of non-nursing preterm infants. *J Hum Lact.* 1999;15(3):209–216.

Hill PD et al. Predictors of preterm infant feeding methods and perceived insufficient milk supply at week 12 postpartum. *J Hum Lact.* 2007;23(1):32–38, 39–43.

Hopkinson JM, Schanler RJ, Garza C. Milk production by mothers of premature infants. *Pediatrics.* 1988;81(6):815–820.

HMBANA. 2006 Best practice for expressing, storing and handling of mother's own milk in hospital and at home: HMBANA; 2006.

Hurst NM et al. Skin-to-skin holding in the neonatal intensive care unit influences maternal milk volume. *J Perinatol.* 1997;17(3):213–217.

Hurst NM, Myatt A, Schanler RJ. Growth and development of a hospital-based lactation program and mother's own milk bank. *J Obstet Gynecol Neonatal Nurs.* 1998;27(5):503–510.

Hurst NM et al. Mothers performing in-home measurement of milk intake during breastfeeding of their preterm infants: maternal reactions and feeding outcomes. *J Hum Lact.* 2004;20(2):178–187.

Hutchens TW et al. Origin of intact lactoferrin and its DNA-binding fragments found in the urine of human milk-fed preterm infants. Evaluation by stable isotopic enrichment. *Pediatr Res.* 1991;29(3): 243–250.

Hylander MA, Strobino DM, Dhanireddy R. Human milk feedings and infection among very low birth weight infants. *Pediatrics.* 1998;102(3):E38.

Hylander MA et al. Association of human milk feedings with a reduction in retinopathy of prematurity among very low birthweight infants. *J Perinatol.* 2001;21(6):356–362.

Jackson K, Ternestedt BM, Schollin J. From alienation to familiarity—experiences of parents of preterm infants during the first 18 months of life. *J Adv Nurs.* 2003;43(2):120–129.

Jaeger MC, Lawson M, Filteau S. The impact of prematurity and neonatal illness on the decision to breastfeed. *J Adv Nurs.* 1997;25(4):729–737.

Jennings T, Meier W, Meier P. High lipid and caloric content in milk from mothers of preterm infants. *Pediatr Res.* 1997;41:233A.

Jenson D, Wallace S, Kelsay P. LATCH: A breastfeeding charting system and documentation tool. *J Gynecol Obstet Neonatal Nurs.* 1994;23:27–32.

Jensen RG. *The Lipids of Human Milk.* Boca Raton, FL: CRC Press; 1989.

Jim WT et al. Transmission of cytomegalovirus from mothers to preterm infants by breast milk. *Pediatr Infect Dis J.* 2004;23(9):848–851.

Jocson MA, Mason EO, Schanler RJ. The effects of nutrient fortification and varying storage conditions on host defense properties of human milk. *Pediatrics.* 1997;100(2 pt1):240–243.

Jones E. Strategies to promote preterm breastfeeding. *Mod Midwife.* 1995;5(3):8–11.

Jones E, Spencer SA. Optimising the provision of human milk for preterm infants. *Arch Dis Child Fetal Neonatal Ed.* 2007;92(4):F236–F238.

Jorgensen MH et al. Visual acuity and erythrocyte docosahexaenoic acid status in breast-fed and formula-fed term infants during the first four months of life. *Lipids.* 1996;31(1):99–105.

Kavanaugh K, Meier PP, Engstrom JL. Reliability of weighing procedures for preterm infants. *Nurs Res.* 1989;38(3):178–179.

Kavanaugh K et al. Getting enough: mothers' concerns about breastfeeding a preterm infant after discharge. *J Obstet Gynecol Neonatal Nurs.* 1995;24(1):23–32.

Kavanaugh K et al. The rewards outweigh the efforts: breastfeeding outcomes for mothers of preterm infants. *J Hum Lact.* 1997;13(1):15–21.

Kent J, Mitoulas L, Cox D, Owens R, Hartmann P. Breast volume and milk production during extended lactation in women. *Exp Phys.* 1999;84: 435–447.

Killersreiter B, Grimmer I, Buhrer C, Dudenhausen JW, Obladen M. Early cessation of breast milk feeding in very low birthweight infants. *Early Hum Dev.* 2001;60(3):193–205.

Kirsten GF, Bergman NJ, Hann FM. Kangaroo mother care in the nursery. *Pediatr Clin North Am.* 2001;48(2):443–452.

Koletzko B et al. Long chain polyunsaturated fatty acids (LC-PUFA) and perinatal development. *Acta Paediatr.* 2001;90:460–464.

Korchazhkina O et al. Effects of exclusive formula or breast milk feeding on oxidative stress in healthy preterm infants. *Arch Dis Child.* 2006;91(4):327–329.

Korja R et al. Mother-infant interaction is influenced by the amount of holding in preterm infants. *Early Hum Dev.* 2008;84(4):257–267.

Kosloske AM. Breastmilk decreases the risk of neonatal necrotizing enterocolitis. *Adv Nutr Res.* 2001; 10:123–137.

Kotiw M et al. Late-onset and recurrent neonatal Group B streptococcal disease associated with breast-milk transmission. *Pediatr Dev Pathol.* 2003;6(3):251–256.

Krouse AM. The family management of breastfeeding low birth weight infants. *J Hum Lact.* 2002;18(2): 155–165.

Kunz C, Rudloff S. Biological functions of oligosaccharides in human milk. *Acta Paediatr.* 1993; 82:903–912.

Kuschel C, Harding J. Multicomponent fortification of human milk for promoting growth in premature infants. *Cochrane Database Syst Rev.* 1998(revised 2003);3. Art. No.: CD000343. DOI: 10.1002/14651858.CD000343.pub2.

Lang S, Lawrence CJ, Orme RL. Cup feeding: an alternative method of infant feeding. *Arch Dis Child.* 1994;71(4):365–369.

Lau C et al. Oral feeding in low birth weight infants. *J Pediatr.* 1997;130(4):561–569.

Lau C, Hurst N. Oral feeding in infants. *Curr Probl Pediatr.* 1999;29(4):105–124.

Lau C et al. Characterization of the developmental stages of sucking in preterm infants during bottle feeding. *Acta Paediatr.* 2000;89(7):846–852.

Lau C, Smith EO, Schanler RJ. Coordination of suck-swallow and swallow respiration in preterm infants. *Acta Paediatr.* 2003;92(6):721–727.

Lau C et al. Ethnic/racial diversity, maternal stress, lactation and very low birthweight infants. *J Perinatol.* 2007;27(7):399–408.

Lauritzen L et al. Maternal fish oil supplementation in lactation: effect on developmental outcome in breast-fed infants. *Reprod Nutr Dev.* 2005;45(5):535–547.

Lawrence RA. Breastfeeding support benefits very low-birth-weight infants. *Arch Pediatr Adolesc Med.* 2001;155(5):543–544.

Legault M, Goulet C. Comparison of kangaroo and traditional methods of removing preterm infants from incubators. *J Obstet Gynecol Neonatal Nurs.* 1995;24(6):501–506.

Lemons JA et al. Differences in the composition of preterm and term human milk during early lactation. *Pediatr Res.* 1982;16(2):113–117.

Lucas A et al. Creamatocrit: simple clinical technique for estimating fat concentration and energy value of human milk. *Br Med J.* 1978;1(6119):1018–1020.

Lucas A, Cole TJ. Breast milk and neonatal necrotising enterocolitis. *Lancet.* 1990;336(8730):1519–1523.

Lucas A et al. A randomised multicentre study of human milk versus formula and later development in preterm infants. *Arch Dis Child Fetal Neonatal Ed.* 1994;70(2):F141–F146.

Lucas A, Morley R. Breastfeeding, dummy use, and adult intelligence. *Lancet.* 1996;347(9017):1765–1766.

Lucas A, Morley R, Cole TJ. Randomised trial of early diet in preterm babies and later intelligence quotient. *BMJ.* 1998;317(7171):1481–1487.

Ludington-Hoe SM et al. Kangaroo care: research results, and practice implications and guidelines. *Neonatal Netw.* 1994;13(1):19–27.

Ludington-Hoe SM, Hosseini R, Torowicz DL. Skin-to-skin contact (Kangaroo Care) analgesia for preterm infant heel stick. *AACN Clin Issues.* 2005;16(3):373–387.

Ludington-Hoe SM et al. Neurophysiologic assessment of neonatal sleep organization: preliminary results of a randomized, controlled trial of skin contact with preterm infants. *Pediatrics.* 2006;117(5):e909–e923.

Lundqvist C, Hafstrom M. Non-nutritive sucking in full-term and preterm infants studied at term conceptional age. *Acta Paediatr.* 1999;88(11):1287–1289.

Luukkainen P, Salo MK, Nikkari T. Changes in the fatty acid composition of preterm and term human milk from 1 week to 6 months of lactation. *J Pediatr Gastroenterol Nutr.* 1994;18(3):355–360.

Luukkainen P et al. Fatty acid composition of plasma and red blood cell phospholipids in preterm infants from 2 weeks to 6 months postpartum. *J Pediatr Gastroenterol Nutr.* 1995;20(3):310–315.

Maas YG et al. Development of macronutrient composition of very preterm human milk. *Br J Nutr.* 1998;80(1):35–40.

Marinelli KA, Burke GS, Dodd VL. A comparison of the safety of cupfeedings and bottlefeedings in premature infants whose mothers intend to breastfeed. *J Perinatol.* 2001;21(6):350–355.

Martell M et al. Suction patterns in preterm infants. *J Perinat Med.* 1993;21(5):363–369.

McGrath JM, Braescu AV. State of the science: feeding readiness in the preterm infant. *J Perinat Neonatal Nurs.* 2004;18(4):353–368, 369–370.

Medoff-Cooper B. Multi-system approach to the assessment of successful feeding. *Acta Paediatr.* 2000;89(4):393–394.

Meier PP, Anderson GC. Responses of small preterm infants to bottle- and breast-feeding. *MCN Am J Matern Child Nurs.* 1987;12(2):97–105.

Meier PP. Bottle and breast-feeding: effects on transcutaneous oxygen pressure and temperature in preterm infants. *Nurs Res.* 1988;37(1):36–41.

Meier PP et al. The accuracy of test weighing for preterm infants. *J Pediatr Gastroenterol Nutr.* 1990;10(1):62–65.

Meier PP et al. Breastfeeding support services in the neonatal intensive-care unit. *J Obstet Gynecol Neonatal Nurs.* 1993;22(4):338–347.

Meier PP et al. A new scale for in-home test-weighing for mothers of preterm and high risk infants. *J Hum Lact.* 1994;10(3):163–168.

Meier PP. Caution needed in extrapolating from term to preterm infants: author's reply. *J Hum Lact.* 1995;11:91.

Meier PP, Brown LP. State of the science. Breastfeeding for mothers and low birth weight infants. *Nurs Clin North Am.* 1996;31(2):351–365.

Meier PP et al. Estimating milk intake of hospitalized preterm infants who breastfeed. *J Hum Lact.* Mar 1996;12(1):21–26.

Meier PP, Brown LP. Defining terminology for improved breastfeeding research. *J Nurse Midwifery.* 1997;42(1):65–66.

Meier PP et al. Nipple shields for preterm infants: effect on milk transfer and duration of breastfeeding. *J Hum Lact.* 2000;16(2):106–114, 129–131.

Meier PP. Breastfeeding in the special care nursery. Prematures and infants with medical problems. *Pediatr Clin North Am.* 2001;48(2):425–442.

Meier PP et al. The Rush Mothers' Milk Club: breast-feeding interventions for mothers with very-low-birth-weight infants. *J Obstet Gynecol Neonatal Nurs.* 2004;33(2):164–174.

Merewood A et al. The effect of peer counselors on breastfeeding rates in the neonatal intensive care unit: results of a randomized controlled trial. *Arch Pediatr Adolesc Med.* 2006;160(7):681–685.

Miller JB et al. The oligosaccharide composition of human milk: temporal and individual variations in monosaccharide components. *J Pediatr Gastroenterol Nutr.* 1994;19(4):371–376.

Milsom SR et al. Potential role for growth hormone in human lactation insufficiency. *Horm Res.* 1998;50(3):147–150.

Miracle DJ, Meier PP, Bennett PA. Mothers' decisions to change from formula to mothers' milk for very-low-birth-weight infants. *J Obstet Gynecol Neonatal Nurs.* 2004;33(6):692–703.

Miron D et al. Incidence and clinical manifestations of breast milk-acquired Cytomegalovirus infection in low birth weight infants. *J Perinatol.* 2005;25(5):299–303.

Moody GJ et al. Feeding tolerance in premature infants fed fortified human milk. *J Pediatr Gastroenterol Nutr.* 2000;30:408–412.

Moro G et al. Growth and plasma amino acid concentrations in very low birthweight infants fed either human milk protein fortified human milk or a whey-predominant formula. *Acta Paediatr Scand.* 1989;78(1):18–22.

Mulford C. The mother-baby assessment (MBA): An "Apgar score" for breastfeeding. *J Hum Lac.* 1992;8:79–82.

Mussi-Pinhata MM et al. Perinatal or early-postnatal cytomegalovirus infection in preterm infants under 34 weeks gestation born to CMV-seropositive mothers within a high-seroprevalence population. *J Pediatr.* 2004;145(5):685–688.

Narayanan I et al. Sucking on the 'emptied' breast: non-nutritive sucking with a difference. *Arch Dis Child.* 1991;66(2):241–244.

Neifert M, Lawrence R, Seacat J. Nipple confusion: toward a formal definition. *J Pediatr.* 1995;126(6):S125–S129.

Newburg DS, Ruiz-Palacios GM, Morrow AL. Human milk glycans protect infants against enteric pathogens. *Annu Rev Nutr.* 2005;25:37–58.

Newburg DS, Walker WA. Protection of the neonate by the innate immune system of developing gut and of human milk. *Pediatr Res.* 2007;61(1):2–8.

Newman TB et al. Prediction and prevention of extreme neonatal hyperbilirubinemia in a mature health maintenance organization. *Arch Pediatr Adolesc Med.* 2000;154(11):1140–1147.

Nicholl RM, Gamsu HR. Changes in growth and metabolism in very low birthweight infants fed with fortified breast milk. *Acta Paediatr.* 1999;88(10):1056–1061.

Novak FR et al. Contamination of expressed human breast milk with an epidemic multiresistant *Staphylococcus aureus* clone. *J Med Microbiol.* 2000;49(12): 1109–1117.

Nowak AJ, Smith WL, Erenberg A. Imaging evaluation of artificial nipples during bottle feeding. *Arch Pediatr Adolesc Med.* 1994;148(1):40–42.

Nowak AJ, Smith WL, Erenberg A. Imaging evaluation of breast-feeding and bottle-feeding systems. *J Pediatr.* 1995;126(6):S130–134.

Nyqvist KH, Ewald U, Sjoden PO. Supporting a preterm infant's behaviour during breastfeeding: a case report. *J Hum Lact.* 1996;12(3):221–228.

Nyqvist KH et al. Development of the Preterm Infant Breastfeeding Behavior Scale (PIBBS): a study of nurse-mother agreement. *J Hum Lact.* 1996;12(3):207–219.

Nyqvist KH, Sjoden PO, Ewald U. The development of preterm infants' breastfeeding behavior. *Early Hum Dev.* 1999;55(3):247–264.

Nyqvist KH et al. Early oral behaviour in preterm infants during breastfeeding: an electromyographic study. *Acta Paediatr.* 2001;90(6):658–663.

Ogechi AA, William O, Fidelia BT. Hindmilk and weight gain in preterm very low-birthweight infants. *Pediatr Int.* 2007;49(2):156–160.

Olver WJ et al. Neonatal group B streptococcal disease associated with infected breast milk. *Arch Dis Child Fetal Neonatal Ed.* 2000;83(1):F48–F49.

Omarsdottir S et al. Transmission of cytomegalovirus to extremely preterm infants through breast milk. *Acta Paediatrica.* 2007;96(4):492–494.

Ortenstrand A et al. Early discharge of preterm infants followed by domiciliary nursing care: parents' anxiety, assessment of infant health and breastfeeding. *Acta Paediatr.* 2001;90(10):1190–1195.

Paramasivam K, Michie C, Opara E, Jewell AP. Human breast milk immunology: a review. *Int J Fertil Womens Med.* 2006;51(5):208–217.

Peterson JA et al. Milk fat globule glycoproteins in human milk and in gastric aspirates of mother's milk-fed preterm infants. *Pediatr Res.* 1998;44(4):499–506.

Pietschnig B, Siklossy H, Gottling A, Posch M, Kafer A, Lischka A. Breastfeeding rates of VLBW infants–influence of professional breastfeeding support. *Adv Exp Med Biol.* 2000;478:429–430.

Pinelli J, Atkinson SA, Saigal S. Randomized trial of breastfeeding support in very low-birth-weight infants. *Arch Pediatr Adolesc Med.* 2001;155(5):548–553.

Pinelli J, Symington A. Non-nutritive sucking for promoting physiologic stability and nutrition in preterm infants. *Cochrane Database Syst Rev.* 2005. Issue 3. Art. No.: CD001071. DOI: 10.1002/14651858.CD001071.pub2.

Polberger S, Lonnerdal B. Simple and rapid macronutrient analysis of human milk for individualized fortification: basis for improved nutritional management of very-low-birth-weight infants. *J Pediatr Gastroenterol Nutr.* 1993;17:283–290.

Premji S, Chessell L. Continuous nasogastric milk feeding versus intermittent bolus milk feeding for premature infants less than 1500 grams. *Cochrane Database Syst Rev.* 2001(1):CD001819.

Preyde M, Ardal F. Effectiveness of a parent "buddy" program for mothers of very preterm infants in a neonatal intensive care unit. *CMAJ.* 2003;168(8): 969–973.

Quan R et al. Effects of microwave radiation on anti-infective factors in human milk. *Pediatrics.* 1992; 89(4 pt1):667–669.

Quan R et al. The effect of nutritional additives on anti-infective factors in human milk. *Clin Pediatr (Phila).* 1994;33(6):325–328.

Qureshi MA et al. Changes in rhythmic suckle feeding patterns in term infants in the first month of life. *Dev Med Child Neurol.* 2002;44(1):34–39.

Raimbault C, Saliba E, Porter RH. The effect of the odour of mother's milk on breastfeeding behaviour of premature neonates. *Acta Paediatr.* 2007;96(3): 368–371.

Rassin DK et al. Feeding the low-birth-weight infant: II. Effects of taurine and cholesterol supplementation on amino acids and cholesterol. *Pediatrics.* 1983; 71:179–186.

Reyna BA, Pickler RH, Thompson A. A descriptive study of mothers' experiences feeding their preterm infants after discharge. *Adv Neonatal Care.* 2006;6(6): 333–340.

Robbins ST, Beker LT, eds. Infant feedings: guidelines for preparation of formula and breastmilk in health care facilities: American Dietetic Association; 2004.

Rocha NM, Martinez FE, Jorge SM. Cup or bottle for preterm infants: effects on oxygen saturation, weight gain, and breastfeeding. *J Hum Lact.* 2002;18(2): 132–138.

Rodriguez NA, Miracle DJ, Meier PP. Sharing the science on human milk feedings with mothers of very-low-birth-weight infants. *J Obstet Gynecol Neonatal Nurs.* 2005;34(1):109–119.

Ross ES, Browne JV. Developmental progression of feeding skills: an approach to supporting feeding in preterm infants. *Semin Neonatol.* 2002;7(6):469–475.

Saarela T, Kokkonen J, Koivisto M. Macronutrient and energy contents of human milk fractions during the first six months of lactation. *Acta Paediatr.* 2005;94(9):1176–1181.

Sangild PT et al. Preterm birth affects the intestinal response to parenteral and enteral nutrition in newborn pigs. *J Nutr.* 2002;132(9):2673–2681.

Sankaran K et al. A randomized, controlled evaluation of two commercially available human breast milk fortifiers in healthy preterm neonates. *J Am Diet Assoc.* 1996;96(11):1145–1149.

Santiago MS et al. Effect of human milk fortifiers on bacterial growth in human milk. *J Perinatol.* 2005; 25(10):647–649.

Schanler RJ. The role of human milk fortification for premature infants. *Clin Perinatol.* 1998;25(3):645–657.

Schanler RJ, Shulman RJ, Lau C. Feeding strategies for premature infants: beneficial outcomes of feeding fortified human milk versus preterm formula. *Pediatrics.* 1999;103(6 pt 1):1150–1157.

Schanler RJ, Atkinson SA. Effects of nutrients in human milk on the recipient premature infant. *J Mammary Gland Biol Neoplasia.* 1999;4(3):297–307.

Schanler RJ, Hurst NM, Lau C. The use of human milk and breastfeeding in premature infants. *Clin Perinatol.* 1999;26(2):379–398.

Schanler RJ. The use of human milk for premature infants. *Pediatr Clin North Am.* 2001;48(1):207–219.

Schmolzer G et al. Multi-modal approach to prophylaxis of necrotizing enterocolitis: clinical report and review of literature. *Pediatr Surg Int.* 2006;22(7): 573–580.

Sharland M, Khare M, Bedford-Russell A. Prevention of postnatal cytomegalovirus infection in preterm infants. *Arch Dis Child Fetal Neonatal Ed.* 2002;86(2):F140.

Shin H, White-Traut R. The conceptual structure of transition to motherhood in the neonatal intensive care unit. *J Adv Nurs.* 2007;58(1):90–98.

Shoji H, Koletzko B. Oxidative stress and antioxidant protection in the perinatal period. *Curr Opin Clin Nutr Metab Care.* 2007;10(3):324–328.

Shulman RJ et al. Early feeding, feeding tolerance, and lactase activity in preterm infants. *J Pediatr.* 1998; 133(5):645–649.

Shulman RJ et al. Early feeding, antenatal glucocorticoids, and human milk decrease intestinal permeability in preterm infants. *Pediatr Res.* 1998;44(4): 519–523.

Simmer K, Metcalf R, Daniels L. The use of breastmilk in a neonatal unit and its relationship to protein and energy intake and growth. *J Paediatr Child Health.* 1997;33(1):55–60.

Singhal A et al. Breastmilk feeding and lipoprotein profile in adolescents born preterm: follow-up of a prospective randomised study. *Lancet.* 2004; 363(9421):1571–1578.

Sisk PM et al. Lactation counseling for mothers of very low birth weight infants: effect on maternal anxiety and infant intake of human milk. *Pediatrics.* 2006;117(1):e67–e75.

Slusher T et al. Promoting the exclusive feeding of own mother's milk through the use of hindmilk and increased maternal milk volume for hospitalized, low birth weight infants (< 1800 grams) in Nigeria: a feasibility study. *J Hum Lact.* 2003;19(2):191–198.

Spatz DL. Report of a Staff Program to Promote and Support Breastfeeding in the Care of Vulnerable Infants at a Children's Hospital. *J Perinat Educ.* 2005;14(1):30–38.

Sweet L. Breastfeeding a preterm infant and the objectification of breastmilk. *Breastfeed Rev.* 2006; 14(1):5–13.

Telang S et al. Fortifying fresh human milk with commercial powdered human milk fortifiers does not affect bacterial growth during 6 hours at room temperature. *J Am Diet Assoc.* 2005;105(10):1567–1572.

Thompson N et al. Contamination in expressed breast milk following breast cleansing. *J Hum Lact.* 1997;13(2):127–130.

Tornhage CJ et al. Plasma somatostatin and cholecystokinin levels in preterm infants during kangaroo care with and without nasogastric tube-feeding. *J Pediatr Endocrinol Metab.* 1998;11(5):645–651.

Tornhage CJ et al. First week kangaroo care in sick very preterm infants. *Acta Paediatr.* 1999;88(12):1402–1404.

Torres AG et al. Polyunsaturated fatty acids and conjugated linoleic acid isomers in breast milk are associated with plasma non-esterified and erythrocyte membrane fatty acid composition in lactating women. *Br J Nutr.* 2006;95(3):517–524.

Tully MR. A year of remarkable growth for donor milk banking in North America. *J Hum Lact.* 2000;16(3):235–236.

Uauy R et al. Visual and brain function measurements in studies of n-3 fatty acid requirements of infants. *J Pediatr.* 1992;120(4 pt2):S168–S180.

Uauy R, Hoffman DR. Essential fat requirements of preterm infants. *Am J Clin Nutr.* 2000;71(1 suppl):245S–250S.

Ustundag B et al. Levels of cytokines (IL-1beta, IL-2, IL-6, IL-8, TNF-alpha) and trace elements (Zn, Cu) in breast milk from mothers of preterm and term infants. *Mediators Inflamm.* 2005;(6):331–336.

Uvnas-Moberg K. Physiological and endocrine effects of social contact. *Ann N Y Acad Sci.* 1997;807:146–163.

Uvnas-Moberg K. Oxytocin may mediate the benefits of positive social interaction and emotions. *Psychoneuroendocrinology.* 1998;23(8):819–835.

Valentine CJ, Hurst NM, Schanler RJ. Hindmilk improves weight gain in low-birth-weight infants fed human milk. *J Pediatr Gastroenterol Nutr.* 1994;18(4):474–477.

van den Berg A et al. A randomized controlled trial of enteral glutamine supplementation in very low birth weight infants: plasma amino acid concentrations. *J Pediatr Gastroenterol Nutr.* 2005;41(1):66–71.

van der Strate BW et al. Viral load in breast milk correlates with transmission of human cytomegalovirus to preterm neonates, but lactoferrin concentrations do not. *Clin Diagn Lab Immunol.* 2001;8(4):818–821.

Vohr BR et al. Beneficial effects of breast milk in the neonatal intensive care unit on the developmental outcome of extremely low birth weight infants at 18 months of age. *Pediatrics.* 2006;118(1):e115–e123.

Vohr BR et al. Persistent beneficial effects of breast milk ingested in the neonatal intensive care unit on outcomes of extremely low birth weight infants at 30 months of age. *Pediatrics.* 2007;120(4):e953–e959.

Walker M. Test weighing and other estimates of breast-milk intake. *J Hum Lact.* 1995;11(2):91–92.

Wang B et al. Brain ganglioside and glycoprotein sialic acid in breastfed compared with formula-fed infants. *Am J Clin Nutr.* 2003;78(5):1024–1029.

Ward PP, Paz E, Conneely OM. Multifunctional roles of lactoferrin: a critical overview. *Cell Mol Life Sci.* 2005;62(22):2540–2548.

Waterland RA et al. Calibrated-orifice nipples for measurement of infant nutritive sucking. *J Pediatr.* 1998;132(3 pt1):523–526.

Wauben IP et al. Growth and body composition of preterm infants: influence of nutrient fortification of mother's milk in hospital and breastfeeding post-hospital discharge. *Acta Paediatr.* 1998;87(7):780–785.

Wauben IP et al. Moderate nutrient supplementation of mother's milk for preterm infants supports adequate bone mass and short-term growth: a randomized, controlled trial. *Am J Clin Nutr.* 1998;67(3):465–472.

Weaver LT, Lucas A. Development of bowel habit in preterm infants. *Arch Dis Child.* 1993;68(3 spec no):317–320.

Wheeler JL et al. Promoting breastfeeding in the neonatal intensive care unit. *Breastfeed Rev.* 1999;7:15–18.

Whitelaw A, Liestol K. Mortality and growth of low birth weight infants on the Kangaroo Mother Program in Bogota, Colombia. *Pediatrics.* 1994;94(6 pt1):931–932.

Williamson MT, Murti PK. Effects of storage, time, temperature, and composition of containers on biologic components of human milk. *J Hum Lact.* 1996;12(1):31–35.

Woltil HA et al. Erythrocyte and plasma cholesterol ester long-chain polyunsaturated fatty acids of low-birth-weight babies fed preterm formula with and without ribonucleotides: comparison with human milk. *Am J Clin Nutr.* 1995;62(5):943–949.

Woodward DR, Rees B, Boon JA. Human milk fat content: within-feed variation. *Early Hum Dev.* 1989;19(1):39–46.

Wooldridge J, Hall WA. Posthospitalization breastfeeding patterns of moderately preterm infants. *J Perinat Neonatal Nurs.* 2003;17(1):50–64.

Xiao X et al. Epidermal growth factor concentrations in human milk, cow's milk and cow's milk-based infant formulas. *Chin Med J (Engl).* 2002;115(3):451–454.

Yasuda A et al. Evaluation of cytomegalovirus infections transmitted via breast milk in preterm infants with a real-time polymerase chain reaction assay. *Pediatrics.* 2003;111(6 pt1):1333–1336.

The Preterm Infant Breastfeeding Behavior Scale (PIBBS)

The PIBBS is used to describe the infant's behavior, as defined by the scale. It does not assess the infant's breastfeeding behavior capacity in a way that can be quantified by a total score.

Scale Items	Maturational Steps	Score
Rooting	Did not root	0
	Showed some rooting behavior	1
	Showed obvious rooting behavior	2
Areolar grasp	None, the mouth only touched the nipple	0
(How much of the breast was inside the baby's mouth?)	Part of the nipple	1
	The whole nipple, not the areola	2
	The nipple and some of the areola	3
Latched-on and fixed to the breast (scored on a continuous scale)	Did not latch on at all so the mother felt it	0
	Latched on for 5 minutes or less	1
	Latched on for 6–10 minutes	2
	Latched on for 11–15 minutes or more	3
Sucking	No sucking or licking	0
	Licking and tasting, but no sucking	1
	Single sucks, occasional short sucking bursts (2–9 sucks)	2
	Repeated short sucking bursts, occasional long bursts (> 10 sucks)	3
	Repeated (2 or more) long sucking bursts	4
Longest sucking burst (in consecutive sucks, scored on a continuous scale)	1–5	1
	6–10	2
	11–15	3
	16–20	4
	21–25	5
	26–30 or more	6
Swallowing	Swallowing was not noticed	0
	Occasional swallowing was noticed	1
	Repeated swallowing was noticed	2

Definition of Terms

1. Rooting: Some rooting (mouth opening, tongue extension, hand-to-mouth movements) and obvious rooting (simultaneous mouth opening and head turning). Examples of suggestions to mothers for stimulation of rooting are touching the infant's lips with the nipple and expressing some milk on the lips.

2. Areolar grasp: Part of the nipple, whole nipple, or nipple and part of the areola. The mother can facilitate this by encouraging the infant to continue rooting until he shows a wide open mouth, by shaping her breast into a form that fits the infant's mouth, and then letting the infant latch-on and pulling him close to her body; in order for successful latching-on to take place the mother should sit in an upright position; with proper support for her back, arms, and feet; and with a pillow under the infant that supports a comfortable position in front of the breast.

3. Duration of latching-on: Momentarily, less than a minute, or several minutes. The infant is assisted in staying fixed at the breast by adjustment of the mother's and infant's position and of the areolar grasp.

4. Sucking: occasional sucks, short or long (10 consecutive sucks or more) sucking bursts, occasional or repeated bursts. The mother can encourage sucking by talking to the infant and by gently depressing the breast tissue in front of the infant's mouth, which makes the nipple touch the hard palate.

5. The longest sucking burst: Maximum number of consecutive sucks, a measure of sucking maturity.

6. Swallowing: Occasional or repeated. When swallowing is noticed, the mother can be asked to commence test weighing (if this is included in the unit policy), and the milk given by alternative methods can be reduced.

Source: Nyqvist, 1996. Reprinted with permission.

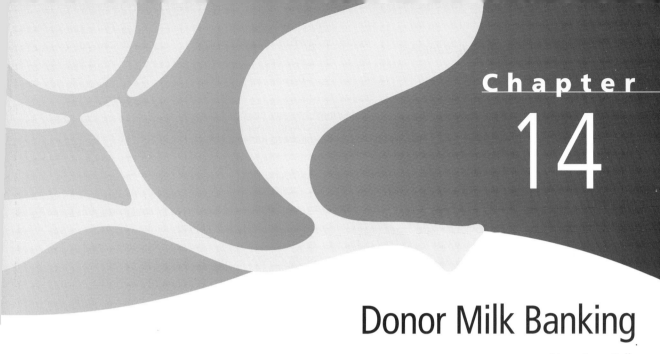

Donor Milk Banking

Mary Rose Tully
Frances Jones

Introduction

Donor human milk banks recruit and screen mothers who have excess milk or are willing to express for the milk bank beyond what their own baby needs. The banks then collect, process, screen, store, and distribute the donated milk to meet the specific needs of individuals for whom human milk is prescribed by a licensed healthcare provider (Human Milk Banking Association of North America [HMBANA], 2008). Donor milk and donor milk banks should not be confused with handling and storage of a mother's own milk for her own infant.

This chapter provides a description and discussion of donor human milk banking and the issues surrounding clinical uses of donor human milk including safety and availability. A history of donor human milk banking is presented, as well as milk-banking procedures. Research regarding donor milk is described and finally, selected case studies are presented to illustrate the benefits of donor milk for a range of conditions in infants.

Use of Donor Milk

Donor milk is never intended to replace mother's own milk but to provide human milk where there is a medical need that the infant's own mother cannot meet (see Figure 14–1). Donor milk is most often used for high-risk premature and ill infants in the hospital setting (see Figure 14–2). It may be used to supplement a mother's own milk or for babies whose mothers are not lactating. There are also several situations in which donor milk is used therapeutically for older babies, including infants who are otherwise healthy but not thriving on human milk substitutes; as a short-term therapy after gut surgery (Rangecroft et al., 1978); for infants with short-gut syndrome; as a source of IgA for an IgA-deficient infant who is not being breastfed; or an older child or adult suffering from IgA deficiency (Merhav et al., 1995; Tully, 1990) (see Table 14–1).

In the United States and Canada, donor milk is also occasionally used for infants whose mothers cannot lactate, such as in cases of adoption. However, when there is no identified medical need for human milk, the processing fee is not covered by health insurance or the healthcare system. Patients and families are responsible for the expense. Milk can only be dispensed for these babies when there is sufficient milk available to provide for recipients with a medical need first (HMBANA, 2008; Tully, 2002). In a few hospitals in North America donor milk is offered when any breastfed baby has

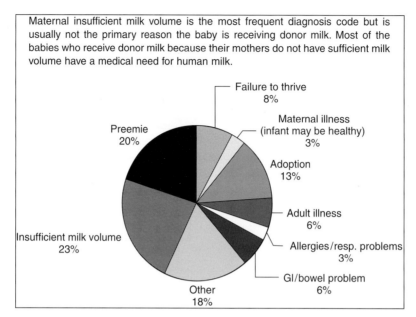

Maternal insufficient milk volume is the most frequent diagnosis code but is usually not the primary reason the baby is receiving donor milk. Most of the babies who receive donor milk because their mothers do not have sufficient milk volume have a medical need for human milk.

FIGURE **14–1** Distribution of diagnosis codes for donor milk orders placed with HMBANA member banks in 2007.

Source: Human Milk Banking Association of North America 2007 Annual Report. Used with permission.

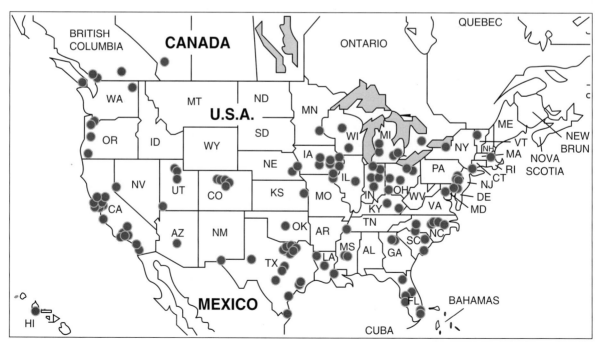

FIGURE **14–2** Cities in North America with hospitals that ordered donor milk in 2007 from HMBANA member banks.

Source: Human Milk Banking Association of North America 2007 Annual Report. Used with permission.

TABLE 14–1	Diagnoses for Which Donor Milk Has Been Ordered from HMBANA Member Banks

- Prematurity
  - *Mother is often pumping, but may have difficulty establishing a supply or have more than one infant.*
- Full-term infant with a medical problem
  - *Some infant problems make breastfeeding difficult such as cleft palate, Pierre Robin syndrome, low muscle tone or a cardiac anomaly.*
- Formula allergy or other feeding intolerance
- IgA deficiency (infant, children, and adults)
- Postsurgical nutrition
- Severe gastrointestinal infections
- Metabolic disorders
- Supplementation of healthy infant
  - *Insufficient maternal milk supply may be temporary or permanent and due to lack of glandular tissue, breast surgery, delayed lactogenesis, health problems (including diabetes), inadequate breast emptying, or adoption.*

Source: Human Milk Banking Association of North America 2007 Annual Report. Used with permission.

medical need of supplementation. Donor milk is mentioned in the most recent infant feeding statements of both the World Health Organization (WHO, 2003) and the American Academy of Pediatrics (AAP) (Gartner et al., 2005) as an alternative when a mother's own milk is not available.

When considering whether to offer donor milk as the first alternative, if a mother's own milk is not available for a preterm or sick infant, the preponderance of evidence supports that there is risk to not feeding human milk (Gartner et al., 2005; Ip et al., 2007; Lucas et al., 1989, 1990, 1992, 1994; Lucas & Morley, 1994). More and more healthcare providers as well as parents and insurers are finding this a compelling argument to support the investment necessary to make donor milk available to every needy infant. Article 25 of the Convention on the Rights of the Child (United Nations, 1990) recognizes the right of every child to "the enjoyment of the highest attainable standard of health and to facilities for the treatment of illness and rehabilitation to health." For healthcare providers, the question becomes one of offering the highest standard of care to all infants regardless of the individual mother's ability to provide milk.

History of Donor Milk Banking

Until the 1900s mothers were encouraged to breastfeed their children (Jefferson, 1954). When a mother was unavailable or had insufficient milk, human milk from another mother was needed. In these situations families used wet nurses (women who nursed children to whom they were not biologically related) or sought donated human milk from friends, relatives, or strangers. Women who wetnursed or provided donor milk were screened for diseases and healthy life styles. In addition, checks were made on the health of their children. These early practices form the foundation upon which modern milk banking is built.

Prior to the late 1800s, attempts at replacing human milk with substances often proved fatal. By the late 1880s, with the advances in science and understanding of food composition, many artificial feeding products were being sold throughout Europe, Australia, and the Americas by a number of companies including Nestlé (Apple, 1986; Wood, 1955). By the beginning of the 1900s, improved sanitation, greater understanding of infant nutrition, and availability of refrigeration resulted in increased success with artificial feeding products using modified animal milk (Baker, 1914; Blackman, 1977; Jefferson, 1954). As the marketing increased, the support for artificial feeding increased, although as one physician stated, "It is difficult to overcome a prejudice in favor of breast milk" (Tow, 1934).

Between 1900 and 1950, a cultural shift occurred and breastfeeding was replaced by artificial feeding as the "norm" in North America and many other developed countries. This shift resulted from changes in physicians' and women's roles, increased belief in science, and aggressive marketing of artificial feeding products. During the first half of the 1900s, mothering came under the purview of physicians with the idea that mothers needed direction from physicians, who were almost exclusively male. In addition, an increasing number of women began working outside the home, which made breastfeeding difficult.

Science held a privileged status in society, and physicians emphasized the close relationship between science and medicine (McHaffie, 1927). The specialty of pediatrics was established in the early 1900s with infant-feeding direction as part of the physician's job. The proprietary companies realized the value of a partnership with the medical community. In the 1930s the American Medical Association (AMA) published specific advertising guidelines for infant foods stating that physicians should provide direction to every mother on infant feeding (Apple, 1980). These guidelines restricted manufacturers from publishing instructions on artificial feeding products. Mothers were directed to visit their physicians who provided instruction sheets supplied by manufacturers of human milk substitutes. By following these guidelines the companies were awarded the American Medical Association seal of approval for their products, allowed to advertise in the *Journal of the American Medical Association* (*JAMA*) and have displays at AMA conferences. These arrangements proved to be financially advantageous to both parties. The companies sold greater amounts of their product, and the physicians had more patient visits. This relationship between health professionals and proprietary companies contributed to the movement of infant feeding from the domestic sphere, in which women helped other women, to the scientific, medical world and from breastfeeding to artificial feeding.

Almost 80 years later, this relationship remains with the product marketing becoming more subtle through funding of journals, newsletters, conferences, meetings, research, gifts, and travel for medical professionals and allied health providers (Moynihan, 2003; Wright & Waterston, 2006). The common marketing themes of best nutrition, physician endorsement, and pseudoscience have remained constant throughout the 100 plus years of artificial feeding marketing.

During this period modern milk banking was born. In 1909, with the technical advances that made artificial feeding products possible, milk banking also became possible and the first milk bank was established in Vienna, Austria. In 1910 two more milk banks were established, one in Boston, Massachusetts, and one in Germany. Interest in milk banking grew as increasingly earlier premature infants and infants with more complex illnesses survived owing to the advances in health care.

The Boston Milk Bank provided education and support to a number of institutions resulting in the establishment of milk banks in both Canada and the United States (Barret & Hiscox, 1939). The arrival of the premature Dionne quintuplets in northern Ontario gave milk banking a boost with the publicity that surrounded sending donor milk to them from Toronto and parts of the northeastern United States (Breton, 1978).

By the 1940s the American Academy of Pediatrics developed guidelines for donor milk banking and by the early 1980s, there were 30 milk banks in the United States and 23 in Canada. Donor milk was dispensed either raw or pasteurized, depending on the preference of the milk bank. It was used primarily for infants in need, particularly those who were premature and ill. The Human Milk Banking Association of North America (HMBANA) was founded in 1985 with an early goal of standardizing donor milk banking operations (HMBANA, 2008).

In the mid 1980s, concern was raised regarding the transmission of cytomegalovirus (CMV) in human milk with potentially serious neurological consequences for preterm infants (Rawls et al., 1984; Yeager et al., 1983), and the world was faced with the plague of acquired immune deficiency syndrome (AIDS) caused by human immunodeficiency virus (HIV), another virus that can be found in human milk. Many milk banks closed as the concern over possible spread of disease decreased the amount of milk that was being ordered. Once requirements for screening of donors, including serum screening, and heat processing of all donor milk were suggested as the appropriate standard, many more banks closed because they had no funding base to support the additional processing. At the same time, the development and marketing of specialty formulas, particularly for preterm infants, convinced many practitioners that human milk could be replaced. By the 1990s donor milk banks in North America reached an all time low (Jones, 2003).

However, the pendulum quickly swung back as smaller and smaller babies were saved and there

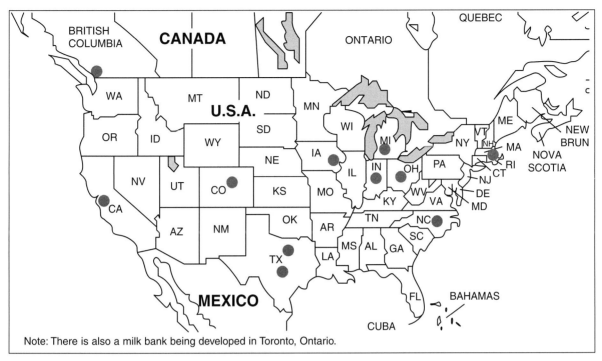

FIGURE 14–3   In 2008, there were 10 donor milk banks in the United States and 1 in Canada.

Source: Human Milk Banking Association of North America. Used with permission.

was increased research on appropriate nutrition for preterm infants. This research led to increased awareness of the many benefits of human milk, and a resurgence of interest in donor milk banking. In North America, the number of banks and the size of some of the banks began to increase dramatically during the late 1990s and early 2000s (see Figure 14–3 and Table 14–2).

Donor Milk Globally

Today, donor milk banking is expanding globally. Milk banks are operating in Africa, Asia, Australia, Central America, North America, South America, and Europe. In a few countries with limited resources for health care, including Russia and China, in-hospital milk banks are supplied primarily by mothers during their postpartum stay, and sharing of mother's milk in informal arrangements is encouraged.

Globally, Brazil leads the world in support of donor milk banking. There are over 173 milk banks in hospitals within the country (Almeida & Dorea, 2006). Donor milk banking is integrated into the promotion, protection, and support of breastfeeding nationally.

Brazil has the most extensive national milk banking standards, a National Human Milk Bank Network, national and international breastfeeding promotion, and donor milk banking conferences (Tully, 2001).

Brazil provides a creative model to countries around the world not only through active support of donor milk banking at the federal, state, and local levels, but also in the way milk banks are operated. For example, there is a national reference milk bank at FIOCRUZ University in Rio de Janeiro that acts as the liaison between the milk banks and the Ministry of Health (Gutiérrez & de Almeida, 1998). It provides mandatory, standardized training for all milk bank personnel across the country and monitors all of the milk banks by reviewing bacteriologic screening of milk prior to and after pasteurization. Communication in the Brazilian system is now done via the Internet. Each milk bank is located in a hospital and provides breastfeeding support and education as well as recruiting donors, screening the milk, and processing it (Giugliani & de Almeida, 2005).

Further integrating breastfeeding into the healthcare system, as part of their emergency medical technician (EMT) training, Brazilian firefighters receive

TABLE 14–2	**Current Member Banks in the Human Milk Banking Association of North America**

United States

California
Mothers' Milk Bank
751 South Bascom Ave
San Jose, CA 95128
Phone (408) 998-4550
Fax (408) 297-9208
mothersmilkbank@hhs.co.santa-clara.ca.us
www.milkbanksj.org

Colorado
Mothers' Milk Bank at Presbyterian St. Luke's
    Medical Center
1719 E. 19th Ave
Denver, CO 80218
Phone (877) 458-5503
Fax (720) 382-2218
mmilkbank@health1cares.com
www.bestfedbabies.org

Indiana
Indiana Mothers' Milk Bank, Inc.
Methodist Medical Plaza II
6820 Parkdale Place, Suite 109
Indianapolis, IN 46254
Phone (317) 329-7146
Fax (317) 329-7151
inmothersmilkbank@clarian.org
www.immilkbank.org

Iowa
Mother's Milk Bank of Iowa
Department of Food and Nutrition Services
University of Iowa Hospitals and Clinics,
    Room C330 GH
200 Hawkins Drive
Iowa City, IA 52242
Phone (319) 356-2652
Fax (319) 356-8674
jean-drulis@uiowa.edu
www.uihealthcare.com/milkbank

Michigan
Bronson Mothers' Milk Bank
601 John St., Box 306
Kalamazoo, MI 49007
Phone (269) 341-8849
Fax (269) 341-8918
Duffc@bronsonhg.org

New England
Mothers' Milk Bank of New England (developing)

PO Box 600091
Newtonville, MA 02460
info@milkbankne.org
www.milkbankne.org

North Carolina
WakeMed Mothers' Milk Bank and Lactation Center
3000 New Bern Ave
Raleigh, NC 27610
Phone (919) 350-8599
Fax (919) 350-8923
BMoore@wakemed.org
Suevans@wakemed.org
www.wakemed.com/body.cfm?id=135

Ohio
Mothers' Milk Bank of Ohio
Grant Medical Center at Victorian Village Health Center
1087 Dennison Avenue
Columbus, OH 43201
Phone (614) 544-0810
Fax (614) 544-0812
gmorrow@ohiohealth.com

Texas
Mothers' Milk Bank at Austin
900 E. 30th St., Suite 214
Austin, TX 78705
Phone (512) 494-0800
Toll-free 1 (877) 813-MILK (6455)
Fax (512) 494-0880
info@mmbaustin.org
www.mmbaustin.org

Mothers' Milk Bank of North Texas
1300 W. Lancaster, Suite 108
Ft. Worth, TX 76102
Phone (817) 810-0071
Toll-free 1 (866) 810-0071
Fax (817) 810-0087
mmbnt@hotmail.com
www.mmbnt.org

Canada

British Columbia
BC Women's Milk Bank
C & W Lactation Services
4500 Oak Street, IU 30
Vancouver, BC V6H 3N1
Phone (604) 875-2282
Fax 604-875-2871
fjones@cw.bc.ca

Source: Human Milk Banking Association of North America. Used with permission.

40 hours of breastfeeding education and clinical training, including time in a donor milk bank. In some states fire fighters also collect milk from donors daily, since few Brazilians have large refrigerators or freezers to accommodate storing the milk for any length of time at home. As EMTs, they also provide breastfeeding advice. Interestingly, letter carriers for the postal service are also trained to promote and support breastfeeding (Personal communication, João Aprigio de Almeida, June 2000). Both of these groups of government employees are well represented at national breastfeeding meetings with several hundred members attending. Brazil also has an annual national donor milk day that recognizes milk bank donors, and well-known local celebrities are featured on posters breastfeeding their children and supporting donor milk banking (Giugliani & de Almeida, 2005).

In the last 5 years the renewed appreciation of donor human milk has led to the establishment of additional regional organizations including those in South America and Europe. These regional groups and individual country organizations have come together under the umbrella of the International Milk Banking Initiative (IMBI) founded by HMBANA and the United Kingdom Association of Milk Banks (UKAMB) for cooperation, collaboration, education, and research.

Safety

Donor milk banks worldwide have an enviable track record of product safety. There has never been a recorded case of a patient becoming seriously ill from donor milk received from a recognized milk bank anywhere in the world. Table 14–3 compares the safety of donor milk from banks following HMBANA or similar guidelines to the safety of human milk substitutes for preterm infants. Despite this outstanding record, there are still some neonatologists who express concerns about the safety of donor milk (Wight et al., 2003). Through education and dissemination of current research, however, more donor milk is being used in healthcare systems.

Availability

As with all donor tissue, donor milk is dispensed only on physician order. Nonprofit donor milk banks provide milk for patients with a medical need. In most countries donor milk is only available in the in-patient setting. However, in North America, donor milk is frequently dispensed to patients at home, who may only be able to remain at home because the human milk provides needed therapeutic properties. Access to donor milk may be restricted due to lack of information on the part of the healthcare provider or the family of the patient.

The expense of screening donors, processing and dispensing the milk, and record keeping require a charge from the milk bank. Many healthcare systems and insurance companies pass the cost of the processing fee on to the patient. Therefore, cost can be a barrier, since the processing fee in 2008 was typically US$3–5 per ounce (30 mL) plus the expense of overnight shipping.

Informal Sharing or Sale of Milk and Wet-Nursing

Human milk carries a very low risk of disease transmission, even in a donor situation. However, human milk, like any other food, needs to be handled and stored appropriately to avoid contamination. It is an excellent growth medium for bacteria if heavily contaminated or if left at room temperature too long. If one purchases human milk directly from a donor mother, there is also the potential risk that the milk may be adulterated to increase volume. With informal milk sharing, there is no easy way for recipients to check whether they are receiving safe human milk.

Wet-nursing, the first form of donor milk banking, is the practice of breastfeeding someone else's child for hire. Wet-nursing has been noted throughout human history (Lawrence & Lawrence, 2005) and continues today. Although it currently is not very common in developed countries, a resurgence of wet-nursing is being reported in the popular press as a service similar to having a nanny. There may be risks for both the wet nurse (donor mother) and her child or the recipient child. For the donor mother, if the recipient child were to become ill, she needs to consider what, if any, her legal liability would be. For the recipient child, disease transmission risk (HIV, HTLV, possibly hepatitis B and other viruses) is low, but it is a risk.

There is also the risk of contamination of the milk if it is not handled appropriately and the potential for a woman who is being paid to dilute her milk to increase volume. Risks for the donor's own child include the potential for inadequate milk intake and exposure to illness. On the other hand, the lactating

TABLE 14–3	The Safety of Donor Human Milk Compared to Human Milk Substitutes (Formula)

Donor Human Milk	Human Milk Substitutes
Screening procedures for donors and banking procedures in North America were developed with input from the Centers for Disease Control (CDC), American Academy of Pediatrics (AAP), and US Food and Drug Administration (FDA) (HMBANA, 2008) and similar governmental bodies around the world (Gutiérrez & de Almeida, 1998; United, 2003; Springer, 2004; Voyer et al., 2000; Morrow, 2006; De Nisi, 2000).	Standards developed by Codex Alimentarius (Codex, 2007), an international commission created by the World Health Organization (WHO) and the Food and Agriculture Organization of the United Nations (UN) are the standards used by the US Food and Drug Administration (FDA).
Banking procedures are reviewed and updated regularly based on current research (HMBANA, 2008; Gutiérrez, 1998; United, 2003; Springer, 2004; Voyer et al., 2000; Morrow, 2006; De Nisi, 2000).	Modifications of infant formulas, even for the preterm infant, are registered with the FDA but do not require clinical trials or other testing for approval (FDA, 2006).
Human milk is designed to meet the needs of human infants (Ip et al., 2007; Schanler, 2007).	"Formula" is bovine milk or soy extract modified to approximate human milk as closely as possible (Codex Alimentarius, 2007).
There has never been a recall for tainted or inadequate formulation of the milk.	There are constant recalls of formula for contamination and incorrect formulation (Codex Alimentarius, 2007; US FDA, 2006; Walker, 2006).
There is no documented morbidity or mortality attributed to donor milk from a recognized donor milk bank following standard screening and processing procedures.	There are regular reports documenting evidence of morbidity and mortality due to contaminated or incorrectly formulated "formula" (Codex Alimentarius, 2007; US FDA, 2006; Walker, 2006; International Food Safety Authorities Network, 2005).

breasts usually increase volume to meet the demand placed on them, and the woman's immune system will be developing antibodies to protect against any bacteria, viruses, or parasites to which she is exposed. In a hospital setting, if the mother wishes to have someone else provide milk for or breastfeed her child, it is essential to document all relevant information in the infant's and mother's chart.

In North American milk banks there are several layers of screening for each donor, the milk is then pasteurized, and a final bacterial screen is done before the milk is released. Each bank has well-trained donor screening personnel with access to a variety of advisors and current tissue banking resources. It would be risky for someone to use the milk banking screening forms, and even the blood testing guideline, to assess suitability of a donor for informal sharing and assume that the milk is equally safe. For healthcare providers, such as physicians, nurses, midwives, and international board-certified lactation consultants (IBCLCs) to involve themselves in an informal exchange of milk raises both ethical and liability questions.

Currently in Canada and the United States there are no federal laws to regulate the sale of human milk. However, Health Canada and the US FDA are monitoring the sale of milk over the Internet, and Health Canada has released a cautionary bulletin regarding this practice (Health Canada, 2006). A few states in the United States, including California, Maryland, New York, and Texas, have either health facility regulations or laws covering donor milk banking, both collecting donor milk and dispensing it, which include adherence to HMBANA's guidelines. It is important for IBCLCs to be aware of any regulations or laws where they are practicing.

Informed Decision Making

Full informed consent for selecting feeding options for infants in a healthcare setting includes information on the availability of donor milk in situations where the mother cannot provide her own (Gartner et al., 2005; WHO, 2003). The evidence that human milk is the most appropriate form of nutrition and immunologic protection for the preterm and full-term infant and that there are risks associated with not breastfeeding or using human milk is becoming more compelling each year (Ip et al., 2007; Schanler, 2007).

For-Profit and Not-for-Profit Milk Banking

When women donate their milk it is important that they clearly understand how it will be used and whether anyone will make a profit from their donation. In North America donors are not paid for their milk or for their efforts. However, there is one for-profit milk bank that pays collection sites by the ounce for collecting milk and also makes a profit when the milk is sold to hospitals.

In the case of HMBANA member banks, donors sign a consent form acknowledging that they know they will not be paid for their milk or for their efforts, and that any of their donation that cannot be fed to recipients may go to research on donor milk (HMBANA, 2008). Recipients are charged a processing fee similar to other tissue banking to cover the expense of screening, processing, and testing the milk, but it is not payment for the milk itself.

With a for-profit milk banking model, the milk becomes a commodity used to generate income for investors, which raises ethical issues. Regardless of whether the for-profit bank is contacting women directly, or through collection sites that are paid for the milk they collect, there is more chance of pressure being applied to the donor to provide a specific volume regardless of her own infant's needs.

Milk Banking Procedures

In 1985 when HMBANA was formed, one of the primary goals included supporting the creation of new banks (Flatau & Bradley, 2006) and developing standards for screening of donors and processing of their milk. *Guidelines for Establishment and Operation of a Donor Human Milk Bank* (available from HMBANA at www.hmbana.org) is updated annually, or more often if needed. Each member bank follows the mandatory guidelines as a minimum. These guidelines have been used as the basis for developing donor milk banking guidelines in countries around the world.

Donor Screening

Donor screening is detailed and involves verbal, written, and serum screening. In some developing countries, serum screening is not done, but all milk is pasteurized, which destroys both viruses and bacteria. When a prospective donor contacts the milk bank, a general conversation covers the requirements for donation as well as the type of screening done and storage requirements for donor milk. If the donor wishes to proceed, the initial screening questionnaire is completed by phone or in person. The mother is then sent a more detailed set of forms asking about health and lifestyle issues as well as consent to contact the mother's and baby's healthcare provider(s). The actual screening forms are not published for the public, because they should not be used by anyone who does not have the appropriate training and references to interpret the information. Generally, any healthy lactating woman who meets the requirements for blood donation and is not on any regular medication is an acceptable donor. Once these forms are received by the milk bank and reviewed, the mother is contacted. A number of questions are asked of the physician focusing on the health and suitability of the mother as a donor. Once the healthcare provider form is received and reviewed, the mother is screened for HIV 1 and 2, human T-lymphoma virus (HTLV), hepatitis B, hepatitis C, and syphilis (HMBANA, 2008). After these results are received and reviewed, the mother is contacted about arrangements for getting her milk delivered to the milk bank. Although a mother can continue breastfeeding her own baby, a donor is *temporarily* disqualified for a period following consumption of medications or alcohol, and during certain short-term medical conditions.

Storage and Handling of Milk

The fundamental principles of good hand hygiene and using clean equipment are emphasized to each donor. All prospective donors are given information about correct cleaning of breast pump equipment.

Each container of milk is marked with the time and date of expression and the mother's name and/or identification number. The milk is stored frozen in an appropriate freezer (one that is cold enough to keep ice cream hard) at home until there is enough accumulated to justify shipping the milk to the milk bank.

Processing of Milk

Once the donor screening is complete, the donor is notified and provided with specific instructions about getting the frozen milk to the milk bank. The frozen milk may be delivered to the milk bank directly (see Figure 14–4) or shipped via overnight express

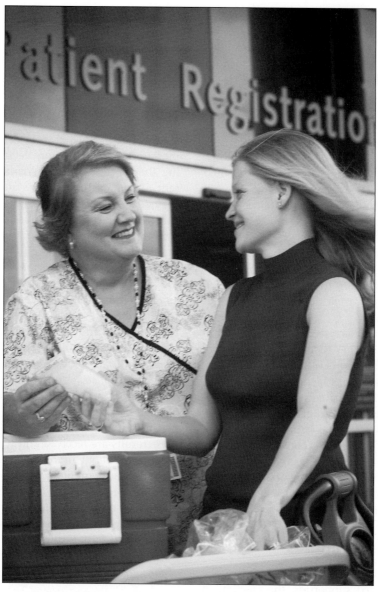

FIGURE 14–4 Donor brings milk to the Mothers' Milk Bank at WakeMed, Raleigh, North Carolina. Mothers who live in the area bring their milk to the bank, and mothers from farther away ship their milk via overnight express at milk bank expense.

Source: © 2008 Mothers' Milk Bank at WakeMed.

(see Figure 14–5). All banks provide instructions for shipping the milk overnight, and US milk banks provide shipping containers and pay the shipping expenses.

Raw milk from screened donors is stored in designated freezers. Prior to processing, the milk is thawed, either by placing it in a refrigerator overnight or by setting it out at room temperature for a few hours. In some banks, the milk is analyzed for protein or total calories and pooled to optimize either caloric or protein content for specific recipients. This is called targeted pooling. Other banks pool milk based on when it was expressed and appearance (i.e., amount of fat that has risen to the top). Milk expressed by mothers whose babies were born at or before 36 weeks gestation is pooled separately for the 4 weeks after birth and referred to as "premie" milk. It is distributed to hospitals for premature infants because research has

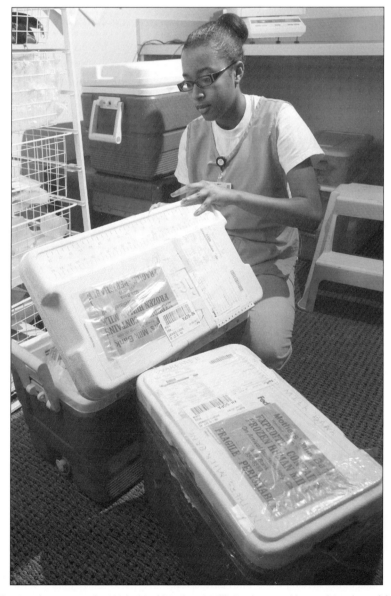

FIGURE 14–5 A volunteer at the WakeMed Mothers' Milk Bank unpacking a shipment of frozen milk.

Source: © 2008 Mothers' Milk Bank at WakeMed.

shown that it has a higher protein and mineral content, which encourages better growth in this population. Before pasteurization, thawed milk is pooled (usually four to six donors), aliquoted into individual bottles, and capped.

Pasteurization

In North American banks pasteurization is done either using a shaking water bath (see Figure 14–6) or a human milk pasteurizer (see Figure 14–7). Both methods are effective and achieve Holder pasteurization. The milk is rapidly heated, and the containers are agitated while the temperature of the milk is held at 62.5°C for 30 minutes. The milk is then rapidly cooled in a slurry of ice water. The bottles are dried, labeled with batch number, date, and name of the milk bank (see Figure 14–8). A sample is drawn from each batch for bacterial screening and the milk frozen. In a few developed countries with a very low incidence of HIV, such as Germany and Norway, donor milk is still screened and dispensed raw, but this is not very common.

Screening Milk

Once the pasteurization is complete, a sample of milk is taken and tested in a Clinical Laboratory Improvement Act (CLIA) certified laboratory to ensure that there is no bacterial growth. When the negative test results are received (after 48 hours), the milk can be dispensed (see Figure 14–9). If any contamination is reported, the milk is retested to assure that the results are not a laboratory error. If bacterial growth is still found, the milk is discarded.

Storage of Milk in the Milk Bank

Milk is stored frozen in separate freezers depending on whether it is raw or processed. The freezers are monitored and equipped with alarms to ensure that the temperature stays within two degrees of –20°C (see Figure 14–10).

Records

Milk bank records are carefully maintained and kept in secure areas. Most banks use both computer and

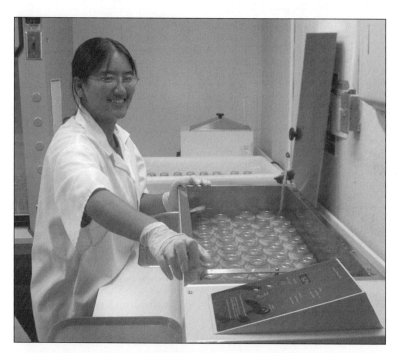

FIGURE 14–6   A milk bank technician at WakeMed Mothers' Milk Bank in San Jose, California placing bottles of milk in the shaking water bath pasteurizer.

Source: © 2008 Mothers' Milk Bank at WakeMed.

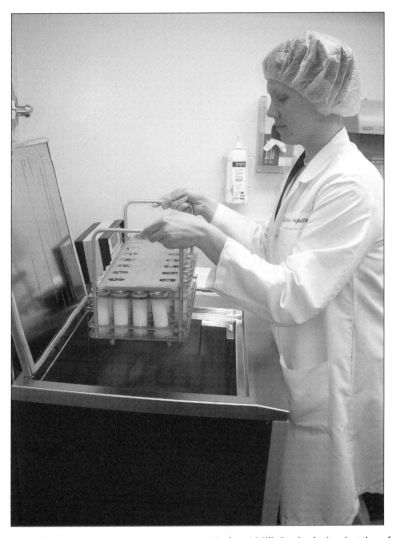

FIGURE **14–7**   A milk bank technician at BC Women's Mothers' Milk Bank placing bottles of milk in the human milk pasteurizer.

Source: © 2008 Mothers' Milk Bank at WakeMed.

written records to document all stages of screening, processing, dispensing, and contact with both donors and recipients. All milk banks are required to keep records for at least 10 years or until all recipients of the milk have reached 21 years of age.

Recalls

Although a recall has never been necessary in an HMBANA member bank, the guidelines require that every bank complete a mock recall every 3 years to ensure their process is workable. Currently HMBANA requires each member bank to complete an annual review form. The organization is currently considering formalizing this review process with peer-review site visits.

Research Findings on Donor Milk

In 1992 Lucas and colleagues published results of a multicenter study involving neonatal intensive care units in the United Kingdom (UK) that found that infants fed at least some human milk in the first month of life (mother's own or donor, all by

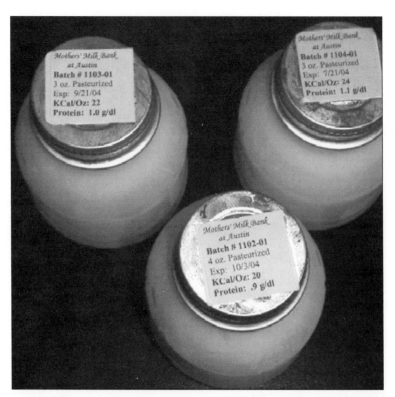

FIGURE **14–8**   Bottles of pasteurized milk from different batches processed at the Mothers' Milk Bank at Austin. Note that the label on each bottle gives identifying information for the milk and lists the calories per ounce and grams of protein per ounce, which is determined using infrared analysis.

Source: © 2008 Mothers' Milk Bank at WakeMed.

gavage) had higher IQs at 7.5–8 years old, even when controlling for psychosocial influences. Interestingly, since this study was done in the late 1980s, at least some of the donor milk was "drip milk," or milk collected in breast shells while a woman breastfed her own child on the opposite breast. Even though this milk has since been shown to have a very low fat content, the babies who received it had good long-term outcomes. Follow-up studies of the multicenter NICU cohort in the UK show that as they reached adolescence the children who were fed human milk, mother's own or donor milk, have lower cholesterol and better HDL to LDL ratios than those children fed preterm formula (Singhal et al., 2004).

A meta-analysis of randomized controlled trials comparing incidence of necrotizing enterocolitis (NEC), a devastating bowel disease that is frequently fatal for preterm infants, showed that use of donor human milk compared to human milk substitutes (formula) was protective (McGuire & Anthony, 2003). Although none of the individual studies showed a significant risk to using formula, aggregating the numbers from the smaller, individual studies showed that infants who were fed donor milk when mother's own was not available were four times less likely to develop confirmed NEC. A paper by Schanler et al. (2005) reported that donor milk, "offered little observed short-term advantage over [preterm formula] for feeding extremely premature infants." However, the authors were careful to qualify that the parameters they measured were *short-term*, and as Wight pointed out (2005), this study did show a significantly lower incidence of chronic lung disease among the babies fed mother's own and donor milk compared to those fed preterm formula as well as a trend toward fewer days on a ventilator.

Another US study by Schanler et al. at a large neonatal unit showed that using fortified mother's own milk was related to decreased infections and

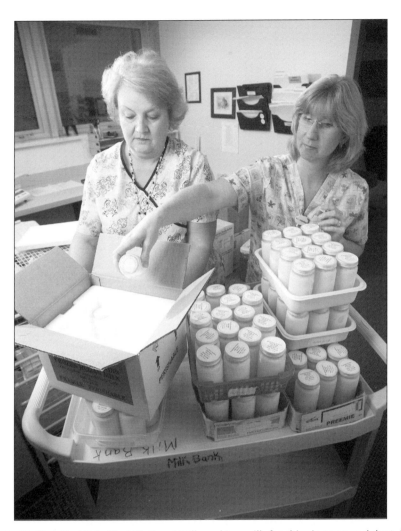

more rapid achievement of full feeds with no untoward effects related to slower weight gain, because the feedings were better tolerated (1999). Many clinicians who regularly use donor milk find the same to be true of babies fed donor milk. Finally, Wight estimated that because of the reduction in length of stay, necrotizing enterocolitis, and sepsis, there is a relative saving of approximately US$11 to the hospital or healthcare plan for each US$1 spent for donor milk obtained from a nonprofit bank (2001).

There are several published case reports describing the use of donor milk for treatment of a variety of conditions or to provide immunologic support and appropriate nutrition to full-term infants and older children (Tully et al., 2004) as well as some adults. Donor milk has been used as adjunct to other therapies in infants with chronic renal failure (Anderson & Arnold, 1993), metabolic disorders (Arnold, 1995), IgA deficiency, and allergy (Tully, 1990).

Although not reported in the literature, milk banks report many cases of feeding intolerance and allergy that have been treated with donor milk, including infants who have failed to thrive on anything but human milk. Donor milk is typically a

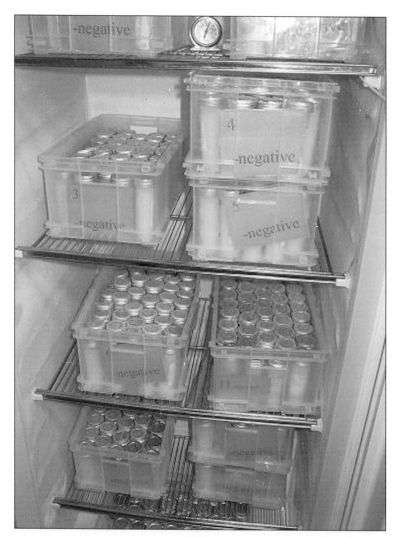

FIGURE **14–10** Milk ready for distribution at the BC Women's Mothers' Milk Bank. The milk is moved to the distribution freezer after the negative culture report is received. Each freezer has a thermometer for continuous temperature monitoring.

Source: © 2008 Mothers' Milk Bank at WakeMed.

treatment of last resort in these cases, both because of the expense and because it is not a commonly used therapy, so fewer clinicians have experience with it.

Some adult conditions respond to human milk, including hemorrhagic conjunctivitis (MMWR, 1982), IgA deficiency in liver transplant recipients (Merhav et al., 1995), and gastrointestinal problems, such as severe reflux (Wiggins & Arnold, 1998). Research from the University of Lund in Sweden first published in 1995 found that human milk contains a unique protein, multimeric alpha-lactalbumin, which

induces apoptosis (programmed cell death) in certain cancer cells (Gustafsson et al., 2005; Hakansson et al., 1995). The group went on to discover that alpha-lactalbumin-oleic acid isolated from human milk is successful as a topical treatment for skin papillomas resistant to traditional treatment (Gustafsson et al., 2004). Further work has been reported using the rat model to investigate the use of HAMLET (human alpha-lactalbumin made lethal to tumor cells), extracted from human milk, as a very specific treatment for human glioblastomas (brain tumors) (Gustafsson et al., 2005).

Selected Case Studies

The vast majority of individual infants receiving donor milk are preterm infants, and in many countries, including Brazil and the UK, they are the only recipients of donor milk. Alternatively, in North America, donor milk has also been used in many other situations. Boxes 14–1 to Box 14–4 illustrate cases in which donor milk was used for mainly older infants with various fairly rare conditions.

BOX 14–1

Baby J Case Study

Baby J was 15 months old suffering from acute lymphatic leukemia (ALL) when she contracted rotovirus and was hospitalized. She had been fed only with hyperalimentation for several months without improvement. She was started on donor milk in very small volumes as a therapy because human milk effectively destroys rotovirus. Within 2 weeks she had improved to the point that she could be discharged home and the hyperalimentation was being weaned down as she increased her intake of donor milk. She continued on donor milk for several months before she was weaned back to an age-appropriate normal diet.

Source: WakeMed Mothers' Milk Bank. Used with permission.

BOX 14–2

Baby L Case Study

Baby boy L was born at 30 weeks gestation and suffered respiratory distress syndrome (RDS), hyperbilirubinemia, apnea of prematurity, bradycardia, anemia, suspected sepsis, and feeding intolerance. He was considered at risk for developing necrotizing enterocolitis. His mother could not continue providing her milk because of her own health issues, and he was put on donor milk as a preventive measure. He was discharged to home with donor milk and continued on it for several months.

Source: San Jose Mothers' Milk Bank. Used with permission.

14–3

Baby P Case Study

Baby girl P was born at 35 weeks due to placental insufficiency. She spent 5 days in NICU, during which her mother was breastfeeding and expressing milk for her. At 2 weeks postpartum her mother's supply was still only at half what P needed, and she began to exhibit signs of feeding intolerance whenever formula was used. Treatment for reflux did not alleviate the symptoms (discomfort and difficulty with stooling). She was tried on six different formulas. She was then referred to a pediatric gastroenterologist, who recommended even more formulas to try. Based on the parents' observation that when she was fed strictly her mother's milk, she was comfortable and happy, the parents went to the Internet seeking donor milk. They found the HMBANA Web site and contacted their nearest milk bank. After discussions with the baby's physicians, donor milk was prescribed and her symptoms began to subside quickly. After 3 weeks, the physician wanted to try two more hypoallergenic formulas. Her symptoms returned with each of them. She had difficulty with stooling and stopped gaining weight well. She was put back on donor milk and began thriving and gaining weight well. Her mother observed that milk from donors on dairy-free diets seemed to agree with her the most. Milk from a pool of three donors on dairy-free diets was tried. Her symptoms increased, so the milk bank created pools from each donor separately. One donor's milk gave her the most relief from symptoms. The milk bank contacted that donor with a request to increase her volume, if possible. She did for several weeks.

During this time Baby P's mother developed mastitis and her milk supply diminished completely, so starting at 5 months Baby P was exclusively on donor milk and thriving, even when she did not get exclusively dairy-free milk. This case is unusual because targeting of a specific donor to a recipient is rarely done, but is possible in situations such as this where a baby is not thriving.

Source: San Jose Mothers' Milk Bank. Used with permission.

BOX	**14–4**

Baby N Case Study

Baby N was put on donor milk at 7 months due to failure to thrive. His mother's milk supply began diminishing at 2 months postpartum due to a subsequent pregnancy. However, he refused formula and exhibited feeding intolerance when he took it. He was failing to thrive and had barely doubled his birth weight at 7 months. Because his mother suffered from Crohn's disease, donor milk was thought to be a good choice. Within a month he had gained a pound and continued to thrive on the donor milk with appropriate complementary feedings for his age.

Source: WakeMed Mothers' Milk Bank. Used with permission.

Summary

Donor milk banking and the use of donor human milk in clinical situations is one significant strategy in the promotion, protection, and support of breastfeeding. The use of banked donor milk is a strong endorsement of the incomparable and irreplaceable nature of human milk. The first choice is always mother's own milk except in very unusual circumstances. The *2002 WHO Global Strategy for Infant and Young Child Feeding* (World, 2003) states:

For those few health situations where infants cannot, or should not, be breastfed, the choice of the best alternative—expressed breast milk from an infant's own mother, breast milk from a healthy wet nurse or a human-milk bank, or a breast milk substitute fed with a cup, which is a safer method than a feeding bottle and teat—depends on individual circumstances [Section 18: [40], p. 10].

Key Concepts

- Donor human milk banks recruit and screen donors, and collect, process, screen, and distribute donated milk to meet the needs of individuals for whom donor milk is prescribed by a licensed healthcare provider.
- The screening process is based on blood and tissue donor screening, with additional criteria unique to human milk.
- Donor milk is provided in situations where mother's own is insufficient or unavailable and there is a medical need for human milk.
- Use of donor milk, when mother's own is not available, ensures the highest standard of care particularly for ill and high-risk infants.

- The first known donor milk bank was established in Vienna in 1909.
- The first known milk bank in North America was established in 1910 in Boston, Massachusetts.
- By the 1940s the American Academy of Pediatrics developed guidelines for donor milk banking.
- During the 1970s and early 1980s there was a proliferation of formal and informal hospital and community-based donor milk banks.
- The Human Milk Banking Association of North America (HMBANA) was founded in 1985 with a goal of standardizing milk banking operations.
- In the mid 1980s with the awareness of CMV and HIV combined with the development and

promotion of specialty preterm formulas, many donor milk banks closed.

- Currently donor milk banking is growing globally as research indicates that human milk, mother's own and donor, is optimal for infants.
- Pasteurized human milk from screened donors has a stronger safety record than products that are used to replace it.
- One of the primary barriers to use of donor milk is the lack of awareness and education among healthcare providers.
- For healthcare professionals to involve themselves in an informal exchange of human milk

raises both ethical and liability questions. Although informal sharing is usually low risk, screening of potential donors needs to be completed by personnel trained to complete milk bank screening.

- HMBANA member banks in North America, as well as donor milk banks everywhere else in the world, are nonprofit, which ensures that the safest product is available at the lowest possible cost.

Internet Resources

American Academy of Pediatrics statement on breastfeeding and human milk: aappolicy.aappublications.org/cgi/content/full/pediatrics;115/2/496

Breastfeeding Committee of Canada (BCC): www.breastfeedingcanada.ca

CDC breastfeeding resources: www.cdc.gov/breastfeeding

Human Milk Banking Association of North America: www.hmbana.org

Journal of Human Lactation: jhl.sagepub.com/archive

United Kingdom Association for Milk Banking: www.ukamb.org

United States Breastfeeding Committee: www.usbreastfeeding.org

References

Almeida SG, Dorea JG. Quality control of banked milk in Brasilia, Brazil. *J Hum Lact.* 2006;22:335–339.

Anderson A, Arnold LD. Use of donor breast milk in the nutrition management of chronic renal failure: three case histories. *J Hum Lact.* 1993;9:263–264.

Apple RD. "To be used only under the direction of a physician": commercial infant feeding and medical practice, 1870–1940. *Bull Hist Med.* 1980;54:402–417.

Apple RD. "Advertised by our loving friends": the infant formula industry and the creation of new pharmaceutical markets, 1870–1910. *J Hist Med Allied Sci.* 1986;41:3–23.

Arnold LD. Use of donor milk in the treatment of metabolic disorders: glycolytic pathway defects. *J Hum Lact.* 1995;11:51–53.

Baker J. The infants' milk stations: their relation to the pediatric clinics and to private physician. *Arch Pediatr.* 1914;31:165–170.

Barret C, Hiscox I. The collection and preservation of breast milk. *Can Nurs.* 1939;1:15–18.

Blackman J. Lessons from history of maternal care and childbirth. *Midwives ChronNurs Notes.* 1977;3:46–49.

Breton P. *The Dionne Years.* New York, NY: WW Norton and Co; 1978.

Buss IH et al. Vitamin C is reduced in human milk after storage. *Acta Paediatr.* 90:813–815.

Codex Alimentarius. *Standard for Infant Formula and Formulas for Special Medical Purposes Intended for Infants.* Geneva, Switzerland: WHO, 2007.

De Nisi G. *La Banca del Latte Materno.* Trento, Italy: New Magazine; 2000.

Flatau G, Bradley S. *Starting a Donor Human Milk Bank: A Practical Guide.* Raleigh, NC: HMBANA; 2006.

Gartner LM et al. Breastfeeding and the use of human milk. *Pediatrics.* 2005;115:496–506.

Giugliani E, de Almeida JA. *The role of donor milk banking in breastfeeding promotion: Brazil's experience.* Alexandria, VA: 2005.

Goldblum RM et al. Human milk banking. II. Relative stability of immunologic factors in stored colostrum. *Acta Paediatr Scand.* 1982;71:143–144.

Goldblum RM et al. Human milk feeding enhances the urinary excretion of immunologic factors in low birth weight infants. *Pediatr Res.* 1989;25:184–188.

Gustafsson L et al. Treatment of skin papillomas with topical alpha-lactalbumin-oleic acid. *N Engl J Med.* 2004;350:2663–2672.

Gustafsson L et al. HAMLET kills tumor cells by apoptosis: structure, cellular mechanisms, and therapy. *J Nutr.* 2005;135:1299–1303.

Gutiérrez D, de Almeida JA. Human milk banks in Brazil. *J Hum Lact*. 1998;14:333–335.

Hakansson A et al. Apoptosis induced by a human milk protein. *Proc Natl Acad Sci USA*. 1995;92: 8064–8068.

Health Canada. *Information Update. Health Canada Raises Concerns About Sale and Distribution of Human Milk*. Ottowa, Canada: Health Canada; 2006.

Hernandez J et al. Effect of storage processes on the bacterial growth-inhibiting activity of human breast milk. *Pediatrics*. 1979;63:597–601.

Human Milk Banking Association of North America (HMBANA). *Guidelines for the Establishment and Operation of a Donor Human Milk Bank*. Raleigh, NC: HMBANA; 2008.

International Food Safety Authorities Network. *Enterobacter sakazakii* in powdered infant formula. http://www.who.int/foodsafety/fs_management/No_01_Esakazakii_Jan05_en.pdf.

Ip S et al. Breastfeeding and maternal and infant health outcomes in developed countries. *Evid Rep Technol Assess (Full Rep)*. 2007;1–186. http://www.AHRQ.gov.

Jefferson DL. Child feeding in the United States in the nineteenth century. *J Am Diet Assoc*. 1954;30: 335–344.

Jones F. History of North American donor milk banking: one hundred years of progress. *J Hum Lact*. 2003;19:313–318.

Jones F, Tully MR. *Best Practice for Expressing, Storing and Handling Human Milk in Hospitals, Homes and Child Care Settings*. Raleigh, NC: HMBANA; 2006.

Lawrence RA, Lawrence RM. *Breastfeeding: A Guide for the Medical Profession*. Philadelphia, PA: Elsevier Mosby; 2005.

Lucas A et al. Early diet in preterm babies and developmental status in infancy. *Arch Dis Child*. 1989;64:1570–1578.

Lucas A et al. Early diet of preterm infants and development of allergic or atopic disease: randomised prospective study. *BMJ*. 1990;300:837–840.

Lucas A et al. Breast milk and subsequent intelligence quotient in children born preterm. *Lancet*. 1992;339:261–264.

Lucas A, Morley R. Does early nutrition in infants born before term programme later blood pressure? *BMJ*. 1994;309:304–308.

Lucas A et al. A randomised multicentre study of human milk versus formula and later development in preterm infants. *Arch Dis Child Fetal Neonatal Ed*. 1994;70:F141–F146.

McGuire W, Anthony MY. Donor human milk versus formula for preventing necrotising enterocolitis in preterm infants: systematic review. *Arch Dis Child Fetal Neonatal Ed*. 2003;88:F11–F14.

McHaffie LP. The artificial feeding of young babies. *Can Nurs*. 1927;23:635–664.

Merhav HJ et al. Treatment of IgA deficiency in liver transplant recipients with human breast milk. *Transpl Int*. 1995;8:327–329.

Morbidity and Mortality Weekly Report (MMWR). Acute hemorrhagic congunctivitis—American Samoa. *MMWR*. 1982;3:1.

Morrow G. *Donor Milk Banking in Norway. HMBANA Matters*, 2006. http://www.hmbana.org/downloads/2006Jan_newsletter.pdf. Accessed Feb. 22, 2008.

Moynihan R. Who pays for the pizza? Redefining the relationships between doctors and drug companies. 1: entanglement. *BMJ*. 2003;326:1189–1192.

Pardou A et al. Human milk banking: influence of storage processes and of bacterial contamination on some milk constituents. *Biol Neonate*. 1994;65: 302–309.

Rangecroft L et al. A comparison of the feeding of the postoperative newborn with banked breast-milk or cow's-milk feeds. *J Pediatr Surg*. 1978;13:11–12.

Rawls WE et al. Neonatal cytomegalovirus infections: the relative role of neonatal blood transfusion and maternal exposure. *Clin Invest Med*. 1984;7:13–19.

Schanler RJ et al. Feeding strategies for premature infants: beneficial outcomes of feeding fortified human milk versus preterm formula. *Pediatrics*. 1999;103:1150–1157.

Schanler RJ et al. Randomized trial of donor human milk versus preterm formula as substitutes for mothers' own milk in the feeding of extremely premature infants. *Pediatrics*. 2005;116:400–406.

Schanler RJ. Evaluation of the evidence to support current recommendations to meet the needs of premature infants: the role of human milk. *Am J Clin Nutr*. 2007;85:625S–628S.

Singhal A et al. Breast milk feeding and lipoprotein profile in adolescents born preterm: follow-up of a prospective randomised study. *Lancet*. 2004;363: 1571–1578.

Sousa R, Barness L. Bacterial growth in refrigerated human milk. *Am J Dis Child*. 1987;141:111–112.

Springer S. Donor milk for preterm and sick children: human milk banking in Germany. *Adv Exp Med Biol*. 2004;554:509–510.

Tow A. Simplified infant feeding. A four hour feeding schedule. *Arch Pediatr*. 1934;51:49–50.

Tully MR. Banked human milk in the treatment of IgA deficiency and allergy symptoms. *J Hum Lact*. 1990;6:75.

Tully MR. Excelencia em bancos de leite humano: uma visao do futuro—the First international congress on human milk banking. *J Hum Lact*. 2001;17:51–53.

Tully MR. Recipient prioritization and use of human milk in the hospital setting. *J Hum Lact*. 2002;18:393–396.

Tully MR et al. Stories of success: the use of donor milk is increasing in North America. *J Hum Lact*. 2004;20:75–77.

US Food and Drug Administration (FDA). Frequently asked questions about FDA's regulation of infant formula. College Park, MD: FDA; 2006.

United Kingdom Milk Banking Association (UKAMB). *Guidelines for the Establishment and Operation of Human Milk Banks in the UK*. London, UK: UKAMB; 2003.

United Nations. *United Nations Convention on the Rights of the Child.* 1990. http://www.unicef.org/crc/index_framework.html. Accessed Feb. 22, 2008.

vom Saal FS, Hughes C. An extensive new literature concerning low-dose effects of bisphenol A shows the need for a new risk assessment. *Environ Health Perspect.* 2005;113:926–933.

Voyer M et al. *Human milk banks organization in France: legal proceedings and their consequences on milk bank activities.* Trento, Italy: New Magazine; 2000.

Walker M. *Recalls of Infant Feeding Products.* Weston, MA: National Alliance for Breastfeeding Advocacy; 2006.

Wiggins PK, Arnold LD. Clinical case history: donor milk use for severe gastroesophageal reflux in an adult. *J Hum Lact.* 1998;14:157–159.

Wight NE. Donor human milk for preterm infants. *J Perinatol.* 2001;21:249–254.

Wight NE et al. *Neonatologists' Attitudes and Practice on the use of Mothers' Own and Pasteurized Donor Human Milk in the NICU.* San Francisco, CA: 2003.

Wight NE. Donor milk: down but not out. *Pediatrics.* 2005;116:1610.

Wood AL. The history of artificial feeding of infants. *J Am Diet Assoc.* 1955;31:474–482.

World Health Organization (WHO). *Global Strategy for Infant and Young Child Feeding.* Geneva, Switzerland: WHO; 2003.

World Health Organization (WHO). *Global Strategy for Infant and Young Child Feeding and Care.* Geneva, Switzerland: WHO; 2003.

Wright CM, Waterston AJ. Relationships between paediatricians and infant formula milk companies. *Arch Dis Child.* 2006;91:383–385.

Yeager AS et al. Sequelae of maternally derived cytomegalovirus infections in premature infants. *J Pediatr.* 1983;102:918–922.

Expressing, Storing, and Handling Human Milk

Human milk is a living tissue. As such, it has many properties that both preserve its integrity and protect the infant. However, it is important to recognize that each step in the collection and storage process may affect the final product. Expression, collection, and storage recommendations may vary somewhat depending on the health of the child or infant, whether premature, full-term, healthy, or ill. Recommendations will also depend on where the milk will be stored and fed, whether in the home, hospital, or child care setting.

To preserve the composition of the milk and maximize the benefit to the infant, freshly expressed milk should be used whenever possible (Goldblum et al., 1989). Providing optimal nutrition is important. As long as human milk has been expressed and stored in a manner that renders the product bacteriologically safe, human milk is far superior to any replacement product except in extremely unusual circumstances. There is limited research on the precise effect of storage on human milk and none to show that at a specific time or temperature the milk *spoils*. In the case of a preterm or ill infant, use of fresh milk is always optimal, and milk that has been refrigerated and not been used within 48 hours probably should be frozen to better preserve the immunologic properties. However, freezing decreases the activity of the digestive enzymes in the milk.

Issues to consider that may affect the immunological function, caloric content, and nutritional value of the milk include the following:

- Careful hand washing and appropriate cleaning of pump parts
- Determining the most appropriate type of expression/pump for the mother's situation and baby's condition
- Type of storage container
  - Clean (sterile is not necessary)
  - Glass or hard plastic containers are preferred for preserving immunologic function of the milk. Note: Scientific concerns have been raised regarding storage or heating of any food in polycarbonate plastics (hard, clear plastics) because they can release bisphenol A, an endocrine disruptor, into the milk or other food (vom Saal & Hughes, 2005).
- Polyethylene bags increase the risk of spillage from tears in the bag, and research has shown that fats tend to stick to the plastic (Goldblum et al., 1982).

Human milk that has been refrigerated retains its antibacterial activity for several days, and data show that bacterial counts in refrigerated expressed milk gradually decrease over time (Pardou et al., 1994; Hernandez et al., 1979; Sousa & Barness, 1987). However, enzymatic activity continues during refrigeration and is significantly slowed by freezing, so the recommendation to freeze preterm infants' milk that has not been used within 48 hours is at least partially based on slowing enzyme activity. Short-term storage for healthy full-term infants or young children who receive most of their nutrition through direct breastfeeding presents a wider range of options when compared to storage for premature or otherwise compromised infants. Optimal handling and storage is far more critical when infants are premature or otherwise compromised and may have implications for nutrient supplementation. When infants are receiving all of their nutrition from expressed milk, every effort must be made to maximize the nutritional and immunologic value of the milk. For example, Buss et al. found that loss of vitamin C is significant during storage (Buss et al., 2001); therefore, babies primarily fed expressed, stored milk require vitamin C supplementation. Even when storage and handling of milk is optimal, premature infants may need additional fortification of their human milk feedings given their individual nutritional needs.

In addition to optimal handling and storage, it is important that each baby receive his or her own mother's milk. Many facilities require two staff members to check the label on the milk container prior to feeding it to the infant to minimize the risk of error. When an infant receives another mother's milk in error, the most commonly expressed concern is disease transmission. Although the chances of this are minimal, follow- up should include an apology to both mothers that the error occurred, blood testing of the unintended donor (or confirmation that it has been done recently), and counseling and reassurance for both the mother whose milk was misappropriated and the parents of the baby given the wrong milk (Jones & Tully, 2006).

Section 4

Beyond Postpartum

The CDC recommendation as set forth in the document entitled *Recommendations to Improve Preconception Health and Health Care—United States* provides a framework for health promotion during the reproductive life span (CDC, 2006; see Chapter 15 references). The CDC model is designed to ensure consideration of adequate social support and health care during preconception, pregnancy, birth, and breastfeeding so that they go well. Most women are healthy during their childbearing years, and it is rare that a mother's nutritional status is detrimental to her health and ability to lactate. Nonetheless, some mothers encounter difficulties, many of which are preventable and nearly all of which can be resolved in a manner that preserves breastfeeding. Major concerns for the breastfeeding woman include her child's health, her employment outside the home, and concerns relating to her fertility and resumption of sexual activity after the birth of her infant. Infant assessment provides the baseline for assisting both the healthy and the ill breastfeeding child.

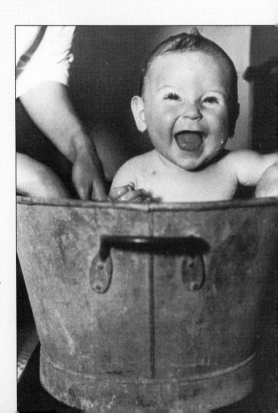

Maternal Nutrition During Lactation

Yvonne L. Bronner

As THE RATES OF BREASTFEEDING continue to increase, this method of infant feeding is becoming the norm in the United States. The American Dietetic Association, the American Academy of Pediatrics, the American College of Obstetricians and Gynecologists, the American Academy of Family Physicians, the Women, Infants, and Children (WIC) Supplemental Food Program, and other public and private organizations strongly encourage breastfeeding. In an effort to clarify nutritional issues related to breastfeeding, this chapter discusses common concerns that lactating women bring to dietitians such as weight change, exercise, and vegetarian diets. In addition, we examine the effect of supplements (used to maintain or add to nutrient intake in the childbearing woman), caffeine, and food flavorings on both mother and breastfeeding baby. We also explore factors associated with allergic reactions during lactation while offering counseling suggestions related to the questions most frequently asked by mothers who are planning to breastfeed or who already are breastfeeding their babies. Finally, we warn against being rigid about the lactating mother's diet and instead incorporate cultural food habits into healthy eating patterns that she enjoys.

Women are beginning to relate nutritional intake to the entire continuum of childbearing—from the preconceptional phase through lactation. Pregnant women have traditionally been more motivated to eat a more healthful and varied diet than they ate before they were pregnant. This increased interest is now being sustained during lactation. Based on recommendations by CDC and in the Institute of Medicine (IOM) report, *Nutrition During Pregnancy and Lactation: An Implementation Guide*, and US Dietary Guidelines 2005, more women and healthcare practitioners recognize the benefits of improving nutritional intake during the preconception period and maintaining these improved habits throughout the life (MMWR, 2006; Institute of Medicine, 1992; USDA, 2005). Thinking about optimal nutrition during pregnancy and lactation is targeted to improved health status throughout life and not limited to this stage of the lifespan. This is similar to the transition seen in the use of the word *diet*, which is time limited, versus *weight management*, which encompasses a larger portion of the lifespan. Pregnancy is a "teachable moment" in the continuum for encouraging good nutrition for a lifetime.

Although the emphasis on achieving and maintaining a "good" diet is important, this message must be tempered by an understanding that the breastfeeding woman can still breastfeed even if her diet is not optimal. Why? Because the body efficiently uses nutrients that are available in the mother even if the mother's diet is limited. Under conditions of chronic malnutrition, nutrients to synthesize breastmilk can be mobilized from maternal stores (Alam et al., 2003; Dewey, 1997).

Worldwide studies support the finding that maternal nutrition has only a modest effect on milk production and milk composition. For example, during the "hunger winter" in Holland between 1944 and 1945, women were severely undernourished as a result of wartime conditions. Dutch infants born during this period were found not to be affected by their mothers' inadequate nutritional intake. Slightly less maternal milk was produced than in previous years when the food supply was more ample, but neither duration of breastfeeding nor infant growth patterns were affected (Smith, 1947). Malnourished Brazilian women produce milk with a slightly higher fat content than do more well-nourished women (Spring et al., 1985). Nepalese women with protein–calorie malnutrition breastfed babies who were in the low-normal range of weight and length for age yet who appeared healthy. And Bangladeshi women who are considered "marginally nourished" maintain an average daily milk production of 750 gm (Brown et al., 1986). Results from a study of 1272 women in Italy found that low prepregnant weight was not associated with either low adoption or shorter duration of breastfeeding (Giovannini et al., 2007).

Maternal Caloric Needs

The goal for caloric intake during lactation is to achieve balance between the amount of energy taken in and the amount of energy expended. The lactating mother need not maintain a markedly higher caloric intake than that prior to pregnancy. In most cases, 500 calories in excess of that which is needed to maintain the mother's body weight is sufficient during the first 6 months and 400 excess calories thereafter. There are no Recommended Dietary Allowance (RDA) levels for energy because energy intake above the estimated energy requirement (EER) would result in energy storage thus contributing to weight gain (IOM, 2005). For several

reasons, a woman might ingest fewer calories during lactation:

- She is attempting to return to her prepregnancy weight while breastfeeding her infant.
- She does not have access to sufficient food in a given day.
- She does not wish to gain weight.
- She did not eat this amount of calories before she became pregnant.
- She is less active.

Basal metabolic rates are higher during lactation but are lower than those during the latter months of pregnancy (Piers et al., 1995). Metabolic efficiency increases during pregnancy, enabling women to use fewer calories more efficiently. This energy efficiency has not been demonstrated as well for lactation although women with a wide variety of energy intakes adequately breastfeed their infants. Two studies make the case for recommending fewer calories as a base against which to evaluate maternal energy intake during the childbearing years (Murphy & Abrams, 1993; Todd & Parnell, 1994). Other studies using new techniques for measuring energy expenditure are now being conducted on lactating women; thus more, and perhaps better, data will be used for future energy intake recommendations.

In their prospective study of 458 pregnant women followed for 1 year, Murphy and Abrams (1993) found that for lactating women in this study the mean energy intake was considerably lower than recommended levels. Among white and higher-income mothers lactating beyond 3 months postpartum, energy levels were lower than in the earlier postpartum period. This pattern was reversed among African-American and lower-income women, who increased their energy intake as the infant aged.

Most striking in this study is the substantial difference between RDAs and reported energy intake, averaging 700 to 900 kcal lower than levels routinely recommended. Murphy and Abrams (1993) offer the following explanation for this disparity: pregnant and postpartum women (whether lactating or not) have lower energy requirements than were previously computed as a result of their lower average energy expenditures. Additional studies are needed to track the energy intake of pregnant and lactating women, and to note the health outcomes of their infants over time. Only with such studies can we be assured that women are able to adequately sustain lactation with lower energy levels at no risk to themselves or the babies for whom they are producing milk.

Todd and Parnell (1994) followed 73 women who provided nutrient intake information with 24-hour recalls for 3 months. Most of the women in this study reported dietary energy intakes approximately two thirds the level of the Australian Recommended Nutrient Intake (RNI). The authors concluded that lactation can be maintained on lower levels of energy intake than currently are recommended, and they suggest reassessment of RNI levels. It should be noted that recommendations are usually set higher than average need; therefore, it is not surprising that reported intakes are less than those recommended.

The efficiency of conversion of food energy into breastmilk appears to be higher than the 80 percent assumed by the FAO/WHO/UNU joint expert consultation (1985), according to Piers et al. (1995). Frigerio et al. (1991) propose that the figure of 95 percent is more appropriate to calculate the energy cost of lactation. However, the consensus of opinion still suggests that 80 percent is the efficiency value of conversion.

Maternal Fluid Needs

The Report of the Dietary Guidelines Advisory Committee on the Dietary Guidelines for Americans 2005 support the position that if the mother drinks to meet her own thirst needs, she will drink enough to sustain lactation (USDA, 2005). The relationship between fluid intake and breastmilk production should not be overemphasized, because excess fluid intake may result in reduced milk production (Dusdieker et al., 1994). What the mother drinks will not markedly affect the fluid content of breastmilk. One easy way to ensure adequate fluid intake is to suggest that the mother have something to drink each time she sits down to breastfeed the baby. If a busy mother forgets to drink enough fluids as she rushes through her day, she may experience more constipation, one of the first signs of dehydration. Additionally, she can check the color of her urine as she voids throughout the day. With the exception of the first-morning urination, if the mother is drinking enough liquid, her urine will be clear to light yellow.

A woman should be encouraged to follow a diet appropriate to her culture, eating foods of different colors, flavors, and textures, and in as natural a state as possible. It should be noted that water intake includes the water present in food. Stumbo et al. (1985) found that on average, about 22 percent of the usual water intake came from the foods that lactating women ate. Mothers who breastfeed should avoid processed foods as much as possible, particularly those containing refined sugars and added salt.

Weight Loss

Well-nourished women are reported to usually lose approximately 0.8 kg/month during the first 6 months of lactation (IOM, 2005). Weight becomes more stable during the next 6 months unless there is a specific effort to reduce caloric intake and/or increase energy expenditure through exercise. Teleologically speaking, fat storage during pregnancy is a normal physiologic adaptation in order to give new mothers a nutrient reserve during times of food deprivation. A portion of the energy stored during pregnancy will be mobilized to accommodate milk production. For example, if a woman gains 24 to 26 lb (11 to 12 kg) during pregnancy, she can expect that a reserve of about 4 to 7 lb (2 to 3 kg) is used at the rate of 100 to 150 kcal/day to support lactation (IOM, 1989). If all goes well, this mobilized fat will be associated with a gradual but steady weight loss until the client reaches her prepregnant weight or "healthy weight" (the weight achieved when the client is eating wholesome foods and engaging in at least 30 minutes of physical activity on most days of the week (Meisler & St. Jeor, 1996; USDA, 2004).

Because being thin is often equated with feminine attractiveness, new mothers are concerned about their weight. They also may want information about dietary regimens that are compatible with breastfeeding, advice about when they can begin an exercise program, and how strenuously they can exercise.

The true effect of lactation on maternal weight after delivery is still unclear despite dozens of international studies on the topic. A review requested by the Department of Health and Human Services (DHHS) office of Women's Health from the Agency for Healthcare Research and Quality (AHRQ) evaluated the relationship between return to prepregnancy weight or postpartum weight change and breastfeeding (AHRQ, 2007). This report found that while average postpartum weight retention is modest, about 1.5 kg, some women retain as much as 26 kg with 14 to 20 percent of women retaining about 5 kg. The AHRQ concluded that the effect of breastfeeding on return to prepregnancy weight was negligible when the women were followed for 1–2 years postpartum based on three prospective cohort studies. The equivocal findings from all seven studies assessed was attributed to the fact that many confounding factors impact weight change, and it is therefore difficult to determine the causal impact of breastfeeding. However, we can make the following evidence-based conclusions about postpartum weight loss and breastfeeding.

Breastfeeding women appear to lose slightly more weight postpartum than do their nonbreastfeeding counterparts (Bradshaw & Pfeiffer, 1988; Dugdale & Eaton-Evans, 1989; Kramer et al., 1993) although the evidence is conflicting, as some studies show no correlation of lactation with weight loss after delivery (Thorsdottir & Birgisdottir, 1998; Walker & Freeland-Greaves, 1998) possibly because of inconsistencies in the definition of breastfeeding and also due to confounding factors that were not taken into consideration (Fraser & Grimes, 2003).

Maternal weight loss is greater in the first 12 months postpartum if mothers breastfed; the weight-loss pattern is less marked in the second 6 months postpartum and is related to both breastfeeding frequency and duration (Dewey et al., 1993). The longer the mother breastfeeds, the more weight she is likely to lose (up to a point) (Dugdale & Eaton-Evans, 1989).

During the recuperative postpartum period, mothers tend to eat less and to be less active than they were prior to delivery. This pattern of lessened activity is more pronounced among breastfeeding than among bottle-feeding mothers. In spite of these differences, breastfeeding women lose more weight than bottle-feeding women throughout the first 6 months postpartum (Dugdale & Eaton-Evans, 1989).

Even moderate dieting during breastfeeding can achieve a 4 to 5 lb weight loss per month (Dewey & McCrory, 1994). Breastfeeding women begin losing body fat from the 15th day postpartum (Fornes & Dorea, 1995).

Gradual weight reduction has no deleterious effect on lactation and is attainable with lower energy intakes than usually are recommended (Butte et al., 1984; van Raaij et al., 1991). Women with a caloric intake of 2600 kcal/day had no weight loss, whereas those taking in fewer than 2200 kcal/day gradually lose weight. Mothers with less than 20 percent body fat do not produce less milk than do heavier mothers; however, they do consume more energy. In addition to weight loss from stored energy reserves, weight loss during lactation is best achieved by lowering the fat content of the diet and exercising (Dewey, 1998; McCrory et al., 1999). Weight loss is more likely to occur when the fat content represents no more than 20 to 25 percent of total calories. Modest weight loss (approximately 1 lb/week) appears to have no adverse effect on the quantity or quality of the breastmilk (Dusdieker et al., 1994). Strode et al. (1986) reported that a modest intake of 1500 kcal/day in the first 6 months postpartum did not adversely affect milk production. With this nutritional intake, prolactin levels remained unaffected, and the nursing mothers lost approximately 1 lb/week.

The mother who chooses to diet while lactating should be encouraged to avoid crash or fad diets that promise marked, rapid weight loss. Fat-soluble environmental contaminants and toxins stored in body fat are released into the milk in larger quantities when caloric intake is severely restricted. Additionally, a marked reduction of caloric intake can result in fussiness in some babies. Modest food intake (1500 kcal/day) does not adversely affect milk production; however, a rapid, severe weight loss may negatively affect infant weight gain.

Motil et al. (1994) reported a case in which a breastfed infant failed to thrive as a result of the mother's seriously fat-restricted dietary regimen. The volume of milk declined markedly, although milk composition was unaffected. A safe maternal weight-loss regimen includes careful analysis of the mother's prepregnancy caloric needs accompanied by a plan that enables her to maintain her own nutritional needs while total calories are gradually reduced. In most cases, a weight loss of no more than 1 to 1.5 lb/week can be sustained during lactation without compromising the baby's total milk supply or cream content.

Exercise

Regular exercise is healthy at any time during life, including during lactation. Exercise does not interfere with the mother's milk supply (Larson-Meyer, 2002; Lovelady et al., 2001; Rooney & Schauberger, 2002) or with the baby's feeding pattern (Dewey et al., 1994; Dewey, 1998). Lovelady et al. (2000) followed 40 overweight breastfeeding women beginning 4 weeks after they gave birth. About half were assigned to a diet-and-exercise group and half to a control group. Women in the diet-and-exercise group lost an average of 10 pounds by the end of 10 weeks. They reported that they seemed to be producing enough milk and that the exercise sessions gave them more energy. Women in the control group, on the other hand, lost an average of only 2 pounds.

In an earlier study, Lovelady et al. (1990) followed eight exercising and eight sedentary women who were exclusively breastfeeding their 9- to 24-week-old infants. No differences in plasma hormones or milk energy, lipid, protein, or lactose content of the milk was noted between the groups. However, the subjects who were exercising gained less weight during their pregnancy, made more milk, expended more energy, and ate more than the nonexercising women. In no way was lactation adversely affected by these women's moderate exercise regimen.

Alternatively, exercising to exhaustion may increase lactic acid levels to the point at which the baby refuses to breastfeed (Wallace et al., 1992). Removing milk from the breasts prior to exercise and giving this milk to the baby might be one way to reduce the likelihood of infant refusal or even difficulty accepting milk with elevated lactic acid. The authors speculated that, when the breasts are not emptied in advance of vigorous exercise, lactic acid increases rapidly and then decreases steadily throughout the postexercise recovery period. Dewey and Lovelady (1993) noted that such elevated lactic acid levels are not seen when moderate exercise is practiced.

Bariatric Surgery

In recent years bariatric surgery has increased as a treatment for morbid obesity. Gastroplasty and gastric bypass are two examples of bariatric surgery. Nutrient absorption is most impacted by gastric bypass surgery because the digestive route does not include the duodenum and part of the jejunum resulting in the need to carefully monitor vitamin and mineral intake and nutritional status (Rolfes et al., 2006). Research is required to determine the exact effects of bariatric surgery on human lactation. However, several reviews provide preliminary recommendations for nutrient intakes including iron, vitamin B_{12}, folate, and calcium for nonlactating and lactating women (Stefanski, 2006). It should be noted that human milk production has proven to be robust in the face of a wide variety of calorie and nutrient intakes (Brown, 1986; Dewey, 1997; Smith, 1947; Spring, 1985). Women who become pregnant and breastfeed following bariatric surgery are recommended to remain under the careful supervision of their healthcare provider and have their nutritional status assessed periodically using appropriate procedures.

Calcium Needs and Bone Loss

Some women fear that breastfeeding will cause sufficient bone loss to place them at risk for developing osteoporosis later in life. These concerns are unfounded. In fact, the opposite is true: bone density is restored after weaning, although the mother suffers slight bone loss while she is lactating (Carranza-Lira & Mera, 2002; Ensom et al., 2002; King, 2001).

Prentice (1994) reviewed the RDAs for calcium in different countries and found that they vary widely. Similarly, calcium intake varies widely with women in Finland having the highest levels, whereas black women in South Africa have the lowest calcium intakes. These findings reflect dietary and supplement differences in these countries. Prentice points out that for postmenopausal osteoporosis to occur, the woman must not have achieved maximum bone mass during her young adult life. Furthermore, calcium intake by the mother is not closely related to her breastmilk calcium secretion. In fact, no relationship has been found between breastmilk calcium concentrations and maternal calcium intake through food or calcium supplements (Kirksey et al., 1979; Vaughn, Weber, & Kemberling, 1979). Increasing calcium intake may result in increased risk of kidney stones and urinary tract infections and may result in reduced absorption of other minerals, including iron, zinc, and magnesium (Prentice, Goldberg, & Prentice, 1994). In fact, additional calcium intake from diet or supplements does not prevent bone loss during lactation nor does it influence the recovery of calcium status after weaning (Kalkwarf & Specker, 2002).

Outcomes of bone-loss studies during lactation are relatively consistent and favor breastfeeding. There is little evidence to justify therapeutic intervention. Specker, Tsang, and Ho (1991) compared 26 lactating women with 32 nonlactating postpartum controls over the first year postpartum. Lactating women were more likely to mobilize bone during lactation and to recover bone mass during and after weaning, whether that occurred before or after 6 months postpartum. Cumming and Klineberg (1993) asked whether there was a relationship between parity, breastfeeding, age at menarche and menopause, and the risk of hip fracture among Australian women aged 65 years and older. As duration of breastfeeding increased, the risk of hip fracture decreased in a dose-response relationship ($P = < .01$). Additionally, parous women who breastfed all their children were at lower risk for hip fracture than were parous women who had never breastfed their children.

In another study (Sowers et al., 1993) women who breastfed longer than 6 months had mean bone mineral density (BMD) losses of 5.1 percent of the lumbar spine and 4.8 percent of the femoral neck. Women who breastfed 1 month or less lost no BMD at either site. Among the women who breastfed 6 months or longer, there was a return to baseline BMD levels at 12 months postpartum. The authors stated that transient bone loss occurs with several months of lactation, but this bone loss is recovered following lactation.

Sowers et al. (1995) reported 5 percent short-term bone loss among breastfeeding women, followed by recovery of lost bone within the first 18 months after parturition. Predictive factors were lactation status and the number of months to resumption of menses. These authors concluded that menstrual activity, rather than diet, dietary calcium intake, or physical activity, is the primary factor in bone mass recovery after initial bone loss during lactation.

Kalkwarf and Specker (1995) followed 65 lactating women and 48 nonlactating women for 5 to 6 months postpartum. The breastfeeding women lost significantly more bone in the total body (2.8 percent versus 1.7 percent) and lumbar spine (3.9 percent versus 1.5 percent) than did the nonbreastfeeding women.

However, after weaning, the breastfeeding women gained significantly more bone in the lumbar spine (5.5 percent versus 1.8 percent) than the nonbreastfeeding women. These investigators also found that earlier resumption of menses was associated with small amounts of bone loss during lactation and with greater increase of bone after weaning. They concluded that lactation may result in a transient loss of bone and that compensation may exceed the level of loss.

Although dietary calcium intake does not explain calcium recovery after lactation, Kalkwarf et al. (1996) suggest that calcium and phosphorus levels are higher in breastfeeding women and that this becomes apparent after weaning and resumption of menses. These researchers suggest that serum calcium concentrations are maintained or elevated by calcium that is metabolized from bone owing to low blood estrogen concentrations. King (2001) contends that calcium needs for milk production are met by decreased urinary excretion of calcium and increased bone resorption.

Vegetarian Diets

Vegetarianism as a nutritional practice continues to be popular in the United States. People choose vegetarianism for religious, economic, cultural, and ecologic reasons. Lacto-ovo vegetarians eat milk, eggs, and plants. Lacto-vegetarians eat milk and plants. Usual vegetarian diets supply a balance of nutrients but may be low in energy owing to their low fat and high fiber content. The milk of breastfeeding vegetarians is generally nutritionally adequate. However the vegan and macrobiotic diets generate concern because they are very restricted, especially limiting sources of vitamin B_{12} if not well planned (Sanders, 1999; Ciani et al., 2000; Walsh, 2001; Shaikh et al., 2003; Rolfes et al., 2006). Some practitioners of these diets are called fruitarians; they eat only fruit, nuts, and honey. Women on a macrobiotic diet who avoid meat, poultry, dairy products, and sometimes fish may produce milk with decreased levels of calcium, magnesium, and vitamin B_{12} (Reghu et al., 2005). Women practicing these forms of vegetarian diets should be encouraged to take in adequate calories and complementary protein combinations. They should consume foods rich in iron, calcium, and vitamins D and B_{12}, as well as riboflavin, to ensure adequate nutritional intake (Specker, 1987a). Special attention should be given to vitamin B_{12} intake because cases of deficiency have recently been reported among infants who were breastfed by mothers who were deficient (MMWR, 2001; Koebnick et al., 2004), and this vitamin is available only from animal sources, fortified soy, meat analogues, or B_{12} supplements (Institute of Medicine, 1998).

Dietary Supplements

Nutrient needs during lactation vary by the volume of breastmilk produced and the mother's postpartum nutritional status. Generally, if the mother is consuming the recommended calories from a variety of foods, her nutrient needs will be met from food alone. If insufficient resources to purchase food of adequate quantity or quality is a problem, WIC and similar programs should be recommended and referrals made. For women whose income level qualifies them, WIC provides food supplements for lactating mothers. This program supports breastfeeding by providing additional food to the breastfeeding mother through the first year of the baby's life, should the mother breastfeed that long. In addition to food, nutrition education and suggestions about how to select and prepare foods for optimal food value are offered. If the mother is restricting her caloric intake to fewer than 1800 kcal/day in order to lose weight while nursing, she should be encouraged to eat nutrient-dense foods—that is, foods that supply a large proportion of nutrients relative to their calorie content. Vegetables and legumes are good examples of nutrient-dense foods.

If a nutrient deficiency is identified, a balanced multivitamin supplement that supplies iron to 100 percent of RDAs may be recommended on an individual basis. Women who avoid dairy products and other calcium-rich food sources may need a calcium supplement of 600 mg/day of elemental calcium taken with meals. In recent years there have been multiple reports of rickets in breastfed infants, both dark and light skinned (Gartner, 2003; Greer, 2004; Ziegler, 2006; Dawodu et al., 2003; Shaikh & Chantry, 2006). Given the amount of interest in the emerging science of vitamin D, a useful description of vitamin D metabolism is presented by Holick (2006). Basile et al. (2006) found that high doses of vitamin D was associated with improved vitamin D status

without signs of toxicity or calcium imbalance. The American Academy of Pediatrics recommends that all breastfed babies be supplemented with 200 IU vitamin D daily to achieve sufficiency (AAP, 2005).

Foods That Pass into Milk

Caffeine

Caffeine-containing foods or fluids have been questioned as an appropriate item for breastfeeding mothers. Some mothers report that their very young babies seem to react when caffeinated beverages or foods are part of the maternal diet. Measurable amounts of caffeine pass into breastmilk. However, the amount of caffeine available to the infant is minimal, only 0.06 to 1.5 percent of the maternal dose, and no caffeine is detected in the infants' urine (Berlin et al., 1984). Breastfeeding women who ingest caffeine in moderate amounts present no significant dose to the normal full-term infant.

Ryu's findings (1985a,b) are also reassuring for parents who regularly consume caffeinated beverages. For young neonates, even 5 cups of coffee ingested daily by the mother over a 5-day period altered neither infant heart rate nor sleep time. Concentrations of caffeine in the term infants' serum were slightly elevated but, by day 9, caffeine levels in the mothers' milk and their babies' serum were below the limits of detectability. LeGuennec and Billon (1987), however, caution that babies born prematurely exhibit a delay in eliminating caffeine. Maternal intake of caffeine may have variable effects on preterm or sick infants.

Food Flavorings

Food flavorings are often the first and most lasting cultural cues that infants receive, potentially expanding the sensory experience of feeding. Mennella and Beauchamp (1991) examined the effects of maternally ingested garlic and reported that breastfeeding babies suckled longer and obtained more milk when it was garlic flavored. They speculated that formula-feeding might represent a deficient sensory experience in that the milk always tastes the same. Sullivan and Birch (1994) (see also Mennella & Beauchamp, 1997) reported that breastfed babies were more accepting of solids at their introduction than were formula-fed infants. These investigators suggested that the varied flavor cues to which breastfeeding babies are exposed might facilitate acceptance of new foods. Furthermore, "learning" the taste of foods acceptable to the mother may also facilitate later independent appropriate food selection by the young child (Mennella, 1995).

Vanilla, a potent food flavoring, also alters infant feeding behavior (Mennella & Beauchamp, 1996). Breastfeeding babies suckled longer when first exposed to vanilla-flavored milk. Bottle-feeding babies similarly exposed fed longer when the milk was flavored but did not continue to do so over time, suggesting that the change in flavor, but not the flavor itself when repeated, may trigger altered feeding behavior. For the breastfeeding baby, continued flavor changes enable the child to become familiar with the flavors represented in his family's foods.

Heavy Metals and Breastmilk

Lead (Pb) and Mercury (Hg) are of concern during lactation owing to their potential toxic effects and their wide availability in the environment. These metals are generally related to maternal dietary habits, and levels in breastmilk reflect prenatal exposure. The World Health Organization (WHO) sets tolerable limits at 1.4–1.7 ng Hg/g and 2–5 ng Pb/g (WHO, 1989). Greater quantities of these metals are transmitted across the placenta during pregnancy when the neurotoxic effects are likely to be more pronounced than into breastmilk during lactation.

The concern with mercury is mainly in fish or amalgam tooth filling. There appears to be an attenuated transfer of mercury to breastmilk such that level of exposure is not well correlated with the amount in breastmilk. Method of preparation is important since the level of mercury can increase from 45 to 75 percent during deep frying. Mercury is found in both muscle and fat tissue; therefore, removing the fat will not significantly decrease the level of mercury in the fish. Farmed salmon does not have less mercury, and the amount in poultry and cow milk is related to that found in the fishmeal-based rations that they are fed. The main approach to decreasing mercury consumption is to observe local fish advisories, decrease fish consumption to recommended levels, and decrease the

consumption of products from animals raised on fishmeal (Dorea, 2004). Exposure to mercury from amalgam tooth fillings is not sufficient to be associated with adverse effects in infants (Drexler & Schaller, 1998).

The concern from lead is in food, water, and the environment (dust, paint, and air). Lead is stored in bone, and the level of absorption is significantly decreased by adequate calcium and phosphorus nutritional status. It should be further noted that the amount of lead in cow milk may be significant due to the bone meal in their diet (Dorea, 2004).

Allergens in Breastmilk

Now and then, infants who are exclusively breastfed and are receiving no solids develop allergic symptoms that appear to be from something they have ingested. In this case, the baby is probably reacting to foods or substances taken by the mother that are being passed through the breastmilk. The most common allergic-producing offenders are cow's milk and milk products. Other foods that tend to produce allergic responses in Western cultures are chocolate, cola, corn, citrus fruit, wheat, and peanuts. Peanut allergy can result in severe, even life-threatening reactions in susceptible babies (Vadas et al., 2001).

Health professionals are beginning to realize that some breastfeeding infants have a sensitivity to certain foods transmitted into breastmilk. When exclusively breastfeeding mothers in a study were asked what foods they ate that they believed caused fussy behavior in their infants, they identified broccoli, cabbage, cauliflower, chocolate, cow's milk, and onion (Lust, Brown, & Thomas, 1996). Allergies and breastfeeding are discussed in greater detail in Chapter 4.

The Goal of the Maternal Diet During Lactation

The goal of the maternal diet during lactation is optimal nutritional intake. Certain demographic, lifestyle, and environmental factors may place a client at increased nutritional risk during lactation. The most important of these factors are listed in Box 15–1.

In 1992, the Institute of Medicine published *Nutrition During Pregnancy and Lactation: An Implementation Guide*, a key document that was developed to help deliver high-quality nutritional care during

BOX **15–1**

Nutritional Risk Factors During Lactation

1. Maternal age younger than 17 years: Teens may often have less-than-adequate dietary habits. Therefore, a careful assessment of their food intake is important. Often such assessment will reveal low intake of calcium-rich food as well as fruits and vegetables rich in vitamins and fiber.

2. Economic deprivation: The WIC program, the Commodity Supplemental Food Program, food stamps, and the Expanded Food and Nutrition Education Program (EFNEP) are examples of federally funded food and nutrition programs that may meet the needs of economically deprived mothers.

3. Past restrictive dietary practices or unsound current dietary practices: Some women severely restrict caloric intake in order to lose weight shortly after pregnancy, even while they are breastfeeding. Screen for less-than-adequate food intake, especially the omission of an entire group of foods (grains, fruits, vegetables, protein rich foods, and dairy products).

4. Multiple babies: The mother of multiples should be encouraged to eat to appetite and drink to thirst while getting as much rest as possible.

5. Maternal weight less than 85 percent of suggested height and weight: Data are provided by the Institute of Medicine (1989).

6. Suboptimal weight gain during pregnancy: This will result in a low postpartum body mass index (< 19.8).

7. Rapid weight loss while breastfeeding: May indicate inadequate caloric intake.

8. Pregnant while breastfeeding: Breastfeeding one infant while pregnant with another necessitates that the mother eat to appetite and drink to thirst while getting as much rest as possible.

Source: Adapted from the American Dietetic Association, 1996.

Note: Items 5 through 7 in this list relating to weight should receive careful assessment by the healthcare team. The screening questions in Box 15–2 might be useful.

lactation (Institute of Medicine, 1992). This guide contains a variety of information:

- A sample nutrition questionnaire to help identify women at nutritional risk (see Box 15–2)
- Answers to questions in the nutrition questionnaire
- General strategies for providing effective nutritional care
- Dietary assessment and nutritional guidance

- Guidance for assessing weight change using the body mass index chart (which helps in evaluating whether the lactating woman is underweight, overweight, or in the average weight range)
- A chart of indications for vitamin and mineral supplementation
- Supplementary information for nutrition referrals and resources to help the clinician meet the comprehensive nutritional needs of clients

Screening Questions Assessing Maternal Nutritional Risk

1. Do you have trouble getting adequate food on a regular or periodic basis? For example, do you run out of food before the end of the month? Do you have problems getting to the store to purchase food? Do you use money allocated for food for other purposes?
2. Does your diet contain calcium-rich foods such as dairy products, fish with edible bones, greens (collards, turnip, etc.), tofu, and broccoli?
3. Are you restricting your food intake in order to lose weight?
4. If you practice vegetarianism, indicate which of the following foods you exclude from the diet: meat, fish, poultry, eggs, and dairy products.

5. Are you on some type of special diet that causes you to limit your food intake?
6. Within a week, do you regularly eat 5 fruits and vegetables?
7. Are you exposed to sunlight on a regular basis? If not, do you regularly consume vitamin D-fortified milk or cereal products?
8. How would you describe your weight status—underweight, overweight, average weight?

Source: Adapted from the Institute of Medicine, 1992.

The nutrition questionnaire will help to evaluate the client's (1) eating behavior (meal patterns, food intake patterns), (2) food security (the ability to get enough food), (3) actual food intake, and (4) lifestyle issues related to nutritional status (smoking, alcohol, and other drug use). Answers provided on the questionnaire will help to focus nutrition counseling. After reviewing the steps to successful dietary counseling in Box 15–3, the lactation consultant can begin the counseling session. She should bear in mind that certain factors place mothers and babies at nutritional risk during lactation.

Nutrition Basics

The term *nutrition* has multiple meanings but consists of several different elements, including energy; macronutrients, such as carbohydrates, protein, and fat; and micronutrients such as vitamins and minerals.

Energy

Energy is the capacity to do work. The sun provides the source of energy through plant photosynthesis. Humans gain energy by eating plants or animals that have eaten plants. Several factors influence the total daily amount of energy needed by the body: (1) the basal metabolic rate (BMR), which represents the amount of energy needed for mechanical activities of the body, such as breathing, heart muscle activity, and maintaining body temperature; (2) physical activity; and (3) the thermal effects of food, such as digestion and metabolism. Energy needs are individualized, and studies suggest that there may be some adaptive conservation adjustments in energy expenditure during lactation (Illingsworth et al., 1986; Paul, Muller, & Whitehead, 1979; Schutz, Lechtig, & Bradfield, 1980).

The 400–500 additional calories recommended during lactation can be obtained in the form of a

---

BOX 15–3

Steps to Successful Dietary Counseling

1. Acknowledge that the client is doing something right.
2. Help the client identify areas of the diet that need to be improved.
3. Let the client help develop a plan to improve her food intake.
4. Work with the client to determine exactly how the plan will be implemented.
5. Identify facilitators to more appropriate food intake and barriers to same.
6. Determine a time for follow-up so that progress toward meeting the dietary goals can be evaluated.

---

sandwich (~300 to 350 kcal), fruit (60 to 80 kcal), and a glass of skim milk (90 kcal). This calculation assumes 10 hours of rest and 14 hours of moderate activity.

Macronutrients

Carbohydrates

Food intake during lactation is designed to provide for the nutritional needs of the mother while enabling her to produce adequate milk for the baby. Therefore, most nutritional needs increase during lactation. Carbohydrates are the main energy source for all body functions. Low carbohydrate intake is associated with fatigue, dehydration, and energy loss. Carbohydrates provide 4 kcal/gm. When carbohydrate is in short supply, protein is broken down to take its place as a source of energy (Mahan & Escott-Stump, 1996).

Carbohydrates should make up 55 percent of total calories, with a minimum intake of 100 gm/day for lactating women. Lactating women should obtain their carbohydrates from foods such as whole-grain breads and cereals, fresh fruit, and vegetables, and avoid simple sugars found in soft drinks and juice products labeled as "drinks."

The diet should also contain 25 gm/day of dietary fiber. The carbohydrates just recommended, in the form of soluble or insoluble fiber, will help lactating women reach this goal. Soluble fiber (found in fruit—apples, citrus fruit, strawberries, etc.) helps reduce serum cholesterol levels and cardiovascular disease. Insoluble fiber (found in fruit and vegetable pulp and skins) helps prevent constipation and reduces the incidence of colon cancer.

Protein

Proteins are the highly complex substances in the body that build muscle tissue, enzymes, hormones, and antibodies. They are made up of 22 amino acids, eight of which are essential for adults. The body cannot produce adequate quantities to meet physiological needs; therefore, they must be supplied from the diet. Food proteins are considered complete and of high quality when they contain all eight of the essential amino acids. Protein from animal sources and combinations of protein from plants such as cereals, legumes, and nuts results in a mixture of amino acids that are adequate for protein synthesis. When caloric intake is adequate, vegetarian diets containing a variety of nutrient-dense foods provide sufficient essential amino acids for protein metabolism.

Rice contains all of the essential amino acids although in less-than-optimal quantities. When rice is mixed with small quantities of meat or fish, amino acids become adequate for protein synthesis. Complete proteins can be mixed with incomplete proteins or with each other to provide adequate amounts of the essential amino acids. Adding milk to cereal is an example (Mahan & Escott-Stump, 1996).

The average daily dietary protein requirement is influenced by many factors such as age, digestibility, rate of protein synthesis, and carbohydrate and fat levels (DeSantiago et al., 1995). The current recommendation is 65 gm/day of protein intake for the mother during lactation during the first 6 months and 62 gm/day during the second 6 months (Institute of Medicine, 1984). Protein provides 4 kcal/gm.

Fat

Of all the nutrients in human milk, lipids are most affected by the mother's food intake (Butte et al., 1984; Nommsen et al., 1991). Fats carry the fat-soluble vitamins A, D, E, and K, as well as the essential fatty acid linoleic and the long-chain omega-3 polyunsaturated fatty acid—docosahexaenoic acid (DHA) (Brenna et al., 2007). DHA is important to brain development in infants and has been noted to be low in American women (Al et al., 1995, 1997; Benisek et al., 2000; Francois et al., 1998; Horwood & Fergusson, 1998). During a recent National Institute of Health workshop, a group of experts recommended an intake of 300 mg/day of DHA as adequate intake for lactating women. This intake is related to adequate DHA levels in breastmilk (Simopoulos et al., 1999; Specker et al., 1987b). DHA supplements are associated with higher breastmilk levels (Fidler et al., 2000; Jensen et al., 2000; Helland et al., 2003). These supplements are being marketed to US women. Fats provide elements for tissue structure, cell metabolism, and nerve impulse transmission. They are a concentrated source of energy— 9 kcal/gm, as compared to 4 kcal/gm from carbohydrates and protein. Fat should make up no more than 30 percent of the total calories consumed daily. No more than 7 to 10 percent of calories should be from saturated fat (available primarily from animal sources such as milk and meat, as well as coconut and palm oils), more than 10 percent should be monounsaturated, and 10 percent should be polyunsaturated fat (from vegetable sources, nuts, and seeds) (Mahan & Escott-Stump, 1996). The overall recommended distribution of calories from the macronutrients for lactating women is as follows:

- Carbohydrates: 50 to 55% of calories
- Protein: 12 to 15% of calories
- Fat: < 30% of calories

Macronutrients are required in large amounts, and they compose most of the body's weight, whereas micronutrients are required in smaller quantities and make up a small percentage of body weight.

Micronutrients

Vitamins

Traditionally, vitamins have been best known by diseases deriving from their deficiencies (e.g., vitamin A deficiency causes blindness; vitamin C deficiency causes scurvy). More recent recommendations for vitamin intake are based on principles of health promotion and disease prevention. An example is increasing folate during the periconceptional period to protect against neural tube defect.

Vitamins are organic, noncalorigenic food substances that are required by the body in small quantities and contribute to the regulation of metabolic processes. Fat-soluble vitamins (A, D, E, and K) are stored by the body in fatty tissue, whereas water-soluble vitamins (B complex and C) are not stored for long periods and need to be supplied in the diet more frequently. As a mother's intake of water-soluble vitamins increases, the vitamin level in her milk will also increase, but it will reach a plateau that is not raised by giving additional vitamin supplements. Water-soluble vitamin levels in human milk are more likely to be associated with maternal diet or supplement intake than are fat-soluble vitamins or minerals. For example, vitamin B_6 is essential to normal neurological development. Concentrations in breastmilk vary with the vitamin B_6 nutritional status of the mother. Therefore, mothers whose dietary intake of vitamin B_6 is low may be at risk of secreting milk with less-than-adequate quantities (Borschel, Kirksey, & Hannemann, 1986; MMWR, 2003).

Even though vitamin K is fat soluble and passes more slowly into human milk, oral supplements of vitamin K in exclusively breastfed infants elevate plasma levels and may be an alternative method of supplementation in situations in which parents refuse intramuscular newborn vitamin K prophylaxis shortly after birth. In addition, maternal oral supplements postpartum should be considered, given the decreased intake of breastmilk during the first few days of life and the risk of hemorrhagic disease of the newborn (Greer et al., 1997).

Minerals

Minerals are inorganic substances that build body tissues and that activate, regulate, and control metabolic processes. They also transmit neurological messages. There is no consensus regarding the exact amount of calcium required during lactation (Prentice et al., 1995). The recommendation for calcium is 1200 mg/day, an amount that can generally be achieved with generous quantities of dairy products and green, leafy vegetables. Since calcium need is linked to level of protein consumption, low levels of calcium intake may be adequate in cultures and circumstances where protein intake is low. Even in countries in which calcium intake is chronically low, Fairweather-Tait et al. (1995) report no effect on the efficiency of calcium absorption by type or amount of calcium supplementation or stage of lactation. This finding suggests that body calcium may be mobilized to meet additional needs during lactation if necessary.

Clinical Implications

Optimal food patterns to maintain health emphasize intake of grains, fruit, vegetables, and small amounts of low-fat meat and legumes and low-fat dairy products. When making recommendations related to eating, the lactation consultant must consider such factors as the client's or family's culture, environment, socioeconomic status, and energy and nutrient needs. Food labels help mothers apply the principles from the US Dietary Guidelines for Americans when purchasing food and planning meals. These guidelines emphasize seven general recommendations, each of which applies to all members of the family:

1. *Eat a variety of foods.* Different foods are rich in varying nutrients. Therefore, it is important to eat foods from each of the five food groups (grains, fruit, vegetables, protein-rich foods, and dairy products) and to explore new foods to increase their variety. Vegetarians can obtain adequate nutrients if they eat a variety of foods and take in adequate calories. Vegans, who eat only foods from plant origin, need to ensure that they take a vitamin B_{12} supplement or eat foods fortified with the vitamin.

2. *Balance the food eaten with physical activity.* Physical activity will help to maintain appropriate weight. Although it is important to select foods wisely, it is also necessary to watch portion sizes. For example, a hamburger roll is 2 servings of bread; 1 cup of raw or cooked vegetable equals 1 serving; 3 oz of meat (about the size of the palm of the adult hand) equals 1 serving. People who restrict their total calorie intake need to eat nutrient-dense foods (high portion of nutrients per calories). Lactating women need to eat a diet rich in calcium (low-fat dairy products, dark-green, leafy vegetables, tofu, canned fish with soft bones) and iron (low-fat meat, fish, and poultry, leafy greens, legumes, and iron-enriched grain products). To maintain a healthy weight, food intake should be balanced with exercise.

3. *Choose a diet with plenty of grain products, vegetables, and fruit.* Most calories should come from grain products, fruit, and vegetables. These foods are high in nutrients and fiber and low in fat.

4. *Choose a diet low in fat, saturated fat, and cholesterol.* Total and saturated fat is highly correlated with serum cholesterol. Therefore, eating low-fat dairy products and meat and increasing the number of meatless meals by using legumes as the main dish are recommended. Monounsaturated and polyunsaturated fats found in olive and canola oils are recommended over butter and fats that are hard at room temperature (such as lard). Limit the number of meals containing egg yolks, organ meats, and other meats to decrease cholesterol intake. Total cholesterol intake should be kept below 300 mg/day.

5. *Choose a diet moderate in sugar.* Sugars alone are not associated with diabetes or becoming overweight, but people who eat large quantities of sweets (foods that are often also high in fat) will consume too many calories, which can lead to obesity.

6. *Choose a diet moderate in salt and sodium.* Processed and prepared foods often contain high amounts of salt and sodium. In addition,

some people add salt at the table and during food preparation. Encourage women to enjoy the natural taste of food by eating fresh fruit and vegetables rather than versions that have added salt or sugar. If a client is salt sensitive, ask her to limit her intake. The daily value for sodium is 2400 mg/day. Reading food labels can help you to determine when a food is high in sodium.

7. *If you choose to consume alcoholic beverages, do so in moderation.* Any alcohol taken during lactation can cross into the milk; the effect on the infant is dose-related. Alcohol is not recommended during lactation but, if it is taken, it should be ingested in small amounts, with meals, and at a time when breastfeeding is less likely to be compromised.

Dietitians have extensive education in infant and maternal nutrition and so are well equipped to educate lactating women; yet they remain a rarely tapped resource in breastfeeding management (Helm, Windham, & Wyse, 1997). The dietitian or clinician who is assisting the breastfeeding family to eat in an optimal fashion may wish to refer them to one or more of many nutrition information resources. In the United States, these resources include the following:

- Institute of Medicine: *Nutrition During Lactation: Report and Summary.* Washington, DC: National Academy Press, 1991
- Institute of Medicine: *Nutrition During Pregnancy and Lactation: An Implementation Guide.* Washington, DC: National Academy Press, 1992
- USDA/DHHS: *US Dietary Guidelines for Americans, 1995*

Questions that mothers commonly ask about nutrition and lactation are reviewed in Box 15–4.

BOX 15–4

Questions Mothers Often Ask About Nutrition and Lactation

1. *Am I at risk for osteoporosis from calcium loss when I breastfeed my baby?* No. Breastfeeding for 6 months or longer is the best protection against bone loss. Although calcium is mobilized during breastfeeding, hormones increase calcium absorption and limit the amount of calcium that is excreted. A diet that includes low-fat dairy products and green, leafy vegetables will provide adequate calcium; taking in plenty of sunshine will ensure an adequate supply of vitamin D, which also is important in bone health.

2. *Can I provide sufficient vitamin D to protect my breastfeeding baby against rickets?* Human milk contains small amounts of vitamin D, and some sunshine exposure is usually sufficient to maintain appropriate levels of vitamin D in the breastfeeding baby. However if you live in an area where sunlight may be severely limited for several months of the year or if your baby's clothing restricts the amount of sunlight he receives, your healthcare provider will probably recommend a vitamin D supplement for your baby.

3. *I am a teen mother. Can I make enough milk for my baby?* Yes. Only minimal differences exist between milk samples from teenage mothers and older mothers (Lipsman, Dewey, & Lönnerdal, 1985). If you are capable

(Continues)

BOX **15–4** (Continued)

of sustaining a pregnancy, you can also make sufficient milk to nourish your baby.

4. *What about folic acid?* I have been told this is important for the growing infant. Folate deficiency and subsequent anemia is highly unlikely in the breastfeeding baby. Breastfeeding babies nearly always have higher folate levels than their formula-feeding age-mates (Salmenpera, Perheentupa, & Siimes, 1986).

5. *If I eat high-fat foods, will I also produce high-fat milk?* To some degree. The specific dietary fatty acids that you consume will be reflected in the milk your baby receives. However, foods low in fat will not prevent you from making milk with sufficient creamy portions.

6. *If I have low levels of vitamin B_6, will this affect my milk supply?* Vitamin B_6 deficiency in a mother may contribute to lethargy in her infant. In one study, a baby with this deficiency also was difficult to console when distressed (McCullough et al., 1990).

7. *What if I am anemic? Will this mean that my baby will have low iron levels too?* Breastfed babies use the iron in their mother's milk more efficiently than do babies who are fed iron-fortified commercial formulas; thus your baby is at lower risk for anemia when breastfed (Duncan et al., 1985).

8. *Is it true that caffeine makes breastfed babies jittery?* Most studies do not support this expectation. The amounts of caffeine found in infants are usually very small; in other cases, they are undetectable (Berlin et al., 1984).

9. *Will I make enough milk if I don't eat "right"?* Your diet does not have to be perfect in order for you to breastfeed. Caloric intake is what enables a mother to make milk. Even if you eat foods high in sugar or fats, you will still make milk that can nourish your baby. Nonetheless, it is to your advantage to select foods wisely not only because you are breastfeeding, but because you are feeding yourself, your body, and your future, and because you are responsible for modeling healthful eating for your baby.

10. *How will I know my milk is "rich" enough or "not too rich" for my baby?* Nature has made the nutritional composition of your breastmilk just right for your baby. In particular, your milk has an abundant supply of the fatty acids that will lead to optimal nerve and brain development in your child. The milk you make will vary slightly from one feeding to the next, throughout the day, and throughout the baby's entire breastfeeding period. Some feedings will be richer than others, but all will meet the baby's needs.

11. *I am a vegetarian. Can I still breastfeed?* People who practice vegetarianism eat a variety of foods, and most of them are healthful. Nutritionists and other health professionals recommend five or more fruit and vegetable servings per day for everyone. As long as you consume enough calories to maintain an appropriate weight and you use a variety of foods, including legumes and other forms of protein, you will do well. If you are a vegan—consuming only plant foods—you may need to take a vitamin B_{12} supplement. If you express milk after eating a large amount of dark green vegetables,

(Continues)

15–4 (Continued)

your milk may have a slight green tinge, but the baby will not care!

12. *I hate to drink milk. Does this mean I cannot breastfeed?* Drinking milk and making breastmilk are not related. Think about the nutrients available from milk and get them from other foods. You can get calcium, for example, from other low-fat dairy products, green, leafy vegetables, and canned fish with soft bones.

13. *What do you mean by "drink to thirst?" How much should I drink?* This depends in part on where you live. A hot, dry climate may cause you to drink more than another climate. Your body needs water to make optimal use of the foods you eat. If you drink sufficiently, your urine will be pale in color. If you are thirsty, drink water; it is a thirst-quencher. Sugar-added fluids tend to make you feel more, not less, thirsty.

14. *How soon can I resume my previous exercise plan now that I am breast-feeding? Is it true that exercise will make my milk sour?* You can begin a previous exercise plan as soon as you feel ready to do so. However, it is wise to breastfeed shortly before doing any exercise that causes the breasts to bounce. Wear a support bra. Your milk will not be affected by exercise unless you are exercising to exhaustion; most women report no effects whatsoever (Dewey & McCrory, 1994).

15. *I was told I could not begin a weight-reduction program while breastfeeding, but I need to lose weight—and more than a few pounds too!* Some of the weight you gained during pregnancy is designed to be used during lactation. Most of the reputable weight-reduction programs

have a plan geared to pregnant and breastfeeding women. They are safe. Increasing fiber and the number of fruit and vegetable servings, using low-fat cooking methods, and decreasing the number of meals that are high in fat, sodium, and calories but low in fiber will also help you lose weight. In addition, daily exercise helps with weight reduction. Frequent breastfeeding has been shown to help women lose weight, particularly in the early weeks and months when the baby is most likely to be fully breastfeeding (Dewey et al., 1993).

16. *I have never been one to take pills, even vitamins. How important are extra vitamins if I breastfeed?* If you eat a healthful diet and you and your baby get plenty of sunshine (30 minutes per week), there should be no need to take extra vitamins.

17. *What special foods should I eat in order to breastfeed?* You do not need to eat any special foods in order to breastfeed. Eating a variety of nutrient-dense foods should be your goal—before, during, and after you are pregnant or lactating.

18. *What foods should I avoid in order to breastfeed?* Most babies and mothers do well with most foods. Sometimes babies will react to certain foods in the mother's diet. Experiment if this happens to you: eliminate the suspected food to determine whether the difficulty goes away. If so, eliminate this food for a while. In most cases, a baby who seems to react to a food when he is very young may not have a problem with that same food when he is older, even if still breast-feeding. Remember too that babies have been found to like highly

(Continues)

flavored milk, such as occurs when the mother uses garlic (Mennella & Beauchamp, 1991). Do not be afraid to enjoy highly flavored foods when you eat. Variety seems to be the spice of life for breastfed babies too!

Summary

Nutrition during the pregnancy continuum has been highlighted as an opportunity to keep in place or begin healthy food intake habits that will lead to optimal health for a lifetime. During pregnancy, what a woman eats will influence her physical well-being and that of her growing fetus. During lactation, how well she eats has less effect on her ability to make milk than on her well-being. Nevertheless, it is appropriate for clinicians who are offering suggestions pertaining to food intake to encourage the breastfeeding mother to eat in a manner that will support her optimal health.

At the same time it is not necessary to emphasize that the lactating mother must stick to a rigid diet of the "right foods" in order to breastfeed. Overemphasis on diet adds to the mother's stress level, and places an unnecessary burden on her; it will likely result in reluctance by some to breastfeed their babies out of fear that their own eating habits are not adequate. Food choices that the client is already making that support and sustain adequate energy intake and optimal health deserve praise; suggestions for change need to be offered within the context of established food patterns.

Food intake—including food selection, meal planning and preparation, and serving size—reflects a social behavior that has significance far beyond its nutritional and life-sustaining roles. Remaining sensitive to this understanding will enable the clinician to make suggestions more likely to be accepted and acted on by the client. Enabling a new mother to breastfeed by encouraging her to view her milk as the optimal food for her growing baby and child may help her to make changes in her own dietary choices that will sustain her health as well as that of her children.

Key Concepts

- Optimal nutrition during pregnancy and lactation encourages good nutrition for a lifetime.
- Although the emphasis on achieving and maintaining a "good" diet is important, the breastfeeding woman can still breastfeed even if her diet is not optimal.
- The lactating woman needs only an extra 400 to 500 calories per day.
- If the mother drinks enough fluids to meet her own thirst needs, she will drink enough to sustain lactation.
- A portion of the energy stored during pregnancy will be mobilized to accommodate milk production. This mobilized fat will be associated with a gradual but steady weight loss. Breastfeeding women lose slightly more weight postpartum although the evidence is conflicting.
- Gradual weight reduction has no deleterious effect on lactation and is attainable with lower energy intakes (fewer than 2200 kcal/day) to gradually lose weight. Modest weight loss (approximately 1 lb/week) appears to have no adverse effect on the quantity or quality of the breastmilk.
- Exercise does not interfere with the mother's milk supply or with the baby's feeding pattern; however, exercising to exhaustion may increase lactic acid levels to the point at which the baby refuses to breastfeed.

- Women have slight bone loss during lactation; this bone density is restored after weaning.
- Breastfeeding women who are vegetarians should consume foods rich in iron, calcium, and vitamins D, B_{12}, and riboflavin to ensure adequate intake. Special attention should be given to vitamin B_{12} intake.
- A balanced multivitamin supplement may be recommended on an individual basis. Women who avoid dairy products and other calcium-rich food sources may need a calcium supplement of 600 mg/day.
- Breastfeeding babies suckle longer and obtain more milk when breastmilk retains the flavor of vanilla or garlic that the mother has eaten. The varied flavors of breastmilk to which babies are exposed contrasts with a deficient sensory experience of babies who are fed formula that always tastes the same.
- Cow's milk and milk products are the most common allergens in breastmilk. Others are chocolate, cola, corn, citrus fruit, wheat, and peanuts. Peanut allergy can result in severe, even life-threatening reactions.
- Alcohol consumed during lactation crosses into the milk; the effect on the infant is dose-related. If taken, alcohol should be ingested in small amounts.
- The lactating mother need not stick to a rigid diet of the "right foods" in order to breastfeed. Overemphasis on diet can cause some mothers to be reluctant to breastfeed out of fear that their eating habits are inadequate.

Internet Resources

American Dietetic Association, breastfeeding promotion:
www.eatright.org

The decade's progress in 44 developing countries, 1989–1999:
www.childinfo.org

A resource guide for breastfeeding mothers:
www.breastfeeding.com

CDC's commitment to increase breastfeeding rates in the United States:
www.cdc.gov/breastfeeding

United States Department of Health and Human Services support site for breastfeeding:
www.womenshealth.gov/breastfeeding/index.cfm?page=home

A service of the US National Library of Medicine and the National Institutes of Health on breastfeeding:
www.nlm.nih.gov/medlineplus/breastfeeding.html

The World Health Organization and breastfeeding:
www.who.int/topics/breastfeeding/en

Resources available from the American Academy of Pediatrics and external organizations to help initiate and successfully continue breastfeeding:
www.aap.org/healthtopics/breastfeeding.cfm

An Internet resource to help empower women to choose to breastfeed and to educate society at large about the importance and benefits of breastfeeding:
www.breastfeedingonline.com

References

Agency for Healthcare Research and Quality. Breastfeeding and maternal and infant health outcomes in developed countries. Evidence Report/Technology Assessment No. 153. AHRQ Publications No. 07-E007. Rockville, MD: AHRQ; 2007.

Al MDM et al. Maternal essential fatty acid patterns during normal pregnancy and their relationship to the neonatal essential fatty acid status. *British J Nutr.* 1995;74:55–68.

Al MDM et al. Relation between birth order and the maternal and neonatal docosahexaenoic acid status. *Eur J Clin Nutr.* 1997;51:548–553.

Alam DS et al. Energy stress during pregnancy and lactation: consequences for maternal nutrition in rural Bangladesh. *Eur J Clin Nutr.* 2003;57:151–156.

American Academy of Pediatrics Section on Breastfeeding. Breastfeeding and the use of human milk. *Pediatrics.* 2005;115:496–506.

American Dietetic Association. *Manual of clinical dietetics.* Chicago, IL: Chicago Dietetic Association and the South Suburban Dietetic Association; 1996.

Basile LA et al. The effect of high-dose vitamin D supplementation on serum vitamin D levels and milk calcium concentration in lactating women and their infants. *Breastfeeding Med.* 2006;1:27.

Benisek D et al. Dietary intake of polyunsaturated fatty acids by pregnant or lactating women in the United States. *Obstet Gynecol.* 2000;95(4 suppl 1): S77–S78.

Berlin CM et al. Disposition of dietary caffeine in milk, saliva, and plasma of lactating women. *Pediatrics.* 1984;73:59–63.

Borschel MW, Kirksey A, Hannemann RE. Effects of vitamin B_6 intake on nutrition and growth of young infants. *Am J Clin Nutr.* 1986;43:7–15.

Bradshaw MK, Pfeiffer S. Feeding mode and anthropometric changes in primiparas. *Hum Biol.* 1988;60:251–261.

Brenna JT et al. Docosahexaenoic and arachidonic acid concentrations in human breast milk worldwide. *Am J Clin Nutr.* 2007;85:1457–1464.

Brown KH et al. Lactation capacity of marginally nourished mothers: infants' milk nutrient consumption and patterns of growth. *Pediatrics.* 1986;78: 920–927.

Butte NF et al. Effect of maternal diet and body composition on lactational performance. *Am J Clin Nutr.* 1984;39:296–306.

Carranza-Lira S, Mera JP. Influence of number of pregnancies and total breast-feeding time on bone mineral density. *Int J Fertil Womens Med.* 2002;47: 169–171.

Casella EB et al. Vitamin B_{12} deficiency in infancy as a cause of developmental regression. *Brain Dev.* 2005;27:592–594.

Centers for Disease Control and Prevention. Recommendations to improve preconception health and health care–United States: a report of the CDC/ATSDR Preconception Care Work Group and the Select Panel on Preconception Care. *MMWR Weekly.* 2006;55:6.

Ciani F et al. Prolonged exclusive breast-feeding from vegan mother causing an acute onset of isolated methylmalonic aciduria due to a mild mutase deficiency. *Clin Nutr.* 2000;19:137–139.

Cumming RG, Klineberg RJ. Breastfeeding and other reproductive factors and the risk of hip fractures in elderly women. *Int J Epidemiol.* 1993;22:684–691.

Dawodu A et al. Hypovitaminosis D and vitamin D deficiency in exclusively breastfeeding infants and their mothers in summer: a justification for vitamin D supplementation of breastfeeding infants. *J Pediatr.* 2003;142:169–173.

DeSantiago S et al. Protein requirements of marginally nourished lactating women. Unidad de Investigacion en Nutricion, Hospital de Pediatria, Centro Medico Nacional. *Am J Clin Nutr.* 1995;62:364–370.

Dewey KG. Energy and protein requirements during lactation. *Annu Rev Nutr.* 1997;17:19–36.

Dewey KG. Effects of maternal caloric restriction and exercise during lactation. *J Nutr.* 1998;128: 386S–389S.

Dewey KG, Lovelady C. Exercise and breast-feeding: a different experience [letter]. *Pediatrics.* 1993;91: 514–515.

Dewey KG, McCrory MA. Effects of dieting and physical activity on pregnancy and lactation. *Am J Clin Nutr.* 1994;49(suppl):446s–448s.

Dewey KG et al. Maternal weight-loss patterns during prolonged lactation. *Am J Clin Nutr.* 1993;58:162–166.

Dewey KG. A randomized study of the effects of aerobic exercise by lactating women on breast-milk volume and composition. *N Engl J Med.* 1994;330:449–453.

Dorea JG. Mercury and lead during breastfeeding. *Br J Nutr.* 2004;92:21–40.

Drexler H, Schaller KH. The mercury concentration in breast milk resulting from amalgam fillings and dietary habits. *Environ Res.* 1998;77:124–129.

Dugdale AE, Eaton-Evans J. The effect of lactation and other factors on post-partum changes in body-weight and triceps skinfold thickness. *Br J Nutr.* 1989;61:149–153.

Duncan B et al. Iron and the exclusively breast-fed infant from birth to six months. *J Pediatr Gastroenterol Nutr.* 1985;4:421–425.

Dusdieker LB et al. Is milk production impaired by dieting during lactation? *Am J Clin Nutr.* 1994;59: 833–840.

Ensom MH et al. Effect of pregnancy on bone mineral density in healthy women. *Obstet Gynecol Survey.* 2002;57:99–111.

Fairweather-Tait S et al. Effect of calcium supplements and stage of lactation on the calcium absorption efficiency of lactating women accustomed to low calcium intakes. *Am J Clin Nutr.* 1995;62: 1188–1192.

FAO/WHO/UNU. *Report of a Joint Expert Consultation: Energy and Protein Requirements.* Geneva, Switzerland: WHO; 1985. Tech. Rep. series 724.

Fidler N et al. Docosahexaenoic acid transfer into human milk after dietary supplementation: a randomized clinical trial. *J Lipid Res.* 2000;41: 1376–1383.

Fornes NS, Dorea JG. Subcutaneous fat changes in low-income lactating mothers and growth of breast-fed infants. *J Am Coll Nutr.* 1995;14:61–65.

Francois CA et al. Acute effects of dietary fatty acids on the fatty acids of human milk. *Am J Clin Nutr.* 1998;67:301–308.

Fraser A, Grimes DA. Effect of lactation on maternal body weight; a systematic review. *Obstet Gynecol Surv.* 2003;58:265–269.

Frigerio C et al. Is human lactation a particularly efficient process? *Eur J Clin Nutr.* 1991;45:459–462.

Gartner LM, Greer FR. Prevention of rickets and vitamin D deficiency: new guidelines for vitamin D intake. *Pediatrics.* 2003;111:908–910.

Giovannini M, Radaelli G, Banderali G, Riva E. Low prepregnant body mass index and breastfeeding practices. *J Hum Lact.* 2007;23:44–51.

Greer F. Issues in establishing vitamin D recommendations for infants and children. *Am J of Clin Nutr.* 2004; 80(suppl):1759S–1762S.

Greer F et al. Improving the vitamin K status of breast-feeding infants with maternal vitamin K supplements. *Pediatrics.* 1997;99:88–92.

Helland IB et al. Maternal supplementation with very-long-chain n-3 fatty acids during pregnancy and lactation augments children's IQ at 4 years of age. *Pediatrics.* 2003;111:e34–e39.

Helm A, Windham CT, Wyse B. Dietitians in breast-feeding management: an untapped resource in the hospital. *J Hum Lact.* 1997;13:221–225.

Holick MF. Resurrection of vitamin D deficiency and rickets. *J Clin Invest.* 2006;116:2062–2072.

Horwood LJ, Fergusson DM. Breastfeeding and later cognitive and academic outcomes. *Pediatrics.* 1998;101:E9.

Illingsworth PJ et al. Diminution in energy expenditure during lactation. *Br Med J.* 1986;292:437–441.

Institute of Medicine (IOM) Committee on Nutritional Status During Pregnancy and Lactation, Food and Nutrition Board. *Nutrition During Pregnancy and Lactation: An Implementation Guide.* Washington, DC: National Academy Press; 1992.

Institute of Medicine (IOM) Food and Nutrition Board, National Research Council. *Recommended Dietary Allowances.* 9th ed. Washington, DC: National Academy Press; 1984.

Institute of Medicine (IOM) Food and Nutrition Board, National Research Council. *Dietary Reference Intakes for Energy, Carbohydrates, Fiber, Fat, Fatty Acids, Cholesterol, Protein, and Amino Acids.* Washington, DC: National Academy Press; 2005.

Institute of Medicine (IOM), Food and Nutrition Board, National Research Council. *Dietary Reference Intakes for Thiamin, Riboflavin, Niacin, Vitamin B6, Folate, Vitamin B12, Pantothenic Acid, Biotin, and Choline.* Washington, DC: National Academy Press; 1998.

Institute of Medicine (IOM), Food and Nutrition Board, National Research Council, National Academy of Sciences. *Recommended Dietary Allowances.* 10th ed. Washington, DC: National Academy Press; 1989.

Institute of Medicine (IOM): *Nutrition During Lactation: Report and Summary.* Washington, DC: National Academy Press; 1991.

Institute of Medicine (IOM): *Nutrition During Pregnancy and Lactation: An Implementation Guide.* Washington, DC: National Academy Press; 1992.

Jensen CL et al. Effect of docosahexaenoic acid supplementation on lactating women on the fatty acid composition of breast milk lipids and maternal and infant plasma phospholipids. *Am J Clin Nutr.* 2000;71:292s–299s.

Kalkwarf HJ, Specker BL. Bone mineral loss during lactation and recovery after weaning. *Obstet Gynecol.* 1995;86:26–32.

Kalkwarf HJ, Specker BL. Bone mineral changes during pregnancy and lactation. *Endocrine.* 2002;17:49–53.

Kalkwarf HJ et al. Intestinal calcium absorption of women during lactation and after weaning. *Am J Clin Nutr.* 1996;63:526–531.

King JC. Effect of reproduction on the bioavailability of calcium, zinc and selenium. *J Nutr.* 2001;131: 1355S–1358S.

Kirksey A et al. Influence of mineral intake and use of oral contraceptives before pregnancy on the mineral content of human colostrum and of more mature milk. *Am J Clin Nutr.* 1979;32:30–39.

Koebnick C et al. Long-term ovo-lacto vegetarian diet impairs vitamin B-12 status in pregnant women. *J Nutr.* 2004;134:3319–3326.

Kramer FM et al. Breast-feeding reduces maternal lower-body fat. *J Am Diet Assoc.* 1993;93:429–433.

Larson-Meyer DE. Effect of postpartum exercise on mothers and their offspring: a review of the literature. *Obstet Res.* 2002;10:841–853.

LeGuennec JC, Billon B. Delay in caffeine elimination in breast-fed infants. *Pediatrics.* 1987;79:264–268.

Lipsman S, Dewey KG, Lönnerdal B. Breast-feeding among teenage mothers: milk composition, infant growth, and maternal dietary intakes. *J Pediatr Gastroenterol Nutr.* 1985;4:426–434.

Lovelady CA et al. Lactation performance of exercising women. *Am J Clin Nutr.* 1990;52:103–109.

Lovelady CA et al. The effect of weight loss in over-weight lactating women on the growth of their infants. *N Engl J Med.* 2000;342:449–453.

Lovelady CA et al. Effect of energy restriction and exercise on vitamin B_6 status of women during lactation. *Med Sci Sports Exerc.* 2001;33:512–518.

Lust KD, Brown JE, Thomas W. Maternal intake of cruciferous vegetables and other foods and colic symptoms in exclusively breast–fed infants. *J Am Diet Assoc.* 1996;96:46–48.

Mahan LK, Escott-Stump S. *Krause's Food, Nutrition, and Diet Therapy.* 9th ed. Philadelphia, PA: Saunders; 1996.

McCrory MA et al. Randomized trial of the short-term effects of dieting compared with dieting plus aerobic exercise on lactation performance. *Am J Clin Nutr.* 1999;69:959–967.

McCullough AL et al. Vitamin B_6 status of Egyptian mothers: relation to infant behavior and maternal-infant interaction. *Am J Clin Nutr.* 1990;51: 1067–1074.

Meisler JG, St. Jeor S. Summary and recommendations from the American Health Foundation's Expert Panel on Healthy Weight. *Am J Clin Nutr.* 1996;63 (suppl):474s–477s.

Mennella JA. Mother's milk: a medium for early flavor experiences. *J Hum Lact.* 1995;11:39–45.

Mennella JA, Beauchamp GK. Maternal diet alters the sensory qualities of human milk and the nursling's behavior. *Pediatrics.* 1991;88:737–744.

Mennella JA, Beauchamp GK. The human infants' response to vanilla flavors in mother's milk and formula. *Infant Behav Dev.* 1996;19:13–19.

Mennella JA, Beauchamp GK. Mothers' milk enhances the acceptance of cereal during weaning. *Pediatr Res.* 1997;41:188–192.

Motil KJ et al. Case report: failure to thrive in a breast-fed infant is associated with maternal dietary protein and energy restriction. *J Am Coll Nutr.* 1994;13:203–208.

Murphy SP, Abrams BF. Changes in energy intakes during pregnancy and lactation in a national sample of US women. *Am J Public Health.* 1993;83:1161–1163.

Nommsen LA et al. Determinants of energy, protein, lipid, and lactose concentrations in human milk during the first 12 months. *Am J Clin Nutr.* 1991;53: 457–465.

Paul AA, Muller EM, Whitehead RG. The quantitative effects of maternal dietary energy intake on pregnancy and lactation in rural Gambian women. *Trans R Soc Trop Med Hyg.* 1979;73:686–692.

Piers LS et al. Changes in energy expenditure, anthropometry, and energy intake during the course of pregnancy and lactation in well-nourished Indian women. *Am J Clin Nutr.* 1995;61:501–513.

Prentice A. Maternal calcium requirements during pregnancy and lactation. *Am J Clin Nutr.* 1994;59 (suppl):477s–483s.

Prentice A et al. Calcium requirements of lactating Gambian mothers: effects of a calcium supplement on breast-milk calcium concentration, maternal bone mineral content, and urinary calcium excretion. *Am J Clin Nutr.* 1995;62:58–67.

Prentice AM, Goldberg GR, Prentice A. Body mass index and lactational performance. *Eur J Clin Nutr.* 1994;48(suppl l3):S78–S89.

Reghu A et al. Vitamin B_{12} deficiency presenting as oedema in infants of vegetarian mothers. *Eur J Pediatr.* 2005;164:257–258.

Rolfes SR, Pinna K, Whitney E. *Understanding Normal and Clinical Nutrition.* 7th ed. Belmont, CA: Thompson/Wadsworth; 2006.

Rooney BL, Schauberger CW. Excess pregnancy weight gain and long-term obesity: one decade later. *Obstet Gynecol.* 2002;100:245–252.

Ryu JE. Caffeine in human milk and in serum of breast-fed infants. *Dev Pharmacol Ther.* 1985a;8:329–337.

Ryu JE. Effect of maternal caffeine consumption on heart rate and sleep time of breast-fed infants. *Dev Pharmacol Ther.* 1985b;8:355–363.

Sanders TAB. Essential fatty acid requirements of vegetarians in pregnancy, lactation and infancy. *Am J Clin Nutr.* 1999;70:555S–559S.

Salmenpera L, Perheentupa J, Siimes MA. Folate nutrition is optimal in exclusively breast-fed infants but inadequate in some of their mothers and in formula-fed infants. *J Pediatr Gastroenterol Nutr.* 1986;5:283–289.

Schutz Y, Lechtig A, Bradfield RB. Energy expenditures and food intakes of lactating women in Guatemala. *Am J Clin Nutr.* 1980;33:892–902.

Shaikh M, Chantry C. Reflections on the American Academy of Pediatrics 2005 policy statement on "breastfeeding and the use of human milk". *J Hum Lact.* 2006;22:108–110.

Shaikh MG et al. Transient neonatal hypothyroidism due to a maternal vegan diet. *J Pediatr Endocrinol Metab.* 2003;16:111–113.

Simopoulos AP et al. Workshop on the essentiality of and recommended dietary intakes for omega-6 and omega-3 fatty acids. *J Am Coll Nutr.* 1999;18:487–489.

Smith CA. Effects of maternal undernutrition upon the newborn infant in Holland (1944–45). *J Pediatr.* 1947;30:229–243.

Sowers MF et al. Changes in bone density with lactation. *JAMA.* 1993;269:3130–3135.

Sowers MF et al. Biochemical markers of bone turnover in lactating and nonlactating postpartum women. *J Clin Endocrinol Metab.* 1995;80:2210–2216.

Specker BL, Tsang RC, Ho ML. Changes in calcium homeostasis over the first year postpartum: effect of lactation and weaning. *Obstet Gynecol.* 1991;78: 56–62.

Specker BL et al. Effect of race and diet on human-milk vitamin D and 25-hydroxyvitamin D. *Am J Dis Child.* 1985;139:1134–1137.

Specker BL et al. Effect of vegetarian diet on serum 1,25-dihydroxyvitamin D concentrations during lactation. *Obstet Gynecol.* 1987a;70:870–874.

Specker BL et al. Differences in fatty acid composition of human milk in vegetarian and non-vegetarian women: long-term effect of diet. *J Ped Gastroent Nutr.* 1987b;6:764–768.

Spring PCM et al. Fat and energy content of breast milk of malnourished and well nourished women, Brazil 1982. *Ann Trop Paediatr.* 1985;5:83–87.

Stefanski J. Breastfeeding after bariatric surgery. *Today's Dietitian.* 2006;8:47.

Strode MA et al. Effects of short-term caloric restriction on lactational performance of well-nourished women. *Acta Paediatr Scand.* 1986;75:222–229.

Stumbo PJ et al. Water intakes of lactating women. *Am J Clin Nutr.* 1985;42:870–876.

Sullivan SA, Birch LL. Infant dietary experience and acceptance of solid foods. *Pediatrics.* 1994;93: 271–277.

Thorsdottir I, Birgisdottir BE. Different weight gain in women of normal weight before pregnancy: postpartum weight and birth weight. *Obstet Gynecol.* 1998;92:377–383.

Todd JM, Parnell WR. Nutrient intakes of women who are breastfeeding. *Eur J Clin Nutr.* 1994;48:567–574.

US Department of Agriculture Department of Health and Human Services. *US Dietary Guidelines for Americans.* Washington, DC: USDA; 2005.

Vadas P et al. Detection of peanut allergens in breast milk of lactating women. *JAMA*. 2001;285:1746–1748.

van Raaij JM et al. Energy cost of lactation, and energy balances of well-nourished Dutch lactating women: reappraisal of the extra energy requirements of lactation. *Am J Clin Nutr*. 1991;53:612–619.

Vaughn LA, Weber CW, Kemberling SR. Longitudinal changes in the mineral content of human milk. *Am J Clin Nutr*. 1979;32:2301–2306.

Walker LO, Freeland-Greaves J. Lifestyle factors related to postpartum weight gain and body image in bottle and breastfeeding women. *JOGN*. 1998;27:151–160.

Wallace JP et al. Infant acceptance of postexercise breast milk. *Pediatrics*. 1992;89:1245–1247.

Walsh S. What every vegan should know about vitamin B_{12}. Available at: http://www.beyondveg.com/walsh-s/vitamin-b12/vegans-1.shtml. Accessed January 9, 2009.

World Health Organization. Minor and trace elements in human milk. *Report of a Joint WHO/IEAE Collaborative Study*. Geneva, Switzerland: WHO; 1989.

Ziegler EE et al. Vitamin D deficiency in breastfed infants in Iowa. *Pediatrics*. 2006;118:603–610.

Women's Health and Breastfeeding

Jan Riordan

THIS CHAPTER DISCUSSES acute and chronic maternal health problems that have an effect on lactation. The health of a mother has a direct effect on her ability (both emotional and physical) to care for her infant. For example, mothers of preterm infants are particularly vulnerable to decreases in their immune function postpartum and have greater anxiety and depression compared to mothers of term infants. The normal immunosuppression of pregnancy recovers slowly over the months postpartum, exacerbating immune-mediated diseases such as rheumatoid arthritis and lupus (Gennaro et al., 1997).

Most lactating women are healthy and fit. Illness is usually episodic, such as a head cold or a case of influenza. Breastfeeding empowers women to stay healthy by providing a variety of such health benefits as a reduction in the likelihood of carcinoma-in-situ of the uterine cervix (Brock et al., 1989), ovarian cancer (Rosenblatt & Thomas, 1993; Siskind et al., 1997), endometrial cancer (Rosenblatt & Thomas, 1995), breast cancer (Newcomb et al., 1999), rheumatoid arthritis (Brun et al., 1995), osteoporosis (Paton et al., 2003), midlife metabolic syndrome (Ram et al., 2008), and obesity (Hammer et al., 1996). Even plasma concentrations of both cholesterol and triglycerides remain significantly lower in breastfeeding mothers

than in bottle-feeding mothers during postpartum (Qureshi et al., 1999).

Maternal health and the ability to breastfeed have monetary value that is ignored in national accounting. In a study that estimated the economic value of human milk in 1992, Smith (2005) calculated that the quantity of human milk from Australian women had a market value of AU$2.0–2.2 billion.

The lactation consultant usually does not see the more serious health conditions described in this chapter. When she does, she needs a working knowledge of these conditions and the ability to develop a plan of care based on the wishes and needs of the breastfeeding mother who has a health problem.

Alterations in Endocrine and Metabolic Functioning

Anything that affects control of the endocrine system can also affect the production of breastmilk. The following discussion of diabetes mellitus, thyroid problems, and pituitary dysfunction explains uncommon conditions that may affect the breastfeeding mother's milk supply. Any woman with symptoms that suggest she might have an altered metabolic functioning should be referred to a physician for further evaluation and treatment.

Diabetes

Diabetes is a chronic disease of impaired carbohydrate metabolism caused by insufficient insulin or the inefficient use of insulin. Pregnant women with diabetes mellitus can be classified into two main categories: women who have (1) prepregnancy diabetes (type I or II), or women who have (2) gestational diabetes. Type I diabetes is a serious disease in which insulin is not being produced as a result of autoimmunity directed at the β cells of the pancreas. Type II diabetes used to be seen infrequently in pregnancy because the age of diagnosis was usually made after the reproductive years. It is much more common in pregnant women today and is part of a metabolic syndrome commonly seen with hypertension, obesity, and dyslipidemia. For each additional year that a woman lactates, she has a 15 percent decrease in the risk of diabetes later in life (Stuebe et al., 2005).

Gestational Diabetes

Gestational diabetes, a glucose intolerance that occurs in 4 percent of all pregnancies, manifests itself only during pregnancy (American Diabetes Association, 2000). Gestational diabetes is far more common than a decade ago because more women (as well as the rest of the population) are obese today. Gestational diabetes is detected in the same ways as other forms of diabetes. Most women with gestational diabetes will revert to normal status. Breastfeeding should be encouraged and proceed normally in these women. In fact, women with gestational diabetes are twice as likely to develop type II diabetes later if they do not lactate following the birth of the baby whose pregnancy provoked gestational diabetes (Kjos et al., 1993). Lactation—even for a short duration—improves glucose metabolism and is a low-cost intervention that may reduce or delay diabetes in these women.

Type I Diabetes

With improvement in the monitoring and control of maternal blood sugar, women with type I diabetes who have well-controlled glucose levels can usually look forward to a safe and relatively healthy pregnancy and birth. It is commonplace today for a woman with diabetes to experience a normal delivery and for the infant to be with the mother from birth and to breastfeed without the need for special care. The current use of subcutaneous insulin infusion pumps and multiple daily insulin doses has decreased the erratic glucose levels once seen, resulting in fewer perinatal complications. During pregnancy, the mother's blood glucose levels should be maintained below 130 mg/dl as much as possible. During labor, delivery, and for some time after delivery, blood glucose levels are closely monitored. Controlling for gestational age and class of maternal diabetes, breastfed infants had fewer episodes of hypoglycemia and less need for supplements than bottle-fed infants according to one study (Taylor et al., 2005).

The woman with type I diabetes not only can, but should, be encouraged to breastfeed her infant. Colostrum helps to stabilize the infant's blood sugar and, although breastfeeding should begin as soon after birth as possible, this is usually not the case. Infants of mothers with diabetes are occasionally placed in the special care unit after delivery. If breastfeeding is delayed, the mother should be encouraged to begin expressing or pumping her milk as soon as she feels able.

Lactating women with type I diabetes have lower milk prolactin concentrations than do women without diabetes (Ostrom & Ferris, 1993), causing a delay of about one day in lactogenesis II, or "coming in" of the milk for mothers (Arthur, Kent, & Hartman, 1994; Bitman et al., 1989; Miyake et al., 1989; Murtaugh et al., 1998). These mothers and their neonates need additional attention and care to establish lactation. In addition to early, frequent feedings, pumping to stimulate the milk supply is advised as well. It may be necessary to supplement the neonate during the first 2 to 3 days. Formula is often given in the interim until the mother's milk comes in, which brings up the issue of a potentially destructive autoimmune response in an infant. Rather than give artificial milk supplements, one pregnant mother with type I diabetes stored donor breastmilk that she later used to supplement her baby during the first few days postpartum.

During the immediate postnatal period, sudden but normal hormonal changes cause marked fluctuation in maternal blood glucose levels. Maternal hypoglycemia can be expected to occur immediately postbirth, lasting 5 to 7 hours after delivery. In addition, lactose excretion in the urine drops to a low level 2 to 5 days after birth and then rises rapidly. These sudden metabolic shifts of erratic blood glucose levels and an increase in insulin reaction require close monitoring. Juggling the feeding schedule of the infant and the amount of milk taken at each feeding are factors to be considered in maintaining good diabetic balance. Nighttime feedings present special challenges to the breastfeeding mother with diabetes. The mother should be encouraged to test her glucose levels during the night. She may need an additional snack at night.

Lactose is reabsorbed from the breast and is normally excreted in the urine; therefore, nurses and mothers should be aware that in testing the urine after delivery, the presence of lactose might result in a false-positive test if copper-reducing urine testing (Clinitest) is used. For this reason, testing with Testape or Diastix, which measure only glucose, are the preferred methods. Once she is physiologically stable, the patient can return to subcutaneous injection insulin or to injection via a portable infusion pump.

Blood glucose meters are reliable for testing blood glucose by the mother at home. By keeping a daily record of blood glucose levels, the mother can self-monitor day-to-day changes. Once the blood glucose level stabilizes, it is generally lower during lactation. Ferris et al. (1988, 1993) compared 30 mothers with type I diabetes with 30 controls and found that fasting plasma glucose levels during the exclusive breastfeeding period were significantly lower than were the glucose levels of the women with type I diabetes who had stopped breastfeeding or who had never breastfed, even in the face of markedly higher caloric intake by the breastfeeding mothers. Women with type I diabetes usually take insulin by injection. Insulin, a large peptide that does not pass into breastmilk, is not a problem medication with breastfeeding.

Given the continuous conversion of glucose to galactose and lactose during milk synthesis, less insulin is required when the mother breastfeeds. Davies et al. (1989) showed that women with diabetes might need to reduce their prepregnancy insulin dose by about 27 percent to avoid hypoglycemic reactions. Breastmilk nutrients, especially

lactose, vary slightly during the first several days postpartum (Lammi-Keefe et al., 1995), but these changes do not affect the mother's ability to produce breastmilk.

In addition to providing the known physiological advantages of breastfeeding for the infant, breastfeeding helps to fulfill the mother's need to feel normal in spite of her diabetic condition. An advantage of working with these women is their keen awareness of their body functions and the importance of diet. They are more knowledgeable than the average woman about physiology and are quick to notice changes that may forewarn of problems.

Mothers with diabetes may be more susceptible to mastitis, especially if they are not well controlled (Ferris et al., 1988; Gagne, Leff, & Jefferis, 1992). Any infection will quickly raise the level of blood glucose. Self-care teaching should emphasize recognizing early symptoms of mastitis and seeking prompt treatment while continuing to breastfeed. Mothers with diabetes are also at risk for candidiasis if blood glucose levels are elevated. Preventing this problem involves careful control of blood glucose, drying the nipple after breastfeeding, and being aware of the early symptoms (see Chapter 15).

Once lactation is established, most women who have diabetes report that their breastfeeding experiences are no different from those of mothers without diabetes. The mother with diabetes needs additional calories while breastfeeding. As her child begins to wean, the mother will again need to make alterations in her diet and insulin intake to compensate for a decrease in milk production. If weaning is gradual, fewer problems and adjustments arise.

Crohn's Disease and Inflammatory Bowel Disease (IBD)

Inflammatory disease is an autoimmune process of unknown origin. It primarily affects the gastrointestinal (GI) tract and has two major forms: ulcerative colitis, which involves the colon, and Crohn's disease which can occur in any part of the GI tract.

Crohn's disease is more common in northern climate and is a chronic, incurable disease where the individual has a lifetime of disease activity and remissions. Both genetics and environment appear to play a role in causation. Symptoms are bleeding, diarrhea, nausea, weight loss, abdominal pain, and fatigue. Drug therapy can include sulfasalazine, mesalamine (acute phase), corticosteroids, and immunosuppressive drugs.

Work in other autoimmune disorders has found that breastfeeding may be associated with an increased risk for developing postpartum disease relapse; however, in a study of 122 women attending an IBD center, breastfeeding did not appear to make any difference in disease activity for either Crohn's or ulcerative colitis. About half of the women attending the center did not breastfeed. The low percentage of those breastfeeding was because of concern about the effect of maternal medications on the breastfeeding infant (Kane & Lemieux, 2005).

Turner's Syndrome

Turner's syndrome is an inherited chromosomal defect that occurs only in women. The main features are a short stature, webbing of the skin of the neck, retarded development of secondary sexual characteristics, and other abnormalities. The treatment is growth hormone replacement therapy started in early adolescence. A single case study reports a 32-year-old woman with Turner's syndrome and associated insulin-dependent diabetes (Parker, 2005). She had been on hormone replacement therapy since adolescence and became pregnant through in vitro fertilization and the donor egg program. Following birth, a nipple shield and complementary feeds were used until the baby learned to suckle at the breast. This remarkable woman had two more pregnancies including a set of twins. With each birth she was able to breastfeed.

Thyroid Disease

The thyroid gland controls the body's metabolism and promotes normal growth of central nervous system development. It produces three hormones: thyrosine (T_4), triiodothyronine (T_3), and calcitonin. T_3 and T_4 are chemically similar and are known as thyroid hormones. Postpartum thyroid dysfunction is a common event, occurring in some 17 percent of women. Thyroid disease is considered an immune-mediated dysfunction. Its connection to the postpartum changes of the immune system is not yet clear (Gennaro et al., 1997). Breastfeeding women who develop disorders of the thyroid gland can be treated and continue to breastfeed.

Hypothyroidism

Maintaining full-term pregnancy is rare in untreated women who suffer from hypothyroidism; therefore, most breastfeeding women with a history of hypothyroidism are on replacement therapy. For the untreated breastfeeding woman, hypothyroidism can result in a reduced milk supply. Other symptoms in the mother are thyroid swelling or nodules (goiter), cold intolerance, dry skin, thinning hair, poor appetite, extreme fatigue, and depression. When the thyroid deficiency is not known, these problems are often attributed to postpartum hormonal changes and changes in lifestyle (notably, constant care of the baby) and remain undiagnosed—at least for a time. When the infant of one mother suddenly and completely weaned, the mother, subsequently receiving a diagnosis of hypothyroidism, reported that she "never experienced any fullness in the breast—it was as though I'd dried up overnight."

These complaints, sometimes coupled with the infant's failure to gain weight satisfactorily on breastmilk alone, should alert the nurse or lactation consultant to the possibility of thyroid deficiency and to the reality that the mother needs further medical diagnostic evaluation. If replacement therapy of thyroid extract with synthetic T_4 (thyroxine, sodium levothyroxine, or Synthroid) or other thyroid preparation is adequate, the relief of the symptoms and an increase in the milk supply can be quite dramatic. The daily replacement dose of thyroid extract is 0.25 to 1.12 mg of sodium levothyroxine or equivalent doses of other thyroid preparation. Women whose replacement therapy was determined before pregnancy should be reevaluated after the baby's birth to determine whether adjustment is necessary. In another case, hypothyroidism developed in a preterm infant whose initial screening thyroid function test results were normal at 2 weeks of life. The infant's mother was packing her Cesarean incision with iodine-soaked gauze, resulting in a markedly increased breast milk iodine concentration. Treatment with oral L-thyroxine normalized thyroid function tests (Smith, Svoren, & Wolfsdorf, 2006).

Postpartum Thyroiditis

Postpartum thyroiditis is an autoimmune disorder that affects women worldwide. Its symptoms—fatigue, depression, and anxiety—may go unrecognized in the postpartum period.

Hyperthyroidism

An excess of thyroid hormone is characterized by loss of weight (despite an increased appetite), nervousness, heart palpitations, and a rapid pulse at rest. A well-developed case of hyperthyroidism with exophthalmos (bulging eyes) is called Graves' disease. Hyperthyroidism, a common disorder thought to affect 2 percent of women typically in their mid 20s or 30s, can develop for the first time postpartum. The ability to lactate does not appear to be affected, although the mother's nervousness may complicate her ability to cope with the daily caregiving of her infant.

Generally, laboratory diagnosis of hyperthyroidism can be established by values from just two laboratory tests: serum TSH and serum free T_4 index. When evaluation of the thyroid using a radioactive substance is deemed essential, technetium-99m pertechnetate is the preferred agent. A listing on the safety of use of isotopes in breastfeeding women from the Nuclear Regulatory Commission can be found at http://neonatal.ttuhsc.edu/lact/html/radio.html.

Pituitary Dysfunction

Severe postpartum hemorrhage and hypotension may result in the pituitary gland's failure to produce gonadotropins, which leads to a condition known as *panhypopituitarism* or *Sheehan's syndrome*. Along with lactation failure, the woman has loss of pubic and axillary hair, intolerance to cold, breast tissue atrophy, low blood pressure, and vaginal tissue atrophy. Milder cases of pituitary disruption may occur, with less severe symptoms and delay in milk synthesis. DeCoopman's report (1993) that lactation continued following pituitary resection suggests that the role of the pituitary gland may be temporary in the early establishment of lactation rather than an essential requirement throughout its course. Prolactinomas (prolactin-secreting adenomas) are pituitary tumors that stimulate the secretion of prolactin and produce secondary amenorrhea and galactorrhea. Women with prolactinomas may breastfeed without restriction.

Polycystic Ovarian Syndrome

Polycystic ovarian syndrome (PCOS) is an endocrine-metabolic disorder in women in which the presence of multiple cysts interferes with ovarian function. The prevalence of PCOS is anywhere from 3 to 20 percent. Originally called Stein-Leventhal syndrome, women with polycystic ovarian syndrome are also likely to have amenorrhea and hirsutism (unusual hair growth), to be obese, and have unusual breast development. A radiographic study of breast tissue noted frequent aberrations that included hypoplasia and large breasts filled primarily with fatty tissue (Balcar et al., 1972). Tissue samples from another study found "gross disorders of the glandular parenchyma" (Fonseca et al., 1985). Marasco (2005) notes that this information has not been reflected in articles on PCOS since then. It was thought that the high level of testosterone associated with PCOS interferes with the hormones necessary for full lactation; however, results of a study of one such hormone, insulin, showed no differences between breastfeeding women with and without PCOS (Maliqueo et al., 2001). Metformin has become one of the first choices for treatment. It improves the endocrinopathy of PCOS, facilitates conception, appears to reduce first trimester miscarriage and gestational diabetes, does not appear to cause birth defects, and appears to be safe in the first 6 months of infancy (Glueck, 2007; Glueck et al., 2006). Clomiphen has been a mainstay of ovulation induction for women with PCOS.

Marasco, Marmet, and Shell (2000) describe three cases of breastfeeding women with PCOS who had insufficient milk supply. While working with a mother who is experiencing a delay with her milk coming in, it is wise to ask questions about menstrual problems, infertility, miscarriages, and ovarian cysts. Marasco (2005) wisely cautions healthcare professionals.

> *When primary lactation failure is evident, great sensitivity is needed in guiding the mother through the process of deciding how she wants to proceed. Remember that she is facing a complex situation that does not offer a guarantee of full results and that she may even have come to us hesitantly, afraid of "fanaticism" that ignores the emotions and realities of her situation. Anything that feels like subtle pressure can heap more guilt upon her, resulting in anger and resentment. (Marasco, 2005)*

self-fulfillment, workplace policy, work motivation, and family or baby motivation (Killien, 1998; Nichols & Roux, 2004). As more women work outside the home, potential conflicts arise between breastfeeding, which demands a woman's unique ability to meet her baby's needs and her efforts to balance the demands of work and family.

Work has played a prominent role in women's lives for centuries. Prior to the Industrial Revolution, women played two active roles: raising a family and working predominantly in the home. In 1800, only 5 percent of white women worked outside the home (Begun, Blair, & Quiram, 1998). Factors influencing married women to seek employment during the early industrial period were caused by wartime demand for labor, mandatory schooling for young children, a decline in fertility rates, and inadequate earnings by men. The proportion of women in the labor force increased from 9.7 percent in 1870 to 20 percent in 1940. The proportion of married women in the labor force increased from 5.6 percent in 1900 to 15.2 percent in 1940 (Marshall & Paulin, 1987). In 1978, working wives contributed only 26 percent to family income. Employment rates for women have increased considerably since 1960 for both single and married women. Based on data from the US Department of Labor, Women's Bureau (2007), between 1940 and 2005, the rate of women working increased from 25 to 59 percent. The growth in labor force participation of single women rose from 55 to 74 percent between 1990 and 2000. In 2006, the rate of mothers working in the labor force was 71 percent, and of this, 69 percent were married (US Department of Labor, 2007).

Examining global employment trends, women's participation in the labor market worldwide grew substantially during the 1980s and 1990s. The total female labor force worldwide was 1.2 billion (52.6 percent of women worldwide) in 2006. The percentage of women in wage and salary work has grown during the last decade from 42.9 percent in 1996 to 47.9 percent in 2006. However, women are more likely to earn less than men for the same type of work and on average contribute less to the family income in all regions of the world (International Labour Office, 2007). Even in high-skill occupations such as accounting and computer programming, the average female wage is only 88 percent of the male wage. Countries with a greater gender wage gap in

high-skill occupations also had a greater gender wage gap in low-skill occupations (International Labour Office, 2007).

The number of working women in the United States varies with the age of the youngest child, marital status, and race. Rates of employment were highest among married women with young children. In 2007, 55.1 percent of all women with children under one year of age returned to the labor force, with 70 percent of those women working full-time (US Bureau of Labor Statistics, 2008). The labor force participation rate for unmarried mothers with children under 1 year old rose by 4.3 percentage points to 59 percent in 2006 (US Department of Labor, 2007). Working mothers usually play multiple roles and share domestic responsibilities such as household chores; thus, they juggle to maintain balance between work and family. Many women report that neither their employers nor public policy adequately recognizes or supports women's family responsibilities (Killien et al., 2001; Killien, 2005). Another study revealed that postpartum mothers experienced many resiliency challenges such as role overload; family stress; and family/child, financial, and psychosocial issues when they returned to work (Nichols & Roux, 2004).

The Effect of Work on Breastfeeding

The National Immunization Survey (NIS) indicates that the prevalence of breastfeeding initiation and duration through 6 months and 1 year of age in the United States has reached its highest recorded levels: 70.9, 36.2, and 17.2 percent respectively (Centers for Disease Control and Prevention [CDC], 2007). Although breastfeeding initiation rates in the United States have been rising over the past decade, the rates at 6 and 12 months are still far below the *Healthy People 2010* goals. The prevalence of continued exclusive breastfeeding for the birth years 2000 to 2004 at 3 and 6 months were 30.5 percent and 11.3 percent respectively (CDC, 2007).

The increasing numbers of women with infants under 1 year of age entering the workforce each year has serious implications as many women will choose to combine breastfeeding and employment. Some empirical evidence suggests that employment has a negative impact on women's decision to initiate breastfeeding especially among those women who plan to return to work in the first few weeks postpartum (Fein & Roe, 1998; Lindberg, 1996; Roe et al., 1999), while other studies found no impact on breastfeeding initiation (Kimbro, 2006; Noble et al., 2001; Ong et al., 2005; Ryan, Zhou, & Arensberg, 2006). Studies outside the United States on maternal employment status and breastfeeding also reported that full-time employed women were less likely to initiate breastfeeding than mothers who were not employed (Chen, Wu, & Chie, 2006; Hawkins et al., 2007; Ong et al., 2005).

However, for many women within and outside the United States, the workplace seems to be incompatible with breastfeeding for a longer period. Lindberg (1996) used a role-incompatibility model to explain why some employed women breastfeed and others do not. She noted that women working part-time were more likely than full-time workers to breastfeed, and that more women quit breastfeeding in the same month that they returned to work, supporting her contention that these two behaviors—breastfeeding and working—are viewed by many as being incompatible. Numerous studies indicate that full-time working mothers breastfeed for a shorter duration than those who work part-time or are unemployed (Arthur, Saenz, & Replogle, 2003; Dodgson & Duckett, 1997; Fein & Roe, 1998; Kimbro, 2006; Roe et al., 1999; Ryan, Zhou, & Acosta, 2002). Ryan, Zhou, and Arensberg (2006) reported that 65.5 percent and 26.1 percent of women who worked full-time were breastfeeding their infants compared to 64.8 percent and 35 percent of those women who did not work at hospital discharge and 6 months respectively. Note that while initiation rates were similar in both groups the continuation rates were measurably different. Fein and Roe (1998) also found that women who worked full-time at 3 months postpartum decreased breastfeeding duration by an average of 8.6 weeks compared to those women who were not employed. Some studies also have suggested that the longer women delayed their return to work, the lower the negative effect of employment on their breastfeeding experience (Arthur et al., 2003; Lindberg, 1996; Roe, Whittington, Fein, & Teisl, 1999; Visness & Kennedy, 1997). Most international studies, particularly those conducted in developing countries, report that working negatively affects breastfeeding (Chen, Wu, & Chie, 2006; Ong et al., 2005; Rea et al., 1999; Yimyam, 1998; Yimyam & Morrow, 1999).

The intensity of breastfeeding has also been associated with duration of breastfeeding. Working mothers who exclusively breastfeed (no formula supplementation), are more likely to continue breastfeeding longer than those who partially breastfeed (Ong et al., 2005; Piper & Parks, 1996). In addition, when a mother was satisfied and viewed breastfeeding as a special time with the baby that she did not want to give up, she was more likely to breastfeed longer (Lindberg, 1996; Rojjanasrirat, 2000).

Types of occupations were also associated with duration of breastfeeding. Women who were classified as professional, administrative, or managerial had a longer duration of breastfeeding than did women in the lower-skill occupations such as clerical and service jobs (Piper & Parks, 1996; Visness & Kennedy, 1997; Whaley et al., 2002). In contrast, a recent study reported that women in service occupations and administrative positions weaned earlier than other women (Kimbro, 2006). In general, there is a need for more research to test interventions and set policies that supports breastfeeding among women in service jobs, as well as in shift work.

Facilitators and Barriers to Breastfeeding in the Workplace

A number of barriers to breastfeeding in the workplace have been identified (Johnston & Esposito, 2007; Meek, 2001; Zinn, 2000). Significant factors and reasons for early weaning among working mothers include insufficient milk supply, lack of knowledge regarding management of breastfeeding in the work place, lack of time to pump, and work facilities that are not conducive to breastfeeding (Arthur et al., 2003; Bar-Yam, 1998; Dodgson & Duckett, 1997; Ong et al., 2005; Roe et al., 1999; Scott et al., 2006; Thompson & Bell, 1997). Arthur et al. (2003) examined the breastfeeding decisions and experiences of female physicians related to employment. They reported that the three major factors contributing to complete discontinuation of breastfeeding were returning to work (45 percent), diminishing milk supply (31 percent), and lack of time to pump (18 percent).

Factors enhancing or facilitating the continuation of breastfeeding in the workplace include on-site child care, long maternity leave, flexible work schedules, availability of a lactation room, types of breast pumps, and supportive environment (coworkers and employers) (Arthur et al., 2003; Stevens & Janke, 2003; Thompson & Bell, 1997; Witters-Green, 2003; Ortiz et al., 2004). Consideration of these barriers and facilitators when planning for combining work and breastfeeding can enhance success. We turn now to strategies to manage breastfeeding and work, beginning with the individual woman's efforts and then moving to a discussion of the other key players in the quest to support the breastfeeding employed woman.

Individual Strategies to Manage Breastfeeding and Work

Prenatal Planning and Preparation

Just as pregnancy is a time of planning that focuses on caring for and feeding a baby, pregnancy is the best time to plan for one's return to employment. Some women have already thought about a plan, often before they become pregnant. Preconception planning, as advocated by Johnson and Esposito (2007), in their review of the literature on barriers and facilitators for breastfeeding among working mothers, suggested healthcare providers use posters, videos, and pamphlets, as well as referral to lactation consultants, to enhance attitudes and commitment to continued breastfeeding after returning to work. Preconception and prenatal planning allows women to sort out existing myths about breastfeeding, especially those saying that combining breastfeeding and employment is difficult and not worth the effort. Thus the healthcare worker who has contact with the employed pregnant woman does her a great service simply by asking how she plans to combine breastfeeding and returning to work. In some cases, the mother's reply to such a question will identify fallacies that need to be corrected and areas of information that need to be shared.

For mothers who are ambivalent or undecided about continued breastfeeding after returning to work, healthcare workers can share information on the benefits of continued breastfeeding in general, and in combination with employment, including: (1) optimal infant health, growth, and development; (2) fewer work absences due to infant illness, lower expenses for infant health care, and increased employee morale (Cohen et al., 1995); (3) lower expenses for infant nutrition; (4) less energy and time spent for purchasing, storing, and preparing formula; (5) feeling more connected and bonded to the baby during the workday when pumping or feelings of enhanced motherliness (Hills-Bonczyk et al., 1993; Rojjanasrirat, 2004; Stevens & Janke, 2003); (6) periodic lactation breaks that restore mother's perspective; and (7) the opportunity to restore feelings of closeness while nursing the baby when back together (Stevens & Janke, 2003).

The healthcare worker should begin by encouraging the pregnant woman, especially the first-time breastfeeding mother, to learn as much as she can about breastfeeding so she can be sure to get off to a smooth start when breastfeeding after returning to work. This includes learning about infant feeding patterns, breast pump alternatives, milk expression and storage, and maintaining the optimal milk supply (Biagioli, 2003; Meek, 2001; Zinn, 2000). Various books, pamphlets, and Web sites may also provide the woman with helpful information (see the Internet resources and other sources of information listed at end of this chapter).

The woman should also talk with women who have combined breastfeeding and employment to learn practical tips. Zinn (2000) suggested that the healthcare practitioner develop a roster of mothers willing to act as listeners and supporters to other mothers wishing to combine breastfeeding and work outside the home. Prenatal breastfeeding classes, especially those with an emphasis on planning for return to work while breastfeeding, can be very helpful and can boost a mother's knowledge and confidence about breastfeeding. Rojjanasrirat (2000) tested a prenatal educational intervention to prepare first-time mothers to combine breastfeeding and employment. The education focused on an individual plan for combining breastfeeding and employment along with involvement of the partner or significant other, and role modeling by employed, breastfeeding women. The researcher found a favorable trend among the experimental group, indicating they breastfed for longer durations than those in the control group.

The healthcare provider can next help the mother to begin planning for breastfeeding when she returns to work. The timing of the return to work should be decided before the baby arrives and in most cases is planned with her family and her employer. The constraints of official maternity leave and family financial needs often determine the timing. However, the longer that a mother can stay at home after birth the better, as demonstrated by research showing a detrimental effect of shorter maternity leave on breastfeeding duration (Arthur, Saenz, & Replogle, 2003; Lindberg, 1996; Piper & Parks, 1996; Roe, Whittington, Fein, & Teisl, 1999).

The employed pregnant woman will want to determine whether her workplace is supportive of breastfeeding so that she can use her work breaks to nurse her baby or to express milk. She must also determine if there is a private and clean space to express her milk and facilities to store it (see Figure 17–1). An open discussion with the employer about the benefits of continued breastfeeding after returning to work—for example, reduced absenteeism (Cohen, Mrtek, & Mrtek, 1995)—may be useful in gaining employer support. There is further discussion about worksite considerations later in this chapter.

The healthcare provider should discuss different work options and the woman's specific plans or goals for breastfeeding while employed. Will she work full-time or part-time? Research indicates that women who work part-time breastfeed longer (Haider, Jacknowitz, & Schoeni, 2003; Hills-Bonczyk, 1993; Lindberg, 1996; Ryan, Zhou, & Acosta, 2002; Ryan, Zhou, & Arensberg, 2006). Therefore, encouraging the woman to work less, if financially possible, is recommended.

Working at Home

Working at home is an option for some mothers, particularly where electronic linking to the job via computer modems, the Internet, and fax machines is possible. Telecommuting offers an opportunity for parents who previously worked elsewhere to continue employment while remaining at home with an infant or young child. It not only enables the new mother to resume an organized way of life, but she also learns that a less structured day that recognizes the baby's needs has its own rewards. However, even these workers will likely need to go

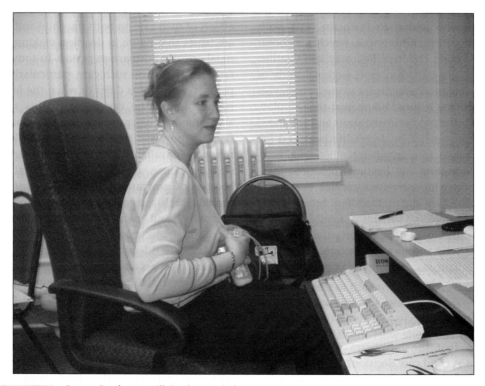

FIGURE **17–1**   Expressing breastmilk in the workplace.

BOX 17–2

General Guidelines for Storing Human Milk

- Always use a clean container.
- Label each container with date and time of the earliest contribution to the container, particularly if "layering" different expressions into the same container. Include baby's name for day care center storage.
- Store milk in the approximate quantities that the baby is likely to need for one feeding.
- If refrigerated within 6 to 8 hours, store in a clean, tightly capped container for the unrefrigerated interim period.
- Milk may be stored in an insulated cooler bag with ice packs for 24 hours.
- If refrigerated, use within 8 days. Store milk in the back of the main body of the refrigerator, where the temperature is the coolest.
- Milk can be stored in a normal refrigerator with other food items. The US Occupational Safety and Health Administration and CDC say human milk does not require special handling or storage in a separate container.
- Freezer compartment located inside the refrigerator (5°F or –15°C): *2 weeks.*
- If frozen in a refrigerator freezer with separate door, use within 3 months.*
- If frozen in a deep-freezer, use within 6 months.*
- Discard any remaining milk that was not used at the feeding for which it was thawed and warmed.
- Use thawed milk within 24 hours.
- Match the "age" of the milk as closely as possible to the baby's age in order to optimize the degree of fit between the baby's needs and the properties of the milk.

---

* Shake while thawing to remix the creamy portion that separates during storage.

should be reminded that human milk is a substance that is matched to the baby's age: milk obtained when the baby was 3 months old will not as completely meet that same baby's needs when he is 6 months old. Therefore she should label the milk with the date expressed and use the milk that was expressed first.

If the mother finds that her milk changes in odor or consistency after storage, or if the baby begins to refuse it, the mother may need to reduce the storage time and freeze rather than refrigerate it in order to avoid possible adverse reactions. Once the milk has been refrigerated or frozen, it should be thawed and warmed to body temperature by placing it under the faucet in a sink and running gradually warmer water over the container. It is inappropriate to thaw milk at room temperature; this practice enables bacteria to multiply in the milk. Neither should it be heated very quickly on a stove or in a microwave oven. Although some research (Carbonare et al., 1996; Ovesen et al., 1996) suggests that microwave heating does not negatively impact immunoglobulins (IgA) and nutrients (vitamins B_1 and E, linoleic and linolenic acids), microwave heating nearly always results in uneven distribution of the heat. This can go unnoticed because the container rarely feels as warm as the center portion of the fluid; thus the milk can be too hot in some spots and substantially cooler in others. Even water-warmed milk should be mixed well and tested on the inside of the caregiver's wrist before offering it to the baby. Mixing should be done not only for heat distribution but also to ensure that the creamy portion of the milk is redistributed.

The fat content of milk is altered with refrigeration as well as when the milk is frozen and then thawed for reuse (Pardou et al., 1994). Loss can be minimized when the container is shaken gently before offering its contents to the baby, and single-serving amounts should be stored to prevent wastage. When giving thawed milk, the unused portion should be discarded to prevent bacterial colonization. Mothers should be told not to refreeze thawed milk. However, small amounts of fresh milk can be added to frozen milk. It is recommended that the fresh milk be refrigerated before adding to the frozen milk.

Fatigue and Loss of Sleep

Sleep deprivation is a fact of life for nearly all parents of very young infants. For women who return to work following childbirth, fatigue and loss of sleep become a bigger concern, and may be compounded in the breastfeeding mother. The relationships between breastfeeding and perceived fatigue have been supported in some studies (McGovern et al., 2006; Pugh & Milligan, 1993; Wambach, 1998), while other studies suggested that perceived fatigue is not dependent on types of feeding (Callahan, Sejourne, & Denis, 2006) and not related to milk volume (Hill et al., 2005). Wambach (1998) examined fatigue levels among first-time breastfeeding mothers over the first 9 weeks postpartum, finding levels were moderate during the first 3 weeks postpartum and then decreased to mild levels at 6 and 9 weeks. It was also demonstrated that women experiencing greater difficulty in combining working and breastfeeding had greater fatigue. A prospective study of 817 working mothers at 5 weeks postpartum revealed that breastfeeding mothers experienced significantly more fatigue than women not breastfeeding (McGovern et al., 2006).

Knowing that fatigue and sleep disturbances may affect breastfeeding can guide healthcare providers and lactation consultants in helping mothers who plan to return to work to manage their own and their infants' sleep patterns. Many employed breastfeeding mothers who work during the day find that their babies' sleep patterns change after their return to work. Instead of taking short naps during the day and sleeping longer at night, the baby begins to sleep for very long periods during the day and remains awake later into the evening. Called "reverse-cycle breastfeeding," this is a coping behavior that enables the baby to tolerate many hours away from his mother. Often, the baby's waking time with his mother may alternate between short breastfeeding episodes and simply nestling in her arms. Such behavior need not mean that the mother loses still more sleep. In fact, what better built-in "excuse" than breastfeeding does a mother have for lying down on the couch when she gets home? Sleep-saving techniques that families have found work well include any one of a variety of cosleeping arrangements:

- Keeping the baby's cradle or crib in the parents' room
- Creating an extension on the parents' bed
- Placing a spare mattress on the floor of the baby's room for late night cuddling and nursing away from other family members (McKenna, Mosho, & Richard, 1997)

Workplace Strategies to Support Breastfeeding and Work

Based on empirical evidence, support for breastfeeding in the workplace requires four essential elements: time, space, person, and policy (Bar-Yam, 1998; Brown, Poag, & Kasprzycki, 2001; Dunn et al., 2004; Ortiz, McGilligan, & Kelley, 2004; Thompson & Bell, 1997). These elements have been included in the definition of support for breastfeeding in the workplace by the CDC (2005) as "several types of employee benefits and services, including writing corporate policies to support breastfeeding women; teaching employees about breastfeeding; providing designated private space for breastfeeding or expressing milk; allowing flexible scheduling to support milk expression during work; giving mothers options for returning to work, such as teleworking, part-time work, and extended maternity leave; providing on-site or near-site child care; providing high-quality breast pumps; and offering professional lactation management services and support" (p. 7). These

Advocacy efforts regarding breastfeeding and employment globally and nationally are abundant. As mentioned earlier in this section the United States Breastfeeding Committee is an overarching group formed to coordinate breastfeeding advocacy activities in the United States. The committee is composed of representatives from health professional associations, breastfeeding support organizations, relevant government departments, and nongovernmental organizations. Approximately 50 member organizations make up the committee and include such notables as the American Academy of Pediatrics; International Lactation Consultant Association; Association of Women's Health, Obstetric, and Neonatal Nurses; the CDC, and Wellstart International. Many of these members have position papers or advocacy programs relative to promoting and supporting breastfeeding and employment. Therefore, strides are being made in the United States, but there is much yet to do in the overall area of protecting and promoting family and maternal interests. In other countries of the world breastfeeding advocacy groups are also prevalent and endorse support and protection of the working mother in her right to breastfeed (see Internet Sources). We turn next to the efforts of the International Labour Organization to support breastfeeding women in the workplace.

International Labour Organization

One of the primary goals of the International Labour Organization (ILO) is to protect the maternity health needs of women workers and their babies and to promote the retention of women in the workforce throughout their childbearing years. The ILO is composed of representatives of governments, workers, and employers, and it is a member of the United Nations. It sets international labor standards through conventions and recommendations. Upon ratification of an ILO convention, its articles are binding on member states through a regulatory mechanism that influences national law and practice. To illustrate this, many African countries have at least 12 weeks of maternity leave, in spite of the fact that only three countries in the region actually ratified the 1952 convention that stipulates 12 weeks as a minimum.

The ILO has issued three conventions related to maternity protection for working women. In 1919,

convention 3 recognized the need to give women workers maternity leave and breastfeeding breaks. In 1952, maternity leave was increased to 12 weeks in convention 103. The latest ILO Maternity Protection Convention 2000 (183) provides for at least 14 weeks of paid maternity leave and the right to one or more breastfeeding breaks daily (see Internet Resources section). The convention also allows for a reduction of working hours, which gives added flexibility in settings where short breaks are not feasible.

The widened scope of convention 183 affects all employed women. Provisions relating specifically to breastfeeding women are health protection at the workplace; paid maternity leave of not less than 14 weeks; 6 weeks of compulsory leave after childbirth; cash benefits at no less than two thirds of previous earnings; and nondiscrimination and employment protection in relation to pregnancy and breastfeeding.

The convention also emphasizes that maternity protection is a social responsibility and that the burden of costs should thus be shared by all of society. Recommendation 191, which accompanies convention 183, further encourages an extension of maternity leave to at least 18 weeks and the adaptation of the frequency and length of nursing breaks to the particular needs of mothers and babies, and promotes the establishment of adequate hygienic facilities at or near the workplace for nursing mothers (see http://www.ilo.org/public/english/employment/skills/hrdr/instr/r_191.htm).

Breastfeeding advocates can make use of several areas within ILO standards where the needs of breastfeeding women are addressed. When national or workplace policies are being created or updated, the ILO works to ensure that, for example, breastfeeding breaks are sufficient in number and frequency and that minimum requirements for a hygienic facility for breastfeeding or expression of milk are met. Flexibility is the key word. In light of the new World Health Organization recommendation of exclusive breastfeeding for 6 months, maternity leave should be long enough to enable working women meet this goal.

Improvements in maternity protection measures for working women can best be achieved by working together with the trade unions and other social partners. Two global trade union bodies—Public Services International (PSI) and the International

Confederation of Free Trade Unions—launched a campaign for ratification of convention 183 in 2001. Campaign materials can be downloaded from the PSI Web site (see Internet Sources at end of chapter). Affiliates of these international bodies can be found in most countries of the world and can be contacted to find out the most appropriate course of action related to ongoing efforts.

Clinical Implications

When providing information about breastfeeding and employment, the lactation consultant (LC) or other healthcare provider is wise to sprinkle such information throughout several discussions of breastfeeding, maintaining a matter-of-fact attitude and establishing a positive expectation that this combination of roles is possible. The LC should discuss breastfeeding with the mother well in advance of her return to work (Bocar, 1997; Meek, 2001; Neifert, 2000). The mother should be encouraged to identify her breastfeeding goals early in pregnancy and be aware of several breastfeeding options available based on the individual work circumstances (see Box 17–3). The combined breastfeeding and work assessment checklist presented earlier in Table 17–1 may be used to assess the important work-related elements so the appropriate planning can be done to fit with a mother's breastfeeding goal.

The role overload of the full-time employed mother necessitates that she learn how to organize her time for maximum efficiency. In breastfeeding, she has found an ideal combination for meeting the physical and psychological needs of her young child. In returning to work, she need not feel that she must shorten the period of lactation that she had planned. Some mothers may choose to breastfeed exclusively whereas some may elect to breastfeed partially and supplement with artificial milk. It is crucial that mothers understand clearly the consequences of each option. Mothers who choose to return to work early and desire to breastfeed exclusively may anticipate pumping frequently to maintain their milk supply.

Other mothers may choose not to express their milk at all. These women will need to know that expressing for comfort, at least during the first week or two, may be necessary if they are to avoid unpredictable, potentially embarrassing leak spots while their body is adjusting to the lack of breast stimulation during the workday. Additionally, these mothers should be encouraged to have someone introduce a bottle or cup of formula to the baby well in advance of her first day at work in case the baby develops an allergic reaction or does not tolerate formula well.

Some mothers will choose to return to work as soon as possible, often because they are financially unable to do otherwise; other women will make every effort to delay returning to work. The type of job that the woman has, the degree of involvement of coworkers and bosses, her relationship with them, her seniority, and a wide array of other factors will influence these decisions. The healthcare worker can provide information about maternal employment and breastfeeding, but only the mother can implement the final plan.

The lactation consultant can share with the mother how other women have coped with similar situations and should answer her questions based on research findings whenever possible. Babies do know when a mother is not available and adapt to her absence by altering sleep patterns. Changes in wakeful and sleepy periods are typical in families in which the mother works at times when the baby has previously been awake a great deal. Increased breastfeeding frequency when the mother is home (reverse-cycle nursing) is a common reaction, particularly in very young babies who breastfeed often. Such a pattern needs to be pointed out to the child care provider; the mother should ask that the provider not wake the baby for feedings. Instead, the provider should let the baby indicate when to be fed during the day. These reverse-cycle nursing episodes do not always increase during the mother's nighttime sleeping hours; rather, they tend to be more frequent during the early daytime hours when she is preparing to leave for work and during the evening hours after she has returned home. Many mothers find that setting the alarm an hour earlier than they plan to be up reminds them to offer the baby the breast before heading for the shower or the kitchen to start the day. If she is encouraged to see this as the baby's touching and social time, the mother is more likely to view such behavior as a sign of the baby's attachment to her.

No "magic bullet" will resolve day care issues. Unlike other countries, in which government

BOX 17–3

Decisions the Employed Breastfeeding Mother Must Make

When to Return to Work

- Work intensity: Women must determine the status or intensity of their employment whether they choose to work part-time or full-time, or to not return to work after childbirth.
- Breastfeeding goals: Breastfeeding goals can be determined by considering factors such as length of maternity leave, breastfeeding intensity (exclusive or partial breastfeeding), work intensity, work circumstances, and amount of support available.

How Long to Breastfeed

- The decision regarding how long to breastfeed depends on a mother's breastfeeding goals and if weaning would occur due to mother-led reasons or baby-led reasons.

How Often to Pump

- The frequency of milk expression or pumping when a mother returns to work depends on the age of the baby and the duration of separation time between the mother and her child.
- The older the baby, the less frequent is the time needed to pump each day.

Generally, mothers should express at least twice within 8 to 10 hours of work to maintain milk supply.

How Much Supplementation to Use

- How much supplementation or breast-milk substitute is used depends on breastfeeding intensity. For mothers who plan to breastfeed exclusively, they should avoid supplementation to prevent decreased milk production.
- Breastmilk substitutes are used for missed breastfeeding when mothers choose to breastfeed partially. The disadvantage of this option is that the mother's milk supply will decline as the baby receives more supplementation.

Child-Care Decisions

- Decisions on using child care services depend on several factors, such as issues of trust, convenience, and finances.
- The options for child care include the following: in the baby's own home, in a neighbor's or friend's home, in the home of someone who provides day care services, or in a day care center.

subsidies enable many mothers to stay home for a substantial period following the birth of their babies, the United States has no federal policy supporting paid maternity leave. At the same time, increasing numbers of families make economic choices that mandate a two-worker household. In addition, day care workers, often because they are so poorly paid, represent a workforce that has a high turnover, inadequate training, and lack of job commitment.

Summary

The role of the healthcare worker is to inform the working mother that she is not alone and that other women have in most cases faced what she is likely to encounter. In some cases, the mothers found partial solutions; in other cases, their solutions enabled them, and will enable others, to proceed with breastfeeding with minimal interruption. Whatever the mother's individual situation, the person providing information needs to do so from a perspective of what has worked for others, recognizing that each mother's situation has unique strengths and pitfalls.

In settings in which institutionalized day care is well organized and carefully supervised, many families' concerns can be set aside. In other day care situations, the increased illness rates and other issues related to meeting the infant's and child's many needs warrant considerable concern. At-home care is both more expensive and more difficult to obtain; in addition, it provides no guarantee that some of the problems that have surfaced in group settings, including child neglect or abuse, will not also occur.

The length of time that a child breastfeeds (even if it is 2 years) represents a very small amount of the total time that the child will live in the parents' home. The length of the mother's employment is likely to last far longer than her child's infancy. The longer the mother is home during the baby's early weeks and months, the shorter the time that breastfeeding is most likely to be negatively affected by that employment.

Key Concepts

- Currently 54 percent of married women return to the labor force while their children are under the age of 1 year.
- More women are choosing to breastfeed, and many will continue to breastfeed after they return to work.
- Research indicates that returning to work does not affect breastfeeding initiation but does adversely affect duration of breastfeeding.
- Working full-time versus part-time affects breastfeeding duration negatively.
- The sooner a mother returns to work, the shorter the duration of breastfeeding.
- The longer a mother stays at home before returning to work, the longer the breastfeeding duration.
- Level of job skill is associated with combining breastfeeding and employment: combined breastfeeding and employment increase as job skills increase.
- Prenatal planning is important to women who choose to combine breastfeeding and employment. Key to planning is learning about breastfeeding and combining it with employment, decisions regarding work options and timing of the return to work, assessing workplace support of breastfeeding, and child care decisions.
- Four elements have been identified as enhancers of breastfeeding in the workplace: time, space, person, and policy.
- Benefits of combined breastfeeding and employment to employers include decreased absenteeism owing to decreased infant illness, which translates into decreased healthcare costs and increased worker productivity.
- There is evidence that lactation support programs in the workplace reduce healthcare costs, absenteeism, and infant illness while increasing breastfeeding duration.
- Breastfeeding problems may depend on the age of the infant and the timing of the return to work.
- Common concerns and issues for women who breastfeed and work outside the home include loss of sleep, fatigue, maintaining an adequate milk supply, and day care issues.
- Decisions regarding exclusive or partial breastfeeding upon returning to work and the baby's age will determine the need and frequency of milk expression.
- There are several factors to consider in breast pump choice including cleanliness, ease of use, comfort, efficiency, and cost.

- Human milk storage guidelines exist to promote safety and are based on research.
- Community resources for the breastfeeding-employed woman include healthcare providers, lactation consultants, La Leche League, breastfeeding support groups, and online information and support.
- Legislative support and public advocacy is increasing to promote and protect women's rights to breastfeed after returning to work.

- The International Labour Organization has been instrumental in protecting maternal rights, including breastfeeding in the workplace, since 1919.

Internet Resources

Breastfeeding position papers
International Lactation Consultant Association:
http://www.ilca.org
American Academy of Family Physicians:
http://www.aafp.org
American Academy of Pediatrics:
http://www.aap.org
Breast pump information
Pumping Moms Information Exchange:
http://www.pumpingmoms.org
Breastfeeding advocacy, consumer information, and discussion forums
Promotion of mothers' milk:
http://www.promom.org
Mother-to-Mother Forum for Working and Breast-feeding Mothers:
http://forums.llli.org/index.php
Breastfeeding Basics—breastfeeding information, questions and answers, and shopping:
http://www.Breastfeedingbasics.com
Medline Plus breastfeeding information for the consumer:
http://www.nlm.nih.gov/medlineplus/breastfeeding.html
The Balancing Act: Breastfeeding and Working, pamphlet on employment and breastfeeding, available from LLLI online store (set of 10 pamphlets $9.50):
http://store.llli.org/public
Transportation Security Administration:
http://www.tsa.dhs.gov/travelers/airtravel/children/formula.shtm
Breastfeeding promotion and support
La Leche League International:
http://www.llli.org

National Women's Health Information Center:
http://www.4women.gov/breastfeeding
Women, Infants, and Children (WIC) Works Resource System:
http://www.nal.usda.gov/wicworks
United States Department of Agriculture National Breastfeeding Promotion Campaign:
http://www.fns.usda.gov/wic/Breastfeeding/lovingsupport.HTM
Breastfeeding and child care
US Department of Agriculture (USDA):
http://www.usda.gov
US Department of Health and Human Services, Maternal and Child Health Bureau (MCHB):
http://www.mchb.hrsa.gov
United States Breastfeeding Committee:
http://www.usbreastfeeding.org
Rhode Island Department of Health. Tips for child care providers:
http://www.health.ri.gov/family/breastfeeding/professionals-guidelines.php
Australian Breastfeeding Association Breastfeeding Workplace Accreditation Program:
http://www.breastfeeding.asn.au/bfinfo/mfwp.html
Other non-USA national initiatives and resources
Breastfeeding Committee of Canada:
http://www.breastfeedingcanada.ca
International Labour Organization:
http://www.ilo.org/global/lang–en/index.htm
Public Services International (PSI):
http://www.world-psi.org/psi.nsf
International Confederation of Free Trade Unions:
http://www.icftu.org

References

Abdulwadud OA, Snow ME. Interventions in the workplace to support breastfeeding for women in employment. *Cochrane Database Syst Rev.* 2007; 18,3:CD006177.

Arthur CR, Saenz RB, Replogle WH. The employment-related breastfeeding decisions of physician mothers. *J MS Med Assoc.* 2003;44:383–387.

Auerbach KG. Employed breastfeeding mothers: problems they encounter. *Birth.* 1984;11:17–20.

Auerbach KG. Assisting the employed breastfeeding mother. *J Nurse Midwifery.* 1984;35:26–34.

Auerbach KG. Sequential and simultaneous breast pumping: a comparison. *Int J Nurs Stud.* 1990b;27:257–265.

Auerbach KG, Guss E. Maternal employment and breastfeeding: a study of 567 women's experiences. *Am J Dis Child.* 1984;138:958–960.

Bar-Yam NB. Workplace lactation support, part 1: a return to work breastfeeding assessment tool. *J Hum Lact.* 1998;14:249–254.

Begun AM, Blair C, Quiram JF. Women's changing roles. Wylie, TX: Information Plus; 1998.

Biagioli F. Returning to work while breastfeeding. *Am Fam Phys.* 2003;68:2199–2206.

Biancuzzo M. Selecting pumps for breastfeeding mothers. *JOGNN.* 1999;28:417–426.

Bocar D. Combining breastfeeding and employment: increasing success. *J Perinat Neonat Nurs.* 1997; 11:23–43.

Bridges CB, Frank DI, Curtin J. Employer attitudes toward breastfeeding in the workplace. *J Hum Lact.* 1997;13:215–219.

Brown CA, Poag S, Kasprzycki C. Exploring large employers' and small employers' knowledge, attitudes, and practices on breastfeeding support in the workplace. *J Hum Lact.* 2001;17:39–46.

Buss IH et al. Vitamin C is reduced in human milk after storage. *Acta Paediatr.* 2001;90:813–815.

Callahan S, Sejourne N, Denis A. Fatigue and breastfeeding: an inevitable partnership? *J Hum Lact.* 2006;22:182–187.

Calnen G. Paid maternity leave and its impact on breastfeeding in the United States: An historic, economic, political and social perspective. *Breastfeeding Med.* 2007;2:34–43.

Carbonare SB et al. Effect of microwave radiation, pasteurization and lyophilization on the ability of human milk to inhibit *Escherichia coli* adherence to Hep-2 cells. *J Diarrhoeal Dis Res.* 1996;14:90–94.

Centers for Disease Control and Prevention (CDC). Support for breastfeeding in the workplace. Department of Human Services. http://www.cdc.gov/breastfeeding/resources/guide.htm. Accessed October 22, 2008.

Centers for Disease Control and Prevention (CDC). Lactation Support Program. Department of Human Services. (2007). http://www.cdc.gov/ nccdphp/dnpa/hwi/toolkits/lactation/index.htm. Accessed October 22, 2008.

Chen YC, Wu YC, Chie WC. Effects of work-related factors on the breastfeeding behavior of working mothers in a Taiwanese semiconductor manufacturer: a cross-sectional survey. *BMC Public Health.* 2006;6:160.

Chezem J, Montgomery P, Fortman T. Maternal feelings after cessation of breastfeeding: influence of factors related to employment and duration. *J Perinat Neonat Nurs.* 1997;11:61–70.

Choplin M. Personal communication. Kansas City, Missouri: February 7, 2003.

Christrup SM. Breastfeeding in the American workplace. *Journal of Gender, Social, Policy, and The Law.* 2001;9:472–503.

Click ER. Developing a worksite lactation program. *MCN.* 2006;31:313–317.

Cohen R, Mrtek MB. The impact of two corporate lactation programs on the incidence and duration of breast-feeding by employed mothers. *Am J Health Prom.* 1994;8:436–441.

Cohen R, Mrtek MB, Mrtek RG. Comparison of maternal absenteeism and infant illness rates among breast-feeding and formula-feeding women in two corporations. *Am J Health Prom.* 1995;10:148–153.

Daly SEJ, Hartmann PE. Infant demand and milk supply: the short-term control of milk synthesis in lactating women. *J Hum Lact.* 1995;11:27–37.

Dodgson JE, Duckett L. Breastfeeding in the workplace: building a support program for nursing mothers. *AAOHN Journal.* 1997;45:290–298.

Dornan BA, Oerman MH. Breastfeeding websites for patient education. *MCN.* 2006;31:18–23.

Dunn BF et al. Breastfeeding practices in Colorado businesses. *J Hum Lact.* 2004;20:170–177.

Eldridge S, Croker A. Breastfeeding friendly workplace accreditation. Creating supportive workplaces for breastfeeding women. *Breastfeed Rev.* 2005;13:17–22.

Fein SB, Roe B. The effect of work status on initiation and duration of breastfeeding. *Am J Pub Health.* 1998;88:1042–1046.

Fetherston C. Risk factors for lactation mastitis. *J Hum Lact.* 1998;14:109.

Galtry J. The impact on breastfeeding of labour market policy and practice in Ireland, Sweden, and the USA. *Soc Sci Med.* 2003;57:167–177.

Gordon RA, Kaestner R, Korenman S. The effects of maternal employment on child injuries and infectious disease. *Demography.* 2007;44:307–333.

Hager WD, Barton JR. Treatment of sporadic acute puerperal mastitis. *Infec Dis Obstet Gyn.* 1996;4:97–101.

Haider SJ, Jacknowitz A, Schoeni RF. Welfare work requirements and child well-being: Evidence from the effects on breast-feeding. *Demography.* 2003; 40:479–497.

Hamosh M et al. Breastfeeding and the working mother: effect of time and temperature of short-term storage on proteolysis, lipolysis, and bacterial growth in milk. *Pediatrics.* 1996;97:492–498.

Hawkins SS et al. Millennium Cohort Study Child Health Group. (2007). Maternal employment and breast-feeding initiation: findings from the Millennium Cohort Study. *Paediatr Perinat Epidemiol.* 2007;21:242–247.

Hills-Bonczyk SG. Women's experiences with combining breastfeeding and employment. *J Nurse Midwifery.* 1993;38:257–266.

Hill et al. Psychological distress and milk volume in lactating mothers. *West J Nurse Res.* 2005;27:676–693.

International Labour Office. Global employment trends for women brief, March 2007. http://www.ilo.org/trends. Accessed October 1, 2007.

International Labour Organization. ABC of women workers' rights and gender equality. Geneva, Switzerland: ILO Bureau of Publications; 2000.

International Labour Organization. C183 Maternity Protection Convention, 2000. http://www.ilo.org/ilolex/cgi-lex/convde.pl?C183. Accessed October 17, 2007.

International Labour Organization. R191 Maternity Protection Recommendation, 2000. http://www.ilo.org/public/english/employment/skills/hrdr/instr/r_191.htm. Accessed October 17, 2007.

Johnston M, Esposito N. Barriers and facilitators for breastfeeding among working women in the United States. *JOGNN.* 2007;36:9–20.

Kelloway EK, Gottlieb BH. The effect of alternative work arrangements on women's well-being: a demand-control model. *Women's Health: Research on Gender, Behavior, and Policy.* 1998;4:1–18.

Killien M, Habermann B, Jarrett M. Influence of employment characteristics on postpartum mothers' health. *Women's Work, Health, and Quality of Life.* 2001;33:63–81.

Killien MG. Postpartum return to work: mothering stress, anxiety, and gratification. *Can J Nurs Res.* 1998;30(3):53–66.

Killien MG. The role of social support in facilitating postpartum women's return to employment. *JOGNN.* 2005;34:639–646.

Kimbro RT. On-the-job Moms: Work and breastfeeding initiation and duration for a sample of low-income women. *Matern Child Health J.* 2006;10(1):19–26.

Libbus MK, Bullock FC. Breastfeeding and employment: an assessment of employer attitudes. *J Hum Lact.* 2002;18:247–251.

Lindberg LD. Women's decisions about breastfeeding and maternal employment. *J Marr Fam.* 1996;58:239–251.

Linnecar A, Yee V. Maternity legislation: protecting women's rights to breastfeed. WABA Activity Sheet 6.

http://www.waba.org.my/resources/activitysheet/acsh6.htm. Accessed October 22, 2008.

Marshall R, Paulin B. Employment and earnings of women: historical perspective. In: Koziara KS, Moskow MH, Tanner LD, eds. *Working Women: Past, Present, Future.* Washington, DC: Bureau of National Affairs; 1987.

McGovern P et al. Postpartum health of employed mothers 5 weeks after childbirth. *Ann Fam Med.* 2006;4:159–167.

McKenna J, Mosho S, Richard C. Bedsharing promoted breastfeeding. *Pediatrics.* 1997;100:214–219.

Meek J. Breastfeeding in the workplace. *Ped Clin N A.* 2001;48:461–474.

Neifert M. *Dr. Mom's Guide to Breastfeeding.* New York, NY: Penguin Putnam; 1998.

Neifert M. Supporting breastfeeding mothers as they return to work. *American Academy of Pediatrics Newsletter,* 2000. http://www.aap.org/healthtopics/breastfeeding.cfm. Accessed October 10, 2007.

Nichols MR, Roux GM. Maternal perspectives on postpartum return to the workplace. *JOGNN.* 2004;33:463–471.

Noble S, ALSPAC Study Team. Maternal employment and the initiation of breastfeeding. *Acta Paediatr.* 2001;90:423–428.

Ogundele MO. Techniques for the storage of human breastmilk: implications for antimicrobial functions and safety of stored milk. *Eur J Pediatr.* 2000;159:793–797.

Ong G et al. Impact of working status on breastfeeding in Singapore. *Eur J Pub Health.* 2005;15:434–430.

Ortiz et al. Duration of breast milk expression among working mothers enrolled in an employer-sponsored lactation program. *Pediatr Nurs.* 2004;30:111–119.

Ovesen L et al. The effect of microwave heating on vitamins B_1 and E, and linoleic and linolenic acids, and immuno-globulins in human milk. *Int J Food Sci Nutr.* 1996;47:427–436.

Pardou et al. Human milk banking: influence of storage processes and of bacterial contamination on some milk constituents. *Biol Neonate.* 1994;65:302–309.

Piper S, Parks PL. Predicting the duration of lactation: evidence from a national survey. *Birth.* 1996;23:7–12.

Potter B. Women's experiences of managing mastitis. *Comm Pract.* 1995;78:209–212.

Prevention Institute. Breastfeeding. http://www.preventioninstitute.org/pdf/CHI_breastfeeding.pdf. Accessed September 22, 2007.

Pugh L, Milligan R. A framework for the study of childbearing fatigue. *Adv Nurs Sci.* 1993;15:60–70.

Rea MF et al. Factors which facilitate and constrain breastfeeding among women working in factories in Sao Paulo, Brazil. *J Hum Lact.* 1999;13:233–239.

Riccitiello R. Corporate efforts: what some companies are doing to accommodate nursing moms.

http://www.breastfeeding.com/reading_room/corporate.html. Accessed October 27, 2007.

Roe B et al. Is there competition between breast-feeding and maternal employment? *Demography.* 1999; 36:157–171.

Rojjanasrirat W. *The Effects of a Nursing Intervention on Breastfeeding Duration Among Primiparous Mothers Planning to Return to Work* [dissertation]. University of Kansas; 2000.

Rojjanasrirat W. Working women's breastfeeding experiences. *MCN.* 2004;29:222–227.

Ryan AS, Zhou W, Acosta A. Breastfeeding continues to increase into the new millennium. *Pediatrics.* 2002;110:1103–1109.

Ryan AS, Zhou W, Arensberg MB. The effect of employment status on breastfeeding in the United States. *Women's Health Iss.* 2006;16:243–251.

Scott JA et al. Predictors of breastfeeding duration: evidence from a cohort study. *Pediatrics.* 2006; 117:646–655.

Slusser WM et al. Breast milk expression in the workplace: a look at frequency and time. *J Hum Lact.* 2004;20:164–169.

Smith K, Downs B, O'Connell M. Maternity leave and employment patterns: 1961–1995, U.S. Census Bureau, Current Population Reports, Washington, DC, 2001.

Stevens KV, Janke J. Breastfeeding experiences of active duty military women. *Mil Med.* 2003; 168:380–384.

Thompsen AC, Espersen T, Maigaard S. Course and treatment of milk stasis, noninfectious inflammation of the breast, and infectious mastitis in nursing women. *Am J Obstet Gynecol.* 1984;149:492–495.

Thompson PE, Bell P. Breast-feeding in the workplace: how to succeed. *Iss Comp Pediatr Nurs.* 1997; 20:1–9.

Tully MR. Recommendations for handling of mother's own milk. *J Hum Lact.* 2000;16:149–151.

United States Breastfeeding Committee. *Breastfeeding and child care* [issue paper]. Raleigh, NC: United States Breastfeeding Committee; 2002.

US Bureau of Labor Statistics. Employment characteristics of families in 2007. http://www.bls.gov/cps/demographics.htm#families. Accessed October 22, 2008.

US Census Bureau. Statistics of United States Businesses: 2004. http://www.census.gov/epcd/susb/2004/mo/MO–.HTM. Accessed October 22, 2008.

US Census Bureau. Who's minding the kids? Child care arrangements: winter 2002. http://www.census.gov/prod/2005pubs/p70-101.pdf. Accessed October 22, 2008.

US Department of Health and Human Services. *HHS Blueprint for Action on Breastfeeding.* Washington, DC: US Department of Health and Human Services, Office on Women's Health; 2000.

US Department of Labor. Employment characteristics of family summary. Washington, DC. http://www.bls.gov/news.release/famee.nr0.htm. Accessed October 22, 2008.

Vanek EP, Vanek JA. Job sharing as an employment alternative in group medical practice. *Med Group Manage J.* 2001;48:24–40.

Visness CM, Kennedy KI. Maternal employment and breast-feeding: findings from the 1988 National Maternal and Infant Health Survey. *Am J Public Health.* 1997;87:945–950.

Waldfogel J. Family and medical leave: evidence from the 2000 surveys. *Monthly Lab Rev.* 2001;124:17–23.

Wambach K. Maternal fatigue in breastfeeding primiparae during the first nine weeks postpartum. *J Hum Lact.* 1998;14:219–229.

Whaley SE et al. Predictors of breastfeeding duration for employees of the Special Supplemental Nutrition Program for Women, Infants, and Children (WIC). *J Amer Diet Assoc.* 2002;102:1290–1293.

Win NN et al. Breastfeeding duration in mothers who express breast milk: a cohort study. *Int Breastfeeding J.* 2006;1:28.

Witters-Green R. Increasing breastfeeding rates in working mothers. *Fam Sys Health.* 2003;21:415–434.

World Alliance for Breastfeeding Action (WABA). Status of maternity protection by country. http://www.waba.org.my/womenwork/MaternityProtectionChart21May2006.pdf. Accessed October 17, 2007.

Wyatt SN. Challenges of the working breastfeeding mother: workplace solutions. *AAOHN J.* 2002; 50:61–66.

Yimyam S. Breastfeeding, work, and women's health among Thai women in Chiang Mai. *Breastfeed Rev.* 1998;6:17–22.

Yimyam S, Morrow M. Breastfeeding practices among employed Thai women in Chiang Mai. *J Hum Lact.* 1999;15:225–232.

Zinn B. Supporting the employed breastfeeding mother. *J Midwifery Women's Health.* 2000;45:216–226.

TABLE 18–1	Studies on Breastfeeding and Children's Intelligence, Development and Motor Skills	
Source	**Method**	**Findings**
Singhal et al., 2007 (United States)	262 children aged 4 to 6 years; breastfeeding benefits on stereoscopic vision maturation and dietary intake of docosahexaenoic acid (DHA). Children assigned either DHA or arachidonic acid (n = 94) or control formula (n = 90) for 6 months. Random dot E test and Sonksen-Silver acuity system used to assess visual responses.	Breastfed children had significantly greater likelihood of foveal stereoacuity ($P = .001$), independent of partial confounding ($P = .005$). Stereoacuity did not differ significantly between children who received DHA supplemented or control formula. Results suggest factors other than DHA in breastmilk account for benefits.
Julvez et al., 2007 (Norway)	Behavioral areas, as related to long term breastfeeding were assessed on 4 year olds, from Menorca (N = 420) and Spain (N = 79). Children assessed for neuropsychological function (McCarthy test), attention-hyperactivity behavior (ADHA Criteria of DSM-IV) and social behavior (California Preschool Competence Scale).	Long-term breast feeding (< 12 and 20 weeks) associated with fewer attention and hyperactivity symptoms, and improvement in neuropsychological and sociobehavioral outcomes. Outcomes remained significant when included as covariates in the regression models.
Martin et al., 2007 (United Kingdom)	Cohort study with a 60 year follow-up of 1414 participants from England and Scotland, assessing breastfeeding with social class mobility.	Participants who breastfed were 41% more likely to move up social class in adulthood ($P = .007$) than bottle-fed infants. Longer breastfeeding duration associated with upward mobility.
Eickmann et al., 2007 (Brazil)	191 infants from low-income population, tested at 12 months, using Bayley Scales of Infant Development II. Controlled for covariates.	Full breastfeeding at 1 month associated with small but significant benefits in mental development (+3.0 points, $P = .02$). No association with breastfeeding longer than 1 month or benefits in motor development.
Vohr et al., 2006 (United States)	1035 extremely low birth weight infants assessed at 18 months, corrected age with three tests: Bayley Mental and Development Indexes and Behavioral Rating Scale	Infants with highest ingestion of breastmilk in NICU scored higher on Bayley tests than infants with lower or no breastmilk intake. For each 10 ml/kg/day breastmilk increase, score points increased: Development by 0.53, Psychomotor by 0.63, Behavioral by 0.82. A 5-point (1/2 SD) increase in IQ suggests long-term benefits of breastfeeding for extremely low birth weight infants.

(Continues)

TABLE 18-1	Studies on Breastfeeding and Children's Intelligence, Development and Motor Skills (Continued)

Source	Method	Findings
Hart et al., 2006 (United States)	Effect of natural docosahexaenoic acid (DHA) levels in breastmilk on neurobehavioral outcomes in newborn infants. Breastmilk from N = 20 mothers collected 9 days postpartum. Tested with Brazelton Neonatal Behavioral Assessment Scale (NBAS).	Pearson correlations revealed positive association between DHA concentrations in breastmilk and infant scores on NBAS. State cluster scores, suggest breastmilk DHA beneficial to neonatal neurobehavioral functioning.
Sacker et al., 2006 (United Kingdom)	Cohort study of 14,660 term singleton infants who weighed > 2500 g at birth.	Infants never breastfed 50% more likely to have gross motor coordination delays than infants who had been breastfed exclusively for 4 months and 40% more likely to have fine motor delays than infants who were breastfed for a prolonged period.
Slykerman et al., 2005 (New Zealand)	550 European children, half small for gestational age (SGA), and half appropriate for gestational age (AGA). IQ assessed at 3.5 years, using Stanford Binet Intelligence Scale, breastfeeding duration assessed by maternal interviews.	SGA children breastfed longer than 12 months had adjusted IQ scores 6.0 points higher ($P = .06$) than nonbreastfed infants. Breastfeeding not significantly related to IQ scores for the total SGA and AGA sample.
Daniels et al., 2005 (Philippines)	Normal birth weight (NBW, n = 1790) and low birth weight (LBW, n = 189 < 2500 g) infants, born close to term, in Philippines, 1983–1984. Cognitive ability assessed at ages 8.5 and 11.5 years with Nonverbal Intelligence Test.	Scores at 8.5 years higher for infants breastfed longer (12 to < 18 months vs < 6 months): NBW (1.6 points), and LBW (9.8 points). Findings indicate importance of both predominant and long-term partial breastfeeding in LBW infants, born close to term.
Rao et al., 2002 (Norway, Sweden)	529 full-term small for gestational age (SGA) and normal weight Norwegian and Swedish infants followed up to 5 years. Norwegian Weschler Intelligence-Revised and Raven Progressive Matrices used to measure IQ.	Total IQ increased linearly with duration of exclusive breastfeeding for durations over 12 weeks giving an 11-point advantage in total IQ for SGA children exclusively breastfed for 24 weeks compared to those exclusively breastfed for 12 weeks.
Wigg et al., 1998 (Australia)	Cognitive assessments on 375 children at 2, 4, 7, and 11 to 13 years. Bayley Mental Development and Wechsler Full-Scale IQ.	Small, nonsignificant effect of breastfeeding on scores. Breastfed children had higher scores on Bayley Mental Development at ages 2 and 4, and higher IQ at ages 7 and 11.

(Continues)

TABLE 18–1	Studies on Breastfeeding and Children's Intelligence, Development and Motor Skills (Continued)	
Source	**Method**	**Findings**
Johnson et al., 1996 (United States)	204 children measured at age 3. Stanford-Binet, Hollingshead Index of Social Status used; controlled for socioeconomic status, mother's intelligence, smoking, gender and birth order.	Initiation of breastfeeding predicted scores on intelligence tests at age 3. Breastfeeding associated with 4.6 higher mean in intelligence.
Floury, Leech, & Blackhall, 1995 (United Kingdom)	592 first-born infants; Bayley Scales of Infant Development used.	Higher mental development (3.7–5.7 points) significantly related to breastfeeding at 2 weeks after discharge after control for social and demographic factors. No differences for psychomotor development or behavior.
Temboury et al., 1994 (Spain)	364 healthy infants measured between 18 and 29 months of age. Bayley Scales of Infant Development used; controlled for maternal and infant variables.	Low results on the Index of Mental Development associated with bottle-fed infants, lower-middle and lower social class, mother education, temper tantrums, and having siblings.
Rogan & Gladen, 1993 (United States)	855 newborns; Bayley Scales of Infant Development and McCarthy Scale used; prospective case control.	Statistically significant but small increases in scores among breastfed children on cognitive skills, not motor skills. Slightly higher English grades on report cards after adjusting for confounding variables.
Lucas et al., 1992 (United Kingdom)	926 low birth weight infants tube-fed with human milk or formula. Measured at 8.5 years of age; Weschler Intelligence Scale for Children used; randomized trial of feeding mode; controlled for maternal contact, social class, education.	Dose-response relationship between proportion of breastmilk and IQ. Breastfed children scored 8.3 points higher.
Morley et al., 1988 (United Kingdom)	771 low birth weight infants; Bayley Mental Scale and Developmental Profile 11 used; measured at 18 months postterm; randomized controlled trial of feeding mode.	Breastfed children had significant 4.3 point advantage on the Bayley Mental Developmental Index over the children who received only formula. ($P < .005$).

have demonstrated improved visual and mental development in infants receiving a formula supplemented with DHA (Birch et al., 2000; Singhal et al., 2007).

Another possible reason for enhanced cognitive function of breastfed children is the high concentration of sialic acid in breastmilk. Maturation of the brain is associated with total sialic concentration.

Breastfed infants have higher brain sialic acid levels than do formula-fed infants because human milk is a rich source of sialic acid containing oligosaccharides, while formula contains very little (Wang et al., 1998).

Growth and Development

Physical Growth

Infant and child growth is affected by genetic makeup, general health, and nutrition. Infants and children vary in their tempo of growth and development, which tends to be marked by spurts of growth separated by plateaus. Still, there are universal patterns of growth for all children. These universal patterns include cephalocaudal growth (growth that proceeds from head to foot), proximodistal growth (growth that occurs from the center outward), and general-to-specific movements. The infant's head accounts for about one fourth of the infant's length at birth and illustrates cephalocaudal direction of growth. Maturation of motor skills also follows the cephalocaudal pattern: an infant masters control of his head before he masters arm and trunk control, which is followed by leg control (Figure 18–1).

Proximodistal and general-to-specific development is illustrated by the sequence of muscle control: infants control large muscles before they control small muscles. For example, the child is able to wave "bye-bye" before he is able to grasp with his whole hand and before he is able to hold a small object with his thumb and forefinger (pincer grasp). There is some evidence that breastfeeding has a beneficial effect on neurological development in children. Lanting et al. (1994) found a small advantageous effect of breastfeeding on the neurological status of children 9 years of age.

Weight and Length

Change, rather than stability, is the hallmark of infancy; weight increases faster in infancy than at any other time of life. The average neonate weighs about 3000 to 4000 gm (6.5–8.5 lb). Because full-term infants are born with excess fluid, they lose 5 to 10 percent of their birth weight following birth and then stabilize within a few days. Generally speaking, infants double their birth weight by about

5 months of age, triple it by 1 year of age, and quadruple it by 2 years of age.

As discussed earlier in this book, weight patterns of formula-fed infants differ from those of infants who are fed exclusively at the breast. Their weights are similar for the first few months, but at 3 to 4 months, formula-fed infants begin to weigh more than do their breastfed counterparts. This appears to hold cross culturally: formula-fed Japanese babies 6 to 8 months old weigh significantly more (135 gm) than do those breastfed (Yoneyama, Nagata, & Asano, 1994). As discussed in Chapter 4, North American breastfed babies gain an average of 35 gm (approximately 1 oz) per day at 1 month and 19 gm (0.6 oz) per day at 4 months, whereas formula-fed infants gain an average of 34.4 gm per day at 1 month and 23 gm per day at 4 months. Despite their slightly slower weight gain, breastfed infants at 4 months have more body fat (Butte et al., 1995).

Length at birth is about 50 to 53 cm (20–21 in) and, on the average, male infants tend to be 5 oz heavier and 0.5 inches longer than females. A baby grows about 1 inch each month for the first 6 months and about 0.5 inches per month for the next 6 months. By the infant's first birthday, his length has increased by 50 percent. Length and head-circumference growth are similar for both breastfed and formula-fed infants (Butte et al., 1990). The weight of the baby's brain increases most rapidly during infancy as nerve cells enlarge, become longer and branched, and gain myelin sheathing. By 18 months of age, the infant's brain is 75 percent of its adult weight. If the infant becomes malnourished, the first growth factor to be affected is weight. Only when malnourishment is severe and long-standing are the infant's length or head circumference compromised.

In 2006 the World Health Organization (WHO) released new International Child Growth Standards, based on research begun in 1997 on over 8,000 children in six countries: Brazil, Ghana, India, Norway, Oman, and the United States. The new growth charts are based on breastfed infants, exclusively breastfed for 6 months, with the addition of complementary foods after 6 months, in addition to continuing breast-feeding. A detailed description of new WHO standards and growth charts can be found in Chapter 10 and online at http://www.who.int/nutrition/edia_page/en

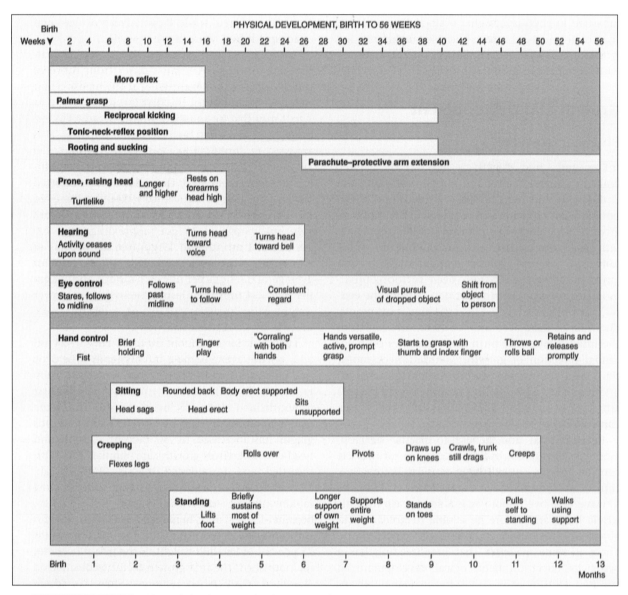

FIGURE 18–1 Physical development, birth to 56 weeks.

and http://www.who.int/childhoodgrowth/standards/chart_catalogue/en/index.html.

Senses

Neonates and young infants have remarkably well-developed sensory capabilities. At birth, the infant's auditory nerve tracts have sufficient myelin sheathing to allow them to hear well; they can differentiate various tastes and smells. This ability to selectively respond through their senses enhances the infant's early attempts to locate and attach to the nipple and to distinguish between his own mother and other individuals.

Within several days after birth, breastfeeding infants respond preferentially to breast or axillary odors from their mother. In striking contrast, bottle-feeders display no evidence of recognizing axillary odors from their mothers. While feeding at the breast, the neonate's nostrils are in close proximity with the mother's bare skin, which provides the opportunity to become familiar with her characteristic odor (Makin & Porter, 1989).

As early as 2 months before birth, hearing develops in the womb. The fetus is already responding to both internal sounds from the mother and to noises outside the mother. Some young infants, for instance, appear to recognize their mother's favorite soap opera when it comes on television. Neonates discriminate between differences in pitch and can detect the direction of the source of sound.

Loud, low sounds are likely to disturb and alarm the infant, whereas soft, high-pitched sounds have a calming effect; therefore, the higher-range tones of the female voice tend to quiet and focus the baby's attention. When one baby starts crying in a nursery, others will do the same. Newborns respond to sound by differentiating the caregiver's voice from that of strangers. They also sense heat, cold, pressure, and pain.

The neonate's vision is less developed because retinal structures and the optic nerve are not yet complete. A neonate focuses mainly on large objects close to his face and sees best at a range of 8 to 12 inches, with 9 inches as the optimum—just about the distance between the baby's face and the mother's face while the baby is being held at the breast level. Neonates are able to follow and track a moving object with their eyes and prefer moving objects to stationary ones.

Babies seem to have an innate visual preference. They prefer more complex stimuli, such as the human face, to a plain surface and will look at a face longer than at other visual patterns. All infants have dark, smoky eyes at birth. Their lids are puffy, and the tear ducts do not function. Eye muscles may occasionally drift to a crossed position.

Reflexes

The fragile appearance of neonates belies the sophistication of their reflexes, which are designed to enhance survival. Reflexes protect the infant and give the central nervous system and brain time to mature and to begin to govern coordinated behaviors (see Chapter 19).

Rooting, suckling, swallowing, and gag reflexes are directly applicable to breastfeeding. The rooting reflex initiates the act of suckling milk from the mother's breast and is considered vital to life. The suck-swallow reflex is presumably developed at 34 weeks of gestation. Synchronized coordination of suckling and swallowing with breathing appears to be achieved consistently by infants of more than 37 weeks postconception age (Bu'Loc, Woolridge, & Baum, 1990), but as discussed in Chapter 13 on prematures, many low birth weight infants can suckle at the breast. By 3 to 4 months after birth, the rooting reflex begins to diminish. In Chapter 3, we described the infant's oral and suckling capabilities as the cockpit of the nervous system. The presence of rooting, sucking, swallowing, and gag reflexes are barometers that indicate an intact, functioning central nervous system.

Levels of Arousal

Young infant behavior can be described by several levels of arousal states (Gill et al., 1988; Prechtl & Beintema, 1975). The Anderson Behavioral State Scale (Gill et al., 1988) lists 15 categories, with states ranging from very quiet sleep to hard crying (Box 18–1). The infant's most complex interaction with his environment is made in the quiet awake state; at this time, the neonate fixates on and follows objects and turns his head toward any sound. The neonate becomes more alert when he senses a new stimulus; if it is repeated, the infant responds less or habituates to the stimulus (Als & Brazelton, 1981). This decrement in response allows the neonate to control his behavioral state. Overactive infants are said to lack this ability to habituate (respond less to repeated stimuli).

Theories of Development

Nature Versus Nurture

Which is more important in a child's development, nature (genes, heredity) or nurture (environment)? At one end of the spectrum, how a child develops is thought to be determined at conception; at the other end, development is seen as a product of the environment. Although we can demonstrate that breastfeeding appears to optimize development, the issue is still complex. For example, are the overall

BOX **18–1**

Anderson Behavioral State Scale: Behavioral States

Sleep
Very quiet sleep
Quiet sleep
Restless sleep
Very restless sleep
Quiet awake
Awake
Drowsy
Alert inactivity

Restless
Restless awake
Very restless awake
Fussing
Crying
Hard crying

Source: Adapted from Gill et al., 1988.

parenting patterns of a woman who chooses to breastfeed different from those of a woman who chooses to bottle-feed? We cannot say that any one aspect of child development is determined exclusively by either nature or nurture; clearly each plays a role. The extent of influences from nature versus nurture differ among developmental theorists. How these two issues interact are addressed in two classic theories about child development.

Erikson's Psychosocial Theory

Eric Erikson (1963, 1968) identified stages of development that center around conflicts. These conflicts are central issues of crucial importance to the personality at each stage of life. Characteristics of the first two stages (infant and toddler) of Erikson's theory are shown in Table 18–2. Each stage requires resolution of its particular conflict, and each stage widens the social radius of the infant's influence. The first conflict is trust versus mistrust. According to Erikson, the first year is when confidence in having one's needs met and feeling physically safe results in the infant's either trusting or mistrusting his environment.

Once trust, as opposed to mistrust, is established, the toddler moves into the next stage, in which autonomy must be mastered over shame and doubt. By then (18 months to 3 years of age), he walks, runs,

and expresses himself verbally, eagerly exploring his exciting new world but still needing reassurance and returning to his mother for "emotional refueling." If an infant is lovingly fed and his biological needs are cared for, he develops a sense of trust in the world. Being left hungry or crying for long periods results in a sense of mistrust of the world. Breastfeeding for nourishment becomes breastfeeding for reassurance and comfort in this stage. The process of individuation, a realization that he is a separate individual, unfolds gradually as the child begins to assert control over his life.

Piaget's Cognitive Theory

Jean Piaget (1952) identified the major periods through which humans pass in the course of intellectual maturation. The first is the sensorimotor stage, in which an infant's knowledge of the world comes primarily through his sensory experiences and motor activities. Its main features are presented in Table 18–3.

As infants experience sensory and motor activities, they construct schemas (concepts or models) for dealing with information and experiences. These schemas are put into play through complementary processes of assimilation and accommodation. Assimilation refers to the process of absorbing new information from the environment and using current structures to deal with

TABLE 18–2	**Theories of Development**	
Theorist	**Infant**	**Toddler**
Erikson (psychosexual)	Trust versus mistrust (birth–1 year)	Autonomy versus shame and doubt (1–3 year)
	Requires basic needs (food, comfort, warmth) to be met	Increasing independence in eating, dressing, toileting, and bathing
	Learns to trust self (and environment)	Father becomes important
	Mutual giving and getting between self and caregivers	Limits (firm and consistent) lead to security
	Mistrust results if needs not met consistently or inadequately	Acquires "will"; feeling of self-control, bias for self-esteem
Piaget (cognitive)		Excessive criticism and expectation of perfection leads to shame and doubt about ability to control self and world
	Sensorimotor (birth–2 years); uses senses, motor skills, reflexes to explore	Proconceptual (2–7 years)
	Object permanence	Self-centered; other centeredness begins
	Trial and error	Perception from own point of view
	"Insight" problem solving	Use of symbols, especially language
	Able to think before acting (18–24 months)	Literal interpretation of works and action
		Judges thing for outcome, consequence to self
		Transductive reasoning

Source: Adapted from Erikson, 1963; Piaget & Inhelder, 1969.

the information. Accommodation refers to the process by which the infant alters his behavior and adjusts existing schemas to the requirements of objects or events to integrate new learning with old (and thus adapt to his ever-expanding environments). For example, if a child is breastfed, and a pacifier is given to him, the pacifier nipple may be sufficiently different so that the old sucking patterns do not work well. When this happens, disequilibrium occurs, and the child must restructure the existing view of suckling so that it fits with the new information or experience.

This process is called *accommodation*. Through these processes, schemas are developed and refined.

The concept of object permanence is a feature of the sensorimotor period. Piaget (1952) suggested that the infant younger than 6 to 9 months of age lacks the ability for mental representation of the unseen. For instance, when an object such as a toy is out of sight, it ceases to exist, and the infant does not search for it. With the ability for mental representation, the infant realizes that an object or person continues to exist when out of sight, and he searches for a hidden object.

Characteristics of Infants' Thinking: Sensorimotor State

TABLE
18–3

Major Task

Conquest of Object
Throughout this stage, infants are unable to think. Intelligence proceeds from directly acting, as a whole, on the environment to more goal-directed attending to and action on particular objects to make specific events occur. All the senses and motor skills are actively used to define and interpret objects and events.

Perception

- *Birth–3 months:* View of world and self undifferentiated; unconscious of self.
- *4–6 months:* View of world centered around body: self-centered.
- *After 6 months:* View of world as centered around objects.
- *6–12 months:* Self seen as separated from objects.
- *12–18 months:* Objects seen to have constancy and permanence.
- *18–24 months:* Represents spatial relationships between objects and between objects and self (e.g., knows smaller things fit inside larger things).

Thought

- *Birth–3 months:* Not present. Uses inborn reflexes and senses.
- *4–6 months:* Questions presence of thought. Uses combination of reflexes and senses purposively. Develops habits.
- *6–12 months:* Knows objects by how he or she uses them. Knows objects have constant size before knows objects have same form; serially acts out two previously separate behaviors in goal-directed sequences.
- *12–24 months:* Object permanence stimulates purposive, intentional use of behaviors to find hidden objects and to cause event via trial and error—problem solve via "insight": can now see effect when given the cause (e.g., knows where train will come out when it goes into tunnel). Symbolism

and memory begin—uses deferred imitation to discover new ways of acting (e.g., when "pretends" sleep means "know" symbolic sleeping).

Reasoning

- *Birth–6 months:* Not present.
- *6–24 months:* Syncretism (1) perceives "whole"—impression without analysis of parts or synthesis of relations, (2) lacks systematic exploratory behavior until end of state, (3) begins to connect series of ideas into a confused whole.

Language

- *Birth–3 months:* Undifferentiated cry. Use of different intensities, patterns, and pitches of cry for different feelings (e.g., pain, hunger, fatigue).
- *6–8 weeks:* Cooing: contented and happy sounds.
- *3–6 months:* Babbling: repeated various sounds for sensation of pleasure. Laughing: when happy or excited.
- *6–12 months:* Spontaneous vocalization: imperfect imitation. Echolalia: conscious imitation of sounds.
- *12–18 months:* Expressive jargon: use of information, rhythms, and pauses to imitate sentence sounds. Holophrases: use of one word to convey meaning. Gestures: substitute for or add meaning to speech.
- *18–24 months:* Telegraphic speech: use of noun and verb to convey many meanings.

Play

- *Birth–6 months:* Exercise play—repetition of actions and sounds for pleasure (e.g., rolling over, babbling).
- *6–12 months:* Exploratory play: pleasure from causing effect and reconfirming skill (e.g., "peek-a-boo," "drop and retrieve," "pat-a-cake").
- *12–24 months:* Deferred imitation—imitates previously observed actions (not reasons for or purposes of actions) from memory (e.g., pretends to be "Daddy" and goes through getting dressed, shaving, then walks outside, and gets in the "car").

Source: Adapted from Servonsky & Opas, 1987, p. 22.

It is now quite certain that person permanency precedes object permanency; an infant does recognize his mother, father, or caretaker long before 8 months and thus experiences loss or anxiety when an all-important person is not present. Later, as the child broadens the ability to recognize a separate existence from his mother, he begins to tolerate brief periods of separation from different caretakers. The ability roughly coincides with diminishing separation anxiety and with Erikson's establishment of trust progressing to the beginnings of autonomy.

Social Development

As infants grow, their periods of waking and socializing lengthen. By 2 to 8 weeks of age, a baby smiles spontaneously to pleasurable stimuli, particularly at human faces. Babies coo and babble to their parents and other fascinated adults who coo and babble back. By 3 months, the infant is interested in his environment and playfully reaches out to grasp objects, including breasts, nipples, noses, and hair. By 6 months of age, the infant reaches out to be picked up, squeals with pleasure at recognition of his mother, and enjoys games such as peek-a-boo.

Language and Communication

Because infants hear well from birth, they are able to discriminate between different intonations and between vowels and consonants. This ability to understand the spoken word is called *passive*, or *receptive*, *language*. The ability to produce meaningful utterances is called *expressive language*. The speech center in the brain borders on the areas of the motor cortex that control both mouth-tongue movement and hand movement. This proximity explains why we tend to express ourselves with both our hands and our mouths. Infants, as well, use many gestures in association with sounds and expressive language. Children consistently acquire language communication in a definable sequence:

- *Crying*—From birth; different rhythms signifying emotions and needs (hunger, anger, pain)
- *Cooing and gooing*—After 2 weeks; a wide variety of meaningless speech sounds (Figure 18–2)
- *Babbling*—3 to 12 months ("mama-mama," "dada-dada")
- *Holophrasing*—12 months; one-word sentences
- *Telegraphic speech*—18 months; subject-verb-object
- *Complete sentences*—2 years

The duration of a baby's crying during the early months of life typically increases until about 6 weeks of age, followed by a gradual decrease until 4 months of age. Infants cry more and are more wakeful during the late afternoon and evening. If the infant is carried during fussy periods, crying and fussing decrease, but the number of feedings and the duration of his sleep do not change (McKenna, Mosko, & Richard, 1997).

Although infants differ in the number of hours of sleep, each baby gets as much sleep as he needs. Newborns sleep an average of 16.5 hours per day; some sleep a total of about 10 hours, others sleep up to 23 hours. Generally, infants fuss and cry before falling asleep. The sleeping pattern of breastfed infants differs from that of formula-fed infants. Breastfed infants wake more often during the night and have shortened sleep patterns (Elias et al., 1986; Mosko et al., 1996, 1997). The expression "He sleeps just like a baby" simply is not true during the first few months of life for any infant. The typical pattern is one of frequent, short periods of sleep interrupted by crying and fussing. This occurs night and day. The so-called infant sleep disorders being diagnosed today are not disorders at all but normal sleep patterns.

Mothers and babies interact with one another using a variety of communications that are visual, vocal, tactile, and postural. Babies coo, goo, and babble whenever they are alert and content. These sounds change from week to week and are elicited by the smiling faces of adults, by voices, or by touch. Any mother who has breastfed knows that feeding at the breast is a prime time for her baby to communicate actively with coos, babbling, and speech sounds as he looks into the eyes of his mother (Figure 18–3). These exquisite sensory interchanges further bond the mother and baby. Epstein (1993) videotaped breastfeeding mothers and their babies during feedings to investigate maternal–infant interactions. These videos were later observed and analyzed.

The interactions between the mother and infants were elaborate and complex, with each breastfeeding dyad interacting with its own individual style. All of the mothers and babies looked at their partners' bodies, not just at their faces, during the breastfeeding session. All of the mothers had happy and affectionate expressions on their faces as they watched their babies, yet the amount of time they maintained the positive expression differed between mothers. Certain babies in the

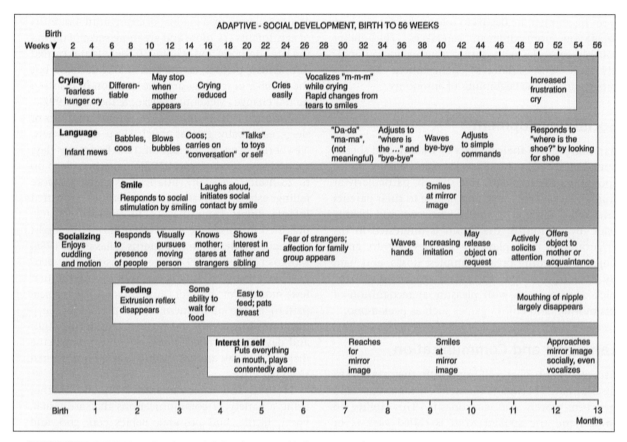

ADAPTIVE - SOCIAL DEVELOPMENT, BIRTH TO 56 WEEKS

Crying Tearless hunger cry	Differentiable	May stop when mother appears

FIGURE 18–2   Adaptive-social development, birth to 56 weeks.

study even smiled and laughed with their mother's nipples in their mouths. Babies and mothers were observed vocalizing to one another. In some dyads, intricate vocal interactions occurred. Babies made sounds that their mothers initiated and this resulted in the babies continuing to make sounds and the mothers continuing to imitate them. In all of these cases, the sounds that the babies made seemed to be expressions of pleasure.

Mothers speak to their infants in a universal dialogue that instinctively uses exaggerated upbeat tones and facial gestures to talk to babies. Mothers use slowly rising crescendo and decrescendo allowing the baby time to process each short vocal package before the next communication arrives. How a mother talks to her baby is more important than what she says.

This sing-song quality of the mother's speech is tailored to the baby's listening abilities. Smiling,

grasping, and talking all play important roles in the attachment process (i.e., the reciprocal development of an affectional tie between the mother or caregiver and the baby) (Pridham & Chang, 1992). During these interactions, the mother not only gives care to

As the mother holds her infant to her breast, assumes the en face position, and talks to her newborn, her eyes are the optimal distance away and her head, mouth, and eyes move slowly and within a closely circumscribed range. Her newborn will also be sending stimuli, such as changes in facial expression, vocalizations, and eye-to-eye contact. The mother's response to such stimuli is immediate.

her infant but the newborn gives care back to his mother. For this reason, Anderson (1977) called the mother and infant "mutual caregivers" (p. 53):

In a review of the theoretical framework for studying factors that affect the maternal role, Mercer (1981) emphasized the role of the infant in his mother's maternal role-taking process. The newborn's ability to see, hear, and track the human face shows socialization capabilities at birth that allow the infant to be an active partner with the mother in the attachment process. Each new infant presents a challenge to maternal adaptation, and previous experience with infants makes little difference to becoming the parent of a new child. Moreover, the transition process of being mother to a new infant is different in the second and third months from the process in the first month (Pridham & Chang, 1992). Breastfeeding plays an important role in a mother's feelings of competence. Tarkka (2003) reported that breastfeeding was a main predictor of a woman's competence as a mother. Competence was measured as the ability to make independent child care decisions, to find pleasure in parenthood, and to meet the demands of being a parent.

The infant uses play as a part of the communication process. During the earliest (sensorimotor) stage of life, infants begin with exercise play, such as repeating newly learned actions for pleasure. Stick out your tongue at a young infant, and he will stick out his tongue at you. Next, infants play in order to explore their skills, crawling backward down the stairs, for example, or pushing a finger into the mother's mouth while breastfeeding and then squealing with glee when she pretends to bite the finger (Figure 18–4). The older baby's playful activities as he breastfeeds are a part of communication and attachment with his mother. Deferred imitation play begins at around 18 months of age, when toddlers begin to imitate the behavior and language they see and hear. For example, little girls, who are already adopting the gender role of their mothers, will very seriously and readily "nurse" their dolls at their breasts (Figure 18–5).

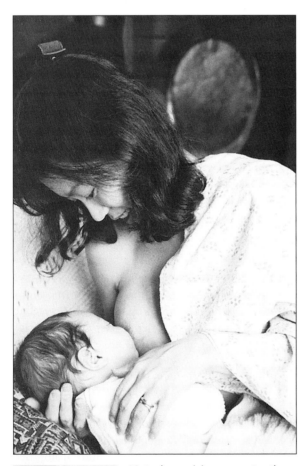

FIGURE **18–3** Mutual caregiving promotes the maternal role-taking process.

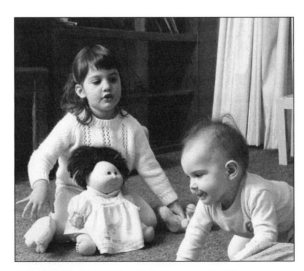

FIGURE **18–4** Developing motor skills by exploring environment.

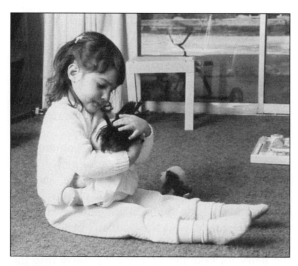

FIGURE 18–5   Child "nursing" doll.

Attachment and Bonding

This exquisite dance of reciprocal reinforcement in the mother–infant dyad leads to the mother's "taking-in" her maternal role, cementing the mother–infant bond. Early theorists paved the way for understanding the processes of bonding and attachment. Konrad Lorenz (1935) noted the behavior and imitation of the mother animal by the young, which is necessary for survival, and labeled it *imprinting*. It is believed that attachment and bonding are the human equivalent of imprinting.

Bowlby's seminal paper (1958), which introduced the principles of attachment theory, emphasized the importance of an infant's developing a primary attachment to a caring, responsible adult. Later, Harlow and Harlow (1965) demonstrated the importance of contact comfort for the attachment and emotional well-being of the newborn rhesus monkey. When presented with "surrogate" mothers—one formed out of unpadded chicken wire and equipped with milk-filled bottles, the other made out of padded terry cloth but without bottles—the baby monkeys spent much more time with the warm, cloth-covered mothers, going only briefly to the bottles for food.

Mothers who room-in with their infants after birth touch their infants' face and head more often than do mothers who have minimal contact with

their newborn (Prodromidis et al., 1995). Rubin (1967) showed a progressive attachment that results from touching: a mother first explores her newborn's extremities with her fingertips, rapidly moves to the baby's arms and legs, and finally caresses the trunk with the palm of her hand. A conceptual model for the maternal-infant bonding might well be like the weaving of a tapestry. Rubin described bonding as:

> *not a cord, nor a bond, nor a welding job, rather a large creative work, framed between the child and the mother's own significant social world, systematically and progressively developed for durability against time and stress to form the substance of her own personal identity and the fabric of her relationship with this particular child.*

Ainsworth et al. (1978) studied brief infant separation from mothers in a laboratory situation to measure the degree of attachment. Mothers defined by the researchers as "securely attached" to their infants were most sensitive to their baby's needs, whereas mothers identified as "insecurely attached" to their infants were less emotionally expressive, felt more aversion to close body contact with the babies, and were more frequently irritated, resentful, and angry. A multitude of circumstances affect the mother–child relationship, which begins before the child is born; even though the baby is unseen, the mother imagines or fantasizes about her child.

The mother's perceptions of the "dream child" and, subsequently, her relationship with that child will not only be influenced by her self-concept but also by her total life experience. Her culture, social relationship, economic status, and state of health can all add to or detract from her relationship with her unborn child. If she experiences social isolation and economic deprivation during her pregnancy, her emotional reserves will be lowered. If she experiences physical discomfort and ill health, her physical stamina may be depleted. Thus the support she receives during pregnancy and from her total environment will affect her acceptance and readiness for mothering.

The infant's birth forces the mother to compare her real-life baby with her dreams, fantasies, and expectations. If reality and expectations are congruent, attachment begins soon after birth; if they are divergent, the mother must first work through the loss of the "dream child" and strive to fall in love with this stranger who bears little resemblance to the child of her fantasies.

Klaus and Kennell (1975) moved the concept of attachment one step further by popularizing the existence of a sensitive period for attachment shortly after birth. Barring excessive medication of the mother during delivery, a newborn will normally be in an alert state for at least 1 hour following birth. During this period, the mother will spend a significant amount of time gazing en face (face to face) into her infant's eyes, touching, and stroking. The neonate is born in a state of readiness for this human interaction. The infant's remarkable perceptual and sensory abilities (hearing, seeing, smelling, and tasting) at birth facilitate the attachment process. As attachment becomes established, the newborn is observed to move his arms and legs in rhythm to the cadences of the mother's voice, in a synchronous pattern that may be the foundation for later speech (Condon & Sander, 1974). Such interaction is known as *entrainment*, and its effects carry over into later life (Figure 18–6).

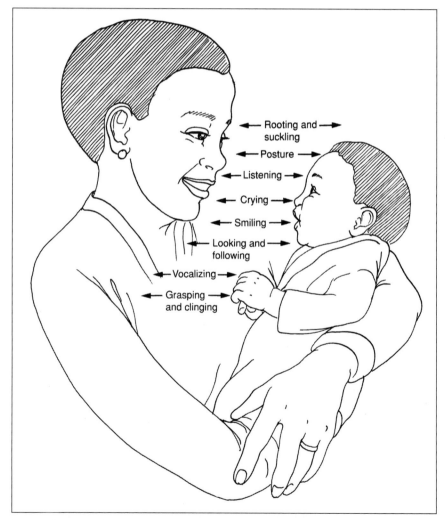

FIGURE 18–6 Components of attachment.

Source: Adapted from Mott S. Nursing care of children and families. Redwood City, CA: Addison-Wesley; 1993:206.

An active partner in the attachment process, the infant initiates about one half of parent–infant interaction. Through predictable and clear-cut transmission of cues or nonverbal signals, neonates are capable of producing the desired behavior in the parent and selectively reinforcing parent behavior. In many ways, the infant is as competent as the parents, perhaps even more so than young, inexperienced parents.

The baby's cry is an impossible-to-ignore cue for attention, and his mother responds by picking up, feeding, or carrying him. The perceptive mother is attuned to her baby's cues and reacts to them appropriately. If he coos and smiles, she reacts happily to his pleasure. The infant's contentment or irritability signal the mother to increase or decrease stimulation. If parents are aware of these cues as a method of communication for their infant, they respond by viewing their infants as individuals. Informing mothers about the behavioral characteristics of their babies is an effective means of enhancing the interaction between mothers and their infants (Anderson, 1981).

Breastfeeding, with its frequent touching, holding, and eye-to-eye contact, offers enhanced opportunities for attachment and responding to infant cues. Certainly, the frequency of subjective verbal responses by mothers who state that they "feel closer" to the breastfed child merits serious consideration. Through breastfeeding, the infant may exert more control: for example, the decision to end the feeding is a shared decision between the mother and baby when the mother "reads" and responds to her baby's behaviors. In bottle-feeding, on the other hand, the mother is chiefly responsible for ending the feeding. Maternal bonding consists of two global aspects: the first is related to preoccupations with infant safety, the second concerns developing a selective and unique bond with the baby. Even mothers of normal healthy babies experience thoughts and worries. Initial separation increases these preoccupations (Feldman et al., 1999).

The common practices today of rooming-in and mother–baby care in maternity care were the result of many studies of maternal–infant attachment and bonding in the 1970s that demonstrated that mother–baby contact was associated with stronger attachment. Now a flurry of research on skin-to-skin touching (kangaroo care) is similarly influencing

this type of care for low birth weight infants (Anderson et al., 2003c). Numerous published reports relating to the safety, efficacy, and feasibility of kangaroo care have associated it with both immediate and long-term effects (Anderson et al., 2003a). In a survey of US neonatal intensive care units, about 80 percent practice some form of kangaroo care in their units (Engler et al., 2002).

Kangaroo care is now commonly practiced in neonatal care units in the United States and worldwide. Case Western Reserve University nurse researchers Gene Cranston Anderson (2001, 2003) and Susan Ludington-Hoe (1996, 2000) have led clinical research teams that study kangaroo care.

The intervention of skin-to-skin contact may be critical for mothers, especially those who have low birth weight babies or are otherwise unable to take their infants home. By promoting skin-to-skin touching, kangaroo care builds the components of bonding and even has been shown to increase the volume of breastmilk production (Hurst, Valentine, & Renfro, 1997). The positive encounter of skin-to-skin provides a bonding experience that helps to offset the mother's experience of loss avoiding bonding failure (Anderson et al., 2003c). Kangaroo care is also discussed in Chapter 13.

Although immediate postpartum mother–child contact is desirable, it is no longer considered critical. Almost all parents are attached to their babies, even if they experience marked disruption of the early parent–child contact, which most healthy mothers and babies now take for granted (see Chapter 9). For example, Hedberg-Nyqvist and Ewald (1997) found that Swedish infants who were separated from their mothers on the first day because they were ill or because of a complicated delivery breastfed for as many months as did those who had immediate contact with their mothers. Parents should be assured that not having the opportunity to interact and bond with their baby soon after birth will not cause irreparable damage to their child.

Temperament

During the past two decades, researchers have studied the temperament of the infant and how it influences parenting. The longitudinal work of Thomas and Chess (1977) suggested that every child exhibits a particular temperament from birth and that (1) infants have individual characteristics even as newborns, (2) these characteristics differentiate infants one from another, and (3) they remain constant over time. Categories of response that influence a child's temperament include activity level, regularity of body functions, adaptability, response to new situations, sensory threshold, intensity of reaction, quality of mood, distractibility, and attention span and persistence. These characteristics were rated for three temperaments: the easy child, the difficult child, and the slow-to-warm-up child. Characteristic temperament styles of each are seen in Table 18–4.

Sears (1987) reduced these three temperament characteristics into two categories in which he identified high-need and low-need babies and popularized the concept for parents to understand and use. High-need babies are fussy, seem to breastfeed "all the time," and cry if put down; low-need babies are content and cuddly and do not need constant carrying or attention. Two questionnaires or tools for assessing the temperament of an infant or child are the Infant Temperament Questionnaire (ITQ) for infants 4 to 12 months of age (Carey & McDevitt, 1978) and the Toddler Temperament Scale for children 1 to 3 years of age (Hegvik, McDevitt, & Carey, 1982). The ITQ scores identify a child's temperamental style; the results may be used as an opportunity for making parents aware of their child's temperament and for suggesting appropriate parenting skills.

Stranger Distress

As the infant grows older, the significance of his major caregiver is recognized and, during the second half of the first year of life, another developmental phenomenon appears: stranger distress. The infant who up to that time has been curious about everything in his environment, including strangers, suddenly frowns and cries and may even attempt physical escape when a stranger approaches. Stranger distress appears quite suddenly as early as 6 months but more commonly at 8 months. It is more pronounced when the mother or primary caretaker is not present. As a consequence, exposure to a variety of strangers is disruptive to an infant at this age. Although stranger distress occurs at about the same period of development as that of separation anxiety, it is a separate phenomenon.

Separation Anxiety

As mother or father leave the room, anxious eyes follow. Almost instantly, the child's face is contorted by rage; he cries loudly and may throw himself wildly about, kicking and screaming. No action brings solace at this point. This behavior is the first phase of separation anxiety, a phenomenon that emerges toward the middle of the first year of life, peaks from 13 to 20 months, and decreases after the second birthday. Separation anxiety, according to psychoanalytic theory, is the painful effect of anxiety engendered by the threat of actual separation from a loved one. Bowlby (1973) and Robertson (1958) delineated three phases of separation anxiety in young children: (1) protest, (2) despair, and (3) denial.

Protest

In an angry and yearning attempt to recover his mother or primary caregiver, the child violently cries and throws himself about, kicking and screaming. He is angry with the world and with his mother for leaving him. He feels that she must be angry with him also, because she left him. The protest phase can last from a few hours to several days, depending on the energy of the child, his age, his relationship with his mother, and the quality of the new environment.

Despair

Gradually, the child moves into quiet grieving and mourning as he begins to accept his fate. He shows little interest in his environment but suffers intensely; his expression is one of great sadness. Regressive behavior, such as thumb sucking, occurs as the child turns inward for solace.

Detachment or Denial

The child develops a defense mechanism to deal with his loss by detaching himself from the importance of his mother's love. He gradually begins to interact with others, approaching anyone and even appearing cheerful. This stage is often misinterpreted as adapting or "settling in." Actually, he is coping with his loss by indiscriminately attaching to caretakers. When he is reunited with his mother at this point, he may appear uninterested and may not seem to recognize her.

| TABLE 18–4 | Characteristics of Temperament Styles in Children | | |

Factor	Easy Child	Slow-to-Warm-Up Child	Difficult Child
Activity level—amount of physical activity during sleep, feeding, play, dressing	High	Medium	Low
Regularity—of body functions in sleep, hunger, bowel movements	Fairly regular	Variable	Fairly irregular
Adaptability to change in routine—ease or difficulty with which initial response can be modified in socially desirable way	Generally adaptable	Variable	Generally slow to adapt
Response to new situations—initial reaction to new stimuli, foods, people, places, toys, or procedures	Approach	Variable	Withdrawal
Level of sensory threshold—amount of external stimulation, such as sounds necessary to or changes in food or people, produce a response	High threshold (much stimulation needed)	Medium threshold	Low threshold (little stimulation needed)
Intensity of response—energy content of responses regardless of their quality	Generally intense	Variable	Generally mild
Positive or negative mood—energy content of responses regardless of their quality	Generally positive	Variable	Generally negative
Distractibility—effectiveness of external stimuli (sounds, toys, people) in interfering with ongoing behavior	Easily distractible	Variable	Nondistractible
Persistence and attention span—duration of maintaining specific activities with or without external obstacles	Persistent	Variable	Nonpersistent
Percentage of all children	40%	15%	10%

Source: Adapted from Carey, 1978; Servonsky & Opas, 1987, p. 180.

Clinical Implications

Deviations from normal patterns of attachment signal that a problem may be present; hence assessing the infant's or child's growth and developmental level—and being able to apply a working knowledge of developmental patterns—is as important as knowing the specifics of a child's health problem. If a baby is being examined, for example, the close proximity of his mother helps to reduce stranger distress. Although clothing that appears "friendly" (nonwhite) helps to ameliorate the baby's distress, by no means does it prevent his crying and avoidance behavior as the examiner approaches him, especially for the first time.

How can healthcare workers who are strangers to the child minimize this fear? First, take advantage of his attachment to his mother by relating to the mother first in the presence of the child. During this interaction with his mother, the child is carefully observing her response to and acceptance of the "stranger" and will take cues from her. Even body position is important; turning slightly sideways away from the child to avoid en face contact while talking with the mother is less threatening to the child. Spitz (1946) demonstrated in one of his films that when a stranger approaches with his back to the child, the child becomes curious and will even reach out after a bit and tug at the stranger. Using a soft, low voice rather than a loud or high-pitched tone is more pleasing to the child and facilitates his acceptance of this new person in his life.

Nursing and medicine have made great progress in recognizing and applying development theories in practice. Because a comprehensive listing and discussion of developmental assessment and screening tools is not within the scope of this book, we refer the reader to the many excellent references that discuss child development in detail. In addition, we remind the reader of the use of assessment tools, such as the Bayley Scales of Infant Development, the Denver Development Screening Test, and the Brazelton Neonatal Behavior Assessment Scale.

Immunizations

Immunizations have greatly reduced the incidence of childhood diseases worldwide. Many infections that contributed to high infant mortality in the past can now be prevented through a series of immunizations. Smallpox, for example, has been eliminated and poliomyelitis, rubella, and rubeola have decreased markedly since the rigorous enforcement of a series of immunizations. Additionally, a number of combination vaccines are available that reduce the number of injections required. The exact timing of the immunizations is not nearly as important as the fact that the child eventually receives all of the immunization doses. The United States Recommended Childhood Immunizations Schedule (2008) is available on the Internet at http://www.cdc/gov/vaccines.

Recommendations for immunizations for young children are the same for breastfed children as for nonbreastfeeding children. In the United States, the recommended age for beginning primary immunizations of infants is at birth, with the hepatitis B (HepB) vaccine prior to hospital discharge, given to all newborns who weigh at least 2 kg (4.4 lbs). The birth dose can only be delayed with physician order and the mother's negative hepatitis surface antigen (HBsAg) documented on the infant's medical record. Only monovalent hepatitis B vaccine can be used for the birth dose. Either monovalent or combination vaccine can be used to complete the series. Infants born to HbsAg-positive mothers should receive the vaccine plus hepatitis B immune globulin (HBIG) within 12 hours after birth, at separate sites. A second dose of HepB vaccine at 1 to 2 months, and a third dose at 6 months, with monovalent vaccine, or a fourth additional dose with combination vaccines, complete the usual series. Infection with hepatitis B has been identified as a major public health problem. In 1992, the American Academy of Pediatrics (AAP) recommended universal immunization of newborns in the United States against HBV. Not everyone agrees with this recommendation, claiming that this decision marks the first time that a vaccine is recommended for children to prevent a disease that primarily occurs in adults.

The primary schedule for DTaP/Hib (diphtheria, tetanus, acellular pertussis) is given at 2, 4, and 6 months of age, with boosters at 15 to 18 months, and DTaP at 4 to 6 years of age. The acellular pertussis has essentially replaced the older pertussis vaccine because it produces fewer side effects. *Haemophilus influenzae* type b vaccine (Hib) is given at 2, 4, and 6 months of age, with a Hib booster at 12 to 18 months

person's risk factors for deficiency (Madhusmitam, Pacaud, Petryk, Collett-Solberg, & Kappy, 2008).

Dental Health and Orofacial Development

The first primary (deciduous) teeth to erupt are the lower central incisors, which appear at about 6 to 8 months of age. By two and a half years of age, children have a full set of primary teeth that will be replaced by permanent teeth. Although breastfeeding helps to protect the teeth, healthy dental practices should in no way be neglected because the child is breastfeeding.

Dental health includes good oral care, cleaning the mouth with soft cloths and soft brushes; fluoride in the water supply, topical fluorides, or tooth sealants/varnishes; and good nutrition. Other factors that lead to poor dental health are iron deficiency, lead exposure, tobacco smoke, sweetened pacifiers, putting babies to bed with a bottle, fruit juices, sodas, sweetened foods, and "sippy" cups. Early childhood caries can be detected by checking the child's teeth for white spots that indicate early caries. Every child should visit the dentist by age 12 months, and have continued dental care (Altshuler, 2006). Xylitol used as a sweetener has been shown to reduce caries. The American Dental Association recommends a level of 0.7–1.2 parts fluoride per million in the water supply and dietary fluoride supplements if needed.

Nursing-bottle caries is a term applied to progressive dental caries aggravated by sucking on a bottle while sleeping and is associated with a high count of lactobacilli in dental plaque, low socioeconomic status, and nutritional deficiencies (Smith & Moffatt, 1998). *Streptococcus mutans* (*S. mutans*) is a major factor in this plaque biofilm on teeth. In developed countries, the prevalence varies between 1 and 12 percent (Milnes, 1996). Decay usually starts with the maxillary (upper) incisors and spares the mandibular (lower) incisors. Several studies suggest that breastfed children have less dental decay than do those who are fed otherwise (Al-Dashti, Williams, & Curzon, 1994; Oulis et al., 1999; Weerheijm et al., 1998; Altshuler, 2006). Probable reasons for this include the mechanical differences between breastfeeding and bottle-feeding. Drawn deep into the child's mouth, the human nipple rests at the junction of the hard and soft palate during breastfeeding, posterior to the child's teeth. A suckle is automatically followed by a swallow, thus preventing the teeth from being bathed in pooled milk. In contrast, the milk from a bottle flows out spontaneously with only the slightest pressure into the anterior part of the mouth, permitting stagnation of the milk on and around the teeth. Brazilian children who were premature and did not breastfeed were at higher risk for developmental enamel defects of primary teeth and tooth decay (Lunardelli and Peres, 2006). A few studies have reported a condition similar to nursing-bottle caries that occurred in breastfed children, especially those who breastfed for 2 to 3 years and have spent long, uninterrupted periods at the breast. Although these cases represent a small percentage of young children who breastfeed, nursing caries is associated with the practice of breastfeeding at night "at will" after 6 months of age (Al-Dashti, Williams, & Curzon, 1994; Matee et al., 1994). A study of 629 Iowa children, ages birth to 4 years (Sptiz et al., 2006) suggests that maternal reports of child temperament may be early indicators of risk factors for caries. Children reported as having "easy" temperaments were more likely to be breastfed throughout the night, while children perceived as "difficult" were more likely to be bottle-fed to sleep. As the numbers of breastfeeding toddlers increase, however, it is reasonable to expect that some of them will develop dental disease, especially after the introduction of solids that often contain sugar.

A lack of methodological consistency in studies on dental caries in breastfed children makes it difficult to draw conclusions. For example, none of the studies reported the dietary habits of the remainder of the children's diet. If a child ingests a sugar-rich food and then breastfeeds, the lips are pressed against the teeth, thus restricting flow of saliva and facilitating caries development (Bowen et al., 1997). As a result, when Valaitis et al. (2000) reviewed 151 articles on caries and breastfeeding, she was unable to come to a conclusion. Erickson (1999) conducted a unique in vitro study on caries development and human milk. She found that when children's teeth were exposed to human milk as the only carbohydrate source, caries did not occur. When breast milk was supplemented with 10 percent sucrose, caries development was rapid.

Dental caries is also thought to be an inherited trait; therefore, these children probably represent a group who are more susceptible, and prolonged nocturnal exposure to human milk becomes a risk factor. It could be argued that some breastfed children develop caries not because they were breastfed but in spite of it. The susceptibility of the child's teeth to decay cannot be clinically predicted, and caries may be extensive before they become evident.

Orofacial development is a health issue in which breastfeeding has a measurable impact (Palmer, 1998). The orofacial development of a child is affected by feeding methods, swallowing patterns, and finger sucking (Sanger & Bystrom, 1982). The mechanisms by which bottle-feeding might contribute to the development of malocclusion include a forward thrusting of the tongue, which in turn leads to underdevelopment of the masseter and buccinator muscles, abnormal swallowing patterns, and increased prevalence of nonnutritive sucking. A study of preschool children in Puerto Rico (Lopez Del Valle et al., 2006) revealed that breastfeeding helped prevent malocclusions, such as space deficiency, open bites and cross-bites, and decreased thumb sucking and pacifier use. In Brazil, children, ages 3 years to 6 years, were studied for the relationship between breastfeeding, nasal breathing, and deleterious oral habits (Trawitzki et al., 2005). The breastfeeding time period was longer among nasal breathers. Mouth breathing children were breastfed for shorter time periods and had statistically significant deleterious oral habits, such as suction ($P = .004$) and biting habits ($P = .0002$).

Solid Foods

Every breastfed infant reaches a point when breastmilk alone no longer fulfills his nutritional needs. If breastfeeding is continued exclusively, the baby will eventually become malnourished. How long exclusive breastfeeding can satisfy the nutrient needs of babies is a crucial public health issue, especially in areas with an unsafe water supply and poor sanitation, where early supplements are likely to be associated with infections.

Introducing Solid Foods

Solid foods are not necessary, nor are they recommended, before a baby is 4 to 6 months of age (AAP, 1997). Developmental cues for introducing solid foods to the infant are the fading of his tongue-extrusion reflex, eruption of teeth, the ability to sit, and purposeful movement of the baby's hands and fingers, all of which normally occur during the middle months of the first year of life. Most infants will at first actively resist the advances of even the most enterprising parent in attempts to spoon-feed them during the early months of life. Before 6 months of age, a baby has a tongue-extrusion reflex and is unable to push food to the back of his mouth. In the full-term baby, the prenatal storage of iron acquired during the last trimester of pregnancy gradually begins to diminish by 4 to 5 months of age, and external sources of iron are needed (Pisacane et al., 1995).

Early introduction of solids is still a common practice in the United States, even though the American Academy of Pediatrics' Committee on Nutrition has consistently held that no nutritional advantage results from the introduction of supplemental foods prior to 4 to 6 months of age. A study of mothers in Kentucky found that by 1 month of age, 12 percent of mothers reported that their infant had received solid food and cereal added to the bottle. Fruit juices were given to one fifth of the study infants by 1 to 2 months of age (Barton, 2001).

In fact, mothers sometimes competitively seek to outdo one another in initiating solid food, as if how soon an infant eats adult food is a measure of his maturity. Despite official recommendations and a concerted effort to teach parents to delay solids, many infants still receive solid foods during their first few months of life. The first solid food is usually cereal, which is given in the evening because some parents wrongly believe or have been told that feeding solids to the baby will help him sleep through the night. However, feeding infants solids prior to bedtime is not related to evening sleep patterns; according to well-controlled studies, babies who receive solids before bedtime have the same sleep patterns as do babies who are not given solids (Keane et al., 1988; Macknin, Medendorp, & Maier, 1989).

Energy-intake patterns between breastfed and formula-fed infants discussed earlier in this book indicate that breastfed infants maintain energy-intake levels below those of formula-fed infants. These patterns persist even after solid foods are introduced. If breastfeeding infants are given solids at from 3 to 6 months, their milk intakes decline significantly; the energy from solids generally replaces that from breastmilk. Although the infant breastfeeds fewer times during the day, the frequency of night feedings remains the same (Heinig et al., 1993). This is not true for formula-fed infants, who continue to take about the same amount of formula when early solids are given. In industrialized countries, infants fed solids early appear to have about the same incidence of illness as do infants who are fed solids later. In developing countries, however, the risk of diarrhea is such that the risks of introducing solids before 6 months outweighs any potential benefits.

Choosing the Diet

If solids are started after 6 months of age, the sequence of foods is not critical. If solids are introduced earlier, the following order is suggested: cereals, yellow vegetables, fruits, meats, and (last) legumes. For cereal that requires mixing with a liquid, breastmilk (rather than cow's milk) avoids any potential allergic reaction. Egg yolk, if carefully separated from the white (which is highly allergenic), is high in protein and iron, is hypoallergenic, and is therefore safe.

Infants need additional water when solids are started because of their added osmolar load. Historically, fruit juice was recommended by pediatricians as a source of vitamin C and water. Because fruit juice tastes sweet, children readily accept it. Although fruit juice has some benefits such as the vitamins and in some cases calcium that it contains, it also has potential detrimental effects (AAP, 2001). Children can become addicted to consuming fruit juices at the expense of eating other foods, especially healthy, fresh foods. It has been recommended that honey not be given to infants under a year of age because there is a highly unlikely but possible chance of contracting botulism from honey (Lawrence & Lawrence, 2005).

A basic rule is to feed the infant foods in as close to a natural state as possible: pieces of raw, peeled apples, slices of banana, toasted whole wheat bread, orange sections, and a chicken leg with the skin removed are all good choices. They can be picked up and held and are tasty, nutritious, and satisfying to chew. Small amounts at first followed by gradually increased amounts (along with continued breastfeeding),

avoids constipation. Mothers should be prepared for changes in consistency, odor, and frequency of stool when solids are begun. Generally, all foods eaten by the family can be given to the infant in a consistency that he can handle. The beginning eater enjoys foods of all kinds and relishes the tactile pleasures of squeezing, smearing, and crushing his food—an activity he should be allowed with impunity because it is also a learning experience. General guidelines for initiating solid foods are found in Table 18–5.

Breastfed babies are exposed to a variety of flavors of whatever is transmitted in their mothers' breastmilk (Mennella, 1995). As a result, it seems likely that they would be more accepting of novel flavors in solid foods than are formula-fed infants who are not so exposed. Likewise, flavors from the mother's diet during pregnancy are transmitted to amniotic fluids and swallowed by the fetus. Consequently, food flavors eaten by women during pregnancy are experienced by infants before their first exposure to solid foods (Mennella, Jagnow, & Beauchamp, 2001). To test this assumption, Sullivan and Birch (1994) compared acceptance of vegetables by 4- to 6-month-old infants. These infants were randomly assigned to be fed one vegetable on 10 occasions for 10 days. They found that breastfeeding infants ate more vegetables than did formula-fed infants. Thus breastmilk may facilitate the acceptance of solid foods during the important transition from suckling to feeding solids. Babies who are given cereal were more accepting of it if it was mixed with mother's milk rather than water (Mennella & Beauchamp, 1997). And, in situations in which families are unable to provide high-quality solids, continued breastfeeding beyond 1 year of age is recommended to enhance linear growth in toddlers (Marquis et al., 1997).

Foods prepared at home are not only more wholesome and nutritious but cost less than do commercially prepared baby foods. Carrots and applesauce, for example, cost about one half the store price when prepared at home, and blended beef or chicken provide more nutrients by weight than do their commercial counterparts, chiefly because they contain less water. With the aid of an electric blender, food mill, or grinder, preparing baby food is easily accomplished. The foods should be selected from high-quality fresh or frozen fruits, vegetables, or meats, with special attention to hygienic preparation and storage. For convenience,

TABLE
18–5
Introducing Solid Foods into a Breastfed Infant's Diet

When to Introduce	Approximate Total Daily Intake of Solids*	Description of Food and Hints Giving Them
6–7 months if infant is breastfed	*Dry cereal:* Start with 1/2 tsp (dry measurement); gradually increase to 2–3 tb. *Vegetables:* Start with 1 tsp; gradually increase to 2 tb. *Fruit:* Start with 1 tsp; gradually increase to 2 tb. Divide food among 4 feedings per day (if possible).	*Cereal:* Offer iron-enriched baby cereal. Begin with single grains. Mix cereal with an equal amount of breastmilk. *Vegetables:* Try a mild-tasting vegetable first (carrots, squash, peas, green beans). Stronger-flavored vegetables (spinach, sweet potatoes) may be tried after infant accepts some mild-tasting ones. *Fruits:* Mashed ripe banana and unsweetened, cooked, bland fruits (apples, peaches, pears) are usually well-liked. Apple juice and grape juice (unsweetened) may be introduced. Initially, dilute juice with an equal amount of water. Introduce one new food at a time and offer it several times before trying another new food. Give a new food once daily for a day or two; increase to twice daily as the infant begins to enjoy the food. Watch for signs of intolerance. Include some foods that are good sources of vitamin C (other than orange juice).
6–7 months if infant is breastfed	*Meat:* Start with 1 tsp and gradually increase to 2 tb. Divide food among 4 feedings per day (if possible). *Dry cereal:* Gradually increase up to 4 tb. *Fruits and vegetables:* Gradually increase up to 3 tb of each.	*Meat:* Offer pureed or milled poultry (chicken or turkey) followed by lean meat (veal, beef); lamb has a stronger flavor and may not be as well-liked initially. Liver is a good source of iron; it may be accepted at the beginning of a meal with a familiar vegetable. Continue introducing new cereals, fruits, and vegetables as the infant indicates he is ready to accept them, but always one at a time; introduce legumes last.
7–9 months if infant is breastfed	*Dry cereal:* Up to 1/2 cup. *Fruits and vegetables:* Up to 1/4 to 1/2 cup of each.	Soft table foods may be introduced—for example, mashed potatoes and squash and small

(Continues)

TABLE 18–5	**Introducing Solid Foods into a Breastfed Infant's Diet (Continued)**	
When to Introduce	**Approximate Total Daily Intake of Solids***	**Description of Food and Hints About Giving Them**
8–12 months if infant is breastfed	*Meats:* Up to 3 tb. Divide food among 4 feedings per day (if possible). *Dry cereal:* Up to 1/2 cup. *Bread:* About 1 slice. *Fruits and vegetables:* Up to 1/2 cup of each. Divide food among 4 feedings per day (if possible).	pieces of soft, peeled fruits. Toasted whole grain or enriched bread may be added when the infant begins chewing. If introduction of solids is delayed until now, it is not necessary to use strained fruits and vegetables. Continue using iron-fortified baby cereals. Table foods cut into small pieces may be added gradually. Start with foods that do not require too much chewing (cooked, cut green beans and carrots, noodles, ground meats, tuna fish, soft cheese, plain yogurt). If fish is offered, check closely to be sure there are no bones in the serving. Mashed, cooked egg yolk and orange juice may be added at about 9 months of age. Sometimes offer peanut butter or thoroughly cooked dried peas and beans in place of meat.

* Some infants do not need or want these amounts of food; some may need a little more food.

small individualized portions can be stored safely in the refrigerator or freezer for reasonable periods. A list of foods that can be quickly and easily prepared appears in Box 18–2.

Some parents prefer to buy commercial baby food rather than to make their own. In addition to being expensive, commercial baby foods are generally produced by pulverizing fruit, grain, vegetable, and meat ingredients with water and adding filler ingredients such as colorings, additives, and preservatives (Randle, 1999).

For families on vegan diets, their infants may need supplements of vitamin B_{12} when dairy products and eggs are excluded from the diet. Older infants may need zinc supplements and reliable sources of iron and vitamin D as well as vitamin B_{12}.

Timing of solid-food introduction is similar to that recommended for nonvegetarians. Tofu, dried beans, and meat analogs are introduced as protein sources around the middle of the first year (Mangels & Messina, 2001).

Choosing Feeding Location

The best place to feed a baby is at the family table at mealtime, in a high chair or on someone's knee. Young children love to be considered one of the family and to sit at the same height as the rest of the family. Even before the infant is ready to take solids, he enjoys being nearby during meals and can "join in" by chewing on such food as a bread crust or a carrot.

BOX 18–2

Quick, Easy-to- Prepare Infant Foods

- Yogurt (low-fat)
- Fresh fruit: cut-up apples, pears, oranges, bananas, grapes, or any fruit in season
- Cheese, cut into chewable pieces
- Toast of whole grain bread, cut into strips
- Chicken: leg, wing, or cut-up pieces
- Egg: soft-boiled; hard-boiled as finger food

- Vegetables: mashed; whole (e.g., peas); in strips or pieces as finger food
- Crackers: whole grain; cheese spread
- Custard
- Cottage cheese
- Dried fruit: apples, dates, figs, prunes (pitted)
- Liver: sauteed and cut into strips
- Tuna: drained; with grated cheese

Delaying Solid Foods

Current recommendations (American Public Health Association, American Academy of Pediatrics, World Health Organization) include exclusive breastfeeding for the first 6 months of life, with continued breastfeeding for at least the first 1 to 2 years, and introduction of complementary foods between 4 to 6 months of age. Reviews of nutritional options during pregnancy, lactation, and the first year of life that addressed dietary management for prevention of atopic disease (atopic dermatitis, asthma, allergic rhinitis, and food allergy) replace previous policy statements from the American Academy of Pediatrics (Greer et al., 2008). There is evidence that breastfeeding for at least 4 months prevents or delays occurrence of atopic dermatitis, cow milk allergy, and wheezing in early childhood. There is scant evidence that delaying the timing of introduction of complementary foods beyond 4 to 6 months of age prevents the occurrence of atopic disease, except for the benefit to infants at high risk of developing allergy (i.e., those with at least 1 first-degree relative—parent or sibling—with allergic disease). Foods considered to be most highly allergic include fish, eggs, and food containing peanut protein.

At age 6 months, the infant produces sufficient IgA antibody to prevent absorption of food antigens through the intestinal wall, thus reducing food allergy. IgE, which is associated with allergy, rises in direct time sequence to the introduction of solid foods. IgE is also associated with allergy verified by a positive skin test later in life. Before the age of 6 months, the infant's intestine lacks the necessary digestive enzymes to completely digest complex proteins and starches down to amino acids and simple sugars. At the same time, the infant's intestinal mucosa is permeable to some intact proteins and starches. These incompletely digested peptides and starches can be absorbed and serve as sensitizing agents to the infant's immune system. IgE is then produced and allergy results in some (perhaps many) infants.

Obesity

Childhood obesity, a growing problem throughout the world, is most commonly measured by body mass index (BMI). Obesity in children is defined as a BMI at or above the 95th percentile, and overweight is defined as a BMI at or above the 85th percentile to the 95th percentile. In the United States 16 percent of 6- to 19-year-olds are obese, and 31 percent are overweight. Obesity is also increasing in the preschool-aged population, with 10 percent obese and 20% overweight children. Significant ethnic differences have been documented, with higher rates of obesity and overweight in non-Hispanic black, Mexican American, Native American, Alaskan Native, and Pacific Islander population (Matheson & Robinson, 2008).

Children are driven to school, and when they come home they watch television and/or play computer games many hours each day. Children of obese parents are more likely to be overweight themselves (Hediger et al., 2001; Maffeis, 1999). In addition to lack of exercise and genetic endowment, early diet plays a role in obesity. Breastfed infants regulate their food intake according to their caloric needs and, at the same time, control their mother's milk production. In contrast, the satiated bottle-fed baby is encouraged to empty the bottle and may not ever develop control over food intake. Are breast-feeding children then less likely to become obese? It depends on who is asked and the culture where a study takes place.

Dewey (2003) and Butte (2001) extensively reviewed breastfeeding and childhood obesity studies worldwide. Dewey concluded that breastfeeding reduces the risk of a child becoming overweight to a moderate extent. Butte found the association to be insignificant. Many large studies have shown that breastfed babies are less likely than bottle-fed infants to become obese (Armstrong & Reilly, 2002; Bergmann et al., 2003; Gillman et al., 2001; Kramer, 1981; Toschke et al., 2002; von Kries et al., 1999; Singhal & Lanigen, 2006; Arnez & von Kries, 2005). Other research showed no such relationship between breastfeeding and later obesity (Baranowski et al., 1992; Li, Parsons, & Power, 2003), and some found that breastfed children were more likely to become fat (Agras et al., 1990; Kersey et al., 2005).

The literature is contradictory in part because many studies are based on small sample sizes, missing data, lack of adequate control for confounding factors (e.g., the mother's nutritional awareness, exercise patterns), and methodological problems (e.g., operational definitions of obesity, the distinction between a "breastfed" infant versus a "bottle-fed" infant, and the timing of feedings). Moreover, differences in exercise patterns of children were not included in studies as a confounding factor. Breastfeeding, along with genetic, racial, socioeconomic, and behavioral factors, affects later obesity and the risks of developing cardiovascular disease,

hypertension, metabolic syndrome, and diabetes mellitus. A large meta-analysis study showed that formula-fed infants had higher plasma-insulin concentrations and higher protein intake compared to breastfed infants, suggesting stimulation of fat deposition and a significant positive relationship between high protein intake early in life and increased risk of obesity later in life (Arnez & von Kries, 2005). A large study review (Owen et al., 2006) concluded that breastfeeding in infancy is associated with lower blood glucose and serum concentrations in infancy, with marginal lower insulin concentrations and reduced risk of type II diabetes mellitus in later life. Policy makers and clinicians cannot ignore the growing body of evidence that breastfeeding lowers the risk of becoming overweight later in life (Gillman, 2002).

Other dietary factors, such as early introduction of sweet drink consumption, when infants are developing taste preferences can lead to excessive sugar intake and the long-term consequences of type II diabetes mellitus, low nutrition, low calcium intake, low bone density, dental caries, and some behavior issues (Saalfield & Jackson-Allen, 2006).

Long-Term Breastfeeding

Long-term breastfeeding is considered "comfort nursing"—a form of nurturance and a special bonding rather than nourishment. Nutritional benefits are considered secondary. The conceptual difference is that breastfeeding is considered as a "process" rather than a "product" (Van Esterik, 1985). Do older breastfeeding children receive sufficient food to grow? Nutrition in long-term breastfeeders in the United States appeared to be adequate in one study. When daily food intake of these children was measured, their nonbreast intake of complementary foods met RDA energy requirements (Buckley, 2001).

Weaning

In the United States, weaning usually takes place during the first year of life. Women who breastfeed longer than this have difficulty with acceptance by relatives, peers, and health professionals (Page-Goertz, 2002). If "baby-led weaning" is practiced, weaning usually takes place between the child's second and fourth birthdays (Sugarman & Kendall-Tackett, 1995). To counteract social pressures for early weaning, women with breastfeeding toddlers find peer support for each other, sometimes changing their circle of friends.

In a study by Wrigley and Hutchinson (1990) of 12 mothers who practiced long-term breastfeeding, one mother reported that her obstetrician told her anyone who breastfed an infant past 6 months of age was "perverted." Another said that her father thought she was "strange." Many healthcare workers, who wholeheartedly support breastfeeding and would never advocate taking a security blanket away from a baby reel in horror when a mother breastfeeds a walking child. Page-Goertz (2002) advises "To avoid embarrassing moments at the mall due to the toddler's increasing language skills, parents may want to teach their child a code word for breastfeeding. Examples are "pillow" and "nums." This can prevent a child from yelling 'BOOBY, mom—now!'"

Ideally, the time for weaning is a joint decision in which both the mother and the baby reach a state of readiness to begin weaning around the same time; however, this is not always the case. The child may be ready before his mother; more often, the mother is ready before her child. In a unique study of weaning times of 36 primates, anthropologist Dettwyler (1995) determined what would be a natural duration of breastfeeding in modern humans. Her evidence suggests that 2.5 years is the minimum duration of time for breastfeeding, and that 4 or 5 years, or longer, is within the normal range for humans.

Sometimes, the decision is made to wean quickly. Although the literature offers considerable advice about gradual weaning, there is little information for the anxious mother in a situation in which weaning must be rapid and will necessarily be traumatic. The following nondrug therapies may make deliberate weaning easier and at the same time avert plugged ducts or mastitis:

- Shower and allow the warm water to run over the breasts, or soak the breasts by lying down in the tub.
- Use a breast pump or manual expression to relieve breast fullness.
- Wear a supportive, comfortable bra.
- Observe for signs of plugged ducts or a breast infection.

- Expect to feel very emotional during this time and seek support from people who will listen sympathetically.
- Give the baby extra cuddling and holding.

It may take several days before the mother finds it is no longer necessary to express breastmilk for comfort. As described earlier in this book, an Australian method for reducing engorged breasts is to wear cool raw cabbage leaves in the bra. Doing so has been reported to quickly relieve engorgement.

Implications for Practice

Care providers assume responsibility for educating families in optimal infant-feeding practices and for providing rationale and support when they are needed. The introduction of foods other than breastmilk is culturally influenced and common worldwide. Some mothers encourage their babies to eat as much as possible, believing that a plump baby represents the picture of health. Competition among mothers can also lead to the early introduction of baby foods. Mothers who feel pressure to give their babies solids may misinterpret the baby's cries as hunger, when the baby merely needs stimulation by holding and interacting. Education is a powerful tool for teaching healthy food practices.

It is not unusual for children, usually from about 2 years of age, to become very fussy about food and to refuse to eat certain items; they may especially dislike vegetables. Children will go through periods of eating very little for a period from as short as a week to as long as a few months; then they gradually start eating more again. The mother should be reassured that "this too shall pass" and that her child will start eating again. Meanwhile, she should make the food he does like easily available and neither force the child to eat nor mask his natural appetite by offering sugary foods.

Choices about weaning should be based on the mother's own wishes rather than on the expectations of others and should call for active listening to her feelings. If the mother enjoys breastfeeding but feels pressure to wean, pointing out the advantages of continued breastfeeding and the cultural differences in weaning practices may be all the reinforcement she needs. On the other hand, if she expresses resentment each time her baby breastfeeds and is impatient for each feeding to end, she is entitled to know options for safe and comfortable weaning techniques. Some women report that after weaning their baby, they experienced improvement in mood and sexuality and felt less fatigue (Forster et al., 1994).

Summary

Imperative to assisting a breastfeeding family is recognition and knowledge of a wide array of areas of child health. Taking the holistic view, breastfeeding is but one aspect of the child's overall health and welfare. This chapter has offered readers basic information derived from research findings and clinical experiences. Teaching parents and incorporating research findings into the daily lives of families are the linchpins of effective practice.

Key Concepts

- Worldwide studies indicate that breastfed infants are more likely to have higher intellectual ability and cognitive development compared with those who were not breastfed.
- Universal child growth patterns include cephalocaudal and proximodistal growth.
- Generally, both breastfed and bottle-fed infants double their birth weight by the middle of the first year of life and triple it by 1 year. Breastfeeding infants weigh slightly more than their formula-fed counterparts for the first 3 to 4 months.
- The infant's brain grows rapidly during infancy.
- Neonates are born with well-developed sensory abilities of hearing, smell, and taste. Visual preference is for human faces and moving objects.
- Theories about early developmental stages include (1) trust versus mistrust and autonomy versus shame and doubt (Erickson), and (2) sensorimotor, assimilation, and accommodation (Piaget).
- Breastfed infants tend to be more wakeful, cry more often during the late afternoon and evening, and wake more frequently during the night.
- Attachment and bonding is a series of physical contact and sensory interactions between mother and baby as "mutual caregivers."
- Stranger distress and separation anxiety, which occur during the second half of the first year of life, is a normal phenomenon where the child fears strangers and being apart from his primary caretaker.

- Developmentally speaking, the ability to tolerate solids offers no evidence that their early introduction is advantageous. In fact, the practice may initiate a chain of disadvantages that include allergies and obesity.
- Recommendations for immunizations are usually the same for breastfed children as for nonbreastfed children.
- The rise in cases of rickets in breastfed infants has led to recommendations for vitamin D supplementation of infants at risk.
- Breastfeeding infants generally have fewer dental caries. Reported cases of dental caries are usually associated with nighttime feedings, genetic predisposition, and dietary sugar.
- Solids foods are not necessary before 4 to 6 months of age. Developmental cues for introducing solid foods are fading of the child's tongue-extrusion reflex, the eruption of teeth, the ability to sit, and purposeful movement of the baby's hands and fingers, all of which normally occur during the middle months of the first year of life. Full-term babies have storage of iron that begins to diminish by 4 to 5 months of age.
- Total solid food elimination for the first 4 to 6 months of life, in addition to exclusive breast-milk feeding, appears to reduce atopic disease in children who are at hereditary risk. Delaying introduction of foods beyond this period does not appear to have a significant protective effect on the development of atopic disease.
- Breastfeeding appears to have a slight protective effect against later obesity, but it appears to

be weaker than genetic, racial, socioeconomic, and behavioral factors.
- Cosleeping facilitates breastfeeding. Safe cosleeping includes bedding that fits tightly to the mattress, no soft pillows or space between the bed and the wall, and placing the baby on his back or side.

- Ideally weaning takes place when both the mother and baby reach a state of readiness around the same time. Cross-culturally, weaning takes place around 2.5 years of age.

Internet Resources

Brian Palmer's Web site, focusing on child health topics: sleep apnea, SIDS, dental caries
http://www.brianpalmerdds.com
American Academy of Pediatrics (AAP)
http://www.aap.org
American Academy of Pediatrics (AAP) Immunizations
http://www.cispimmunize.org
American Academy of Pediatric Dentistry
http://www.aapd.org
Academy of General Dentristry
http://www.agd.org
American Dental Association
http://www.ada.org
Bright Futures at Georgetown University: A national resource for child health promotion
http://www.brightfutures.org
Calgary Health Region: Early Childhood Caries: Search for "Lift the Lip" screening
http://www.calgaryhealthregion.ca
Centers for Disease Control
http://www.cdc.gov
Centers for Disease Control (CDC) Immunizations
http://www.cdc.gov/vaccines
Immunization Action Coalition
http://www.immunization.org

Healthy Steps: Focus on first 3 years of life
http://www.healthysteps.org
National Association of Pediatric Nurse Practitioners (NAPNAP): Information resource for child health promotion special initiatives
KySS: Keep your children/yourself Safe and Secure (mental health)
HEAT: Healthy Eating and Activity Together (childhood obesity)
http://www.napnap.org
World Health Organization
http://www.who.int/en
New growth standard information
http://www.who.int/nutrition/media_page/en
New growth charts
http://www.who.int/childgrowth/standards/chart_catalogue/en/index.html
UNICEF
Information and statistical data for professionals and researchers. Brochures and pamphlets for family and community members:
www.unicef.org
UNICEF Breastfeeding and Complementary Feeding:
www.childinfo.org/eddb/brfeed/test/database.htm

References

Agras WS et al. Influence of early feeding style on adiposity at 6 years of age. *J Pediatr.* 1990;116: 805–811.

Ainsworth MDS et al. *Patterns of Attachment.* Hillsdale, NJ: Lawrence Erlbaum; 1978.

Al-Dashti AA, Williams SA, Curzon MEJ. Breast feeding, bottle feeding and dental caries in Kuwait, a country with low-fluoride levels in the water supply. *Community Dent Health.* 1994;12:42–47.

Als H, Brazelton TB. A new model of assessing the behavioral organization in preterm and full-term infants. *J Am Acad Child Psychol.* 1981;20:239.

Altshuler A. Early childood caries: new knowledge has implications for breastfeeding families. *Leaven.* April-May-June, 2006.

American Academy of Pediatrics (AAP). Work Group on Breastfeeding. Breastfeeding and the use of human milk. *Pediatrics.* 1997;100:1035–1039.

American Academy of Pediatrics (AAP). The use and misuse of fruit juice in pediatrics. *Pediatrics.* 2001;107:1210–1213.

American Academy of Pediatrics. Policy Statement. http://aappolicy.aappublications.org/cgi/content/abstract/pediatrics;97/3/413. Accessed March 3, 2008.

American Academy of Pediatrics (AAP). Prevention of rickets and vitamin D deficiency: new guidelines for vitamin D intake. *Pediatrics.* 2003;111:908.

Anderson GC. The mother and her newborn: mutual caregivers. *JOGNN.* 1977;6:50–55.

Anderson GC. Enhancing reciprocity between mother and neonate. *Nurs Res.* 1981;30:89–93.

Anderson GC, Dombrowski MA, Swinth JY. Kangaroo Care: not just for stable preemies anymore. *Reflect Nurs Leadership.* 2001;27:32–34.

Anderson GC et al. Early skin-to-skin contact for mothers and their healthy newborn infants. (Cochrane Review). In: *The Cochrane Library*, Oxford, England: Update Software; Issue 2, 2003a.

Anderson GC et al. Mother-newborn contact in a randomized trial of kangaroo (skin-to-skin) care. *JOGNN.* 2003b;32:604–611.

Anderson GC et al. Skin-to-skin for breastfeeding difficulties postbirth. In: Field T, ed. *Advances in Touch.* New Brunswick, NJ: Johnson & Johnson; 2003c.

Armstrong J, Reilly JJ. Breastfeeding and lowering the risk of childhood obesity. *Lancet.* 2002; 359:2003–2004.

Arnez F, von Kries R. Protective effect of breast-feeding against obesity in childhood. *Adv Exp Med Biol.* 2005;569:40–48.

Arshad SH. Food allergen avoidance in primary prevention of food allergy. *Allergy.* 2001;56(suppl 67): 113–116.

Ball HL. Breastfeeding, bed-sharing, and infant sleep. *Birth.* 2003;30:181–188.

Baranowski T et al. Height, infant-feeding practices and cardiovascular functioning among 3 or 4 year old children in three ethnic groups. *J Clin Epidemiol.* 1992;45:513–518.

Barton SJ. Infant feeding practices of low-income rural mothers. *MCN.* 2001;26:93–98.

Bergmann KE et al. Early determinants of childhood overweight and adiposity in a birth cohort study: role of breastfeeding. *Int J Obesity.* 2003;27: 162–172.

Birch EE et al. A randomized controlled trial of early dietary supply of long-chain polyunsaturated fatty acids and mental development in term infants. *Dev Med Child Neurol.* 2000;41:174–181.

Bowen WH et al. Assessing the carcinogenic potential of some infant formulas, milk and sugar solution. *JADA.* 1997;128:865–871.

Bowlby J. The nature of the child's tie to his mother. *Int J Psychoanal.* 1958;39:350–372.

Bowlby J. *Attachment and Loss: Separation.* Vol 2. New York, NY: Basic Books; 1973.

Buckley KM. Long-term breastfeeding: nourishment or nurturance? *J Hum Lact.* 2001;17:304–312.

Bu'Loc F, Woolridge MW, Baum JD. Development of co-ordination of sucking, swallowing and breathing: ultrasound study of term and preterm infants. *Dev Med Child Neurol.* 1990;32:669–678.

Butte NF. The role of breastfeeding in obesity. In: Schanler R, ed. Breastfeeding 2000, part 1. *Pediatr Clin North Am.* 2001;48:189–198.

Butte NF et al. Energy utilization of breast-fed and formula-fed infants. *Am J Clin Nutr.* 1990;51:350–358.

Butte NF et al. Influence of early feeding mode on body composition of infants. *Bio Neonate.* 1995; 67:414–424.

Carey WB, McDevitt SC. Revision of the infant temperament questionnaire. *Pediatrics.* 1978;61:735–739.

Centers for Disease Control and Prevention (CDC). Influenza vaccination coverage among children—United States. *MMWR.* 2008;57(38).

Centers for Disease Control and Prevention (CDC). Recommended childhood immunization schedule—United States, 2002. *MMWR.* 2002;287(6):70–78.

Condon WS, Sander LW. Neonate movement is synchronized with adult speech: interaction participation and language acquisition. *Science.* 1974;183:99.

Daniels MC et al. Breast-Feeding influences cognitive development in Filipino children. *J Nutr.* 2005;135: 2589–2595.

Dettwyler KA. A time to wean. In: Stuart-Macadam P, Dettwyler KA, eds. *Breastfeeding: Biocultural Perspectives.* New York, NY: Aldine de Gruyter; 1995:39–73.

Dewey KG. Is breastfeeding protective against child obesity? *J Hum Lact.* 2003;19:9–18.

Efe E, Ozer ZC. The use of breast-feeding for pain relief during neonatal immunization injections. *Appl Nurs Res.* 2007;20:10–16.

Eickmann SH et al. Breast feeding and mental and motor development at 12 months in a low-income population in northeast Brazil. *Paediatr Perinat Epidemiol.* 2007;21:129–137.

Elias F et al. Sleep/wake patterns of breast-fed infants in the first 2 years of life. *Pediatrics.* 1986;77:322–329.

Engler AJ et al. Kangaroo Care: national survey of practice, knowledge, barriers and perceptions. *MCN.* 2002;27:146–152.

Epstein K. The interactions between breastfeeding mothers and their babies during the breastfeeding session. *Early Child Dev Care.* 1993;87:93–104.

Erikson EH. *Childhood and Society.* 2nd ed. New York, NY: Norton; 1963.

Erikson EH. *Identity, Youth and Crisis.* New York, NY: Norton; 1968.

Erickson PR. Investigation of the role of human breast-milk in caries development. *Pediatr Dentistry.* 1999;21:86–90.

Farquharson J et al. Infant cerebral cortex phospholipid fatty-acid composition and diet. *Lancet.* 1992; 340:810–813.

Feldman R et al. The nature of the mother's tie to her infant: maternal bonding under conditions of proximity, separation, and potential loss. *J Child Psychol Psychiatry.* 1999;40:929–939.

Floury CV, Leech AM, Blackhall A. Infant feeding and mental and motor development at 18 months of age in first-born singletons. *Int J Epidemiol.* 1995;24(3)(suppl 1):S21–S26.

Forster et al. Psychological and sexual changes after the cessation of breast-feeding. *Obstet Gynecol.* 1994;84:872–876.

Gill NE et al. Effect of nonnutritive sucking on behavioral state in preterm infants before feeding. *Nurs Res.* 1988;37:347–350.

Gillman MW. Breast-feeding and obesity [editorial]. *J Pediatr.* 2002;141:749–750.

Gillman MW et al. Risk of overweight among adolescents who were breastfed as infants. *JAMA.* 2001;285:2453–2460.

Greer FR et al. Effects of early nutritional interventions on the development of a topic disease in infants and children: the role of maternal dietary restriction, breastfeeding, timing of introduction of complementary foods, and hydrolyzed formulas. *Pediatrics.* 2008; 121:183–191.

Harlow HF, Harlow M. The affectional systems. In: Schrier A, Harlow H, Stollnitz F, eds. *Behavior of Nonhuman Primates.* Vol. 2. New York, NY: Academic; 1965.

Hart SL et al. Brief report: newborn behavior differs with docosahexaenoic acid levels in breast milk. *J Pediatr Psychol.* 2006;31:221–226.

Hedberg-Nyqvist K, Ewald U. Successful breast feeding in spite of early mother-baby separation for neonatal care. *Midwifery.* 1997;13:24–31.

Hediger ML et al. Association between infant breastfeeding and overweight in young children. *JAMA.* 2001;285:2453–2460.

Hegvik R, McDevitt SC, Carey W. The middle childhood temperament questionnaire. *J Dev Behav Pediatr.* 1982;3:197–200.

Heinig MJ et al. Intake and growth of breast-fed and formula-fed infants in relation to the timing of introduction of complementary foods: the DARLING study. *Acta Paediatr.* 1993;82:999–1006.

Hurst N, Valentine CK, Renfro L. Skin-to-skin holding in the neonatal intensive care unit influences maternal milk volume. *J Perinatol.* 1997;27: 213–217.

Johnson DL et al. Breast feeding and children's intelligence. *Psychol Rep.* 1996;79:1179–1185.

Julvez J et al. Attention behavior and hyperactivity at age 4 and duration of breast-feeding. *Acta Paediatr.* 2007;96:842–847.

Keane V et al. Do solids help baby sleep through the night? *Am J Dis Child.* 1988;142:404–405.

Kersey M et al. Breast-feeding history and overweight in Latino preschoolers. *Ambulatory Pediatr.* 2005;5: 355–358.

Klaus MH, Kennell JH. *Maternal-Infant bonding: The Impact of Early Separation and Loss on Family Development.* St Louis, MO: Mosby; 1975.

Kramer MS. Do breast-feeding and delayed introduction of solid foods protect against subsequent obesity? *J Pediatr.* 1981;98:883–887.

Krogh V et al. Postpartum immunization with rubella virus vaccine and antibody response in breast-feeding infants. *J Lab Clin Med.* 1989;113:695–699.

Lanting CI et al. Neurological differences between 9-year-old children fed breast-milk or formula-milk as babies. *Lancet.* 1994;344:1319–1322.

Latz S, Wolf AW, Lozoff B. Co-sleeping in context. *Arch Pediatr Adolesc Med.* 1999;153:339–346.

Lawrence R, Lawrence RM. *Breastfeeding: A Guide for the Medical Profession,* 6th ed. Philadelphia, PA: Mosby; 2005:634.

Li L, Parsons TJ, Power C. Breastfeeding and obesity in childhood: cross sectional study. *BMJ.* 2003; 327:904–905.

Lopez Del Valle L et al. Associations between a history of breast feeding, malocclusion and parafunctional habits in Puerto Rican children. *P R Health Sci J.* 2006;25:31.

Lorenz KZ. The companion in the environment of the bird. *J Ornithol.* 1935;83:137–215, 289–413.

Lucas A et al. Breastmilk and subsequent intelligence quotient in children born preterm. *Lancet.* 1992;339:261–264.

Ludington-Hoe S, Swinth JY. Developmental aspects of Kangaroo Care. *JOGNN.* 1996;25:692–703.

Ludington-Hoe S et al. Kangaroo Care compared to incubators in maintaining body warmth in preterm infants. *Biol Res Nurs.* 2000;260–273.

Lunardelli SE, Peres MA. Breast-feeding and other mother-child factors associated with developmental enamel defects in the primary teeth of Brazilian children. *J Dent Child.* 2006;73(2):70–78.

Macknin ML, Medendorp SV, Maier MC. Infant sleep and bedtime cereal. *Am J Dis Child.* 1989;143:1066–1068.

Madhusmitam, M, Pacaud D, Petryk A, Collett-Solberg P, Kappy M. Vitamin D deficiency in children and its management: review of current knowledge and recommendations. *Pediatrics.* 2008;122:398–417.

Maffeis C. Childhood obesity: the genetic–environmental interface. *Endocrinol Metab.* 1999;13:31.

Makin JW, Porter RH. Attractiveness of lactating females' breast odors to neonates. *Child Dev.* 1989;60:803–810.

Mangels AR, Messina BV. Considerations in planning vegan diets: infants. *J Am Diet Assoc.* 2001; 101:670–677.

Marquis GS et al. Breastmilk or animal-products foods improve linear growth of Peruvian toddlers consuming marginal diets. *Am J Clin Nutr.* 1997;66: 1102–1109.

Martin RM et al. Breast feeding in infancy and social mobility: 60-year follow-up of the Boyd Orr cohort. *Arch Dis Child.* 2007;92:317–321.

Matee MIN et al. Nursing caries, linear hypoplasia, and nursing and weaning habits in Tanzanian infants. *Community Dent Oral Epidemiol.* 1994;22:289–293.

Matheson D, Robinson T. Obesity in Young Children. In: Birch L, Dietz W, eds. *Eating Behaviors of the Young Child: Prenatal and Postnatal Influences on Healthy Eating.* Elk Village, IL: Am Acad Pediatr. 2008:33–58.

McKenna J, Mosko S, Richard C. Bedsharing promotes breastfeeding. *Pediatrics.* 1997;100:214–219.

Mennella JA. Mothers' milk: a medium for early flavor experiences. *J Hum Lact.* 1995;11:39–45.

Mennella JA, Beauchamp GK. Mothers' milk enhances the acceptance of cereal during weaning. *Pediatr Res.* 1997;41:188–192.

Mennella JA, Jagnow CP, Beauchamp GK. Prenatal and postnatal flavor learning by human infants. *Pediatrics.* 2001;107:E88.

Mercer R. A theoretical framework for studying factors that impact on the maternal role. *Nurs Res.* 1981; 30:73–77.

Milnes AR. Description and epidemiology of nursing caries. *J Public Dent.* 1996;56:38–50.

Moon MA. Studies link gene on chromosome 7 to autism. *Pediatr News.* 2008;42:33.

Morley R et al. Mother's choice to provide breastmilk and developmental outcome. *Arch Dis Child.* 1988;63:1382–1385.

Mortensen EL et al. The association between duration of breastfeeding and adult intelligence. *JAMA.* 2002;287:2365–2371.

Mosko S et al. Infant sleep architecture during bedsharing and possible implications for SIDS. *Sleep.* 1996;19:677–684.

Mosko S et al. Infant arousals in the bedsharing environment: implications for infant sleep development and SIDS. *Pediatrics.* 1997;100:841–849.

Oulis CJ et al. Feeding practices of Greek children with and without nursing caries. *Pediatr Dent.* 1999; 21:409–416.

Owen CG et al. Does breastfeeding influence risk of type 2 diabetes in later life? A quantitative analysis of published evidence. *Am J Clin Nutr.* 2006; 84:1043–1054.

Pabst HF et al. Effect of breast-feeding on immune response to BCG vaccination. *Lancet.* 1989;1(11): 295–296.

Page-Goertz S. Breastfeeding beyond 6 months. *Adv Nurs Pract.* 2002;45–48.

Palmer B. The influence of breastfeeding on the development of the oral cavity: a commentary. *J Hum Lact.* 1998;14:93–98.

Piaget J. *The Origins of Intelligence in Children.* Cook M, trans. New York, NY: International Universities Press; 1952.

Piaget J, Inhelder B. *Psychology of the Child.* New York, NY: Basic Books; 1969.

Pisacane A et al. Iron status in breast-fed infants. *J Pediatr.* 1995;127:429–431.

Pollard K et al. Night-time non-nutritive sucking in infants aged 1 to 5 months: relationship with infant stage, breastfeeding, and bed-sharing versus room-sharing. *Early Hum Dev.* 1999;56:185–204.

Prechtl J, Beintema D. *The Neurological Examination of the Full Term Infant* (child development medical series, 12). Philadelphia, PA: Lippincott; 1975.

Pridham KF, Chang AS. Transition to being the mother of a new infant in the first 3 months: maternal problem solving and self-appraisals. *J Adv Nurs.* 1992; 17:204–216.

Prodromidis M et al. Mothers touching newborns: a comparison of rooming-in versus minimal contact. *Birth.* 1995;22:196–2000.

Randle J. Starting solids. *New Beginnings.* La Leche League International, May-June, 1999.

Rao MR et al. Effect of breastfeeding on cognitive development of infants born small for gestational age. *Acta Paediatr.* 2002;91:267–274.

Rennels MB. Influence of breast-feeding and oral poliovirus vaccine on the immunogenicity and efficacy of rotavirus vaccine. *J Infect Dis.* 1996; 174(suppl 1):S107–S111.

Robertson J. *Young Children in Hospital.* New York, NY: Basic Books; 1958.

Rogan WJ, Gladen BC. Breast-feeding and cognitive development. *Early Hum Dev.* 1993;31:181–193.

Rubin R. Attainment of the maternal role. *Nurs Res.* 1967;16:237, 342.

Saalfield S, Jackson-Allen P. Biopsychosocial consequences of sweetened drink consumption in children 0–6 years of age. *Pediatr Nurs.* 2006;32: 460–461.

Sacker A, Quigley MA, Kelly Y. Breastfeeding and developmental delay: findings from the millennium cohort study. *Pediatrics.* 2006;111:3.

Sanger R, Bystrom E. Breastfeeding: does it affect oral facial growth? *Dent Hygiene.* 1982;56:44–47.

Sears W. *Growing together.* Franklin Park, IL: La Leche League International; 1987:30, 71.

Servonsky J, Opas SR. *Nursing Management of Children.* Boston, MA: Jones and Bartlett; 1987.

Singhal A et al. Infant nutrition and stereoacuity at age 4–6 years. *Am J Clin Nutr.* 2007;85:152–159.

Singhal A, Lanigan J. Breastfeeding, early growth and later obesity. *Obesity Rev.* 2006;8:51–54. http:// www.blackwell-synergy.com. Accessed February 12, 2009.

Slykerman RE et al. Breastfeeding and intelligence of preschool children. *Acta Paediatr.* 2005;94: 832–837.

Smith PJ, Moffatt ME. Baby-bottle decay: Are we on the right track? *Int J Circumpolar Health.* 1998;57(suppl 1): 155–162.

Spitz R. Anaclitic depression. *Psychoanal Study Child.* 1946;2:313–342.

Spitz AS et al. Child temperament and risk factors for early childhood caries. *J Dent Child.* 2006;73(2): 98–104.

Sugarman J, Kendall-Tackett KA. Weaning ages in a sample of American women who practice extended breastfeeding. *Clin Pediatr.* 1995;34:642–647.

Sullivan SA, Birch LL. Infant dietary experience and acceptance of solid foods. *Pediatrics.* 1994;93:271–277.

Tarkka MT. Predictors of maternal competence by first-time mothers when the child is 8 months old. *J Adv Nurs.* 2003;41:233–240.

Temboury MC et al. Influence of breast-feeding on the infant's intellectual development. *J Pediatr Gastroenterol Nutr.* 1994;18:32–36.

Thomas A, Chess S. *Temperament and Development.* New York, NY: Brunner/Mazel; 1977.

Toschke AM et al. Overweight and obesity in 6 to 14 year old Czech children in 1991: protective effect of breast-feeding. *J Pediatr.* 2002;141:764–769.

Trawitzki LV et al. Breastfeeding and deleterious oral habits in mouth and nose breathers. *Rev Bras Otorrinolaringol.* 2005;71:747–751.

Valaitis R et al. A systematic review of the relationships between breastfeeding and early childhood caries. *Can J Pub Health.* 2000;91:411–417.

Van Esterick P. Commentary: an anthropological perspective on infant feeding in Oceania. In: Marshall LB, ed. *Infant Care and Feeding in the South Pacific.* New York, NY: Gordon & Breach Science Publishers; 1985:331–343.

Vesikari T, Glaquinto C, Huppertz H. Clinical trials of rotavirus vaccines in Europe. *Pediatr Infect Dis.* 2006; 25:S42–S47.

Vohr BR et al. Beneficial effects of breast milk in the neonatal intensive care unit on the developmental outcome of extremely low birth weight infants at 18 months of age. *Pediatrics.* 2005;118:e115–e123.

von Kries R et al. Breast feeding and obesity: cross sectional study. *BMJ.* 1999;319:147.

Wang B et al. Sialic acid concentration of brain gangliosides: Variation among eight mammalian species. *Comp Biochem Physiol.* 1998;119:435–439.

Weerheijm KL et al. Prolonged demand breast-feeding and nursing caries. *Caries Res.* 1998;32:46–50.

Welch TR et al. Vitamin D-deficient rickets: the reemergence of a once-conquered disease [editorial]. *J Pediatr.* 2000;137:143–145.

Wigg NR et al. Does breastfeeding at six months predict cognitive development? *Aust N Z J Pub Health.* 1998; 22:232–236.

Willinger M et al. Trends in infant bed sharing in the United States, 1993–2000: the national infant sleep study. *Arch Pediatr Adolesc Med.* 2003;157:43–48.

Wolfe MS. Vaccine for foreign travel. *Pediatr Clin North Am.* 1990;37:757–769.

World Health Organization. Collaborative study group on oral poliovirus vaccine: factors affecting the immunogenicity of oral poliovirus vaccines: a prospective evaluation in Brazil and the Gambia. *J Infect Dis.* 1995;171:1097–1106.

Wrigley EA, Hutchinson SA. Long-term breastfeeding: the secret bond. *J Nur Midwifery.* 1990;35:35–41.

Yoneyama K, Nagata H, Asano H. Growth of Japanese breast-fed and bottle-fed infants from birth to 20 months. *Ann Hum Biol.* 1994;21:597–608.

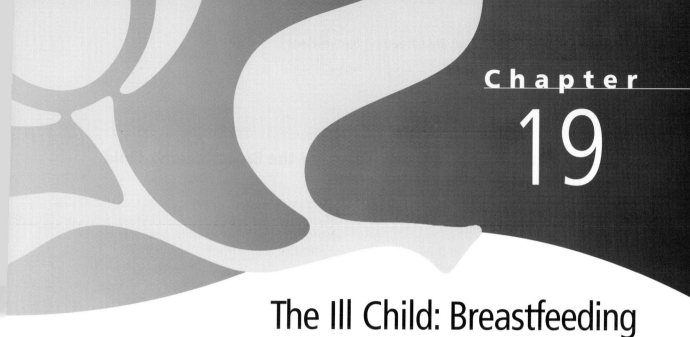

Chapter

19

The Ill Child: Breastfeeding Implications

Sallie Page-Goertz and Jan Riordan

BREASTFEEDING IS MUCH MORE than nutrition—it is comfort and love shared between a mother and her baby. Breastfeeding provides important comfort and security for the baby. Regrettably, babies born with congenital defects are less likely to ever be breastfed (Rendon-Macias et al., 2002). For ill or hospitalized children who have established breastfeeding, the breastfeeding relationship can be threatened. When illness or other health problems makes the breastfeeding relationship difficult or impossible, nurses and other healthcare providers can help families by providing both practical and emotional support and encouragement to establish lactation, facilitate direct breastfeeding when possible, and prevent unnecessary weaning. This chapter presents strategies for helping parents of breastfeeding children who need special breastfeeding support due to health problems beyond the newborn period.

Team Care for the Child with Feeding Difficulties

A variety of healthcare specialists participate in assessment and treatment of a child who has ongoing feeding difficulties. A team might include a physical or occupational therapist, neurologist, developmental medicine specialist, lactation consul-

tant, speech-language pathologist, dentist, social worker, psychologist, and dietitian. Box 19–1 describes the services that each has to offer the child and family. When several people are involved in the child's care, one of them should serve as the coordinator to facilitate communication with the family and the child's primary healthcare provider, and among the health team members themselves. Families will need both verbal and written instructions, and they should be encouraged to perform return demonstrations of recommended feeding techniques. Videotaping the breastfeeding mother and child while teaching special techniques allows the family to have a customized teaching aid.

Feeding Behaviors of the Ill Infant/Child

A child who is not feeling well commonly has a diminished appetite. A nursing infant may feed less vigorously and less often or more frequently but in brief bouts; the magnitude of the change in feeding routine varies with the severity of the illness. The child's condition may impair ability to suckle vigorously or frequently enough to take in sufficient calories to meet requirements for growth. In the face of illness such as congenital heart defect (Ripmeester &

BOX 19–1

Members of the Healthcare Team for the Breastfeeding Child with Special Healthcare Problems

Nurse
Assesses the global needs of child and family
Assists in identification of referral needs
Provides initial assessment of breastfeeding status
Ensures that the healthcare plan is implemented
Provides family education
Provides direct nursing care to the child as needed

Lactation Consultant
Assesses the breastfeeding dyad
Identifies strengths and weaknesses
Identifies referral needs for the child with complex oral-motor difficulties
Develops a breastfeeding plan of care

Physician/Subspecialist
Diagnoses underlying illness/condition
Develops medical plan of care
Refers to other professionals as needed
Refers to neurologist or developmental specialist to assist in evaluation

Physical Therapist
Assesses gross motor capabilities
Develops plan of care to optimize baby's skills

Geneticist/Genetic Counselor
Provides risk counseling related to inherited conditions

Occupational Therapist
Assesses oral-motor/feeding capability as well as fine and gross motor skills as needed
Works with the mother to identify optimal positioning for the baby at breast

If breastfeeding is not possible, helps identify a preferred alternative feeding method
Develops plan of care to optimize baby's skills

Speech-Language Pathologist
Assesses oral-motor/feeding capabilities
May provide similar services to the OT related to oral-motor issues
Develops plan of care to optimize baby's skills

Dietitian
Assesses nutritional status of child
Develops plan of nutrition care
Identifies preferred supplements if needed

Mental Health Therapist
Assists families with the adaptation to a child with acute or chronic healthcare problem

Social Worker
Assesses family's needs for practical and psychosocial support
May provide counseling services

Dunn, 2002), the metabolic needs of the child may increase beyond the normal recommended daily allowances for age and height.

Milk supply may diminish fairly quickly with waning demand. Mothers may have uncomfortable breast fullness if the child is breastfeeding less frequently or effectively. Any time that a baby has diminished appetite or is unable to maintain normal weight gain with direct breastfeeding, the mother must augment breast stimulation by expressing breastmilk by hand or pump (see Chapter 12) to maintain her milk supply and to prevent engorgement. Milk obtained in excess of a baby's immediate need can be stored for use at a later date. Box 19–2 provides milk collection and storage guidelines for the hospitalized infant.

The infant who is unable to feed orally for prolonged periods of time (days or weeks), needs oral stimulation by other means—typically a pacifier, despite the concern that sucking on an artificial teat may create problems in getting the baby back to the breast. Suckling the empty breast is an alternative. The baby who experiences uncomfortable procedures in and around the mouth such as suctioning, intubation, or operative intervention may be reluctant to breastfeed and requires special attention.

Skilled feeding assessment of the child with special healthcare needs is vital. Assessment includes observation of at least one complete breastfeeding and monitoring of the infant's weight in order to determine the adequacy of milk transfer and caloric intake. If the child is not gaining weight normally, the amount of milk ingested is inadequate, regardless of what that amount might be. Even if before- and after-feed weights indicate good intake for age (e.g., 3 oz/90 ml feeding in a 7 pound/3.2 kg infant), this volume may not be adequate for a daily weight gain of 1/2 to 1 oz (15–30 gm), or 1 percent of the child's weight). An ill infant may have well-developed, effective oral-motor skills but may lack the energy to maintain suckling long enough to obtain sufficient calories for normal weight gain, as in the case of complex congenital heart disease.

What to Do If Weight Gain Is Inadequate

If a child is not gaining sufficiently, several strategies can be tried. General strategies will be discussed in this section, and the condition-specific sections will address specific strategies and techniques.

The first suggestion is to simply change the baby's position at the breast. The upright posture shown in Figure 19–1 increases the baby's alertness through stimulation of the vestibular system and may increase breastfeeding vigor. Providing extra support for the baby's cheeks and jaw using the "Dancer" hand position (Figure 19–2) may also help. "Burp and bother" and other techniques are described in Chapter 10. Strategies for helping the child with abnormal tone (see Box 19–5, discussed later in this chapter) are useful for a baby who is neurologically normal but has a weak suckle. Trying to feed a soundly sleeping baby usually results only in frustration for both baby and mother, and it is not recommended. Supplementation with mother's milk, particularly high calorie hindmilk, or calorie-enriched mother's milk may be needed to improve weight gain. For the child with greatly increased metabolic demands, such as the infant with congenital heart disease, continuous or intermittent feeding with higher calorie milk through a nasogastric tube is often necessary to meet the increased caloric requirements for growth (Figure 19–3).

What to Do When Direct Breastfeeding Is Not Sufficient

When a child is incapable of or does not thrive with direct breastfeeding, healthcare providers are faced with two challenges: (1) they must develop a feeding plan that will lead to optimal weight gain, and (2) they must help a family come to a peaceful acceptance of at least a temporary change in their breastfeeding dreams. The health provider can make a difference in how a family comes to view these early experiences with their child. Some will remember brusque interactions and feelings that the provider had no understanding of the important nurturing aspect of breastfeeding. Other families may work with professionals who are so enthusiastic about breastfeeding that they lose sight of the importance of the infant's growth and development, even putting children at risk for severe dehydration or failure to thrive. The fortunate family interacts with professionals who are skilled in feeding assessment, understand the importance of optimal growth, and know when the child needs something different than exclusive or direct breastfeeding—and who can communicate this with sensitivity.

BOX **19–2**

Milk Collection and Storage Guidelines for the Hospitalized Nursling

- Wash hands before initiating milk expression, giving careful attention to fingernails and nail beds.
- A hospital grade electric breast pump is preferred.
- Each mother must use her own collection kit.
- Cleaning collection kits:
  - Take apart the kit.
  - Rinse parts with cool water to remove milk residue.
  - Wash with warm, soapy water, then thoroughly rinse.
  - Air dry on a clean paper towel.
  - Alternatively, rinsed parts can be cleaned in a dishwasher.
  - If water is contaminated, boiled or bottled water must be used for cleaning pump kits.
- Labeling containers:
  - Label with the date of expression, date of freezing, mother and baby's name, and baby's hospital identification number.
- Preparing milk for storage:
  - Storage containers:
    - Use either feeding bottles or food storage containers made of glass, polybutylene plastic, or polypropylene plastic with leak-proof lids.
    - Use of polyethylene bags is associated with up to 60% decrease of the SIgA.
  - Containers do *not* need to be sterile.
  - Store in single feeding portions; aliquots larger than 8 oz should not be used.

- Fill container only 3/4 full to allow room for expansion with freezing.
- Use a new container for each pumping for the hospitalized/ill child.
- Temperature for storage:
  - Refrigerator temperature: 39°F/4°C
  - Freezer temperature: –4°F/–20°C
- No need for bacteriologic screening of milk unless it is donor milk, or if a high-risk infant receiving mother's pumped milk develops sepsis.
- Fresh milk should be used preferentially.
- Otherwise, use "oldest" frozen milk first.
- Storage:
  - Fresh milk—4–6 hours at room temperature
    - Store up to 24 hours at 15°C (cooler with frozen gel packs).
    - Refrigerate for up to 8 days.
    - Freeze up to 12 months at –20°C (milk stored less than 3 months is preferred for the ill/preterm infant).
  - Thawed milk—Refrigerate after thawing, and use within 24 hours.
    - Do *not* leave at room temperature.
    - Do *not* refreeze.
- Once infant has started feeding, any milk remaining in the feeding container is to be discarded.

Source: Adapted from Human Milk Banking Association of North America, 2005.

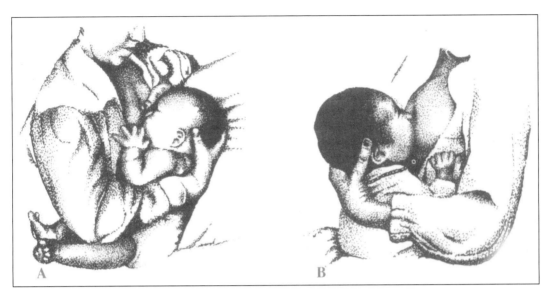

FIGURE **19–1** Upright positioning. Either (A) side sitting, or (B) straddling the mother's thigh may serve to maximize the baby's breastfeeding efficiency.

Source: Provided courtesy of the Cleft Palate Foundation, 1-800-24 CLEFT, http://www.cleftline.org.

When families of children with chronic conditions are interviewed about their experiences, they express appreciation for advice that is straightforward and, most importantly, accurate. Mothers of babies with cleft palate report how frustrating it was to realize that the enthusiasm of the pamphlets and the professionals they spoke to about the possibility of exclusive breastfeeding were in fact extraordinarily misleading (Miller, 1998). These mothers experienced feelings of failure, because their babies did not breastfeed "like the story in the pamphlet." Such pressure often leads to unrealistic, exhausting breastfeeding efforts that undermine the developing relationship between mother and baby.

When it is evident that direct or exclusive breastfeeding is not working, the skilled lactation consultant needs to acknowledge the disappointment a mother may feel. Do point out other strengths that the child has. For example "Look how the baby is watching you." "Isn't it wonderful how she follows your voice?" "What a wonderful snuggler you have." The goal is to reframe what's happening: Mothers and babies aren't breastfeeding failures—rather they're presented with a special challenge. It is also helpful to separate the two components of breastfeeding: the milk (nutrition) and the love (nurture) that happens with breastfeeding. The milk

can continue to be offered, or saved until the baby can have oral feedings; the love continues on without interruption.

Alternative Feeding Methods

Breastfeeding specialists disagree about how to supplement children with special feeding needs. Unfortunately, there is insufficient data upon which to base the majority of recommendations, especially for infants and for children who are failing to thrive owing to a myriad of other underlying health problems or conditions. Lacking such evidence, we base the recommendations presented here on understanding the child's condition, the anatomy and physiology of breastfeeding, the occasional case report, discussions with colleagues, and one's best clinical judgment. Consultation with an occupational therapist, physical therapist, and speech-language pathologist, as well as a dietitian, should be considered when working with a child who is not thriving with direct breastfeeding. These professionals provide valuable input into the assessment of how a particular child's strengths and weaknesses determine a plan of care that will optimize feeding and growth. If the child is not taking in sufficient volume of the mother's milk to thrive, the dietitian

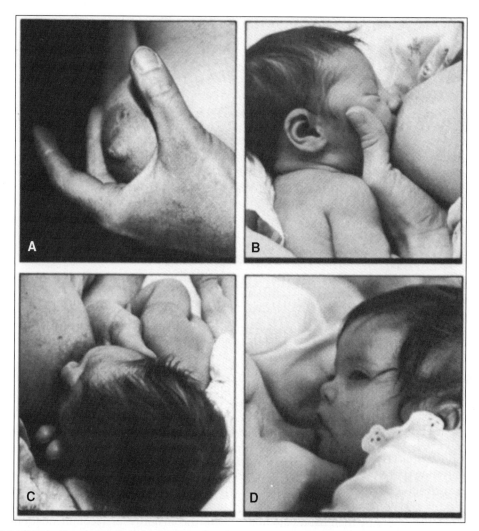

FIGURE 19–2   Dancer-hand support. Dancer-hand positioning provides stability to the baby's jaw and support to weak masseter muscles. (A) The hand under the breast slides forward so that the breast is supported by three fingers rather than four. A "U" is formed with thumb and index finger. (B) The baby's head rests in the U where the jaw is supported, and cheeks are gently squeezed. (C) View from over the mother's shoulder shows how the hand supports both the mother's breast and the baby's head. (D) A modified dancer-hand position can provide just chin support, with the index finger applying pressure behind the mandible to support the tongue.

Source: © Childbirth Graphics Ltd., Rochester, NY.

provides input as to the preferred way to enrich the caloric content of the milk. Hindmilk or the addition of carbohydrate, fat, and/or protein supplements to breastmilk may be preferred, depending on the particular child's health condition.

Replacement feeding methods and supplementation devices such as cup, finger, and syringe feeding are discussed in detail in Chapters 7 and 10.

Although a supplementation device is suitable for a prolonged period, the infant must be able to generate sufficient negative intraoral pressure to pull milk from the device. If the reservoir of the device is flexible, the mother can squeeze it so that a bolus of milk goes directly into the child's mouth and normal suckling skills may not be needed to accomplish sufficient intake. If the baby can latch

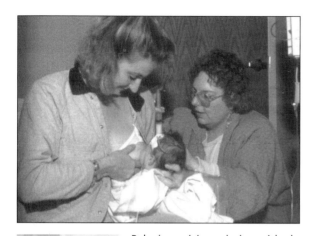

onto the breast, supplementing at the breast is always the preferred way to provide extra calories. If the child is unable to gain adequate weight, other feeding methods need to be explored. Neither cup, or finger, or syringe feeding is conducive to long-term provision of large volumes of milk. Dowling et al. (2002) found that with cup-feeding, volumes of milk ingested were small and about one third of the amount taken from the cup was recovered on the bib.

For some children, bottle-feeding may be the best alternative feeding method. The feeding bottle can be used in ways that help develop or mimic breastfeeding skills (Kassing, 2002; Noble & Bovey, 1997). Gromada and Sandora (2007) describe "paced feeding" techniques, an approach to bottle-feeding that assures that the baby's feeding cues are respected and that milk flow does not overwhelm the infant. The feeding bottle is held horizontally to reduce speed of flow. When baby exhibits stress cues, the baby is allowed to rest briefly, either by removing the nipple from the mouth or leaving the nipple in place, but tipping the baby forward so that milk cannot flow into the mouth. A squeezable bottle allows the caregiver to deliver a milk bolus into the baby's oral pharynx for swallowing, even when the baby is unable to generate negative intraoral pressure to accomplish milk flow. Higher volumes of milk or

normal volumes of calorie-enriched milk can be provided to maximize weight gain for many children who are not thriving with direct breastfeeding.

Choice of feeding bottle and teat depends on a particular infant's need. Some children will be successful with a standard baby bottle—a firm reservoir with a variety of teats. Figure 19–4 illustrates one such bottle, which has a teat with a very wide base that encourages a wide-open latch. In general, it is best to select a wide-based teat that encourages latch with a wide-open mouth, that has a soft texture like the breast, and that has a nipple length that goes deep into the child's mouth but does not cause the child to gag. Longer teats may be helpful for the child with cleft lip/palate to avoid milk going directly into the cleft. Bottles that have been recommended for children who are not thriving with direct breastfeeding or use of a traditional feeding bottle include the Haberman feeder and the Mead-Johnson cleft palate feeder (Figure 19–5). Each of these bottles has a flexible reservoir allowing the caregiver to release a bolus of milk into the child's mouth. The Haberman has a specially designed valve and teat that allows the feeder to adjust milk flow to suit the baby's needs. There is a slit in the nipple, rather than a hole, which closes when the baby is not compressing/sucking the teat, preventing the flow of an unexpected bolus of milk into the mouth. The Pigeon nipple (Figure 19–6) has a flow valve that reduces the amount of negative intraoral pressure needed for milk transfer, similar to the Haberman feeder; the Pigeon nipple is softer and more flexible. It can be used on any standard infant feeding bottle. Fadavi et al. (1997) found that the Playtex nipple set flowed faster with less negative pressure and thus represented an increase in risk of choking and decreased oxygenation because of interrupted breathing patterns, particularly in hypotonic and preterm babies.

The baby can be fed with a bottle in ways to maximize closeness that naturally occurs with breastfeeding. Mothers and children need to be comfortable; babies can be skin to skin with their mothers or other caregivers during feeding. Eye contact, singing, and reading of stories are not precluded with bottle-feeding. Families should be taught to alternate holding the baby in the left and right arms to provide equal visual stimulation, as normally happens with breastfeeding. When

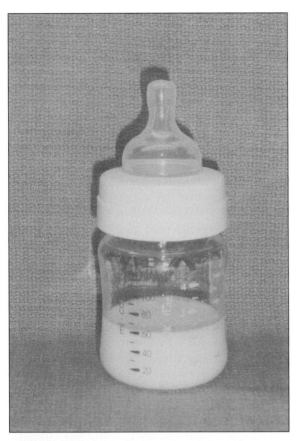

FIGURE 19–4   The Avent bottle has a wide-based teat to encourage a wide-open mouth.

Source: Courtesy of Sallie Page-Goertz.

presenting the bottle to the baby, touch the lips to stimulate root/gape, and if possible, allow the baby to draw the teat deeply into the oral cavity. If the baby is unable to draw in sufficient milk to form a bolus to stimulate swallowing, use a flexible bottle, or feeders using nurser bags to squeeze intermittent small boluses into the baby's pharynx for swallowing.

If bottle-feeding, even with calorie-enriched milk, is not sufficient for improving weight gain, more invasive feeding methods must be considered. Nasogastric feeding with a feeding tube, either by bolus or continuous drip for part or all of the day with regular or enriched milk, may need to be added to breast- or bottle-feedings. If oral feedings are not possible, enteral feedings can be given via gastrostomy or jejeunostomy tube.

Pain Management Concerns

Children with acquired or congenital conditions may be faced with pain related to their illness, surgery, or other procedures. Breastfeeding needs to be considered in the armamentarium of strategies for assisting with procedural pain. Infants breastfed during painful procedures have less pain. A Cochrane review evaluated the effectiveness of breastfeeding in reducing procedural pain such as immunizations and heel sticks for blood sampling. Infants breastfed during such procedures had greater reductions in heart rate, duration of crying, and lower pain scores than did infants who were not breastfed during the procedure (Shah et al., 2006). However, it is not known to what extent breastfeeding might contribute to alleviating other types of pain.

Care of the Hospitalized Breastfeeding Infant/Child

Hospitalization—whether it is planned or an emergency—disrupts family equilibrium. Unexpected admission to a pediatric intensive care unit of a previously healthy child causes parents to be near a panic level of anxiety (Huckabay & Tilem-Kessler, 1999). Parents find that the hospital setting presents uncertain boundaries regarding their roles and responsibilities for their own children. Tomlinson, Swiggum, and Harbaugh (1999) found that these uncertainties were lessened in an environment where the child was treated as a normal child and where the parent was free to continue to provide comfort care. Melnyk et al. (2004) implemented an educational behavioral intervention program within hours of PICU admission that taught families what specific behaviors to expect from their critically ill child and how to respond. Mothers and children in the treatment group demonstrated better outcomes than the group who did not receive the intervention.

The goal for the hospitalized infant or child is to minimize disruption of normal routine. A secondary goal is to maintain and strengthen family unity. Families of breastfeeding children have a unique set of needs. Box 19–3 lists key characteristics of breastfeeding-friendly pediatric units. The stress of dealing with an ill child, perhaps hospitalization,

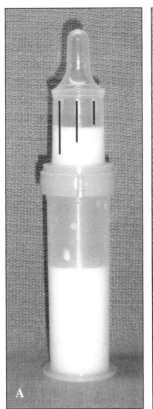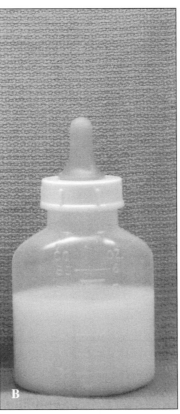

FIGURE 19–5   Bottles recommended for children not thriving with direct breastfeeding. (A) The Haberman feeder allows the caregiver to adjust the flow for the baby by aligning the marks with the baby's nose—the longer line provides greater flow. The one-way valve limits the negative pressure required to withdraw milk, and the flexible nipple reservoir allows the caregiver to squeeze a bolus of milk into the baby's mouth. (B) The Mead-Johnson cleft palate feeder has a flexible reservoir allowing the caregiver to squeeze milk into the baby's mouth. The nipple is somewhat flattened and long so that milk can be released well into the baby's oral cavity.

Source: Courtesy of Sallie Page-Goertz.

and unexpected diagnoses makes intake of new information challenging for family members. Popper (1998) relates that families appreciate having a customized folder containing helpful information regarding the child's condition. Contents might include specific information about the child's illness and medications, breastfeeding tips, support group contacts, and the names of healthcare team members. They can also include important family contact information, self-adhesive notes to use for communicating to staff when family members are away from the bedside, and blank paper to jot down questions or concerns for the healthcare team. The AAP breastfeeding policy statement includes a recommendation related to support of breastfeeding

should hospitalization be necessary (Section on Breastfeeding, 2005). For the child who is breastfed, feeding and nurturing patterns should approximate as closely as possible the normal home situation. Only by acquiring information can personalized and individualized care be given to families. Box 19–4 lists elements of the admission history that focus on breastfeeding issues. If the breastfeeding child is old enough to talk, the family may use a "code" word for breastfeeding, such as *nummies, yum-yum, nursie, snugglies, night-night,* or *side.* Acceptance of the normalcy of a walking and talking child who breastfeeds is discussed in Chapter 24.

If the infant is not feeding effectively, the hospital will ideally provide the mother with access to a

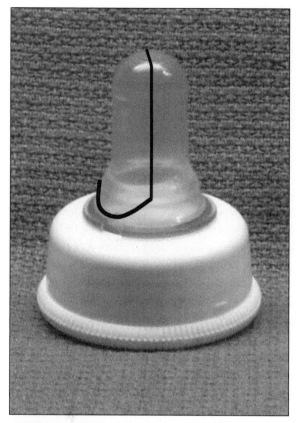

FIGURE 19-6 The Pigeon nipple has a one-way valve that decreases the amount of negative pressure required to withdraw milk. The outlined area of the nipple is slightly firmer and is positioned against the roof of the mouth.

Source: Courtesy of Sallie Page-Goertz.

hospital-grade electric pump and the maternal attachments that allow for dual collection, to maximize effectiveness of milk expression. Healthcare workers should assist mothers in initiating milk expression as soon as it is noted that the infant's suckling abilities are not sufficient to maintain weight or when oral feedings are not possible. Mothers may initially need assistance in negotiating any monitoring or therapeutic paraphernalia that is attached to her baby as she puts the child to breast (Figure 19-7).

Spatz (2006) provides a clinical pathway designed to protect breastfeeding in the hospitalized infant, targeted at the readmitted newborn infant with complications of ineffective breastfeeding. This can serve the bedside nurse as a guide for providing evidence-based patient care. It calls for breastfeeding assessment, use of before- and after-breastfeeding test weights, steps to assist women to increase their milk supply, and calls for development of an alternative feeding plan for babies unable to take sufficient volume/calories.

Home from the Hospital: The Rebound Effect

The child's reactions following hospitalization depend on the extent of trauma that has been experienced and the availability of coping mechanisms for self-protection. Almost all hospitals now encourage a parent to stay with the child during hospitalization. When parents room-in with the child, very few behavior changes occur on returning home. The young child who has experienced a painful separation may withdraw as a coping strategy, refusing to breastfeed and showing little interest in family members. The baby may cry a great deal and want to be held and breastfed exceptionally often, vigorously protesting having the mother out of sight for even a moment. For toddlers, emotional upheaval, including nightmares and insomnia, is common in the first few weeks following hospitalization. Helping parents to recognize their child's normal response to the stress of hospitalization, and how to ameliorate their distress is a critical element of comprehensive nursing care.

Perioperative Care of the Breastfeeding Infant/Child

Perioperative issues include the preoperative fasting period and postoperative recovery. The purpose of fasting is to avoid pulmonary aspiration. The fasting period should be as short as physiologically appropriate for reducing anesthesia risk due to aspiration, risk of dehydration, and risk of hypoglycemia. Cook-Sather and Litman (2006) report that the risk of aspiration in infants less than 6 months of age is 3:9266, using the "liberalized" fasting guidelines published in 1999 by the American Society of Anesthesiologists (ASA). These guidelines are as follows: clear liquids—2 hours; breastmilk—4 hours; formula, other nonhuman

---

BOX 19–3

Characteristics of a Breastfeeding-Friendly Pediatric Unit

- Has written breastfeeding policies in place.
- Employs or trains staff capable of skilled breastfeeding assessment and breastfeeding intervention when needed.
- Provides parents with written and verbal information about the benefits of breastfeeding and breastmilk.
- Facilitates unrestricted breastfeeding.
- Facilitates milk expression by mothers who wish to provide milk for infants who are unable to breastfeed. The following services should be available:
  - Breast pump and privacy for pumping.
  - Storage place for expressed milk.
  - Referral to lactation services and pump rental sources if needed.
- Provides breastfed children only age-appropriate or medically indicated supplementation of food or drink.

- Uses alternative feeding methods most conducive to successful breastfeeding and appropriate weight gain.
- Provides 24-hour rooming-in of parents and their children.
- Provides meals and snacks for the breastfeeding mother.
- Plans medication schedule and procedures to avoid interfering with the breastfeeding relationship.
- Provides information about breastfeeding support available in the hospital and the community.
- Assesses compliance with policies through quality assurance activities and research.

Source: Adapted from Minchin et al., 1996 and Popper, 1998.

---

milks, or light meal—6 hours; full meal—8 hours (American Society of Anesthesiologists, 1999). The preoperative patient who is breastfeeding does *not* need to be NPO (nothing by oral route) for as long as the formula-fed infant because human milk is digested more quickly. Kosko's meta-analysis summary states that for the infant at low risk for aspiration, there is no reason not to offer ad lib clear fluids until 2 hours prior to surgery, and that there is insufficient data to comment on what period is safe for offering milk feedings, or what period might be appropriate for high-risk infants (2006). Although some feel even shorter fasting periods for breastfeeding infants are safe, Lawrence (2005) reviewed current research and concurs with the

1999 ASA guidelines that fasting for breastfed infants should be 4 hours. A baby can be offered ad libitum clear fluids up to 2 hours before surgery according to current guidelines.

Separation of child and family should be minimized to reduce stress on all. Anticipating ways to comfort a distressed breastfeeding baby during the fasting period is important. If another family member can be with the baby, rather than the mother, this may reduce the child's desire for breastfeeding. A pacifier can be offered as well as a clear-liquid feeding up to 2 hours preoperatively. Following surgery, breastfeeding should resume as soon as the physician indicates oral feeds can safely begin. There is no need for a first glucose-water feeding.

BOX **19–4**

Admission History for the Breastfeeding Patient

- Usual feeding routine
  - Frequency of breastfeeding
  - Length of breastfeeding
  - Behavior of the baby during and after feeding
  - Special equipment needs
  - Preferred positioning for feedings
  - Special words for breastfeeding
  - If parent not present, preferred alternative feeding method

- Use of supplements
  - How much is given per feeding and during a 24-hour period?
  - What is used for supplementation?

- How is it given?
- When is it given?

- Use of herbal or other complementary therapies for mother or baby
- Solid foods
  - Preferred foods
  - Schedule for solid foods

- Recent changes in feeding routine
- Recent changes in weight gain
- Other approaches to feeding that have been used
- Solitary or cosleeper

The mother may need to express milk until her infant is ready to resume breastfeeding.

Emergency Room

Nurses in the emergency room environment face the need to respond with split-second reactions and require a thorough background in a wide range of areas. Often, emergency room providers do not have basic knowledge regarding breastfeeding. We are frequently told of situations where mothers were counseled to suspend or stop breastfeeding when there was in fact no medical indication to do so. For example, when the child presents with gastroenteritis, typical advice is to suspend all milk feedings and begin an oral electrolyte solution, as the physicians may be unaware that guidelines recommend continuation of breastfeeding during diarrheal illness. Or, a newborn with hematemesis (bloody vomit) is given an invasive gastrointestinal workup before someone thinks to ask if the mother's nipples are sore and bleeding. Or a breastfeeding mother is prescribed pain medication or antibiotic and told that

she needs to stop breastfeeding to protect the baby. Having a nurse in the emergency room who is aware of breastfeeding management concerns for the ill child or mother may prevent inappropriate treatment or unnecessary interruption of breastfeeding.

Care of Children with Selected Conditions

Infection

Numerous research studies demonstrate that breastfeeding—even short-term, nonexclusive breastfeeding—reduces the risk of a variety of infections, both minor and major (Ip et al., 2006). Protection from infection is afforded in a dose-response manner—the greater the dose, the greater the protection (Raisler, Alexander, & O'Campo, 1999; Scariati, Grummer-Strawn, & Fein, 1997). The reduction in risk is most dramatic in resource-poor countries, but it is also significant in developed countries. Nonetheless, any child may

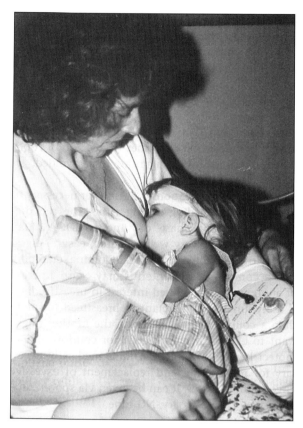

FIGURE **19–7** Breastfeeding with intravenous infusion. Mother may need some help negotiating the baby's equipment at first so baby can settle into the comfort of breastfeeding.

Source: Courtesy of Debi Leslie Bocar.

experience infection at some point during the breastfeeding period. Breastfed children lose less weight during an infectious illness and are less likely to require hospitalization than if they are not breastfed. Lopez-Alarcon et al. (2004) postulate that DHA in human milk contributes to the decreased anorectic response of breastfed infants who have infection. There is no reason to interrupt breastfeeding during infectious illnesses. However, the infant occasionally may be so severely ill that feeding capability is temporarily impaired. In these situations, the mother can express her breastmilk and save it until the baby resumes breastfeeding. Expressed milk can be provided to the child via nasogastric feeding when appropriate or stored for use at a later date.

Gastroenteritis

Gastroenteritis is caused by a number of viral and bacterial pathogens. Symptoms include vomiting, diarrhea, fever, anorexia, and fussiness presumably due to nausea and abdominal cramping. Sometimes new parents mistakenly believe that the normally loose breastmilk stools they observe in their newborn or the normal spitting up that babies do are signs of illness. (The emergency room physician might think so as well!) Viral gastroenteritis is responsible for more than 1.5–2.5 million deaths annually worldwide, primarily in resource-poor areas; in the United States it is estimated that there are about 300 deaths and 200,000 hospitalizations for treatment of dehydration (Iovino, 2003; Centers for Disease Control [CDC], 2003). In the United States, rotavirus gastroenteritis infection, the most common cause of gastroenteritis, leads to an estimated 500,000 office or emergency room visits and 50,000 hospitalizations. Breastfeeding is associated with reduced hospitalization, with exclusive breastfeeding to 6 months providing the most potent benefit (Quigley, 2007). Risk factors for hospitalization for rotavirus infection in US children include lack of breastfeeding, day care attendance, siblings in the home, and economic disadvantage (Dennehy, 2006). Rotavirus vaccine is now available to reduce incidence and severity of rotavirus-associated gastroenteritis.

The acute danger with gastroenteritis is dehydration when the infant takes in less fluid than is lost through vomiting and diarrhea. With repeated gastrointestinal infections, the child also risks becoming chronically malnourished, increasing the probability of significant morbidity and mortality from other causes. Infants are at greater risk for dehydration than older children or adults due to increased body surface area and therefore greater evaporative losses. Diarrhea and vomiting can also result in electrolyte imbalance caused by the losses of sodium and potassium. Electrolyte imbalance may be more severe if families have been supplementing with either high-sodium fluids, such as broth, or very low-sodium fluids such as water or soda pop, transforming a straightforward isotonic dehydration to a more complex hypotonic or hypertonic dehydration (Eliason & Lewan, 1998).

Assessment and management of the child with gastroenteritis should follow the CDC guidelines for

---

BOX 19–7

Interventions for the Infant with Symptomatic Gastroesophageal Reflux

- Feed the baby in a more upright position, avoiding abdominal compression.
- Use one breast per feeding to reduce the volume of each feeding and increase access to higher calorie hindmilk.
- Feed more frequently.
- Elevate the bed to a 30 to 45 degree angle. (A baby who is sleeping on the parent's chest is in this position.)
- Avoid placing child in an infant seat or car seat after feedings. This compresses the stomach, increasing reflux episodes.

- Avoid using cereal to thicken feedings, a commonly advised treatment that does not help (Bailey et al., 1987).
- Avoid prone positioning for sleep. Due to the association with increased risk of SIDS, this is not recommended by pediatric gastroenterologists (GER Guidelines Committee, 2001).
- Left-lateral positioning significantly reduces reflux frequency and duration (Tobin et al., 1997; Ewer, James, & Tobin, 1999).

---

laparoscopic techniques (Aspelund & Langer, 2007). Feeding resumes once the infant has recovered from anesthesia. Vomiting may occur irrespective of post-op feeding regimen, and families need to know to expect this (Adibe et al., 2007).

Breastfeeding Implications. Lactation consultants should have PS on their list of concerns for any baby that they see who is struggling with weight gain and is spitting up—remembering there are lots of causes for vomiting in infants in addition to GER. Ad libitum breastfeeding once the child has recovered from anesthesia is safe (Adibe et al., 2007), decreases length of hospital stay, and saves an average of $400 per patient compared to a more lengthy fasting period with incremental feedings (Garza et al., 2002). Mothers will need to express their milk for the few feeds that are missed during the perioperative period.

Chylothorax

Chylothorax occurs when the lymphatic system is obstructed due to congenital anomalies in the development of the lymphatic system, or sec-

ondary to traumatic injury as a complication of thoracic surgery (Helin et al., 2006). Chylous fluid accumulates in the chest cavity. This fluid is formed of lymph and fat cells secreted from the intestine. Management includes drainage of the chest cavity via chest tubes, as well as dietary management including low-fat, high-protein oral feedings using special formulas with medium-chain triglycerides, or total parenteral nutrition. Ocreotide is the only medication that may hasten the resolution of a chylothorax. It reduces lymph fluid production by a number of mechanisms, including decreasing the volume of gastric, pancreatic, and biliary secretions so that the volume and protein content of fluid within the thoracic duct is reduced (Helin, 2006). Pediatric use of ocreotide is limited; however, it is reported to reduce the number of days of chylous effusion and to have a low side effect profile.

Breastfeeding Implications. Until recently, human milk was not given to infants with chylothorax because of its high long-chain fatty acid content. However, in an initial case report, Whitehouse

(2003) described how a mother of a baby with chylothorax discovered that by centrifuging her breastmilk she was able to skim off the fat to obtain low-fat breastmilk for her baby. The child began to thrive and is 3 years old at this writing. Recently, Chan and Lechtenberg (2007) reported the successful use of fat-free human milk in seven infants with chylous pleural effusion. The fat portion of the milk was skimmed off using a special centrifuging technique. The skim human milk then must be supplemented with calories, fats, and fat-soluble vitamins under the guidance of a pediatric dietician. Once the drainage ceases, the baby will eventually be able to receive unaltered breastmilk/breastfeeding.

Imperforate Anus

Imperforate anus ranges from no opening at all to a normal-appearing rectum that ends in a blind rectal pouch just above the opening. Presence of an imperforate anus is confirmed only by careful examination and by a diagnostic x-ray examination. As with EA/TEF, there is an association of a number of other VACTERL defects. Thus careful examination of the baby is critical to establish the presence of associated anomalies. Depending on the severity of the defect, anal reconstruction may be done in the immediate newborn period. More commonly, a three-step approach is required—colostomy, anal reconstruction, and colostomy reversal (Sydorak, 2002). After colostomy placement surgery, feeding can begin as soon as bowel sounds are present—usually within 24 hours. When the colostomy is reversed, enteral feedings are suspended for 4 to 7 days—until nasogastric tube drainage is clear, and the child begins passing gastric secretions from the anus.

Breastfeeding Implications. The baby cannot have enteral feedings until there is either a reconstructed anus or a functioning colostomy. Parenteral nutrition is usually required for a period of time both pre- and postoperatively. Mothers will need to express their milk until the child can have oral feedings. The normally loose stools of the breastfed infant lessen the risk of constipation with subsequent breakdown of the surgical area and local infection.

Metabolic Dysfunction

More than 100 metabolic diseases can be detected in infancy. Diseases for which screening is performed vary from region to region, based in part on ethnic, financial, and political issues. Newborn screening for phenylketonuria (PKU) and congenital hypothyroidism is done in all 50 US states and in most western countries (Clague & Thomas, 2002). Other metabolic disorders for which screening is commonly performed include galactosemia, amino and organic acidemias, and cystic fibrosis. Private companies now make extensive newborn screening available directly to parents. Other acquired metabolic conditions such as diabetes are not screened for in the newborn period and may not become symptomatic until much later in infancy or childhood.

Rare Amino and Organic Acidemias

With the exception of PKU and galactosemia, there is very limited information regarding breastfeeding in the rare inborn metabolic diseases (IMD). PKU is the only disorder for which there are consensus guidelines for including breastfeeding as part of the child's diet. Dietary control is critical in order to reduce the risk of the devastating permanent consequences of these disorders. Gokcay et al. (2006) report on a handful of infants with a variety of organic acidemias. Babies who received breastfeeding had fewer infections, metabolic episodes, and hospital admissions related to their metabolic disease. MacDonald et al. (2006) surveyed IMD centers worldwide regarding their experience with breastfeeding for their patients. Breastfeeding, in combination with special complementary formulas, was reportedly successful in a very small number of children with a variety of inborn errors of metabolism. Exclusive breastfeeding is rarely safe for children with these disorders. However, combination of breastfeeding with a specifically prescribed formula can be accomplished and is recommended by some (MacDonald et al., 2006; Gokcay et al., 2006). When a decision is made to include breastmilk in the diet, more frequent monitoring of clinical parameters and biochemistry is required. Huner et al. (2005) report on a small group of children with a variety of inborn errors of metabolism. Not all of these children fared well with breastmilk as part of their diet, experiencing more frequent metabolic crises. Parents will need help to balance the risk and benefits of including breastmilk as part of their baby's diet if this can be done safely. If one is providing support for a family, close collaboration with the medical team is a must to avoid metabolic crises.

Phenylketonuria

Phenylketonuria (PKU) is an autosomal recessive inherited metabolic disorder of phenylalanine (PHE) metabolism. A defect in the enzyme phenylalanine hydroxylase decreases conversion of phenylalanine to tyrosine. Abnormal metabolites accumulate in blood and tissues, including the brain, interfering with central nervous system development. To prevent brain damage, the amount of dietary PHE must be strictly limited, beginning in the first days of life. Delay in dietary treatment is associated with developmental problems. PHE blood levels are monitored very closely, with adjustment of the diet accordingly. Current research concerns include the risk of micronutrient deficiency in children who are on the prescribed PKU diet; therefore, assessment of the effects of supplementation with specific nutrients is underway (Giovannini et al., 2007). Current thinking is that it is best to be on a special PKU diet for life.

Breastfeeding Implications.   Human milk has lower levels of PHE than does any commercial infant formula. Infants with PKU who are breastfed, along with special low-PHE or PHE-free formula have significantly higher intelligence quotient scores—a 12.9-point advantage even after adjusting for social and maternal education status (Riva et al., 1996). Breastfed infants who receive a daily amount of 362 ml (first month) to 464 ml (fourth month) of breastmilk each day, in addition to supplemental PHE-free formula, have a lower PHE intake than do infants who are fed exclusively on low-PHE formula during their first 6 months of life (McCabe et al., 1989). Thus fluctuations in the volume of breastmilk the baby takes are less worrisome than in formulas with higher PHE levels.

The lactation consultant needs to work closely with a physician and dietician who specialize in metabolic disorders to manage the dietary plan for the infant with PKU. In the United States, there is at least one medical center in each state designated to serve as a consultant and treatment facility for metabolic defects, including PKU (Duncan & Elder, 1997).

Breastfeeding along with supplemental use of PHE-free formula is prescribed. There are a number of approaches to manipulating the child's diet to maintain the low PHE levels required for normal brain development. Recommendations for incorporating breastfeeding into a PKU diet include weighing of infants before and after breastfeeding to ensure correct dietary intake, a time-consuming task that may not be accurate. Greve et al. (1994) developed a less cumbersome method of calculating the low-PHE dietary prescription (see Box 19–8). The child's healthcare provider uses this information to calculate the daily amount of PHE-free formula that is needed to keep PHE at the appropriate level. The child receives the prescribed amount of PHE-free formula, along with breastfeeding. The PHE-free formula can be provided either via supplementer at the breast or with some other alternative method prior to breastfeeding. In 2003, van Rijn et al. reported on a series of nine infants fed with alternating breastfeeds and PKU formula-feeds. With each feeding, the baby was allowed to feed to satiety. Outcomes of these infants were compared with infants who only had formula-feeding. There were no differences in growth or PHE levels between the groups. Women who have PKU should be on a diet prior to conception and throughout the pregnancy to reduce the chances of harming the developing fetus. Fox-Bacon et al. (1997) reported on the PHE levels in milk of identical twins with PKU breastfeeding women, and the PHE status of their infants. They found that high maternal PHE serum levels and high milk PHE levels did not result in abnormal PHE levels in their breastfeeding infants who did not have PKU.

Galactosemia

Galactosemia, a disorder of the metabolism of galactose-1-phosphate that is transmitted as an autosomal recessive trait, occurs in only one in about every 60,000 to 80,000 births. The liver enzyme that changes galactose to glucose is absent and as a result, the infant is unable to metabolize lactose. Any intake of galactose results in liver dysfunction. These infants appear normal at birth but soon start having feeding

BOX 19–8

Calculating Breastmilk and PHE-Free Formula Intake for the Infant with PKU

Given: Maximum phenylalanine (PHE) intake allowed is 25 to 45 mg/kg/day depending on the age of the infant. Mature breastmilk has .41 mg/ml PHE.

Calculate the amount of PHE-free formula supplementation for the breastfed baby:

1. Find the estimated volume of daily milk intake in ml (110 kcal/kg/day):
   (Infant weight in kg) times 110 = total calories/day
   (Total calories) divided by 20 = total number of oz/day
   (Total number of oz) times 30 = total volume in ml/day

2. Calculate the maximum allowable PHE/day (breastmilk has 0.41 mg PHE/ml):
   45 mg times infant weight in kg = total number of mg PHE allowed
   Total mg divided by .41 = total volume in ml of breastmilk allowed

3. Calculate amount of replacement PHE-free formula required:
   Total daily volume minus maximum volume allowed = amount of replacement feeding needed

Below are the calculations for a 4.0 kg infant:

1. Estimate volume of daily intake in ml:
   110 kcal times 4.0 = 440 calories
   440 divided by 20 = 22 oz
   22 oz times 30 = 660 ml

2. Calculate maximum allowable breastmilk/24 hours:

45 mg times 4.0 kg = 180 mg PHE maximum per day
180 times 0.41 = 439 ml of breastmilk

3. Calculate amount of PHE-free replacement feedings needed in order for infant to not drink more breastmilk than allowed:
   660 ml minus 439 ml = 221 ml replacement PHE-free formula required daily

The PHE-free formula can be given via a nursing supplementer during breastfeeds or with a bottle prior to breastfeeding. The total daily amount needed can be divided into several aliquots. For example, the baby above needs about 220 ml/day of PHE-free formula. This could be given in 30 ml aliquots with each breastfeeding for 8 feedings. The PHE-free formula should be offered prior to the breastfeeding, or along with the breastfeeding using a supplementer, rather than being offered after the breastfeeding.

difficulties. Other symptoms include vomiting, poor weight gain, jaundice, hepatosplenomegaly, and bleeding. Without treatment, liver failure and mental retardation follow. Untreated galactosemia leads to fatal liver disease. Treatment within the first 10 days of life is associated with the best neurodevelopmental outcomes.

Breastfeeding Implications. Abrupt weaning is necessary due to the galactose content of human milk. Avoidance of all galactose is required to prevent irreversible damage to the infant. Positive newborn screening tests are not always accurate, so results should be confirmed before recommending that women stop expressing milk while awaiting confirmation. Nurses and lactation consultants working with babies that have jaundice and poor weight gain need to remember to check newborn screening results, as galactosemia as well as congenital hypothyroidism can also cause these symptoms. If the diagnosis is confirmed, the mother will need instruction for relief of engorgement as well as emotional support for the loss of the breastfeeding relationship (see Box 19–9).

It is safe for women who have galactosemia to breastfeed. A case study reported that although the mother had galactosemia, her milk was normal in nearly all respects; her baby thrived on exclusive breastfeeding for 5 months and continued to breastfeed while receiving solids thereafter (Forbes et al., 1988).

Congenital Hypothyroidism

Congenital hypothyroidism (CH) is caused by a lack of thyroid secretion, either because the thyroid gland is absent or because there is an inborn enzymatic deficiency in the synthesis of thyroxine. Routine screening results show that congenital hypothyroidism occurs in one of every 3500 births (VanVliet, 2001). A transient form of hypothyroidism can occur from transfer in utero or during breastfeeding of antithyroid drugs or topical application of povidone-iodine on the mother at the time of delivery (Bartalena et al., 2001; Casteels, Punt, & Bramswig, 2000). Prompt treatment is required to prevent irreversible developmental delay and growth problems. Hypothyroidism is rarely diagnosed based on clinical findings in the early weeks—yet this is

when the child is most vulnerable to irreversible brain damage. In the early weeks, parents of an untreated infant may praise their "good baby" because he cries so little. Without treatment, the symptoms of hypothyroidism become noticeable in 3 to 6 months: coarse, brittle hair; anemia; a large, protruding tongue; a wide forehead; and lack of skeletal growth. Untreated cases result in severe mental retardation. Treatment for congenital hypothyroidism is daily thyroid replacement for life. Blood levels are monitored periodically to adjust the dose as the child grows. Synthetic levothyroxine sodium (Synthroid or Levothyroid) is usually given.

Breastfeeding Implications. Lactation consultants involved with newborns who are jaundiced or not thriving need to make sure that neonatal thyroid screening results are normal—as nonspecific early symptoms of CH may include feeding difficulties and hyperbilirubinemia.

Type I Diabetes

The delayed exposure to cow's milk protein provided with exclusive breastfeeding may reduce incidence of type I diabetes in the at-risk individual (Kimpimaki et al., 2001). It is very unusual for the onset of type I diabetes to occur during infancy. Diabetes management for the infant and toddler is challenging as feeding schedules and activity level are not predictable, and the child is not able to communicate symptoms of low blood glucose to parents or caregivers. This increases the risk of severe hypoglycemia, which could result in coma, seizures, and subsequent learning and behavioral disorders. Target blood sugars are in the range of 100 to 200 mg/dL (5.56 to 11.11 mmol/L). Insulin administration is tailored to the child's feeding schedule—usually given 2 to 4 times per day. Insulin doses are quite low. Berhe et al. (2006) reported the effective use of insulin pumps in the diabetic management of toddlers and young children. The children had improved hemoglobin A_{1c} levels, and fewer episodes of hypoglycemia, and parents felt much more confident in their ability to manage their child's diabetes.

Breastfeeding Implications. No research has been found that discusses breastfeeding and management of the infant with diabetes; however, the most

BOX 19–9

A Mother's Guide to Saying Goodbye to Breastfeeding/Milk Expression

- When the time comes to stop breast-feeding or milk expression, you may have very mixed emotions. The following are all normal responses when saying goodbye to breastfeeding.
  - If you are not ready to give up breastfeeding or the hope for a breastfeeding relationship, you may feel regret or sadness.
  - If you are so tired, you may feel a bit glad that the time committed to milk expression is available for other demands.
  - You may be glad to have your body back to yourself, but you may feel guilty that you have those feelings.
  - Your hormones will also be changing, and that may affect your mood.
- As you stop breastfeeding/milk expression, you can express a small amount of milk to make you com-fortable. This will keep your breasts from being uncomfortably full, and reduce your risk of developing a breast infection.
- A firm, but not tight, bra may provide comfort.
- Cold compresses may be soothing, and pain medication such as aceta-minophen or ibuprofen can provide pain relief if your breasts become uncomfortably engorged.
- If you find yourself feeling unbearably sad, please call on your healthcare provider for advice.
- Know that you gave your baby a wonderful gift of love.

important considerations for insulin dosing would be estimating the quantity of breastmilk the baby is taking. Nighttime breastfeedings and demand breastfeedings are difficult to measure. Newer rapid-acting insulin can be given after feedings (contrary to the usual method of giving insulin prior to feed-ings), which facilitates incorporating breastfeeding into the diabetes management plan. If the health-care team finds it critical to quantify the amount of breastmilk ingested per feeding in order to develop a treatment plan, the child could be weighed before and after feedings for a day or two using a rented scale. This would assist in estimating the contribu-tion of breastmilk to the child's total caloric intake, as well as to quantify carbohydrate, fat, and protein points. Another way to make sure the milk is mea-sured is to have the mother pump and give the breastmilk via a bottle or other feeding device. Weaning would not be advised.

Celiac Disease

Celiac disease (CD) is an autoimmune condition triggered by gluten. Complete removal of gluten from the diet in a patient with celiac disease should result in symptomatic, serologic, and histologic remission. CD is characterized by changes in the intestinal mucosa or villi that prevent the absorption of foods, mainly fat. The mucosal damage appears to stem from sensitivity to gliadin, the protein fraction of gluten found in wheat, rye, barley, and other grains. Formula-feeding and the early introduction of solids accelerate the appearance of symptoms of celiac disease (Akobeng et al., 2006). It has been thought that CD was rare in the United States; however, more recent case finding indicates 0.5–1 percent of children may have CD, and that many with more subtle symptoms are not being diagnosed (D'Amico et al., 2005). The infant with this disorder is asymptomatic until solids containing gluten are introduced into the diet. Clinical symptoms are insidious and chronic. Fatigue, diarrhea, and failure to thrive are the most common presenting symptoms, with later onset observed in breastfed children (D'Amico et al., 2005). Because fat is not absorbed, the child's stools become frothy appearing, foul smelling, and excessive. Deficiencies of the fat-soluble vitamins (A, D, K, and E) appear. If the disease progresses without treatment, abdominal distension and general wasting are evident. The affected child's diet must be modified lifelong and vigorously maintained to exclude gluten, thus improving food absorption and preventing malnutrition.

Breastfeeding Implications. The impact on breastfeeding in the prevention of CD remains uncertain. Farrell (2006) reminds us that it is not certain what the role of breastfeeding might be—is it the delay of exposure to glutens or the modulation of the child's immune response to gluten that is altered due to breastmilk's effect on the gut? Introduction of gluten both before 3 months and after 7 months is associated with increased risk of symptoms in at-risk children (Norris et al., 2006). Exclusive breastfeeding for 6 months and continued breastfeeding during the introduction of gluten may prevent or delay onset of symptomatic CD (Chertok, 2007).

Cystic Fibrosis

Cystic fibrosis (CF) is a genetic disorder caused by a defect in a single gene on chromosome 7. This leads to abnormalities in the apical membrane of epithelial cells that line the airways, biliary tree, intestines, vas deferens, sweat ducts, and pancreatic ducts. Secretions of these sites become more viscid and obstruct

ducts, leading to dysfunction at the organ level. The exocrine glands of the affected child produce abnormally thick and sticky secretions that block the flow of pancreatic digestive enzymes, clog hepatic ducts, and impede the movement of cilia in the lungs. The increased sodium chloride in the child's sweat provides an important diagnostic clue: the family reports that the child tastes salty when kissed. In the newborn, CF may present as a meconium ileus (intestinal obstruction caused by a plug of meconium). Signs of intestinal obstruction include abdominal distension, vomiting, and failure to pass stools. This is a surgical emergency. At birth, about half of the affected children are already pancreatic insufficient. Nutrient absorption—particularly of fat-soluble vitamins—is thus impaired from the beginning. Because of problems with fat absorption, the infant fails to gain weight, despite reports of a voracious appetite. When solid foods are introduced, the stools become bulky, more frequent, foul smelling, and frothy. Pulmonary complications are almost always present, and the child often has persistent, severe respiratory infections because of inability to clear thick secretions.

Prevention of respiratory complications and malnutrition are the mainstay of management for the child with CF. Protection from and aggressive treatment for respiratory infection is accomplished by airway clearance procedures (postural drainage and percussion, chest vest, and others), aerosol therapy, and medications, such as bronchodilators, inhaled corticosteroids, and antibiotics. The use of aerosolized recombinant human DNase to decrease the viscosity of secretions was a breakthrough in CF treatment (Jackson & Vessey, 1996).

Nutrition management includes promoting breastfeeding, providing fat-soluble vitamin supplements, and prescribing pancreatic enzyme replacement, pancrease (Koletzko & Reinhardt, 2001). The enzyme microspheres are mixed in a tiny amount of applesauce. The enzyme dose is based on estimated fat intake, not abdominal symptoms such as bloating or cramping, or on weight of the infant (Anthony et al., 1999). Because salt content in the infant diet is very low, salt supplementation may be recommended. For breastfed children, this is especially important during hot weather or periods of increased fluid losses (diarrheal illness, fever). If the child is not gaining weight well, or presents with failure to thrive at the time of late diagnosis, calorie supplementation may be needed. Extra calories may be added in a number of different ways—for example, with glucose polymers or fat added to breastmilk. The child's medical provider will ensure that enzyme replacement dose is sufficient. Other comorbid problems, such as GERD or cow's milk protein allergy, may also interfere with weight gain.

Breastfeeding Implications. Breastfeeding offers the protection from infection as well as the easy digestibility of breastmilk that are particularly important for this high-risk group. Parker et al. (2004) found that infants who received exclusive breastfeeding through 6 months of age had significantly decreased disease severity based on recent IV antibiotic use. However, they did not find differences in symptom onset as related to feeding history. Children with CF who were exclusively breastfed were found to be taller and heavier than those who were exclusively formula-fed (Holliday et al., 1991). A survey of CF centers in the United States found that most of them recommended breastfeeding alone or combined with pancreatic enzyme supplement or hydrolyzed formula (Luder et al., 1990). Babies with CF produce normal levels of gastric lipase, which is an important digestive enzyme. This enzyme, together with milk lipase in breastmilk, may help the infant with CF to absorb fat more efficiently. Human milk contains appreciably greater amounts of lipase than cow's milk.

Allergies

The issue of the preventive nature of breastfeeding for allergic disease continues to be controversial. At present, there is no consensus about whether breastfeeding protects against the development of asthma and allergy. There are studies documenting that breastfeeding reduces risk, ameliorates severity, or delays onset of atopic conditions (Bloch et al., 2002; Tarini et al., 2006). However there are also those finding that breastfeeding either has no effect on risk or even increases risk (Bergmann et al., 2002; Sears et al., 2002).

Allergic disease is multifactorial, with incidence related to family history, sensitization, and triggers. Family history has the best predictive value for identifying at-risk neonates who should be targeted for

allergy prevention (Zieger, 2000). The atopy-prone infant is at increased risk to sensitization to allergens prior to birth and early after birth. Antigen exposure is evident as early as the 22nd week of gestation (Jones et al., 1996).

Food allergy is generally defined as an adverse reaction to a foreign substance or antigen accompanied by immunological changes, notably a rise in IgE. It occurs in about 4 to 6 percent of children (Zieger, 2000). As shown in Table 19–3, the most common offending foods in the United States are cow's milk, peanuts, nuts, chicken eggs, soy, and fish (Zieger, 2000). The initial exposure is sensitization, which does not usually result in allergic symptoms. With a subsequent exposure, however, allergic symptoms may become evident. This distinction helps to make it clear why a baby given a routine cow's milk formula in the hospital may not experience a reaction until the next exposure several days or weeks later. If the mother is not informed that supplement was given in the nursery, she may not recognize that a sensitizing event occurred. This is one reason why parents must be asked for permission before any supplementation is given to their baby.

Breastfeeding Implications. When someone asks if an infant can be allergic to breastmilk, the answer is "yes." Proteins of foods ingested by the mother pass into the breastmilk, where they may trigger an allergic response in the at-risk child who has been sensitized. Antigens in human milk have been detected for peanuts, lactoalbumin, and ovoalbumin (Casas et al., 2000; Vadas et al., 2001). Furthermore, there can be cross-reactivity between cow's milk and human milk proteins (Bernard et al., 2000). The amount of allergen needed to sensitize or trigger symptoms is minute. For bovine beta-lactoalbumin, only 1 ng (that's 1 nanogram, which is one billionth of a gram!) is required for sensitization. The amount of bovine b-lactoalbumin in mother's milk ranges from 0.5 to 32 ng/L. A 40-ml feeding of cow's milk formula contains bovine lactoalbumin in the equivalent to the amount found in 21 years of breastfeeding (Businco, Bruno, & Giampietro, 1999).

The list of symptoms caused by food allergy is long: vomiting, diarrhea, colic, colitis, bloody stools (hematochezia), eczema, urticaria, rhinitis, fussiness, and poor sleep patterns are among them. Some exclusively breastfed infants develop allergic

TABLE 19–3	Selected Sources of Allergenic Foods that May Affect the Nursling
Food*	**Sources**
Cow's milk in any form	Butter, bread, pudding, yogurt, cheese, baked goods, sherbet, ice cream, creamed soups, powdered-milk drinks, gravies, casein or whey used as additives
Eggs	Baked goods, custard, French toast, root beer, mayonnaise, breaded foods, some cake icings, meatloaf, noodles
Wheat	Bread, baked goods with wheat flour, pasta, hot dogs, bologna, some canned soups, some puddings and gravies, textured vegetable protein
Peanuts, legumes	Peanut butter, beans, peas, lentils as well as foods containing soy protein, soy flour, or oil
Nuts, kola nut	Candy, granola, baked goods, chocolate, cocoa, cola beverages
Corn	Cereal, chips, Cracker Jacks, corn tortillas and other Mexican foods with corn masa, popcorn, cornstarch, cornmeal
Fish, shell fish	Fish sticks, appetizers
Citrus fruits	Orange, lemon, lime, grapefruit, fruit deserts, fruit punch, sorbet
Tomatoes	Ketchup, tomato juice, meatloaf, stew or other mixed dishes, spaghetti sauce, pizza sauce

* This is not an exhaustive list of foods containing allergens. Patients need to be provided with detailed written information to allow them to avoid a particular allergen.

symptoms following exposure to cow's milk or other proteins because they have been sensitized to them transplacentally, through inadvertent exposure via supplementation, or through their own mother's milk (Fukushima et al., 1997). Individual infants may respond differently to allergenic foods. Cow's milk protein allergy is the most common food allergy during infancy. Two studies have reported a series of children with proctocolitis during exclusive breastfeeding, which resolved within 48 to 72 hours with maternal dietary exclusion of cow's milk protein (Patenaude et al., 2000; Pumberger, Pomberger, & Geissler, 2001). When a child's symptoms are suspected to be due to allergies, maternal elimination diets may be prescribed. If the offending food has been eliminated, symptoms should improve within 48 to 72 hours, though some recommend a full 2-week elimination trial (Mohrbacher & Stock, 2003).

Clinicians approach this problem in a variety of ways. One is to have the mother begin an extreme diet, eliminating a list of common offenders. Food groups can then be reintroduced one at a time, from the least likely suspect to the most suspect food group. Others will have the mother begin with a more "simple" elimination diet (no elimination diet is really simple) of omitting all dairy products, as that is the most common offending food group. If the elimination diet is to be of any value, it has to be carefully followed and clearly spelled out: written instructions are the most helpful, and scrupulous reading of labels on packaged foods helps to avoid inadvertent consumption of foods that should be eliminated. Especially if several foods are contributing to the baby's adverse reaction, the mother may find food-elimination plans difficult to implement (de Boissieu et al., 1997). It is necessary in some cases to remove all dairy foods.

Repucci (1999) and Schach and Haight (2002) report success of a novel approach to helping the allergic breastfeeding dyad when the child's symptoms do not resolve with maternal elimination diets. Mothers of infants with severe bloody stools due to allergic colitis were prescribed Pancrease MT4, digestive enzymes normally used in the treatment of cystic fibrosis for improving breakdown of foods in the gastrointestinal tract. With more thorough food digestion, fewer intact proteins would be available to enter the mother's milk. In these two reports, colitis symptoms in the infants resolved in most of the treated dyads.

Occasionally, the healthcare provider recommends the interruption of breastfeeding, substituting a hypoallergenic formula for a short or long period of time to relieve severe symptoms (severe colic, significant gastrointestinal bleeding, severe eczema) before reintroducing breastfeeding. Soy-based formulas are not appropriate breastmilk substitutes for the atopic child (AAP, 2004).

Allergy prevention should be targeted to high-risk infants—those whose parents have allergies. There is disagreement among experts as to the role of maternal allergy avoidance during pregnancy. The *AAP's Nutrition Handbook* (2004) recommends this, while others feel that there is not sufficient evidence to do so (Muraro et al., 2004). There is more consensus as to how to approach prevention for the *high-risk* infant (AAP, 2004; Muraro et al., 2004; Fiocchi et al., 2006):

- Exclusively breastfeed for 6 months, with continued breastfeeding during the addition of complementary foods.
- If supplement is needed, use hydrolyzed or partially hydrolyzed breastmilk substitutes.
- Delay potentially allergenic foods until after 12 months.
- Avoid dairy until after 12 months.
- Avoid hen's eggs until 24 months.
- Avoid peanuts, tree nuts, fish, and seafood until 36 months.

Recommendations for other infants include exclusive breastfeeding for 6 months, with continued breastfeeding during addition of complementary foods and cautious introduction of egg, peanut, tree nuts, fish, and seafood. For all infants, introduction of one ingredient at a time is recommended (AAP, 2004; Muraro et al., 2004; Fiocchi et al., 2006).

Common offenders (Table 19–3) should be avoided if possible during the first year of life. If the mother removes dairy products and other foods from her diet, she must take sufficient calcium from other foods or from calcium supplements, and monitor her nutritional status (Holmberg-Marttila et al., 2001).

Food Intolerance

Most children do not care at all what their mothers eat or drink. This is why it is not necessary to provide mothers with a list of foods to avoid. However the occasional child may have a consistent uncomfortable response to the food ingested by the mother. Children who do not tolerate specific foods, but do not have true allergic responses, may have gastrointestinal and dermatologic symptoms that are difficult to distinguish from an allergic response. Typical offenders according to retrospective maternal reports include chocolate, onion, and cruciferous vegetables such as broccoli or cauliflower (Lust et al., 1996). Some babies are sensitive to caffeine and become irritable when their mothers drink too much. Mothers can be instructed to titrate their caffeine intake to their baby's behavior. If a mother notes that her baby is always excessively cranky after she has a huge serving of chocolate cake, then she can decide to reduce the size of the portion next time and see if the baby is happier.

Lactose Intolerance

Fortunately, primary lactase deficiency is a rare problem in infancy as lactose is the carbohydrate in human milk. Humans normally produce sufficient lactase for lactose digestion until childhood, when selected populations begin to have problems with insufficiency. However, infants may experience symptoms related to secondary lactase deficiency following gastrointestinal illness or antibiotic use, or as a result of feeding mismanagement. Symptoms of lactose intolerance include escalating fussiness, excessive gassiness, and bright green, irritating, slimy stools.

Woolridge and Fisher (1988) describe very clearly the problem of colicky symptoms and feeding mismanagement. When mothers rather than babies control the child's time at the breast, the child may receive high-volume, low-fat feedings that result in a higher than normal lactose load for the baby to digest. When a baby is allowed to nurse as long as desired on the first breast before being moved to the second, the feeding is more likely to have the appropriate balance of volume, fat, and lactose. Following gastrointestinal illness, or antibiotic administration, the brush border of the gastrointestinal tract where lactase is located may be damaged, leading to transient lactose intolerance.

Psychosocial Concerns

Anytime families face the unexpected with their children, the myriad of feelings and concerns that bombard them can be overwhelming. Nurses have an absolutely instrumental role in supporting a family's adaptation to whatever is facing them. Each family differs in their response to the birth of a child with a defect or who is diagnosed with a serious or chronic illness, and each will need support from their healthcare team. It is important for professionals to have a working knowledge of crisis and grief theories to support their clinical work with families.

Family Stress

Issues that challenge families include financial concerns, caretaking, fatigue, depression, altered family image, and goal diffusion. However, these stresses are not fixed or predictable (Burke et al., 1998). Reframing these burdens as tasks that need to be mastered can give families direction to take rather than seeing themselves as victims (Burke et al., 1999). The degree of stress may relate more to issues of social support rather than to the specific health problem that the child faces (Smith, Oliver, & Innocenti, 2001; Visconti et al., 2002). Pelchat et al. (1999) compared parents of children with congenital heart disease, Down syndrome, cleft lip and palate, and children without disabilities. They discovered that parents with Down syndrome and congenital heart disease reported higher levels of parenting and psychological stress and that parents of babies with cleft lip and palate and nondisabled children had lower stress levels.

The family's response to a chronic illness involves their definition or perception of the event as well as the family's resources—social, financial, and emotional. A family with no health insurance and limited financial resources may perceive their child's chronic illness as more stressful than would a family with sufficient resources. Parents may harbor feelings of guilt for bringing on the illness or for not recognizing how sick the child was in early stages. Hospitalization brings about a disruption of lifestyle and environment to the family tantamount to culture shock. A barrage of unfamiliar stimuli is thrust on them: infusion pumps that periodically sound an alarm, mist tents, and a constantly rotating staff of new faces all place tremendous stress on the family. Normally affable people can become demanding and even hostile as a by-product of their stress and guilt, and perceived or actual unmet needs. These defensive behaviors are part of the parents' coping strategies for managing their feelings and help to protect families from painful realities. They are not necessarily maladaptive. Although it can be difficult and even painful to deal with such parents, it is far preferable to work with these concerned parents than with those who are unconcerned or passive. Sympathetic listening and simple, understanding statements, such as "I can see you are upset," or "This is such a difficult time," can help parents through this trying time. If hospital nurses rationally assess parents' behaviors and use of defenses, their interactions with parents will be more therapeutic.

Parents who are many miles from home during their child's hospitalization must arrange for sleeping accommodations in the area if both are not allowed to stay overnight at the hospital. Fortunately, many cities now have Ronald McDonald Houses that shelter these families. Support groups of other parents experiencing a similar life crisis are effective, because each person in the group understands the day-to-day issues and problems of caring for an ill child or rearing one with a chronic disease. Nevertheless, support groups are not for all parents; some are so overwhelmed by their own problems that they are not able to reach out and support others.

Chronic Grief and Loss

When the breastfeeding child is chronically ill or has a disabling defect, the disappointment, sorrow, and frustration of parents can be overwhelming. Instead of the perfect child expected during the pregnancy, there is an intense feeling of loss. If the child requires indefinite special care and attention, there is a persistent effect that is described in Olshansky's classic work, *Chronic Sorrow* (1962). Unlike acute grief, which is limited in time, chronic sorrow is prolonged and recurrent. Over time, coping processes evolve and parents can find satisfaction and joy from their child: "The shock and numbness linger for days, even months. . . . It is only after you have gotten over that first crisis that you begin to realize a life and soul have been given into your care" (Good, 1980). The onset of chronic sorrow is variable among families and sometimes difficult to identify; however, this condition is a natural outgrowth of parenting and is an adaptive response. Breastfeeding may have an ameliorating effect for both the child and the parents when chronic illness is involved. The mother of a breastfed baby has the satisfaction of giving something special to her child, which may help her deal with her feelings of loss.

The Empty Cradle . . . When a Child Dies

Parents must face the tremendous task of coping and somehow continuing with life when their child dies. Our understanding of so-called stages of grief is incomplete (Davies, 2004). There is almost no empirical research on what many consider the classical stages of grief proposed by Elizabeth Kübler-Ross. Every person responds differently. In addition, there are cultural traditions and expectations that may dictate a family's response to their child's death. Parents need to be able to express their feelings any way they desire—by crying, yelling, quietly talking about how they feel, or remaining silent. Compassionate care assists families to cope with death. Giving the parents the opportunity to hold the body of their child and to say goodbye may or may not help this process. This is a very common practice and a recent meta-analysis of bereavement indicated that families appreciated the opportunity to have contact with their child's body. However, Hughes and Riches (2003) found that women who had contact with their deceased infant had more difficulty with grieving, and further, that the intensity of their difficulty was correlated with the "dose" of contact with their infant's body. This is clearly an area where we need more knowledge to guide both our own actions as healers, as well as to provide counsel to families we care for.

The assumption that mothers and fathers respond very differently to the death of their child is not validated by recent research. Seecharan (2004)

did *not* find significant differences in mothers' and fathers' responses to the death of their child. Mothers had more intense reactions when a death was unexpected (Seecharan, 2004). The breastfeeding mother may have to cope with the physical discomfort of breast fullness and leaking and needs advice for management of involution (see Box 19–9). Occasionally, a mother will continue to pump her milk, donating it to a milk bank so that other children may benefit from it. Doing so is her way of coping by maintaining visible evidence of the existence of the lost child. When she offers to do so, the best approach is to put her in touch with a milk bank whose staff members can assist her.

Caring for Bereaved Families

When an infant dies, memories that tie the parents to the child are very important to families. Parents should never be denied the right to their sorrow. Remarks such as "It just wasn't meant to be," or "You can always have another baby," are hurtful. They provide no consolation whatsoever regarding the loss of this baby. The following suggestions for healthcare providers who are assisting parents and families through the grief process are based on the authors' experiences as well as those of other healthcare professionals:

- Call the baby by name.
- If the mother was lactating, help her to remain comfortable. Mothers who lose a baby after 20 weeks of gestation may become engorged. This sometimes comes as a complete shock. Often, women are reluctant to relieve their discomfort by expressing milk for fear of stimulating milk production (see Box 19–9).
- Help parents anticipate how to share the bad news with other children and family members.
- Refer the parents to bereavement support groups such as AMEND (Aiding Mothers and Fathers Experiencing Neonatal Death).
- Acknowledge the parents' loss by sending a card or calling. If you do not know the parents well, anything more may be too much.
- Attend the funeral if it seems like the right thing to do.
- Allow parents to verbalize feelings of anger, fear, guilt, and anxiety.
- Feel your way through the conversation, getting feedback from the parent; wait for him or

her to lead the way. Most parents appreciate a chance to talk about their baby and their experience with someone who will understand. Ensure that they know you are available to talk whenever needed.

- Families should have the opportunity to participate in a postdeath debriefing with the child's healthcare provider. Such a conference serves to review the events that lead to the child's death, to respond to questions/concerns that the family may have about the events, or about the medical care provided. Timing of such a conference is at the family's request, but it may be more helpful weeks to months after the death, in addition to a conference at the time of death.

S u m m a r y

There are unique considerations for helping the breastfeeding family when their infant or young child has special healthcare needs or illness. These special needs can be met by recognizing the developmental stage, assessing family lifestyle, reducing parental stress, involving parents in direct care of their child, and most of all, minimizing separation between family members. Discontinuing breastfeeding is rarely necessary for the child with a health problem. However, feeding patterns may need to be modified. Too often, weaning from the breast is assumed to be necessary. This is rarely the case.

Each family is unique. The experience of one situation can never be duplicated; therefore, care providers helping families must be versatile and have solid knowledge about the nature of the health problem so that the best possible care can be provided. Competent care, and then compassionate care, are the top priorities. Informing the parents about every aspect of the health problem, including them in decision making, and developing a working relationship between the healthcare team members and the family is what creates mutual respect and allows for effective breastfeeding problem management.

K e y   C o n c e p t s

- The health, nutrition, and growth of the infant with special healthcare needs are of primary concern.
- Breastfeeding may be adversely affected when a child is ill or has special healthcare needs.
- Infants with certain special healthcare needs may not thrive on only direct breastfeeding.
- Babies and their mothers can often experience a better breastfeeding experience with the help of competent nurses and lactation consultants.
- Supplementation and alternative feeding methods may be needed to provide optimal nutrition in selected situations.
- The use of adaptive devices and positioning techniques can maximize breastfeeding effectiveness.
- The milk supply can be maintained and supported until the child is able to breastfeed directly, or for as long as is necessary.

- Direct breastfeeding rarely requires suspension or cessation.
- Galactosemia is the only condition requiring complete cessation of human milk feeding.
- Children with other inborn errors of metabolism (phenylketonuria, and amino or organic acidemias) may have human milk in addition to special dietary formulas.
- Families who have a child with special healthcare needs face many stressful issues and may be chronically grieving for the loss of the healthy baby they dreamed of.
- The loss of a "normal" breastfeeding experience may add to family stress.
- The breastfeeding mother whose child has died requires sensitive support.
- Breastfeeding-friendly pediatric hospital units can ease the unique stresses of the breastfeeding family.

Internet Resources

Parents and Families

International Birth Defects Information System (links to information and support about many congenital problems in multiple languages): www.ibis-birthdefects.org

March of Dimes Birth Defects Foundation (information and support about birth defects): www.modimes.org

Mothers Overcoming Breastfeeding Issues - MOBI (support and advice for women who are/were unable to breastfeed, feel unsuccessful in breastfeeding, are/were experiencing severe breastfeeding problems, or experienced untimely weaning): www.mobimotherhood.org

National Organization for Rare Disorders (information for families and professionals): www.rarediseases.org

Allergies

Food Allergy & Anaphylaxis Network (information, recipes, support): www.foodallergy.org

Milk Soy Protein Intolerance Guide (information on maternal dietary restriction for babies with milk and soy protein allergies, ordering information for cookbook for MSP restricted diets): www.mspiguide.org

Celiac Disease

Celiac Disease Foundation: www.celiac.org

Celiac Sprue Association (family support and information): www.csaceliacs.org

Congenital Heart Disease

American Heart Association: www.americanheart.org

Congenital Heart Information Network (information, parent support): www.tchin.org

Diabetes Mellitus

American Diabetes Association (information and support): www.diabetes.org

Learning About Diabetes (information, patient education materials in English/Spanish): www.learningaboutdiabetes.org

Juvenile Diabetes Research Foundation International (information and support): www.jdrf.org

Down Syndrome

National Association for Down Syndrome (parent support and information): www.nads.org

National Down Syndrome Congress (parent support): www.ndsccenter.org

National Down Syndrome Society (parent support and information in English and Spanish): www.ndss.org

Gastrointestinal Disorders

Esophageal Atresia/Tracheoesophageal Fistula (child and family support connection): www.eatef.org

International Association of Reflux Parents (information and support): www.geocities.com/HotSprings/Villa/2193

International Foundation for Gastrointestinal Disorders (information and support): www.aboutkidsgi.org

PAGER (Pediatric and Adolescent Gastroesophageal Reflux Association) information and support: www.reflux.org

Metabolic Problems

Children Living with Inherited Metabolic Disease (information and support): www.climb.org.uk

Parents of Galactosemic Children (parent information and support): www.galactosemia.org

PKU News (information and support):
www.pkunews.org

Neural-Tube Defects

National Hydrocephalus Foundation (information and support):
www.hydroassoc.org
Spinal Bifida Association of America (information and support):
www.sbaa.org

Oral-Facial Anomalies

Cleft Palate Foundation (information for families and professionals):
www.cleftline.org
FACES (support group of the National Craniofacial Association):
www.faces-cranio.org
Pierre Robin Network (connects families of children with Pierre Robin sequence):
www.pierrerobin.org
Wide Smiles (parent-to-parent support):
www.widesmiles.org

References

Adibe O et al. Ad libitum feeds after laparoscopic pyloromyotomy: a retrospective comparison with a standardized feeding regimen in 225 infants. *J Laparoendosc Adv Surg Tech.* 2007;17(2):235–237.

Akobeng A et al. Effect of breast feeding on risk of coeliac disease: a systematic review and meta-analysis of observational studies. *Arch Dis Child.* 2006; 91(1):39–43.

Albrich W et al. Changing characteristics of invasive pneumococcal disease in metropolitan Atlanta, Georgia, after introduction of a 7-valent pneumococcal conjugate vaccine. *Clin Infect Dis.* 2007;44(12):1569–1576.

American Academy of Pediatrics. Managing acute gastroenteritis among children: oral rehydration, maintenance and nutritional therapy. *Pediatrics.* 2004; 114(2):507.

American Academy of Pediatrics Committee on Nutrition and Kleinman, RE. *Pediatric Nutrition Handbook.* Elk Grove, Illinois: AAP; 2004.

American Academy of Pediatrics Subcommittee on Management of Otitis Media. Diagnosis and management of acute otitis media. *Pediatrics.* 2004; 113:1451–1465.

American Society of Anesthesiologists. Practice guidelines for preoperative fasting and the use of pharmacologic agents to reduce the risk of pulmonary aspiration: application to healthy patients undergoing elective procedure—a report by the American Society of Anesthesiologists. Task Force on Preoperative Fasting. *Anesthesiology.* 1999;90(3):896–905.

Aniansson G et al. Otitis media with breast milk of children with cleft palate. *Scand J Plast Reconstr Surg Hand Surg.* 2002;36(1):9–15.

Anthony H et al. Pancreatic enzyme replacement therapy in cystic fibrosis: Australian guidelines. *J Paediatr Child Health.* 1999;35:125–129.

Armon K et al. An evidence and consensus-based guideline for acute diarrhoea management. *Arch Dis Child.* 1999;85:132–142.

Aspelund G, Langer J. Current management of hypertrophic pyloric stenosis. *Seminars in Pediatr Surg.* 2007;16:27–33.

Aumonier ME, Cunningham CC. Breastfeeding in infants with Down's syndrome. *Child Care Health Dev.* 1983;9:247–255.

Bailey DJ et al. Lack of efficacy of thickened feeding as treatment for gastroesophageal reflux. *J Pediatr.* 1987;110:187–189.

Bartalena L et al. Effects of amiodarone administration during pregnancy on neonatal thyroid function and subsequent neurodevelopment. *J Endocrinol Invest.* 2001;24(2):116–130.

Baudon JJ et al. Motor dysfunction of the upper digestive tract in Pierre Robin sequence as assessed by sucking-swallowing electromyography and esophageal manometry. *J Pediatr.* 2002;140:719–723.

Baujat G et al. Oroesophageal motor disorders in Pierre Robin syndrome. *JPGN.* 2001;32:297–302.

Bergmann RL et al. Breastfeeding is a risk factor for atopic eczema. *Clin Exp All.* 2002;32:205–209.

Berhe T et al. Feasibility and safety of insulin pump therapy in children aged 2–7 years with type 1 diabetes: a retrospective study. *Pediatrics.* 2006;117(6):2132–2137.

Bernard H et al. Molecular basis of IgE cross-reactivity between human beta-casein and bovine beta-casein, a major allergy in milk. *Mol Immunol.* 2000;37:161–167.

Bloch AM et al. Does breastfeeding protect against allergic rhinitis during childhood? A meta-analysis of prospective studies. *Actae Paediatr.* 2002;91:275–279.

Boctor DL, Pillo-Blocka F, McCrindle BW. Nutrition after cardiac surgery for infants with congenital heart disease. *Nutr Clin Pract.* 1999;14:111–115.

Bodley V, Powers D. Long-term nipple shield use—a positive perspective. *J Hum Lact.* 1996;12(4):301–304.

Bovey A, Noble R, Noble M. Orofacial exercises for babies with breastfeeding problems? *Breastfeed Rev.* 1999;7(1):23–28.

Brigham M. Mothers' reports of the outcome of nipple shield use. *J Hum Lact.* 1996;12(4):291–297.

Bruner J et al. Intrauterine repair of spina bifida: preoperative predictors of shunt-dependent hydrocephalus. *Am J Obstet and Gynecol.* 2004;190(5): 1305–1312.

Burke SO et al. Stressors in families with a child with a chronic condition: an analysis of qualitative studies and a framework. *Can J Nurs Res.* 1998;30: 71–95.

Burke SO et al. Assessment of stressors in families with a child who has a chronic condition. *MCH.* 1999;24:98–106.

Businco L, Bruno G, Giampietro PG. Prevention and management of food allergy. *Acta Paediatr Suppl.* 1999;88(430):104–109.

Casas R et al. Detection of IgA antibodies to cat, beta-lactoalbumin and ovoalbumin antigens in human milk. *J Allergy Clin Immunol.* 2000;105:1236–1240.

Casteels K, Punt S, Bramswig J. Transient neonatal hypothyroidism during breastfeeding after postnatal maternal topical iodine treatment. *Eur J Pediatr.* 2000;159(9):716–717.

Centers for Disease Control and Prevention. Managing acute gastroenteritis among children: oral rehydration, maintenance, and nutritional therapy. *MMWR.* 2003;52(16):1–16.

Chan GM, Lechtenberg E. The use of fat-free human milk in infants with chylous pleural effusion. *J Perinatol.* 2007;27(7):434–436.

Chantry C, Howard C, Auinger P. Full breastfeeding duration and associated decrease in respiratory tract infection in US children. *Pediatrics.* 2006;17(2): 425–432.

Chertok I. The importance of exclusive breastfeeding in infants at risk for celiac disease. *MCN.* 2007; 32(1):50–54.

Clague A, Thomas A. Neonatal biochemical screening for disease. *Clin Chim Acta.* 2002;315(1–2):99–110.

Cohen R et al. Impact of pneumococcal conjugate vaccine and of reduction in antibiotic use on nasopharyngeal carriage of nonsusceptible pneumococci in children with otitis media. *J Pediatr Infect Dis.* 2006;25(11):1001–1007.

Cohen M. Immediate unrestricted feeding of infants following cleft lip and palate repair. *Br J Plast Surg.* 1997;50:143.

Colombo JL, Hopkins RL, Waring WW. Steam vaporizer injuries. *Pediatrics.* 1981;67:661–663.

Combs VL, Marino BL. A comparison of growth patterns in breast and bottle-fed infants with congenital heart disease. *Pediatr Nurs.* 1993;19:175–179.

Cook-Sather SD, Litman RS. Modern fasting guidelines in children. *Best Pract Res Clin Anaesthesiol.* 2006; 20(3):471–481.

Coy K, Speltz ML, Jones K. Facial appearance and attachment in infants with orofacial clefts: a replication. *Cleft Palate Craniofac J.* 2002;39(1):66–71.

D'Amico M et al. Presentation of pediatric celiac disease in the United States: prominent effect of breastfeeding. *Clin Pediatr.* 2005;44:249–260.

Danner SC. Breastfeeding the infant with a cleft defect. *Clin Iss Perin Wom Health Nurs.* 1992;3: 634–639.

Darzi MA, Chowdri NA, Bhat AN. Breast feeding or spoon feeding after cleft lip repair: a prospective, randomized study. *Br J Plastic Surg.* 1996;49:24–26.

Davies R. New understandings of parental grief: literature review. *J Adv Nurs.* 2004;46(5):506–513.

de Boissieu D et al. Multiple food allergy: a possible diagnosis in breastfed infants. *Acta Paediatr.* 1997; 86:1042–1046.

Denk MJ. Advances in neonatal surgery. *Ped Clin No Amer.* 1998;45(6):1479–1506.

Dennehy P et al. A case-control study to determine risk factors for hospitalization for rotavirus gastroenteritis in U.S. children. *Pediatr Infect Dis J.* 2006; 25(12):1123–1131.

Denny A, Amm C. New technique for airway correction in neonates with severe Pierre Robin Sequence. *J Pediatr.* 2005;147:97–101.

Dowling D et al. Cup-feeding for preterm infants: mechanics and safety. *J Hum Lact.* 2002;18(1):12–20.

Duncan LL, Elder SB. Breastfeeding the infant with PKU. *J Hum Lact.* 1997;13:231–235.

Eliason BC, Lewan RB. Gastroenteritis in children: principles of diagnosis and treatment. *Am Fam Physician.* 1998;58:1769–1776.

Ewer AK, James ME, Tobin JM. Prone and left lateral positioning reduce gastro-esophageal reflux in preterm infants. *Arch Dis Child Fetal Neonatal Ed.* 1999;81:F201–F205.

Fadavi S et al. Mechanics and energetics of nutritive suckling: a functional comparison of commercially available nipples. *J Pediatr.* 1997;130:740–745.

Farrell R. Infant gluten and celiac disease: too early, too late, too much, too many questions. *JAMA.* 2006; 293(19):2410–2412.

Fiocchi A et al. Food allergy and the introduction of solid foods to infants: a consensus document. *Ann Allergy Asthma Immunol.* 2006;97:10–21.

Forbes GB et al. Composition of milk produced by a mother with galactosemia. *J Pediatr.* 1988;113:90–91.

Fox-Bacon C et al. Maternal PKU and breastfeeding: case report of identical twin mothers. *Clin Pediatr.* 1997;36(9):539–542.

Fukushima Y et al. Consumption of cow milk and egg by lactating women and the presence of beta-lactoglobulin and ovalbumin in breast milk. *Am J Clin Nutr.* 1997;65:30–35.

Garza JJ et al. Ad libitum feeding decreases hospital stay for neonates after pyloromyotomy. *J Pediatr Surg.* 2002;37(3):493–495.

GER Guidelines Committee, North American Society for Pediatric Gastroenterology and Nutrition. Pediatric GE reflux clinical practice guidelines. *J Pediatr Gastoenterol Nutr.* 2001;32 (suppl):2.

Gervasio MR, Buchanan CN. Malnutrition in the pediatric cardiology patient. *Crit Care Q.* 1985; 8:49–56.

Ghaem M et al. The sleep patterns of infants and young children with gastrooesophageal reflux. *J Paediatr Child Health.* 1998;34(2):160–163.

Giovannini M et al. Phenylketonuria: dietary and therapeutic challenges. *J Inherit Metab Dis.* 2007;30: 145–152.

Gokcay G et al. Breast feeding in organic acidaemias. *J Inherit Metab Dis.* 2006;29:2–3, 304–310.

Good J. *Breastfeeding the Down's syndrome baby.* Franklin Park, IL: La Leche League International; 1980.

Gorelick MH, Shaw KN, Murphy KO. Validity and reliability of clinical signs in the diagnosis of dehydration in children. *Pediatrics.* 1997;99(5):E6.

Goyal A et al. Oesophageal atresia and tracheo-oesophageal fistula. *Arch Dis Child Fetal Neonatal Ed.* 2006;91:F381–F384.

Greve L et al. Breast-feeding in the management of the newborn with phenylketonuria: a practical approach to dietary therapy. *J Am Diet Assoc.* 1994;94:305–309.

Gromada K, Sandora L. Safe and breastfeeding compatible oral behaviors for the infant receiving a bottle. ILCA 2007 Conference. San Diego, CA. August 17, 2007.

Habbick BF. Infantile hypertrophic pyloric stenosis: a study of feeding practices and other possible causes. *Clin Commun Stud.* 1989;140:401–404.

Harabuchi Y et al. Nasopharyngeal colonization with nontypeable Haemophilus influenzae and recurrent otitis media. *J Infect Dis.* 1994;170(4):862–866.

Heacock HJ et al. Influence of breast versus formula milk on physiological gastroesophageal reflux in healthy, newborn infants. *J Pediatr Gastroenterol Nutr.* 1992;14:41–46.

Helin R, Angeles ST, Bhat R. Octreotide therapy for chylothorax in infants and children: a brief review. *Pediatr Crit Care Med.* 2006;7(6):576–579.

Hernell O, Ivaarsson A, Persson LA. Coeliac disease: effect of early feeding on the incidence of the disease. *Early Hum Dev.* 2001;65(suppl):S153–S160.

Hitchcock NE et al. Pyloric stenosis in western Australia 1971–1984. *Arch Dis Child.* 1987;62(5):512–513.

Holliday KE et al. Growth of human milk-fed and formula-fed infants with cystic fibrosis. *J Pediatr.* 1991;118:77–79.

Holmberg-Marttila D et al. Do combined elimination diet and prolonged breastfeeding of an atopic infant jeopardize maternal bone health? *Clin Exp Allergy* 2001;31:88–94.

Huckabay LM, Tilem-Kessler D. Patterns of parental stress in PICU emergency admission. *Dimens Crit Care Nurs.* 1999;18(2):36–42.

Hughes P, Riches S. Psychological aspects of perinatal loss. *Curr Opin Obstet Gynecol.* 2003;15(2):107–111.

Human Milk Banking Association of North America. Best Practice for Expressing, Storing and Handling Human Milk in Hospitals, Homes and Child Care Settings. Raleigh, NC. 2005.

Huner G et al. Breastfeeding experience in inborn errors of metabolism other than phenylketonuria. *J Inherit Metab Dis.* 2005;28:457–465.

Hurtekant K, Spatz D. Special considerations for breastfeeding the infant with spina bifida. *J Perinat Neonatal Nurs.* 2007;21(1):69–75.

Iovino LA. Astroviruses are now a significant source of gastroenteritis in children. *Infect Dis Child* 2003; 16(2):35.

Ip S et al. *Breastfeeding and Maternal and Infant Health Outcomes in Developed Countries* [Evidence Report/Technology Assessment No. 153]. Rockville, Maryland: Agency for Healthcare Research and Quality; 2007. AHRQ Publications No. 07-E007

Jackson PL, Vessey KJ. *Child With A Chronic Condition.* 2nd ed. St Louis, MO: Mosby; 1996.

Jones AC et al. Fetal peripheral blood mononuclear cell proliferative responses to mitogenic and allergenic stimuli during gestation. *Pediatr Allergy Immunol* 1996;7:109–116.

Kassing D. Bottle-feeding as a tool to reinforce breastfeeding. *J Hum Lact.* 2002;18(1):56–60.

Kimpimaki T et al. Short-term exclusive breastfeeding predisposes young children with increased genetic risk of Type I diabetes to progressive beta-cell autoimmunity. *Diabetologia.* 2001;44(1):63–69.

Kleinman L et al. The infant gastroesophageal reflux questionnaire revised: development and validation as an evaluative instrument. *Clin Gastroenterol hepatol.* 2006;4(5):588–596.

Kogo J et al. Breast feeding for cleft lip and palate patients, using the Hotz-type plate. *Cleft-Palate Craniofac J.* 1997;34:351–353.

Koletzko S, Reinhardt D. Nutritional challenges of infants with cystic fibrosis. *Early Hum Dev.* 2001;65 (suppl):S53–S61.

Korppi M, Hiltunen J. Pertussis is common in nonvaccinated infants hospitalized for respiratory syncytial virus infection. *Pediatr Infect Dis J.* 2007;26(4): 316–318.

Kosko J, EBCH European editorial base. Summary of preoperative fasting for preventing perioperative complications in children. *Evidence-based Child Health: A Cochrane Review Journal* 2006;1:281–284.

Kuzik BA et al. Nebulized hypertonic saline in the treatment of viral bronchiolitis in infants. *J Pediatr.* 2007;151(3):266–270.

Lammer EJ, Edmonds LD. Trends in pyloric stenosis incidence, Atlanta, GA: 1968–1982. *J Med Genet.* 1987;24(8):482–487.

Lawrence R. Lactation support when the infant will require general anesthesia: assisting the breastfeeding dyad in remaining content through the preoperative fasting period. *J Hum Lact.* 2005;21(3): 355–357.

Lawrence RA, Lawrence RM. *Breastfeeding A Guide for the Medical Profession,* 6th ed. p. 288. Philadelphia, PA: Elsevier Mosby; 2005.

Lopez-Alarcon M et al. Breastfeeding protects against the anorectic response to infection in infants: possible role of DHA. *Adv Exp Med Biol.* 2004;554: 371–374.

Luder E et al. Current recommendations for breastfeeding in cystic fibrosis centers. *Am J Dis Child.* 1990;144:1153–1156.

Lust K et al. Maternal intake of cruciferous vegetables and other foods and colic symptoms in exclusively breast-fed infants. *Am Diet Assoc.* 1996;96(1):46–48.

MacDonald A et al. Breastfeeding in IMD. *J Inherit Metab Dis.* 2006;29:299–303.

MacMahon B. The continuing enigma of pyloric stenosis of infancy: a review. *Epidemiology.* 2006;17(2):195–201.

Manoha C et al. Epidemiological and clinical features of hMPV, RSV and RVs infections in young children. *J Clin Virol.* 2007;38:221–226.

Marcellus L. The infant with Pierre Robin sequence: review and implications for nursing practice. *J Ped Nurs.* 2001;15(1):23–33.

Marino BL, O'Brien P, LoRe H. Oxygen saturations during breast and bottle-feedings in infants with congenital heart disease. *J Pediatr Nurs.* 1995;10(6):360–364.

Marques IL et al. Clinical experience with infants with Robin Sequence: a prospective study. *Cleft Palate Craniofac J.* 2001;38(2):171–178.

Masarei A et al. The nature of feeding in infants with unrepaired cleft lip and/or palate compared with healthy noncleft infants. *Cleft Palate Craniofac J.* 2007;44(3):21–28.

Mathisen B et al. Feeding problems in infants with gastrooesophageal reflux disease: a case controlled study. *J Paediatr Child Health.* 1999;35:163–169.

McBride MC, Danner SC. Sucking disorders in neurologically impaired infants. *Clin Perinatol.* 1987;14:109–130.

McCabe L et al. The management of breastfeeding among infants with phenylketonuria. *J Inherit Metal Dis.* 1989;12:467–474.

McIntosh K. Community-acquired pneumonia in children. *N Engl J Med.* 2002;346(6):429–437.

Meier P. Nipple shields for preterm infants: effect of milk transfer and duration of breastfeeding. *J Hum Lact.* 2000;16(2):106–114.

Melnyk B et al. Creating opportunities for parent empowerment: program effects on the mental health and coping outcomes of critically ill young children and their mothers. *Pediatrics.* 2004;113(6):e597–e607.

Merewood A, Philipp BL. *Breastfeeding: Conditions and Diseases.* Amarillo, TX: Pharmasoft Publishing; 2002.

Michail S. Gastroesophageal reflux. *Pediatr Rev.* 2007;28(3):109.

Miller JH. *The Controversial Issue of Breastfeeding Cleft-Affected Infants.* AB, Canada: InfoMed Publications; 1998.

Minchin M et al. Expanding the WHO/UNICEF Baby Friendly Hospital Initiative: eleven steps to optimal infant feeding in a pediatric unit. *Breastfeeding Rev.* 1996;4:87–91.

Mizuno K, Ueda A. Development of sucking behavior in infants with Down's syndrome. *Acta Paediatr.* 2002;90:1384–1388.

Mizuno K, Ueda A, Takeuchi T. Effects of different fluids on the relationship between swallowing and breathing during nutritive sucking in neonates. *Biol Neonate.* 2002;81(1):45–50.

Mohrbacher N, Stock J. *The Breastfeeding Answer Book.* 3rd ed. Schaumburg, IL: La Leche League International; 2003.

Montagnoli L et al. Growth impairment of children with different types of lip and palate clefts in the first 2 years of life: a cross-sectional study. *J Pediatr.* 2005;81(6):461–465.

Muraro A et al. Dietary prevention of allergic diseases in infants and small children, part III: critical review of published peer-reviewed observational and interventional studies and final recommendations. *Pediatr Allergy Immunol.* 2004;15:291–307.

National Center on Birth Defects and Developmental Disabilities CDC. Neural tube defects (NTDs) rates, 1995–1999. *Teratology.* 2002;66(suppl 1):s212–s217.

Nelson S et al. Prevalence of symptoms of gastroesophageal reflux during infancy: a pediatric practice-based survey. *Arch Pediatr Adolesc Med.* 1997;151:569–572.

Niemela M et al. Pacifier as a risk factor for acute otitis media: a randomized, controlled trial of parent counseling. *Pediatrics.* 2000;106(3):483–488.

Noble R, Bovey A. Therapeutic teat use for babies who breastfeed poorly. *Breastfeed Rev.* 1997;5(2):37–42.

Norris J et al. Risk of celiac disease autoimmunity and the timing of gluten introduction in the diet of infants at increased risk of disease. *JAMA.* 2006;293(19):2343–2351.

Oddy W. A review of the effects of breastfeeding on respiratory infections, atopy and childhood asthma. *J Asthma.* 2004;4(6):605–621.

Olshansky S. Chronic sorrow: a response to having a mentally defective child. *Soc Casework.* 1962;43:190–193.

Orenstein SR, Shalaby TM, Putnam PE. Thickened feedings as a cause of increased coughing when used as therapy for gastroesophageal reflux in infants. *J Pediatr.* 1992;121:913–915.

Pandya AN, Boorman JG. Failure to thrive in babies with cleft lip and palate. *Br J Plast Surg.* 2001;54(6):471–475.

Paradise JL et al. Evidence in infants with cleft palate that breast milk protects against otitis media. *Pediatrics.* 1994;94:853–860.

Parker E et al. Survey of breastfeeding practices and outcomes in the cystic fibrosis population. *Pediatr Pulmonol.* 2004;37(4):362–267.

Patenaude Y et al. Cow's milk-induced allergic colitis in an exclusively breast-fed infant: diagnosed with ultrasound. *Pediatr Radiol.* 2000;30:379–382.

Pediatric Toxicology Committee and Data Committee, National Association of Medical Examiners, Srinivasan A, Budnitz DM, Shehab N, Cohen A. Infant deaths associated with cough and cold medications—two states, 2005. *MMWR.* 2007;56(1):1–4.

Pelchat D et al. Longitudinal effects of an early family intervention programme on the adaptation of parents of children with a disability. *Int J Nurs Stud.* 1999;36(6):465–477.

Pinnington LL et al. Feeding efficiency and respiratory integration in infants with acute viral bronchiolitis. *J Pediatr.* 2000;137:523–526.

Piscane A et al. Breast feeding and hypertrophic pyloric stenosis: population based case-control study. *BMJ.* 1996;312(7033):745–747.

Piscane A et al. Down syndrome and breastfeeding. *Acta Paediatr.* 2003;92;1479–1481.

Popper PK. *The Hospitalized Nursing Baby* [Unit I/Lactation Consultant Series Two]. Schaumburg, IL: La Leche League International; 1998.

Prahl C et al. Infant orthopedics in UCLP: effect on feeding, weight, and length: a randomized clinical trial (Dutchcleft). *Cleft Palate Craniofac J.* 2005;42(2):171–177.

Pumberger W et al. Proctocolitis in breast-fed infants: a contribution to differential diagnosis of haematochezia in early childhood. *Postgrad Med.* 2001;77(906):252–254.

Quigley M, Kelly Y, Sacker A. Breastfeeding and hospitalization for diarrheal and respiratory infection in the United Kingdom millennium cohort study. *Pediatrics.* 2007;119(4):e837–e842.

Raisler J, Alexander C, O'Campo P. Breastfeeding and infant illness: a dose-response relationship. *Am J Public Health.* 1999;89:25–30.

Reid J, Reilly S, Kilpatrick N. Sucking performance of babies with cleft conditions. *Cleft Palate Craniofac J.* 2007;44(3):312–320.

Reilly S, Reid J, Skeat J. ABM clinical protocol #17: guidelines for breastfeeding infants with cleft lip, cleft palate, or cleft lip and palate. *Breastfeeding Med.* 2007;2(4):243–250.

Rendon-Macias M et al. Breastfeeding among patients with congenital malformations. *Arch Med Res.* 2002;33(3):269–275.

Repucci A. Resolution of stool blood in breast-fed infants with maternal ingestion of pancreatic enzymes. *J Ped Gastro Nutr.* 1999;84:353–360.

Ribeiro G et al. Haemophilus meningitis 5 years after introduction of the haemophilus influenzae type b conjugate vaccine. *Vaccine.* 2007;25(22):4420–4428.

Ripmeester P, Dunn S. Against all odds: breastfeeding a baby with Harlequin Ichthyosis. *JOGNN.* 2002;31:521–525.

Riva E et al. Early breastfeeding is linked to higher intelligence quotient scores in dietary treated phenylketonuric children. *Acta Paediatr.* 1996;85:56–58.

Rovers MM, de Kok IM, Schilder AG. Risk factors for otitis media: an international perspective. *Int J Pediatr Otorhinolaryngol.* 2006;70(7):1251–1256.

Rutter M. Evaluation and management of upper airway disorders in children. *Seminars in Pediatr Surg.* 2006;15:116–123.

Sandberg D, Magee W, Denk M. Neonatal cleft lip and cleft palate repair. *AORN J.* 2002;75(3):490–506.

Sandler A. *Living With Spina Bifida: A Guide for Families and Professionals.* Chapel Hill, NC: University of North Carolina Press; 1997.

Scariati PD, Grummer-Strawn LM, Fein SB. A longitudinal analysis of infant morbidity and the extent of breastfeeding in the United States. *Pediatrics.* 1997;99:E5.

Schach B, Haight M. Colic and food allergy in the breast-fed infant: is it possible for the exclusively breast-fed infant to suffer from food allergy? *J Hum Lact.* 2002;18(1):50–52.

Sears MR et al. Long-term relation between breastfeeding and development of atopy and asthma in children and young adults: a longitudinal study. *Lancet.* 2002;360:901–907.

Seecharan G et al. Parents' assessment of quality of care and grief following a child's death. *Arch Pediatr Med.* 2004;158:515–520.

Section on breastfeeding. Breastfeeding and the use of human milk. *Pediatrics.* 2005;115(2):496–506.

Seitz G et al. Primary repair of esophageal atresia in extremely low birth weight infants: a single-center experience and review of the literature. *Biol Neonate.* 2006;90(4):247–251.

Shah PS et al. Breastfeeding or breast milk for procedural pain in neonates. Cochrane Database Syst Rev 3:CD004950; 2006.

Shaw WC, Bannister RP, Roberts CT. Assisted feeding is more reliable for infants with clefts—a randomized trial. *Cleft Palate Craniofac J.* 1999;36:262–268.

Sinaniotis C, Sinaniotis A. Community-acquired pneumonia in children. *Curr Opin Pul Med.* 2005;11(3):218–225.

Smith TB, Oliver MN, Innocenti MS. Parenting stress in families of children with disabilities. *Am J Orthopsychiatry.* 2001;71(2):257–261.

Smith M, Saunders C. Prognosis of airway obstruction and feeding difficulty in the Robin sequence. *Int J Pediatr Otorhinolaryngol.* 2006;70:319–324.

Spatz D. Preserving breastfeeding for the rehospitalized infant: a clinical pathway. *MCN.* 2006;31(1):45–51.

Sydorak R, Albanese C. Laparoscopic repair of high imperforate anus. *Seminars in Pediatr Surg.* 2002;11(4):217–225.

Tarini B et al. Systematic review of the relationship between early introduction of solid foods to infants and the development of allergic disease. *Arch Pediatr Adolesc Med.* 2006;160:502–507.

Thomas J et al. ABM clinical protocol #16: breastfeeding the hypotonic infant. *Breastfeeding Med.* 2007;2(2):112–118.

Tobin JM, McCloud P, Cameron DJS. Posture and gastroesophageal reflux: a case for left lateral positioning. *Arch Dis Child.* 1997;7:254–258.

Tomlinson PS, Swiggum P, Harbaugh BL. Identification of nurse-family intervention sites to decrease health-related family boundary ambiguity in PICU. *Issues Compr Pediatr Nurs*. 1999;22(1):27–47.

Tubbs R et al. Late gestational intrauterine myelomeningocele repair does not improve lower extremity function. *Pediatr Neurosurg*. 2003;38(3):128–132.

Turner L et al. The effects of lactation education and a prosthetic obturator appliance on feeding efficiency in infants with cleft lip and palate. *Cleft Palate Craniofac J*. 2001;38(5):S510–S524.

Vadas P et al. Detection of peanut allergens in breast milk of lactating women. *JAMA*. 2001;285:1746–1748.

van Rijn M et al. A different approach to breastfeeding of the infant with phenylketonuria. *Eur J Pediatr*. 2003;162:323–326.

VanVliet G. Treatment of congenital hypothyroidism. *Lancet*. 2001;358(9276):86–87.

Visconti KJ et al. Influence of parental stress and social support on the behavioral adjustment of children with transposition of the great arteries. *J Dev Behav Pediatr*. 2002;23(5):314–321.

White M et al. Sensitivity and cost minimization analysis of radiology versus palpation for the diagnosis of hypertrophic pyloric stenosis. *J Pediatr Surg*. 1998;33:913–917.

Whitehouse T. Bobby's diary: nursing a baby with chylothorax. La Leche League International. *Leaven*. 2003;39(2):27–30.

Wilson-Clay B. Clefts. Personal communication, December 12, 1995.

Woolridge M, Fisher C. Colic, "overfeeding" and symptoms of lactose malabsorption in the breast-fed baby: a possible effect of feed management? *Lancet*. 1988;2(8605):382–384.

Young JL et al. What information do parents of newborns with cleft lip, palate, or both want to know? *Cleft Palate Craniofac J*. 2001;38(1):55–58.

Zieger RS. Dietary aspects of food allergy prevention in infants and children. *J Pediatr Gastroenterol Nutr*. 2000;30:S77–S86.

TABLE 20-1	**Essential Components of the Perinatal History**

Component	Required Data
Family history	• Family history of genetic disorders such as cystic fibrosis, sickle cell anemia, trisomy, phenylketonuria • Family history of diseases such as diabetes, seizures, chronic disorders
Psychosocial history	• Marital status and support systems • Substance abuse • Tobacco use • Exposure to environmental hazards • Inadequate finances • Poor nutrition • Inadequate housing • Psychiatric history • Maternal age < 16 or > 35 years • Education < 11 years • Domestic violence
Maternal medical history	• Surgical procedures, particularly involving reproductive organs • Hospitalizations • Endocrine disorders (diabetes, thyroid) • Cardiovascular disorders (hypertension, heart disease) • Respiratory disorders (asthma, pneumonia) • Renal (frequent infections, chronic kidney disease) • Hematologic (sickle, blood type and Rh factor, blood disorders, Rh isoimmunization) • Cancer • Infections • Sexually transmitted diseases • Medications taken prior to pregnancy
Maternal reproductive history	• Gravidity, parity • Infertility • History of abnormal Pap smear • Previous perinatal loss • Last birth < 1 year before present conception • Previous cesarean birth • Infant with congenital anomaly, birth injury, neurologic deficit • Spontaneous or elective abortions • Malformations of cervix, uterus
Pregnancy history	• Last known menstrual period • EDC (estimated date of confinement) • Nutrition and general health • Prenatal care (when first obtained and frequency) • Prenatal laboratory tests (VDRL; screening for hepatitis B, HIV, STDs, rubella) • Weight gain during pregnancy • Results of prenatal testing (ultrasonography, amniocentesis, chorionic villus testing, alpha-fetoprotein, triple screen) • Medications (prescription, over-the-counter, recreational)

(Continues)

TABLE 20–1	Essential Components of the Perinatal History (Continued)

Component	Required Data
Intrapartum history	• Length of labor • Type of birth (vaginal or cesarean) • Rupture of membrane (spontaneous or artificial, time from rupture until birth) • Appearance of amniotic fluid • Complications • Instrumentation • Analgesia and anesthesia • Apgar scores and resuscitation of infant
Breastfeeding history	• Previous maternal breastfeeding experience • Desire to breastfeed • Anticipated duration of breastfeeding • Exposure to breastfeeding education • Cultural influences related to breastfeeding • Maternal support system

Source: Barron, 2008; Orr, 2004.

The following classification terms are used to describe the developmental status of the newborn (Askin & Wilson, 2007):

- Classification according to size
  - *Extremely low birth weight (ELBW):* An infant whose birth weight is less than 1000 grams
  - *Very low birth weight (VLBW):* An infant whose birth weight is less than 1500 grams
  - *Low birth weight (LBW):* An infant whose birth weight is less than 2500 grams
  - *Small for date (SFD) or small for gestational age (SGA):* An infant whose birth weight is below the 10th percentile on intrauterine growth curves
  - *Appropriate for gestational age (AGA):* An infant whose birth weight falls between the 10th and 90th percentiles on intrauterine growth curves
  - *Large for gestational age (LGA):* An infant whose birth weight is above the 90th percentile on intrauterine growth curves
  - *Intrauterine growth restriction (IUGR):* An infant whose intrauterine growth curve is retarded
- Classification according to gestational age
  - *Preterm (premature):* An infant born at less than 37 weeks' gestation, regardless of weight
  - *Full-term:* An infant born between 37 and 42 weeks' gestation, regardless of weight
  - *Postterm (postmature):* An infant born after 42 weeks' gestation, regardless of birth weight

The New Ballard Score

The New Ballard Score (Ballard et al., 1991) is a commonly used objective tool that includes the assessment of six external physical characteristics and six neurologic signs to estimate the gestational age of the infant. This scoring system has its highest reliability when performed within 48 hours of birth and is considered accurate within 2 weeks of actual gestation (Ballard et al.). Although the New Ballard Score has been expanded to include extremely premature infants, the Donovan et al. study (1999) failed to demonstrate a close relationship between gestational age and fetal maturation, as measured by this scoring system, in infants less than 28 weeks gestation. Thus, possible inaccuracies in gestational age based on New Ballard Scores should be considered when implementing treatment for infants less than 28 weeks.

Each item is scored from –1 to 4 (or 5 with two of the signs) by comparing the infant with the descriptor on the scoring sheet (Figure 20–1). The numbers

TABLE 20–2	Physiologic Characteristics Associated with Gestational Age and Size That Affect Feeding/Nutrition	
Gestational Age/Size Classification	**Characteristic**	**Risk**
Low birth weight Prematurity	• Coordination of sucking and swallowing not present until 32–34 weeks, full coordination after 36–37 weeks • Immature gag reflex < 36 weeks	Aspiration
	• Higher extracellular water content (90% vs. 70% in full-term infant)	Inadequate hydration
	• Poor muscle tone in the area of the lower esophageal sphincter < 37 weeks	Regurgitation into the esophagus, which can cause vagal stimulation—apnea, bradycardia, aspiration
	• Limited stomach capacity	Over distension; compromises respiration
	• Carbohydrates and fat less tolerated • Secretion of lactase low < 34 weeks • Inefficient in digesting and absorbing lipids—low levels of pancreatic lipase and low bile acid • Low reserve of calcium, iron, phosphorus, proteins, and vitamins A and C • Absent, weak, or ineffectual sucking	Inadequate nutrition
	• Decreased muscle mass; decreased deposits of brown fat • Lack of subcutaneous fat • Poor reflex control of skin capillaries	Thermoregulation Hypoglycemia
Postmaturity	• Decreased efficiency of the placenta • Macrosomia • Meconium aspiration • Polycemia	Respiratory distress Hypoglycemia Hyperbilirubinemia
LGA	Transient hyperinsulinism	Hypoglycemia
SGA	Intrauterine malnutrition	Hypoglycemia

Source: Askin & Wilson, 2007; Putman, 2004.

of points assigned per item are added to obtain a total score. The total score is then used to determine an estimate of gestational age in weeks by comparing the infant's score with the maturity rating score on the New Ballard Score. The following neuromuscular and physical signs are used for scoring (Cheffer & Rannalli, 2004; Creehan, 2008):

• Neuromuscular signs of maturity
  • *Posture:* Observe the posture when the infant is quiet. A term newborn's arms and legs are

flexed with good body muscle tone. A preterm infant's arms and legs are extended with the body flaccid (Figure 20–2).
• *Square window:* Flex the infant's wrist down toward the ventral forearm and estimate the angle between the hand and forearm. Do not rotate the wrist. Measure the degree of flexion against the New Ballard Score chart. There is no downward angle with the full-term infant (i.e., a score of 3 or 4). The angle decreases with decreasing gestational age.

MATURATIONAL ASSESSMENT OF GESTATIONAL AGE (New Ballard Score)

NAME_____ DATE/TIME OF BIRTH_____ SEX _____

HOSPITAL NO. _____ DATE/TIME OF EXAM_____ BIRTH WEIGHT_____

RACE _____ AGE WHEN EXAMINED _____ LENGTH_____

APGAR SCORE: 1 MINUTE_____ 5 MINUTES_____ 10 MINUTES_____ HEAD CIRC. _____

EXAMINER _____

NEUROMUSCULAR MATURITY

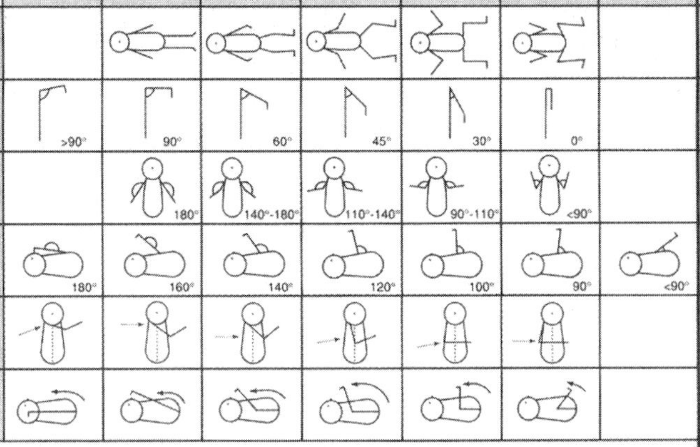

NEUROMUSCULAR MATURITY SIGN	SCORE -1	0	1	2	3	4	5	RECORD SCORE HERE
POSTURE								
SQUARE WINDOW (Wrist)	>90°	90°	60°	45°	30°	0°		
ARM RECOIL		180°	140°-180°	110°-140°	90°-110°	<90°		
POPLITEAL ANGLE	180°	160°	140°	120°	100°	90°	<90°	
SCARF SIGN								
HEEL TO EAR								

TOTAL NEUROMUSCULAR MATURITY SCORE

PHYSICAL MATURITY

PHYSICAL MATURITY SIGN	-1	0	1	2	3	4	5	RECORD SCORE HERE
SKIN	sticky friable transparent	gelatinous red translucent	smooth pink visible veins	superficial peeling &/or rash, few veins	cracking pale areas rare veins	parchment deep cracking no vessels	leathery cracked wrinkled	
LANUGO	none	sparse	abundant	thinning	bald areas	mostly bald		
PLANTAR SURFACE	heel-toe 40-50 mm:-1 <40 mm:-2	>50 mm no crease	faint red marks	anterior transverse crease only	creases ant. 2/3	creases over entire sole		
BREAST	imperceptible	barely perceptible	flat areola no bud	stippled areola 1-2 mm bud	raised areola 3-4 mm bud	full areola 5-10 mm bud		
EYE/EAR	lids fused loosely: -1 tightly: -2	lids open pinna flat stays folded	sl. curved pinna; soft; slow recoil	well-curved pinna; soft but ready recoil	formed & firm instant recoil	thick cartilage ear stiff		
GENITALS (Male)	scrotum flat, smooth	scrotum empty faint rugae	testes in upper canal rare rugae	testes descending few rugae	testes down good rugae	testes pendulous deep rugae		
GENITALS (Female)	clitoris prominent & labia flat	prominent clitoris & small labia minora	prominent clitoris & enlarging minora	majora & minora equally prominent	majora large minora small	majora cover clitoris & minora		

TOTAL PHYSICAL MATURITY SCORE

SCORE

Neuromuscular_____
Physical _____
Total _____

MATURITY RATING

score	weeks
-10	20
-5	22
0	24
5	26
10	28
15	30
20	32
25	34
30	36
35	38
40	40
45	42
50	44

GESTATIONAL AGE (weeks)

By dates_____
By ultrasound_____
By exam_____

FIGURE 20–1 New Ballard Score.

Source: Reprinted from *Journal of Pediatrics*, Vol. 119, No. 3, Ballard et al., "Maturational Assessment of Gestational Age (New Ballard Score)," pp. 417–423, Copyright 1991, with permission from Elsevier.

- *Arm recoil:* Fully flex the infant's arms for 5 seconds. Release. Score the degree of immediate return of arm flexion against the score sheet. A vigorous, fully flexed response is a score of 4. A slow response receives a lower score.
- *Popliteal angle:* With the infant's hips flat on the examining table, place one of the infant's thighs on the abdomen. Slowly, attempt to straighten the leg towards the infant's head. Do not force. Stop when resistance is met. Score the angle of the flexed leg according to the chart. A full-term infant will usually score a 3 or 4.
- *Scarf sign:* Pull the infant's arm across the chest and around the neck. Observe the infant's elbow in relation to the midline of the body. Score according to the chart. A full-term infant will usually score 2, 3, or 4.

- *Heel to ear:* With the infant's hips on the examining table, slowly pull the heel toward the ear until resistance is felt. Observe the distance between the foot and the head as well as the degree of knee extension. Score according to the chart. A full-term infant will usually score 3 or 4.
- Physical signs of maturity
  - *Skin:* Observe the skin for color and texture. Observe the trunk area for opacity. With increasing gestational age, the skin becomes less transparent and develops more texture. Blood vessels are generally not visible on the trunk of a full-term infant. Some peeling of the hands and feet is common in full-term infants. A preterm infant's skin is thin and smooth with visible vessels. Score the infant according to the chart. A full-term infant will usually score a 3 or 4.
  - *Lanugo:* Observe the skin for this fine, downy hair. Lanugo covers the body of the fetus from about 24 to 28 weeks. After 28 weeks, it begins to disappear. Score the infant according to the descriptors on the chart. Note that a very premature infant will have no lanugo or it is sparse, thus scoring a 0 or –1. A full-term infant will usually score 3 or 4.

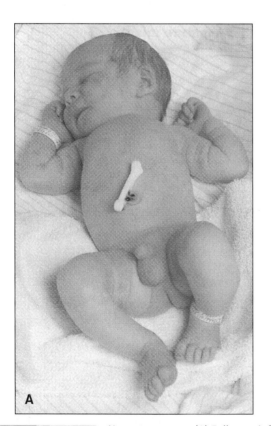
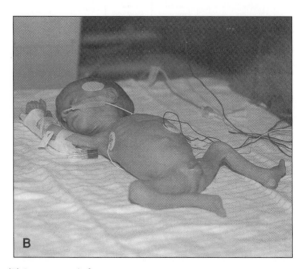

FIGURE **20–2**   Neonate posture. (A) Full-term infant. (B) Premature infant.

Source: Moore ML, Nichols FH, Zwelling E, eds. *Maternal-newborn nursing: theory and practice.* Philadelphia: W. B. Saunders, 1080-1131, 1997. Reprinted with permission of Elsevier Publications.

- *Plantar surface:* Observe the soles of the feet for creases. The creases on the anterior surface of the foot begin to appear between 28 and 30 weeks. As gestational age increases so do the number and depth of creases. Score according to the descriptors on the chart. A full-term infant will usually score a 3 or 4. Note that after 12 hours, the validity of plantar creases as an indicator of gestational age decreases because the skin begins to dry.
- *Breast:* Place two fingers of one hand on either side of the areola bud tissue. Measure (in millimeters) the diameter of the bud with a tape measure. Score according to the chart. A full-term infant will usually score a 3 or 4.
- *Eye/Ear:* Prior to 26–30 weeks gestation, the eyelids are fused. After the eyes are open, there is no maturity scoring on the New Ballard Score. The ears are assessed for formation and amount of cartilage that is present in the pinna. Examine the pinna between the thumb and forefinger for amount of cartilage that is present. Fold the ear anteriorly. After approximately 36 weeks when some cartilage has developed, the pinna will spring back from being folded. Score according to the chart. A full-term infant will usually score 3 or 4.
- *Genitalia (male):* Gently feel for the presence of the testes by examining the scrotum between the thumb and fingers of one hand. Observe the degree of descent into the scrotum and the development of rugae. The testes begin to descend at 28 weeks and descent is normally complete by 40 weeks. The scrotum of a full-term infant is also covered with deep rugae.
- *Genitalia (female):* Observe the genitalia of the female infant without spreading the labia majora. At full term, the infant's labia majora covers the labia minora. The premature infant will have a more prominent clitoris with small, widely separated labia.

After these assessments, complete the scoring by adding the total neuromuscular maturity score to the total physical maturity score. Compare that score, found on the left side of the maturity rating scale, with the corresponding gestational age on the right side of the rating scale. To complete the assessment of gestational age, plot the infant's weight, length, and head circumference in relation to maturity rating from the New Ballard Score on the Classification of Newborn by intrauterine growth and gestational age (Figure 20–3). The infant's maturity level can then be classified according to the previously defined classification terms.

Indicators of Effective Breastfeeding and Assessment Scales

This section defines behaviors that indicate whether breastfeeding is going well and reviews several breastfeeding assessment scales.

Breastfeeding Behaviors and Indicators

Breastfeeding is not a single behavior of suckling but a series of behaviors that can be described, assessed, and measured. Historically a lack of consistency in defining breastfeeding behaviors had resulted in difficulty comparing breastfeeding studies, thus limiting their use; however, generally speaking, breastfeeding infants who are feeding effectively spontaneously turn their mouth to their mothers' nipples when put to breast, grasp the nipple firmly, suckle rhythmically, and pause to rest between bursts of suckling while continuing to hold the nipple in the mouth. Swallowing is observed during the first 3 days postpartum; swallowing is both observed and heard beginning 4 days postpartum or earlier for some mothers.

A concept analysis is necessary in development of any tool. In the case of breastfeeding tools, we must agree upon operational definitions of interactive breastfeeding behaviors before we can evaluate relationships between breastfeeding behaviors and breastfeeding outcomes (Mulder, 2006). Mulder further points out "To be considered essential attributes or behaviors of effective breastfeeding the characteristics must occur and be present in all examples of the concept and be required to achieve the transfer of milk between the mother and infant adequate to meet both maternal and infant needs." As a starting point, the authors of this chapter define commonly used breastfeeding concepts.

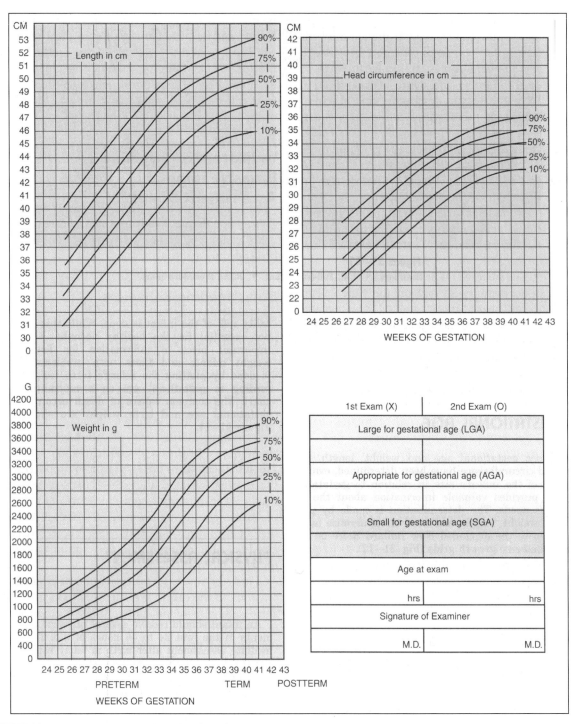

24 25 26 27 28 29 30 31 32 33 34 35 36 37 38 39 40 41 42 43
WEEKS OF GESTATION

FIGURE 20–3 Intrauterine growth grids.

Source: Adapted from Lubchenko, Hansman, & Boyd, 1996.

Rooting. Rooting is a reflexive behavior in which the infant turns his head in the direction of the stimulus and opens his mouth wide anticipating feeding. Rooting enables the infant to "catch" the mother's nipple and keeps the infant's tongue on the bottom of the mouth, important for compressing milk ducts (Figure 20–4). Licking movements typically precede and follow rooting in the early neonatal period.

Length of Time Before Latch-On. The time before latch-on is the amount of time in minutes before the infant latches on and remains on the breast.

Latch-On. Latch-on refers to the ability of the infant to grasp the nipple, flange the upper and lower lips outward against the breast areola, and remain firmly on the breast between bursts of suckling.

Suckling. Coordinated and rhythmic suckling, swallowing, and breathing characterized by a pattern of suckling burst, pause, suckling burst, pause: that is, alternating between nutritive (milk ingested) and non-nutritive (no milk ingested) suckling. The infant's lips should be visibly flanged outward during suckling to prevent friction and abrasion of the mother's areolar

tissue and to provide the seal that allows negative intraoral pressure. The distance between the nipple and the infant's hard-soft palate junction makes no difference in the amount of milk transfer. The nipple does not need to be level with the junction as previously thought (Jacobs et al., 2007).

Swallowing. In swallowing, the back of the tongue elevates and presses against the posterior pharyngeal wall. The soft palate rises and closes off the nasal passageways. The larynx then moves up and forward to close the trachea and propels the milk into the esophagus, thus initiating the baby's swallow reflex. Afterward, the larynx returns to its previous position. A sufficient volume of milk is needed to trigger swallowing. Swallowing can usually be observed during the first several days following birth and becomes audible following lactogenesis at approximately 4 days postpartum (or earlier). Swallowing produces observable movements of the infant's jaw (long, rhythmic jaw excursions) and throat muscles. Audible swallowing was the only significant predictor of how much breastmilk transfers from mother to baby at any feeding (Riordan, Gill-Hopple, & Angeron, 2005).

Other Behaviors. Positioning or alignment is commonly named as an essential attribute for breastfeeding to be "correct" (Shrago & Bocar, 1990). A number of authors suggest that good positioning prevents breastfeeding problems and may be the only assistance the mothers needs for optimal breastfeeding. However, there is a conspicuous lack of evidence and agreement on what constitutes optimal positions of the mother and baby during a feed despite considerable attention paid to it. For example, experienced lactation consultants Chele Marmet and Ellen Shell (2008) describe about 30 therapeutic positions for breastfeeding. Among them:

- Straddle sit
- Side saddle sit
- Clutch V position
- Physiologic flex
- "Fake position"
- Prone suck
- Over the shoulder prone suck

Obviously work must be done before we reach an agreement about the attributes of positioning.

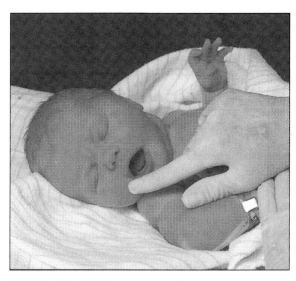

FIGURE 20–4   Rooting reflex.

Source: Moore ML, Nichols FH, Zwelling E, eds. *Maternal-newborn nursing: theory and practice.* Philadelphia: W. B. Saunders, 1080-1131, 1997. Reprinted with permission of Elsevier Publications.

Experienced lactation specialists quickly assess when the feeding is going well without a tool. A baby may not look technically perfect but if the sucking is strong and regular and the mother is pain free, chances are that the positioning is right for that mother and baby.

Breastfeeding Scales and Tools

Early feeding assessment scales were developed for and tested on infants who were bottle-fed. When breastfeeding became more common, hospital nurses documented breastfeedings with subjective phrases such as "breastfed well" or "breastfed poorly." Since then, breastfeeding assessment has evolved to use quantitative scales also known as "tools." Matthews (1988) separated and labeled indicators of infant feedings at the breast into the first scored assessment tool for breastfeeding. Around the same time, Shrago and Bocar (1990) published a list of breastfeeding behaviors for assessing feedings; however, they did not add a scoring system. Since then, several other scales have been developed; their description is below. The tools are shown in Appendix 20-A through 20-D. In addition to assessing feedings at the breast, a breastfeeding scale can serve as an outcome measure for research, as a method of documentation and communication among healthcare workers, and as a teaching tool for mothers to show them normal breastfeeding patterns of their babies (Riordan, 1998).

Infant Breastfeeding Assessment Tool (IBFAT). A Canadian midwife developed the IBFAT, the first such scale, as her master's thesis (Matthews, 1988). The IBFAT has four indicators: (1) readiness to feed, (2) rooting, (3) fixing, and (4) sucking. A numerical score (0 to 3) is given for each indicator; the total score can range from 0 to 12. Breastfeeding is considered to be effective when scores range from 9 to 12. Reliability and validity of the IBFAT is supported. Matthews (1988) found that the observer and mother agreed on the breastfeeding score 91 percent of the time and that the higher the score, the more pleased the mother was with the feeding (Matthews, 1990). Riordan et al. (2001) found the same high agreement in another study. Low IBFAT scores have been associated with the use of labor analgesia (Crowell, Hill, & Humenick, 1994; Riordan et al., 2000). Mothers with low IBFAT scores breastfed for a

significantly shorter period than those with medium or high scores ($P < .001$) (Riordan et al., 2000). Furman and Minish (2006) tested the use of the IBFAT to assess breastfeeding in very low weight infants. Although the IBFAT scores did not identify feeding sessions with adequate intake, most infants in the study took very small volumes.

Mother-Baby Assessment Tool (MBA). The MBA scoring system divides the process of breastfeeding into five steps: (1) signaling, (2) positioning, (3) fixing, (4) milk transfer, and (5) ending (Mulford, 1992). For each step, both a maternal and an infant behavior are scored. Ten is the highest possible feeding score: 5 for infant indicators and 5 for maternal indicators. Reliability and validity testing had mixed results. Percentage of agreement among the nurses rating videotapes of breastfeeds using the MBA ranged from 37 to 95 percent. The indicator receiving the greatest agreement was readiness of the baby and mother to feed (97 percent); the lowest was the milk transfer indicator (37 percent) (Riordan & Koehn, 1997). Morrison et al. (2002) reported a strong correlation between the MBA and the next tool described here—the LATCH Tool.

LATCH Assessment Tool. The LATCH tool (Jensen, Wallace, & Kelsay, 1994) evaluates five indicators of breastfeeding. A numerical score (0, 1, or 2) is assigned to each measure for a possible total score of 10. Each letter of the acronym title denotes a category. *L* represents how well the infant latches onto the breast, *A* represents audible swallowing, *T* describes the mother's nipple type, *C* represents the mother's degree of breast or nipple comfort, and *H* evaluates the amount of help the mother needs to position her baby at breast. The LATCH scale appears to measure different aspects of breastfeeding behavior than the IBFAT, because another study found that the correlations between the two scales were not significant (Schlomer, Kemmerer, & Twiss, 1999).

When LATCH scores were compared with the overall duration of breastfeeding, women still breastfeeding at 6 weeks postpartum had significantly higher LATCH scores than those who had weaned (Riordan et al., 2001). Although this finding supports the scale's validity overall, it should be noted that this prediction was due to the item "comfort of nipples." Mothers who had very sore nipples stopped breastfeeding early. In other testing of the LATCH tool, scores of lactation consultants, scores determined by raters, and scores determined by mothers were positively correlated (r = .53 to .67) (Adams & Hewell, 1997), an indication of reliability.

Via Christi Breastfeeding Assessment Tool. The Via Christi Breastfeeding Assessment Tool is modified from the LATCH and IBFAT scales. It is a combination of indicators from other assessment scales that were selected because they demonstrated positive correlation with mother's evaluation and amount of breastmilk ingested during feedings—indicators of reliability and validity—in previous studies (Adams & Hewell, 1997; Riordan et al., 2001; Riordan & Koehn, 1997; Schlomer, Kemmerer, & Twiss, 1999). Mothers' evaluations of the feedings were added to the scale because of a high positive correlation with other indicators. Mothers can gauge the effectiveness of the feed; only they can feel sensations of breastfeeding (baby's firm latch on the breast, letdown, uterine contractions, etc.). Audible swallowing was included because it predicts the amount of breastmilk taken by the baby (Riordan, Gill-Hopple, & Angeron, 2005).

Preterm Infant Breastfeeding Assessment Scale (PIBBS). The Preterm Infant Breastfeeding Behavior Scale was developed as an observational tool to study preterm infant feeding behavior (Hedberg-Nyqvist & Ewald, 1999). Hedberg-Nyqvist, Rubertsson, and Ewald (1996) found acceptable agreement of scores between nurses and raters but not as satisfactory agreement between nurses and mothers. The score of PIBBS predicted 75 percent of the variance for the amount of milk the baby ingested in breastfeedings (Radzyminski, 2005). This tool appears in Chapter 13.

Neonatal Oral-Motor Assessment Scale. The Neonatal Oral-Motor Assessment Scale (NOMAS) was originally developed to assess feedings in premature and medically compromised newborns (Palmer, Crawley, & Blanco, 1999). NOMAS is a nonnutritive sucking assessment done with the examiner's finger in the infant's mouth. The revised version has four parts that test normal and abnormal characteristics of the jaw and tongue. The examiner assesses and rates the newborn for these characteristics. The rating ranges from 0 to 16 (MacMullen & Dulski, 2000).

NOMAS has some evidence of validity (Case-Smith, Cooper, & Scala, 1988).

Summary of Breastfeeding Assessment Scales

As more women choose to breastfeed and are discharged early with uncertain breastfeeding support we need valid and reliable tools that measure breastfeeding. Because the scoring must take place quickly in busy maternity units by overworked nurses, the scale should be short and easy to use. Which scales are best for assessing feedings of full-term babies? At the time of this writing, these tools have support for their clinical use: (1) the IBFAT, (2) the LATCH, (3) the Via Christi, and (4) the PIBBS. In addition to having evidence of validity and reliability, all are brief and are being successfully used in clinical settings. The PIBBs Tool can be used to assess feeding readiness of both low birth weight and full-term babies (Hedberg-Nygvist, Rubertsson, & Ewald, 1996). The PIBBS Tool is the only tool that has been shown to significantly predict the amount of breastmilk ingested by the infant during a feeding (Radzyminski, 2005). The only single behavior found that predicted milk intake is audible swallowing (Riordan, Gill-Hopple, & Angeron, 2005).

NOMAS is seldom used for routine breastfeeding assessment because of its complexity, intrusiveness, and required training. Finally, the journey to find the "best" breastfeeding assessment scale has only begun. Existing tools will be revised and new tools developed as new knowledge becomes available.

Physical Assessment

Transitional Assessment

During the first 24 hours of life, the newborn undergoes a typical pattern of adjustment indicating normal adaptation to extrauterine life. The first several hours after birth are considered the first period of reactivity (Davidson et al., 2008). During the first 30 minutes of this time, the healthy full-term newborn is alert, (unless affected by maternal medication), cries spontaneously, and when put to the mother's breast will root, lick, and otherwise nuzzle the mother's breast. This is followed by hand-to-mouth movements and later latching-on to the nipple and suckling. This is an ideal time to begin breastfeeding, as the newborn is wide-eyed, alert, and responsive to environmental cues.

Physiologic changes during this time include rapid respiration and heart rate, and increased mucus secretions. There may be a transient episode of tachypnea and nasal flaring, but this should resolve spontaneously within the first 30 minutes. The next phase of this period begins when the infant falls into a deep sleep. Heart and respiratory rate decrease, temperature continues to be unstable, and mucus production decreases. Stimulation of the newborn at this time usually results in little response. This is normal neonatal behavior but can be upsetting to parents and nurses who are anxious for the baby to breastfeed sooner than the baby is ready for it. Some acrocyanosis may still be evident, although it usually shows a steady improvement. Bowels sounds may become audible at this time.

The second stage of reactivity occurs when the newborn awakens from a deep sleep state, alert and responsive (Davidson et al., 2008). The newborn's heart and respiratory rate increase; however, the baby can have periods of apnea associated with a decrease in heart rate. Tactile stimulation is used to improve the heart and respiratory rate. When apneic periods are associated with skin color changes further evaluation is necessary. It is not unusual for the newborn to gag, choke, and regurgitate as gastric and respiratory secretions increase. The gastrointestinal system is active, and most newborns will pass the first meconium stool within 8 to 24 hours of birth. Many newborns void immediately after birth. If the infant was not fed during the first period of reactivity this is an ideal time to initiate a feeding.

When performing a head-to-toe physical assessment (Table 20–3) a warm surface must be provided for the newborn. Exposing the newborn's body to uncontrolled temperatures increases the risk of hypothermia. Placing the baby in a radiant warmer for the initial examination after the birth avoids this problem. For subsequent examinations, expose one area of the body at a time to minimize the amount of time the newborn is exposed to cold air. The Moro or startle reflex is elicited by loud noise or sudden movement of the surface the infant is lying on (Figure 20–5).

Skin

Observe the condition of the skin for color, opacity, thickness, and consistency. Dryness, cracking and peeling are signs of full- or postterm maturity. A full-term newborn is likely to have flaking skin in the major creases at the ankles. Vernix caseosa—a combination of discarded epithelial cells, lanugo, and sebaceous gland secretions—is evident on term newborns and usually becomes less visible after 40 weeks gestation. Vessels should not be visible over the trunk of the body of the full-term newborn. Inspect the skin for color as well as bruises, lesions, rashes, or discolorations in natural light.

The skin should be warm, dry, and smooth. Skin color of the newborn will depend on the ethnicity of the parents. African-American newborns may appear pink or yellow-brown. Asian descent newborns may have a tan or rose color. Caucasian newborns are usually pink to red, and Hispanic newborns may have pink skin with an olive or yellow tint. Native American newborns may vary from pink to light brown or darker brown. Blanch the skin by gently pressing a finger over the chest or forehead. The skin should show its own color as the finger is removed. The skin should not be jaundiced or yellow tinged during the first 24 hours of life (see Chapter 11). Jaundice usually appears on the head first and progresses to the lower portion of the body and extremities as the bilirubin level rises. This abnormal finding requires documentation and a

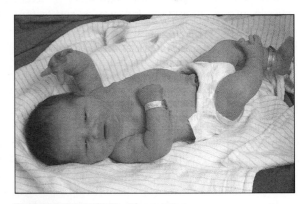

FIGURE **20–5** Moro reflex.

Source: Moore ML, Nichols FH, Zwelling E, eds. *Maternal-newborn nursing: theory and practice.* Philadelphia: W. B. Saunders, 1080-1131, 1997. Reprinted with permission of Elsevier Publications.

TABLE 20–3	**Newborn Physical Assessment**		

	Normal	**Normal Variations**	**Abnormal**
Vital Signs	• Temperature Axillary • 36.5–37.4°C • 97.9–98°F		• < 36.5°C • > 37.4°C
	• Pulse 120–140 beats/minute	• Increased with crying • Decreased when sleeping	• Tachycardia • Bradycardia < 80 to 100 • Associated with color changes
	• Respirations 30–60/minute	• Increased during first period of reactivity and with crying • Decreased when sleeping	
Measurement	• Head circumference 33–35 cm (13–14 in.) • Chest circumference 30.5–33 cm (12–13 in.) • Head to heel length 48–53 cm (19–21 in.)	• Molding may decrease head circumference	• Head < 10th or > 90th percentile
	• Birth weight 2700–4000 gm (6–9 lb)		• Weight < 10th or > 90th percentile
Skin	• Bright red, smooth at birth • Vernix caseosa, lanugo	• Acrocyanosis • Cutis marmorata—mottling when exposed to low temperature, stress or overstimulation • Milia • Erythema toxicum • Mongolian spots • Telangiectatic nevi • Harlequin color changes • Jaundice after first 24 hours	• Jaundice in the first 24 hours • Central or generalized cyanosis • Pallor • Mottling • Plethora • Persistent petechiae or hemorrhage or ecchymosis • Café au lait spots • Nevus flammeus
Head	• Anterior fontanelle 2.5–4.0 cm (1–1.75 in.), diamond-shaped	• Molding after vaginal birth • Fontanelle bulging when crying • Caput succedaneum • Cephalhematoma	• Fused sutures • Depressed or bulging fontanelles when quiet

(Continues)

TABLE 20–3	**Newborn Physical Assessment (Continued)**		

	Normal	Normal Variations	Abnormal
	• Posterior fontanelle 0.5–1 cm (0.2–0.4 in.), triangular-shaped • Soft, flat fontanelles		
Eyes	• Edematous lids • Absence of tears • Slate gray, dark blue, or brown • Positive red, corneal, pupillary, and blink reflex • Fixes on objects, follows to midline	• Subconjunctival hemorrhages • Epicanthal folds in Asian newborns	• Purulent discharge • Upward slant of eyes • Iris pink color • Constricted or dilated pupil • Absence of red, corneal, papillary reflex • Inability to follow objects to the midline • Sclera yellow
Ears	• Pinna flexible, well formed level with outer canthus of the eye	• Pinna flat against the head • Irregular shape, size • Skin tags	• Low placement of ears
Nose	• Patent • Thin, white nasal discharge	• Flattened, bruised, or slightly deviated	• Nonpatent • Thick, bloody discharge • Nasal flaring
Mouth/Throat	• Intact, arched palate • Midline uvula • Tongue centered in the mouth • Reflexes: sucking, rooting, gagging extrusion • Vigorous cry	• Natal teeth • Epstein's pearls	• Cleft lip • Cleft palate • Large, protruding tongue • Drooling or copious salivation • Candidiasis– white, adherent, thick patches on tongue, palate, buccal surfaces • Weak, high-pitched cry

(Continues)

TABLE 20–3	**Newborn Physical Assessment (Continued)**		
	Normal	**Normal Variations**	**Abnormal**
Neck	• Short, thick • Tonic neck reflex	• Torticollis	• Extra skinfolds or webbing • Resistant to flexion • Absence of tonic neck reflex
Chest	• Equal anteroposterior and lateral diameter • Smooth clavicles • Breast enlargement	• Supernumerary nipples • Thin breast secretions	• Crepitus or asymmetry over clavicle • Depressed sternum • Marked retractions • Asymmetrical expansion • Wide-spaced nipples
Lungs	• Bilateral bronchial breath sounds • Periodic breathing	• Crackles immediately after birth	• Inspiratory stridor • Expiratory grunting • Retractions • Unequal breath sounds • Apnea • Persistent fine crackles or wheezing • Peristaltic sounds
Abdomen	• Cylindrical shape • Soft to palpation • Umbilical cord bluish white at birth, with 2 arteries and 1 vein • Bowel sounds present • Femoral pulses equal bilaterally	• Firm to palpation when crying • Umbilical hernia • Diastasis recti	• Abdominal distension • Localized bulging • Absent bowel sounds • Drainage or blood at umbilical cord • Absent or unequal femoral pulses • Visible peristaltic waves

(Continues)

TABLE **20-3**	**Newborn Physical Assessment (Continued)**		
	Normal	**Normal Variations**	**Abnormal**
Genitalia	*Female* • Labia majora and clitoris edematous • Urethral meatus behind clitoris • Vernix caseosa between labia • Urination within first 24 hours	• Blood-tinged, mucous discharge • Hymenal tag	• Fused labia • Absence of vaginal opening • Masses in labia • Enlarged clitoris with urethral meatus at tip • Ambiguous genitalia • No urination within first 24 hours
	Male • Urethral opening at tip of penis • Palpable testes • Scrotum: rugae edematous, pendulous, deeply pigmented in dark-skinned newborns • Smegma • Urination within first 24 hours	• Nonretractable foreskin • Urethral opening covered by prepuce • Testes palpable in inguinal canal • Small scrotum	• Hypospadius • Epispadius • Chordee • Testes nonpalpable in scrotum or inguinal canal • Hypoplastic scrotum • Hydrocele • Masses in scrotum • Discoloration of testes • Ambiguous genitalia • No urination within first 24 hours
Back/Rectum	• Spine intact, no deviations, openings, or masses • Trunk incurvation reflex • Patent anal opening • Anal reflex • Meconium passed within first 24 hours		• Anal fissures or fistulas • Imperforate anus • Absent anal reflex • No meconium within 36–48 hours • Pilonidal cyst or sinus • Tuft of hair • Spina bifida
Extremities	• Ten fingers and toes • Full range of motion	• Partial syndactyly between second and third toes	• Polydactyly • Syndactyly (webbing)

(Continues)

TABLE	**Newborn Physical Assessment (Continued)**

20–3

Normal	Normal Variations	Abnormal
• Pink nail beds • Creases on anterior two thirds of sole • Symmetrical extremeties • Equal muscle tone bilaterally • Equal bilateral brachial pulses • Equal leg and gluteal folds	• Second toe overlapping third toe • Wide gap between hallux and second toes • Asymmetric length of toes • Dorsiflexion and shortness of hallux	• Persistent nail bed cyanosis • Nail beds yellowed • Transverse palmar crease • Fractures • Decreased or absent range of motion • Unequal leg or gluteal folds • Limited hip abduction • Audible click with abduction • Asymmetry

report to the physician. In Hispanic and African-American babies, the color of the mucous membranes is used to assess for jaundice.

The color of the skin changes with the activity state of the newborn. When the newborn is crying the skin is likely to be darker in color. Within the first few hours of birth the newborn may have brief periods of cyanosis, not associated with heart rate changes or apnea. Generally, this resolves within the first few hours of life. Transient mottling may be apparent, especially when the newborn is exposed to cool temperatures. A common variation in the first 24 to 48 hours of life is acrocyanosis, a bluish discoloration of the hands and feet. As peripheral circulation improves this will resolve and disappear within a few days after birth. Acrocyanosis lasting longer than the first 48 hours after birth should be investigated. Newborns with plethora, a ruddy color, have an excess of red blood cells contributing to the bright red skin color. This occurs more often in infants of diabetic mothers. Plethora is one sign of polycythemia, and thus, a complete blood count should be obtained. Polycythemia is defined as a hematocrit of 65 percent or higher. These infants should be monitored closely for other signs of polycythemia, which include peripheral cyanosis, respiratory distress, lethargy, hypoglycemia, and

hyperbilirubinemia (Fuloria et al., 2002; Askin & Wilson, 2007). Pallor is most often associated with anemia, hypoxia, or poor peripheral perfusion, and needs to be evaluated. Harlequin color changes may occur as the result of the dependent half of the newborn's body reacting to a temporary autonomic imbalance of the cutaneous vessels. The skin on the dependent portion of the body becomes deep red, while the upper portion appears pale. When the newborn is turned to the opposite side the color variation reverses. This is a benign condition occurring more often in low birth weight infants (Lund & Kuller, 2003).

Observe and note the location of petechiae, pinpoint superficial hemorrhages that occur due to pressure during descent and rotation through the birth canal. Petechiae are more likely to be seen if there has been a nuchal cord; they will usually fade within 24 to 48 hours after birth.

Skin turgor is the result of the outward pressure of interstitial fluid on the cells. Assess skin turgor by gently grasping and lifting the skin of the chest, abdomen or thigh between the thumb and finger. Skin that readily springs back to its original shape indicates the newborn has adequate skin turgor, a sign of appropriate hydration. Dimpling, wrinkling or folding of the skin indicates possible dehydration.

Milia are common variations that may occur on the skin of the newborn, commonly visible over the nose, cheeks, and brow. Milia are sebaceous glands that have swollen under the influence of maternal hormones. Treatment is not required for milia, as they resolve spontaneously within the few weeks after birth. A common newborn rash, erythema toxicum, is a pink, papular rash with vesicles occurring first on the face then spreading to the chest, abdomen, back and buttocks that is often visible by the first or second day. This will disappear within one week. The rash may reappear and dissipate spontaneously without treatment.

Birthmarks

A bluish-black area of pigmentation over the buttocks and back of the newborn with dark skin may be apparent. This can easily be confused with bruising, however it is a common variation known as a Mongolian spot caused by a collection of melanocytes in the dermal layer (Figure 20–6). Mongolian spots are most often observed in African-American, Asian, Hispanic, and other dark-skinned races (Davidson et al., 2008). The macular lesion or patch may also be seen on the legs or flank of the newborn, appearing gray or blue-green and usually fades over time. Café au lait spots are light brown or tan macular areas with well-defined edges. As long as there are fewer than six spots, and are less than 3 cm in length they do not hold significance. Infants with larger or numerous spots may have cutaneous neurofibromatosis (McCord, 2007).

Telangiectatic nevi, "stork bites" are flat, deep pink areas over the eyelids or on the forehead or bridge of the nose that blanch with pressure. Most nevi fade with time, although they may become brighter in color when the newborn is crying. Nevus flammeus, "port wine nevus", is a reddish or flat pink lesion that does not blanch with pressure, caused by dilated capillaries below the epidermal surface. This lesion usually remains constant in size and does not fade with time. It often appears over the face, but may also be observed over the upper body.

Approximately 1 to 3 percent of newborns have hemangiomas present at birth, and another 10 percent will develop hemangiomas within the first 3 to 4 weeks (Lund & Kuller, 2003). Strawberry hemangiomas are soft, raised, lobed tumors with a

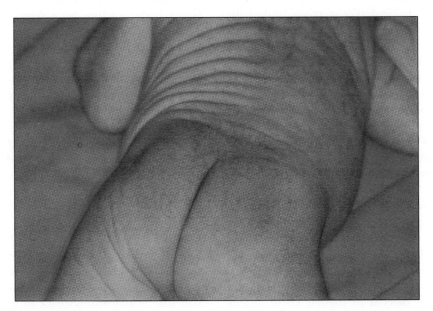

FIGURE 20–6 Mongolian spot.

Source: Moore ML, Nichols FH, Zwelling E, eds. *Maternal-newborn nursing: theory and practice.* Philadelphia: W. B. Saunders, 1080-1131, 1997. Reprinted with permission of Elsevier Publications.

bright red color, usually occurring on the head, neck, trunk or extremities. The red color is caused by the dilated mass of capillaries formed in the dermal and subdermal layers of the skin. Although spontaneous regression usually occurs, it may take several years. There will be no permanent scars if these lesions are left alone. Tumors that interfere with feeding, respiration, and vision require treatment. Infection, bleeding, ulceration, and compression of the vital organs are rare complications of strawberry hemangiomas.

Head

Observe the head for shape, symmetry, bruises, and lesions. Palpation of the head may reveal swelling, masses, or bony defects. Common variations are molding, caput succedaneum, and cephalhematoma. The negative pressure created when the amniotic sac ruptures and draws a portion of the scalp into the cervical os causes a caput succedaneum. Dilated capillaries cause the edema and bruising that occurs over the occipitoparietal area of the head. Swelling usually resolves within 24 hours after birth. Overriding suture lines are common in the infant born vaginally in a vertex position. This irregular shape resolves within a few days in the full-term infant and may persist for several weeks in premature infant. A soft area over the suture lines indicates the sutures are separated.

The intersections of the cranial sutures are called fontanelles. The anterior fontanelle, diamond in shape, is the largest and most important for assessment (Figure 20–7). The anterior fontanelle is normally described as soft and flat but may appear to be bulging when the infant is crying vigorously, coughs, or vomits. Palpate the tension in the fontanelle with the infant in an upright and a recumbent position. A newborn with a soft sunken fontanelle in the prone position is dehydrated. The anterior fontanelle usually closes around 18 months of age. The posterior fontanelle—triangular shaped at the junction of the sagittal and lambdoidal suture—is small, 0.5–1 cm (0.25–0.5 in.) and closes between 2 to 4 months of age (Creehan, 2008).

Move the head through its full range of motion to assess flexion, extension, bending, and rotation. The normal newborn's head is easily mobile in all directions, although the infant is not able to turn its head from side to side until 2 weeks of age. Assess for signs of torticollis as these may indicate feeding difficulties: pliagocephaly (a flattening of the occiput), misalignment of the eyes, asymmetry of the ears, a depression of the side of the neck under the ear, flattening of the mandible, upward tilting of the lower jaw, limited neck movement, and occasional asymmetries associated with the back, chest, hips, and feet (Stellwegen et al., 2004). These signs/symptoms may appear in varying degrees. The differences between two types of torticollis were described by van Vlimmeren et al. (2004):

- Congenital muscular torticollis
  - The incidence is less than 0.4 percent
  - A palpable mass noted in the sternocleidomastoid muscle 2 to 3 weeks after birth
  - The male/female ratio is 3:2
  - The mass persists for 2 to 3 months and slowly disappears within 4 to 8 months
  - Progressive and persistent torticollis in 25 percent of cases
- Positional torticollis
  - More common: 7.6–8.2 percent

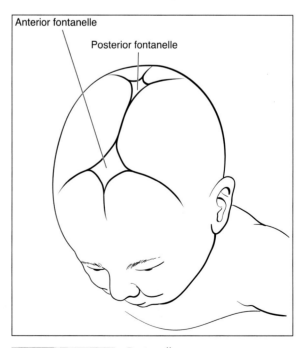

Anterior fontanelle

Posterior fontanelle

FIGURE 20–7   Fontanelles.

- No morphological changes in the sternocleidomastoid muscle
- Active range of motion restricted

Infants with asymmetry of the mandible (crooked jaw) may have difficulty with successfully latching onto the breast with resultant excessive weight loss. Mothers of these infants frequently report nipple pain with breastfeeding attempts (Wall & Glass, 2006). Assessment techniques include the following:

- Positioning: Assess if infant consistently turns to one side
- Eyes: Assess for one eye that is smaller and higher
- Ears: Assess for one ear that is cupped forward with the other ear flat
- Lips: Assess for symmetry at rest, crying, or yawning
- Gum lines: Assess for parallel upper and lower jaw

Newborns have varying degrees of head control. When held in a supine position and pulled forward from the arms into a sitting position by the examiner, hyperextension and head lag are normal. While in a supported sitting position the newborn may attempt to raise the head. The head will be in a straight line with the spine when the newborn is held in a ventral suspension position (Wheeler & Wilson, 2007).

Ears and Eyes

Inspect facial features for symmetry, shape, bruising, or dysmorphic features. Asymmetry may result from compression of the fetal head in the uterus or from nerve injury related to birth trauma. The sclera of the eyes should be white and without drainage. The eyelids are usually edematous immediately after birth, with no tears present. Scleral and small conjunctival hemorrhages may be present.

Able to fix on objects and follow objects to the midline the newborn can focus on objects 8 to 10 inches (20 to 25 cm) away, the distance of the mother's face when the infant is at the breast. At this time, visual acuity ranges from 20/100 to 20/400. It is common in the newborn for the eyes to remain fixed when the head is moved through full range of motion (doll's eye reflex). By 4 weeks, the infant can intently watch when spoken to by the parent.

Convergence on near objects begins at 6 weeks and is well established by 4 months of age (Wilson, 2007).

The ear should be horizontal with the outer canthus of the eye. The pinna is flexible and well formed in the full-term infant. There should be no drainage from the ears. Fold the ear forward to examine the undersurface of the ear for skin tags. Assessment of hearing can begin early in the infant's life with simple observation of reaction to auditory stimuli. The newborn should respond with a startle reflex, head turning, eye blinking, and a pause in body movements, particularly when a familiar voice is heard. The degree of the infant's alertness will affect response; however, it is wise to be observant for signs of normal behavior. Practice standards vary by geographic area, although routine auditory screening of all newborns is common.

Nose

Inspect the nose for shape, symmetry, patency, and skin lesions. Observe each naris for a visual opening and gently occlude one side of the naris to observe breathing through the other side. Repeat the same process for the other naris. Newborns are often nose breathers but should be able to tolerate occluding one naris during assessment. There should be no visible drainage from either naris. The nose may be misshapen at birth, due to uterine or vaginal compression, but resolves within a few days. Obstructions or deformities, such as choanal atresia, may indicate congenital syndromes or anatomic malformations. Since clefting of the oral area may include the nose, close assessment is necessary.

Mouth

Inspect the mouth for size, shape, symmetry, color, and presence of abnormal structures and masses when the newborn is both at rest and crying. Birth trauma may result in facial asymmetry due to nerve damage. The midline region between the nose and the lips, the philtrum, should be well defined. The lips are fully formed and the maxilla rounded. Newborns with at least two dysmorphological characteristics of the face may have fetal alcohol syndrome or effects: microcephaly (head circumference below the tenth percentile), short palpebral fissures, thinned upper lip, hypoplastic or smooth philtrum (vertical ridge in upper lip), short, upturned nose (Askin & Wilson, 2007).

The sucking reflex, so important for breast-feeding, can be elicited right after birth by stimulating the mucous membranes of the mouth with a gloved finger (Figure 20–8). Assess the buccal pads on the sides of the mouth. A full-term newborn has adequate buccal pads that assist in the negative pressure created when suckling at the breast. Preterm or malnourished newborns may not have full buccal pads. The mucous membranes and tongue are pink and moist, and the tongue protrudes symmetrically over the alveolar ridge (gum line) when the mouth is open. The tongue fits easily within the mouth when closed. Macroglossia, an abnormally large tongue, may be seen in some congenital syndromes such as Beckwith-Wiedeman syndrome and in hypothyroidism. Underdevelopment of the jaw, micrognathia, may be seen in certain malformation syndromes such as Pierre-Robin sequence.

The lingual frenulum has a consistency that may vary from thick and fibrous to very thin. The frenulum may be attached at the tip or midway along the undersurface of the tongue. Ankyloglossia (tongue-tie) occurs when the frenulum is unusually thick, tight, or short. Variations and differing degrees of severity occur. During breastfeeding, as opposed to bottle-feeding, the tongue is projected further forward causing the nipple to elongate. During normal feeding the nipple, along with some of the breast tissue, is held in the mouth with the tongue covering the lower gum ridge. The infant's lower jaw elevates compressing the breast behind the nipple, while the front of the tongue moves up to compress the milk ducts under the areola (Hall & Renfrew, 2005). Ankyloglossia prohibits tongue extension beyond the lower gum and resultant problems with latching on, nipple trauma, and continued breastfeeding. However, there is a lack of a uniform definition for ankyloglossia and therefore, a lack of sufficient evidence to support the best treatment: intensive lactation support or frenotomy (Griffiths, 2004; Hall & Renfrew et al., 2005).

Along the gums—which are smooth and raised— or the palate there may be retention cysts known as Epstein's pearls, which are yellow or white in color and occasionally mistaken for teeth. However, they resolve spontaneously within a few weeks (Creehan, 2008). Occasionally an infant will be born with supernumerary teeth that are soft with no enamel and are usually shed spontaneously. Primary teeth will normally erupt in a wide range of ages. At age 10 months, most Anglo infants have two upper and two lower central incisors. Approximately every 4 months four more teeth will erupt, so that there will be eight teeth by 14 months of age, 12 by 18 months, 16 by 22 months, and 20 by 26 months.

Palpate the soft and the hard palate, which should be smooth, gently arched and intact with the uvula in the midline. While a gloved finger is in the mouth assess the suck reflex. It should be strong and coordinated in the full-term newborn. The newborn should be able to completely form a seal around the examiner's finger. Saliva will be either minimal or absent. Excessive drooling or oral secretions indicate an inability to swallow, or the presence of a pharyngeal or esophageal obstruction.

Neck

The newborn's neck is short and thick, which makes it difficult to observe swallowing, a cardinal sign of breastmilk intake. Palpate the clavicles for crepitus or shortening which may indicate fracture. The tonic reflex elicited by rotating the baby's head to one side (Figure 20–9) is seen as early as 35 weeks.

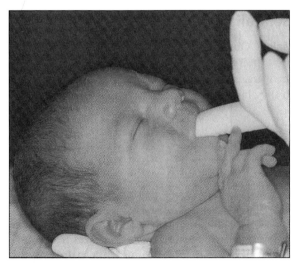

FIGURE 20–8 Suckling reflex.

Source: Moore ML, Nichols FH, Zwelling E, eds. *Maternal-newborn nursing: theory and practice.* Philadelphia: W. B. Saunders, 1080-1131, 1997. Reprinted with permission of Elsevier Publications.

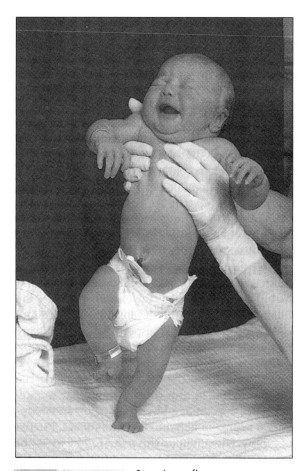

FIGURE 20–11   Stepping reflex.

Source: Moore ML, Nichols FH, Zwelling E, eds. *Maternal-newborn nursing: theory and practice.* Philadelphia: W. B. Saunders, 1080-1131, 1997. Reprinted with permission of Elsevier Publications.

newborn will void two to six times per day for the first 2 days, up to 20 times per day after 2 days, owing to the kidneys' inability to concentrate urine, and later on five to eight times per day. By the end of the first week the newborn's output is approximately 200 to 300 ml per 24 hours (Wheeler & Wilson, 2007). The presence of uric acid crystals, pink or red stains in the diaper, while usually insignificant during the first week of life, indicate the importance of a complete assessment of hydration.

Stool progression in the newborn follows a fairly predictable pattern relative to feedings. The first stool, meconium, usually occurs within the first 24 hours. Composed of intestinal secretions, mucosal cells, and other fluids, the stool will appear black, thick, and tarry. Within two to three days the stools will appear greenish black to greenish brown, then yellow or golden in color. These transitional stools may be watery or thick in texture, and they are odorless and less sticky than meconium (see Color Plate 53).

Behavioral Assessment

The infant's behavior is a reflection of his capacity for self-organization (Brazelton, 1984). Self-organization refers to the infant's ability to control reactions, motor responses, responses to people and events associated with external stressors, and the ability to maintain an appropriate degree of alertness (Blackburn & Loper, 1992). An infant's reaction to stimuli affects how mothers as well as other caregivers react to him or her. This has important implications for breastfeeding as well as parent–child relationships.

Infant state is the foundation for interpreting an infant's behavior. Initially, newborns exhibit a period of alertness (2 to 4 hours) followed by a longer period of sleep. A newborn may sleep most of the next 2 to 3 postbirth days, most likely to recover from the birth experience. Subsequently, infants will demonstrate more organization of behavioral states. Infant behavior is state dependent. Infant behaviors while feeding at the breast follow a pattern as the baby develops. Table 20–4 shows infant behaviors at certain points of development.

Sleep–Wake States

The normal, healthy infant demonstrates six sleep–wake states (Table 20–5; Figure 20–12). The first two are sleep states. In the first, "deep sleep," the infant cannot be easily aroused even when stimulated. While in the second state, "quiet sleep," the infant exhibits some bodily movements and facial expressions. In this state, the infant is more easily aroused by stimuli, either internal or external. The newborn infant may spend as much as 18 hours per day in a combination of these sleep states. Consequently, the infant will not easily latch on to the breast when in one of these two sleep states.

The third state, "drowsy," is a transitional state. In this state, the infant is relaxed; he exhibits irregular breathing and his eyes are either open or closed.

TABLE 20–4	Infant Psychosocial and Breastfeeding Behaviors by Age	
Age	**Psychosocial Behavior**	**Breastfeeding Behavior**
First day postpartum	• Quiet alert state after birth, followed by long sleep.	• May or may not feed following delivery; sleepy, learning how to suckle.
1 month	• Follows objects with eyes; reacts to noise by stopping behavior or crying.	• Becoming efficient at suckling; feedings last approximately 17 minutes. • Feedings now 8–16 times per day.
2 months	• Smiles; vocalizes in response to interactions.	• Easily pacified by frequent breastfeeding.
3 months	• Shows increased interest in surroundings; voluntarily grasps objects. • Vocalizes when spoken to. • Turns head as well as eyes in response to moving objects.	• Will interrupt feeding to turn to look at father or other familiar person coming into room and to smile at mother.
4–5 months	• Shows interest in strange settings. • Smiles at mirror image.	• Continues to enjoy frequent feedings at the breast.
6 months	• Laughs aloud. • Shows increased awareness of caregivers versus strangers. • May become distressed if mother or caregiver leaves.	• Solids offered; fewer feedings. • Feeds longer before sleep for the night. • May begin waking to nurse more often at night.
7–8 months	• Imitates actions and noises. • Responds to name. • Responds to "no." • Enjoys peek-a-boo games. • Reaches for toys that are out of reach.	• Will breastfeed anytime, anywhere. • Actively attempts to get to breast (i.e., will try to unbutton mother's blouse).
9–10 months	• Distressed by new situations or people. • Waves bye-bye. • Reaches for toys that are out of reach.	• Easily distracted by surroundings and interrupts feedings frequently. • May hold breast with one or both hands while feeding.
11–12 months	• Drops objects deliberately to be picked up by other people. • Rolls ball to another person. • Speaks a few words. • Appears interested in picture books. • Shakes head for "no."	• Tries "acrobatic" breastfeeding (i.e., assumes different positions while keeping nipple in mouth).
12–15 months	• Fears unfamiliar situations but will leave mother's side to explore familiar surroundings.	• Uses top hand to play while feeding: forces finger into mother's mouth, plays with

(Continues)

TABLE 20–4	Infant Psychosocial and Breastfeeding Behaviors by Age (Continued)	

Age	Psychosocial Behavior	Breastfeeding Behavior
	• Shows emotions (e.g., love, anger, fear). • Speaks several words. • Understands meanings of many words.	her hair, and pinches her other nipple. • Pats mother's chest when wants to breastfeed. • Hums or vocalizes while feeding. • Verbalizes need to breastfeed; may use "code" word.
16–20 months	• Has frequent temper tantrums. • Increasingly imitates parents. • Enjoys solitary play or observing others. • Speaks 6 to 10 words.	• Verbalizes delight with breastfeeding. • Takes mother by the hand and leads her to favorite nursing chair.
20–24 months	• Helps with simple tasks. • Has fewer temper tantrums. • Engages in parallel play. • Combines 2 or 3 words. • Speaks 15 to 20 words.	• Stands up while nursing at times. • Nurses mostly for comfort. • Feeding before bedtime is usually last feeding before weaning. • When asked to do so by mother, willing to wait for feeding until later.

The infant is more reactive to stimuli and may either return to a sleep state or progress to one of the three awake states.

In the fourth state, "quiet alert," the infant is attentive to external stimuli but exhibits little bodily movement. Because the infant is calm in this state, this is an excellent time for breastfeeding. If a stimulus is presented at this point, such as the stroking of the cheek or the lips, the infant will become more alert and search for the stimulus. As the infant moves into the "active alert" state, he will become more sensitive to external stimuli, such as increased handling, diaper changing, or bathing, or internal stimuli such as hunger. The last state, "crying," is a state of much activity with crying and color change (pink to red). The infant is highly sensitive to external and internal stimuli and may need to be calmed and comforted before he will latch on to the breast. Comforting interventions such as swaddling, rocking, and softly singing or talking may help the infant return to the quiet alert or active alert state.

As part of the complete infant assessment, assess the infant's ability to move from one state to another. Observe for any self-quieting activities, such as the infant sucking on his own hand. Also, observe the infant's response to a caregiver's voice or other calming interventions. Is the infant able to move from a crying state to one of the alert states? As the infant matures, he should show increasing ability to move from one state to another.

Neurobehavioral Cues

The cues that an infant gives about his self-organizational abilities assist the caregiver in recognizing the infant's readiness for interactions. Early and late cues that indicate the baby is hungry are

	TABLE 20–5	Infant Sleep/Wake States with Implications for Breastfeeding

Infant State	Description	Implications for Breastfeeding
Deep or quiet sleep	• Closed eyes with no eye movement; regular breathing • Relaxed • Absent body movements with occasional isolated startles	• Only intense stimuli will arouse • Do not attempt to feed
Light or active sleep	• Closed eyes with rapid eye movements • Irregular breathing • Sucking, smiling, grimacing, yawning • Some slight muscular twitching of the body • Most infant's sleep is in this state	• More easily aroused by stimuli • Not alert enough to feed
Drowsy	• May have eyes open • Irregular breathing • Variable body movements with mild startles • Relaxed	• Stimuli may arouse infant but may return to sleep • May enjoy nonnutritive sucking
Quiet alert	• Eyes bright and wide open • Responsive to stimuli • Minimal body activity	• Interacts with others • Excellent time to initiate breastfeeding before becomes fussy and agitated
Active alert	• Eyes open • Rapid and irregular breathing • More sensitive to stimuli and discomfort • Active	• Comfort (change diaper, hold, talk quietly) • Initiate breastfeeding before progression to crying
Crying	• Eyes open or tightly closed • Irregular breathing • Crying, very active • Uncoordinated, thrashing movements of extremities	• Comfort (hold, swaddle, talk quietly, rock) before attempting to breastfeed

seen in Table 20–6. For example, if the infant displays disengagement cues such as yawning, facial grimacing, arching, or rapid state change, he may be indicating a lack of self-organization and the need for a period of rest. That is, instead of playing with the infant or attempting to breastfeed, it may be better to swaddle, hold, rock, or otherwise provide comfort. On the other hand, engagement cues such as alertness, sucking, mouthing, smiling, or smooth movements indicates good self-organization and readiness for interaction or feeding (Blackburn & Loper, 1992) (Figure 20–13). Neonatal reflexes that have important implications for breastfeeding are seen in Table 20–7.

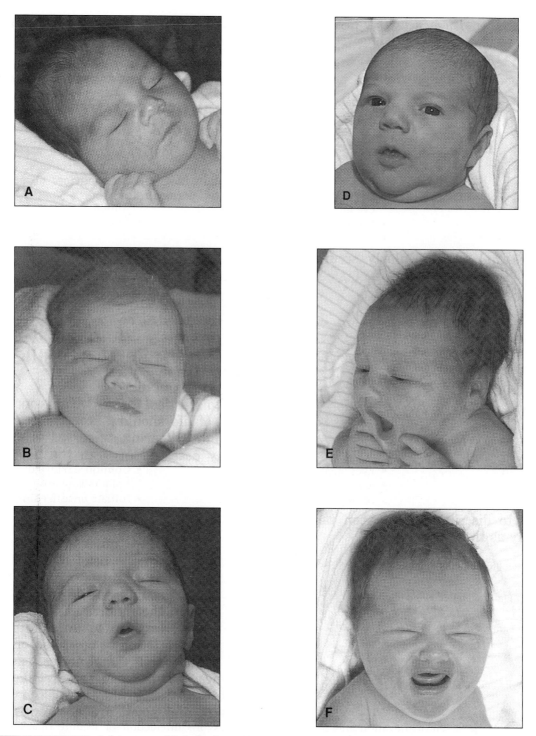

FIGURE 20–12   Infant states. (A) Deep sleep. (B) Light sleep. (C) Drowsy. (D) Quiet alert. (E) Active alert. (F) Crying.

Source: Moore ML, Nichols FH, Zwelling E, eds. *Maternal-newborn nursing: theory and practice.* Philadelphia: W. B. Saunders, 1080-1131, 1997. Reprinted with permission of Elsevier Publications.

TABLE 20–6	**Early and Late Feeding Cues**

Early Feeding Cues

- Body wriggling
- Hand and foot clasping
- Bringing hands to mouth or face
- Light sucking motions followed by more vigorous sucking
- Rooting behavior
- Tongue extension
- Light sounds or whimpering
- Body flexion
- Turning head to the side

Late Feeding Cues

- Crying
- Exhaustion
- Falls asleep

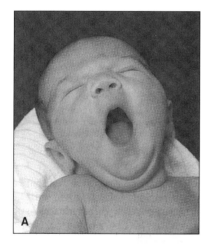 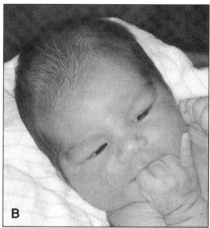

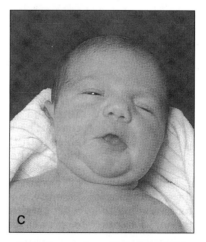

FIGURE 20–13	Infant behaviors. (A) Self-consoling. (B) Social. (C) Disengagement.

Source: Moore ML, Nichols FH, Zwelling E, eds. *Maternal-newborn nursing: theory and practice.* Philadelphia: W. B. Saunders, 1080-1131, 1997. Reprinted with permission of Elsevier Publications.

TABLE 20–7	Developmental Infant Reflexes and Implications for Breastfeeding	

Reflex	Description	Implications for Breastfeeding
Moro (Startle)	• Elicited by any sudden noise or motion such as a handclap or jarring of the crib or cradle. • Extension of arm and opening of hands followed by flexion of arms on the chest and closing of hands. • Present by 34 weeks gestation. • Disappears at approximately 6 months of age.	• If the infant is exhibiting the Moro reflex, handle the infant more gently • Avoid exposure to sudden, loud noises.
Sucking	• Elicited by stimulating the mouth/lips. • Infant will open the mouth and begin to suck. • Appears at 28 weeks gestation (weak and uncoordinated). • Mature at 34 weeks gestation. • Disappears at approximately 4 months of age.	• Cue for feeding (in quiet alert state). • Nutritive sucking: long, deep, suck-swallow-breathe pattern; audible. • Nonnutritive sucking: light, no audible sucking.
Rooting	• Elicited by lightly stroking the infant's cheek. • Infant will turn head in direction of stimulus. • Appears at 28 weeks gestation (immature). • Mature at 34 weeks gestation. • Disappears at approximately 4 months of age.	• May be difficult to elicit in a recently fed infant or one in a state of deep sleep. • Lightly stroking the mother's nipple on the center of the infant's lower lip will cause the infant to turn toward the breast. • Facilitates latch-on.

Summary

In summary, a complete infant assessment includes the perinatal history, gestational age assessment, breastfeeding assessment, physical assessment, and behavioral assessment. The purpose is to identify prenatal influences on the health status of the infant, provide a baseline of the infant's health status, and provide early identification of actual or potential problems. Finally, a complete assessment is important when initiating breastfeeding, as well as educating and assisting the parents in understanding how to best meet the needs of their infant.

Key Concepts

- The perinatal history provides the context for the physical and behavioral assessment.
- The New Ballard Scoring System has its highest reliability when performed within 48 hours of birth.
- The infant's gestational age classification is useful for determining the infant's vulnerability to feeding or nutritional problems.
- The quiet alert state is the most appropriate time to initiate breastfeeding.
- Behavioral assessment is useful for helping families understand how to meet their infant's needs as well as how to foster positive attachment.
- Providing a warm surface when performing physical assessment is necessary to maintain thermoregulation.

- Inspect the mouth for size, shape, symmetry, color, and the presence of abnormal structures and/or masses both when the newborn is at rest and crying.
- The tongue is pink and moist and protrudes symmetrically over the alveolar ridge when the mouth is open.

- Bowel sounds should be audible within the first hour after birth.
- The first stool, meconium, usually occurs within the first 24 hours.
- Transitional stools may be watery or thick in texture, and are odorless and less sticky than meconium.

References

Adams D, Hewell SD. Maternal and professional assessment of breastfeeding. *J Hum Lact.* 1997;113:279–283.

American Academy of Pediatrics and American College of Obstetricians and Gynecologists. *Guidelines for Perinatal Care.* 5th ed. Washington, DC: Author; 2002.

Askin DF, Wilson D. The high-risk newborn and family. In: Hockenberry MJ, Wilson D, eds. *Wong's Nursing Care of Infants and Children.* 8th ed. St. Louis, MO: Mosby; 2007:344–419.

Ballard J et al. New Ballard Score, expanded to include extremely premature infants. *J Pediatr.* 1991; 119:417–423.

Barron ML. Antenatal care. In: Simpson KR, Creehan PA. *AWHONN's Perinatal Nursing.* 3rd ed. Philadelphia, PA: Wolters Kluwer/Lippincott Williams & Wilkins; 2008:88–124.

Blackburn ST, Loper DL. The neuromuscular and sensory systems. In: Blackburn ST, Loper DL, eds. *Maternal, Fetal, and Neonatal Physiology: A Clinical Perspective.* Philadelphia, PA: WB Saunders; 1992:522–580.

Brazelton TB. Neonatal Assessment Scale. 2nd ed. Philadelphia, PA: JB Lippincott; 1984.

Buschbach D. Physical assessment of the newborn infant. In: Deason J, O'Neill P, eds. *Core Curriculum for Neonatal Intensive Care Nursing.* 2nd ed. Philadelphia, PA: WB Saunders; 1999:74–100.

Case-Smith J, Cooper P, Scala V. Feeding efficiency of premature infants. *Am J Occup Ther.* 1988; 43:245–250.

Cheffer ND, Rannalli DA. Newborn biologic/behavioral characteristics and psychosocial adaptations. In: *Core Curriculum for Maternal-Newborn Nursing.* 3rd ed. St. Louis, MO: Elsevier Saunders; 2004:437–464.

Creehan PA. Newborn physical assessment. In: Simpson KR, Creehan PA. *AWHONN's Perinatal Nursing.* 3rd ed. Philadelphia, PA: Wolters Kluwer/Lippincott Williams & Wilkins; 2008:546–579.

Crowell MK, Hill PD, Humenick SS. Relationship between obstetric analgesia and time of effective breastfeeding. *J Nurse Midwifery.* 1994;39:150–156.

Davidson MR, London ML, Ladewig PA. *Maternal-Newborn Nursing and Women's Health Across the Lifespan.* 8th ed. Upper Saddle River, NJ: Pearson/Prentice Hall; 2008.

Donovan EF et al. Inaccuracy of Ballard scores before 28 weeks' gestation. *J Pediatr.* 1999;135:147–152.

Evans JC et al. Newborn assessment. In: Fox JA, ed. *Primary Health Care of Infant, Children, and Adolescents.* St. Louis, MO: Mosby; 2002:107–136.

Fuloria M, Kreiter S. The newborn examination: part 1. Emergencies and common abnormalities involving the skin, head, neck, chest, and respiratory and cardiovascular systems. *Am Fam Physician.* 2002; 65:61–68.

Furman L, Minich NM. Evaluation of breastfeeding of very low birth weight infants: Can we use the infant breastfeeding assessment tool? *J Hum Lact.* 2006; 22:175–181.

Griffiths DM. Do tongue ties affect breastfeeding? *J Hum Lact.* 2004;20:409–414.

Hall DMB, Renfrew MJ. Tongue tie. *Arch Dis Child.* 2005;90:1211–1215.

Hedberg-Nyqvist K, Ewald U. Infant and maternal factors in the development of breastfeeding behaviour and breastfeeding outcome in preterm infants. *Acta Paediatr.* 1999;88:1194–1203.

Hedberg-Nyqvist K, Rubertsson C, Ewald U. Development of the preterm infant breastfeeding behavior scale (PIBBS): a study of nurse–mother agreement. *J Hum Lact.* 1996;12:207–219.

Jacobs LA et al. Normal nipple position in term infants measured on breastfeeding ultrasound. *J Hum Lact.* 2007;23:52–59.

Jensen D, Wallace S, Kelsay P. LATCH: a breastfeeding charting system and documentation tool. *JOGNN.* 1994;23:27–32.

Kenner CD, D'Apolito K. Outcomes of children exposed to drugs in utero. *JOGNN.* 1997;26:595–603.

Landau M, Krafchik B. The diagnostic values of café au lait macules. *J Am Acad Dermatol.* 1999;40:877–890.

Lubchenko LO, Hansman C, Boyd E. Intrauterine growth in length and head circumference as estimated from live births at gestational ages from 26 to 42 weeks. *Pediatrics.* 1996;37:403–408.

Lund CH, Kuller JM. Assessment and management of the integumentary system. In: Kenner C, Lott JW, eds. *Comprehensive Neonatal Nursing.* Philadelphia, PA: WB Saunders; 2003:700–724.

McCord SS. Health problems of middle childhood. In: Hockenberry MJ, Wilson D, eds. *Wong's Nursing Care of Infants and Children.* 8th ed. St. Louis, MO: Mosby; 2007:752–810.

MacMullen NJ, Dulski LA. Factors related to sucking ability in health newborns. *JOGNN*. 2000; 29:390–396.

Marmet C, Shell E. Therapeutic positioning for breastfeeding. In: Genna CW, ed. *Supporting Sucking Skills in Breastfeeding Infants*. Sudbury, Mass: Jones and Bartlett; 2008:305–325.

Matthews MK. Developing an instrument to assess infant breastfeeding behaviour in the early neonatal period. *Midwifery*. 1988;4:154–165.

Matthews MK. Mothers' satisfaction with their neonates' breastfeeding behaviors. *JOGNN*. 1990;20:49–55.

Moore ML, Nichols FH. Neonatal assessment. In: Nichols FH, Zwelling E, eds. *Maternal-Newborn nursing: Theory and Practice*. Philadelphia, PA: WB Saunders; 1997:1080–1131.

Morrison B et al. Psychometric validation of the mother–baby assessment instrument. Presented at: State of the Nursing Science Congress, Washington, DC, September 29, 2002.

Mulder PJ. A concept analysis of effective breastfeeding. *JOGNN*. 2006;35:332–339.

Mulford C. The mother-baby assessment (MBA): an "Apgar Score" for breastfeeding. *J Hum Lact*. 1992; 8:79–82.

Palmer MM, Crawley K, Blanco IA. Neonatal oral-motor assessment scale. *J Perinatol*. 1999;13:28–34.

Radzyminski S. Neurobehavioral functioning and breastfeeding behavior in the newborn. *JOGNN*. 2005;34:335–341.

Riordan J, Gill-Hopple K, Angeron J. Indicators of effective breastfeeding and estimates of breast milk intake. *J Hum Lact*. 2005;21:406–412.

Riordan J. Predicting breastfeeding problems. *AWHONN Lifelines*, 1998;2(6):31–33.

Riordan J. The effect of labor pain relief medication on neonatal suckling and breastfeeding duration. *J Hum Lact*. 2000;16:7–12.

Riordan J, Riordan S. The effect of labor epidurals on breastfeeding. Unit 4: lactation consultant series 2. Schaumburg, IL: La Leche League, International; 1999:8.

Riordan J, Koehn M. Reliability and validity testing of three breastfeeding assessment tools. *JOGNN*. 1997; 26:181–187.

Riordan J et al. Predicting breastfeeding duration using the LATCH tool. *J Hum Lact*. 2001;17:20–23.

Schlomer JA, Kemmerer J, Twiss, J. Evaluating the association of two breastfeeding assessment tools with breastfeeding problems and breastfeeding satisfaction. *J Hum Lact*. 1999;15:35–39.

Shrago LC, Bocar DL. The infant's contribution to breastfeeding. *JOGNN*. 1990;19:211–217.

Stellwegen LM, Hubbard LM, Vaux E. Look for the "stuck baby" to identify congenital torticollis. *Contemp Pediatr*. 2004;21:55–65.

van Vlimmeren LA et al. Diagnostic strategies for the evaluation of asymmetry in infancy: a review. *Eur J Pediatr*. 2004;163:185–191.

Wall V, Glass R. Mandibular asymmetry and breastfeeding problems: experience from 11 cases. *J Hum Lact*. 2006;22:328–334.

Wheeler B, Wilson D. Health promotion of the newborn and family. In: Hockenberry MJ, Wilson D, eds. *Wong's Nursing Care of Infants and Children*. 8th ed. St. Louis, MO: Mosby; 2007:257–309.

Wilson D. Health promotion of the infant and family. In: Hockenberry MJ, Wilson D, eds. *Wong's Nursing Care of Infants and Children*. 8th ed. St. Louis, MO: Mosby; 2007:499–606.

Infant Breastfeeding Assessment Tool (IBFAT)*

Indicator	3	2	1	0
Readiness to feed	No effort needed	Needs mild stimulation	Need more stimulation to rouse	Cannot be roused
Rooting	Roots effectively at once	Needs coaxing, prompting, or encouragement	Roots poorly, even with coaxing	Did not root
Fixing/latch-on	Latches on immediately	Takes 3–10 minutes	Takes over 10 minutes	Did not latch-on
Suckling	Suckles well on one or both breasts	Suckles on and off but needs encouragement	Weak suckle, suckles on and off	Did not suckle

* Scored 0–12.

Source: Matthews, 1988.

LATCH Assessment Tool*

Indicator	0	1	2
Latch-on	Too sleepy, reluctant, no latch	Repeated attempts; holds nipple in mouth; needs stimulus to suck	Grasps breast; tongue down; lips flanged; rhythmic suckling
Audible swallowing	None	A few with stimulation	Spontaneous and intermittent, 24 hours old; spontaneous and frequent > 24 hours old
Type of nipple	Inverted	Flat	Everted after stimulation
Comfort (breast/nipple)	Engorged, cracked, bleeding, blisters, bruises	Filling; reddened; small blisters or bruises; moderate discomfort	Soft; tender
Hold (positioning)	Full assistance needed	Minimal assistance; teach one side, mother does other; staff holds, mother takes over	No assistance needed; mother able to position/hold infant

* Scored 0–10.

Source: Jensen, Wallace, & Kelsay, 1994.

Mother–Baby Assessment Scale

Indicator	Mother Score = 1	Baby Score = 1	Score 0–10
Signaling	Watches and listens for baby's cues; holds, strokes, rocks, talks to baby; stimulates baby if he is asleep, calms if he is fussy.	Gives readiness cues: stirring, alertness, rooting, suckling, hand-to-mouth, cries.	
Positioning	Holds baby in good alignment within latch-on range of nipple; body is slightly flexed; entire ventral surface facing mother's body; head and shoulders are supported.	Roots well; opens mouth wide, tongue cupped and covering lower gum.	
Fixing	Holds her breast to assist baby; brings baby in close when his mouth is wide open; may express drops of milk.	Latches on, takes all of nipple and about 2 cm (1 in.) of areola into mouth, then suckles, has burst-pause suckling pattern.	
Milk transfer	Reports feeling any of the following: uterine cramps, increased lochia, breast ache or tingling, relaxation, sleepiness; milk leaks from opposite breast.	Swallow audibly; milk is observed in baby's mouth; may spit up milk when burping. Rapid "call-up suckling" rate (2 suckles/ second); changes to nutritive suckling, about 1 suckle/second.	
Ending	Breasts are comfortable; lets baby suckle until he is finished. After nursing, breasts feel softer; has no lumps, engorgement, or nipple soreness.	Releases breast spontaneously; appears satiated. Does not root when stimulated. Face, arms, and hands relaxed; may fall asleep.	

Source: Mulford, 1992.

Mother–Baby Assessment Scale

Fertility, Sexuality, and Contraception During Lactation

Kathy I. Kennedy

FERTILITY, SEXUALITY, AND CONTRACEPTION are interrelated aspects of reproduction. Breastfeeding affects each of these entities; thus the reproductive aspects of women's lives are more complex during lactation than during the nonlactating state (Figure 21–1). Although breastfeeding clearly has a fertility-reducing effect on the nursing mother, the nature of this effect is not fully understood. In general, the child's suckling initiates a cycle of neuroendocrinologic events that results in the inhibition of ovulation. One consequence of this inhibition is the creation of the hypoestrogenic state in the woman. Consequently, the dry, sometimes atrophic, vaginal mucosa may result in pain upon intercourse. Because of this and other circumstances, many breastfeeding women have sexual relationships infrequently and are thus at reduced risk of pregnancy for behavioral reasons. Emotions related to motherhood, such as intensive (albeit normal) involvement with the infant, and feelings of undesirability on the part of a woman who has not recovered her prepregnancy body, may affect her sexual behavior as well. Fear of subsequent pregnancy may also play a role in coital behavior and therefore risk of pregnancy. Since some contraceptives may relieve the vaginal symptoms of hypoestrogenicity as well as lessen the fear of pregnancy, coital frequency may also be related to family-planning choice. These are but a few

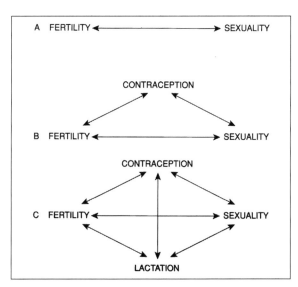

FIGURE 21–1 The interrelationships among fertility, sexuality, contraception, and lactation. (A) In the absence of a family planning intention, the phenomena of reproduction and sexual behavior (fertility and sexuality) are related in the most simple and direct manner. (B) When a family planning method is used for spacing or limiting pregnancies, it clearly affects fertility, and sometimes also sexual behavior (e.g., coitus-dependent methods). (C) Lactation can have independent effects on fertility, sexual behavior, and contraceptive decisions and patterns of use.

705

BOX **21-1**

Factors Related to Duration of Amenorrhea

Nonfeeding Variables

1. (High) number of live births = longer amenorrhea***
2. (High) maternal body mass index at 6 to 8 weeks postpartum = shorter amenorrhea***
3. (High) percent follow-up visits in which infant was ill = longer amenorrhea***

Feeding Variables

4. (Long) time from delivery to first breastfeed = shorter amenorrhea**
5. (Yes) regular supplementation with any food or drink = shorter amenorrhea**
6. (High) total 24-hour duration of breastfeeding = longer amenorrhea*

7. (High) percent of feeds constituted by breastmilk = longer amenorrhea***
8. (High) frequency of water/noncaloric supplements = longer amenorrhea***
9. (Yes) weaned = shorter amenorrhea***
10. (Yes) supplements comprise 50 percent of feeds = shorter amenorrhea**

* $p < 0.05$
** $p < 0.01$
*** $p < 0.001$

Source: Adapted from World Health Organization, 1998a, 1998b.

The Repetitive Nature of the Recovery of Fertility

Unpublished studies in France, the Philippines, Australia, and Canada (reviewed in Kennedy, 1993) found that a significant association exists between the duration of lactational infertility after one pregnancy and the duration in the same woman after her next pregnancy. These and anecdotal observations prompted the secondary analyses of large, existing datasets about the relationship between the durations of lactational amenorrhea reported in consecutive pregnancies.

In a large prospective study of Bangladeshi women, 418 women were observed through the course of breastfeeding two consecutive babies. The length of amenorrhea while breastfeeding the first child had significant predictive value for the subsequent length of amenorrhea. The author concluded that information on previous experience with lactational amenorrhea should be incorporated

into guidelines for the introduction of family planning during lactation (Ford, 1992).

In the WHO Multinational Study of Breastfeeding and Lactational Amenorrhea (WHO 1998b), the duration of lactational amenorrhea after the previous pregnancy was recorded at the time of admission. This single predictor was so highly significant and explained so much of the variance in the duration of lactational amenorrhea in the prospective study that no other factor in a multivariate analysis was significantly associated with the duration of lactational amenorrhea.

If a woman is to experience the same duration of infertility (or of amenorrhea) while breastfeeding two consecutive babies, the breastfeeding behavior is presumed to be roughly similar in both cases. Then the amount of neurosensory stimulation received by the mother through suckling would be roughly the same, eliciting roughly the same fertility repressing effect in the woman. We can suppose that this is likely to happen in many cases because

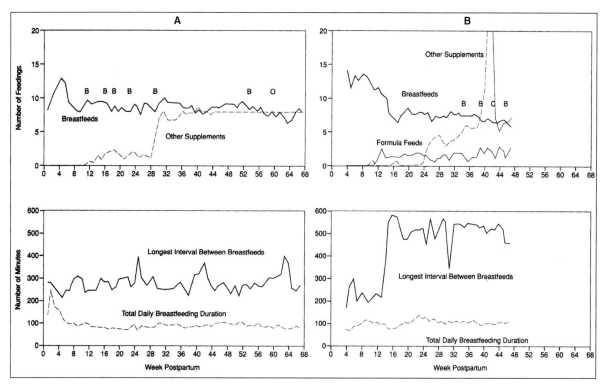

FIGURE **21–4** The effect of supplementation on breastfeeding. (A) In one example, the introduction of supplements at postpartum week 28 had no effect on breastfeeding frequency, duration, or the interval between feedings. (B) In another example, the introduction of supplements at about week 9 coincided with a decrease in breastfeeding frequency and an increase in the longest interval between breastfeeds. Ovulation was still postponed for about 10 months, probably because breastfeeding frequency and duration were high enough.

Source: Rivera, 1988.

two factors would be roughly the same in both breastfeeding couplets:

- The organism of the woman is the same; that is, her basic physiology is roughly the same. (If many years have passed between the pregnancies, then the woman's organismic responses to reproductive hormones may have changed somewhat with age.)
- The woman's orientation to infant feeding, and her ideas and habits about breastfeeding, probably remained constant across the two experiences. Differences also are likely to occur if her pattern of breastfeeding has also changed markedly. However, the research to date suggests that women generally can expect a similar pattern of recovery of fertility from one birth to the

next, provided that the breastfeeding pattern does not change dramatically.

Of course, two infants with markedly different feeding needs and personalities could cause different effects on the mother's return to fertility.

In a later section, the timing of the introduction of postpartum contraception will be addressed. As suggested by Ford (1992), when the duration of the previous length of lactational amenorrhea is known, this may be a useful factor when making an individual decision about the commencement of postpartum contraception. In whole communities, information about the average duration of lactational amenorrhea may inform programs as to the most effective community approaches to postpartum contraception (Weiss, 1993).

The Bellagio Consensus

By the late 1980s, researchers on five continents had completed prospective studies of the changes in ovarian hormones in breastfeeding women. Many of these researchers assembled in Bellagio, Italy, to determine whether their various findings about women with vastly different patterns of breast-feeding behavior could be synthesized into a state-ment about how breastfeeding women might predict their recovery of fertility (Box 21–2).

The basis for the consensus in 1988 was a body of published and unpublished studies of the pregnancy rates (3 studies in two countries), as well as data on the probability of a recognizable pregnancy from prospective studies of the recovery of ovulation dur-ing lactation (10 studies in seven countries). Among these studies, the highest pregnancy rate reported in fully breastfeeding amenorrheic women during the first 6 months postpartum was lower than 2 percent (Family Health International, 1988; Kennedy, Rivera, & McNeilly, 1989).

The Bellagio Consensus states that bleeding in the first 56 days postpartum can be ignored. This claim is supported by a prospective study of postpartum bleeding in 477 experienced breastfeeding women in the Philippines. A median duration of postpartum

bleeding of 27 days was reported, which did not vary by age, parity, breastfeeding frequency, or level of supplementation. Furthermore, more than a quarter of these women experienced a subsequent bleeding episode beginning not later than postpartum day 56. Only 10 women may have had their first cyclic menses before day 56. None became pregnant, although not all were yet sexually active (Visness, Kennedy, & Ramos, 1997). A prospective study of 72 fully breastfeeding women in developed countries found that nearly half experienced some bleeding or spotting between the sixth and eighth weeks post-partum. Despite ovarian follicular development in seven of the 72 cases, there was no ovulation in any woman in the first 8 weeks postpartum (Visness et al., 1997). Findings from the WHO Multinational Study of Breastfeeding and the return of menses are consistent with the advice to ignore bleeding prior to postpartum day 56 (WHO, 1999a).

The Bellagio Consensus is important because it reflects principles that are believed to be applicable across cultures. Yet this aspect of the consensus is also one of its weaknesses: by making generaliza-tions that apply to a range of breastfeeding pat-terns and practices, some possible situations could not be accommodated. For example, in societies in which a child is breastfed for 2 years or more, or

---

BOX 21–2

The Bellagio Consensus

Lactational amenorrhea should be regarded as a potential family planning method in all maternal and child health programs in developing and developed countries.

Postpartum women should be offered a choice of using breastfeeding as a means of family planning, either to help achieve opti-mal birth spacing of at least 2 years, or as a way of delaying the introduction of other contraceptives. They should be informed of how to maximize the antifertility effects of breastfeeding to prevent pregnancy.

Breastfeeding provides more than 98 percent protection from pregnancy during the first 6 months postpartum if the mother is "fully" or nearly fully breastfeeding and has not experi-enced vaginal bleeding after the 56th day postpartum.

Source: Family Health International, 1988; Kennedy, Rivera, & McNeilly, 1989.

among La Leche League mothers in industrialized countries who choose to breastfeed for these longer periods, lactational amenorrhea alone may be a viable marker of returning fertility. Cognizant of this, Kennedy, Rivera, and McNeilly (1989, p. 485) cautioned as follows:

> *Guidelines specific to a particular country or population for using breastfeeding as a postpartum family-planning method can be developed based on this consensus. Local infant feeding practices, the average duration of amenorrhea, and the ongoing changes in women's status and health practices should be considered in adapting these general guidelines.*

The consensus is also important because it represents the framework for the actual use of lactational amenorrhea as a method of contraception. Guidelines on how to integrate the Lactational Amenorrhea Method (LAM) into family planning and breastfeeding support programs have been developed based on the Bellagio Consensus (Labbok et al., 1994).

During the 8 years after the Bellagio Consensus, a new body of research was undertaken to test the consensus prospectively. Four clinical trials of the contraceptive efficacy of LAM were conducted in Chile (Perez, Labbok, & Queenan, 1992), Pakistan (Kazi et al., 1995), the Philippines (Ramos, Kennedy, & Visness, 1996), and in a multinational study (Labbok et al., 1997). These studies found cumulative 6-month life-table rates of pregnancy during correct use of the method of 1.0, 0.5, 1.5, and 0.6 percent, respectively. These studies observed women who chose to use LAM as their postpartum contraceptive method and were taught and actually used the method. Other researchers conducted secondary data analyses on existing datasets (Short et al., 1991; Weiss, 1993; Rojnik, Kosmelj, & Andolsek-Jeras, 1995), and found that the protection from pregnancy under the LAM conditions can outlast the parameters set in the Bellagio Consensus. The largest secondary analysis is from the WHO Multinational Study of Breastfeeding and the Return of Menses in which the findings on pregnancy during lactation also uphold the Bellagio Consensus (WHO, 1999b).

On the basis of these studies, as well as unpublished research from a variety of sources, scientists who reconvened at Bellagio in 1995 were able to conclude "the Bellagio Consensus has clearly been confirmed" (Kennedy, Labbok, & Van Look, 1996).

Having accumulated data and experience from prospective clinical trials, the group at "Bellagio II" was able to draw conclusions about the modification of LAM on a local level:

1. It is not possible to eliminate the amenorrhea criterion.

Once menstruation has resumed, fertility is returning, or already has returned. Menses is an absolute indication of the need for another contraceptive method if continued protection is desired.

2. It may be possible to relax the full- or nearly full-breastfeeding criterion.

If breastfeeding behaviors are sound and the introduction of weaning foods is not accompanied by a decline in any breastfeeding parameter, then theoretically the full- or nearly full-breastfeeding criterion may be relaxed. However, this possibility requires more research since the breastfeeding stimulus is what causes lactational amenorrhea, and supplementation can (but does not always) affect that stimulus.

3. It may be possible to extend LAM beyond 6 months postpartum.

In the clinical trials and the secondary analyses, the protection provided by lactational amenorrhea beyond the 6th postpartum month—and hence during supplemented breastfeeding—was found to be relatively low in some settings—for example, 4–9 percent in the multinational study (Labbok et al., 1997) and 0–5 percent in the Philippine clinical trial (Ramos, Kennedy, & Visness, 1996). These rates are not surprising since decades of retrospective research reviewed above showed that 3–10 percent of women conceive during lactational amenorrhea. While these rates indicate significant protection among successfully breastfeeding women using LAM, many other modern contraceptives used correctly can provide better protection in the second 6 months postpartum. Although programmatic experience with the extension of LAM beyond 6 months has produced some useful observations (Wade, Sevilla, & Labbok, 1994; Cooney et al., 1996), no rigorous, prospective data on "extended LAM" from clinical trials are yet available.

A study of the efficacy of LAM among working women in Chile reported a 6-month cumulative pregnancy rate of 5.2 percent (Valdes et al., 2000). This elevated pregnancy rate was among fully breastfeeding women and suggests that despite adequate milk production, frequent suckling as well as full breastfeeding may be necessary to obtain the full protection from LAM.

Challenges to the healthfulness of 6 months of exclusive breastfeeding have been levied and more recently countered by reviews of the literature and position papers. The American Dietetic Association, the American Academy of Pediatrics, and the World Health Organization have all concluded that exclusive breastfeeding is normally sufficient to provide for optimal growth and development in the infant through 6 months (ADA, 2005; AAP, 2005, Kramer & Kakuma, 2002). The International Lactation Consultants Association publishes *Clinical Guidelines for the Establishment of Exclusive Breastfeeding* (ILCA, 2005).

Sexuality

Today, human sexuality is as complex as ever. Although the following discussion will presuppose a stable union between a breastfeeding woman and her male partner, this presupposition is simply for convenience. Nevertheless, the majority of lactating mothers are heterosexual, and there is little if any research about the sexuality of breastfeeding single and lesbian women. It is likely that much of the following discussion will apply to all women.

This discussion is also based on the assumption that libido or sexual desire is the main driving force or motivation for sexual expression (although the desire to please one's partner is also recognized as a motivation). Yet many women have intercourse against their will and/or without sexual desire. This chapter does not consider the role of breastfeeding in coercive or indifferent sexual relationships.

Libido

There are at least five categories of factors that may influence sexual drive or desire during lactation:

- Common situational factors unrelated to breastfeeding

- Libido-inhibiting influences related to parturition
- Libido-inhibiting influences of lactation
- Libido-enhancing factors related to pregnancy, birth, and lactation
- Lactation factors related to the breastfeeding woman's partner

Common Situational Factors Unrelated to Breastfeeding

Many preexisting factors that either facilitated or inhibited sexual arousal before pregnancy or birth will remain a part of a woman's living experience, family routine, or personal preference after the birth of the child. Preexisting factors that inhibit libido—such as the chronic illness of one of the partners, fear of pregnancy, or lack of privacy—persist and are unrelated to breastfeeding. If a couple has a dysfunctional or unsatisfying sexual rapport, this is no more likely to be spontaneously remedied by lactation than a faltering marriage is to be "saved" by adding a child to the family chemistry.

Conversely, there is no reason to assume that individualized stimuli per se, such as a preferred cologne, a special song, or candlelight, should lose their excitatory effects because a baby joins the family. Opportunity to attend to the old stimuli, however, is another matter. Some of the preexisting sexual stimuli or circumstances associated with sexual opportunity may be decreased due to having a young baby in the home. For example, the couple may find that they now lack time alone and that they endure constant interruptions—especially, it seems, at night. The quiet evening at home may seem gone forever.

Libido-Inhibiting Influences Related to Parturition

Much of the natural process of physical recovery from vaginal delivery takes about 6 weeks, although there is some variation across women. Postpartum abstinence is sensible until the woman decides that she has sufficient physical comfort to resume sexual intercourse.

The tenderness from episiotomy or vulvo-vaginal or perineal stress following vaginal delivery usually lasts for several months. Although the woman's stitches may have healed, she may still experience discomfort upon intercourse. A study in London found that 62 percent of 403 primiparas reported dyspareunia (pain upon intercourse) in the first 3 months after birth, dropping to half that percentage by 6 months (Barrett et al., 2000). In a study of 93 parturients in New South Wales, Australia, the median time required to achieve comfort during intercourse was 3 months, with a range of from 1 month to more than 12 months. Whether or not the women had episiotomies (58 yes, 35 no) did not affect the time until pain-free intercourse was experienced, but this may be because of the commonness of tearing (69 percent) of the vulval tissues, which required sutures in the women who did not have an episiotomy (Abraham et al., 1990). In a longitudinal study of 119 primiparous women attended at a London teaching hospital, 40 percent complained of soreness and occasionally painful intercourse at 3 months postpartum (Robson, Brant, & Kumar, 1981). Another study of British women reported dyspareunia during the first postpartum intercourse in 40 percent of mothers; of these, 64 percent refrained from further coitus after the initial distressing event (Grudzinskas & Atkinson, 1984). The anticipation of pain during intercourse may cause the woman to avoid sexual suggestion. A clear understanding of feelings and ongoing communication may help the couple to defer intercourse until some future time and to express their love and caring in other ways.

Soon after delivery, women experience a precipitous decline in ovarian steroid levels. This drastic hormonal change is sometimes associated with noticeable mood changes. The immediate effect is usually temporary and probably overlaps with the period of postpartum abstinence. In some women, postpartum depression can follow delivery immediately or occur after a few days or weeks. Although the etiology of postpartum depression is not well understood, this depression probably has both endogenous and exogenous sources. Some women experience emotional vulnerability when their progesterone levels are low, as happens during the postpartum period. (By way of analogy, the symptoms of premenstrual syndrome in the nonpregnant woman are often relieved by progesterone administration.) The overwhelming needs of the new baby plus other familial and extrafamilial responsibilities are more than enough to make a normal person weary (Figure 21–5). Thus exogenous

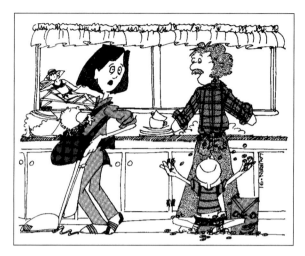

FIGURE 21–5 The postpartum domestic scene. The overwhelming needs of the new baby plus other familial and extrafamilial responsibilities are more than enough to make a normal person weary.

sources of postpartum depression should not be underestimated. Depression is commonly characterized by a lack of sexual drive, and postpartum depression is no exception.

Even if the mother does not experience postpartum depression, she will probably be spending most of her emotional energy caring for and bonding with her newborn. This process is sometimes likened to a love affair in which infatuation with one's beloved is like an obsession. It is difficult to refrain from thinking about and doing things for the object of one's affection. Between mother and child, this bonding serves exceedingly important functions by creating an enduring parental talent and commitment in the mother and a sense of trust and security in the infant. However, this process can preclude opportunity and emotional availability for the partner.

Psychological factors unrelated to hormones or to attachment can also be strong inhibitors of libido. Fear of pregnancy can be an important inhibitor of sexual drive. If the new baby was unplanned, especially if a contraceptive failure occurred, sexual inhibition could understandably be great. Parents of a firstborn sometimes have trouble synthesizing the roles of lover and mother or father, because the parental role was previously understood subconsciously to be asexual. Colic or

Therefore to some people, having given birth and becoming nonpregnant again may be less sexually stimulating than being "great with child." Because each person and each couple is unique, any discussion of sexuality during lactation must be couched in generalities, recognizing that individual expression varies widely.

Barrett et al. (2000) reported that most women experience change in their sexual practices after delivery. The frequencies of intercourse and oral sex were reportedly lower after delivery, but 10 percent of women reported better quality in their sex lives. Very few women talk to their healthcare professional about their sexual health. It seems possible that many couples could have better sexual satisfaction equipped with a few simple facts and some lubricant.

Factors Related to the Breastfeeding Woman's Partner

The possibility of role conflict has already been mentioned and is a reminder that men also experience psychological adjustments to accommodate the major life event of birth. No doubt the experience is most profound the first time that a man becomes a father. While the male partner is often assumed to be ever ready, willing, and wanting sex, this is an overgeneralization, possibly reflecting the relative lack of a cycle in the male capacity to fertilize. Men are subject to libidinal influences in everyday life, and, analogous to the female perspective discussed at the beginning of this section, these facilitators and inhibitors do not disappear with the birth of a child or during the lactation course of a partner.

When the man has witnessed his pregnant partner's metamorphosis into lactating mother, this may affect his perception of her as a sex partner, either because of her body's obvious changes or because of the meaning he ascribes to her maternity. Motherhood or lactation may make her more or less sexually appealing to him.

Fear of hurting a postpartum woman during vaginal intercourse may inhibit male sexual expression. A man may feel guilty for desiring his breastfeeding partner if he perceives that she has "more important" maternal matters. Identifying and talking about their sexual feelings, desires, and inhibitions, while earnestly caring for the welfare of each other, can help the couple through this sometimes awkward period.

Sexual Behavior During Lactation

To measure a level of sexual functioning or behavior in breastfeeding women, researchers have studied the resumption of postpartum intercourse and coital frequency. First, intercourse and coital frequency are relatively easy variables to quantify, although they certainly do not yield a complete understanding of sexual practices during lactation. Unfortunately, little qualitative information about sexual behavior during lactation is reported in the scientific literature. Few studies of sexual behavior during lactation contain large numbers of subjects, and the results of the studies are sometimes contradictory.

First Postpartum Intercourse

In one study in the postnatal hospital clinic of a city in England, 328 women were interviewed. By the time of the postnatal visit, 51 percent had already resumed intercourse, which was most frequently (the mode) during the fifth week postpartum (Grudzinskas & Atkinson, 1984). In the London study, 62 percent of women resumed sexual intercourse by the 7th or 8th week postpartum (Barrett et al., 2000). An intensive study of 25 breastfeeding women in Edinburgh, Scotland, found that 6 to 7 weeks was the mean time preceding initial postpartum intercourse. In a prospective study of 130 breastfeeding women in Santiago, Chile, the participants had "usually" resumed sexual relations by the beginning of the second month (Diaz et al., 1982).

A population-based survey of 3080 parturients was conducted in Cebu, the Philippines, where breastfeeding is the norm. The study included all identified pregnancies in 27 administrative districts in and around metropolitan Cebu. Sixty percent of women returned to coitus by 8 weeks postpartum (Udry & Deang, 1993). A study of 485 LAM users in Manila, the Philippines, reported a median time to the resumption of coitus of 7 weeks (Ramos, Kennedy, & Visness, 1996). In a study involving 27 breastfeeding women in Bangkok, Thailand, the mean time until the first postpartum coitus was 7.8 weeks, although the range of time until the first coitus was from 3 weeks to more than 21 weeks postpartum (Israngkura et al., 1989). Although this is a small and nonrepresentative sample, the women recorded coitus data prospectively, unlike the methodology used in population-based surveys. In a study of 399 LAM users in Pakistan, three quarters of the volunteers were from the city of Karachi. By the end of the second month, 80 percent reported that they were sexually active, up from 14 percent in the first month (Kazi et al., 1995). The Cebu, Manila, Bangkok, and Karachi studies show that the postpartum resumption of sexual activity in urban areas of Asian developing countries typically occurs by 7 to 8 weeks.

Whether the average time to the resumption of sexual relations during breastfeeding is 4 weeks or 8 weeks, large numbers of women are sexually active before the traditional time of the postpartum checkup (i.e., 6 weeks postpartum). As will be discussed below, an argument can be made to schedule the postpartum visit on the basis of the time that the woman needs a provider to deliver her chosen contraceptive method. Of course, the new mother should always have access to care in the event of unexpected pain, vaginal discharge, or other physical concerns. Given that the majority of women have some sexual discomfort or concerns postpartum, health professionals should discuss sexual issues—actual or potential—when counseling on contraception.

Postpartum Coital Frequency

An analysis of retrospective and prospective data on coital frequency was performed using information provided by 91 nonpregnant, nonlactating women in North Carolina who were married or living with a male partner as if married. First, the women reported from memory their "usual" weekly frequency of sexual intercourse. Then they recorded each morning, for 1 to 3 months, whether they had intercourse during the previous 24 hours. The women reported a significantly higher frequency of coitus for the period prior to the first interview (2.5 times per week) compared with their later prospective recordings (1.7 times per week)—an average of 0.8 episodes per week. This overestimate occurred uniformly in subgroups of women and was thought to be caused by the women's tendency to report a frequency that would exist in the absence of travel, illness, menses, and other influencing factors. The prospective data showed trends toward decreased coital frequency with increasing age, education, income, and duration of relationship. Also, women currently using an

intrauterine device (IUD) or who had had a tubal ligation had intercourse twice as often (2.0 times per week) as women with "no" contraceptive use (1.1 times per week) (Hornsby & Wilcox, 1989). Although the North Carolina analysis is a study of the methodology for obtaining information about coital frequency, it offers a clear example of the potential bias incurred with the use of retrospective data. Furthermore, while it is a study of normally cycling women, it provides a good context in which to view studies of coital frequency during lactation.

In the aforementioned study in Santiago, Chile, the reported coital frequency ranged from one to six times per week in the first 6 months postpartum among breastfeeding women (Diaz et al., 1982). Conversely, the Cebu study found a remarkable lack of variance in coital frequency in the first 6 months postpartum. These women were asked every 2 months about the frequency of intercourse in the previous week. After controlling for a large number of potentially influential factors, coital frequency of 0.5 to 0.6 times per week did not vary meaningfully with any of the demographic or situational factors observed (Udry & Deang, 1993).

The variability in coital frequency in the Cebu study could not be well explained by factors such as age and education. Other factors, such as fear of pregnancy, may be stronger correlates of sexual behavior, as may psychological factors, such as perceived locus of control (the perception that one is in control of one's life and fate rather than the victim of forces outside oneself).

In the aforementioned study in Manila, coital frequency averaged three times per month among LAM users (Visness & Kennedy, 1997). In this study of breastfeeding women, the number of living children was unrelated to coital frequency, while maternal age was related in two ways: younger women reported an increase in frequency with time postpartum, and their overall frequency was greater than that reported by older women.

On an individual basis, coital frequency may only be important to know so that it may be compared with frequency before the pregnancy and/or the birth. An Edinburgh study prospectively measured coital frequency during weeks 12 to 24 postpartum and found a mean frequency of 1.2 times per week. The recalled prepregnancy frequency was 2.6 times per week ($P < .01$) (Alder et al., 1986). In light of the findings of Hornsby and Wilcox (1989), it is possible that the retrospectively generated prepregnancy frequency was an overestimate. Also, it is not clear whether the prepregnancy period being recalled is a time in which pregnancy was actively sought, which could inflate sexual frequency above previous or later levels for the couple.

Does breastfeeding affect the resumption of sexual activity or coital frequency? Survey data from Bangladesh (Islam & Khan, 1993) and the Philippines (Udry, 1993) show lower coital frequencies among breastfeeding than nonbreastfeeding women. Alder and Bancroft (1988) reported that, when compared with bottle-feeders, breastfeeding women showed a lower preferred frequency of intercourse; delayed the resumption of coitus for a longer period; had a greater reduction in sexual interest and enjoyment compared with prepregnancy levels; experienced more pain during intercourse; and were slightly more depressed at 3 months postpartum. All of these differences disappeared by 6 months except for dyspareunia. The findings of Barrett et al. (2000) corroborate this conclusion.

By contrast, works by Masters and Johnson (1966) and by Kenny (1973) reported a more prompt return of sexual desire, plus a return to higher levels of sexual functioning, among breastfeeding women than among bottle-feeders. These earlier works were conducted during a time and at locations in which breastfeeding was not popular. It is unknown whether women who were less sexually inhibited were the ones who breastfed.

Robson, Brant, and Kumar (1981) reported that breastfeeding showed no influence over several indices of maternal sexuality in 119 primiparas in London. Grudzinskas and Atkinson (1984) reported that breastfeeding was not related to the resumption of coitus in their sample of 328 women. Nationally representative data from Thailand show that there is no overall difference in coital frequency between breastfeeders and nonbreastfeeders, except for a reduced frequency among women who breastfeed six or more times at night (Knodel & Chayovan, 1991).

What do these conflicting results mean? Does breastfeeding stifle sexual experience, accelerate it, or neither? Conflicting results can be due to differences in research methodology or to cultural norms. Additional psychological, behavioral, and biological hypotheses are needed. Can breastfeeding have either an inhibiting or a stimulating effect? Perhaps breastfeeding is a swing factor, sometimes enhancing sexual feelings and sometimes acting as the obstacle to their expression.

Contraception

During lactation, the choice of whether to practice contraception, and if so which method, requires different considerations compared with the same choice during the nonlactating state (Figure 21–7). The array of available family-planning methods has been put into a hierarchy according to their general advisability for use during breastfeeding (Labbok et al., 1994). The hierarchy of family-planning options (Table 21–1) places nonhormonal methods as the first choice, progestin-only methods as the

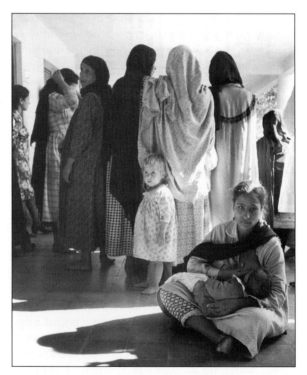

FIGURE 21–7 Family planning care at an Egyptian health center, where maternal and child health services are also included. According to the WHO perspective, family planning is concerned with the quality of life. It is a way of thinking and living that promotes the health and welfare of the family group and thus contributes to economic and social development.

Source: World Health Organization. Used with permission.

TABLE 21–1	**Family-Planning Options as They Relate to the Specific Concerns of Breastfeeding Women**		

Method	Advantages	Disadvantages	Comments
First Choice: Nonhormonal Methods			
Condoms	No effect on breastfeeding; very effective if used correctly.	May be irritating to vagina and require additional lubrication.	Offers some protection against sexually transmitted diseases. No risks to mother or child.
Diaphragms	No effect on breastfeeding; effective if used correctly.	Diaphragm must be refitted postpartum after uterus has returned to prepregnancy size.	Not widely available. Effectiveness depends on use with a spermicide.
Spermicides	No effect on breastfeeding; effective if used correctly.	May be irritating to genital area and to the male partner.	Small amount may be absorbed into maternal blood and some passage into milk: no known effect on infant.
Intrauterine devices (IUDs)	No effect from IUD itself on breastfeeding; effective.	Possible risk of expulsion and uterine perforation if not properly placed or if inserted prior to 6 weeks postpartum.	Delay insertion until after 6 weeks postpartum.
Natural family planning (periodic abstinence)	No effect on breastfeeding; effective if used correctly.	May require extended periods of abstinence. Requires ability to interpret fertility signs during breastfeeding.	Additional training may be necessary to interpret signs and symptoms of fertility during lactation. Calendar rhythm method alone has little value prior to first ovulation.
Vasectomy (voluntary male surgical sterilization)	No effect on breastfeeding; nearly 100% effective.	Minor surgery with chance of side effects; irreversible.	Recommended if no more children are desired. Counseling for couples. No risk to mother or child.
Tubal ligation (voluntary female sterilization)	No direct effect on breastfeeding; nearly 100% effective.	Minor surgery with chance of side effects; irreversible. Possible short-term mother–infant separation. Anesthesia can pass into milk in small amounts.	Recommended if no more children are desired. Counseling for couples.
Second Choice: Progestin-only Methods			
Progestin-only methods (mini-pill, injectables, implants)	Effective; may increase milk volume.	Some hormone passes into breastmilk.	No evidence of adverse effect on

(Continues)

| TABLE 21–1 | **Family-Planning Options as They Relate to the Specific Concerns of Breastfeeding Women (Continued)** | | |

Method	Advantages	Disadvantages	Comments
	Effectiveness during breastfeeding approaches that of combined pill.		infant from small amount of hormone that passes into breastmilk.
Third Choice: Methods Containing Estrogen			
Combined oral contraceptives (estrogen and progestin)	Very effective.	Estrogens reduce milk supply. Some hormone passes into breastmilk.	No evidence of direct negative effect on infant; however, does suppress milk supply and leads to earlier cessation of breastfeeding. If these methods can not be avoided, breastfeeding can and should continue.

Source: Labbok et al., 1994. Adapted with permission of the Institute for Reproductive Health, Georgetown University.

second choice, and methods containing estrogen as a distant third to be used only when other methods are unavailable. This hierarchy is consistent with guidelines published by the World Health Organization (2004a,b) and the International Planned Parenthood Federation (1996).

The Contraceptive Methods

The following discussion describes the advantages and disadvantages of various contraceptive methods used during lactation. It is not intended to be an exhaustive exposition of the methods. Instead it emphasizes the implications of the use of the methods for the breastfeeding mother and baby. A fully detailed discussion of instructions for use, as well as the contraindications of each method unrelated to breastfeeding, can be found in the most recent edition of *Contraceptive Technology* (Hatcher et al., 2004).

Almost every method of family planning can be used during breastfeeding, but the timing of the introduction of the methods can vary profoundly. The question of when to start using a contraceptive

will be revisited at the end of this section, and is also an integral aspect of LAM.

Nonhormonal Methods

The permanent methods of family planning—now the most popular category of methods in the United States—all fall under the nonhormonal method category. They are highly appropriate methods provided that a couple wishes to prevent any future pregnancy, has been properly counseled, fully appreciates the irreversibility of the procedure, and is fully satisfied with the decision to use a permanent method.

When a permanent method is indicated, vasectomy is one of the most appropriate alternatives available, because it is safe and effective and should have no effect whatsoever on lactation. After the vasectomy, the male reproductive tract continues to clear itself of sperm during about 20 ejaculations. If the woman is not pregnant, the couple needs to use a second method of contraception for a period of time in order to be fully protected. The couple may feel that the vasectomy is ideally timed either during the pregnancy itself or in the first few months postpartum, especially if the current pregnancy was unplanned. In an era of only one or two children per family, however, the presumed final pregnancy often is highly planned. If so, couples may feel more comfortable postponing vasectomy until after the pregnancy, in case a miscarriage should occur, or even until after the infancy period of the child.

Female sterilization carries several advantages. It is safe, effective, and relatively convenient since it can be performed on the delivery table. Contrary to previous assumptions, a small risk of female sterilization failure can persist for at least a decade, but this risk is smallest after partial salpingectomy compared with other methods of tubal occlusion (Peterson et al., 1996).

Care should be taken to maintain breastfeeding around the time of the procedure. Drowsiness or any pain the woman feels may temporarily reduce her ability or desire to breastfeed, and it may limit her options for comfortably positioning herself or her infant for breastfeeding. If the mother is experienced and/or well counseled, and if hospital staff does not interfere by bottle-feeding the baby, this interruption of early breastfeeding should not have serious consequences for lactation. The mother should breastfeed just before the administration of the anesthetic, and delay somewhat the breastfeed after the procedure, to minimize the infant's exposure to the anesthetic agent (American Academy of Pediatrics, 2001).

Studies reviewed in the early 1980s have reported that up to 7 percent of women express regret about tubal sterilizations (Divers, 1984; Grubb et al., 1985). In general, regret over the procedure and/or desire for reversal has been associated with younger age (e.g., under 30) or low parity at the time of the procedure, as well as remarriage, the death of a child after the procedure, and having the procedure with a concurrent cesarean section or during the puerperal or postabortion period. Occasionally, lower socioeconomic class and lack of having a child of a specific gender have also been associated with regret over having the procedure. It is possible that regret is intensified when pre-, post-, and intraprocedural factors interact—for example, when a young woman with few children is sterilized immediately postpartum, and she later remarries.

Counseling is crucially important when helping women or couples to select the best family-planning approach for them. When a permanent method is a serious consideration, counseling must begin long before the procedure and be repetitive. This may be especially important when younger women of low parity express an interest in the procedure during the puerperium, as well as when young men under the same conditions consider vasectomy.

The Lactational Amenorrhea Method (LAM) is the proactive use of lactational infertility as a contraceptive method during the period of lactational amenorrhea, under very specific circumstances: (1) the woman is breastfeeding her child exclusively (or nearly exclusively)—meaning no supplemental feedings; (2) the woman has experienced no vaginal bleeding or spotting after lochia ends (all bleeding, spotting, or bloody vaginal discharge before postpartum day 56 can be ignored); and (3) the child is less than 6 months of age. LAM is based on the Bellagio Consensus (Kennedy, Rivera, & McNeilly, 1989; Labbok et al., 1994). LAM is a temporary method of family planning. Another contraceptive method should be used immediately when LAM expires for continued pregnancy protection (Kennedy, Labbok, & Van Look, 1996; Van Look, 1996). Experience with LAM is growing, but it is still limited in the United States. LAM may prove to be a useful stopgap method for women who are delaying the use of a hormonal or a permanent method, but access to continuing protection should be ensured.

Nonhormonal intrauterine devices (IUDs) have been shown to have either no effect or a positive effect on lactation (Koetsawang, 1987). One study found Copper T-380A IUD insertion easier and less painful during lactation, with possibly higher continuation rates than in nonlactating women (Chi et al., 1989a,b). IUDs inserted during the postpartum period tend to be expelled more frequently than IUDs inserted at other times. However, insertion immediately after delivery of the placenta (within 10 minutes) by an experienced person who places the device high in the fundus significantly reduces the chance of expulsion (Chi & Farr, 1989). IUDs inserted within 10 minutes of placental expulsion have not been associated with excessive bleeding or endometritis (Welkovic et al., 2001). Still, a small study of IUD insertion within 10 minutes of placental delivery found that half of IUDs were expelled in vaginally delivered women and women delivered by cesarean section with the IUD inserted through the uterine incision (Muller et. al., 2005). Breastfeeding has not been found to increase the risk of expulsion when the device is inserted at this time or after the postpartum period (Chi et al., 1989a; Cole et al., 1983). Ideally, the IUD should be inserted immediately after placental delivery, or within 48 hours, or after 6 to 8 weeks, or with care and infection prophylaxis after 4 to 6 weeks, in this order (O'Hanley & Huber, 1992).

Because of the advantages of immediate postplacental insertion, contraceptive counseling and informed consent to IUD insertion should occur long before labor and delivery. Counseling on postinsertion care is also important. Women should be encouraged to have early postpartum checkups and to return if the IUD thread is missing, because expulsion, if it occurs, often does so soon after insertion.

A study of US women found the risk of uterine perforation to be significantly elevated in women who were breastfeeding at the time of insertion (Heartwell & Schlesselman, 1983). A small, noncomparative study in Sweden drew the same conclusion (Andersson et al., 1998). However, large studies have been unable to confirm this (Chi, Feldblum, & Rogers, 1984; Farr & Rivera, 1992). Insertion by an experienced person is thought to minimize the risk of perforation.

Little research has been conducted on the effectiveness of barrier methods used during lactation. Clinical trials of contraceptive efficacy have deliberately excluded breastfeeding women because their naturally subfertile state may influence pregnancy rates. The relative effectiveness of the various barrier methods vis-à-vis each other is probably maintained during lactation.

Barrier and/or spermicidal methods are widely used contraceptives among lactating US women. Several characteristics of these methods make them particularly attractive during the breastfeeding period. Condoms, diaphragms, and spermicides are all coitus-dependent methods. Even if couples prefer other methods, they may find these methods useful if they are having intercourse less frequently than before the pregnancy. The lubricative effect of the spermicide can be welcome if the woman experiences vaginal symptoms from estrogen suppression. The contraceptive diaphragm and the cervical cap should not be used in the first 6 weeks postpartum

and may not be able to be fitted properly earlier. The condom is a good barrier method choice during the early postpartum period. Condoms can be purchased with or without a lubricant coating and/or a spermicide in the reservoir. A condom used with a spermicide, whether applied by the user or as part of the condom itself, should have better contraceptive efficacy than the condom alone.

The diaphragm that a woman used prior to her pregnancy is apt to be unsuitable in size after childbirth. A new diaphragm can usually be properly fitted at 6 weeks postpartum (and in some cases sooner), but some breastfeeding women may find the fitting process to be too uncomfortable for many weeks. In this case the couple may wish to abstain or to use lubricated condoms, a spermicide, or LAM until vaginal lubrication is more normal. If the woman will be sexually active before her diaphragm can be sized, she should use another method—such as condoms or LAM—in the interim. With the gain or loss of every 10 pounds, a new diaphragm may need to be sized in order to achieve effective protection, and a clinical gynecologic visit should be sought for this purpose. The diaphragm should always be used with a spermicidal cream or jelly.

Spermicidal cream, jelly, foam, or foaming tablets used alone are not as effective in preventing pregnancy as a spermicide used with a barrier, such as a sponge, diaphragm, or condom. However, spermicides used during breastfeeding, especially during the period of LAM protection, should result in a higher level of effectiveness due to double protection. They also represent a significant improvement over unprotected intercourse, and they have the advantage of being widely available and can be purchased over the counter.

The Billings' Ovulation Method and the Symptothermal Method are considered to be modern natural family-planning (NFP) methods because they are based on sound scientific research. The methods require abstinence from intercourse during the fertile period, which is identified by observing the woman's physical signs and symptoms—e.g., volume, color, stretchiness, sensation, and clarity of cervical mucus; basal body temperature; cervical position; and breast tenderness. The modern natural methods are highly effective when used correctly, but most studies observe a great deal of incorrect use. Incorrect use is usually the failure to abstain from intercourse during the fertile period rather than a misunderstanding of the method or how to use it. Knowledge of the fertile period is also useful for achieving pregnancy.

Modern NFP methods have been adapted for use during lactation. A basic infertile pattern (BIP) of fertility symptoms (such as cervical mucus) is established during a 2-week period of abstinence. Thereafter, alternating nights are available for intercourse unless there is a change in the BIP, which then requires additional abstinence according to method-specific rules (Parenteau-Carreau & Cooney, 1994).

The effectiveness of NFP methods during breastfeeding has seldom been systematically evaluated. As with the study of other contraceptives, most previous efficacy research has excluded all but ostensibly normally cycling women. One study of breastfeeding women observed a poor association between estrogen metabolite excretion and women's reports of the cervical mucus symptom that is regulated by estrogen (Brown, Harrison, & Smith, 1985). Basal body temperature is unknowable unless the woman has at least 6 hours of uninterrupted sleep; this requirement excludes many fully breastfeeding women, particularly in the early months of lactation. One prospective study of the symptothermal method used during breastfeeding found that the method is highly sensitive although not very specific in its ability to determine which days are fertile. That is, fertile days are identified very well, but the method also requires abstinence on many days that probably are not fertile. Thus, correct use of the method during breastfeeding should result in a high degree of protection from pregnancy, but requires more abstinence than is necessary to prevent pregnancy (Kennedy et al., 1995). The requirement for somewhat more abstinence than is absolutely necessary is intentionally built into the method in order to err on the side of pregnancy avoidance. It is not at all clear whether the amount of abstinence required by NFP methods used during breastfeeding is a hardship on couples. If coital frequency is low at this time anyway, and if the BIP is clear and consistent, abstinence may not be a problem. Under opposite circumstances abstinence may be difficult. Thus, NFP leaders recommend that breastfeeding users first apply the rules of LAM in order to eliminate the need for abstinence for up to 6 months postpartum (Parenteau-Carreau & Cooney, 1994). A "2-day"

fertility awareness method has been proposed that may require fewer days of abstinence in the early postpartum period for breastfeeding women (Arevalo, Jennings & Sinai, 2002). Although NFP methods can be taught and learned in simple terms (and illiterate women in many countries have learned to use the modern NFP methods), learning apparently is easier during normal cycles compared with the hypoestrogenic period of lactation. There may be an excess risk of unplanned pregnancy after the first postpartum menses in new users, since the changing fertility symptoms may be especially difficult to interpret (Labbok et al., 1991). Therefore, couples who wish to use natural methods to space or limit pregnancies during lactation are at an advantage if they have learned how to use their NFP method of choice prior to conception and subsequent lactation. However, one ovulation method study in Chile found a 12-month pregnancy rate of 11.1 percent during breastfeeding, but only 2 percent at 12 months were determined to be method failures (Perez et al., 1988).

Hormonal Methods

Hormonal contraceptive methods are not the category of first choice for breastfeeding women (International Planned Parenthood Federation [IPPF], 2002; WHO, 2004b). The main reason is that steroid hormones, natural or synthetic, are transferred into the breastmilk to various degrees (Johansson & Odlind, 1987). The effect of the infant's exposure to exogenous hormones is presumed to be minor because very small amounts of hormone are excreted in the milk or absorbed by the infant. Since the fetus is exposed to very high levels of progesterone in utero, exposure to small quantities of progestins in breastmilk may be of no consequence. Nevertheless, the degree to which exogenous hormones can be cleared by the neonate is unknown. Plasma does not bind steroids well, the immature liver does not metabolize them well, and newborn kidneys are assumed to excrete inefficiently. Excess steroids or their metabolites may attach to receptor sites in the brain or reproductive organs (Harlap, 1987), which may be especially concerning in the first few months of life when extrauterine central nervous system growth is most rapid (Diaz, 2002). The long-term effects of consumption of exogenous steroid hormones on development are as yet unknown. Although the concern about infant exposure to exogenous hormones is theoretical, avoidance of exposure in the early weeks or months is urged because its effects are unknown, and other contraceptive methods are available.

Progestin-only Hormonal Methods. It is recommended that the use of progestin-only hormonal methods be delayed for at least 6 weeks postpartum (IPPF, 1996, 2002; WHO, 2004a,b) to avoid neonatal exposure to the steroid hormone. Since other temporary methods, such as barriers and LAM, should be available to the breastfeeding woman, and since coital frequency can be low during the first 6 weeks postpartum, the use of a stopgap method in the early postpartum period is a reasonable approach.

Progestin transfer to the infant varies across formulations of progestin-only methods. The estimated dose consumed by the infant is much smaller with pills and implants than with injectables. An implant that delivers orally inactive progesterone (i.e., Nesterone or Elcometrine) is available in some countries and would be a better progestin-only alternative than Norplant or Implanon during breastfeeding (Diaz, 2002).

The levonorgestrel-releasing IUD has been found to perform the same as the Copper T-380A during lactation. IUD continuation, breastfeeding continuation, and infant outcomes were the same in a randomized study (Shaamash et. al., 2005).

Progestin-only pills (McCann et al., 1989; Moggia et al., 1991; Sinchai et al., 1995), injections (Hannon et al., 1997; Halderman & Nelson, 2002), vaginal rings (Massai et al., 2005), and subdermal implants (Coutinho et al., 1999; Reinprayoon et al., 2000; Massai et al., 2001; Schiappacasse et al., 2002; Taneepanichskul et al., 2006) are not associated with reduced milk production, breastfeeding frequency, or impaired infant growth or early development, even if initiated before 6 weeks postpartum. (Diaz, 2002; Curtis et al., 2002; WHO, 1994a,b).

Although progestin-only methods should not interfere with breastfeeding (and may actually enhance lactation), anecdotal accounts of lactation failure associated with the very early use of progestin-only contraceptives are of concern. Despite the caution of experts to delay initiating progestin use for at least 6 weeks, some women receive progestin injections on the delivery table, or within 72 hours of delivery prior to hospital discharge. It seems likely that this early bolus of exogenous progestin could interfere with the establishment of lactation, since the physiological trigger for lactogenesis is the precipitous withdrawal of natural progesterone, which does not occur in humans until 2 to 3 days postpartum (Cowie, Forsyth, & Hart, 1980). Accordingly, progestin contraceptive initiation should be delayed for at least 3 full days (Kennedy, Short, & Tully, 1997), and preferably until after the mature milk has come in and lactation is rather well established. Two studies of the initiation of progestin-only pills during the first week postpartum found no deleterious effect on milk production (McCann et al., 1989; Moggia et al., 1991). However, the pill dose is relatively small compared with the injected amount, and pill consumption may have begun later than 3 days postpartum.

Progestin-only pills are marginally less effective than combined estrogen-progesterone formulations, but they are still highly effective when taken consistently and correctly. Progestin-only pills are somewhat unforgiving of incorrect use—e.g., missing a pill—although when used during breastfeeding their effectiveness is close to that of combined pills. Their lower effectiveness can be reasonably compensated by good counseling on method use (Chi, 1993).

Women who use the 3-month progestin-only injectable product Depo-Provera often experience amenorrhea after an interval of irregular bleeding/ spotting. Studies in Bolivia and China have found that breastfeeding women tolerated this common side effect better than nonbreastfeeding women and were more likely to continue using the method (Hubacher et al., 2000; Danli, Qingxiang, & Guowei, 2000).

Combined Estrogen-Progestin Hormonal Methods. Hormone formulations containing estrogen have been observed to decrease the milk supply in several studies (Koetsawang, 1987; WHO, 1988). Therefore, combined estrogen-progesterone pills or injectables should not be used during breastfeeding unless there is no other acceptable alternative. If combined pills (including low-dose formulations) are the only choice, the World Health Organization (2000) and the International Planned Parenthood Federation (2002) recommend that they be avoided, or postponed for at least 6 months or until weaning, whichever comes first. Due to the elevated risk of thrombosis in the first few weeks postpartum, methods containing estrogen should be avoided for about 3 weeks regardless of breastfeeding status (WHO, 2004a,b).

There are important detractors from the consensus view of WHO and IPPF on the use of hormonal contraceptive methods during lactation. A review of the literature concluded that studies of the effects of hormonal methods on breastfeeding are flawed and that no recommendations can be made (Truitt et al., 2003, 2005). (Unfortunately, publications prior to the 1990s did not require all of the details of their methodologies to be printed. Some if not all of the studies reviewed were actually quite robust.) The American College of Obstetrics and Gynecology has made "practical recommendations" for the use of hormonal methods by breastfeeding women that differ from the recommendations of IPPF and WHO (ACOG 2007). Also, the British Faculty of Family Planning and Reproductive Health Care Clinical Effectiveness Unit believes that it is unnecessary to delay progestin-only methods for 6 weeks postpartum, but cannot agree among themselves when it is safe to start (Faculty, 2004). A study in South Africa found that when women were given appropriate information about the controversy over early versus delayed progestin injections, they were able to make their own decisions about when to start (Hani et al., 2003). It seems appropriate to involve women in their own contraceptive decisions given that it is unethical to randomize neonates to early versus late exposure to contraceptive hormones (among other reasons).

Emergency Contraception

Nursing mothers may need to use a method of emergency contraception. Guidance is available for emergency contraceptive approaches during breastfeeding, but no studies of emergency contraception during breastfeeding have been published. Before the 21st day post partum, there is no need for a breastfeeding woman with a contraceptive failure or unprotected sex to use an emergency method. Thereafter, if she is using a hormonal method, a potential contraceptive failure should be managed in the same way as a woman who is not breastfeeding. Beginning at 4 weeks postpartum, an IUD can be offered as an emergency method, especially if the woman wishes to continue using this method, but

the chance of expulsion can also be high. A single 1.5 mg dose of levonorgestrel can be taken as an emergency method after a breastfeed (WHO 2004a,b; Faculty, 2004). Following the dose, mothers should refrain from breastfeeding for at least 8 hours, but not more than 24 hours (Gainer, 2007).

Clinical Implications

When a woman or couple makes a legitimate family-planning decision and/or chooses a method for achieving their family-planning ideal based on full and accurate information and reflection, that person or couple has maximized the likelihood of being satisfied with the decision or choice and of using the chosen method correctly and effectively.

Informed choice has been defined as "effective access to information on reproductive choices and to the necessary counseling, services, and supplies to help individuals choose and use an appropriate method of family planning, if desired" (Piotrow, 1989, p. 2).

Informed choice should be viewed as a continuing process that parallels changing procreative desire and phase of life, as well as personal changes over time. Family-planning intentions do not remain fixed throughout life, and one type of contraceptive is usually not appropriate for the same person throughout all the reproductive years. An appropriate range of available methods includes both male and female methods—and permanent methods as well as long- and short-acting temporary ones. If only a limited range of methods is available to the healthcare provider, he or she should be prepared to offer referrals to help meet the patient's needs.

Information can be shared with patients in different ways, using the written word through pamphlets, books, and posters, or the spoken word through videos, audiovisual presentations, or "class style" (part lecture, part participatory) discussions. Providing information, however, is not sufficient. An interpersonal exchange is necessary to ensure that effective communication of information has been achieved and also to provide clarification and counseling. The desired result of counseling is a patient or couple who has made a choice based on full understanding of the alternatives—and who has made that choice freely, unaffected by the counselor. Information should flow freely between the provider/counselor and the woman/couple. This circumstance exists, ideally, between the lactation consultant and the breastfeeding woman. Accordingly, the lactation consultant needs to be well versed in available family-planning services and alternatives in her community. Perhaps most important, the healthcare provider should be aware of the possible interaction of various contraceptives with breastfeeding as discussed in this chapter. Both lactation consultants and family-planning providers should be prepared to discuss common sexual issues as well.

A review of the literature concluded that the effectiveness of postpartum education about contraception is not known (Hiller, Griffith, & Jenner, 2005). One study found that less than 30 percent of pregnant women discussed family planning with their provider, and long-term options were inadequately explored among women who chose sterilization (Cwiak, Gellasch, & Zieman, 2004). A study in

---

BOX 21–3

Issues to Consider When Discussing Family Planning with the Breastfeeding Woman

Questions

1. Does the mother wish to limit or space any future pregnancies? If so, what method(s) of family planning does she prefer?
2. If she has breastfed a previous child, how long did she remain amenorrheic? What factors may have influenced the duration of her lactational amenorrhea?
3. If she has not breastfed before, how does she plan to do so? Is she familiar with the factors that can reduce the duration of lactational amenorrhea?
4. If she wishes to have no more children, how will her family be affected if a temporary method of contraception fails and she becomes pregnant before she had planned, or in the face of a desire to have no more children?

Information to Share

1. Discuss the effectiveness of the mother's preferred method(s) and offer additional information about other contraceptives as well. Include information about the effect of each method on lactation and on the suckling child.
2. This information may predict the degree of double protection she may experience by using both a contraceptive and breastfeeding to reduce the risk of an unplanned pregnancy.
3. Review the factors that reduce the duration of lactational amenorrhea and increase the early resumption of fertility. Pay particular attention to what is meant by exclusive or nearly exclusive breastfeeding, the impact of pacifier use, regular use of solid foods in the infant's diet, and supplementary bottle-feedings.
4. When the reproductive intention is to prevent any future pregnancies, it is especially important that a highly effective contraceptive method be chosen. Double protection is not an issue under this circumstance.

Scotland showed that postpartum counseling about family planning during the hospital stay after delivery is ineffective (Glasier, Logan, & McGlew, 1996). However, for the immediate postpartum insertion of an IUD or for postpartum sterilization, counseling is essential before delivery. A large multicenter study compared antenatal family-planning counseling with standard postpartum counseling and found no difference in pregnancy and continuation rates at 1 year postpartum, except in Edinburgh where significantly more women counseled antenatally chose sterilization (Smith et al., 2002).

Ideally, a plan for postpartum contraception is decided before delivery, with postpartum follow-up timed to match the requirements of the chosen method. A postpartum checkup with an obstetrician/gynecologist is advised and can probably occur at any time from the 3rd to the 8th week after delivery. The longer the consultation is delayed, the more comfortable a pelvic examination is likely to be for a breastfeeding woman. However, the woman should insist on seeing her clinician earlier than the traditional 6 weeks in the event of abnormal vaginal discharge or pain, or if she needs a contraceptive method before the sixth week or needs help with a postpartum sexual issue. All women who wish to avoid pregnancy should be ensured of a method for doing so before hospital discharge, but preferably before delivery. If a woman's method is not one that can be appropriately delivered in the hospital, then condoms or progestin-only pills—and clear instructions for their use—should be distributed generously at hospital discharge, and LAM should be taught prior to delivery with reinforcement at hospital discharge. Some kind of family-planning follow-up (for example, by phone) should occur in the third to fourth week postpartum to revisit and support the chosen contraceptive strategy. Since the lactation consultant is one of the most likely healthcare providers in the first month postpartum, the lactation consultant can check that a plan is in place, and facilitate or support the couple in procuring their contraceptive method.

Accurate information is an essential tool for lactation consultants, and posing the questions in Box 21–3 will help the LC ascertain some essential information. Additionally, such information will influence the ability of the woman or couple to make a decision without undue influence from the consultant. When the couple freely makes informed choices, the lactation consultant is better able to support the woman and her family in their choices.

Summary

Fertility, sexuality, and contraception are normally related, but each of these aspects of reproduction also affects or is affected by lactation. A clear understanding of the interrelationships of these elements is essential if the healthcare provider is to discuss issues and concerns of the lactating mother as she seeks to determine her fertility in concert with her sexual self. The healthcare provider benefits from an understanding of the relationship between physiological responses to suckling stimulation and the resumption of fertility. Additionally, the breastfeeding woman needs to be prepared for the ways in which her own breastfeeding experience may alter her sexual experience as well as her fertility—in the early weeks after birth as well as when her breastfeeding child is weaning.

Nearly all modern contraceptive methods can be used during breastfeeding, but the timing of the introduction of the methods can vary profoundly. Permanent, long-term, short-term, nonhormonal, and hormonal methods are all viable options when introduced appropriately. Temporary, stopgap methods, such as condoms and LAM, may be a suitable bridge in the early weeks or months of breastfeeding—especially if coital frequency is low—until another method of the couple's choosing is appropriate. All breastfeeding women who wish to avoid pregnancy can be helped to do so, and should plan to do so from the first postpartum coitus. Lactation consultants are well positioned to ensure that a family-planning strategy is in place within the first few weeks postpartum.

To best serve the breastfeeding family, the healthcare provider who is assisting the lactating mother should be thoroughly familiar with how lactation, fertility, sexuality, and contraception are intertwined threads in the cord of life experience.

Key Concepts

- The child's suckling initiates a cycle of neuroendocrinologic events that result in the inhibition of ovulation.
- Anything that decreases the child's suckling behavior or the need to suckle will be a secondary cause of the recovery of fertility. Supplementation may have the effect of decreasing hunger, thirst, and possibly the emotional need for comfort, thereby reducing suckling at the breast.
- A significant association exists between the duration of lactational infertility after one pregnancy and the duration in the same woman after her next pregnancy.
- Breastfeeding provides more than 98 percent protection from pregnancy during the first 6 months postpartum if the mother is "fully" or nearly fully breastfeeding and has not experienced vaginal bleeding after the 56th day postpartum.
- Once menstruation has resumed, fertility is returning or already has returned. Menses is an absolute indication of the need for another contraceptive method if continued protection is desired.
- The tenderness from episiotomy or vulvovaginal or perineal stress following vaginal delivery usually lasts for several months and can cause pain or discomfort during intercourse.
- Postpartum women produce low levels of estrogen until they begin to recover fertility. Among breastfeeding women, this period of hypoestrogenemia can endure for the entire lactation course, and it can cause the vaginal epithelium to be very thin and to secrete little fluid during arousal, which may be remedied by the use of inert, water-based lubricants.
- Most women experience change in their sexual practices after delivery. The frequency of sex is often lower, although some women report better quality in their sex lives.
- Very few women talk to their healthcare professional about their sexual health.
- During breastfeeding, nonhormonal methods are the first-choice category of contraceptives and progestin-only methods are the second choice. Methods containing estrogen should be avoided during breastfeeding, especially in the first 6 months.
- Counseling is crucially important when helping women or couples to select the best family-planning approach. When a permanent method is a serious consideration, counseling must begin long before the procedure and be repetitive.
- Nonhormonal intrauterine devices (IUDs) have been shown to have either no effect or a positive effect on lactation.
- Contraceptive steroid hormones, natural or synthetic, are transferred into the breastmilk to various degrees. Since the fetus is exposed to very high levels of progesterone in utero, exposure to small quantities of progestins in breastmilk may be of no consequence. Nevertheless, the degree to which exogenous hormones can be cleared by the neonate is unknown.
- It is recommended that the use of progestin-only hormonal methods be delayed for at least 6 weeks postpartum to avoid neonatal exposure. Other temporary methods, such as barriers and LAM, can be used, especially since coital frequency can be low during the first 6 weeks postpartum.
- The physiological trigger for lactogenesis is the precipitous withdrawal of natural progesterone at about 2 to 3 days postpartum. Accordingly, progestin contraceptive initiation should be delayed for at least 3 full days and preferably until after the mature milk has come in and lactation is rather well established.
- Progestin-only pills, injections, and subdermal implants are not associated with reduced milk production, breastfeeding frequency, or impaired infant growth or early development.
- Hormone formulations containing estrogen have been observed to decrease the milk supply. Therefore, combined estrogen-progesterone pills or injectables should not be used during breastfeeding unless there is no other acceptable alternative.
- Serving as one of the most likely healthcare providers in the first month postpartum, the lactation consultant can check that a plan for family planning is in place, and facilitate or support the couple in procuring their contraceptive method.

References

Abraham S. Recovery after childbirth. *Med J Aust.* 1990;152:387.

Abraham S et al. Recovery after childbirth: a preliminary prospective study. *Med J Aust.* 1990;152:9–12.

American College of Obstetricians and Gynecologists. Breastfeeding: maternal and infant aspects. *ACOG Clin Rev.* 2007;12(1):1S–16S.

Alder E, Bancroft J. The relationship between breastfeeding persistence, sexuality, and mood in postpartum women. *Psychol Med.* 1988;18:389–396.

Alder EM et al. Hormones, mood and sexuality in lactating women. *Br J Psychiatry.* 1986;148:74–79.

American Academy of Pediatrics, Committee on Drugs. The transfer of drugs and other chemicals into human milk. *Pediatrics.* 2001;108(3):776–789.

American Academy of Pediatrics. Breastfeeding and the use of human milk. *Pediatrics.* 2005;115:496–506.

American Dietetic Association. Position of the American Dietetic Association: promoting and supporting breastfeeding. *J Am Diet Assoc.* 2005;105:810–818.

Andersen AN, Schioler V. Influence of breastfeeding pattern on pituitary-ovarian axis of women in an industrialized community. *Am J Obstet Gynecol.* 1982;143:673–677.

Andersson K et al. Perforations with intrauterine devices—report from a Swedish study. *Contraception.* 1998;57:251–255.

Arevalo M et al. Efficacy of a new method of family planning: the Standard Days Method. *Contraception.* 2002;65:333–338.

Badroui MHH, Hefnawi F. Ovarian function during lactation. In: Hafez ESE, ed. *Human ovulation.* Amsterdam, Holland: Elsevier-North Holland Biomedical Press; 1979:233–241.

Barrett G et al. Women's sexual health after childbirth. *BJOG.* 2000;107(2):186–195.

Becker S et al. Estimation of births averted due to breast-feeding and increases in levels of contraception needed to substitute for breast-feeding. *J Biosoc Sci.* 2003;35:559–74.

Benitez I et al. Extending lactational amenorrhea in Manila: a successful breast-feeding education program. *J Biosoc Sci.* 1992;24:211–231.

Bongaarts J, Menken J. *Determinants of Fertility in Developing Countries.* New York: Academic Press; 1983.

Bongaarts J, Potter RG. *Fertility, Biology and Behavior.* New York, NY: Academic Press; 1983.

Bottorff JL. Persistence in breastfeeding: a phenomenologic investigation. *J Adv Nurs.* 1990;15:201–209.

Brown JB, Harrison P, Smith MA. A study of returning fertility after childbirth and during lactation by measurement of urinary estrogen and pregnanediol excretion and cervical mucus production. *J Biosoc Sci.* 1985;9(suppl.):5–23.

Chi IC. The safety and efficacy issues of progestin-only oral contraceptives—an epidemiologic perspective. *Contraception.* 1993;44:1–21.

Chi IC, Farr G. Postpartum IUD contraception—a review of an international experience. *Adv Contraception.* 5:127–146, 1989.

Chi IC, Feldblum PJ, Rogers SM. IUD-related uterine perforation: an epidemiologic analysis of a rare event using an international dataset. *Contracept Deliv Syst.* 1984;5:123–130.

Chi IC et al. Performance of the Copper T-380A intrauterine device in breastfeeding women. *Contraception.* 1989a;39:603–618.

Chi IC et al. Insertional pain and other IUD insertion-related rare events for breastfeeding and non-breastfeeding women—a decade's experience in developing countries. *Adv Contraception.* 1989b;5:101–119.

Chi IC et al. Tubal ligation at cesarean delivery in five Asian centers: a comparison with tubal ligation soon after vaginal delivery. *Int J Gynecol Obstet.* 1989c;30:257–265.

Cole LP et al. Effects of breastfeeding on IUD performance. *Am J Public Health.* 1983;73:384–388.

Cooney KA et al. An assessment of the nine month lactational amenorrhea method in Rwanda. *Stud Fam Plann.* 1996;27:162–171.

Coutinho EM et al. Use of a single implant of Elcometrine (ST-1435), a nonorally active progestin, as a long-acting contraceptive for postpartum nursing women. *Contraception.* 1999;59:115–122.

Cowie AT, Forsyth IA, Hart IC. *Hormonal Control of Lactation.* Berlin, Germany: Springer-Verlag; 1980.

Curtis KM et al. Contraception for women in selected circumstances. *Obstet Gynecol.* 2002;99:1100–1112.

Cwiak C, Gellasch T, Zieman M. Peripartum contraceptive attitudes and practices. *Contraception.* 2004;70:383–386.

Danli S, Qingxiang S, Guowei S. A multicentered clinical trial of the long-acting injectable contraceptive Depo Provera in Chinese women. *Contraception.* 2000;62:15–18.

Delvoye P et al. The influence of the frequency of nursing and of previous lactation experience on serum prolactin in lactating mothers. *J Biosoc Sci.* 1977;9:447–451.

Diaz S. Contraceptive implants and lactation. *Contraception.* 2002;65:39–46.

Diaz S et al. Fertility regulation in nursing women: I. The probability of conception in full nursing women living in an urban setting. *J Biosoc Sci.* 1982;14:329–341.

Diaz S et al. Contraceptive efficacy of lactational amenorrhea in urban Chilean women. *Contraception.* 1991;43:335–352.

Diaz S et al. Neuroendocrine mechanisms of lactational infertility in women. *Biol Res.* 1995;28:155–163.

Divers WA. Characteristics of women requesting reversal of sterilization. *Fertil Steril.* 1984;41:233–236.

Elias MF et al. Nursing practices and lactational amenorrhea. *J Biosoc Sci.* 1986;18:1–10.

Eslami SS et al. The reliability of menses to indicate the return of ovulation in breastfeeding women in Manila, the Philippines. *Stud Fam Plann.* 1990;21:243–250.

Faculty of Family Planning and Reproductive Health Care Clinical Effectiveness Unit. Contraceptive choices for breastfeeding women. *J Fam Plan Reprod Health Care.* 2004;30:181–189.

Family Health International. Breastfeeding as a family planning method. *Lancet.* 1988;2:(8621):1204–1205.

Farr G, Rivera, R. Interactions between IUD and breast-feeding status at time of IUD insertion: analysis of PCU 380A acceptors in developing countries. *Am J Obstet Gynecol.* 1992;167:2027–2031.

Ford K. Correlation between subsequent lengths of post-partum amenorrhea in a prospective study of breastfeeding women in rural Bangladesh. *J Biosoc Sci.* 1992;24:89–95.

Gainer E et al. Levonorgestrel pharmacokinetics in plasma and milk of lactating women who take 1.5 mg for emergency contraception. *Hum Reprod.* 2007;22(6):1578–1584.

Glasier AF, Logan J, McGlew TJ. Who gives advice about postpartum family planning? *Contraception.* 1996;53:217–220.

Glasier A, McNeilly AS, Baird DT. Induction of ovarian activity by pulsatile infusion of LHRH in women with lactational amenorrhea. *Clin Endocrinol.* 1986;24:243–252.

Gray RH et al. Risk of ovulation during lactation. *Lancet.* 1990;335:25–29.

Gross BA, Eastman CJ. Prolactin and the return of ovulation in breastfeeding women. *J Biosoc Sci Suppl.* 1985;9:25–42.

Grubb GS et al. Regret after decision to have a tubal sterilization. *Fertil Steril.* 1985;44:248–253.

Grudzinskas JG, Atkinson L. Sexual function during the puerperium. *Arch Sex Behav.* 1984;13:85–91.

Halderman LD, Nelson AL. Impact of early postpartum administration of progestin-only hormonal contraceptives compared with nonhormonal contraceptives on short-term breastfeeding patterns. *Am J Obstet Gynecol.* 2002;186:1250–1258.

Hani A et al. Informed choice—the timing of postpartum contraceptive initiation. *S Afr Med J.* 2003;93:862–864.

Hannon PR et al. The influence of medroxyprogesterone on the duration of breastfeeding in mothers in an urban community. *Arch Pediatr Adolesc Med.* 1997;151:490–496.

Harlap S. Exposure to contraceptive hormones through breast milk: Are there long-term health and behavioral consequences? *Int J Gynaecol Obstet.* 1987;25(suppl):47–55.

Hatcher RA et al. *Contraceptive Technology.* 18th ed. New York, NY: Ardent Media; 2004.

Heartwell SF, Schlesselman S. Risk of uterine perforation among users of intrauterine devices. *Obstet Gynecol.* 1983;61:31–36.

Hiller JE, Griffith E, Jenner F. Education for contraceptive use by women after childbirth. *Cochrane Database Syst Rev.* 2005;4.

Hornsby PP, Wilcox AJ. Validity of questionnaire information on frequency of coitus. *Am J Epidemiol.* 1989;130:94–99.

Howie PW et al. Effect of supplementary food on suckling patterns and ovarian activity during lactation. *Br Med J.* 1981;283:757–759.

Howie PW et al. Fertility after childbirth: adequacy of postpartum luteal phases. *Clin Endocrinol.* 1982a;17:609–615.

Howie PW et al. Fertility after childbirth: postpartum ovulation and menstruation in bottle and breast-feeding mothers. *Clin Endocrinol.* 1982b;17:323–332.

Hubacher D et al. Factors affecting continuation rates of DMPA. *Contraception.* 2000;60:345–351.

International Lactation Consultant Association (ILCA). *Clinical Guidelines for the Establishment of Exclusive Breastfeeding.* Raleigh, NC: ILCA; June 2005.

International Planned Parenthood Federation (IPPF). IMAP statement on breastfeeding, fertility, and postpartum contraception. *IPPF Med Bull.* 1996;30:1–3.

International Planned Parenthood Federation (IPPF). IMAP statement on hormonal methods of contraception. *IPPF Med Bull.* 2002;36(5):1–8.

Islam MM, Khan HTA. Pattern of coital frequency in rural Bangladesh. *J Fam Welfare.* 1993;39:38–43.

Israngkura B et al. Breastfeeding and return to ovulation in Bangkok. *Int J Gynaecol Obstet.* 1989;30:335–342.

Johansson E, Odlind V. The passage of exogenous hormones into breastmilk: possible effects. *Int J Gynaecol Obstet.* 1987;25(suppl):111–114.

Jones RE. A hazards model analysis of breastfeeding variables and maternal age on return to menses postpartum in rural Indonesian women. *Hum Biol.* 1988;60:853–871.

Jones RE. Breastfeeding and postpartum amenorrhea in Indonesia. *J Biosoc Sci.* 1989;21:83–100.

Kazi A et al. Effectiveness of the lactational amenorrhea method in Pakistan. *Fertil Steril.* 1995;64:717–723.

Kennedy KI. Fertility, sexuality and contraception during lactation. In: Riordan J, Auerbach K, eds. *Breastfeeding and human milk.* Sudbury, MA: Jones and Bartlett; 1993.

Kennedy KI, Labbok MH, Van Look PFA. Consensus statement—lactational amenonorrhea method for family planning. *Int J Gynecol Obstet.* 1996;54:55–57.

Kennedy KI, Rivera R, McNeilly AS. Consensus statement on the use of breastfeeding as a family planning method. *Contraception.* 1989;39:477–496.

Kennedy KI, Short RV, Tully MR. Premature introduction of progestin-only contraceptive methods during lactation. *Contraception.* 1997;55:347–350.

Kennedy KI, Visness CV. Contraceptive efficacy of lactational amenorrheoa. *Lancet.* 1992;339(8787):227–230.

Kennedy KI et al. Breastfeeding and the symptothermal method. *Stud Fam Plann.* 1995;26:107–115.

Kenny JA. Sexuality of pregnant and breastfeeding women. *Arch Sex Behav.* 1973;2:215–229.

Khan T et al. A study of breastfeeding and the return of menses and pregnancy in Karachi, Pakistan. *Contraception.* 1989;40:365–376.

Knodel J, Chayovan N. Coital activity among married Thai women. In: *Demographic and Health Surveys World Conference Proceedings*, Vol. 2. Columbia, MD IRD/MacroInternational; 1991:925–945.

Koetsawang S. The effects of contraceptive methods on the quality and quantity of breastmilk. *Int J Gynaecol Obstet.* 1987;25(suppl):115–128.

Kramer MS, Kakuma R. The optimal duration of exclusive breastfeeding: a systematic review. WHO, Geneva, Switzerland: WHO, 2002: WHO/FCH/CAH/01.23. http://www.who.int/child-adolescent-health/publications/NUTRITION/WHO_FCH_CAH_01.23.htm. Accessed January 14, 2006.

Labbok MH et al. Ovulation method use during breastfeeding: is there increased risk of unplanned pregnancy? *Am J Obstet Gynecol.* 1991;165:2031–2036.

Labbok MH et al. *Guidelines: Breastfeeding, Family Planning and the Lactational Amenorrhea Method—LAM.* Washington, DC: Institute for Reproductive Health; 1994.

Labbok MH et al. I. Multicenter study of the lactational amenorrhea method (LAM): duration and implications for clinical guidance. *Contraception.* 1997;55:327–336.

Lewis PR et al. The resumption of ovulation and menstruation in a well-nourished population of women breastfeeding for an extended period of time. *Fertil Steril.* 1991;55:529–536.

Massai MR et al. Contraceptive efficacy and clinical performance of Nesterone implants in postpartum women. *Contraception.* 64:369–376, 2001.

Massai R et al. Extended use of a progesterone-releasing vaginal ring in nursing women: a phase II clinical trial. *Contraception.* 2005;72:352–357.

Masters WH, Johnson VE. *Human Sexual Response.* Boston, MA: Little, Brown, and Co.; 1966.

McCann MF et al. The effects of a progestin-only oral contraceptive (levonorgestrel 0.03 mg) on breastfeeding. *Contraception.* 1989;40:635–648.

McNeilly AS. Lactational control of reproduction. *Reprod Fertil Dev.* 2001a;13:583–590.

McNeilly AS. Neuroendocrine changes and fertility in breastfeeding women. *Prog Brain Res.* 2001b;113:207–214.

McNeilly AS, Glasier A, Howie PW. Endocrine control of lactational infertility-I. In: Dobbing J, ed. *Maternal Nutrition and Lactational Infertility.* New York, NY: Raven Press; 1985.

McNeilly AS et al. Fertility after childbirth: pregnancy associated with breastfeeding. *Clin Endocrinol.* 1983;18:167–173.

Moggia AV et al. A comparative study of a progestin-only oral contraceptive versus nonhormonal methods in lactating women in Buenos Aires, Argentina. *Contraception.* 1991;44:31–43.

Muller AL et al. Transvaginal ultrasonographic assessment of the expulsion rate of intrauterine devices inserted in the immediate postpartum period: a pilot study. *Contraception.* 2005;72:192–195.

O'Hanley K, Huber DH. Postpartum IUDs: keys for success. *Contraception.* 1992;45:351–361.

Parenteau-Carreau S, Cooney KA. *Breastfeeding, Lactational Amenorrhea Method and Natural Family Planning Interface: Teaching Guide.* Washington, DC: Institute for Reproductive Health; 1994.

Perez A, Labbok MH, Queenan JT. Clinical study of the lactational amenorrhoea method for family planning. *Lancet.* 1992;339:968–970.

Perez A et al. First ovulation after childbirth: the effect of breastfeeding. *Am J Obstet Gynecol.* 1972;114:1014–1047.

Perez A et al. Use-effectiveness of the ovulation method initiated during postpartum breastfeeding. *Contraception.* 1988;38:499–508.

Peterson HB et al. The risk of pregnancy after tubal sterilization. *Am J Obstet Gynecol.* 1996;174:1161–1170.

Piotrow PT. Informed choice: report of the Cooperating Agencies Task Force. Baltimore, MD: Johns Hopkins University, Center for Communication Programs; 1989.

Ramos R, Kennedy K, Visness C. Effectiveness of lactational amenorrhea in prevention of pregnancy in Manila, the Philippines: non-comparative prospective trial. *Br Med J.* 1996;313:909–912.

Reinprayoon D et al. Effects of the etonogestrel-releasing contraceptive implant (Implanon) on parameters of breastfeeding compared to those of an intrauterine device. *Contraception.* 2000;62:239–246.

Riordan J. *A Practical Guide to Breastfeeding.* St. Louis, MO: Mosby; 1983.

Rivera R et al. Breastfeeding and the return to ovulation in Durango, Mexico. *Fertil Steril.* 1988;49:780–787.

Robson KM, Brant HA, Kumar R. Maternal sexuality during first pregnancy and after childbirth. *Br J Obstet Gynaecol.* 1981;88:882–889.

Rojnik B, Kosmelj K, Andolsek-Jeras L. Initiation of contraception postpartum. *Contraception.* 1995;51:75–81.

Rolland R. Bibliography (with review) on contraceptive effects of breastfeeding. *Biblio Reprod.* 1976;28:1–4, 93.

Schiappacasse V et al. Health and growth of infants breastfed by Norplant contraceptive users: a six-year follow-up study. *Contraception.* 2002;66:57–65.

Shaaban MM et al. The recovery of fertility during breastfeeding in Assiut, Egypt. *J Biosoc Sci.* 1990;22:19–32.

Shaamash AH et al. A comparative study of the levonorgestrel-releasing intrauterine system Mirena® versus the Copper T380A intrauterine device during lactation: breastfeeding performance, infant growth and infant development. *Contraception.* 2005;72: 346–351.

Short RV. Breastfeeding. *Sci Am.* 1984;250(4):35–41.

Short RV et al. Contraceptive effects of extended lactational amenorrhea: beyond the Bellagio consensus. *Lancet.* 1991;337:715–717.

Simpson-Hebert M, Huffman SL. The contraceptive effect of breastfeeding. *Stud Fam Plann.* 1981;12: 125–133.

Sinchai W et al. Effects of a progestin-only pill (Exluton) and an intrauterine device (Multiload Cu250) on breastfeeding. *Adv Contraception.* 1995;11:143–155.

Smith KB et al. Is postpartum contraceptive advice given antenatally of value? *Contraception.* 2002;65: 237–243.

Taneepanichskul S et al. Effects of the etonogestrel-releasing implant Implanon and a nonmedicated intrauterine device on the growth of breast-fed infants. *Contraception.* 2006;73:368–371.

Thapa S, Short RV, Potts M. Breastfeeding, birthspacing and their effects on child survival. *Nature.* 1988; 335(6192):679–682.

Truitt ST, Fraser AB, Grimes DA et al. Combined hormonal versus nonhormonal versus progestin-only contraception in lactation. *Cochrane Database Syst Rev.* 2005;4.

Truitt ST, Fraser AB, Grimes DA et al. Hormonal contraception during lactation: systematic review of randomized controlled trials. *Contraception.* 2003; 68:233–238.

Trussell J et al. Contraceptive failure in the US: an update. *Stud Fam Plann.* 1990;21:51–54.

Udry JR. Coitus as demographic behaviour. In: Gray R, ed. *Biomedical and Demographic Determinants of Reproduction.* Oxford, England: Clarendon Press; 1993.

Udry JR, Deang L. Determinants of coitus after childbirth. *J Biosoc Sci.* 1993;25:117–125.

Valdes V et al. The efficacy of the lactational amenorrhea method (LAM) among working women. *Contraception.* 2000;62:217–219.

Van Ginnekin JK. Prolonged breastfeeding as a birth spacing method. *Stud Fam Plann.* 1974;5:201–20.

Van Look PFA. Lactational amenorrhea method for family planning. *Br Med J.* 1996;313:893–894.

Virden SF. The relationship between infant feeding method and maternal role adjustment. *J Nurs Midwifery.* 1988;33:31–35.

Visness CM, Kennedy KI. The frequency of coitus during breastfeeding. *Birth.* 1997;24(4):253–257.

Visness CM, Kennedy KI, Ramos R. The duration and character of postpartum bleeding among breastfeeding women. *Obstet Gynecol.* 1997;89:159–163.

Visness CM et al. Fertility of fully breastfeeding women in the early postpartum period. *Obstet Gynecol.* 1997;89:164–167.

Wade KB, Sevilla F, Labbok MH. Integrating the lactational amenorrhea method into a family planning program in Ecuador. *Stud Fam Plann.* 1994;25: 162–174.

Weiss P. The contraceptive potential of breastfeeding in Bangladesh. *Stud Fam Plann.* 1993;22:294–307.

Welkovic S et al. Postpartum bleeding and infection after post-placental IUD insertion. *Contraception.* 2001;63:155–158.

Wisniewski PM, Wilkinson EJ. Postpartum vaginal atrophy. *Am J Obstet Gynecol.* 1991;165:1249–1254.

World Health Organization. Effects of hormonal contraceptives on breast milk composition and infant growth. *Stud Fam Plann.* 1988;19:36–69.

World Health Organization. Progestin-only contraceptives during lactation: I. Infant growth. *Contraception.* 1994a;50:35–53.

World Health Organization. Progestin-only contraceptives during lactation: II. Infant development. *Contraception.* 1994b;50:55–68.

World Health Organization. The WHO multinational study of breastfeeding and lactational amenorrhea: I. Description of infant feeding patterns and the return of menses. *Fertil Steril.* 1998a;70:448–460.

World Health Organization. The WHO multinational study of breastfeeding and lactational amenorrhea: II. Factors associated with the length of amenorrhea. *Fertil Steril.* 1998b;70:461–471.

World Health Organization. The WHO multinational study of breastfeeding and lactational amenorrhea: IV. Postpartum bleeding and lochia in breastfeeding women. *Fertil Steril.* 1999a;72(3):441–447.

World Health Organization. The WHO multinational study of breastfeeding and lactational amenorrhea: III. Pregnancy during breastfeeding. *Fertil Steril.* 1999b;72(3):431–440.

World Health Organization. *Medical Eligibility Criteria for Contraceptive Use.* 3rd ed. Geneva, Switzerland: WHO Reproductive Health Research Division. 2004a.

World Health Organization. *Selected Practice Recommendations for Contraceptive Use.* 2nd ed. Geneva, Switzerland: WHO Reproductive Health Research Division. 2004b.

Wrigley EA, Hutchinson SA. Long-term breastfeeding: the secret bond. *J Nurs Midwifery.* 1990;35:35–41.

Section 5

Sociocultural and Research Issues

Breastfeeding exists within the constraints of each culture. Theoretical constructs that allow us to examine the family, its members, and their roles also enable us to identify issues around breastfeeding and to understand breastfeeding women of all cultures. Breastfeeding education, interwoven within the threads of a culture, leads to better care and a more satisfying experience.

As the trend continues toward evidence-based health care, caring for breastfeeding mothers and infants also means measuring clinical outcomes. Thus, lactation consultants need to know about research methods. In addition, they need more research to expand the knowledge of lactation and the variations in breastfeeding behavior. Only with such research will myths about breastfeeding be put to rest.

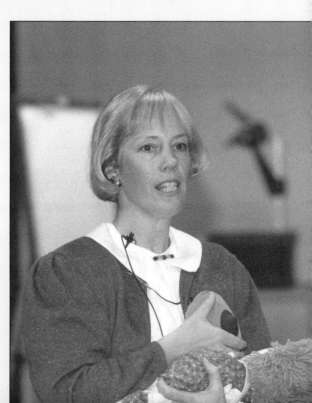

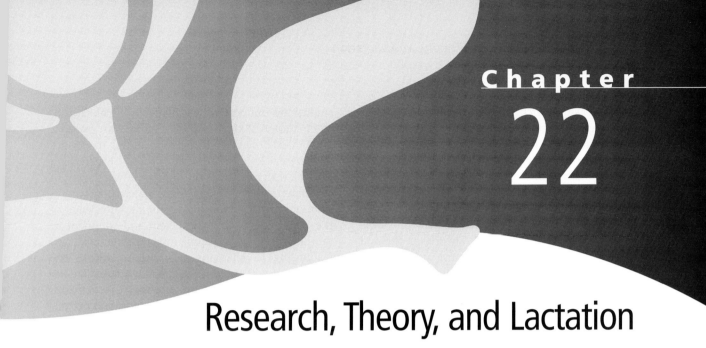

Chapter
22

Research, Theory, and Lactation

Roberta J. Hewat

EXPECTATIONS FOR LACTATION CONSULTANTS, and other healthcare professionals who work with breastfeeding mothers, to base their practice on evidence derived from research findings continue to increase. Intuition, gut reaction, and use of traditional procedures are no longer a sufficient base for accountable and responsible professional practice. Practice and education is founded on knowledge generated or validated from data gathered and interpreted by systematic methods that practitioners continually question, study, and expand. Theories provide the structure for systematically organizing and synthesizing knowledge derived from many sources in order to facilitate its use in research and to guide clinical practice. Both a body of knowledge founded on research and a practice based on the best available evidence legitimizes professional care.

The intent of this chapter is to assist lactation practitioners to develop an interest in—and understanding of—lactation research and theories that support them in their role as research consumers. This entails a complex process: reading articles to learn about current practices, understanding research methods to evaluate and determine whether study findings are relevant, incorporating appropriate findings into practice, and consistently questioning practices to develop questions for further research.

Theories Related to Lactation Practice

Lactation consultant practice draws on an abundance of rich and diverse literature generated in the disciplines of medicine, nursing, immunology, and psychosocial sciences, among other areas. This specialized and in-depth body of knowledge, increasingly based on scientific findings, is the foundation of lactation practice. Theories are conceptual constructions of concepts and their relationships that can be tested through research as well as a guide to practice. Theories provide structure for systematically organizing and synthesizing knowledge that may be from many sources, to facilitate its use in research, and to guide clinical practice. As the specialty advances, assumptions about breastfeeding and lactation are tested using theoretical frameworks and theories to guide the studies.

A *theoretical framework* is a representation of the concepts and relationships inherent in a theory that is the underpinning of a study. Other terms used—often interchangeably, which can be confusing—are *conceptual frameworks* and *models*. All are conceptual structures made up of concepts relevant to a phenomenon that are useful in organizing studies and

739

which make research results more meaningful for applying to clinical practice (Polit & Beck, 2004).

Theories range from those that are exceptionally broad in scope such as grand theories to those that are very narrow in scope, such as as microtheories. The grand theories are complex, often comprising several smaller theories; microtheories are a limited set of propositions about a well-defined phenomenon (Tomey & Alligood, 1998). Theories in the middle range are considered to be most useful to both practice and research, and for highlighting the links between theory, practice, and research (Lenz et al., 1995). The majority of the theories presented in this chapter are middle-range theories. Their selection is based on the interest they have generated among researchers and their historical relationship to lactation and the care of childbearing families.

Maternal Role Attainment Theory and Becoming a Mother

Rubin (1967a,b) attempted to explain the process of taking on the maternal role as a learned rather than an intuitive experience. Based on role theory described by Sarbin (1954) and Mead (1934) and observations of and interviews with women throughout pregnancy and the postpartum period, Rubin proposed two fundamental processes of maternal role attainment: (1) acquisition of the maternal role, and (2) identification of the partner—the infant—through psychological processes such as mimicry, role-play, fantasy, introjection-projection-rejection, and the grief work of letting go of a former role until a new identity or sense of self in the maternal role is recognized. In 1984 Rubin updated her perspectives, replacing the term *maternal role attainment* with *maternal identity* and *maternal experience* and postulating that the maternal identity evolves and changes with the birth of each child.

Rubin's work provided a foundation for Mercer (1981, 1985, 2004) who developed a theoretical framework for studying maternal role attainment during the first year after delivery. Initially Mercer postulated that "maternal role attainment is a process by which mothers achieve competence in the mothering role, integrating their mothering behaviors into their established roles so that they achieve confidence and harmony with their new identities" (Mercer & Ferketich, 1994). Findings from ongoing studies by numerous researchers (Koniak-Griffin, 1993; Martell, 2001; McBride & Shore, 2001; Nelson, 2003) have provided a base for expanding the theory of Maternal Role Attainment to that of Becoming a Mother, which captures the ongoing advancement of the maternal self (Mercer, 2004). Maternal identity is associated with establishing intimate knowledge of the infant and feeling competent and confident in mothering activities, feeling love for the infant, and readjusting to changing relationships within the family and with friends. Mercer advocates that the ongoing transitions of motherhood (e.g., when children are school age, adolescents, adults, and becoming a grandmother) should be investigated to expand the theory throughout a woman's lifespan (Mercer, 2004). Studies conducted by Mercer and associates showed that links between a mother's breastfeeding experience and maternal role attainment are highly relevant. For many, successful breastfeeding is viewed as part of the mothering role, and when feeding problems occur many mothers question their competence and mothering abilities.

Parent–Child Interaction Model

Based on empirical research showing that mother–infant interactions influence the mother–child relationship and the psychosocial development of the child, and that characteristics of each of the interactive partners affect the interaction, the Barnard model was developed to represent the caregiver–infant interaction system (Barnard & Eyres, 1978; Sumner & Spietz, 1994). The interaction is influenced by characteristics of the caregiver and the infant.

Caregiver/parent/mother characteristics important for positive interactions are showing sensitivity to the infant's cues, acting to alleviate the infant's distress, and using strategies that provide experiences that foster growth for the infant. The infant/child characteristics are clarity of cues and responsiveness to the caregiver or parent. Feeding is considered an excellent context for viewing mother–infant interactions. Practitioners throughout the world use the Nursing Child Assessment Feeding Scale (NCAFS) (Sumner & Spietz, 1994) for assessing parent–child interactions during feeding. Certification is required to ensure that assessments and interpretations are correctly made.

The Child Health Assessment Interaction Model (Barnard & Eyres, 1978; Sumner & Spietz, 1994) is an overall framework that is exceptionally useful for practitioner assessments and as a guide for research. In this model, three concentric, overlapping circles represent the environment, the caregiver, and the infant/child. For use in breastfeeding assessments, the largest circle represents the environment, which can include breastfeeding support from family, friends, and health professionals as well as cultural influences, physical surroundings, and all other extrinsic factors influencing the breastfeeding dyad. The second largest circle, representing the mother, can include factors influencing breastfeeding such as maternal age, education, intent to breastfeed, physical attributes for breastfeeding, and postpartum depressive state. The smallest circle represents the infant, and it includes what the infant brings to the interaction such as physical attributes and abilities for breastfeeding and interactional behaviors. A small area where all circles overlap represents the interaction of the infant, mother, and environment and the potential influence each has on the other.

Although numerous infant feeding studies using these conceptualizations have been done, those specific to breastfeeding are few. Furr and Kiregis (1982) examined the quality of mother–infant interactions in an intervention study in which breastfeeding mothers received education on neonatal behaviors, and Hewat (1998) examined and compared mother–infant interactions during breastfeeding for dyads whose infants were perceived as problem breastfeeders and dyads whose infants were perceived to feed well.

Bonding and Attachment Theory

The concept of maternal attachment in healthcare literature is generally founded in Bonding theory proposed by Klaus and Kennell (1976). This theory attempts to explain maternal attachment to the infant as well as disruption in that attachment. Based on a study that compared women who had extended contact with their infant at birth and for the first 3 postpartum days with women whose contact with their infant was limited during this time, the findings showed the mothers with greater access responded differently to their infants, having more eye contact and positive interactions with their infant. Klaus and Kennell postulated that close parent–infant contact soon after birth was critical for optimal child development. In 1982 these claims were modified to include the premise that attachment can occur at a later period because of the adaptability of humans. In spite of critical reviews, this theory was the basis for recognizing the importance of parent–infant ties at delivery and in the early postpartum period (Klaus, Kennell, & Klaus, 1995). This has led to the following changes in hospital practices that support breastfeeding and mother–infant attachment: mother and newborn skin-to-skin contact immediately following birth, keeping mother and infant together throughout hospitalization, and the practice of kangaroo care in neonatal intensive care nurseries (Anderson et al., 2003; Kennell & McGrath, 2005).

Theory of Darwinian and Evolutionary Medicine

The tenets of Darwinian medicine are founded in the theory of natural selection postulated by Charles Darwin in his 1859 publication, *On the Origin of Species by Means of Natural Selection*. The process of natural selection occurs whenever genetically influenced variation among individuals affects their survival and reproduction. Darwinian medicine is the application of Darwin's theory of natural selection to the understanding of human diseases. Emerging in the early 1980s, this biomedical research approach aims at finding evolutionary explanations of vulnerabilities of disease such as infection, injuries and toxins, genetic factors, and abnormal environments (Williams & Nesse, 1991). Evolutionary medicine has the same underpinnings and beliefs, but allows for greater breadth in scope in application. For the breastfeeding dyad it is the basis for focus on the uniqueness of the infant and the mother–infant dyad as the true unit of study (McKenna & Gettler, 2007). This view suggests that "many contemporary social, psychological, and physical ills are related to incompatibilities between the lifestyles and environments in which humans currently live and the conditions under which human biology evolved" (Trevathan, Smith, & McKenna, 1999, p. 1).

Evolutionary theory was the basis for a study conducted by McKenna, Mosko, and Richard (1999) on the association of sudden infant death syndrome (SIDS) and breastfeeding and mother–infant cosleeping. Findings suggest that the interactive responses between mother and infant throughout the night support optimal breastfeeding activities and are a protective mechanism for decreasing the occurrence of SIDS although this latter finding remains controversial. McKenna et al. also concluded that the notion of infants sleeping alone meets the beliefs and values of Western culture rather than the biological needs of the infant.

Two other evolutionary explorations and interpretations of interest to the field of lactation are the questioning of whether neonatal jaundice is a disease or an adaptive process (Brett & Niermeyer, 1999) and infant crying behavior and colic (Barr, 1999). The conclusions of these explorations question conventional knowledge and treatments for both conditions.

Self-Care Theory

Self-care is the basis of Orem's self-care deficit theory of nursing (1983), which includes self-care requisites (a mother's abilities), self-care demand or measures of care required and acted on during times of transitions or to maintain well-being, and actions taken by a nurse (or health professional such as a lactation consultant) to assist in meeting self-care deficits. In the self-care approach to breastfeeding, the lactation consultant assists, encourages, and nurtures the mother and her family toward effective use of their own resources for achieving an optimal breastfeeding experience. Professional assistance is needed only when a problem prevents or hinders normal breastfeeding. This orientation is congruent with healthcare consumer participation. Self-care theory provides a framework that is especially appropriate for lactation practice where the clients are usually in a healthy state.

Self-Efficacy Theory

The basic proposition of self-efficacy theory, derived from social learning theory (Bandura, 1977, 1982), is described as an ongoing cognitive process in which individuals determine their confidence or their perceived ability for performing a specific behavior. The factors influencing this ability are their motivation, emotional state, and social environment. For measuring self-efficacy, a behavior-specific, task-related approach is suggested.

Dennis and Faux (1999; Dennis, 1999) used this theory for developing a breastfeeding self-efficacy scale (BSES) that reflects maternal confidence in breastfeeding. In keeping with the theory, researchers postulate that self-efficacy expectancies are based on the mother's previous breastfeeding experience, observations of successful breastfeeding, encouragement received from others, and her state of wellness. The initial 40-item scale has been shortened to 14 items (BSES-SF) (Dennis, 2003) and both are internally consistent and have construct validity. For mothers completing the scale before hospital discharge, the scores on the scale predicted breastfeeding patterns, which were defined as exclusive breastfeeding, breastfeeding and bottle-feeding, and exclusive bottle-feeding at 6 weeks postpartum and revealed that the scale scores for mothers who were exclusive breastfeeding were significantly different than mothers who were bottle-feeding. Findings in a study by Blyth et al. (2002) showed that mothers who scored high in the self-efficacy scale were significantly more likely to breastfeed and to breastfeed exclusively than mothers with low breastfeeding self-efficacy, exemplifying the use of this theory and scale for predicting which mothers may terminate breastfeeding early because of lack of confidence in their ability to breastfeed.

Theory of Planned Behavior and Theory of Reasoned Action

The origins of the theory of planned behavior (TPB) is an expansion of the theory of reasoned action (TRA) (Ajzen & Fishbein, 1980). TRA and TPB are a function of intention to perform a behavior, and the intention is the main factor in predicting behavior. The original theory constructs are attitudes and social norms, and control was added to the revised theory, TPB. Intention, as the antecedent to behavior, includes an individual's determination as to whether a behavior is worthwhile performing (attitude), the perception about what others think one should do with respect to a certain behavior (social norm), and assessment as to whether or not a behavior is considered easy to perform (control). Both theories have been used to predict breastfeeding behavioral intentions.

TRA was used in a study that examined nurses' support of breastfeeding mothers (Bernaix, 2000). Findings showed that the nurses' knowledge and attitudes were the best predictors of the support they provided to mothers, but that a relationship between intentions and behavior were not found, thereby not supporting the major premise of this theory.

TPB has been used as the theoretical underpinnings in several studies that have used different methods. In a study of infant feeding decision making among economically disadvantaged pregnant adolescents, Wambach and Koehn (2004) used TPB to develop questions for focus groups. The TPB theory is also the basis of the BAPT tool developed by Janke (1992, 1994), later revised by other researchers including Dick et al. (2002). Study results using the revised BAPT tool indicated that it effectively predicted 78 percent of mothers who had stopped breastfeeding at 8 weeks and 68 percent of those that continued to breastfeed, concluding that it is a useful tool for clinicians to use in determining women at risk for premature termination of breastfeeding.

Theories that provide a base for lactation research and practice have been described. Incorporating theory into practice demonstrates cognitive awareness as to the meaning of the *what* and the *why* of practices used, which is a contributing factor to legitimizing a profession.

Origins of Research Methodologies

Research can be conducted in many ways, and the basis of these diversities is often referred to as research paradigms (Polit & Beck, 2004). Paradigms are worldviews that represent belief systems based on philosophical foundations and assumptions (Crotty, 1998). The type of research conducted by an individual is often closely linked to their beliefs in that they frame research questions congruent with how they view the world. The associated assumptions guide investigators in the research methods used and establish the parameters for conducting the study and interpreting the findings. Perspectives used for developing knowledge in healthcare disciplines are the positivist and postpositivist perspective; the naturalistic, humanistic, or interpretive perspective; and the critical or emancipatory

perspective (Gillis & Jackson, 2002; Jacox et al., 1999). Extending the kinds of research perspectives contributes to developing a broader knowledge base for providing relevant health care.

Positivist and Postpositive Perspective

Positivism is the foundation of traditional science methods that are based on objectivity, precision, and a search for accurate, valid, and absolute truth. Often referred to as quantitative research, the ascribed methods are characterized by objectivity, measurement, and control that are context free and void of investigator bias. Investigators use these methods to examine specific variables, control intervening variables, and determine associations or cause and effect relationships among variables using statistical procedures. The goal is to explain, predict, and generalize. Scientists with this worldview claim that new knowledge is attained only through traditional methods. As philosophers and social scientists challenged these claims during the 1900s, the postpositivist perspective emerged. Based on the same worldview and scientific principles, this perspective is tempered in that certainties have changed to probabilities, and truth seeking is approximate rather than a totality. Greater flexibility in use of methods and adherence to philosophical assumptions is evident, although the debate continues between scientists who hold on to the conservative view and those who accept multimethods to understand a phenomenon under study. This perspective dominated health science inquiry throughout the 1900s.

Naturalistic, Humanistic, or Interpretive Perspective

The naturalistic, humanistic, or interpretive perspective constructs understanding of the meaning that human values, beliefs, practices, or life experiences and events have for individuals. Through interactions between the investigator and participants, new information or a new perspective of a phenomenon, and its meaning, is created. Generally conducted in naturalistic settings, all possible variables that influence individuals' perspectives are considered data, and these data are broad and frequently complex. Often referred to as qualitative research, this humanistic approach is congruent with a holistic philosophy of providing health care.

The outcomes of qualitative studies are mainly twofold, theory generation and/or rich descriptions that provide a deeper understanding of the meaning of experiences, events, or practices of individuals. Theory is generated primarily by the process of inductive reasoning, which means that specific ideas progress to more generalized statements. Thus, from the study of an everyday life phenomenon, variables and how they relate are identified. Further interpretation of the data can lead to a conceptualization of an experience from which theories are developed (Morse & Field, 1995). Or in some studies a rich, linguistic construction of the essence of a human experience showing meaning in a deeper manner can provide greater understanding of a phenomenon (van Manen, 1984).

Critical or Emancipatory Perspective

The critical or emancipatory perspective is based on both postpositivist and humanistic perspectives, as well as sociopolitical and cultural factors that influence experience (Jacox et al., 1999). It includes critical theory, action research, feminist research, and ethnocentric approaches of minority groups. The aim of emancipatory methods is to engender social change through or as a result of the research process for individuals or groups that are often unrecognized or considered oppressed. This perspective accentuates growth, change, and empowerment of individuals or groups as well as barriers that limit social change. Participant involvement and equity in every phase of the research process is critical. Research designs and methods may be combined and variable. The methods thought to have the greatest potential to generate the greatest amount of change for a particular group and situation are generally chosen.

It is important to understand and recognize these different perspectives as the underpinnings to research, but the perspectives themselves are not necessarily method specific. Recently, there is greater use of multimethods, particularly in large studies, to answer the research questions and study goals. In addition, increasing numbers of studies are undertaken by teams with representatives from different disciplines, academics to maintain the rigor of the research, and practitioners—and at times patients—to enhance clinical relevance. This trend of research teams conducting studies and the use of multimethods not only broadens the purpose and outcomes of studies but also contributes to greater research complexity.

Types of Research Methods

Research methods are based on philosophical foundations. Quantitative methods emanate from positivism and postpositivism paradigm and utilize the traditional scientific method. This is a process for controlling and systematically collecting, analyzing, and interpreting data about a topic of interest. Qualitative methods originate from the naturalistic paradigm or human science. The focus is on human experience that is holistic and occurs within a specific context. Collection of information, analysis, and interpretation is generally a concurrent process leading to emergence of new insights. These methods, as well as observational, historical, and feminist research that are suitable for breastfeeding research, are described.

Qualitative Methods

The origins of qualitative methods are inherent in philosophy and the social sciences. Phenomenology, ethnography, and grounded theory are three methods commonly used, but studies using other methods, such as discourse analysis, and narrative and interpretive descriptions, are increasing.

Phenomenology and grounded theory methods emanate from philosophy and sociology; ethnographic methods originate from anthropology; discourse analysis from sociolinguistics and cognitive psychology; and interpretive descriptions from nursing. Depending on the origin, there are variations of each method as well as specific practices and procedures for conducting the research.

Phenomenology

Phenomenology is a philosophy, research method, and humanistic scientific approach. The objective is to understand the meaning or nature of everyday life experiences or events from the perspective of those living the experiences. As the science developed, variations in phenomenological methods emerged.

An existential–phenomenological approach includes in-depth interviews with individuals who have lived the experience of interest, then reflection to grasp the essential meaning, followed by written articulation using the form and language specific to phenomenological writing. These rich descriptions attempt to show how these experiences are lived in the everyday world (Colaizzi, 1978; van Manen, 1990). Examples of studies using this approach are "Persistence in breastfeeding: A phenomenological investigation" (Bottorff, 1990), "The experience of living with an incessantly crying infant (Hewat, 1992), "Maternal-newborn nurses' experiences of inconsistent professional breastfeeding support" (Nelson, 2007), and "Breastfeeding in chronic illness: The voices of women with fibromyalgia" (Schaefer, 2004). The deeper understanding that practitioners gain from reading these studies should contribute to more humanistic care when working with individuals who are living these experiences.

A more structured process for conducting and analyzing phenomenological research is proposed by Giorgi (1985). A study using this structured method addresses women's perceptions of the breastfeeding experience (Hewat & Ellis, 1984). The findings describe similarities and differences of women who breastfeed for short and long durations and discuss a conceptualization of the mother–infant breastfeeding relationship. The complexity of the breastfeeding experience is explained and direction is provided for breastfeeding practitioners.

Ethnography

Ethnography is a method used to explain the beliefs, practices, and patterns of behavior from the perspective of the individuals of a culture or subculture within the context of their environment. A traditional ethnography describes the many facets of an entire culture or subculture, whereas a focused ethnography portrays one aspect of a culture (Morse, 1991a). The purpose is to understand, from the study participants, the cultural meanings and perceptions they use to organize and interpret their experiences (Spradley, 1979).

Dykes (2005) conducted a focused ethnography that describes 61 women's breastfeeding experiences in hospital postpartum units in Northern England but findings are applicable to western industrialized and medicalized countries. The identified themes of providing, supplying, demanding, and controlling are based on industrial model, mechanistic illustrations of breastfeeding initiation within the context of the factory-like environment of many hospitals. Findings support the need to shift emphasis from the nutritional aspects of breastmilk to the relational importance of breastfeeding as well as introducing strategies that assist women to regain confidence in their bodies and abilities to breastfeed.

Grounded Theory

Grounded theory is a research method for "generating explanatory theory that furthers the understanding of social and psychological phenomena" (Chenitz & Swanson, 1986). Using a rigorous and structured process, data based on individuals' realities are simultaneously collected and analyzed to develop theoretical constructs (Glaser, 1978; Strauss & Corbin, 1990). The emerging theory represents reality because it is "grounded" in the data. From this new understanding, relevant interventions for clinical practice can evolve.

Using grounded theory Leff, Jefferis, and Gagne (1994a) interviewed 26 mothers concerning successful and unsuccessful breastfeeding. The categories of successful breastfeeding were infant health, infant satisfaction, maternal enjoyment, desired maternal role attainment, and lifestyle compatibility. The overall theme or core concept was "working in harmony." The mothers described successful breastfeeding as a "complex interactive process resulting in mutual satisfaction of maternal and infant needs"(p. 99).

Nelson and Sethi (2005) also used this method to examine the breastfeeding experiences of Canadian teenage mothers. The core concept, "teenage mothers: continuously committing to breastfeeding" was supported by four categories described as deciding, learning, adjusting, and ending breastfeeding and the subcategories of vacillating between the good things and hard things about breastfeeding and social support and other social influences. The authors concluded that teenage mothers' breastfeeding experiences were similar to adult women's experiences but that teenage mothers need additional support.

Discourse Analysis

Discourse analysis examines language and how it is communicated in order to interpret and construct underlying meanings of participants' experiences, events, or practices (Potter & Wetherall, 1987). Accounts are critically analyzed in order to understand the social and cultural influences on the participants' perspectives and behaviors. Rich descriptions constructed to represent the meaning of the participants' dominant discourses lead to a deeper understanding of their experience.

This method was used by Schmied (1999) to examine the experiences of 25 women breastfeeding for 6 months following their infant's birth. The overall theme was that breastfeeding is an embodied experience, and for 35 percent of the study participants' experience was "connected, harmonious, and intimate embodiment" (p. 328). Mixed feelings were revealed by 40 percent of the women, and the remaining 25 percent found breastfeeding as "disrupted, distorted, and a disconnected experience" (p. 329). It was concluded that recognition of the variance of women's personal experiences is important for practitioners working with breastfeeding women.

Quantitative Methods

The major types of quantitative research are nonexperimental and experimental studies. Nonexperimental studies include descriptive and correlational studies that describe or compare conditions or relationships. Experimental and quasi-experimental studies focus on causal relationships and test interventions to determine if an intervention causes a change in a specific outcome. The type of inquiry chosen depends on the current state of knowledge of the study topic and the purpose of the research.

Descriptive Studies

Descriptive studies are appropriate when there is little knowledge about a topic of interest and specific information is desired. For example, the research questions may address characteristics, influencing factors, or knowledge deficits related to a topic. Findings describe the studied phenomenon and may identify relationships among variables.

A study by Zimmerman and Guttman (2001) examined beliefs about breastfeeding and formula-feeding among 94 breastfeeding and 60 formula-feeding women. Major findings revealed that women in both groups rated breastfeeding higher than formula-feeding for health benefits,

enhancement of the infant's development, and creation of a special bond between mother and infant, but breastfeeding was also viewed as restricting a mother's activity. Those who chose formula-feeding did so for lifestyle reasons in spite of their belief that breastfeeding is beneficial to an infant's health. The authors conclude that lifestyle issues should be part of breastfeeding promotion. The findings of some descriptive studies may identify relationships between variables that form the basis for further study.

Correlational or Association Studies

Correlational studies examine relationships between two or more variables and the type (negative or positive) and strength of the relationship(s). These studies require greater type of control than descriptive studies. The data collected is structured in order to allow for numerical representation for correlational analysis to determine if the relationships between variables are statistically significant.

A study by Oddy et al. (2003) that illustrates this method was conducted prospectively to examine the association between the duration of full breastfeeding and cognitive abilities measured by verbal IQ at 6 years of age and performance abilities at 8 years of age. Full breastfeeding was defined as breastfeeding "up to the introduction of milk other than breast milk and did not preclude the intake of solid foods" (p. 82). Data were categorized as never breastfed, full breastfeeding for less than 4 months, full breastfeeding from 4 to 6 months, and full breastfeeding for more than 6 months. Of the 2024 participants, longer periods of full breastfeeding were significantly associated with higher verbal IQ for children tested at 6 years and intellectual performance of children tested at 8 years. An interactive effect of longer breastfeeding and higher maternal education was a finding for the verbal IQ score but not for the performance score. These study findings add to the growing evidence that breastfeeding is positively associated with children's intelligence in the early school years.

Experimental Studies

Experimental studies examine hypothesized relationships between variables to determine cause (often an intervention or treatment) and effect (the outcome). Rigorous control of variables is integral to conducting these studies. Several criteria are essential for a true experimental study:

- *Manipulation* of an experimental intervention or treatment (the independent variable) by the investigator
- *Control* of the experimental situation to eliminate interference or confounding effect of extraneous variables (additional influencing factors) on the outcome (dependent variable)
- *Randomization* so that subjects are systematically allocated with all having an equal chance of participating in the experimental or control study groups (Burns & Grove, 1997)

Noel-Weiss et al. (2006) conducted an experimental study that was a randomized control trial to determine the effects of a prenatal breastfeeding workshop on maternal breastfeeding self-efficacy and breastfeeding duration. The 110 participants were randomly assigned to a control or an intervention group and 92 completed the study. The intervention group attended a 2.5-hour prenatal breastfeeding workshop. A short form of the Breastfeeding Self-Efficacy Scale (BSES) (Dennis, 2003) was used to measure maternal self-efficacy prenatally and at 4 and 8 months postpartum and type of infant feeding defined by eight categories (see section of this chapter on operational definitions) were assessed and compared at the same postpartum periods. Findings revealed that for mothers who attended the workshop self-efficacy scores were significantly higher at 4 weeks postpartum and a higher proportion were exclusively breastfeeding at 8 weeks postpartum. The results of this study support home visits by peer counselors to increase exclusive breastfeeding rates for longer durations. Additional studies that are similar and have comparable outcomes, however, are needed. Research is an ongoing process and many experimental studies about a topic are often necessary before conclusions are accepted as definitive.

The involvement of human subjects does not always permit the rigor necessary for a true experiment. In many situations it is not always practical, efficient, ethical, or feasible to randomly select subjects or to expose them to a specific treatment or experience. When an experimental method is used to study an intervention but only one of the two additional criteria for conducting a true experiment can be met, the research design is quasi-experimental. A study by Martens (2000) to determine the effectiveness of a 1-hour breastfeeding education intervention provided to nursing staff in a small rural hospital illustrates this method. Another hospital in a community of similar size was selected as a control because of similarities to the intervention site but randomization of sites was unfeasible. Hypothesized outcomes for the intervention site were to *increase* exclusive breastfeeding rates for infants at hospital discharge, positive beliefs and attitudes among nursing staff, and compliance with the 10 steps of the Baby-Friendly Hospital Initiative. In a 7-month period, the intervention hospital showed significant increases over the control site in all outcome measures except breastfeeding attitudes, demonstrating that a short and relatively inexpensive education session for nurses contributed to improved breastfeeding care and outcomes for mothers and infants.

Additional Methods and Approaches for Breastfeeding Research

Other research approaches suitable for breastfeeding studies that do not fit precisely into the qualitative or quantitative classification are observational, historical, participatory action, and feminist research. Either quantitative or qualitative methods or a combination of them may be used to conduct these studies.

Observational Research

Observational research is important for studying human behavior or events that cannot be captured through interviews or self-report questionnaires. Originating in the discipline of biology and anthropology, ethology is an observational method that explores and examines animal behaviors within natural settings. Behavioristic psychology also contributed structured methods for conducting observational research. Study outcomes can include frequencies of behavioral occurrences, timing of specific behaviors, and/or sequences of behaviors. Types and timing of behaviors during experiences, practices, and events can add a new perspective and greater understanding of a phenomenon.

Ethology was used in an observational study conducted by Hewat (1998). Videotapes examined and compared mother–infant interactions during breastfeeding between two sets of dyads: those whose infants were perceived by their mothers as problematic breastfeeders and those whose mothers perceived their infants as nonproblematic breastfeeders. From the initial assessment of the interactions, ethograms—detailed descriptions of behaviors and patterns—were created, hypotheses were generated, and a guide was developed for coding behaviors to further examine and compare the mother–infant interactions of the two groups. Differences in tempo and rhythm of the mother–infant interaction patterns were delineated as harmonic attunement, disharmonic attunement, and disattunement. The proportions of interactions that were disharmonically attuned and disattuned were significantly higher among the dyads whose infants were problematic breastfeeders. These findings provide insights for observing mother–infant interactions during breastfeeding and assisting mothers whose breastfeeding sessions are often active and disruptive rather than calm and restful.

Historical Research

Historical research methods are valuable for exploring past practices, examining patterns and trends during specific periods, discovering relationships, and drawing inferences. Past revelations can increase understanding of traditions and practices and guide decision making. Historical inquiry entails identifying, collecting, categorizing, and determining validity of evidence, critical analysis, synthesis, and writing to present meaningful discussion of the subject (Shafer, 1980).

Millard's work (1990) illustrates the value of historical research. Pediatric literature between 1897 and 1987 showed that although breastfeeding was advocated, advice centered on regimes and schedules. Even as flexibility in feeding times became more acceptable, advice including time limitations continued. Study findings suggest that emphasis on time in regard to breastfeeding and the allocation of control in breastfeeding to medical experts undermined breastfeeding during this 90-year period.

Participatory Action

Participatory action is a type of research method for conducting studies aimed at social action and change. It is based on a partnership between individuals and groups most closely affected by and involved with the phenomenon under study. All participants contribute and work together through all stages of the research process. Recognition, increased knowledge, and empowerment for those most affected by an unacceptable or substandard situation contribute to eventual change. This method is often used for community development to establish programs with those who desire and will attend a service. An example is an intervention study conducted in rural northeast Scotland where breastfeeding rates were low (Hoddinott, Lee, & Pill, 2006). In four geographical areas group-based or one-to-one peer coaching breastfeeding interventions were provided that were specific to the needs of participants living in each area. Breastfeeding initiation and duration increased among participants. At 2 weeks postpartum breastfeeding increased from 34.3 to 41.1 percent and remained higher at all time points examined (1, 2, and 6 weeks, and 4 and 8 months postpartum). Establishing working relationships and "equal" partnerships with participants and community representatives is complex and challenging but often worthwhile in establishing meaningful programs in a community setting.

Feminist Research

Feminist research is an approach that is congruent with but not overtly evident in current breastfeeding research. Whether there is a "feminist method" or whether any research method can be conducted from a feminist perspective is an unresolved issue (Kelly, Burton, & Regan, 1994). Feminist research is guided by the following principles: it is about women, for women, and done with, not to, women; it should be empowering for participants; it is directed toward positive social change; and it generally uses qualitative methods. A feminist perspective encourages the researcher to focus on women in a societal and political context and to consider cultural influences and attitudes within society as central to the experience of the women involved (Harding, 1987). Feminist researchers recognize the negotiated social act between the researcher and the participants. The researcher defines the study and interprets the findings and the participants decide what information they will share with the researcher (Maynard & Purvis, 1994).

Multimethod studies that use both qualitative and quantitative approaches simultaneously are an emerging trend. Those who support this approach argue that using several methods can enhance theoretical insights, facilitate incremental growth of knowledge, augment validity of studies, and force investigators to reflect and find new views when, for example, findings from one method are incongruent with another method used. Challenges include the ability of the investigator(s) to reconcile differences in philosophical underpinnings of differing approaches; expense; investigator knowledge about and skills for working with two approaches; analytic challenges; and acceptance of manuscripts by journals that publish studies (Polit & Beck, 2004). Studies using multimethods are complex and should be conducted by an experienced researcher.

Elements of Research

The elements of research are essential to writing proposals and reports, conducting research, and evaluating studies. The major elements include the research problem and purpose, the review of literature, the protection of human subjects, the method, the analysis, and the results and discussion. Although the elements are similar for both qualitative and quantitative research approaches, the content and processes vary. The following section describes the elements and discusses the differences between qualitative and quantitative methods.

Research Problem and Purpose

The research problem is a critical component of a study. It identifies *what* is studied and with *whom*. The purpose delineates *why* the study is conducted. There are many sources for generating research problems. Questioning clinical practice, observing clinical and societal patterns and trends, building on findings from previous studies, and examining theoretical propositions are ways of developing research questions.

A problem that is suitable for study should be important to the topic of breastfeeding and amenable to investigation by scientific inquiry. It should be meaningful to many individuals or have a distinct influence on a few. A study examining the effect of labor pain relief medication on neonatal suckling and breastfeeding duration conducted by Riordan et al. (2001b) illustrates the importance to all childbearing women and their infants. In

contrast, a study about the effect of sequential and simultaneous breast pumping on milk volume and prolactin levels among women who express milk for a prolonged period of time (Hill, Aldag, & Chatterton, 1996) has important implications for a few. Criteria that render a problem appropriate for scientific inquiry include the following:

- *Suitability* of the research design for the research question
- *Accessibility* of study participants
- *Feasibility* of the study with regard to time, funding, and equipment
- *Potentiality* of adhering to ethical requirements throughout all study phases

Reviewing the literature about a study topic provides direction for asking a relevant question and selecting an appropriate method. A qualitative method is indicated when literature is limited about a phenomenon or when more in-depth knowledge is desired. When many studies about a topic have been undertaken, however, the findings often provide a base and focus for further study, and a quantitative method may be most appropriate.

Research problems can be written as questions or declarative statements. Clearly identifying the topic, population, and variables for study is essential for quantitative methods. In qualitative studies, less is known about the topic of interest; therefore, the research question is broader. The purpose is to describe and interpret meanings of a phenomenon, to gain an in-depth understanding of an experience or situation, or to discover variables relevant to a topic rather than to examine variables previously identified. Examples of research questions that can be applied to specific methods are shown in Table 22–1. All questions pertain to breastfeeding following a caesarean birth. For quantitative methods, variables specific to breastfeeding duration and a scheduled lactation consultant visit have been specified.

Variables, Hypotheses, and Operational Definitions

Variables

Variables are defined as "qualities, properties, or characteristics of persons, things, or situations that change or vary and are manipulated or measured in

examine social meanings and cultural biases or norms that guide the actions of individuals within the identified culture (Morse & Field, 1995).

Grounded theory research follows an exceptionally systematic analytic process. Data from transcribed interviews are coded and categorized, and connections between categories are made; a tentative conceptualization or theory is formulated, and the examination continues until a core variable emerges that is the focus of the theory. Concept modification and integration continue through two processes called *memoing* and *theoretical coding*. The process of analysis is not linear. Throughout the data analysis, codes, categories, conceptualizations, and theory are constantly compared, and the researcher moves between inductive and deductive reasoning. Conceptualizations of relationships are deductively proposed, and these are inductively examined for verification. The analytic process is ongoing until a theory, substantiated by the data, is generated (Glaser, 1978; Strauss & Corbin, 1990).

Trustworthiness of Qualitative Research

Ensuring that study findings are trustworthy and reflect the truth is an essential component of qualitative research. This requires ongoing examination by the investigator throughout the research process. Sources of error can occur in sampling, data collection, and analysis. Factors to evaluate throughout the process include the integrity of key informants in providing accurate data, the interviewer's skill in obtaining the participants' true perspectives, the accuracy of field observations, the generation of codes or units of analysis that represent data accurately within a social context, and the interpretations of the data to determine whether they represent true meanings.

Criteria for assessing trustworthiness are outlined by Lincoln and Guba (1985) as credibility, dependability, confirmability, and transferability. *Credibility* is achieved by implementing and demonstrating that the processes in conducting the research are plausible. There are several practices that demonstrate study credibility: engaging in data collection and analyses for a sufficient length of time to ensure the aspects of participants' experiences are understood; using multiple data sources; engaging others to read and interpret transcripts; involving participants to review data, interpretations, and emerging theories for correctness; and illustrating the experience of the research conducting the study. *Dependability* reflects the reality, that is, the representations reflect the participants' views and situations. It is shown through an inquiry audit, which entails having another researcher review the data, process, and rigor undertaken during analysis. *Confirmability* is achieved by developing an audit trail of the data and recording interpretations and their meanings for review by another person. *Transferability* is the extent that findings can be transferred to another group or setting. Rich descriptions of the participants, settings, and experiences allow others to judge if study findings can be transferred to similar settings or populations (Polit & Beck, 2004).

Application of Methods to Quantitative Approaches

Sampling and Sample Size

Probability sampling methods, particularly for correlational and experimental studies, are preferred, so that the study findings can be generalized to a larger population. However, as previously discussed, many studies involving human subjects must employ non-probability sampling methods.

Deciding on the sample size is a critical issue in quantitative studies. Factors to consider include the study purpose, level of inquiry, design, and type of analysis, as well as the availability of subjects, research funds, and the time frame of the study. For descriptive studies that identify and describe characteristics of a population, sample size will generally not affect study outcomes to the same degree as it will for other quantitative methods. Recommendations are to recruit as large a sample as possible after considering the previously described factors.

Sample size is critical in experimental and quasi-experimental studies that statistically test hypotheses. If the sample size is too small, group differences may not be detected when they actually exist, and a null hypothesis (no difference between groups) is not rejected. The result is that an intervention or treatment that is effective is not recognized as making a difference.

For these kinds of studies, a sample size that is adequate to show true differences between groups can be estimated using a *power analysis* (Cohen, 1988; Kramer & Thiemann, 1987). Computer software programs are available for statistically computing an adequate sample size, and investigators generally recruit additional participants to account for those who do not complete a study (i.e., subject attrition). When a research proposal is being developed, researchers frequently consult with a statistician for advice about sample size, study design, and analyses procedures.

In experimental or quasi-experimental studies, *random assignment* of subjects to experimental and control groups is advised but should not be confused with random selection (previously discussed), which allows findings to be generalized to the population from which the sample was selected. This type of study is called a *randomized control trial* (RCT), and random assignment has two purposes: all subjects have an equal and independent chance of receiving the treatment, and it increases the probability that each group is similar in regard to background characteristics. The latter serves as a control of extraneous variables that may influence the effect of treatment. Many of these studies also use a procedure called *intention to treat* (ITT) in data analysis, which means that all participants are included in the analysis of the data even if they did not complete the study. Depending on the number of participants lost, study results may be compromised.

Correlational studies and those using survey questionnaires generally require large samples. The size is reflected in the number of variables to be examined and/or subgroups to be compared. As each of these factors increase, so must the sample size. If numbers are insufficient, statistical analyses and study findings can be compromised.

Two types of epidemiological studies examine associations between variables such as exposure (risk factors) and a disease or health condition: (1) case-control and (2) cohort studies. In case-control studies, subjects with a specific condition are compared, generally retrospectively, with a control group that does not have the condition. Differences between the two groups in the subjects' past experiences or life events are examined to identify factors that may lead to the onset of the condition. Cohort studies are similar except that they are generally follow-up studies of subjects who are exposed or not exposed to a risk factor that is assumed to be associated with the onset of an identified health problem. During the past decade, there has been increasing interest in the relationship of breastfeeding exclusivity and duration and diseases such as infant and childhood leukemia, diabetes, lower respiratory tract infections, and gastroenteritis, as well as the effect of breastfeeding on maternal risks of type 2 diabetes and breast and ovarian cancers (Ip et al., 2007). Case-control studies are a method for providing this information.

Data Collection

All methods of data collection previously described are applicable to quantitative studies if they are applied consistently and objectively. Descriptive studies gather data that are broader in scope or more subjective than correlational or experimental studies. However, questionnaires, interview schedules, and observation criteria must be structured so that the same data are collected in the same manner from all subjects. Measurement studies, such as correlational, quasi-experimental, and experimental studies, require data that can be reduced to numbers in order to apply statistical procedures. Reliable and valid questionnaires and observation checklists used for measuring variable relationships often take years to develop. Once established, they may be used in numerous studies.

Reliability and validity estimates of existing breastfeeding questionnaires and tools are limited. Table 22–2 presents an overview of these tools and what is known about their reliability and validity. Some of the tools can be found in Chapter 20. For correlational and experimental studies, it is recommended that the questionnaires or measures used for data collection are reliable and valid.

Reliability and Validity

Reliability and validity are central issues concerned with measurement error in research. Occurrence of error at any stage of the research process can affect study outcomes and limits the usefulness of the study findings. Reliability refers to the accuracy, consistency, precision, and stability of measurement or data collection. Validity reflects truth, accuracy,

TABLE 22-2	Breastfeeding Questionnaires and Assessment Tools

Title	Purpose	Reliability	Validity
Breastfeeding Attrition Prediction Tool (BAPT) (Janke 1992, 1994; Riordan & Koehn, 1997). Modified BAPT Tool (Dick et al., 2002)	To identify women at risk for early, unintended weaning. Four factors measure negative and positive breastfeeding attitude, perceived maternal control, and social and professional support.	Cronbach alphas for all scales: .79–.85 (Janke, 1992, 1994); .90–1.93 (Riordan & Koehn, 1997); .81–.86 (Dick et al., 2002).	Predictive validity: Three of four scales related to 8-week feeding outcome and negative sentiment scale predicted early unintended weaning (Janke, 1992, 1994). Modified BAPT: Two scales predicted 78% women who discontinued breastfeeding at 8-weeks and 68% of those still breastfeeding (Dick et al., 2002).
Maternal Breastfeeding Evaluation Scale (MBFES) (Leff, Jefferis, & Gagne, 1994b; Riordan, Woodley, & Heaton, 1994).	To measure a mother's overall evaluation of the breastfeeding experience using a 30-item Likert scale. Subscales include: maternal enjoyment; role attainment, infant satisfaction/growth, and lifestyle/maternal body image.	Test-retest correlations: .82–.93 Cronbach alphas for subscales: .80–.93 (Leff et al., 1994b) and .73–.83 (Riordan et al., 1994).	Items developed from qualitative study (Leff et al., 1994a). Predictive validity: Significant positive correlation of total scale and subscales with maternal satisfaction and breastfeeding intent and duration (Leff et al., 1994b; Riordan et al., 1994).
Breastfeeding Self-Efficacy Scale (32 items) (BSES) (Dennis & Faux, 1999) Modified Short form (14 items) (BSES-SF) (Dennis, 2003)	To determine breastfeeding self-efficacy and to identify breastfeeding mothers at high risk, and assess breastfeeding behaviors and cognitions to individualize confidence-building strategies (Dennis, 2003).	Both forms, Cronbach alpha: .96	Content validity. Predictive validity: significant differences between breastfeeding and bottle-feeding at 4 and 8 weeks postpartum. Construct validity; contrasts and correlations with similar construct measures.
LATCH Breastfeeding Assessment Tool (Jensen, Wallace, & Kelsay, 1994)	To assess effective breastfeeding in first week for latch-on, audible swallowing, nipple type, comfort of breast/nipple, and help needed to position baby.	Interrater reliability: Mothers' and nurses' total scores positively correlated (Riordan et al., 2001a).	Requires further testing, but mothers' total scores positively correlated with breastfeeding at 8 weeks postpartum (Riordan et al., 2001a; Kumar et al., 2006).

(Continues)

TABLE 22–2	**Breastfeeding Questionnaires and Assessment Tools (Continued)**		
Title	**Purpose**	**Reliability**	**Validity**
Infant Breastfeeding Assessment Tool (IBFAT) (Matthews, 1988)	To assess and measure infant breastfeeding competence. Four subscales: readiness to feed, rooting, fixing, and sucking.	Interrater reliability: 1% agreement in coassessed feeds (Matthews, 1988). Pairwise correlations of raters .58 (Riordan & Koehn, 1997).	Content validity and observation in clinical practice (Matthews, 1988).

and reality. To be valid, measures and methods of data collection must also be reliable.

Reliability

Accuracy and consistency in the way data are collected, as well as the tools or instruments used, are essential in quantitative studies. Several types of reliability should be addressed.

Interrater reliability refers to accuracy and consistency in data collection when more than one individual or instrument (such as a thermometer) is used for data collection. In such instances the probability of error between the individuals or instruments increases. To control this aspect, checks are made. Similar instruments should be calibrated until measurement is consistent. For individuals making similar observations, the degree of their accuracy can be statistically determined. Acceptable levels of reliability are dependent on the statistical method used—for example, for interobserver reliability an agreement of 90 percent is adequate. When using a Cohen's kappa statistic, a procedure that corrects for level of chance agreement, an acceptable level is .70 (Bakeman & Gottman, 1986). For the Infant Breastfeeding Assessment Tool (IBFAT) described in Table 22–2, interrater reliability was determined by Matthews (1988, 1991) by comparing agreement of the mother's and the investigator's breastfeeding assessments. Overall, agreement was 91 percent accurate, although it was noted that infants who fed well or poorly were easier to assess than those who rated in the middle range and were classified as moderate feeders. Johnson, Mulder, and Strube (2007) report percent agreement among three health

professionals as the following: over 90 percent for responsiveness to feeding cues, timing of feeding, and nutritive sucking bursts; 80 to 88 percent range for position and latch factors; and 79 percent agreement for maternal nipple trauma.

Intrarater reliability refers to accuracy and consistency of observations from one rater over time. For example, when data are collected for more than 6 months, investigators may want to check the accuracy of the individual who is making the observations—and/or the instrument(s) used—every few months. Likewise, repeated observations over short periods of time by the same rater warrant assessment of intrarater reliability. Calculations and acceptability are similar to interrater reliability.

Test-retest reliability indicates the stability of a measure, such as a questionnaire, over time. Results of two questionnaire administrations to the same subjects, occurring approximately 2 to 3 weeks apart, are statistically compared. A coefficient reported as .80 or above is generally acceptable for measurement questionnaires that reflect attitudes or feelings. For some events, however, such as postpartum adjustment, a low correlation coefficient (such as .40 or .50) may be desired since differences in individual scores over a period of time reflect inconsistency and are then a possible indication that the individual is changing or adjusting to a different lifestyle. In such a case, test-retest reliability would not be an appropriate measure of reliability. The Maternal Breastfeeding Evaluation Scale (MBFES) presented in Table 22–2 shows that this tool is highly reliable over time.

Internal consistency refers to the statistical agreement of several items on a questionnaire that reflect the meaning of a concept—for example, satisfaction with breastfeeding. Similarity in meaning or internal consistency of the items can be statistically determined. Cronbach's alpha, based on the average correlation among items and the number of items, is a reliability coefficient frequently computed to determine internal consistency. A coefficient of .70 to .80 is generally acceptable for a questionnaire measuring a construct (Nunnally, 1978). Therefore, the Breastfeeding Attrition Prediction Tool (BAPT), the MBFES, and the Breastfeeding Self-Efficacy Scale (BSES) described in Table 22–2 are all internally consistent questionnaires for data collection.

Validity

Validity addresses the extent to which a questionnaire or measurement instrument reflects the meaning of the concept that is being measured or does what it is intended to do (Waltz, Strickland, & Lenz, 2005). Types of validity referred to in quantitative studies are content, criterion, and construct validity. Questionnaires and interview schedules used for descriptive studies should have *content validity,* which means that the questions or items adequately represent the study concepts. In developing questionnaires, investigators review the literature to include dimensions of the concept being studied and then submit the questionnaire to individuals who are considered experts on the research topic for review. This validation of content with literature and experts is known as content validity. Formalized procedures for assessing content validity and calculation of a content validity index (CVI) of measures has come to be an expected and very important part of the overall instrument development process (Polit & Beck, 2006).

Criterion-related validity is of importance when one wants to infer from a measure an individual's probable standing on some other outside measure, generally a higher order operationalization of the construct. *Predictive validity,* a form of criterion-related validity, ascertains whether a measure at one time can predict future outcomes. *Concurrent validity*, another form of criterion-related validity, determines whether a measure may be used to estimate present standing on the criterion. *Construct validity* assesses the degree to which a tool measures what it is intended to measure and is done so in the context of the theoretical basis of the measure. In

Table 22–2 the BAPT, MBFES, and BFES-SF all show evidence of predictive validity for breastfeeding outcomes, as well as construct validity based on the support of theoretical relationships undergirding the concepts. The use of questionnaires and tools with these types of validity enhances the credibility of study findings.

Data Analysis

Data analysis is the process of organizing, summarizing, examining, and synthesizing the data collected in order to reach conclusions about the research question. Numerical analysis of data is central to quantitative studies. The data collected is converted to numerical values in a variety of ways. Table 22–3 defines levels of measurement and provides examples. The level of measurement has implications for the statistical procedures applied.

Statistical procedures used for correlational, experimental, or quasi-experimental studies can be classified as parametric or nonparametric. Parametric tests are more powerful and preferred because they permit inferences to be made from findings of the study sample to the larger population. The use of parametric procedures requires three assumptions be met: (1) random selection of the sample; (2) variables are normally distributed among the study groups; and (3) measurement of the dependent variable(s) at an interval level. Nonparametric statistics are more suitably used in situations when the following characteristics are evident: (1) the sample size is small; (2) normal distribution of variables in the sample cannot be assumed; (3) parameters of the population are unknown; and (4) the level of measurement of variables is at a nominal or ordinal level.

The selection of an appropriate statistical procedure is dependent on the type of study, sample size, sampling procedure, and level or type of data to be analyzed. Table 22–4 indicates commonly used procedures for study type and level of data. In experimental or quasi-experimental studies, the level of data of the dependent variable dictates the type of statistical testing that can be done. The purpose of this table is to assist research novices to recognize the appropriate use of statistics for reviewing studies. Extensive information about statistical procedures is beyond the scope of this chapter.

TABLE 22–3	**Levels of Measurement**		
	Nominal	**Ordinal**	**Interval/Ratio**
Definitions	Discreet categories of data that do not have any implied order.	Assigned categories of data that can be ranked in order; intervals between categories are not equal.	Categories of data that are ordered and are equal distances apart. Ratio also has a known zero point.
Examples	Gender: male/female Breastfed/not breastfed Marital status	Most Likert-type scales BAPT, MBFES, BSES, and IBFAT scales (see Table 22–2)	Body temperature Blood pressure Weight or length Duration of breastfeeding measured in specified days, weeks, months, or years.

The choice of interval versus ordinal data is controversial. Human feelings and perceptions do not fit the interval scale, and most psychosocial variables can only be superimposed on an ordinal scale. Therefore, statistical procedures that traditionally require interval data are sometimes used with ordinal data based on human responses.

Descriptive Studies

Data collected to describe variables and their relationships are generally subjected to content analysis and descriptive statistics. Content analysis consists of examining the data, identifying similar content or meanings, and classifying those that are identified into mutually exclusive categories. These nominal data can then be used with the descriptive statistics identified in Table 22–4. Findings may be reported as frequencies, percentages, or modes; they may be displayed as bar graphs, pie charts, or contingency tables.

Correlational Studies

Correlation coefficients are the outcomes of statistical procedures for determining the relationship between two variables. The type of relationship is reported as positive (as one variable increases so does the other), negative (variables both decrease), or inverse (as one variable increases the other decreases). The strength of the relationship is reported as a number between +1 and −1; stronger relationships are near 1 (positive) or 1 (negative), and 0 indicates no relationship.

Associations in epidemiological studies are estimated using relative risk (or risk ratio) (RR) and odds ratio (OR). Studies in which a subpopulation is followed and examined in regard to specific health factors can determine the probability or rate of incidence of developing a specific condition for a group exposed to an identified factor. An example is the rate of incidence of infants developing otitis media among those exclusively breastfed compared to those who are fed breastmilk substitutes. The incidence rate for one group (breastfed infants) is divided by the incidence rate for the other group (infants fed breastmilk substitutes) to determine the relative risk (Polit & Beck, 2004). For some studies, such as case-control studies, incidence rate is not possible to determine, but an odds ratio (OR) can be estimated by calculating the ratio of the odds of exposure among the cases (e.g., the exclusively breastfed infants) to that among the control group (e.g., infants fed breastmilk substitutes) (Hennekens, Buring, & Mayrent, 1987).

A relative risk or odds ratio of 1.0 suggests that the incidence rate of disease is the same for both the exposed and nonexposed groups. However, a value above 1—for example, 1.5—indicates an increased risk of 1.5 times or 50 percent higher among those exposed to the factor. Ratios less than 1 indicate decreased risk among those exposed. Odds ratios are often reported with confidence intervals, which "represent the range within which the true magnitude of effect lies with a certain degree of assurance" (Hennekens et al., 1987).

TABLE 22–4	**Statistical Tests Appropriate for Level of Measurement: A Basic Guide**

Numerical Descriptors for Univariate Analysis (One Variable)

Descriptors or Measures of Central Tendency

Numerical Descriptor	Function	Level of Measurement
Mode	Indicates most common value/score	Nominal
Median	Indicates value that is the middle position of a distribution of values	Ordinal
Mean	Indicates the average score	Interval or ratio

Descriptors or Measures of Variability

Range	Shows values/scores in a distribution; highest to lowest	
Standard Deviation	Indicates average deviation values from the mean	Interval or ratio

Descriptors for Bivariate Studies or Two Variables

Contingency table	Shows cross-tabulation of frequency distributions of two variables	Nominal or ordinal (two variables)

Commonly Used Statistical Tests for Bivariate Analysis (Two Variables)

Nonparametric Tests

Test & Test Statistic	Test Function	Measurement Level of IV	Measurement Level of DV
Chi square (χ^2)	Differences in proportions (frequency data) between two or more independent groups	Nominal or ordinal*	Nominal
Fisher exact test	Differences in proportions between two or more independent groups—used when samples sizes are small or < 5 per cell	Nominal	Nominal
Median test (χ^2)	Differences between medians of two independent groups	Nominal	Ordinal
Mann-Whitney U (U)	Differences in ranks of scores/values of two independent groups	Nominal	Ordinal
McNemar's test (χ^2)	Differences in proportions within paired samples	Nominal	Nominal
Wilcoxon paired signed-rank test	Differences in ranks of scores within two dependent groups	Nominal	Ordinal

(Continues)

TABLE 22–4	Statistical Tests Appropriate for Level of Measurement: A Basic Guide (Continued)		
Kruskal Wallis	Differences in ranks of scores of three or more independent groups	Nominal	Ordinal
Spearman's rho (ρ)	Determines correlation between two variables	Ordinal	Ordinal
Kendall's tau (τ)	Determines correlation between two variables	Ordinal	Ordinal

Parametric Tests

Pearson's product moment correlation (r)	Determines correlation between two variables	Interval or ratio	Interval or ratio
t-test (t)	Differences between two independent group means	Nominal	Interval or ratio
t-test, pooled (t)	Differences between two related group means	Nominal	Interval or ratio
Analysis of variance (ANOVA) (F)	Differences between three or more independent groups	Nominal	Interval or ratio
Repeated measures ANOVA (F)	Differences between three or more related groups or scores	Nominal	Interval or ratio

Commonly Used Statistical Tests for Multivariate Analysis

Test	Test Function	Measurement Level and Number of IDs	Measurement Level and Number of DVs
Analysis of covariance (ANCOVA)	Differences between means of two or more groups and controls for one or more covariates	Nominal, one or more variables	Interval or ratio, one variable
Multivariate analysis of variance (MANOVA)	Differences between means of two or more groups for two or more dependent variables	Nominal, one or more variables	Interval or ratio, two or more variables
Multivariate analysis of covariance (MANCOVA)	Differences between means of two or more groups for two or more DVs. Controls for one or more covariates	Nominal, one or more variables	Interval or ratio, two or more variables
Multiple regression	Determine relationship between two or more IVs and one DV	Nominal, interval, or ratio, two or more variables	Interval or ratio, one variable
Canonical correlation	Determine relationship between two sets of variables	Nominal, interval, or ratio, two or more variables	Nominal, interval, or ratio, two or more variables
Logistic regression	Determine relationship between two or more IVs and one DV	Nominal, interval, or ratio, two or more variables	Nominal, one variable

(Continues)

TABLE 22–4	**Statistical Tests Appropriate for Level of Measurement: A Basic Guide (Continued)**		
Test	**Test Function**	**Measurement Level and Number of IDs**	**Measurement Level and Number of DVs**
Discriminant function analysis	Determine relationships between two or more IVs and one DV and identify group membership	Nominal, interval, or ratio, two or more variables	Nominal, one variable
Factor analysis	Examines interrelationships among numerous variables to identify clusters of variables that are similar		

Experimental and Quasi-Experimental Studies

The statistical procedure used to determine differences between groups depends on the number of groups and the level of measurement of the dependent variable, as shown in Table 22–4. Statistical differences are calculated using probability theory. Before analysis, the investigator decides on a level of significance—or a *P* value—that will be used to accept that a statistically significant result indicates true differences between groups. The *P* value reflects the probability that the statistical result can occur by chance, and it establishes the risk of the investigator making a type I error. This means that a null hypothesis is rejected when in reality the hypothesis is true, leading to an incorrect interpretation that an intervention was successful. Conversely, a type II error is the acceptance of a null hypothesis when in fact it is false, and in this situation an intervention that is successful is not recognized as such. In research, *P* values of .01 or .05 are most commonly used. A 0.01 *P* value means that 1 chance out of 100 a type I error could occur; a .05 *P* value means that 5 chances out of 100 a type I error could be made. Reducing the chance of a type I error, however, increases the probability of a type II error. For this reason, most investigators conducting breastfeeding research elect to use a *P* value of .05.

As well as a *P* value, differences between groups, such as the outcomes of two groups exposed to different care interventions, are based on a critical value of the statistical procedure used. Results may be reported numerically as a confidence interval (CI), which comprises a range of values and shows that an investigator is either 95 or 99 percent confident that values for a population falls within the specified range. A CI that is small in range is more precise than a CI with a wide range of values.

Multivariate Analysis

Multivariate analysis is the concurrent analysis of three or more variables to determine patterns of relationships between variables. These advanced statistical procedures are suitable for analyzing complex correlational and experimental studies that have several independent and/or several dependent variables (Tabachnick & Fidell, 1989). Generally, large sample sizes are required to accommodate analysis of increasing numbers of variables. The procedures commonly used include multiple regression, path analysis, analysis of covariance (ANCOVA), factor analysis, discriminate analysis, canonical correlation, and multivariate analysis of variance (MANOVA) (see Table 22–4). As research becomes more sophisticated, the use of multivariate statistics in studies increases. This is a dilemma for beginning researchers and research consumers because studies using complex analytic procedures may be more difficult to evaluate.

Results, Discussion, Conclusions, and Dissemination

Study results or findings should be clear, concise, and congruent with the research question(s) asked and the methods used. The presentation of results varies for the type of study conducted. Qualitative studies are descriptive narratives, which include participants' verbatim accounts that provide evidence of the researcher's data interpretations. The results may be rich descriptions or new constructions of the study phenomenon, hypothetical propositions generated from the data, or a proposed theory.

Quantitative studies frequently use tables and graphs to display results. Variables examined in descriptive studies should be precisely described, and responses should be numerically reported. Relationships of variables investigated in correlational studies and the procedures used to determine relationships must be clear. In studies that test hypotheses, the statistical procedures used, the results, and the decision for supporting or not supporting the hypothesized relationships must be evident for each hypothesis stated. Significant, nonsignificant, and unexpected results must be reported. Findings in studies that are not what the investigator anticipates also contribute knowledge about the study topic; they can be an impetus for asking more relevant or more detailed research questions for future studies.

Interpreting study results is an intellectual process that gives meaning to the study and addresses the implications of the study outcomes. The investigator considers the study results with regard to the study process as well as findings from other studies that support or contradict results of the current study. These can be addressed with the presentation of the results or separately in a section discussing the findings.

Limitations of a study acknowledge factors that may affect study outcomes. Compromises are often necessary in the study process for pragmatic and ethical reasons. These can create weaknesses in design, sampling process, sample size, methods of data collection, or data analysis techniques, and should be reported. The extent to which study findings can be generalized to populations beyond the study sample should also be discussed. Stating limitations assists readers to evaluate the scientific merits of the study and enhances the credibility of the investigator.

Conclusions are concise statements that synthesize the findings; they provide an overall account of the importance of the study and an understanding of the phenomenon in question. The conclusions must be pertinent to the findings and not expanded beyond the study parameters. Following the conclusions, implications of the findings for clinical practice are generally described, and suggestions for further research are identified.

Communicating the results of the study is the final step of conducting research. This is done through research reports, journal articles, and presentations at conferences, workshops, and educational rounds in institutions. Dissemination of research solicits review by peers and facilitates the likelihood of study findings contributing to improved clinical practice.

Evaluating Research for Use in Practice

Evaluation is an analytical appraisal that makes judgments about the scientific merits of a study. The analysis objectively addresses the study's strengths and weaknesses, poses questions about the research, and makes constructive recommendations. Purposes for evaluating studies include determining if study findings are useful to clinical decision making, contributing to knowledge that could change clinical practice, or concluding whether further study of a topic is indicated.

Evaluation begins with reading the research report or journal article several times to become familiar with the study. Analysis of the research elements can then proceed. This chapter can serve as a base for understanding the research process as well as expectations for research approaches and specific methods. A key issue in reviewing a study is congruency. All elements—the research question, purpose, design, sampling procedures, methods of data collection, analysis, interpretation of the findings, and discussion—should be consistent with one another. Table 22–5 lists questions to ask when evaluating qualitative and quantitative studies. Although not exhaustive, the guidelines will assist in the systematic review of studies.

Following examination of the research elements, the reviewer identifies the strengths and weaknesses of the study. All studies have limitations; therefore, weaknesses are considered in relation to how they affect outcomes and the overall meaning of the study. Judgments are made regarding the relevancy of knowledge generated and the usefulness of findings to clinical practice. Legitimate criticisms of a study should be presented with rational and constructive recommendations. Evaluating studies is a skill that develops with practice, increased knowledge and understanding of the research process, and an awareness of the studies related to a specific topic.

Research articles published in professional journals are the most common source of research

TABLE 22–5	Guidelines for Evaluating Quantitative and Qualitative Studies

General Guidelines	Quantitative Studies	Qualitative Studies
1. **Problem and purpose** • Clearly stated? • Amenable to scientific investigation? • Significant to breastfeeding knowledge?	• Provides direction for study?	• Broadly stated? • Exploratory
2. **Review of literature** • Pertinent? • Well organized?	• Includes recent and classic references? • Theoretical base or conceptual framework evident?	• Acknowledges the existence of (or lack of) literature on the topic?
3. **Protection of human rights** • Subject's protection from harm ensured? • Subject suitably informed by a written informed-consent? • Reviewed by an ethics board? • Means for ensuring privacy, confidentiality, or anonymity are explained?		
4. **Method** • Design congruent with research question? • Sampling procedure appropriate for research method? • Method of data collection relevant for design?	• Deductive approach? • Variables identified and defined? • Sample representative of population and adequate size? • Measuring tools suitable, reliable, and valid? • Control of extraneous variables is evident?	• Inductive approach used? • Key informants and theoretical sampling addressed? • Data collection and analysis concurrent? • Process for data collection and analysis described? • Data saturated? • Credibility, dependability, confirmability, and transferability are evident?
5. **Results and discussion** • Analysis suitable for method and design? • Results clearly presented? • Interpretations clear and based on data? • Research question answered? • Limitations of study identified? • Conclusions based on results? • Implications for practice and research described?	• Statistical procedures used suitable for data and sample size? • Tables clear and represent the data? • Successful and unanticipated results reported?	• Examples of informants' accounts displayed? • Rich descriptions or theory presented? • Findings compared with literature? • Theory logical and complete?

reports. The limitations, particularly the length of the report, must be considered in the appraisal. Journal articles lack the detail of full research reports. Studies in refereed journals are subject to review before publication. Members of journal review boards, generally regarded as experts in the field, critique articles to judge them for their scientific merit and make recommendations regarding whether they should be published. The beliefs that members of review boards have regarding the scientific value of qualitative research can influence their decision about publication.

Breastfeeding encompasses many disciplines in the natural, social, and health sciences; therefore, breastfeeding practitioners must consult numerous and varied journals to remain current with new knowledge. Although a challenging task, remaining current is essential for professional practice.

Using Research in Clinical Practice

Bridging the gap between generating and utilizing knowledge is an ongoing process that takes motivation, commitment, persistence, and patience. Implementing research findings into clinical practice is a challenge for researchers and practitioners. The process is facilitated when researchers and practitioners work together to achieve the goal of implementing evidence-based practice. Researchers have the following responsibilities in assisting this process:

- Disseminating study findings directly to practitioners as soon as a study is completed through informal discussions; local, regional, and national presentations; and publications
- Replicating studies that may improve clinical practice; changes are seldom made following the outcomes of one small study
- Encouraging and assisting practitioners to participate in research to develop their interest and awareness
- Listening to concerns about practice in order to generate problems for study that are relevant to a particular practice area; collaborating with practitioners in research projects
- Assisting practitioners with evaluation of research articles so they may increase their

knowledge and competence in judging research findings

Practitioners have the following responsibilities in translating research findings to the practice field:

- Developing a questioning attitude and openness to change
- Sharing concerns about practice with researchers to develop pertinent clinical studies
- Collaborating with researchers and participating in research projects
- Critically reading and evaluating research articles and using relevant findings in practice
- Attending professional conferences where research is presented and discussed
- Telling other clinicians about study findings that reflect, assist, or may alter practice

Evidence-based practice is endorsed as the gold standard for care for healthcare professionals. It is the practice of making clinical decisions that are based on the best research evidence available, clinical knowledge and expertise of the practitioner, and in consultation with the individual receiving care. Findings from studies provide the research evidence; however, changes in clinical practice are not generally made on findings from one study. This should only happen if the study is exceptionally large and the findings are definitive regarding improved practice. Randomized control clinical trials that examine interventions can be systematically combined and summarized using a statistical technique called meta-analysis. These "studies of studies" are useful in providing insights into the effectiveness of interventions or showing that more research is needed. The Cochrane Collaboration (http://www.cochrane.org) of systematic reviews of the effects of healthcare interventions is internationally recognized and increasingly used by healthcare professionals. The amalgamation of qualitative studies on similar topics is called meta-synthesis; however, findings are an interpretation of the interpretations of the individual studies. A broad base of scientific evidence from studies using different approaches and methods are relevant and can expand scientific knowledge related to breastfeeding to optimum practice that benefits mothers, infants, families, and society.

Summary

Research is a process and theory is a base for developing knowledge that serves as a foundation for accountable and responsible practice. The approaches and methods involved in conducting research originate from various philosophical systems: the positivist/postpositivist perspective; the natural science, human science, and interpretation perspective; and the critical and emancipatory perspective. These perspectives give rise to research approaches and methods used in qualitative, quantitative, observational, historical, and feminist research. The research question asked—and whether knowledge is generated inductively or deductively—directs the approach used.

The qualitative approach generates an understanding of the "meaning" that reflects human values, beliefs, practices, and life experiences or events. The three qualitative methods commonly used are phenomenology, ethnography, and grounded theory. The quantitative approach is characterized by objectivity, measurement, and control. The quantitative methods commonly used are descriptive, correlational, experimental, and quasi-experimental studies. The simultaneous use of qualitative and quantitative methods in one study is an increasing trend.

The major elements of research are the problem and purpose, review of literature, protection of human subjects, method, and results and discussion. The research problem identifies *what* is studied and with *whom*, and the purpose delineates *why* the study is conducted. Research questions for quantitative methods are more specific than those of qualitative studies. In quantitative studies, variables are delineated and operationally defined. How breastfeeding and the duration of breastfeeding are defined is of particular importance when conducting or evaluating studies.

Reviewing literature about a study topic assists in formulating the research problem and directs the research method. Qualitative methods are frequently used when little is known about a topic.

Research that involves human subjects must ensure the study participants of basic rights. Ethical review boards or committees help protect subjects by reviewing the informed consent document and evaluating the study before it is conducted.

Study methods address setting, sample, data collection, and data analysis. The setting indicates the location of the study or the source of the participants. The sample is a subset of a larger population or group of individuals in whom the investigator is interested. Sampling is a process for selecting the sample from the population; the two types of sampling are probability and nonprobability. Nonprobability sampling is used in qualitative studies. Probability sampling is preferred in quantitative studies because findings can then be generalized from the study sample to the target population. This method requires random selection of subjects, which is not always possible; therefore, many quantitative studies involving human subjects use nonprobability sampling.

Data are collected when the researcher asks questions, makes observations, and/or measures key variables identified in the research question. In-depth interviews and observations are the most common methods used for qualitative studies, and data collection and analysis occur simultaneously. Systematic and rigorous methods for collecting and analyzing data are developed for all qualitative methods. Methods for data collection in quantitative studies are highly structured and must be the same for every subject.

Reliability and validity issues must be addressed for all research. Reliability refers to accuracy, consistency, precision, and stability of data collected; validity reflects the true meaning of data. In qualitative studies this aspect is referred to as trustworthiness. This includes building in checks in the data collection and analysis process. In quantitative studies, reliability of measurement tools and investigators collecting data can be statistically estimated, as can the validity of the measurements used.

Data analysis is the process of organizing, summarizing, examining, and synthesizing the data collected to identify study findings. Qualitative studies generate rich descriptions and posit hypotheses and/or theory. Descriptive narratives of participants' verbatim accounts support the investigator's interpretations. In quantitative studies, data are translated to numerical terms for statistical analysis. Depending on the type of study and the level of measurement of the data collected, a variety of statistical procedures can be employed. Results are displayed in tables and graphs.

Study results should be clear, concise, and congruent with the method used, and they should answer the research question(s). Significant, nonsignificant, and unexpected results are reported. Limitations of the study and the extent to which findings can be generalized to additional populations must also be addressed. Study conclusions should reflect only the study findings.

Research reports or articles are evaluated to make judgments about their scientific merit and the usefulness of findings for clinical practice. A key issue in evaluation is study congruency.

Implementing research findings into clinical practice is a challenge for researchers and practitioners. This process can be expedited when both work together. Although findings from current studies are not generally definitive and further study is frequently recommended, using relevant findings in practice often serves to question effects and generate new studies. Breastfeeding research is an ongoing process that expands knowledge and facilitates evidence-based practice. The benefactors of health professionals who draw from a scientific body of knowledge and establish practices based on best evidence are mothers, children, families, and society.

Key Concepts

- Research is the systematic and logical inquiry of a phenomenon to discover new knowledge or to validate existing knowledge.
- Theory is a conceptual construction of a view of reality that describes, explains, or predicts something. It includes concepts and their relationships.
- Middle-range theories include well-defined concepts and relationships, but the propositions are more easily tested than those of grand theories. They are amenable to theories used in clinical practice.
- Inductive reasoning is the process of reasoning from specific observations or abstractions to a general premise.
- Deductive reasoning is the process of reasoning from a general premise to the concrete and specific.
- A conceptual framework is a basic structure representing concepts and relationships but not a specific theory that explains the relationships.
- A theoretical framework is a basic structure representing theories, concepts, and propositions that are the underpinnings of a study and in which the propositions can be tested.
- A core concept is the overall theme of a grounded theory study. It is central to and interrelates the themes and categories identified in the study.
- A key informant is an individual who is most knowledgeable and who best articulates the meaning of the phenomenon under study.

- Bias is any factor, action, or influence that distorts the results of a study.
- Control is specific to quantitative research. It is the process of eliminating the influence of confounding variables that could compromise the research findings.
- An operational definition is an explicit description of a concept or variable of interest. For quantitative studies, they are expressed in measurable terms.
- The dependent or outcome variable is the variable the investigator measures in response to the independent or treatment variable; the outcome variable is affected by the independent variable.
- The independent variable is the treatment or invention that is manipulated by the investigator to influence the dependent variable.
- Power is the probability that a statistical test will reject a null hypothesis when it should be rejected, or in other words, detect a significant difference that does exist.
- Reliability is the degree to which collected data are accurate, consistent, precise, and stable over time.
- Validity is the degree to which collected data are true and represent reality, and a measuring instrument reflects what it is intended to measure.
- Trustworthiness is the process of establishing the credibility of qualitative research.

Internet Resources

Canadian Medical Association Infobase (Canada)— Clinical practice guidelines produced or endorsed in Canada by a national, provincial/territorial, or regional medical or health organization, professional society, government agency or expert panel: http://mdm.ca/cpgsnew/cpgs/index.asp

The Cochrane Collaboration—Cochrane database of systematic research reviews: http://www.cochrane.org

Federal US health databases and research articles (PubMed): http://www.ncbi.nlm.nih.gov/pubmed

References

Ajzen I, Fishbein M. *Understanding Attitudes and Predicting Behavior*. Englewood Cliffs, NJ: Prentice Hall; 1980.

Anderson GC et al. Early skin-to-skin contact for mothers and their healthy newborn infants. *Cochrane Database of Systematic Reviews* 2003, Issue 2. Art. No.: CD003519. DOI: 10.1002/14651858.CD003519.

Armstrong HC. International recommendations for consistent breastfeeding definitions. *J Hum Lact.* 1991;7:51–54.

Bakeman R, Gottman JM. *Observing Interaction: An Introduction to Sequential Analysis*. Cambridge, England: Cambridge University Press; 1986.

Bandura A. Self-efficacy: toward a unifying theory of behavioural change. *Psych Rev.* 1977;84:191–215.

Bandura A. Self-efficacy mechanism in human agency. *Am Psychol.* 1982;37:122–147.

Barnard K, Eyres S. Overview of the nursing child assessment project. In: Barnard K, ed. *Nursing Child Assessment Training Learning Resource Manual*. Seattle, WA: University of Washington School of Nursing; 1978:16–21.

Barr RG. Infant crying behavior and colic: an interpretation in evolutionary perspective. In: Trevathan WO, Smith EO, McKenna JJ, eds. *Evolutionary Medicine*. Oxford, England: Oxford University Press; 1999:27–51.

Bernaix LW. Nurses' attitudes, subjective norms, and behavioural intentions toward support of breastfeeding mothers. *J Hum Lact.* 2000;16:201–209.

Blyth R et al. Effect of maternal confidence on breastfeeding duration: An application of breastfeeding self-efficacy theory. *Birth.* 2002;29:278–284.

Bottorff J. Persistence in breastfeeding: a phenomenological investigation. *J Adv Nurs.* 1990;15:201–209.

Breastfeeding definition and algorithms. Breastfeeding Committee for Canada. http://breastfeedingcanada.ca/BCC. Accessed December 27, 2007.

Brett J, Niermeyer S. Is neonatal jaundice a disease or an adaptive process? In: Trevathan WR, Smith EO, McKenna JJ, eds. *Evolutionary Medicine*. Oxford, England: Oxford University Press; 1999:7–25.

Burns N, Grove SK. *The Practice of Nursing Research: Conduct, Critique and Utilization*. 3rd ed. Philadelphia, PA: WB Saunders; 1997.

Chenitz WC, Swanson JM. *From Practice to Grounded Theory*. Menlo Park, CA: Addison-Wesley; 1986:96–98.

Cohen J. *Statistical Power Analysis for the Behavioural Sciences*. 2nd ed. New York, NY: Academic Press; 1988.

Colaizzi P. Psychological research as the phenomenologist views it. In: Valle R, King M, eds. *Existential Phenomenological Alternative for Psychology*. New York, NY: Oxford University Press; 1978.

Crotty M. *The Foundations of Social Research*. Thousand Oaks, CA: Sage Publications; 1998.

Dennis CL. Theoretical underpinnings of breastfeeding confidence: a self-efficacy framework. *J Hum Lact.* 1999;15:195–201.

Dennis CL. The breastfeeding self-efficacy scale: psychometric assessment of the short form. *JOGNN.* 2003;32:734–744.

Dennis CL, Faux S. Development and psychometric testing of the breastfeeding self-efficacy scale. *Res Nurs Health.* 1999;22:399–409.

Dick MJ et al. Predicting early breastfeeding attrition. *J Hum Lact.* 2002;18:21–28.

Dykes F. 'Supply and demand': breastfeeding as labour. *Soc Sci Med.* 2005;60:2283–2293.

Furr PA, Kiregis CA. A nurse-midwifery approach to early mother–infant acquaintance. *J Nurse Midwifery* 1982;27:10–14.

Gillis A, Jackson W. *Research for Nurses: Methods and Interpretation*. Philadelphia, PA: FA Davis Company; 2002.

Giorgi A. Sketch of a psychological phenomenological method. In: Giorgi A, ed. *Phenomenology and Psychological Research*. Pittsburgh, PA: Duquesne University Press; 1985:8–22.

Glaser BG. *Theoretical Sensitivity*. Mill Valley, CA: Sociology Press; 1978.

Haisma H et al. Breast milk and energy intake in exclusively, predominantly, and partially breast-fed infants. *Eur J Clin Nutr.* 2003:57(12);1633–1642.

Harding S, ed. *Feminism and Methodology*. Bloomington: Indiana University Press; 1987.

Hennekens CH, Buring JE, Mayrent S. *Epidemiology in Medicine*. Boston, MA: Little, Brown, and Co.; 1987.

Hewat RJ. Living with an incessantly crying infant. *Phenomenology Pedagogy*. 1992;10:160–171.

Hewat RJ. *Mother-Infant Interaction During Breastfeeding: A Comparison Between Problematic and Nonproblematic Breastfeeders* [dissertation]. Edmonton, AB: University of Alberta; 1998.

Hewat RJ, Ellis DJ. Breastfeeding as a maternal-child team effort: women's perceptions. *Health Care Wom Int*. 1984;5:437–452.

Hill PD, Aldag JC, Chatterton RT. The effect of sequential and simultaneous breast pumping milk volume and prolactin levels: a pilot study. *J Hum Lact*. 1996;12:193–199.

Hoddinott P, Lee AJ, Pill R. Effectiveness of a breastfeeding peer coaching intervention in rural Scotland. *Birth*. 2006;33:27–33.

Ip S et al. Breastfeeding and maternal and infant health outcomes in developed countries. Evidence Report/Technology Assessment No. 153. Rockville, MD: Agency for Health Care Research and Quality; 2007. AHRQ Publication No. 07-E007.

Jacox A et al. Diversity in philosophical approaches. In: Hinshaw AS, Feetham SL, Shaver JIF, eds. *Handbook of Clinical Nursing Research*. Thousand Oaks, CA: Sage Publication; 1999:3–17.

Janke J. Prediction of breast-feeding attrition: instrument development. *Applied Nurs Res*. 1992;5:48–63.

Janke J. Development of the breastfeeding attrition prediction tool. *Nurs Res*. 1994;34:100–104.

Jensen D, Wallace S, Kelsay P. LATCH: a breastfeeding charting system and documentation tool. *JOGNN*. 1994;26:181–187.

Johnson TS, Mulder PJ, Strube K. Mother-infant breastfeeding progress tool: a guide for education and support of the breastfeeding dyad. *JOGNN*. 2007;36:319–327.

Kelly L, Burton S, Regan L. Researching women's lives or studying women's oppression? Reflections on what constitutes feminist research. In: Maynard M, Purvis J, eds. *Researching Women's Lives from a Feminist Perspective*. London, England: Taylor and Francis; 1994:27–48.

Kennell J, McGrath S. Starting the process of mother-infant bonding. *Acta Paediatr*. 2005;94:775–778.

Klaus MH, Kennell JH. *Maternal-Infant Bonding*. St Louis, MO: Mosby; 1976.

Klaus MH, Kennell JH. *Maternal-Infant Bonding*. 2nd ed. St Louis, MO: Mosby; 1982.

Klaus M, Kennell JH, Klaus PH. *Bonding: Building the Foundations of Secure Attachment and Independence*. New York, NY: Addison Wesley; 1995:54–92.

Koniak-Griffin D. Maternal role attainment image. *J Nurs Sch*. 1993;25:257–262.

Kramer HC, Thiemann S. *How Many Subjects? Statistical Power Analysis in Research*. Newbury Park, CA: Sage Publications; 1987.

Kumar SP et al. The LATCH scoring system and prediction of breastfeeding duration. *J Hum Lact*. 2006;22:391–397.

Labbok M. What is the definition of breastfeeding? *Breastfeeding Abstracts*. 2000;19:19–21.

Labbok MH, Coffin CJ. A call for consistency in definition of breastfeeding behaviors. *Soc Sci Med*. 1997;44:1931–1932.

Labbok M, Krasovec K. Toward consistency in breastfeeding definitions. *Stud Fam Plann*. 1990;21:226–230.

Leff EW, Jefferis SC, Gagne MP. Maternal perceptions of successful breastfeeding. *J Hum Lact*. 1994a;10:99–104.

Leff EW, Jefferis SC, Gagne MP. The development of the maternal breastfeeding evaluation scale. *J Hum Lact*. 1994b;10:105–111.

Lenz ER et al. Collaborative development of middle-range nursing theories: Toward a theory of unpleasant symptoms. *Adv Nurs Sci*. 1995;17:1–13.

Lincoln YS, Guba EG. *Naturalistic Inquiry*. Newbury Park, CA: Sage Publications; 1985.

Martell LK. Heading toward the new normal: a contemporary postpartum experience. *JOGNN*. 2001;30:496–506.

Martens PJ. Does breastfeeding education affect nursing staff beliefs, exclusive breastfeeding rates, and Baby-Friendly Hospital Initiative compliance? The experience of a small, rural Canadian hospital. *J Hum Lact*. 2000;16:309–318.

Matthews MK. Developing an instrument to assess infant breastfeeding behavior in the early neonatal period. *Midwifery*. 1988;4:154–165.

Matthews MK. Mothers' satisfaction with their neonates' breastfeeding behaviors. *JOGNN*. 1991;20:49–55.

Maynard M, Purvis J. *Researching Women's Lives from a Feminist Perspective*. London, England: Taylor and Francis; 1994.

McBride AB, Shore CP. Women as mothers and grandmothers. *Annu Rev Nurs Res*. 2001;19:63–85.

McKenna JJ, Gettler LT. Mother-infant cosleeping with breastfeeding in the Western industrialized context: a bio-cultural perspective. In: Hale TW, Hartmann P, eds. *Textbook of Human Lactation*. 1st ed. Amarillo, Texas: Hale Publishing; 2007;271–302.

McKenna J, Mosko S, Richard C. Breastfeeding and mother-infant cosleeping in relation to SIDS prevention. In: Trevathan WR, Smith EO, McKenna JJ, eds. *Evolutionary Medicine*. Oxford, England: Oxford University Press; 1999:53–74.

Mead GH. In: Morris CW, ed. *Mind, Self and Society*. Chicago, IL: University of Chicago Press; 1934.

Mercer RT. A theoretical framework for studying factors that impact on the maternal role. *Nurs Res*. 1981;30:73–77.

Mercer RT. The process of maternal role attainment over the first year. *Nurs Res*. 1985;34:198–204.

Mercer RT. Becoming a mother versus maternal role attainment. *J Nurs Sch*. 2004;36:226–232.

Hospitals, clinics, health maintenance organizations, and medical practice groups increasingly offer classes of all types to parents, siblings, and grandparents. Although the primary purpose of these programs is educational, they are also effective public relations techniques for attracting families to those institutions. In an era in which healthcare agencies are increasingly competitive, patient–client education can be an effective marketing strategy. Shifts in the US healthcare industry affect breastfeeding education of parents. Third-party reimbursement rewards birth settings from which patients are discharged quickly. When families leave the hospital or birthing center within hours or days after birth, teaching opportunities shift to prenatal education or postdischarge follow-up.

Educational programs for health professionals and lactation consultants have proliferated along with parent education. Privately owned continuing education companies, medical centers, and academic institutions regularly offer training in lactation management to health professionals.

Improving infant feeding knowledge is an effective strategy to increase breastfeeding rates. The key seems to be normalizing breastfeeding by social marketing or public health education campaigns aimed at modifying societal perceptions of what is considered normal infant feeding (Tarrant & Dodgson, 2007).

Some programs offer completion certificates or titles, such as breastfeeding educator or counselor. These programs, as well as seminars offered throughout the world, are useful preparation for individuals seeking to improve their knowledge of breastfeeding. Many individuals attend educational offerings not only for professional development but also to qualify for sitting for the certification examination by the International Board of Lactation Consultant Examiners (IBLCE). A current listing of lactation courses can be found on the Web site of the International Lactation Consultant Association (www.ilca.org).

The Internet

We are in the midst of an incredible media revolution: the Internet. As with all topics, the Internet has transformed lactation education. People go to the Internet for information on health issues and for support. They join chat groups, read about health concerns, and learn about treatment options. The Internet has partially replaced patient education provided by health professionals. As the amount of information available to us grows exponentially, powerful search engines make it possible for us to capture it and make sense of it and use it. Information given on Web sites can potentially affect breastfeeding success, especially if the parents have little access to other forms of support.

It is difficult to evaluate Web sites since they are frequently updated or removed. When Shaikh and Scott (2005) evaluated 40 Web sites related to breastfeeding they found that only half complied with standards of medical Internet publishing. They repeated the study a few months later and found that 20 percent of the top Web sites were different from the first list obtained. Given the changing nature of the World Wide Web, lactation specialists should be familiar with at least a few credible Web sites that they can suggest to patients as well as provide some guidelines to judge the credibility of the sites and caution them against potential bias of commercially sponsored Web sites.

The goal of Google and other search engine companies is to provide people with information and make it useful to them. On January 1, 2008, a search of two popular search engines (Google, Yahoo) using the key word *breastfeeding* each yielded over 16 million Web sites. Internet searches offer opportunities for qualitative research.

In addition to finding information, the Internet offers a way for people worldwide to "attend" a course without leaving their home area. Internet courses online are the solution to the problem of a lack of sufficient numbers of students interested in taking such a specialty course, especially for those living in rural areas. The first Internet course on breastfeeding came online in 1997 from Wichita State University School of Nursing (Riordan, 2000). E-learning, a company based in Australia, offers staff education and courses needed to take IBCLC certification. With the rapid proliferation of online education other Web-based breastfeeding courses are becoming available. Outside of formal breastfeeding courses, lactation consultants also can take part in an Internet discussion group called LACTNET. In daily posts, LACTNET participants seek and receive help with clinical cases and discuss current issues that relate to breastfeeding.

Learning Principles

Learning is most effective when individuals are ready to learn (i.e., when they feel a need to know something). "Teachable moments" refer to those periods when learners perceive the need for information and skills. Motivation is further enhanced when the material to be learned is organized in a manner that makes it meaningful to the learner. Activities that are novel and interesting to learners encourage learning. Active, rather than passive, participation is associated with more meaningful and permanent learning (Brillinger, 1990). Learning is divided into three domains, and breastfeeding education incorporates all three (Bloom, 1956):

- Cognitive skills (gathering information, linking concepts, problem solving)
- Psychomotor skills (listening to instructions, observing skills, repetitive practice, mastery of skill performance)
- Affective learning (modifying attitudes, values, and preferences)

Individual learning styles need to be considered when planning teaching strategies (Lauwers & Shinskie, 2000). Some participants learn primarily through auditory perceptions; they listen intently and remember what they hear. Others learn best visually and retain information about what they see. These learners benefit from visual aids and printed materials (Figure 23–1). A third mode of learning is kinesthetic or psychomotor learning. Kinesthetic learners benefit from touching and handling equipment and models. Most learners use all three modalities. Therefore, in teaching about breast pumps, learning is strengthened by discussion coupled with the showing of slides that demonstrate how pumps work and by having the learners manipulate the equipment themselves.

Because success is predictably more motivating than failure, dividing tasks and information into easily mastered segments keeps the adult learners motivated to continue the program. Learners respond to specific descriptions of their positive performance. Praise enhances feelings of self-confidence and conveys respect for the learner.

Adult Education

Adult learners differ widely from children in their learning styles. Unlike children, who are required to attend school, adults are self-directed when they choose to attend educational activities (Knowles, 1980). Adults perceive time as one of their most

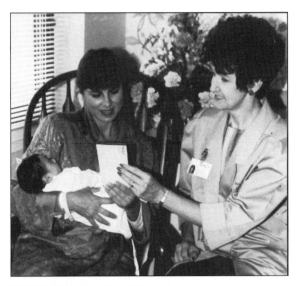

FIGURE 23–1 DVDs and written materials reinforce one-to-one teaching.

Source: Courtesy of Shira L. Bocar.

valued and scarce assets, and they are not willing to spend it in meaningless activity. Education programs must, therefore, demonstrate a clear applicability to the adult's everyday life. For example, discussion of the anatomy of the breast and the physiology of breastfeeding is more meaningful when related directly to practical skills, such as latch-on techniques and how often to feed the baby.

Adult learners have a rich variety of backgrounds and motivations for participating in educational programs. They appreciate and expect respect as unique individuals. If the instructor identifies what these personal learning needs are and fulfills them, learning occurs quickly and easily. Adult learning should be self-directed and provide feedback about the learner's progress toward achieving these goals (Figure 23–2). Parents should be considered colearners in that they teach each other as well as the instructor, who will invariably learn at least one new piece of information at every class. Principles of adult education are easily applied to breastfeeding education using these approaches:

- Ensure that content and timing of teaching coincides with parents' readiness to learn (prior to conception, during pregnancy, immediately postbirth, later postpartum).
- Prioritize and present information in easily understood and easily mastered segments.

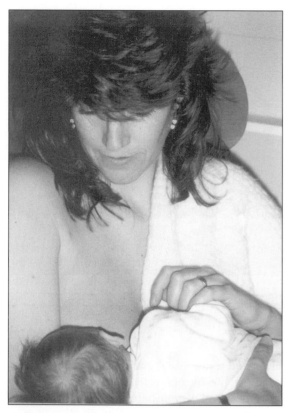

FIGURE **23–2** Adults are self-directed and have individual learning needs.

- Organize activities in increments to increase the likelihood of success.
- Give explicit instructions so that participants clearly understand what they are being asked to do.
- Provide specific, immediate feedback following each activity.
- Recognize the importance of body language and nonverbal communication.
- Use handouts and other media to reinforce and augment rather than to replace individualized assessment and teaching.
- Identify breastfeeding support resources, including telephone numbers of local resources.

There are several factors that enhance a positive learning climate for adult learners. Lighting, temperature, seating, the availability of writing surfaces furnished with paper and pencils, and the ability to view learning materials comfortably have a tremendous impact on learning. Adults appreciate physical comfort and knowing where drinks, food, and restroom facilities are located.

Adult education programs tend to be a social as well as a learning activity, because they afford opportunities to become acquainted with other adults. Greet each person warmly; demonstrate genuine concern for each one as an individual. It is a good idea to structure break periods with refreshments to encourage socializing. Adults enjoy sharing informal learning activities with others, and successful programs encourage adults to have fun as they learn. Adults also expect teachers to value student opinions about the usefulness of learning activities. One way to find out what areas of the program were helpful is to request informal verbal feedback or formal written evaluations. Evaluations are important data to modify and improve programs.

Curriculum Development

Assessing learning needs is mandatory when working with adult learners. There must be a match between what the learner needs to know and what the teacher presents. If the teacher erroneously assumes that learners already possess a high level of knowledge, learners can be frustrated because the information is too complex. Conversely, learners may be offended if the instructor assumes they have minimal knowledge.

To assess levels of knowledge when working with small groups, the facilitator can ask nonthreatening questions—such as, "What are some of the myths about breastfeeding you have heard?" In larger class settings, the content cannot be customized to each participant. Asking participants at the beginning of class what specific topics they would like to discuss helps assess their learning needs and involves them in establishing the curriculum. The importance of a topic should be reflected in the time given to it, taking into consideration how frequently the information will be used. For example, positioning and latch-on are fundamental to breastfeeding and so deserve a more thorough discussion than adoptive nursing, which is relevant to a much smaller group of learners.

Too much information at one time is overwhelming, and prioritizing teaching is critical. Basic physiologic requirements (e.g., adequacy of the infant's nutrient intake) help guide prioritization. Healthcare providers also must be aware of additional family resources and defer some teaching for later health visits. Thus, when a family is in the birth setting, the healthcare provider may share with the mother that breastfeeding can continue when she is employed outside the home. However, specific techniques for doing so will be taught after breastfeeding is established.

Health Professional Curricula

Most people agree that there is a lack of comprehensive breastfeeding content in health professional curricula whether the profession is nursing, medicine or other professions. Later in this chapter we discuss the importance of a team approach to parent education whereby breastfeeding information given to parents is consistent. To that end Spatz, Pugh, and the American Academy of Nursing Expert Panel on Breastfeeding have developed a model breastfeeding curricula for health professionals (2007). Although the model was originally developed for nursing curricula, it can be used for any healthcare curricula (see Box 23–1). They suggest that it is better if the knowledge is integrated in existing curricula, if possible. Several elective courses are available for college credit in US universities, such as the University of Pennsylvania, Johns Hopkins, LaSalle University, and Wichita State University. More are planned.

Student Attitudes

The types of attitudes and beliefs about breastfeeding that the students bring with them when they enter a health profession will determine what and how breastfeeding information is taught to their patients. Graduate students who take an elective course on lactation will have a more positive attitude about breastfeeding than those students who are taking a mandatory maternal–child course in a baccalaureate or associate degree nursing program. When Cricco-Lizza (2006) studied the attitudes of students coming into a school of nursing in the northeastern United States she uncovered and described students' vivid accounts of shocked reactions to women breastfeeding. Students generally believed that breastfeeding offered benefits for babies and mothers, but the beliefs were stronger for those who grew up where breastfeeding was the norm. Many felt that formula was equivalent to human milk. Most were

ambivalent about whether promoting breastfeeding would be forcing their personal views upon mothers and felt that nurses had more of an educational role with patients. If these concerns about ambivalence and past experiences are explored at the beginning of a course it is less likely that they will negatively influence the students' ability to promote breastfeeding in their professional role.

Case Studies

Case studies are an effective way to integrate experiences and knowledge in any topic but especially so in graduate education where students have prior clinical experience. I use case studies extensively in my online course. Each student in the class must present a real case related to breastfeeding from their own experience to a classmate. The classmate, in turn, responds with a plan of care for intervening and helping the breastfeeding dyad. Others in the class are then invited to comment on the case and care plan giving suggestions and criticism. Students are encouraged to save the case studies for future reference.

The University of Pennsylvania School of Nursing offers a course titled "A case study in breastfeeding and lactation." It is one of several case study courses offered to junior and senior nursing students. Students have the option of choosing which case study best meets their career goals (Spatz, 2005).

Textbooks

Instructors in nursing and medical schools should critically review breastfeeding information in textbooks used in their courses before selecting them as course texts. Breastfeeding information in textbooks used by nurses, pediatricians, and obstetricians needs to be consistent, accurate, and evidence based. Unfortunately, recent studies found breastfeeding information in textbooks used by each specialty to be highly variable and at times inaccurate and inconsistent with significant omissions (Davies, 2006; Merewood et al., 2006).

Parent Education

Facilitating the learning experience for parents requires an understanding of the tasks of adulthood. People seeking breastfeeding assistance are couples

BOX **23–1**

Sample Course Content for Elective Course in Lactation

Week	Content
1	Historical overview and policy implication and role of culture and families
2	Anatomy and physiology—maternal–infant roles
3	Biologic specificity of human milk, benefits of breastfeeding
4	Drugs and viruses in human milk
5	Breastfeeding process: antepartum, intrapartum, and postpartum
6	Maternal issues
7	Infant issues
8	Use of human milk and breastfeeding for preterm or other hospitalized infant
9	Maternal issues panel (guest mothers and infants)
10	Contraception
11	Maternal nutrition
12	Technology to support breastfeeding
13	Human milk banking
14	Translation of lactation research into clinical practice

Source: Adapted from Spatz, Pugh and the American Academy of Nursing Expert Panel on Breastfeeding, 2007.

involved in a major life change: acquisition of the parental role. There are four stages of transition into parenthood: anticipatory, formal, informal, and personal. During the *anticipatory stage,* before the birth of the infant, expectant parents benefit from realistic information about infant care. It is important for parents to understand that, in the first weeks after the baby is born, they will experience loss of sleep, fatigue, and episodes of crying (by baby, mom, and possibly dad). In this phase, parents should be encouraged to perform in certain ways:

- Form realistic expectations of infant care.
- Identify responsibilities that they can relinquish to devote time and energy to infant care.
- Learn practical aspects of infant care (including psychomotor experiences with dolls or infants).
- Begin to identify philosophical approaches to child care (such as how they will respond to a crying infant).

- Learn about typical emotional responses to new parenthood so that their experiences can be placed in perspective.
- Review previous personal successful experiences to support self-confidence.
- Socialize with other new families to increase opportunities for incidental learning and for developing a support network.
- Identify community resources that can facilitate the transition into parenthood.

The *formal stage* begins with the birth of the infant. Parents are often surprised at their intense feelings about the responsibilities of parenthood. Although forming attachment bonds with their infant, they are simultaneously achieving parental roles. Attachment is enhanced if parents have rooming-in, which enables them to get acquainted with their baby (Anderson, 1989). Healthcare providers can also use the infant's given name frequently to personalize the infant.

Parental caretaking behavior is often characterized by rigidity as parents seek to perform psychomotor tasks "the one best way." They are often overwhelmed if given too many equally attractive alternatives in child care. They may become noticeably frustrated if they receive conflicting information during this phase of role acquisition. New parents often feel awkward and inadequate because they lack experience and confidence in caretaking skills. They often equate their performance of infant care with their ability to parent effectively. During this stage, new parents are extremely vulnerable to implied judgment of their caretaking abilities. They are quite sensitive to nonverbal communication regarding their performance. Healthcare providers and experienced parents are particularly powerful role models as the self-image of the new parents emerges. The most persistent feelings during such role transition are those of inadequacy and lack of self-confidence.

During this time, mothers are fatigued and feel overwhelmed. In the days immediately after giving birth, women have impaired cognitive function, particularly in memory function (Eidelman, Hoffmann, & Kaitz, 1993). Therefore, new parents benefit from simple, concrete instructions divided into easily mastered segments. Specific, positive feedback about their performance, coupled with an expression of confidence by someone whose opinion is important to them, can greatly enhance their self-confidence. They need frequent assistance in placing their experiences in perspective.

The *informal stage* begins when parents feel that they have mastered child care tasks. Self-confidence increases as a person accrues successful experiences. Several weeks or months are required by most parents to amass adequate positive experiences so that they can proceed to the informal stage of role acquisition. Healthcare providers are in a unique position to enhance parental self-confidence by providing enthusiastic praise of performance and reviewing positive experiences. The relatively restrictive behavior of the formal stage is replaced by a willingness to consider options. Behavior becomes more spontaneous, and there is less fear of imperfection. A reassuring environment that supports experimentation and provides stimulation through a variety of role models enables parents to progress to the final stage of parental role acquisition.

During the *personal stage* behaviors are further modified, so that a parental role style evolves that is consistent with the parents' personalities. Relinquishing the fantasy of being the "perfect parent" frees parents to develop a unique set of behaviors with which they are comfortable. Support groups and classes provide ideal social settings in which parents can share their personal child care techniques and approaches with other parents, thus integrating their new parental role into their personalities (Figure 23–3).

Prenatal Education

Most mothers make decisions about how they will feed their baby before they become pregnant or during pregnancy. Pregnancy is an appropriate time to support a mother's decision to breastfeed, to correct inaccurate information, to add to the information she already has about breastfeeding, and to encourage undecided expectant mothers to consider breastfeeding. Infant feeding should be discussed before mothers start feeling the baby's movements. (Quickening usually occurs around the fifth month of pregnancy.) When mothers begin to perceive their babies as separate beings, they start making concrete plans for care, including how they will feed their babies. Mothers need information about infant feeding before being asked, "How are you going to feed your baby?" Because of the influence of the baby's father or the mother's partner and other family members, breastfeeding education programs should include support persons by encouraging their attendance at classes and group meetings and by providing educational materials specifically directed to them.

Early Breastfeeding Education

Toward the end of pregnancy, breastfeeding education appropriately focuses on the basics of breastfeeding initiation and management during the early days and weeks following the baby's birth. Classes should be accessible (with parking) and offered at times convenient to families. Patients can read pamphlets and view videos while they are waiting for appointments. Healthcare providers can also assess and add to the patients' knowledge during appointments. It is generally better to have frequent, short discussions about breastfeeding throughout

23–3

Sample Content for "How-To" Breastfeeding Class (Based on Common Concerns of Mothers)

How Do I Get Off to a Good Start?

- Best time for breastfeeding: within first hour after birth (importance of colostrum)
- Rooming-in
- What if separation is medically necessary?
- How often to breastfeed
  - Baby-led feedings
  - Identify early hunger cues
  - Feed at least every 3 hours during day (8–12 feedings each 24 hours)
  - Feed at least 5–10 minutes each side
  - Listen for swallowing
  - Watch infant for satiety cues
  - Avoid intense clock watching

Will I Have Enough Milk?

- What causes decreased milk production?
  - Long intervals between feedings
  - Formula or water supplements
  - Smoking
- Do I have to change my lifestyle?
- Nutrition, fluids, rest
  - Listen to your body: eat when hungry, drink when thirsty, rest when tired
- Medications, drugs, alcohol, nicotine
- If mother gets a cold

Will Breastfeeding Hurt?

- Do I have to prepare my nipples?
  - Check for nipple protrusion
- Do I need special supplies or equipment?
- Positioning and latch-on
  - Alerting infants: techniques

- Avoid overuse of swaddling
- Mother's position and breast support
- Infant's position (cradle hold, football hold, side-lying)
- Demonstrate with visual aids, doll
- What is a good latch?
  - Wide-open mouth
  - Lips flanged
  - Nose and chin to breast
  - No sharp pain
- Can I prevent sore nipples?
  - Break latch if it hurts, breastfeed frequently, start on less sore side
  - Creams and ointments (not always helpful)
- What is engorgement? How do I manage engorgement?
  - Breastfeed frequently
  - Cold packs to breasts
  - Use breast pump if necessary
  - Softer, smaller breasts (after engorgement) do not mean lost milk supply

Where Can I Get Help?

- Dad's special role (or primary support person)
- Types of help: practical help, emotional help, skilled assistance
- Dealing with advice and opinions
- Sources for expert help with breastfeeding
- How do I know if baby is getting enough?
  - Can hear baby swallowing regularly
  - Bowel movements (at least four per 24 hours)
  - Satisfied between feedings

(Continues)

- Feeding at least eight times each 24 hours
- Family life with baby: enjoying baby, consoling baby, and fear of "spoiling"
- When to call for help
  - Baby feeding every hour
  - Feedings lasting > 1 hour
  - Baby sleeping for > 4–5 hours more than once each 24 hours

- Baby feeds fewer than seven times in 24 hours
- Baby has fewer than four bowel movements in 24 hours
- Severe nipple pain
- Tender, swollen area in breast
- Learn and respond to baby's cues
- Use expert resources

learning need, whereas only half of the mothers agreed. In a qualitative study, hospital nurses felt the provision of interpersonal and informational support was adequate for successful breastfeeding. The mothers at this facility, on the other hand, wanted encouragement as well as interpersonal and informational support (Gill, 2001).

In addition to needing information and assistance with solving breastfeeding challenges, mothers need support and encouragement to continue breastfeeding (see Box 23–4). Family, peers, and community resources are often her primary sources of support. However, healthcare professionals have a role to play in assessing and augmenting or creating support systems.

How Effective Is Breastfeeding Education?

With short hospital stays and tight hospital budgets, we need to know what strategies work most effectively. Because education can change only those elements that are modifiable, we first need to identify what *can* be changed. When Janke (1993) extensively reviewed the research literature a few years age, she found only six modifiable variables that predict breastfeeding outcomes:

- Mother intends to breastfeed a long time.
- Mother is strongly committed to breastfeeding.

- Mother and family have a strong support system.
- Mother expresses a positive attitude toward breastfeeding.
- Baby has an early first feeding.
- Mother avoids supplemental feedings of water or formula.

Focusing on these modifiable factors and the timing of their contact with expectant parents can maximize the influence of healthcare professionals. How the mother will feed her baby is a decision that often is made prior to conception. Therefore, educational efforts may have to target future parents prior to conception through the elementary and secondary school systems, the mass media, churches, community organizations, and other influential institutions.

Studies summarized in Table 23–1 and in the table of randomized trials in Chapter 1, Table 1–1, show that education and professional interventions make a positive difference in breastfeeding outcomes.

Teaching Strategies

Good teaching involves organizing learning experiences that keep the participant's interest and use the facilitator's time efficiently. The lecture format yields an efficient use of the instructor's time; however, it requires that participants remain passive, and it is associated with decreased retention.

23–4

Recommended Topics for an Ongoing Breastfeeding Support Class

Newborn Adjustment

- Parental fatigue, time management
- Physical changes during postpartum
- Maternal mood changes
- Management of fussiness, crying
  - Concerns about "spoiling" infants
  - Consoling techniques
- Infant sleeping issues, nighttime parenting
- Transition from two to three (feeling left out)
  - Being a person and partner as well as a parent
  - Sexuality and contraception
- Dealing with unsolicited advice
- Blended families, sibling or pet adjustments

Breastfeeding Concerns

- Milk supply concerns
- Assessing adequacy of infant intake
- Strategies to increase milk supply
- Appetite and growth spurts
- Frequency of breastfeeding as baby gets older
- Involving family members
- Obstructed ducts and mastitis
- Weaning

Returning to an Employment Setting

- Feasibility of combining breastfeeding and employment outside the home
- Feeding options
- Childcare considerations
- Time management
- Selecting a breastmilk expression technique (hand expression and breast pump options)
- Expressing and storing breastmilk
- Maintaining milk supply; maintaining baby's interest in breastfeeding
- Keeping breastfeeding in perspective

An effective strategy is to vary the teaching format. Team presentations, small group discussions, demonstrations, role playing, question-and-answer sessions with teacher-led or student-led questioning, observations and comments by participants, group projects, and individualized instruction modules are effective ways to break the monotony of lecture presentations.

Each teaching session should include an introduction, learning experience, and conclusion or summary. A fundamental axiom is to "explain what you're going to teach, teach, and then describe what you have taught." When using the lecture format, remember certain essential guidelines:

- Use a conversational tone (avoid reading notes word for word).
- Vary speech (inflection, speed, and tone).
- Wear bright, interesting clothing.
- Move around while lecturing and use gestures for emphasis.
- Use visual aids liberally (slides, charts, models, portions of videotapes and films).
- Use humor.

TABLE 23–1	**Outcomes of Breastfeeding Education**

Author, Year, Country	Description and Results
Adams et al,, 2001 Ontario, Canada	Hospital-based lactation services offered to all mothers in community. Open hours for outpatient visits. Mothers highly rated service. Positive association between number of visits and breastfeeding duration.
Akram et al., 1997 N = 140 Pakistan	Group discussions and home visits until 6 mo. Significantly higher percent full breastfeeding at 4 mo in intervention group (94 vs. 7%).
Alvarado et al., 1996 N = 138 Chili	Prenatal home visits, hospital visit, group sessions, individual consultation until 6 mo, posters and pamphlets. Significantly higher percent full breastfeeding at 5 mo in intervention group (53 vs. 3%).
Davies-Adetugbo, 1996 N = 256 Nigeria	One-to-one counseling, posters, monthly home visits until 4 mo. Significantly higher percent full breastfeeding at 4 mo in intervention group (40 vs. 14%).
Fallon et al., 2005 N = 696 Australia	Compared breastfeeding outcomes before and after initiating postpartum telephone support service. Improved exclusive breastfeeding duration for 4.5 weeks women in private hospital. No improved rates by women in public hospital.
Greiner & Mitra, 1999 N = 10,128 Bangladesh	Home visits, radio jingles, printed matter, advertisements. No significant results of any breastfeeding 12–23 mo (93 vs. 92%).
Houston et al., 1981 N = 80 Scotland	Hospital and home visits in 1st week and q 2 wks until 24 wks. Significantly higher percent breastfeeding at 20 wk in intervention group (89 vs. 65%).
Martens, 2000 Canada	Education program for nursing staff (1.5 hr). Increase in breastfeeding beliefs ($p < .01$), exclusive breastfeeding rates ($p < .05$), but no change in breastfeeding attitudes.
Noel-Weiss et al., 2006 N = 110 Ontario, Canada	Hospital prenatal breastfeeding workshop 2.5 hours. Higher proportion of exclusive breastfeeding by women attending workshop compared with those not attending. Little difference in duration.
Palti et al., 1988 N = 310 Israel	Individual session from 7th mo of pregnancy until 6 mo postpartum. Full breastfeeding at 6 mo 29 intervention vs. control 18%.
Pugin et al., 1996 N = 422 Chili	Group session 3–5 times during last trimester. Significantly higher percent full breastfeeding at 6 mo in intervention group (80 vs. 65%).
Shinwell et al., 2006 N = 835 Israel	Intensive course on breastfeeding for neonatal nurses and midwives in general hospital. Rate of breastfeeding rose from 84% to 93%.
Valdes et al., 1993 N = 735 Chili	Individual consultation at d 7–10 and monthly until 6 mo. Significantly higher percent full breastfeeding at 6 mo in intervention group (67 vs. 32%).

(Continues)

TABLE 23–1	Outcomes of Breastfeeding Education (Continued)
Author, Year, Country	**Description and Results**
Vega-Franco et al., 1985 N = 50 Mexico	Group session 4 times: 30 min + pamphlet (after 6th mo). Significantly higher percent any breastfeeding at 4 wk in intervention group (72 vs. 16%).
Westphal et al., 1995 Brazil	Improved knowledge of healthcare provider and improved institutional scores related to WHO/UNICEF Ten Steps to Successful Breastfeeding after training course.
Zimmerman, 1999 United States	Prenatal education, support groups, discharge packets. Breastfeeding at 2 weeks increased from 35 to 57%.

- Demonstrate psychomotor tasks.
- Encourage the audience to participate by practicing psychomotor skills and with questions, comments, and small group discussion.
- Schedule breaks every 50 minutes for maximum retention.

PowerPoint computerized slides, video clips, and role playing are useful in dividing a psychomotor skill, such as positioning and latch-on, into understandable steps. If the facilitator previews audiovisual materials and is knowledgeable about equipment operation, it avoids equipment breakdown and wasting time. Warning: computerized video clips are notorious for not working.

Small Group Dynamics

Formal classes and educational media might provide information to large numbers of people, but teaching small groups is a much more powerful method for behavior change. Group discussions enhance peer support, decision making, and decrease dependence on healthcare professionals. A group is two or more people who interact and influence each other, accomplish common goals, and derive satisfaction from maintaining membership in the group. The ideal group size ranges from 8 to 12 people. More than 10 people in a subgroup decreases productivity (Tubbs, 1984).

Small group interaction has the advantage of stimulating a free flow of information and encouragement among participants as different questions are asked and new topics are raised. Small groups meet human needs for companionship, knowledge, and identity. Discussion in a small group is more likely to answer participants' information needs, because they usually feel more comfortable asking questions and changing the topic than when they are in a large group.

An informal, relaxed setting encourages participation. The group leader needs to be expert in the subject content area and skilled in group dynamics. Familiarity with the different roles played by group members enhances the group leader's effectiveness in moving the group in a fruitful direction.

Although the group leader may have to actively guide the discussion initially, the goal is to act as a resource for information, encouraging participants to develop their own creative and problem-solving abilities (Nichols & Edwards, 1988). When participants share their personal experiences, it enhances learning and increases self-worth as individuals' efforts are reinforced and supported by the group.

Multimedia Presentations

Education programs must compete with television, videos, computer disks (CDs), DVDs, and the Internet. Visual enhancements are almost mandatory for educational programs. In an age of television and computers, people expect visual and auditory stimulation. Speakers feel compelled to produce multimedia extravaganzas to compete. Some say our current expectations harken back to humankind's original visual communication style, before language and the printing press. The following items offer ways to present breastfeeding information visually:

- Use computer technology, such as PowerPoint software and LCDs (computerized projectors). PowerPoint presentations are the norm for presentations. It is easy to print professional-looking outlines of your talk for handouts and to make speaker's notes for each slide.
- Arrange for all necessary equipment (projectors, screens, video equipment, tape recorder, pointer, podium light, chart stands) well in advance of the presentation. If using the Internet on the LCD, ensure that the facility has access to the Internet. It is wise best to bring an extra copy of your talk just in case.
- Identify light switches and sound control panels; make certain that a responsible person is available to operate them.
- Adjust the volume of the microphone so that persons in the back of the room can hear easily. Make adjustments before beginning the presentation.
- Tape extension cords and cables to the floor to reduce the likelihood of an accident.
- Adjust the location of the slide projector so that images fill the entire screen and can be seen clearly by all participants.
- Adjust the position of equipment so that all participants can see.
- Adjust the lighting in the room to enhance the visual presentation and still allow for taking notes.
- When showing part of a videotape, preset the tape to the place where it is to begin.
- Meet with the equipment operator, review the audiovisual component of the presentation, and explain what the operator will need to do during the presentation.
- Screen visual aids before the presentation (e.g., are PowerPoint slides in order?).
- Avoid facing the audiovisual aids when speaking or standing between them and the audience.

Audiovisual aids that are presented effectively greatly enhance teaching. Learners are frustrated when such aids are poorly presented or the instructor talks about a wonderful component that is not available. Adequate planning and preparation are the best assurance for an effective presentation.

Electronic Slides

Computer-generated slides are the standard for presentations. Presentation software such as Power-Point creates electronic slides that can be easily modified, so there is little or no expense in revising and updating slides. Some lucky lactation consultants working in hospitals and healthcare agencies have access to audiovisual staff whose sole job is to produce audiovisual aids.

Transparencies

Transparencies or overhead projections are easy to make and the least expensive of all the media options. However, transparencies are easily damaged, are difficult to combine with slide presentations, and may require a second person at the overhead projector. Transparencies are generally limited to charts and words (photographs do not reproduce well) and appear to be less "professional" than other formats in this technology laden world.

Videos and DVDs

DVDs and video clips are excellent for demonstrating live-action psychomotor skills (e.g., positioning mother and baby for breastfeeding) and are easily transported and stored. Maternity facilities that provide a television set in mothers' rooms often have a closed "Newborn Channel" that airs teaching programs on early newborn care including breastfeeding. Almost all households in the United States have videotape and/or DVD players. Many videos and DVDs with breastfeeding information are now available. Search for breastfeeding videos on the Internet. The *Journal of Human Lactation* regularly publishes reviews on breastfeeding-related visuals.

Visuals

When developing a presentation using a visual format, apply these principles:

- Identify key concepts to be emphasized. Develop a story board—a sequence of the presentation's main points. Drawing boxes on a paper pad and filling them in with the secondary points works just fine for a story board first draft. Pictures and drawings can be added later.
- Keep the content simple: one idea per slide; limit to six points related to the main point.

- Ensure that all lettering is large enough to be read in the back of the room.
- Insist that all lettering, artwork, and photography are of professional quality.
- Use multiple colors to maintain interest.
- Use video clips (make sure they work).
- Avoid overuse of clip art. It can distract learners.
- Use simple, clearly labeled graphs and drawings.
- Avoid complicated, detailed artwork that is more suitable for print publications.
- Choose photographs that are sharp, clear, visually appealing, uncluttered, and convey a single key point. Well-selected photographs help viewers to see how information can be used in their lives.
- Use attractive photos of breastfeeding mothers and infants (your presentation will be rated higher by participants than one in which no such photos are used).
- Delete photos with distracting outdated hair or clothing styles.

Educational Materials

People retain new information a shorter period of time when they are under stress. After the physical and emotional stress of childbirth, families benefit from written materials that reinforce verbal teaching throughout pregnancy and after childbirth in addition to one-on-one individualized teaching. Points to remember for creating and using written materials include the following:

- Adults retain only about 30 percent of the information they hear, but a multimodal approach (seeing and hearing) increases their retention to 50 percent. For example, if a mother practices positioning at the breast or assembles a breast pump in addition to reading printed matter, her retention is improved.
- Materials must be scrutinized closely for their accuracy to determine that no outdated information is included. Information must be consistent. New parents are frustrated by conflicting recommendations. Because nonverbal messages have a more profound impact on behavior than do verbal instructions, materials must be carefully reviewed before using them. Mothers need

to make informed decisions about how they will feed their babies.

- New mothers do not need to know how to manage every potential breastfeeding difficulty. Materials that dwell on the management of complications (e.g., breast abscess) may be frightening to mothers still considering how they will feed their baby.
- Materials should always include a local resource telephone number.
- Printed matter should be attractively packaged. Families from a variety of socioeconomic backgrounds have access to sophisticated printed materials and commercial television programs; they expect similar quality in materials about breastfeeding.
- Pamphlets must be inviting, easy to read, and organized with bold headings and generous amounts of white space. Too many words on a page can overwhelm a reader.
- Pictorial learning is superior to verbal learning for recognition and recall. Pictures and drawings make materials more interesting.
- Assess the mother's interest in reading before making recommendations about written materials. Although some mothers welcome books on breastfeeding, women who do not like to read a book or do not speak English may think that if they have to read a book, breastfeeding may be too difficult for them.
- More is not always better when presenting printed materials. If families are bombarded with thick stacks of pamphlets and materials, the likelihood of their use is decreased. A few carefully selected pamphlets can convey the idea that breastfeeding is uncomplicated and enjoyable. Pamphlets and short audiovisual programs are preferable to lengthy materials that attempt to cover the gamut of breastfeeding experiences.

Brief, focused materials should address the issues that the family perceives as meaningful and that they are motivated to learn. This concept applies especially to mothers and families in special circumstances (such as prematurity, birth anomalies, and relactation). Books that are divided into small segments and have detailed indexes help families to locate needed information. Visual materials are more effective if they depict parents with ethnic, socioeconomic, and cultural backgrounds that are similar to the target audience. For example, teenage mothers respond most favorably to visual representations of adolescent mothers. A lending library of books and videotapes conveys a commitment to empowering families.

The source of materials must be considered in evaluating educational materials. Organizations whose purpose is to promote and sell formula cannot be expected to genuinely promote breastfeeding (Valaitis & Shea, 1993). Underlying messages may communicate that bottle-feeding is the cultural norm and that breastfeeding is difficult, complicated, uncomfortable, immodest, and inconvenient. There is often an explicit message that when families begin using formula, the product of that company is optimal.

The target audience should be considered in evaluating educational information. Materials must be written at a reading level that the reader can understand. Most word-processing programs can calculate the reading level of material by a simple push of a button. Box 23–5 lists the criteria for evaluation of education materials.

Continuing Education

Almost all medical centers now offer at least some staff continuing education related to breastfeeding. Some of these programs are highly successful and bring in welcome revenue (Box 23–6). Others less financially successful are considered "loss leaders." The strategy is to attract young families to a particular healthcare system that employs nurses and other providers who are knowledgeable in and supportive of breastfeeding. As birth settings that support breastfeeding are recognized and rewarded by the community, families will, in turn, become lifelong paying "customers" of the healthcare system offering them. Core components of developing and presenting continuing education programs follow these sequential steps:

- Assess the learning needs of the participants.
- Assess participants' motivation and readiness to learn.
- Plan and develop learning objectives, curriculum content, and teaching methods.

- Implement teaching strategies and assist participants in focusing attention on learning tasks.
- Evaluate the outcome of teaching activities.

Managers become aware of learning needs and deficits in the clinical staff through feedback from families and from other healthcare providers. In addition to gaining administrative input regarding learning needs, potential participants of the educational program should be involved in assessing their own learning needs. Their involvement in the planning stage will enhance their belief that the program will benefit them in their clinical practice. Staff may attend educational programs either because their employer requires attendance or because they need to attend a certain number of continuing-education offerings to maintain their professional registration or certification (extrinsic motivation). However, if participants are there because they want to be (intrinsic motivation), they are self-directed learners who have identified their learning goals and are enthusiastic about learning. Relating the curriculum content directly to a clinician's practice is a key strategy for arousing and maintaining interest in the program. Teaching strategies for staff or continuing professional education are similar to those used with breastfeeding families.

Evaluating professional educational programs includes the staff's own assessment of the usefulness of the program to their clinical practices and an appraisal of the speaker and the content. This information is invaluable in modifying future programs; it also helps to convey the goal of clinical applicability and communicates respect for participants as valuable individuals.

Objectives and Outcomes

In developing education programs for healthcare professionals, it is useful to clearly identify what the learner is expected to master. Writing behavioral objectives is one concrete way of identifying learning goals. A behavioral objective states what the student will be able to do at the end of the session. See Table 23–2 for examples of the correct way and the incorrect way to write behavioral objectives.

Program outcomes are different from objectives. Objectives have to do with what a learner is

BOX 23–5

Criteria for Evaluating Educational Material

Content

- Specific to family's needs?
- Accurate, reliable information based on valid research reports?
- Accepted principles of anatomy and physiology?
- Up-to-date recommendations?
- Consistency between narrative and visual aids?
- Simple, uncomplicated approach?
- Avoids dwelling on difficulties or potential complications?

Presentation

- Attractive, inviting?
- Organized for easy scanning: bold headings, short paragraphs, and ample white space?
- Appropriate reading level?
  - *Less than high school education (grade 3).* Need more visuals, less narrative.
  - *High school graduate (grades 5–7).* Newspapers are written at this level.
  - *College graduate (grades 12–13).* Professional journals are written at this level.
- Generous use of appropriate pictures, drawings, and graphs that are consistent with the narrative?

- Visual aids depict families from similar backgrounds of audience?
- Appropriate length to maintain interest?

Promotional Materials

- Enthusiastically discusses benefits of breastfeeding?
- Includes risks of bottle-feeding?
- Culturally appropriate breastfeeding is modeled?
- Includes practical tips for successful breastfeeding?
- Provides information for additional resources?

Source of Materials

- No underlying or hidden messages about the use of formula?
- Breastfeeding presented as complicated, uncomfortable, immodest, and inconvenient?
- Complies with WHO Code, which precludes healthcare providers from distributing materials provided by formula companies?

able to do as a result of an education program whereas outcomes are the *results* of clinical practice that may be an indirect result of educational programs. An example is staff nurses who become more knowledgeable about breastfeeding after attending a series of continuing-education programs, and this new knowledge ultimately results in fewer mothers weaning early. Outcomes must be relevant and measurable and a logical result of clinical practices or of institutional effort. Examples of breastfeeding outcomes of breastfeeding education are many:

- Number and percent of mothers who initiate breastfeeding
- Length of time the mothers breastfed

BOX 23–6

Sample Continuing-Education Program

Program Title: Insufficient Lactation and Infant Weight Gain

Description: This two-hour course reviews the characteristics and interventions of a situation where infant is gaining weight at below acceptable levels owing to apparent maternal lactation insufficiency.

Objectives:

1. Correlate normal growth with expected nutritional intake.
2. Assess the mother–infant to determine probable causes of insufficient milk supply.
3. Identify variation in the lactating breast that may potentially impact a mother's milk supply.
4. Distinguish between primary and secondary lactation insufficiency.
5. Describe effective interventions, supplementation of the infant while maintaining lactation and feedings at the breast.

(Three objectives can usually be adequately covered in one hour.)

Teaching Methodology: Lecture, slides, videotape, case study for discussion

Instructor: Jane Smith, RN, BSN, IBCLC

References:
Hillervik-Lindquist C. Studies on perceived breastmilk insufficiency. A prospective study in a group of Swedish women. *Acta Paediatr Scand.* 1991;Suppl 376:1–27, 1991.
Livingstone V. Problem-solving formula for failure-to-thrive infants. *Can Physician.* 1990;36:1541–1545.
Powers, N. How to assess slow growth in the breastfed infant. In: Schanler RJ, ed. Breastfeeding 2001, Part 11. *Pediatr Clin No Amer.* 2001;48(2):345–363.

Evaluation: Program will be evaluated by participants using the standardized form, The Comprehensive Evaluation Tool for Continuing Health Education Programs. The faculty/presenter will receive evaluation results and participant comments.

- Rate of ER visits for breastfeeding infants with dehydration
- Cost savings to the managed care organization due to the better health of infants because they were breastfed.

All of these outcomes are relevant, measurable and they reflect staff and institutional knowledge and effort. Most managed care organizations now require periodic reports of clinical outcomes periodically. An Excel spreadsheet is available to almost all health agencies. Setting up a database of

breastfeeding outcomes that reflect the effect of educational programs is one more way to document the importance and effectiveness of education.

The Team Approach

A team approach to breastfeeding education enhances the learning experiences of childbearing families by providing a comprehensive approach. The fragmented care that often typifies women's healthcare today is not conducive to effective

TABLE 23–2	Examples of Behavioral Objectives

Incorrect	Correct
The participant will understand the relationship between breastfeeding and jaundice. (Note: the student's "understanding" is not observable.)	The learner will list the types of neonatal jaundice and will describe the relationship of each type to breastfeeding.

Not Observable	Observable
Understand, know, appreciate, learn, perceive, recognize, be aware of, comprehend, grasp the significance of, gain a working knowledge of	State, list, define, identify, describe, compare, critique, rate, demonstrate, plan, design, choose, discuss, match, relate, categorize, distinguish between, select, locate

breastfeeding education. Consistent information shared by a variety of providers on multiple occasions strengthens the impact of each breastfeeding education encounter. The breastfeeding team's exposure to current information (workshops, articles, etc.) strengthens consistency of education. To avoid unintentional contradiction, documenting what has been discussed with teaching checklists and care maps allows the educator to build on that foundation and to reinforce key points. Each healthcare provider develops a unique relationship with a breastfeeding family and can make unique contributions to the family's education (Bocar, 1992).

Childbirth Educators

Childbirth educators develop rapport with breastfeeding families during their multisession classes. They provide invaluable anticipatory guidance by including breastfeeding information in general childbirth education programs. Following childbirth, families frequently seek breastfeeding assistance from childbirth instructors.

Nurses

Most certified lactation consultants are also nurses. Staff nurses not certified as specialists refer more complex cases to lactation consultants. Breastfeeding educators, or lactation counselors, are titles that indicate completion of a study of breastfeeding basics (Figure 23–4).

Lactation Consultants

Lactation consultants are healthcare providers whose primary focus is providing breastfeeding assistance. They provide a variety of specialized services, including individual consultations for unusual breastfeeding situations, care plans developed in collaboration with other healthcare providers, breastfeeding class sessions, and instruction in the use of specific breastfeeding products. They also serve as a resource for information and data, develop special programs or projects related to breastfeeding, provide continuing education programs for healthcare providers, and conduct research. Lactation consultants have received certification from the International Board of Lactation Consultants (IBLCE), the internationally recognized certification body for this specialty area (see Chapter 1).

Physicians

Physicians can serve as powerful breastfeeding promoters. Their support of breastfeeding can be a potent force in a family's decision to begin and continue breastfeeding. About half of new physicians are young women who are likely to choose to breastfeed because of the health benefits and later become strong advocates for breastfeeding. Physicians often refer families to lactation consultants for time-intensive treatment of breastfeeding difficulties or follow-up. Some physicians are certified as lactation consultants and may have practices that are limited to breastfeeding families.

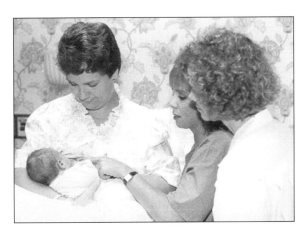

FIGURE 23–4   Perinatal nurse learning new skills from a lactation consultant.

Source: Courtesy of Debi Leslie Bocar.

Dietitians

The responsibilities of dietitians include nutritional counseling for childbearing families. They can describe the influence of breastfeeding on maternal and infant nutrition needs. Many dietitians working with breastfeeding families are employed by WIC programs and in other community health settings.

Community Support Groups

Mother-to-mother support groups create an invaluable social support network for breastfeeding families. Practical tips and much incidental learning about parenting are derived from these important support groups. The largest and most effective self-care group for breastfeeding support is La Leche League International (LLLI). Founded in 1956, LLLI's core service is mother-to-mother support and information provided through small neighborhood-based groups.

Leaders are available between meetings for individual assistance and problem solving. The relaxed, friendly interchange between women with common interests in breastfeeding, childbearing, and childrearing is a basic strength of this highly successful organization. LLLI is effective in meeting the educational and support needs of breastfeeding women worldwide.

Summary

Breastfeeding families are empowered for self-sufficiency when healthcare providers furnish information in an accurate, well-organized manner. When good information is coupled with identification of the family's goals and assistance with problem solving, parents have greater self-confidence and self-reliance.

Developing and presenting educational programs for healthcare providers who assist breastfeeding families requires significant time and energy. One needs to remember the ripple effect related to education; enormous numbers of breastfeeding families benefit from the enhanced knowledge of healthcare providers. A successful education program—regardless of its subject matter—entails positive experiences for learners and educators. Identifying the components of effective breastfeeding education programs can assist healthcare providers who are involved in planning, implementing, and evaluating breastfeeding services.

Key Concepts

- Learning is most effective when individuals are ready to learn (the teachable moment) and the material to be learned is organized in a manner that makes it meaningful to the learner.
- Learning is divided into three domains (cognitive skills, psychomotor skills, and affective learning). Breastfeeding education incorporates all of them.
- Adults are self-directed and perceive time as one of their most valued and scarce assets, and they are not willing to spend it in meaningless activity. Education programs must, therefore, demonstrate a clear applicability to the adult's everyday life.
- The Internet is now a major source for health education including breastfeeding information. Web

- sites should be evaluated before recommending to parents.
- Online courses for continuing education and for college credit are available, and more are planned.
- Using case studies is an effective method for students to integrate knowledge and clinical experience in graduate level courses.
- Assessing learning needs of adults is mandatory. There must be a match between what the learner needs to know, what the teacher presents, and the time taken for important topics.
- Facilitating the learning experience for parents requires an understanding of acquisition of the parental role as one of the tasks of adulthood.
- Families with special needs benefit from individualized teaching, assistance, and ongoing group support. Individualize the content based on family concerns and not what healthcare providers *think* they should have.
- When special circumstances, such as prematurity, multiple births, congenital anomalies, or neurological impairment, affect the initiation of breastfeeding, the learning needs of the parents are complicated by the emotional ramifications of the experience. It is hard for parents to retain information when they are under stress. Prioritize content so that only important information is given and repeated.
- Numerous studies show that education and professional interventions extend the length of breastfeeding.
- A fundamental axiom is to "explain what you're going to teach, teach, and then describe what you have taught."
- Small group teaching is a powerful method for changing behavior. The ideal small group size is 8 to 12 people.
- To develop slides, identify key concepts, write them out on a story board, a sequence of the presentation's main points and secondary points: one idea and six points per slide.
- Adults retain only about 30 percent of the information they hear but 50 percent of a multimodal approach (both seeing and hearing).

Internet Resources

Videos, print materials, links to books, article, support groups, chat rooms:
www.lalecheleague.org
www.promom.org
www.breastfeedingbasics.com
www.aap.org/healthtopics/breastfeeding.cfm
www.babycenter.com
www.breastfeeding.co.uk

www.wrsgroup.com
www.injoyvideos.com
www.noodlesoup.com
Courses on breastfeeding:
www.ilca.org
www.breastfeedingbasic.org
www.health-e-learning.com
www.wichita.edu

References

Adams C et al. Breastfeeding trends at a community breastfeeding center: an evaluative survey. *JOGNN*. 2001;30:392–400.

Akram DS, Agboatwalla M, Shamshad S. Effect of intervention on promotion of exclusive breastfeeding. *J Pak Med Assoc*. 1997;47:46–48.

Alvarado R et al. Evaluation of a breastfeeding support programme with health promoters' participation. *Food Nutr Bull*. 1996;17:49–53.

Anderson GC. Risk in mother-infant separation postbirth. *Image*. 1989;21:196–199.

Bender DE, McCann MF. The influence of maternal intergenerational education on health behaviors of women in peri-urban Bolivia. *Soc Sci Med*. 2000;50:1189–1196.

Berger D, Cook CA. Postpartum teaching priorities: the viewpoints of nurses and mothers. *JOGNN*. 1998;27:161–168.

Bloom BS. *Taxonomy of Educational Objectives*. New York, NY: David McKay Co; 1956:7–8.

Bocar DL. The lactation consultant: part of the health care team. *NAACOG's Clin Iss Perin Wom Health Nurs*. 1992;3(4):731–737.

Brillinger MF. Helping adults learn. *J Hum Lact*. 1990; 6:171–175.

Cricco-Lizza R. Student attitudes and beliefs about breastfeeding. *J Prof Nurs*. 2006;22:314–321.

Davies S et al. Breastfeeding information in nursing textbooks needs improvement. Presented at International

Lactation Consultant Association Annual Conference, San Diego, CA; July, 2006.

Davies-Adetugbo AA. Promotion of breast feeding in the community: impact of health education programme in rural communities in Nigeria. *J Diarrhoeal Dis Res*. 1996;14:5–11.

Eidelman A, Hoffmann N, Kaitz M. Cognitive deficits in women after childbirth. *Obstet Gynecol*. 1993; 81:764–767.

Fallon AB et al. An evaluation of a telephone-based postnatal support intervention for infant feeding in a regional Australian city. *Birth*. 2005;32:291–297.

Gill SL. The little things: perception of breastfeeding support. *JOGNN*. 2001;30:401–409.

Greiner T, Mitra SN. Evaluation of the effect of a breastfeeding message integrated into a larger communication project. *J Trop Pediatr*. 1999;45:351–357.

Houston MJ et al. Do breastfeeding mothers get the home support they need? *Health Bull*. 1981; 39:166–172.

Janke JR. The incidence, benefits, and variables associated with breastfeeding: implications for practice. *Nurse Pract*. 1993;18(6):22–32.

Knowles M. *The Modern Practice of Adult Education*. New York, NY: Cambridge University; 1980.

Lauwers J, Shinskie D. *Counseling the Nursing Mother*. 3rd ed. Sudbury, MA: Jones and Bartlett; 2000.

Martens PJ. Does breastfeeding education affect nursing staff beliefs, exclusive breastfeeding rates, and Baby Friendly Hospital Initiative compliance? The experience of a small, rural Canadian hospital. *J Hum Lact*. 2000;16:309–318.

Merewood A et al. Breastfeeding information in Ob/Gyn textbooks needs improvement. Presented at International Lactation Consultant Association Annual Conference, San Diego, CA; July, 2006.

Nichols FH, Edwards MR. Are your group process skills up to par? *Nurs Health Care*. 1988;9:205–208.

Noel-Weiss et al. Randomized controlled trial to determine effects of prenatal breastfeeding workshop on maternal breastfeeding self-efficacy and breastfeeding duration. *JOGNN*. 2006;35:616–624.

Palti H et al. Evaluation of the effectiveness of a structured breastfeeding promotion program integrated into a maternal and child health service in Jerusalem. *Isr J Med Sci*. 1988;24:342–348.

Pugin E et al. Does prenatal breastfeeding skills group education increase the effectiveness of a comprehensive breastfeeding promotion program? *J Hum Lact*. 1996;12:15–19.

Riordan J. Teaching breastfeeding on the Web. *J Hum Lact*. 2000;16:231–234.

Schlickau J. Development and testing of a prenatal breastfeeding education intervention for Hispanic women. *J Perinat Ed*. 2005;14:24–35.

Shaikh U, Scott BJ. Extent, accuracy, and credibility of breastfeeding information on the Internet. *J Hum Lact*. 2005;21:175–183.

Shinwell ES et al. The effect of training nursery staff in breastfeeding guidance on the duration of breastfeeding in healthy term infants. *Breastfeeding Med*. 2006;1:247–252.

Spatz DL. The breastfeeding case study: a model for educating nursing students. *J Nurs Ed*. 2005;44:432.

Spatz DL, Pugh LC. The American Academy of Nursing Expert Panel on Breastfeeding. The integration of the use of human milk and breastfeeding in baccalaureate nursing curricula. *Nurs Outlook*. 2007;55:257–263.

Tarrant M, Dodgson JE. Knowledge, attitudes, exposure and future intentions of Hong Kong University students toward infant feeding. *JOGNN*. 2007;36:243–254.

Tubbs SL. *A Systems Approach to Small Group Interaction*. Reading, MA: Addison-Wesley; 1984.

Valaitis RK, Shea E. An evaluation of breastfeeding promotion literature: does it really promote breastfeeding? *Can J Public Health*. 1993;84:24–27.

Valdes V et al. The impact of a hospital and clinic-based breastfeeding promotion programme in a middle class urban environment. *J Trop Pediatr*. 1993;38:142–151.

Vega-Franco L, Gordillo LC, Meijerink J. Prenatal education or breast-feeding [spanish]. *Boletin Medico del Hospital Infantil de Mexico*. 1985;42:470–475.

Westphal MF et al. Breastfeeding training for health professionals and resultant institutional changes. *Bull WHO*. 1995;73:461–468.

Zimmerman DR. You can make a difference: increasing breastfeeding rates in an inner-city clinic. *J Hum Lact*. 1999;15:217–219.

The Cultural Context of Breastfeeding

Karen Wambach and Jan Riordan

CULTURE EXERTS A MAJOR INFLUENCE on a mother's attitude toward breastfeeding that crosses the boundary between private and public. Attitudes and patterns of infant feeding cannot be understood without placing them in their specific cultural context. This chapter looks at breastfeeding as a human behavior that is sensitive to cultural influence and social change.

The fastest growing segments of the US population are minorities. Non-European ethnic minorities are fast becoming an aggregate majority. For example, Hispanics compose the fastest growing minority population in the United States (Schlickau, 2005). Currently, Hispanics/Latinos make up 14.8 percent of the total population of the United States, and between 2000 and 2006 they made up one half of the population growth. The Hispanic growth rate (24.3 percent) was more than three times the growth rate of the total population (6.1 percent) (United States Census Bureau, 2006). The increase in the US Hispanic population is driven by high fertility rates. In 2003, the fertility rate for Hispanic women was 96.9 births per 1000 women ages 15–44, compared with 60.5 for non-Hispanic women (Martin et al., 2005). In 2003, 912,329 of the 4,089,950 US births were to Hispanic women accounting for almost one in four live births. Fortunately, according to the 1999–2006 National Health and Nutrition Examination Surveys (NHANES), the rate of breastfeeding among Hispanic women (Mexican American) is higher than among non-Hispanic black or white women in the United States (McDowell, Wang, & Kennedy-Stephenson, 2008), but this also magnifies the need for support from lactation professionals.

Culture is defined as the values, beliefs, norms, and practices of a particular group, which are learned and shared and that guide thinking, decisions, and actions in a patterned way (Leininger, 1985). Culture provides implicit and explicit codes of behavior:

- It is *learned* both through language and socialization.
- It is *shared*, often unconsciously, by all members of a cultural group who are then bound together under one identity.
- It is an *adaptation* to specific conditions related to environmental and technical factors and to the availability of natural resources.
- It is a *dynamic,* ongoing process.

From a practical standpoint, a society's culture consists of whatever one has to know or believe in order to operate in a manner acceptable to the

799

culture's members. Culture is a blueprint for human behavior, a guide that helps us to gain a clearer understanding of individual behaviors. The new mother is the product of all of her history: what she has learned about infants and infant feeding, and what she has seen. If she grows up in a breastfeeding culture, she has many opportunities to observe how infants are fed and knows that her female relatives and neighbors with breastfeeding experience will support her when she becomes a mother (Mulford, 1995). Women and their families have a right to expect that their cultural needs will be met as they are helped with breastfeeding and lactation. Without an understanding of a mother's cultural practices, the care and intervention of healthcare professionals can do more harm than good (Figure 24–1).

The Dominant Culture

Every society has a dominant culture, the values of which are shared by the majority of its members as a result of early common experiences. Although there are approximately 100 ethnic groups in the United States, the dominant cultural group is that of white, middle-class Protestants, descendants of northern Europeans who immigrated to the United States

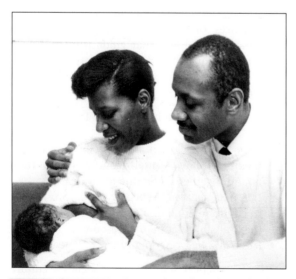

FIGURE 24–1 Expectations about breastfeeding. Each family has its own ideas, which are based in part on culture.

several generations ago. Norms characteristic of this group are a conservative value system, family orientation, commitment to higher education for one's children, a work ethic, materialism, a personal faith in God, the quest for physical beauty, cleanliness, high technology, punctuality, independence, and free enterprise. Given these prevailing values, it may be relevant to consider women's roles, their contribution to the economy, and the extent to which breastfeeding is perceived to hinder this.

The dominant health culture in the United States views birth as dangerous for the mother and neonate. Breastfeeding is seen as the optimal method of infant feeding but as difficult to accomplish and as a private act not to be practiced in public. These norms are slowly changing as waves of immigrating Asians and Hispanics become the "new" Americans. In the United States, Western allopathic medicine is viewed as "professional" health care; any medical tradition outside this system is considered traditional folk medicine with its accompanying connotations of primitive, "useless," "lay," and "outdated." The dominant US health system marketplace is composed of the hospital, the health worker's office, and the community health department. The folk belief system marketplace centers on the home of the clients or of their extended kin.

The role of women in a culture may also define the experience of breastfeeding. In some societies, male control (male physicians, for example) over breastfeeding serves to weaken the woman's role as mother and to emphasize her role as wife. Rather than viewing insufficient milk supply and early weaning as problems in themselves, these factors could be interpreted as reflecting insecurity about the abilities of women's bodies and the precariousness of their lives and as a symptom of broader self-questioning (Obermeyer & Castle, 1997). In 2002, Dykes echoed that sentiment based on her phenomenological study of 10 women's breastfeeding experience, noting that Westernized medicine and a preoccupation on breast milk as a product undermined women's confidence in their ability to breastfeed. She cautioned healthcare providers not to rely solely on empirical parameters of success in breastfeeding such as infant weight gain, but to treat breastfeeding as a holistic process and relationship between mother and child.

Ethnocentrism vs. Relativism

Ethnocentrism may be defined as being centered in one's ethnic or cultural system (i.e., judging the world by one's standards or in the vernacular believing that "my group is best"). When caring for culturally diverse groups, nurses and healthcare workers at first tend toward ethnocentricity, believing that their professional, scientifically based practices are superior. Many of the healthcare workers reading this book have been socialized into their profession within the framework of a Western healthcare system that emphasizes the biomedical model and is based on the white, working- and middle-class value system. If this system is the only model used to evaluate and implement care, the nurse or lactation consultant is ethnocentric. When healthcare workers are exposed to other cultures, they may begin to appreciate why certain behaviors and values are effective in that culture, and the healthcare worker may move beyond ethnocentric behaviors.

The opposite of ethnocentrism is *cultural relativism*, in which the healthcare provider recognizes and appreciates cultural differences and treats individual clients with deference to their cultural backgrounds—building on and using cultural variations rather than seeing them as obstacles. To provide optimal assistance, caregivers must first understand their personal reactions to cultural differences and then appreciate how these cultural values affect the lives of their clients. By discovering areas of commonality between themselves and their patients, nurses or care providers will be better able to recognize and deal with cultural similarities and variations between the clients and themselves. This process is illustrated in Figure 24–2.

Cultural relativism likewise recognizes variation within cultures, such as the diverse ethnic groups in the United States. At one time, people expected and hoped that these ethnic and cultural groups would blend into one common whole: the melting-pot approach. It has not worked out that way; many third- and fourth-generation Americans proudly claim and identify with their original ethnic heritage. The tendency to label subpopulations to explain behaviors is responsible for many myths about new Americans.

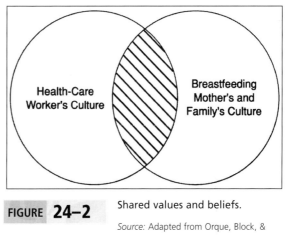

FIGURE 24–2 Shared values and beliefs.

Source: Adapted from Orque, Block, & Monrroy, 1983.

Assessing Cultural Practices

A cultural assessment elicits shared beliefs and customs that affect how nursing care is given (Mattson, 2000). When a nurse or lactation consultant examines cultural traditions, it is helpful to ask questions that indicate respect for cultural practices. A practice that seemingly does not provide any immediately visible benefit may be important to the mothers, and its value should be acknowledged. Nurses and lactation consultants who show that they respect the mothers' practices will gain respect in turn and better adherence to teaching. The following three questions can be used to examine cultural values:

- Are they helpful? All cultures have beliefs, myths, and rituals that may help breastfeeding. For example, the Lusi people in Papua New Guinea prohibit the lactating mother from having intercourse because it is believed that semen poisons her breastmilk (Maher, 1992). One result of this practice is eliminating the likelihood of a superimposed pregnancy. Such beliefs ensure that infants continue to be breastfed and are well nourished and nurtured. Cultural practices such as carrying a baby close, breastfeeding on demand, and spacing children by long-term breastfeeding are likewise considered beneficial.
- Are they harmless? Placing an amulet or charm of garlic around the baby's neck to protect him from harm or pinning a bellyband around his abdomen to prevent an umbilical hernia are harmless practices, assuming that such items

are kept clean. If the mother eats garlic to prevent illness, the practice is harmless to her baby even though her milk will be garlic flavored (Mennella & Beauchamp, 1991).

- Are they harmful? Unlike most of the rest of the world's people, white Europeans put mother and baby in separate sleeping rooms, sometimes even in the hospital, which hinders the establishment of breastfeeding. In rural southern Senegal the mother expresses and discards her colostrum and the infant is fed only water with sugar or honey until the "true" milk comes in, thereby depriving the baby of the concentrated immune properties of colostrum (Whittemore & Beverly, 1996).

Language Barriers

When working with families who speak a different language, the healthcare provider ideally can understand and speak that language. If she cannot, she should study the language spoken by the breastfeeding families that she frequently serves. Rapport is difficult when language differences form a barrier.

Healthcare workers who can speak Spanish are desperately needed in the southwestern United States and in many other large cities where Hispanics/Latinos are fast becoming ethnic majorities (Mattson, 2000). Health agencies with large Hispanic/Latino populations should provide courses in Spanish for their employees (Berry, 1999; Hernandez, 2006). In towns with a high population of Hmong women, Hmong nurses are needed. In the northeast Canadian-border area, French is appropriate. When it is necessary to find someone fluent in a language, a trained interpreter is best able to rephrase words so that they are understandable and more acceptable to the member of the culture. When a translator is available, care providers should speak slowly in a normal voice and should avoid using slang and subjectives (e.g., *would* and *if*). It may also be wise to record the discussion with the mother, so that the discussion may be referred to again. Even with a translator, there may be problems, because there are different dialects within some countries. Vietnamese, for example, is a language with many regional dialects. Also, a word may have different shades of meaning in different regions of the country. In preparing a flip chart and audiocassette for encouraging breastfeeding among mothers in the Dominican Republic, one of the authors (JR) used the word *amamantar* to mean *breastfeeding,* as it is used in many Spanish-speaking countries. This provided much amusement to the Dominican mothers, to whom it meant, "milk the cow."

Most people who are new to a culture are shy. Out of respect for the people with whom they are dealing, they may nod their head and say yes even though they may disagree or not understand what is being said. Whenever possible, printed materials regarding breastfeeding should be written in the family's language. Information sheets on breastfeeding in many different languages may be ordered from La Leche League International. Phrases that are frequently used when helping mothers breastfeed are presented in Spanish in Table 24–1.

The Effects of Culture on Breastfeeding

Immigrants tend to adopt the cultural practices of their new country; for newcomers to the United States, adaptation means bottle-feeding instead of breastfeeding. These mothers were breastfed themselves as infants and breastfed those children born in their native land; however, in their eagerness to fit in with American cultural norms, these women turn away from their heritage of breastfeeding—hardly a surprise in a country where toy baby dolls are sold with formula bottles and women pump milk for their babies in the room reserved for evacuating bodily wastes (Morse, 1989). The longer a newly immigrated woman lives in the United States, the more likely she will choose to bottle-feed, even though she may come from a country where the breastfeeding rate is high. Mexican women in the United States are an example—the least acculturated are more likely to breastfeed than the more acculturated (Libbus, 2000). Breastfeeding becomes a choice for them, neither a cultural norm nor an economic necessity. The women may be wrongly told that it is the custom in the United States to bottle-feed babies.

Perception of breastfeeding support can be different for immigrants compared with women of the

TABLE 24–1	Commonly Used Phrases When Speaking with Spanish-Speaking Women About Breastfeeding

Spanish	English
Leche materna	Breastmilk
Calostro	Colostrum
Madre	Mother
Bebé	Baby
Consultor de lactancia	Lactation consultant
Consejera	Nurse
Masaje del pecho	Breast massage
Expresión manual	Hand expression
No usar chupetes	Do not use pacifiers
No usar biberones	Do not use bottles
Succionar los pechos	Pump breasts
Alimentación suplementaria	Supplemental feeding
Alimentación de pecho	Breastfeeding
Amamantar a su bebé	Breastfeeding
Pecho	Breast
Pezón	Nipple
Ya puede amammantar a su niño(a).	You can breastfeed your baby now.
¿Le va bien cuando da pecho?	How is breastfeeding going?
¿Cada cáundo el niño come cada ves que le da pecho?	How often does the baby breastfeed each day?
¿Esta recibiendo suficiente? Cinco a seis pañales mojados al día?	Getting enough? Five or six wet diapers each day?
¿Esta recibiendo suficiente? Cuatro o más deposiciónes al día?	Getting enough? Four or more bowel movements a day?
¿Cuantas veces hace pupu el niño al día?	How many dirty diapers does the baby have each day?
Le da pecho las veces que el niño quiere, usualmente ocho a doce veces al día.	Breastfeed as often as the baby wants, usually eight to twelve times a day.
Usted puede comer lo que quiera al menos que el niño se ponga malo después de que come algo en particular.	You can eat what you want unless you notice the baby is fussy after you eat certain foods.
Sus pezónes van a estar un paquito enflamados. Pero en unos cuantos dias se le va a quitar.	Your nipples may be sore for a few days. But the soreness will go away.

dominant culture. For example, immigrant mothers in Canada experienced more hospital practices detrimental to breastfeeding than did Canadian-born mothers. But they also received better professional support in the community (Loiselle et al., 2001).

In the 1990s US and Australian care providers' worked increasingly with Asian families who immigrated in search of a new life and opportunities. Few of the women chose to breastfeed (Rasbridge & Kulig, 1995; Rossiter, 1994). These mothers were breastfed as infants, and they breastfed those children born in their native land. However, in what was attributed to their eagerness to acculturate, these women turned away from their cultural heritage of breastfeeding. A local community health nurse asked a Vietnamese mother, "But didn't your mother breastfeed you?" The woman replied, "Yes, but that's the old way. We're in a new land now." More recent research with Vietnamese immigrants in Quebec, Canada, also found that few of the women initiated breastfeeding, and none of the primiparae in the sample breastfed (Groleau, Souliere, & Kirmayer, 2006). However, acculturation to a bottle-feeding culture was not the reason for bottle-feeding. Rather, women's narratives revealed that their new home and separation from family prevented the traditional support and rituals that nurture the new mother, restore her health, and promote healthy breast milk production.

Hmong women living in Wisconsin stated that they bottle-fed rather than breastfed for the following reasons: "not enough milk in breasts," "can go someplace without taking a baby," "going back to school," "stale milk in breasts" (Jambunathan & Stewart, 1995). The father of the baby is likely to agree with his wife, especially if their baby is a boy, in the belief that their son will grow to be physically larger (and more like American men) and to have "harder bones" if he is fed formula.

Consider the influences of a new culture when a mother receives a formula discharge pack from the hospital and free formula through the WIC program in the land "where babies don't die." The WIC office in a Dallas Cambodian community was universally referred to as the *kinlaeng baek tuk dah ko*, "the place to get formula" (Rasbridge & Kulig, 1995). Consider, too, the messages the mother receives when she sees the stacks of formula in the supermarket and the magazine pictures of attractive mothers bottle-feeding their babies. Rossiter (1994) noted that when breastfeeding classes for Vietnamese women living in Australia are geared to their language and their culture, these women have more positive attitudes toward breastfeeding and are more likely to breastfeed.

Why do African-American women choose to breastfeed less often? In a qualitative study by Corbett (2000) an African-American woman described the curiosity of friends who wanted to watch her because they had never seen a woman breastfeed. Breastfeeding seemed to be an unfamiliar and uncertain activity, as is reflected in the lower rate of breastfeeding than among other groups. According to the 1999–2006 National Health and Nutrition Examination Surveys (NHANES) black non-Hispanic women currently have the lowest rates of breastfeeding in the United States (65 percent), compared to white non-Hispanic (79 percent) and Hispanic/Mexican American women (80 percent). Fortunately, like the rest of the United States in general, breastfeeding rates have increased among black women from 36 percent in 1993–1994 to 65 percent in 2005–2006 (McDowell et al., 2008).

When African-American women were asked why they chose bottle-feeding, they acknowledged that breastfeeding is more healthful than formula-feeding (Riordan & Gill-Hopple, 2001), but they offered many reasons for not doing so: "If you've got a job you've got to pump," "It ties women down," "You've got formula given to you from WIC," "It hurt too much and I couldn't take the pain," and "I thought it was just a turn-off." Others said they chose not to breastfeed because they believed that the baby would be "spoiled" and also that the baby would not receive enough milk. Are there other, deeper, unstated reasons why African-American women turn away from breastfeeding? Blum (1999) thinks so and attributes their history of slavery and the common practice of Southern black women wet-nursing white infants, a legacy of embodied exploitation where their sexuality and reproduction were appropriated by white men. Breastfeeding, in which the black baby was denied its mother's milk as she nursed the white infant, is a particularly charged symbol (Blum, 1999).

The baby's grandmother plays a key role in an African-American woman's decision to breastfeed and in when to introduce complementary foods and replacement feedings. Younger mothers in urban settings are often single and living at home with their own mother. The grandmother, the decision maker in the family, wields the authority and experience (Bentley, Dee, & Jensen, 2003; Masvie, 2006). For any breastfeeding promotion in these groups to be successful, it must first educate and convince the grandmothers.

Newer research indicates that origin of birth (outside the United States) was predictive of breastfeeding intention among black and Hispanic women in New York City (Bonuck et al., 2005). In contrast to previous research, the researchers found that black (non-Hispanic) and Hispanic women's breastfeeding plans were similar. This shift was attributed to a dramatic increase in the study locale of blacks from West Indian countries in which breastfeeding is the norm. The research highlights the importance of subcultural differences among ethnic minority groups.

Healthcare provider influence is also important to black women's decision making regarding infant-feeding method. Cricco-Lizza (2006), in her ethnographic investigation of 11 black women enrolled in

WIC clinics, found that healthcare providers offered limited breastfeeding education and support during pregnancy, child birth stay in neonatal intensive care unit, postpartum, and recovery in the community. They also expressed trust/distrust concerns and varying degrees of anxiety about the ways they were treated by nurses and physicians. The researcher concluded that healthcare professionals can improve disparities in breastfeeding rates among blacks, but their efforts in education and support must be coupled with development of trusting relationships and continuity of care.

Cricco-Lizza (2005), in the same sample of women as the preceding study that was described, found that when the WIC clinic environment set a positive tone for service that WIC employees treated the women with caring and respect, and in general the women believed that WIC was a source of support in time of need, and that personalized breastfeeding promotion with trusting relationships influenced the breastfeeding decisions for about half of the women. However the availability of free formula in the WIC clinic facilitated bottle-feeding. Thus, social institutions and healthcare providers do have influence on breastfeeding decisions, and cultural awareness is important in working with ethnic groups that have lower rates of breastfeeding traditionally.

The US view of the breast as erotic and society's notion that motherhood is incompatible with sexuality also have negative ramifications for breastfeeding among immigrants or ethnic minority groups. For example, native Ojibwe women in Canada expressed that they believed breastfeeding is the "right way to feed the baby," yet they were uncomfortable about breastfeeding being related to their view of the breast as sexual (Dodgson et al., 2002).

Breastfeeding in a public place or in the presence of friends is an activity that is extremely sensitive to cultural norms (Figure 24–3). For instance, in Saudi Arabia it is not uncommon to see a totally veiled woman baring her breast to feed her infant in public with no one taking notice—except, perhaps, a foreigner. In France, women in topless swimsuits are perfectly acceptable on certain beaches. However, a French woman would hesitate, or at least cover herself carefully, while breastfeeding in public, even in a restaurant near the "topless" beach. Modesty is

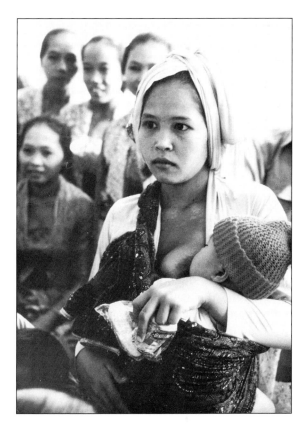

FIGURE 24–3 Well-nourished woman and breastfeeding infant in Searo. Breastfeeding is a basic part of the life process in this part of the world.

Source: Courtesy of World Health Organization.

important for the Mexican-American mother and may be viewed as inconsistent with breastfeeding in public. Breastfeeding in public is becoming a more accepted practice in North America. When Canadian women tested public reaction by breastfeeding in a restaurant and a shopping mall, they received very little notice from passersby (Sheeshka et al., 2001).

Rituals and Meaning

Rituals and cultural meanings associated with infant feeding are critical elements in assessing the culture's infant-feeding practices. Unfortunately, the word *ritual* has come to connote a meaningless ceremonial act. Actually, rituals can have a significant effect if the individual believes in them. Eating a special food or praying to a patron saint to increase the milk supply are cultural rituals that work for some people, just as taking a pill on the advice of a Western-trained doctor may have a positive effect, even if the medicine is a sugar pill. Researchers call this the *placebo effect*, which is based on the observation that if one believes that a particular action will have a desired effect, it will.

In the Philippines, the ritual of *lihi* ensures a good flow of rich milk. The ceremony involves stroking the mother's breasts with broken papaya leaves and stalks of sugar cane. The white sap of the papaya ensures that the mother's milk will be copious, thick, and white, whereas the cane guarantees that it will be sweet. In certain rural areas of Japan, figurines and paintings depicting a woman with a bounteous milk supply are displayed in the belief that they increase the mother's milk (Figure 24–4). A picture of a breastfeeding mother seated in front of a waterfall has been used in the United States for similar effect. The use of nipple creams, popular in some Western countries, could be considered a ritual that is a comfort measure, even if it is not necessary from a physiological point of view.

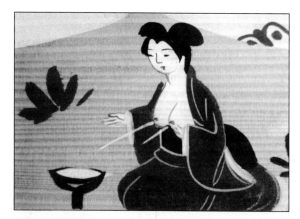

FIGURE 24–4 Votive picture (*ema* in Japanese). This wooden plaque is given to the breastfeeding mother by the temple. She in turn prays to the plaque for sufficient milk. If her wish is fulfilled, she writes her name and age on the plaque and dedicates it to the temple.

Source: Courtesy of K. Sawada.

Colostrum

In many cultures throughout the world, colostrum is accepted and encouraged as the first food for infants. In some cultures, however, colostrum is considered to be "old" milk that has been in the breasts for months and is unfit for the newborn and thus should be expressed and thrown away until the "true" milk appears on the second or third day (Conton, 1985; Fishman, Evans, & Jenks, 1988). In many developing countries, mothers do not give their babies this first milk because they fear it to be pus or poison. This belief exists among people in countries thousands of miles apart, including the native peoples of Guatemala and Korea, and Africans in Sierra Leone and Lesotho. Lactation consultants have the opportunity and responsibility to encourage women to breastfeed their baby early by explaining that colostrum is "special" early milk made just for their baby and will help keep their baby healthy.

Sexual Relations

We are sexual beings, and the breastfeeding woman is no exception. Although breastfeeding is usually a rich meaningful experience, its effect on a woman's sexuality is generally ignored. Historically, sex during the lactation period has been fraught with myths and prescribed behaviors. For example, the notion that semen contaminates breastmilk, a vestige of medieval European thought, is still widespread in many developing countries. It assumes that there is a physiological connection between the uterus and the breast and that the mother's milk may become contaminated by sexual contact. One negative result of a taboo against having sexual intercourse while lactating is that men pressure women to shorten breastfeeding so they can resume sexual relations and that women, concerned that their milk may be "contaminated" by sperm, are more likely to wean early (Maher, 1992). On the positive side, the taboo is an effective means of birth spacing.

When Avery, Duckett, and Frantzich (2000) surveyed 576 breastfeeding women in Minnesota about their sex life, overall they reported that breastfeeding had a slightly negative impact on some aspects of sexuality but did not greatly affect the woman's sexual relationship with her partner. The striking thing was their wide range of experiences. When asked if the sensations of suckling elicited arousal, most of the women (60 percent) reported negatively. Based on the information from this study, caregivers can help mothers deal with sexuality during the breastfeeding by doing the following:

- Teaching normal (and wide) variations of experiences of sexuality
- Discussing resumption of intercourse when she feels ready
- Providing good information about safe and efficacious contraceptives
- Describing methods of reducing perineal pain, such as vaginal lubricants
- Emphasizing that a priority should be placed on time for sleep
- Reminding couples that the window of time devoted to breastfeeding is relatively short compared to their total life together

Wet-Nursing

Wet-nursing, a historic practice worldwide, may provide for a child whose mother has died or who is otherwise unable to breastfeed. Among Japanese, Chinese, and Thai mothers, breastmilk can be shared between infants of the same sex but not those of the opposite sex. Infants who had the same wet-nurse cannot marry in Arabic Moslem countries. In cultures that view breastmilk as a conduit for ancestral power, it is not unusual for wet-nurses to be restricted to women from the mother's or father's clan or lineage (van Esterik & Elliott, 1986). Americans practiced wet-nursing up until recent times; for example, Southern women sometimes used black slaves to wet-nurse their babies. Wet-nursing is now discouraged because of concerns about AIDS transmission. However, a few women still practice wet-nursing; for example, mothers in Northwest Indian tribes, especially sisters, regularly practice wet-nursing secretly.

The practice of wet-nursing by sisters is more accurately labeled cross-feeding or cross-nursing according to Thorley (2008). She described cross-feeding as the practice of informal sharing of breastfeeding between equals, and that it is often of a reciprocal nature. Describing the practice within the context of Australia, Thorley reviewed the literature and found only sporadic written reports of the practice in the 1900s, due to the informal nature of the practice and because of public sentiment against the practice. She did however, point out that there had been "popular press and media" reports about cross-nursing in the United States, Britain, and Canada, with women reporting satisfaction with the experience. Anecdotally, she reported that lesbian couples practice cross-nursing, and advised that lactation consultants inquire sensitively about both partners breastfeeding.

Other Practices

A seclusion period of about 40 days after giving birth is common in many cultures. This time of support from female kin and seclusion for the mother and baby varies according to the culture. Generally, it permits a mother to become acquainted with her baby, to establish her milk supply, and to reduce both her and her infant's exposure to infectious disease. In Bedouin Arab society, female relatives visit the new mother and baby and bring small gifts of money to mark the birth of the baby (Forman et al., 1990).

In Korea, the mother's mother-in-law traditionally takes care of her after the child's birth and serves as her "doula." During pregnancy, Korean women undergo *Thae Kyo* or education-teaching of the fetus. In this ancient tradition a mother-in-law trains her daughter-in-law to be a mother. *Thae Kyo* instructs the expectant mother that to avoid bad luck in having her baby, she should not see fires or fights, she must think pure thoughts and eat "pretty" foods, and she must always walk in a straight line. During the postpartum period, which lasts about 3 to 4 weeks, the woman is also cared for by her own mother and her husband. This perception that the mother is "sick" and requires care runs counter to the expectations of US-trained nurses and to discharge early from the hospital.

Contraception

Methods of contraception used by breastfeeding mothers of any culture should not interfere with lactation. Nurses who advise ethnic minority women in community family planning services play a key role in monitoring the type of oral contraceptive dispensed. Combination pills that contain both progestin and estrogen (Lo/Ovral, Ortho-Novum, Triphasil, Nordette) seriously diminish breastmilk production, and they almost invariably lead to giving formula supplements and weaning (American College of Obstetricians and Gynecologists [ACOG], 2000). If the mother does not speak English or if she is an illegal immigrant, she may hesitate to ask questions as to why her milk supply suddenly dried up after she started taking a combined oral contraceptive pill.

On the other hand, progestin-only oral contraceptives (Micronor, Nor-QD, Ovrette) and long-acting progestin-only injectables (Depo-Provera, Norplant) do not affect the quality of breastmilk and may increase the volume of milk (ACOG, 2000), especially if they are not started until 6 weeks postpartum when lactation is well established (Diaz & Croxatto, 1993). For nonhormonal contraception during the first 6 months after delivery, ACOG (2000) recommends exclusive breastfeeding meeting lactational amenorrhea method criteria and, if desired, using additional protection such as condoms and other barrier methods. (See Chapter 21 for a detailed discussion.)

Infant Care

Swaddling or bundling is an ancient practice still used today to soothe the infant and maintain his body temperature. Swaddling and carrying the baby on the mother's side or back also frees her hands for other tasks. In many parts of rural Nigeria, an infant is wrapped on the mother's back all day and sleeps with her at night. During the first 40 days, the baby is snugly wrapped, a practice that ensures that the infant stays warm and reduces his energy requirements (Omuloulu, 1982).

In parts of the world that do not have intensive care nurseries, premature infants who are clinically stable go directly to the mother as early as 2 to 3 hours after birth. By being held in an upright position, skin-to-skin between their mother's breasts, they are kept warm (Anderson, Marks, & Wahlberg, 1986; Anderson, 1992). This practice has spread to intensive care units worldwide in many countries and is now known as "kangaroo care" (Figure 24–5).

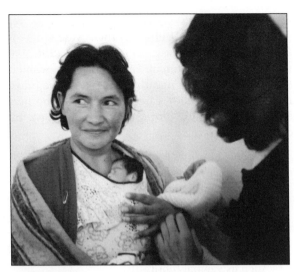

FIGURE 24–5 A premature infant in Bogota goes home. Twelve hours after birth, the baby cradled skin-to-skin with his mother.

Source: Courtesy of G.C. Anderson.

In any culture, swaddling and carrying the baby close typifies mothers who practice unrestricted breastfeeding. As early as 24 hours after delivery, the Zambian infant is secured to his mother's body with a *dashica,* or long piece of cloth. The baby rides on the mother's hip in the *dashica,* and his head is not supported. As a result, the Zambian infant maintains a strong shoulder girdle to keep his head steady and thereby develops early head control. The *aquawo*—a specially woven, strong cotton cloth folded in a special way—is the infant carrier in Bolivia. The *aquawo* can be turned around to several positions to facilitate breastfeeding. In Mexico, a woman uses a long, wide shawl called a *rebozo* for carrying her infant while she goes about her daily activities.

Many different types of baby carriers are used worldwide. Mothers and fathers, regardless of their cultural backgrounds, recognize and enjoy the convenience these carriers afford. Carrying the infant swaddled to his mother's body develops the child's muscle tone and seems to encourage alertness. Being carried about during daily activities offers many opportunities for tactile, visual, and social stimulation.

Babies in the Dominican Republic are not secured to their mother in any fashion but are carried in their arms in a horizontal position until they are old enough to sit up by themselves. Because it is believed that a baby can break his or her neck easily if the head is not held, a mother will become visibly anxious when the nurse assesses her baby's head control.

Diseases recognized only in a particular culture may affect an infant. In Spanish-speaking cultures, the most common is *mollera caida* (fallen fontanel). The health professional interprets a depressed fontanel in the baby as a symptom of dehydration, whereas a Hispanic mother may see it as curable illness caused by removing her nipple while the baby is still suckling, or by the baby falling.

Another Hispanic and Puerto Rican folk disease is *mal de ojo,* or evil eye, which is presumably caused by someone casting very strong glances at the baby or by someone who admired the baby but did not touch him. Symptoms of *mal de ojo* are sometimes vague, but the baby is usually very unhappy, cries continuously, cannot sleep, and may even die (Lacay, 1981). The cure is to find the person who is thought to have given the infant the evil eye and have her or him touch the baby. Lactation consultants working with such clients should take care to touch the baby when admiring him or her to avoid being thought of as the cause of a later case of *mal de ojo.*

Babies often are outfitted with special ornaments or bands that have a specific purpose. Hispanic grandmothers often worry a great deal about the infant's umbilicus and may insist that the baby wear a bellyband (*fajita*) to prevent an umbilical hernia. A traditional necklace protects the Laotian newborn. Babies in Papua New Guinea are protected from disease by special rituals, such as blackening the top of the baby's head with burnt coconut husk (Lepowsky, 1985).

Maternal Foods

Whether she lives on a mountaintop in remote Tibet, in a dusty Mexican village, or in an American suburb or urban high-rise apartment, the lactating woman produces milk that is amazingly homogeneous in composition, despite the wide diversity of foods she consumes. Only the milk of a woman who is severely malnourished will be measurably diminished in its nutrient content and volume because body nutrients are depleted before the milk suffers.

Part of understanding a culture involves becoming acquainted with its foodways—the way in which a distinct group selects, prepares, consumes, and otherwise uses portions of the available food supply. For more than half the inhabitants of this planet, including lactating women, beans, rice, and grains are daily fare. Fruits and vegetables appear seasonally, and meat is found in the family cooking pot only on special occasions. When it does appear, it is usually poultry, goat, horse, or dog, rather than beef. In most cultures, meat plays a minor part in flavoring rice, beans, and vegetables, not the major role it has served in affluent Western industrialized countries.

The daily food pattern of a breastfeeding Mexican mother who eats very little meat might concern us if we did not have a basic knowledge of amino acids and complementary proteins. Beans, a staple item in Mexican foodways, provide an incomplete protein when served alone, because they are low in methionine, an essential amino acid. This deficiency, however, is completely corrected when beans are served with a food high in methionine, such as whole grain breads or cereals. Complementary proteins can be obtained by numerous combinations. For example, eggs or a milk product will balance the protein and amino acids of a meal consisting primarily of plant proteins. However, two protein foods cannot complement each other if they have similar amino acids in their composition. For this reason, nuts and black-eyed peas are not complementary proteins, because both legumes lack the same amino acids.

"Hot" and "Cold" Foods

For many cultural groups, foods involve a balance that must be maintained to sustain health or be restored when illness occurs. Balance between opposing energy forces is based on the Greek theory of body humors. After centuries of dissemination throughout the world, this theory now appears as the hot (*caliente*) and cold (*frio* or *fresco*) system in Hispanic cultures. Other people, such as the Vietnamese, Chinese, East Indians, and Arabs, also use a hot–cold designation to some extent. Classifying foods as hot or cold in a given culture has little to do with their form, color, texture, or temperature, although hot foods are believed to be more easily digested than are cold foods. Instead, the classification is based on the food's effect on an illness or condition, which is itself categorized as hot or cold. During the last trimester of pregnancy, the unborn child is believed to be hot; therefore the mother is in a hot state. Once the child is born, accompanied by a loss of blood, a cold condition exists for both. To correct this imbalance, women believe that they need hot drinks and foods and to keep warm to replace heat and energy (Davis, 2001). Baths are taboo as exposure to water cools the body. Birthing in a hospital where postpartum showers are expected poses serious concerns for these mothers.

Traditional Chinese consider chicken, squash, and broccoli to be hot. Cold foods include melon, fruits, soybean sprouts, and bamboo shoots. In India, milk may be hot or cold, depending on where a person lives. In Hispanic cultures, cold foods include most fresh vegetables, tropical fruits, dairy products, beans, squash, and some meats. Hot foods—cereal grains, chili peppers, temperate-zone fruits, goat's milk, oils, and beef—serve to balance the cold foods. Because the potential listing of hot and cold foods in any particular culture is almost endless, health providers must do their ethnographic homework regarding the belief system of the cultures with whose members they are working. Among Southeast Asian women who delivered infants in the United States in the late 1990s, foods restricted after childbirth included all fruit. Postpartum foods are mainly rice and some boiled chicken. Garlic, black pepper, and ginger create warmth in the body and are encouraged (Davis, 2001).

Another belief system concerning food balance is the Chinese *yin-yang* theory. In America, people who use macrobiotics practice this system. Like the hot–cold theory, the basis of the *yin-yang* belief rests on a proper balance between opposing energy forces. On one side, yin represents "female," a negative force (cold, emptiness, darkness); on the other side, yang represents "male," a positive force (warmth, fullness, light). Too much of either yin or yang food is considered threatening to health. Whether a food is considered yin or yang depends on the effect it is thought to have on the body; the designation is not associated with color, texture, or other obvious characteristics. Without an extensive orientation for things Chinese, it is difficult to understand the "yin-ness" or "yang-ness" of food.

Herbs and Galactogogues

Almost all cultures abound with an array of certain foods for lactating women. In the past, beer and brewer's yeast have been touted as galactogogues— foods that are thought to increase milk secretion and improve let-down. Rice, gruel, soup, vegetables, and medicinal herbs may be used extensively by many cultures during the immediate postpartum period to promote the secretion of milk. Fenugreek tea is a popular galactogogue in the United States but is also used in many other parts of the world. Northern Mexicans make special teas from "hot" plants such as sesame and absinthe, and in some parts of Latin America herbal teas are drunk in the evening to stimulate milk for the morning (Baumslag, 1987). Herbs taken by the breastfeeding mother may have pharmacological effects on her baby, including irritation of the mucosal lining of the intestine and an increase in the release of flatus. Unless these symptoms become troublesome, it is more important for the mother to continue enjoying her favorite herbs in moderation than to stop using them because of her baby's minor stool changes. If the mothers within a particular ethnic group believe that certain foods can promote lactation, encourage these women to eat those foods. This practice gives a clear signal that the healthcare system supports breastfeeding and respects these cultural beliefs.

Weaning

Weaning is a time when childhood illness and death are more likely in developing countries; thus it is a key issue in studies of cross-cultural child care practices. Cultural assessment includes the timing of feeding, types of foods given to infants, and weaning practices. When a substantial proportion of dietary intake comes from food other than breastmilk, growth rates falter, and the effects of morbidity come into play. Woolridge (1991) suggests, as a rule of thumb, that when 25 to 50 percent of a baby's kilocalories come from breastmilk, the milk will protect the baby from environmental pathogens. At the same time, every breastfed infant reaches a point at which breastmilk alone can no longer meet its nutritional needs and solid foods are necessary.

Early solid and semisolid infant foods given by mothers vary widely across cultures, as does the timing of their introduction. Worldwide, there is a high rate of both the initiation of breastfeeding and early supplementation with other foods, even in maternity units certified as Baby Friendly (Alikasifoglu et al., 2001). Although infants in Papua New Guinea are not introduced to supplemental foods until 6 months (Lepowsky, 1985) (an optimal age), this is not a usual pattern. In a comparison study of how mothers feed their infants in four diverse countries, Winikoff, Castle, and Laukaran (1988) noted that early introduction of other foods is common. The majority of Kenyan babies are given foods other than breastmilk before they are 4 months old (Dimond & Ashworth, 1987; van Esterik & Elliott, 1986); in East Java, force-feeding by hand is a common practice from as early as few days after birth (van Steenbergen et al., 1991). Clearly, much has to be done before reaching the goal of exclusive breastfeeding.

Types of Weaning

Weaning from the breast is a process during which mothers gradually introduce their babies to cultur-ally assigned foods as they continue to breastfeed. Weaning begins with the introduction of sources of food other than breastmilk and ends with the last breastfeeding. Three types of weaning have been described:

- *Gradual weaning* that takes place over several weeks or months
- *Deliberate weaning*, a conscious effort initiated by the mother to end breastfeeding at a particular point
- *Abrupt weaning*, an immediate cessation of breastfeeding, which may be forced on the baby by the mother or on mother and baby by others.

Examples of gradual, deliberate, or abrupt weaning may be found in any culture. Gradual weaning, however, is the least traumatic, to both the infant and the mother.

Weaning practice can affect infant health, partic-ularly in developing countries or in inner-city areas in which weaning diarrhea is prevalent. In cultures in which food is available sporadically or is meager,

kwashiorkor, a severe form of protein deficiency, appears during the transition from breastmilk to other foods. In Ga, the language of Ghana, the term *kwashiorkor* means "the disease of the deposed baby." Identifying the reasons for women weaning early sheds considerable light on the beliefs and attitudes that influence the continuation of breastfeeding.

Various stages in infant development are sometimes used as cues to begin deliberate weaning. A common belief among African cultures is that the child should be walking before weaning is attempted. Some kind of independence is implicit in the concept of weaning, so it seems reasonable that the child be self-sufficient in locomotion before leaving the dependency of his mother's breast. In many Western cultures, teething is a developmental reference point thought to signal readiness to wean. In others, subsequent pregnancy signals the time to wean (Bohler & Ingstad, 1996). Usually a toddler or child will spontaneously wean with a new pregnancy. The reasons include a diminished milk supply, changes in the milk composition, and a less desirable taste.

For mammals, the length of lactation is positively correlated with adult female mass. Generally, larger mammals have long lactation periods (Hayssen, 1993). What is the "natural" age for weaning in humans? Dettwyler (1995) suggests four criteria associated with age at weaning in primates that range from 27 months to 7 years:

- *Weaning according to tripling or quadrupling of birth weight:* Using US data, male infants quadruple their birth weight by about 27 months and female infants by around 30 months.
- *Weaning according to attainment of one-third adult weight:* Weaning for the human would be predicted at between 4 and 7 years of age.
- *Weaning according to adult body size:* Using this comparison predicts the age for weaning in humans at between 2.8 and 3.7 years, with larger-bodied populations breastfeeding for the longest time.
- *Weaning according to time of dental eruption of permanent molars:* Modern humans' first molar eruption occurs around 5.5 to 6.0 years of age (the same time as that for adult immune competence).

Some rather harsh techniques have been used to bring about abrupt weaning. One time-honored method calls for pepper, garlic, ginger, or onion to be applied to the mother's breasts to discourage the baby from breastfeeding. In the Fiji Islands, weaning of kali ("to separate") is a 4-day period during which the breast is denied to the infant and the baby's food is specially cooked in a separate pot. The infant is not allowed to sleep with the mother until after weaning and is sometimes cared for by one of the mother's female relatives in another household for this period.

In cultures in which early weaning is a common practice, a minority of people accept long-term breastfeeding. The sight of a walking child calmly sliding onto the mother's lap for milk and deftly opening her buttons to gain access to her breasts is considered shocking and subject to ridicule in some cultures. The term *closet nursing* describes a practice that has evolved in the United States in response to criticism of breastfeeding that extends beyond the culture's expectations. In closet nursing, breastfeeding continues by mutual consent of mother and child, but only in secret. The mother and baby usually have a code word for breastfeeding that can be used in public (Wrigley & Hutchinson, 1990). In many Western cultures, teething is a developmental reference point thought to signal readiness to wean. In others, subsequent pregnancy signals the time to wean. Many toddlers will spontaneously wean with a new pregnancy because of a diminished milk supply and a less desirable taste (Bohler & Ingstad, 1996). Regardless of the culture, weaning is ideally a collaborative effort in which

---

BOX 24–1

Specific Folkways and Ways to Handle Them

- Touching the baby of a Spanish-speaking family while admiring him helps avoid giving the baby *mal de ojo*—the evil eye.
- An anemic breastfeeding mother who is not vegetarian believes that anemia is a yin condition. Suggest that she consume more meat, a yang food, to improve her iron status.
- A Korean mother refuses a cold pack for engorged breasts or for pain resulting from an episiotomy. Offer her cool water from a washcloth or from a peri bottle.
- A mother expects a 40-day period of special care postpartum. Respect the tradition and help her through early discharge with one or more home visits.

- A baby burps during feedings. According to some Hispanic mothers, this air goes to the breast and stops the flow of milk, causing her milk duct to become plugged. Ask her to switch to the other breast and then back to the first breast to release the "air."
- A mother believes that colostrum is "bad." Suggest that she express the first few drops of "impure" milk and discard it before putting the baby to breast, then say, "the sooner you breastfeed, the better the milk."
- Avoid serving ice water or cold drinks to a new mother from Southeast Asia.

both the mother and baby reach a state of readiness to begin weaning.

Implications for Practice

Every culture has its visible elements (housing, clothing, food) and its invisible elements (attitudes, tradition, values); an understanding of both contributes significantly to communication between the breastfeeding client and the healthcare provider. Some Spanish-speaking folkways and how to handle them are seen in Box 24–1. Immigrant mothers may be served foods that traditionally are forbidden to postpartum women, such as raw vegetables and fruit for Vietnamese mothers. Lactation consultants working in these birthing areas can make sure that alternate foods are provided to these women.

Many Indochinese women living in the United States formula-feed their infant, at least while in the hospital, and then both breastfeed and bottle-feed after leaving the hospital; therefore, formula discharge packs are not appropriate. It is advisable to have women health workers care for these mothers, because they regard it as improper for men to touch a woman's body (especially the breasts). If mothers in any culture believe that certain foods can promote lactation, these women should be encouraged to bring these foods to the postpartum unit. This practice will enhance breastfeeding and provide a clear signal that the healthcare system supports breastfeeding and is respectful of these cultural beliefs.

Regardless of the culture, weaning is ideally a collaborative effort in which both the mother and baby reach a state of readiness to begin weaning. In a culture in which unrestricted breastfeeding is practiced and in which the child breastfeeds for a prolonged period, the mother has very little ambivalence when she decides to wean and says, "You, child, have had enough milk!" (Mead & Newton, 1967).

Though weaning practices vary from culture to culture, weaning is thought to be the least traumatic when it is slow, gradual, and related to the needs of the child. It is essential to identify factors that influence continuation or early termination of breastfeeding so as to develop appropriate programs to assist the mother who wishes to maintain breastfeeding. Women involved in long-term breastfeeding develop a special bond with their baby. The mother's choice of how long she wishes to breastfeed is an individual right that may not mesh with others' expectations. All breastfeeding families deserve to be treated in a nonjudgmental manner that accepts the cultural diversity that they represent.

Summary

The study of child-rearing patterns of a given culture is crucial to all healthcare professionals who work with new and growing families. The seeds of a culture are planted, grow, and thrive in child-rearing patterns. Cultural awareness provides liberation from egocentric views in which one looks at the universe and sees only one's beliefs in the center. The study of any culture begins with critical self-reflection and awareness of the differences between one's cultural values and those of other people. By becoming aware of these differences, we begin a process of partnership in which all groups have something to contribute and something to learn. Although acculturation to the United States generally has a negative effect on breastfeeding, it can be offset if the mother receives support from healthcare providers, friends and family, and other social institutions (Cricco-Lizza, 2005; Thiel de Bocanegra, 1998).

Analysis of infant feeding within its cultural context is critically linked to social action and policy decisions regarding breastfeeding promotion and teaching. For those who examine cultural issues carefully, so-called cultural obstacles to solving problems usually include the solutions, too. Within the cultural context of underlying infant-feeding problems, solutions must ultimately emerge. If changes are to last, they must originate from within a culture, rather than being imposed from without.

Thiel de Bocanegra H. Breast-feeding in immigrant women: the role of social support and acculturation. *Hispani J Behav Sci.* 2008;20(4):448–467.

Thorley V. Sharing breastmilk: wet-nursing, cross-feeding, and milk donations. *Breastfeeding Rev.* 2008;16:25–29.

United States Census Bureau. Population estimates July 1, 2000-July 1, 2006. http://www.census.gov/population/www/socdemo/hispanic/hispanic.html. Accessed May 10, 2008.

van Esterik P, Elliott T. Infant feeding style in urban Kenya. *Ecol Food Nutr.* 1986;18:183–195.

van Steenbergen WM et al. Nutritional transition during pregnancy in East Java, Indonesia: I. A longitudinal study of feeding pattern, breastmilk intake and the consumption of additional foods. *Eur J Clin Nurs.* 1991;45:67–75.

Whittemore RD, Beverly EA. Mandinka mothers and nurslings: power and reproduction. *Med Anthropol Q.* 1996;10:45–62.

Winikoff B, Castle MA, Laukaran VH, eds. *Feeding Infants in Four Societies: Causes and Consequences of Mothers' Choices.* New York, NY: Greenwood Press; 1988:187–201.

Woolridge M. *Breastfeeding in the US and Thailand* [presentation]. Miami, FL: International Lactation Consultant Association; 1991.

Wrigley EA, Hutchinson S. Long-term breastfeeding: the secret bond. *J Nurse Midwifery.* 1990;35:35–41.

The Familial and Social Context of Breastfeeding

Karen Wambach and Jan Riordan

WHEN HEALTHCARE PROFESSIONALS help a breastfeeding mother and baby, they help a family. The breastfeeding family exists in a social context; therefore, care providers must recognize "family" as a group that is variously defined and experienced. They need to know about the family from which the mother comes and into which her child will be born and reared. Although every family is expected to perform similar functions, the ways in which those functions are recognized and accomplished will vary.

This chapter examines the family from a developmental perspective. The birth of a baby has rightly been described as a crisis because it forces new ways of behavior on all family members. This chapter discusses issues pertaining to the development of spousal–partner and parent–child attachment, paying particular attention to the father's role as a helpmate and supporter of his partner's role as mother and as breastfeeder. It also addresses the special needs of the adolescent mother, the adoptive mother and family, women living in poverty and finally, considers certain negative family experiences, including violence against women and children.

Family Forms and Functions

Every individual experiences many family forms during a lifetime. Each form meets different needs and serves different functions. A *traditional family* is one in which the mother is a full-time homemaker and primarily responsible for rearing the children, while her husband is a full-time worker outside the home. He is committed to seeing that the children are raised to adulthood, but his role in child rearing is seen as secondary to that of his wife. Although this form has often been viewed as ideal, it is experienced by a much smaller percentage of families than in the mid-1900s (US Department of Labor, 2007). A *nuclear family* includes one or both parents and their children, either born to or adopted by them. An *extended family* usually contains lateral kin (such as aunts, uncles, or cousins) who occupy the same generational status as the parents and children in a nuclear family; or vertical kin (such as grandparents or grandchildren), who represent generations different from the parents and children in the nuclear family. In some cases, an extended family may include "fictive" kin, individuals who cannot trace lineage through blood or marriage ties to the nuclear family members but who act, and are treated, as if they were related (Friedman, Bowden & Jones, 2003).

Examining how different family forms are likely to be experienced throughout an individual's lifetime can provide insight into the stresses that an individual is likely to encounter. It also reveals the people on whom an individual will lean as he or she attempts to cope with those stresses.

Today's families increasingly recognize that child rearing will occupy only a portion of the entire life experience of a couple (regardless of the number of relationships experienced). Though a baby may be the outcome and reflection of the love its parents feel for one another, the presence of a baby nearly always adds stress to the new family unit (Cox, Paley, Burchinal, & Payne, 1999; Rovine & Belsky, 1990; Twenge, Campbell, & Foster, 2003).

One way to identify how babies represent potential and ongoing stress for the couple is to recognize how family interaction patterns are affected by the addition of a new member. The couple relationship is easy to understand. Each member of the couple relates to the other. Add one child and two new relationships are added: one linking mother to child and one linking father to child. In addition, the couple is now husband and wife and mother and father. In assuming these roles, each partner may view the other in new ways that are not always supportive of a continued spousal role. When another child is added, the relationships become even more complex. The mother and the father each have a new relationship with the new baby. And a sibling relationship is added. Thus, in a two-person household, two relationships exist. In a three-person household, three relationships exist; in a four-person household, six relationships exist (Figure 25–1). With each new person added to the family, more than one new relationship is also added, because each person interacts with all other family members.

Family Theory

Numerous types of theories have been applied to understanding how families work, what influences them to work effectively, and how best to offer assistance when they do not. A developmental approach seems particularly appropriate to healthcare providers assisting families by recognizing that they expand and

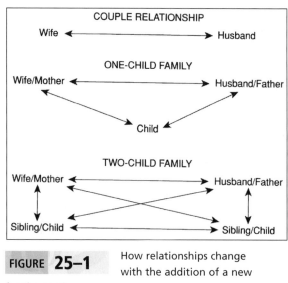

FIGURE 25–1 How relationships change with the addition of a new family member.

contract at different times, based on the addition or launching of children (Rodgers & White, 1993). Thus, over time and based on a stage approach, a given family is likely to experience a couple stage, an expansion stage, a stable stage, and a launching stage.

Most families begin as *couples* and then move to the *expansion stage,* which begins with the first pregnancy and continues until the birth of the last child. In some families, this stage may be very brief, the duration of one pregnancy only; in other families, it might last more than two decades as new infants are added to the family. The *stable stage* occurs when members are neither added nor taken away. This stage is followed by the *launching stage,* which begins when the oldest child leaves home, and it continues until the only individuals remaining in the home are the original couple or their replacements in the family (if one or both of the original couple has remarried). However one views the family from a developmental perspective, the number of stages identified is not nearly as important as are the tasks expected of the family at different times in the family career or family life course.

The healthcare worker assisting breastfeeding mothers is most likely to interact with members of families during the expansion phase of the family's life course. It is important to recognize that varying tasks characterize this phase of the family in order to identify how those tasks will influence decision making and behavior related to infant feeding and other aspects of the early mother–child relationship.

Social Factors that Influence Breastfeeding

The role of supportive significant others in the breastfeeding mother's life cannot be overemphasized. Social support is the mobilization and access to interpersonal resources when an individual attempts to deal with the stress and strains of life. Social support includes emotional support, instrumental support, appraisal support, and informational support (House, 1981; Hughes, 1984). Freedom of choice regarding infant-feeding decisions is always couched within the social context in which it occurs. Thus, for example, in a family in which extended breastfeeding is viewed as aberrant behavior, it is unlikely that the mother will choose to continue breastfeeding unless she receives a preponderance of positive, or at least neutral, reactions from her significant others. In another family in which breastfeeding is viewed as just another activity of 2- or 3-year-olds, extended breastfeeding is far more likely to occur. The interaction of mother and baby with significant others and their acceptance and/or approval of such breastfeeding behavior must be taken into account when determining how best to assist her (Hills-Bonczyk et al., 1994; Rempel, 2004).

In addition to social support, Table 25–1 summarizes some of the variables that affect breastfeeding and can be influenced by the healthcare provider. The results of numerous studies have consistently revealed that the mother's *intention* to breastfeed is the single most important factor in deciding whether she will start breastfeeding and how long she will continue. Research findings have also shown us that intention is linked to social support and influence, the mother's attitude, and her confidence in herself regarding breastfeeding. For example, most lactation consultants can report that they have worked with women whose firm intention to breastfeed resulted in their overcoming all types of adversity in order to continue nursing; conversely, LCs can also describe cases where a mother has plenty of breastmilk and the baby is gaining weight well, yet for no obvious reason she weans the baby. We may possibly assume that her intention was not to breastfeed (at least not for very long). Intention is

invisible, but it can be measured with research tools (see Chapter 22).

Coupled with intention to breastfeed and maternal attitude toward breastfeeding, support systems influence choices (e.g., Kessler et al., 1995). In an older study, Kaufman and Hall (1989) found that women who gave birth to preterm babies and who identified no source of support were six times more likely to stop breastfeeding than were women with a support system. Those most likely to continue breastfeeding could identify several persons who supported their feeding decision. As with mothers of preterm infants, research reveals that teenage mothers also tend to breastfeed longer when they have a support system whose members affirm, aid, and affect in specific practical ways their mothering behavior, including breastfeeding (Nelson & Sethi, 2005; Wambach & Cole, 2000).

Social support also influences the timing of weaning the baby from the breast (Kendall-Tackett & Sugarman, 1995; Morse & Harrison, 1987; Rempel, 2004). Usually pressure from family members to wean and others is more likely as the baby approaches or exceeds the age of 12 months. The support of others moves gradually from actively supporting breastfeeding in the first few months of the baby's life, to tolerating breastfeeding, to ignoring breastfeeding, to actively encouraging weaning. This last stage usually is manifested sometime after the baby's 6th month and may grow markedly stronger after the baby's 12th month in the developed world, when others view the baby as too old to breastfeed.

Social support is especially important in the period immediately following any life stress. As noted previously, one such stress, insofar as it necessitates changes in relationships and life patterns, is childbirth. Another is breastfeeding, particularly if the mother has not breastfed an older child, or if she is the first in her family or group of friends to do so. Very often, mothers and others assume that the mode of feeding is the cause of other infant behaviors. Lower-income, first-time mothers are more likely to breastfeed, and to remain feeding the baby mother's milk when the mothers received support and information before, during, and after the baby's birth. Disadvantaged and younger American mothers tend to follow the advice of their own mothers, especially if the two live in the same house

TABLE 25–1	**How Healthcare Providers Can Influence Factors That Affect Breastfeeding**	
Factor	**Influence**	**Studies**
Social support, social approval, social stigma	Women with greater access to support choose to breastfeed more frequently and breastfeed longer. Support is manifested differently across ethnic and social groups. Support and social approval decrease and social stigma increases with long-term breastfeeding in Western societies.	Balcazar, Trier, & Cobas, 1995; Bar-Yam & Darby, 1997; Kaufman & Hall, 1989; Kendall-Tackett & Sugarman, 1995; Kessler et al., 1995; Hills-Bonczyk et al., 1994; Rempel, 2004
Intention to breastfeed	The majority of pregnant women decide how they will feed their baby before or early in pregnancy. A consistent positive association exists between intended and actual duration of breastfeeding.	Blyth et al., 2004; Chapman & Perez-Escamilla, 2000; Grossman et al., 1990; Losch, Dungy, & Russell, 1995; Rempel, 2004; Wambach, 1997
Attitude toward breastfeeding	There is increased breastfeeding initiation and duration by women with a positive attitude.	Avery et al., 1998; Janke, 1994; Rempel, 2004; Tarkka, Paunonen, & Laippala, 1999
Mother's confidence, breastfeeding self-efficacy, perceived behavioral control	Women with high confidence breastfeed longer than women with low confidence.	Blyth et al., 2004; Boettcher et al., 1999; Chezem, Friesen, & Boettcher, 2003; Dennis & Faux, 1999; O'Campo et al., 1992; Rempel, 2004
Staff knowledge and attitudes toward breastfeeding	Lack of appropriate breastfeeding knowledge in hospital staff is a barrier to assistance from nurses and breastfeeding support.	Balcazar, Trier, & Cobas, 1995; Bernaix, 2000; Coreil et al., 1995; Freed et al., 1996; Lazzaro, Anderson, & Auld, 1995

(Wiemann et al., 1998). Healthcare workers should recognize the grandmother as a key informant and network person and involve her in health care and advice giving.

Mothers who choose to combine breastfeeding and bottle-feeding have not been studied well but may make this choice to reap the infant health benefits of breastfeeding and to avoid embarrassment if they are not able to provide sufficiently for their infants (Boettcher et al., 1999), or it may be due to ambivalence associated with their own developmental or confidence levels, as in teenage mothers (Wambach & Koehn, 2004). Lactation consultants may have the greatest influence on the mother who is undecided about infant feeding. Early studies indicated that healthcare workers are not viewed as consistent support resources for breastfeeding. However, newer research and secondary analysis of these older data found that prenatal education was a strong predictor of intentions to breastfeed (Dennis, 2001).

The racial or ethnic group with which the mother identifies influences whose advice she seeks and follows relating to childbearing and breastfeeding. For example, among low-income Anglo-American women, the male partner, the mother's own mother, the grandmother, and the best friend tend to support breastfeeding. This pattern, with the exception of the best friend, is seen among Mexican-Americans as well. However, in a study of 100 breastfeeding and 100 bottle-feeding women, Giugliani et al. (1994) concluded that, regardless of maternal age, education level, ethnicity, and marital status, women who indicated that their partners preferred breastfeeding were significantly more likely to initiate breastfeeding when compared with women whose partners were ambivalent or preferred bottle-feeding (OR = 32.8, 95% CI = 6.7–159.5).

In contrast, there is some evidence that black women choose breastfeeding because of the information and encouragement they received from their physician during prenatal care (Bentley et al., 1999) or bottle-feeding because of lack of encouragement from healthcare providers (Wiemann et al., 1998), and they reported minimal support from family members. In a qualitative study based on interviews (Corbett, 2000), an African-American woman told of the curiosity of friends who wanted to watch her because they had never seen a woman breastfeed. Breastfeeding seemed to them to be an unfamiliar and uncertain activity. This was reflected in a lower rate of breastfeeding than other groups. A more recent study in the southern United States validated the influence of family and personal experiences with the choice to initiate and continue breastfeeding (Meyerink & Marquis, 2002). Among a random sample of 150 mothers (93 percent African-American) at a county health clinic in Birmingham, Alabama, only 41 percent of women initiated breastfeeding, 24 percent breastfed for at least 1 month, and 8.3 percent breastfed for 3 months or more. Initiation of breastfeeding was positively associated with the mother having been breastfed herself and having breastfed a previous infant. Breastfeeding at and beyond 1 month was more likely among older women and women with close relatives who breastfed, and the mother having been breastfed and having breastfed a previous infant, respectively. These findings highlight that family influence and role modeling are important to choices, and that such support could potentially come from a peer counselor or "surrogate mother" as suggested by these researchers.

For many Southeast Asian women, the mother-in-law is traditionally the person who makes decisions and gives advice about childbearing and child raising, including breastfeeding (Schneiderman, 1996). Most of the Vietnamese women who chose to breastfeed were encouraged by the experiences of significant others: "My mum breastfed all her nine children in Vietnam. She said breastmilk is good for a baby," and "My mother-in-law and my husband both wanted me to breastfeed, particularly because this is our first child" (Rossiter & Yam, 2000).

Generally, the more support a mother has for breastfeeding, the more likely she is to initiate and continue. Healthcare workers should make clear their support of breastfeeding and encourage other family members to support this choice as well. After discharge from the hospital, the degree of support that new mothers have at home is critical. It is imperative that the healthcare provider learns whether the new mother will have someone to whom she can turn once she is at home. If she does not, steps need to be taken to provide follow-up support or to arrange for home visitation by a hospital or social service organizations that provide such assistance. In addition, much of the teaching that is viewed as appropriate during the postpartum period may have to be shifted to a prenatal setting in order to free what little time is available at discharge for key planning issues.

Studies tell us that certain characteristics are associated with breastfeeding over which healthcare providers have no control, but it is helpful to be knowledgeable about their effects. Furthermore, these characteristics are often associated with vulnerable populations and can be targeted for breastfeeding promotion and support efforts (Table 25–2). When attempting to provide ongoing information and help, particularly when that help is provided outside an institutional setting, the healthcare provider and LC need to be aware of the social support system, whether familial or community based, that the mother can tap.

Fathers

Fathers are often the most influential support persons prior to birth in feeding decisions and throughout the breastfeeding period (Bar-Yam & Darby, 1997; Gorman, Byrd, & VanDerslice, 1995; Giugliani et al., 1994; Pavill, 2002). In a study of culturally diverse fathers, 81 percent wanted their babies to be breastfed; more African-American men indicated they preferred their infants to be breastfed than had been reported in any previous study (Pollock, Bustamante-Forest, & Giaratano, 2002). Similarly, Preston (2004) reported in her qualitative study of infant feeding among African-American teenage mothers, that the adolescent fathers were pleased with the participants choosing to breastfeed their infants.

When helping to care for a family breastfeeding a new baby, the healthcare provider and/or lactation consultant can gather information by paying attention to the father. Fathers' reactions to their breastfeeding

TABLE 25–2	**Factors That Affect Breastfeeding Over Which Healthcare Providers Have No Influence**	

Factor	Influence	Studies
Maternal age	Older women are more likely to choose to breastfeed and to breastfeed for a longer period.	Callen & Pinelli, 2004; Chapman & Perez-Escamilla, 2000; Nolan & Goel, 1995
Socioeconomic status	Varies by culture; women in higher SES levels in United States are more likely to breastfeed.	Callen & Pinelli, 2004; Raisler, 2000
Maternal education	Women with more education are more likely to breastfeed; varies according to culture.	Callen & Pinelli, 2004; Nolan & Goel, 1995
Maternal employment	Although not associated with breastfeeding initiation, employment is likely to shorten breastfeeding duration.	Arthur, Saenz, & Replogle, 2003; Chapman & Perez-Escamilla, 2000; Dodgson & Duckett, 1997; Fein & Roe, 1998; Kimbro, 2006; Novotny et al., 2000; Roe et al., 1999; Ryan et al., 2006; Visness & Kennedy, 1997
Previous breastfeeding	Experienced breastfeeders are more likely to breastfeed longer than those without previous experience.	Boettcher et al., 1999; Meyerink & Marquis, 2002; Wambach, 1997

babies vary a great deal. Some will enthusiastically participate in putting the baby to breast, making suggestions, and generally helping. Others, often first-time fathers, will hang back and observe but not interact. A few of these first-time dads look shell-shocked with the first few breastfeedings—perhaps partly due to the unfamiliarity of having their wife's breasts exposed. Alternatively, fathers may feel like they have little control in the situation in which mothers and infants are the focus of attention. In a recent study of transition to first-time fatherhood it was suggested that early postpartum experiences, with the afore-mentioned focus on mother and infant, could compound feelings of inadequacy in new fathers (Buist et al., 2003). Thus, informing expectant and new fathers of their expected roles relative to the care of the infant, as well as support of the mother, is important to their feelings of adequacy, paternal role development, and subsequent mental well-being.

When fathers enter into caregiving roles from the first with their infants, they are more likely to feel that they are an important part of the baby's life and have bonded more readily (Goodman, 2005; Pavill,

2002). See Figure 25–2. When teaching the mother how to put the baby to breast, involve the father by asking him to help with the breastfeeding—meaning placing the baby, helping to control the baby's hands and arms, burping, and so on. Likewise, when giving discharge instructions, address the father as well as the mother. The mother, already overloaded with stress, may not remember what you are saying, but fathers often pay close attention to what is said, sometimes adding questions of their own to the mother's questions.

Examinations of the ways in which men evolve into fathers suggests that the role remains relatively invisible to others; it is a relatively passive reflection of what is happening to the pregnant wife until after the baby's birth. When the baby begins to interact with the father directly, the father's role becomes more explicit—in his own mind as well as in the awareness of others (Goodman, 2005; Jordan & Wall, 1993). Nurturing is a fundamental human quality that need not be gender specific. That many view it as feminine must be seen as a cultural artifact rather than a reflection of inherent differences between males and females.

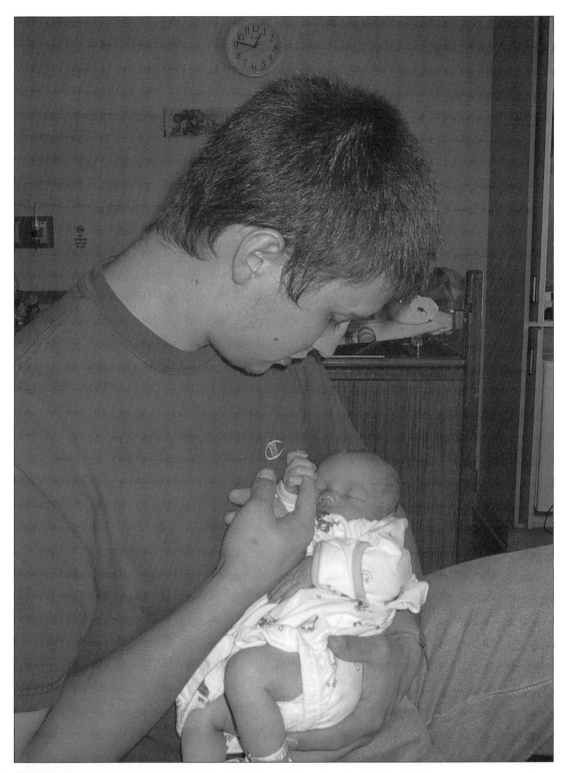

FIGURE 25–2 A father attaches to his baby in much the same way as the mother.

Fathers play a vital role as a supporter of breast-feeding, particularly when they have a positive mind-set relating to breastfeeding (Earle, 2000; Pavill, 2002). Thus prenatal discussions of infant feeding in childbirth and breastfeeding classes are effective in allaying concerns and dispelling myths. Humor is a perfect way to reach and help allay the father's anxieties about the coming baby and their role in the breastfeeding experience. The use of Neil Matterson's cartoons in prenatal classes gets fathers to open up to discuss issues related to breastfeeding (see Other Resources at the end of this chapter). Prenatal classes are also ideal for teaching fathers the benefits of breastfeeding, the physiology of lactation, and for informing a father of how he can help his breastfeeding wife without having to feed the baby. Jordan and Wall (1994) suggested father-only classes in which fathers could communicate openly with one another and have experiences in practicing skills that would be important for them in the care of their infants. The early days of fathering can be as stressful and disruptive to the father as mothering is to the mother (St. John et al., 2005). A synthesis of qualitative study findings indicated that the birth of an infant strains the couple relationship (Goodman, 2005). Furthermore, some fathers report jealousy of the physical and emotional closeness of mother and infant, feelings of uselessness during breast-feeding, sexual frustration, and repulsion from the sight of full, dripping breasts. Some fathers feel ashamed of these emotions and tend not to talk about them, or they may joke about being jealous of the new baby (Gamble & Morse, 1993; Jordan & Wall, 1990).

The most comfortable place for fathers to express these feelings is with other new fathers, many of whom may conceal the same feelings. Childbirth education classes, La Leche League groups, and online discussions for fathers (see Other Resources at end of chapter) provide communication outlets in which new fathers can openly share their feelings and perceptions about the realities of parenthood in an atmosphere of unconditional acceptance. Experienced fathers can help one another realize that they are not alone in having ambivalent feelings about the close-ness between their breastfeeding wives and babies and about giving up certain pleasures in exchange for new responsibilities. One such father offered this report:

If I'd been more prepared that they would be this complete unit unto themselves, it would have been easier. For a while I felt left out, like I was around only to bring home the money and wasn't a part of it. I felt bad, then guilty about feeling bad. Before the baby came, my wife really spoiled me, you know, really adored and lavished attention on me. Then, whammo, she was pregnant 3 months after we were married and I wasn't getting that kind of treatment anymore. I resented it. Things really broke loose and we had a showdown; I finally had to open up and let her know how I really felt. After that, when it was all in the open, things got better. With the next baby, I don't think I'll go through those feelings again.

Support groups for new fathers validate a commitment to recognize the needs of new fathers—to help them develop coping strategies for optimal and involved parenting of their breastfed baby. These father groups tend to attract men who are having more difficulty or who are more open in admitting to feeling stressed by making adjustments. These actions can potentially strengthen family relationships in the years ahead.

Implicit in the notion that breastfeeding prevents father–child closeness is acceptance of the assumption that the most (perhaps the only) significant way in which a father can interact with his child is by feeding her or him. Encourage the father to consider the many ways in which he can interact with the baby, particularly during the very early period when artificial feeding may increase the risk of breastfeeding failure (Figure 25–3). Several options are available:

- *Burping the baby after a feeding:* The necessity of burping is less an issue than is the opportunity to frequently hold the baby when the infant is likely to be relaxed and somnolent; if a burp is obtained, the father also gains a sense of having accomplished something tangible that can be translated to mean "I am a good father."
- *Changing the baby's wet diapers:* This activity occurs frequently.
- *Changing the baby's soiled diapers:* This, too, occurs frequently and, in breastfed infants, is

far less unpleasant because the odor is less noxious than are the soiled diapers of a formula-fed baby.

- *Giving the baby a massage:* Fathers who massage their babies often find that they can put a baby to sleep with little effort; such activity can assist an over-stimulated or colicky baby to relax sufficiently to fall asleep.
- *Bathing the baby:* Assisting with the baby's bath is usually most happily accomplished after the baby begins to enjoy the bath.
- *Rocking the baby:* The father's involvement with the baby frees the mother to engage in other activities.
- *Singing or reading to the baby:* This activity can begin as soon after birth as the father wishes. Often, repeating the same songs that were played during the pregnancy will result in clear signals of recognition by the baby.
- *Playing with the baby:* Generally occurs as the infant ages and is more alert and receptive to interaction.

The Adolescent Mother

Adolescent motherhood presents many social and personal challenges to the individual mother, her family, and society. Although fewer adolescents in the United States are becoming pregnant than in the early 1990s, US rates remain higher than many other industrialized countries (Allan Guttmacher Institute, 2006). Breastfeeding rates among adolescent mothers, although improving according to recent surveys generally are lower than adult women (Li et al., 2005; Scanlon et al., 2007), and they often breastfeed for a much shorter period of time. Older adolescents are more likely to breastfeed than younger ones (Wambach & Cole, 2000).

Many caregivers assume that the young mother is neither interested in giving nor ready to give to another person by breastfeeding. On the contrary, a significant percentage of adolescents consider breastfeeding an option even if they ultimately bottle-feed (Leffler, 2000; Wiemann et al., 1998; Wambach & Koehn, 2004). Many of those who breastfeed make their decision before pregnancy or in the early stages of pregnancy, which suggests that adolescent mothers may be responsive to prenatal

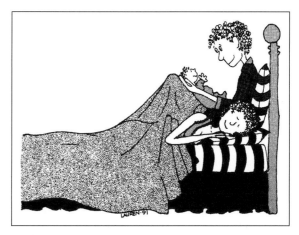

FIGURE **25-3** One of the many ways a dad helps with the care of a new baby.

intervention to promote breastfeeding (Wambach & Cole, 2000; Wambach & Cohen, in press). The volume and properties in breastmilk of adolescents and adults are almost the same. Study data that report that adolescents produce less milk than women beyond the teen years are drawn from adolescent subjects who typically breastfeed less frequently and introduce formula earlier than do adult mothers (Motil, Kertz, & Thotathuchery, 1997).

Role modeling and peer influence are powerful tools for altering adolescent behavior. Not surprisingly, Wiemann, DuBois, and Berenson (1998) found that using a breastfeeding video geared to teens was a key intervention to help adolescents overcome perceived barriers to breastfeeding. Likewise when Volpe and Bear (2000) started a Breastfeeding Educated and Supported Teen (BEST) Club, more teenagers subsequently breastfed than those preceding the implementation of the club. Martens (2001) randomized breastfeeding education sessions that included a video to Canadian Ojibwa adolescents whose beliefs about breastfeeding subsequently improved. In another study, almost all (82 percent) participants in an Australian program for pregnant teenagers decided to breastfeed after attending prenatal classes (Greenwood & Littlejohn, 2002). Most recently, Wambach and colleagues have completed the first randomized control trial in the United States to promote and support breastfeeding in 15–18-year-olds using education and support from an LC and peer counselor team, and have found significant differences in initiation and duration of breastfeeding between the experimental and control group subjects (unpublished data).

Concern about keeping their figure and not gaining weight concerns new mothers of all ages, but it is of particular concern to adolescents (Wambach & Cole, 2000). A study of Korean adolescents tested an intervention using a video that explained misconceptions about breastfeeding including body changes. Apparently the video did not positively impact the adolescents' views, reporting that breastfeeding might make them gain weight and "lose" their figure (Kim, 1998). As in other studies (Wambach & Koehn, 2004; Hannon et al., 2000), these adolescents reported that "embarrassment" was a major barrier to breastfeeding. Fear of pain related to breastfeeding also is a major factor in deciding whether or not to breastfeed. Wambach and Koehn (2004) encouraged healthcare providers to assist pregnant teens with the overall decision-making process by evaluating developmental level of the teen as well as knowledge level. These are important aspects of adolescent decision-making processes (Mann et al., 1989).

Teen mothers, when asked to identify their needs after the birth of their baby, identified the infant's health and medical needs first, followed by daily physical care of the infant, psychosocial needs of mothers and babies, and, finally, the mother's physical care. Mothers rated information about how to breastfeed and care for the breasts as important or very important. This high level of interest in meeting their baby's needs suggests that teen mothers are likely to be motivated to follow advice when it is offered. However, because many teenage mothers often share social characteristics that are linked with the choice not to breastfeed—such as lower educational attainment, low income, and unmarried status—fewer of these young women will choose to breastfeed (Peterson & Da Vanzo, 1992).

Usually, questions of new adolescent mothers are no different from those of older, more experienced women except for concerns about embarrassment with public exposure (Hannon et al., 2000; Wambach & Cohen, in press). Most new mothers are concerned about how to help a baby grasp the breast, how to avoid sore nipples, and how to provide sufficient milk. In contrast, the kind of assistance offered to teens depends on their life

situation. The teen mother living alone may need more frequent assistance and referral to a breastfeeding support group. The teen mother living with her own mother—who may be caring for the baby while the teen is in school—may need to know about resources on which she can draw for additional information and support about breastfeeding. The teen mother living with the baby's father or another male adult needs to know how to balance her baby's needs and needs of the couple relationship. In general, support needs of teenage mothers are as great, or greater than the older mothers, and developmental and social status may impede the teen's ability to reach out for assistance when needed (Dykes et al., 2003; Nelson & Sethi, 2004; Wambach & Cohen, in press). Therefore, the healthcare provider and/or lactation consultant must anticipate needs more accurately and efficiently and also teach the teen how to solicit help when needed. Finally, to facilitate longer duration of breastfeeding (e.g., continued breastfeeding after return to school), resources for obtaining a breast pump are important for the healthcare provider to assist the teenage mother (Hannon et al., 2000; Wambach et al., 2007). The breastfeeding experience of the teenage mother, of whatever duration, helps her to progress toward adulthood with a stronger and more positive sense of self and motherhood and will likely influence a repeat breastfeeding decision for future children.

The Adoptive Mother and Family

Little is written regarding the breastfeeding experience of the adoptive mother who induces lactation (Cheales-Siebenaler, 1999). Obviously the woman who induces lactation for the nourishment of her adoptive child faces several challenges physically. More adoptive mothers are choosing to induce lactation given the process of inducing lactation has been improved. Yet some women may not know the opportunity to induce lactation is a possibility. In describing her experience with nursing her adoptive daughter, Lorraine Hawke commented that initially she did not know about induced lactation and she actually questioned its naturalness (Hawke et al., 2005). However, knowing the nutritional benefits of human milk for the infant convinced this 40-year-old woman that it was the right thing to do. Family support was necessary for the decision as exemplified by this quote:

> My husband said he would fully support whatever I decided. My brothers' and sisters' responses differed from disbelief, to thinking I was nuts, to wondering how it would work and why I would want to do it, to excitement. In the end, they all supported my actions. Afterwards, the key response was fascination that I really could breastfeed without having been pregnant (p. 18).

The story further describes the challenges of inducing lactation beginning one month before the birth using breast stimulation via pumping and use of domperidone and oxytocin spray. A lactation consultant, a midwife, and the birth mother, who was a relative, supported this mother during the rigorous process. The benefits of nursing proved to be much more than nutritional for this mother. Like birth mothers who breastfeed, Lorraine Hawke described a deep bond was developed through breastfeeding with her adopted daughter. Lactation consultants play an important role in supporting the adoptive mother in this important process.

The Low-Income Family

In the United States and other developed countries, fewer low-income mothers than their more affluent countrywomen choose to breastfeed. Poor women, whose babies most need the benefits of human milk, including its far lower production cost and its marked safety as compared to artificial baby milk, are least likely to breastfeed. As more women in the developing world seek to emulate women in the developed world, the cost to these women and the countries in which they live will be even higher.

Background variables can predict whether a low-income woman will breastfeed. Grossman et al. (1989) found that if a poor woman was married, if she had at least a high school education, if she began prenatal care in the first trimester, and if she was white or Hispanic, she was more likely to breastfeed. Libbus and Kolostov (1994) report that if the maternal grandmother breastfed and if the male

partner endorsed breastfeeding, the low-income women in their study were more likely to intend to breastfeed and to view it as a positive experience. As described earlier in this chapter, role modeling and the mother's own previous breastfeeding experiences are very strong predictors of breastfeeding among low-income African-American women (Meyerink & Marquis, 2002).

Environmental efforts to support low-income women's efforts to breastfeed are important to decreasing breastfeeding disparities across race and income levels. Cricco-Lizza (2004) interviewed 109 low-income black women enrolled in a WIC clinic in New York City and found that trusting and respectful relationships between WIC personnel and these women influenced their breastfeeding decision positively.

Lack of Information

Sometimes the reasons for not breastfeeding are related to lack of information. In fact the major assumption behind providing childbirth and breastfeeding education classes prenatally is that women and families need information regarding these events to make informed choices (i.e., knowledge is power). However, research has indicated that low-income women do not attend childbirth education classes as much as higher-income women, and that childbirth education classes are highly associated with breastfeeding initiation (Lu et al., 2003). Kistin, Abramson, and Dublin (1994) studied low-income black women in the United States and found that prenatal education sessions that included in-depth discussions about breastfeeding not only increased the likelihood that the women would choose to breastfeed but also the likelihood that they would act on their choice when the baby was born. These sessions also positively influenced the duration of breastfeeding. The investigators concluded, "Greater educational efforts in institutions and offices serving black, low-income, urban women might yield significant changes in breastfeeding rates." Brent, Redd, and Dworetz (1995) found that prenatal and postpartum instruction from a lactation consultant resulted in more low-income women choosing breastfeeding. One-on-one intervention by a lactation consultant has positive impact on breastfeeding for mothers of all income levels (see Chapter 1).

Hospital Practices

Sometimes the reasons for choosing not to breastfeed are related to hospital factors. Overall, hospital practices concerning breastfeeding have improved in the last decade. Much of this improvement comes from two sources: consumer demand and the Baby-Friendly Hospital Initiative (BFHI), an international program created by the World Health Organization and UNICEF. BFHI has successfully incorporated practices that support breastfeeding into hundreds of hospitals across the world (Turner-Maffei, 2002). As noted in Chapter 2, the Baby-Friendly Hospital Initiative highlights 10 steps by which any institution caring for new postpartum mothers and their neonates can assist the initiation of breastfeeding. As of this writing, certifying records of Baby-Friendly USA, the certifying body for BFHI in the United States, showed that 61 US hospitals and birthing centers had achieved Baby-Friendly Hospital designation, about 1.2 percent of the approximately 5000 hospitals in the United States. Administrators' concerns about the added cost of buying formula (a hospital cannot receive free formula and qualify for Baby-Friendly designation) and lack of professional support from community physicians and nursing staff present barriers to pursuing Baby-Friendly certification.

When the 10 steps recommended by the BFHI are part of the caregiving offered in a given institution, the mothers who give birth and begin breastfeeding there are more likely to have an optimal experience. Three studies in particular have identified the ways in which implementation (or the failure of implementation) of these 10 steps has influenced the breastfeeding experiences of the mothers who gave birth and subsequently received care in the hospitals whose care patterns were examined.

A leading example is the PROBIT study, a large randomized trial carried out in Belarus. Hospitals and clinics were randomized into two groups: an intervention group where the Baby-Friendly 10 steps were implemented and a control group where no practice changes were made. Infants ($n = 17,000$) born at the intervention sites were breastfed significantly more often and had fewer gastrointestinal infections and atopic eczema than infants at the control sites (Kramer et al., 2001).

Merewood and Philipp (2001) overcame numerous obstacles in an inner-city teaching hospital in Boston to become the first Baby-Friendly hospital in Massachusetts. Receiving free formula was a major roadblock. After 2 years of work, 9 of the 10 steps were in place except for dealing with the estimated cost ($72,000) for buying formula instead of receiving it free. Further investigation showed that the quantity of formula listed by the formula company was far in excess of the amount actually used by the hospital. Using a standard figure of 20 cents per bottle of formula, the estimated annual cost of formula came to only $20,000, a far cry from the original $72,000 figure and a proportionately small amount of money for a large hospital with 1800 births per year. Merewood and colleagues also (2005) conducted a large US survey of all Baby-Friendly hospitals in the United States in 2001 and determined that breastfeeding initiation (83.8 percent versus 69.5 percent) and exclusivity rates (78.4 percent versus 46.3 percent) were higher than the national rates at the time, providing further evidence of the impact of the BFHI.

Which of the 10 steps have the greatest impact on breastfeeding? Wright, Rice, and Wells (1996) compared the effects of these steps on the likelihood that the women were fully breastfeeding at 4 months postpartum. The duration and exclusivity of breastfeeding was longer for women who did not receive formula in the hospital, who were not given discharge packs and/or coupons, who roomed-in more than 60 percent of the time, who gave no pacifiers, and who received referral to breastfeeding support organizations.

The Importance of Peer Counselors

The availability of an outside source of support in the first 6 weeks postpartum nearly always lengthens breastfeeding duration in a group of low-income women. Generally, the more breastfeeding friends the mother has, the longer she is likely to breastfeed.

Peer counseling programs, where breastfeeding support is given by trained lay female advisors knowledgeable about breastfeeding, is an effective intervention (Bronner, Barber, & Vogelhut, 2001; Dennis, 2001; Martens, 2002; Anderson, 2005). Women who receive support from trained peer counselors are more likely to initiate breastfeeding and to breastfeed longer than those who do not. Peer counselors know current information, establish supportive personal relationships with low-income women, many of whom are enrolled in the WIC program, refer women to breastfeeding specialists for problems, show enthusiasm, and facilitate breastfeeding (Raisler, 2000). The message that "Breast Is Best" has reached most low-income mothers. Regardless of how they choose to feed their baby, low-income women acknowledge the health benefits from breastfeeding. The choice not to breastfeed is often accompanied by a nagging feeling of guilt (Guttman & Zimmerman, 2000). Although younger low-income women in this same study believed that their community viewed breastfeeding as the optimal feeding method, they reported that friends and peers thought it "nasty." In addition, some of the low-income mothers associated breastfeeding with socioeconomic privilege. When poor women do breastfeed, the empowerment these women gain from the breastfeeding experience is an overlooked secondary effect that has potentially long-term impacts on other aspects of these women's lives (Locklin, 1995). These programs should be supported and expanded. Studies of the effectiveness of peer counseling are listed in Table 25–3.

The Downside of Family Experience

Not all families meander into the sunset "happily ever after." When a marriage dies, the death of that relationship affects not only the spouses but also any children they may have, as well as other relatives and friends. When the mother is breastfeeding, issues surrounding custody may be colored by the fact that she feels (rightly or wrongly) that the court should take her feeding method into consideration in deciding on custody arrangements and contacts of her children with her soon-to-be former husband.

The role of the lactation consultant in such a situation must necessarily be limited to advocacy for breastfeeding. Unless the LC is an attorney, points of law are not her concern. Instead, she can perform a valuable service by educating the judge and the mother's (and perhaps the father's) attorney about the importance of breastfeeding for the child's continued physical and psychological health (Suhler, Bornmann, & Scott, 1991). Questions may surface pertaining to how the father's attachment to the child is enhanced when breast-

feeding is protected. Questions relating to the frequency of breastfeeding may not arise. In most cases, if the child is older than a few months, short periods of time with the father (away from the mother) are unlikely to place the breastfeeding relationship at risk. In addition, maintaining the child's attachment with both parents requires that child and parent are together as often (as much as possible) as they would have been if the marriage and joint parenting experience had remained intact. Prior to her death, Elizabeth Baldwin, a family lawyer, assisted many lactation consultants and their clients in custody and breastfeeding cases (Neely, 2003). LaLeche League International's Web site offers resources regarding breastfeeding in child custody situations such as divorce, many from the late Elizabeth Baldwin. Also on the LLLI Web site is information on state legislation that has been enacted in Hawaii, Maine, Michigan, and Utah regarding custody and breastfeeding.

When the mother is seeking to maintain breastfeeding beyond the time when most people in her society—including the judge and the attorneys—are likely to find it acceptable, the lactation consultant can provide information that again focuses on the health-preserving aspects of breastfeeding (Wilson-Clay, 1990). Such longer-term breastfeeding does not necessarily limit reasonable visitation periods with the noncustodial parent, nor does it prevent periods of separation of the child from the mother. It does place the issue squarely where it must remain: preserving the best interests of the child.

Violence

The lactation consultant may become involved if a woman wishes to breastfeed or is breastfeeding and living in a situation in which she or her children are being threatened or assaulted. Whenever the lactation consultant believes that such violence is occurring, she has a responsibility to report this to relevant authorities who are in a position to intervene and to provide a safe haven for the mother and her children if she chooses to use it. Assisting with breastfeeding in abusive households need not be any different from assisting any other woman, although sensitivity to the abuse situation is necessary.

TABLE 25–3	Studies of Peer Counselors
Arlotti et al., 1998 (N = 36)	Women in Florida WIC program contacted by telephone, letter, or in person five times postpartum. Significant difference between groups in breastfeeding exclusivity but not in overall duration.
Caulfield et al., 1998 (N = 548)	Low-income pregnant women in Baltimore WIC program. Prenatal and postnatal weekly contact. Peer support associated with breastfeeding initiation but not duration at 7 to 10 days postpartum.
Anderson et al., 2005 (N = 162)	Randomized control trial in low-income, mainly Hispanic, pregnant women in Hartford, Connecticut. Exclusive breastfeeding peer counseling support was offered through three prenatal home visits, daily perinatal visits, nine postpartum home visits, and telephone counseling as needed. The likelihood of nonexclusive breastfeeding throughout the first 3 months was significantly higher for the control group than the PC group. The likelihood of having 1 or more diarrheal episodes in infants was cut in half in the PC group.
Dennis et al., 2002 (N = 256)	Randomized trial of primiparous postpartum women near Toronto. Telephone contact occurred within 48 hours postdischarge and as needed. Significant statistical difference between groups in breastfeeding duration and exclusivity at 12 weeks.
Gross et al., 1998 (N = 115)	African-American WIC recipients in four Baltimore, Maryland, clinics. Two-by-two factorial design. Interventions: video and/or peer counseling vs. control group. Higher proportion of breastfeeding in intervention groups vs. control.
Grummer-Strawn et al., 1997	1989–1993 Pediatric Nutrition Surveillance System data were analyzed to compare breastfeeding rates in Mississippi WIC clinics with and without peer-counseling programs. The peer-counseling program significantly increased the incidence of breastfeeding, particularly in clinics with lactation specialists and consultants.
Haider et al., 2000 (N = 720)	Prenatal and postnatal home visits for pregnant women in Bangladesh. Significant differences between initiation and duration of exclusive breastfeeding (70% vs. 6%).
Kistin, Abramson, & Dublin, 1994 (N = 102)	Low-income US women who received support from peer counselors had significantly greater breastfeeding initiation, exclusivity, and duration than those who did not.
Long et al., 1995 (N = 141)	Pregnant Native American women in Utah WIC program. Prenatal and postpartum contact by home and clinic visits and by telephone. Significantly higher breastfeeding initiation (84% vs. 70%) in intervention group but not duration at 12 weeks (49% vs. 36%).
Martens, 2002 (N = 283)	Non-WIC, Canadian Sankeeng First Nation community. Prenatal community health nurse and postpartum PC approach at breastfeeding education and support. Designated points of contact by the PC were once a week for the first month, and once every 2 weeks for months 2 and 3 (at weeks 1, 2, 3, 4, 6, 8, 10, and 12 postpartum). PC clients were half as likely to wean, with 61% still breastfeeding at 2 months (vs. 48% nonclients) and 56% at 6 months (vs. 19%). PC clients had fewer problems and greater satisfaction with breastfeeding.

(Continues)

TABLE 25–3	**Studies of Peer Counselors (Continued)**
Mongeon & Allard, 1995 (N = 194)	Prenatal and postnatal telephone contact with 194 pregnant women in Montreal. No significant difference between control and intervention groups in breastfeeding duration.
Morrow et al., 1999 (N = 130)	Low-income women in Mexico City. Prenatal and postnatal home visits. One control and two intervention groups (Group I: 6 home visits; Group II: 3 home visits). Significant difference between groups in breastfeeding exclusivity (6 visits = 67%; 3 visits = 50%; control = 12%) and duration at 12 weeks.
Pugh et al., 2002 (N = 41)	Community health nurse and peer counselor support starting during postpartum hospitalization. Randomized trial. The intervention group received visits from the team including daily hospital visits, visits at home during weeks 1, 2, and 4, and peer counselor telephone support twice weekly through week 8 and weekly through month 6. Breastfeeding duration was longer among the experimental group.
Schafer et al., 1998 (N = 134)	Prenatal and postnatal face-to-face and telephone contact for rural, low-income women in Iowa. Significant differences between intervention and control groups in breastfeeding initiation (82% vs. 32%) and duration.
Shaw & Kaczorowski, 1999 (N = 192)	Prenatal clinic visit and postnatal phone contact for low-income women in Tennessee WIC program. Significant higher breastfeeding initiation and duration for the intervention group.
Wambach et al., (Unpublished data) (N = 289)	Randomized clinical trial. Midwestern United States. Three-group longitudinal design focusing on urban disadvantaged teenagers (15–18 years old). Experimental interventions: Two prenatal breastfeeding education classes facilitated by lactation consultant (LC) and peer counselors (PC); PC prenatal telephone support; in-patient/postbirth PC and LC support; and postpartum telephone support by PC and LC through 4 weeks. Significant difference between groups on breastfeeding initiation ($P < .05$) and duration ($P < .001$).

The number of breastfeeding women who are in homes in which they are being abused is not known. Acheson (1995) reported that lack of breastfeeding was associated with physical and sexual abuse of the woman or her children or both. In her retrospective review of 800 pregnancies and births in one family practice, Acheson noted that postpartum depression occurred more frequently in the absence of breastfeeding, as did marital problems and domestic violence. The author suggested that the striking 38-fold decrease in frequency of violence against women or their children (or both) when breastfeeding is practiced warrants careful scrutiny. One must ask the question: what is it about the decision to breastfeed, or its practice, that is related to nonviolent households? In other words, is the social dynamic in families in which violence occurs such that breastfeeding is also unlikely and, if so, what factors compose that social dynamic?

Childhood Sexual Abuse

A history of abuse during childhood, including sexual abuse, is likely to result in a variety of reactions to the breastfeeding experience. For example, if a mother wishes to breastfeed but cannot bring herself to allow the baby to latch onto the breast, and if issues such as breast tenderness are not immediately evident, the consultant must consider the possibility that the breast area was involved in the sexual abuse that the mother may have suffered years earlier.

Depending on one's definition of sexual abuse, as many as 20 percent of US women were sexually abused as children (Prentice et al., 2002). Given such a high incidence of abuse, beliefs surrounding the breasts' function and emotions pertaining to these beliefs are very likely to include fears that stem from experiences outside the realm of most lactation consultants' field of expertise.

Sexual abuse can have both short-term and long-term effects on the victim. Those effects may be expressed in various ways, including symptoms of post-traumatic stress disorder, cognitive distortions, emotional distress, impaired sense of self, interpersonal difficulties, health problems, and numerous kinds of avoidance behavior (including amnesia for the abuse-related events, dissociation, and self-destructive behaviors such as drug abuse). Sometimes, pregnancy (Grant, 1992) or childbirth (Courtois & Riley, 1992; Kitzinger, 1992; Rose, 1992) or breastfeeding can trigger recall that has previously been suppressed. One woman first regained memories of her abuse when she tried to breastfeed her infant. Because she was so unprepared for the sensations and the accompanying memories, she was unable to tolerate putting the baby to breast (Heritage, 1998). Coping mechanisms will vary from one woman to the next and may or may not be manifested during pregnancy, childbirth, or breastfeeding (Kendall-Tuckett, 1998).

When she has established rapport with the lactation consultant and feels safe, the mother may admit that she has been a victim of childhood abuse. In many cases, however, she may be unaware of the reason for her extreme discomfort, owing to brain changes that occur as a result of abuse and the coping mechanisms, including amnesia relating to the abusive events, that she may have practiced for years in order to maintain a facade of normalcy (Mukerjee, 1995). Additionally, if the mother recalls the abuse, she may or may not view it as being connected in any way with her current situation, including difficulties she may be having with breastfeeding.

Bowman (2007) conducted a review of the literature on the mental health impact of childhood sexual abuse (CSA) on breastfeeding decision making in adolescent mothers and concluded that healthcare providers need to be aware that a history of CSA may affect the decision to breastfeed in the teenage mother. She pointed out that CSA victims are more likely than non-CSA victims to become sexually active earlier and more likely to become pregnant as a teenager. These mothers are more likely to have issues with establishing an intimate relationship with their infants, and breastfeeding may be considered an intimate parenting behavior. Therefore the provider needs to be sensitive to the possibility of CSA in the pregnant teenager.

Survivors of past sexual abuse may have symptoms of post-traumatic stress disorder. These survivors frequently reexperience the traumatic event through nightmares or intrusive thoughts, such as sudden flashbacks of the abuse experience. If breastfeeding triggers sudden recall, nurturing her baby in this manner may be frightening to the mother. See Box 25–1 for suggestions on how to deal with a new mother who may have been sexually abused.

One mother had no recall of being abused until she put her baby to her breast for the first time. This action triggered a flashback so frightening to her that she screamed and immediately dropped the baby onto her bed. By the time hospital staff reached her, she was weeping and begged them to take the baby to the nursery. She subsequently cried uncontrollably each time she attempted to put her baby to her breast. The staff began helping her by giving her permission to pump her breasts to give her baby her milk. This action was something she could completely control. Being able to determine the degree of suction the pump exerted was important to her. After a week of pumping, during which time she gradually increased the pump pressure, she was willing to "try the baby again." She gradually was able to tolerate feedings without fearing that she would harm her baby.

Despite incidences such as these, the evidence is actually contrary to what may be expected. At least one research group (Prentice et al., 2002) found that mothers who self-identify sexual abuse as a child are *more* likely, not less, to initiate breastfeeding than women who report no such abuse. Could it be possible that women who were sexually abused as children are more concerned about parenting? If this is true, then these women may be more likely to breastfeed because it is a healthier way to feed a baby.

Kendall-Tackett (2007) cautioned that little research has been conducted to accurately describe the breastfeeding experiences and outcome of

Interventions for Helping Sexual Abuse Survivors

- Be gentle and respectful when asking questions about sexual abuse. Whether the LC should ask directly depends on the rapport established with the mother.
- Teach the normal course of lactation, including the normalcy of pleasurable aspects of breastfeeding. Offer suggestions to make breastfeeding more comfortable.
- Suggest that the mother express her milk if she is unable or unwilling to feed at breast. This may be the most

comfortable way for the mother to provide her milk to her baby while protecting herself from what she perceives emotionally (consciously or unconsciously) as an assault on her person.
- Make a referral to a mental healthcare provider. Be cautious about becoming the main source of emotional support.

Source: Adapted from Kendall-Tackett, 1998.

women with a history of physical or sexual abuse. Cortisol levels are known to be higher or lower in abuse victims. Does the response to current stressors, such as those following birth, impact lactogenesis? Do perceptions of insufficient milk supply hamper breastfeeding success? Prentice et al. found that at 1 month after birth, more mothers without CSA histories (82%, $n = 517$) were breastfeeding than mothers with CSA histories (73%, $n = 41$), but the difference was not statistically significant. Clearly more research is needed in this area.

Acceptance of each woman's decision to breastfeed—however that is defined at a given time—may enable her to move closer to a full breastfeeding relationship with her baby and to further cement a healthy ongoing relationship with all of her children, something she may not have enjoyed in her family of origin.

Summary

Different family forms reflect different members' needs. Family developmental theories enable the healthcare worker to identify specific family functions throughout the life cycle. The goal of the healthcare provider should be to help the family to meet its own needs without her or his assistance. Key issues related to family functioning are the family's place within the support system and larger community. The early parenting period is characterized by patterns of attachment behavior and ways that these reflect the growing competence of the parents as parents. In some cases, the father may be the mother's single and most constant supporter; in other situations, he may be less involved in the family and unlikely to support breastfeeding.

Key Concepts

- Examining how different family forms and relationships are likely to be experienced throughout a lifetime can provide insight into the stresses that a family with a new baby is likely to encounter.
- How families interact with healthcare workers in a hospital or clinic setting often is related to the family structure, stage, and tasks related to childbearing.

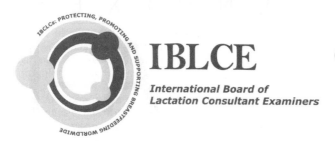

APPENDIX A

IBLCE
International Board of Lactation Consultant Examiners

CLINICAL COMPETENCIES FOR IBCLC PRACTICE*

Much of the clinical practice of the International Board Certified Lactation Consultant (IBCLC) consists of systematic problem solving in collaboration with breastfeeding mothers and other members of the health-care team. This checklist includes most of the clinical and practical skills that an entry-level IBCLC needs in order to be satisfactorily proficient to provide safe and effective care for breastfeeding mothers and babies. The list is designed to encompass common breastfeeding situations and the challenges that are encountered most frequently by lactation consultants. Clinical instructors will be able to use this checklist as an appropriate guide in providing individualized education. A list of possible sites for obtaining clinical and practical experience appears at the end of the list of competencies.

Students are encouraged to become familiar with other documents that address the role of the IBCLC. The knowledge, skills, and attitude inherent in the role of an IBCLC are summarized in a list of 16 Competency Statements contained in the *International Board of Lactation Consultant Examiners Candidate Information Guide*. A more detailed description of the role is provided in the *Standards of Practice for IBCLC Lactation Consultants* published by the International Lactation Consultant Association (ILCA). Optimal breastfeeding care is clearly presented with rationales and references in the *2005 Clinical Guidelines for the Establishment of Exclusive Breastfeeding*, also published by ILCA, www.ilca.org.

Communication and Counseling Skills

In all interactions with mothers, families, health care professionals, and peers, the student will demonstrate effective communication skills to maintain collaborative and supportive relationships.

The student will:

- Identify factors that might affect communication (i.e., age, cultural/language differences, hearing or visual impairment, mental ability, etc.)

- Demonstrate appropriate body language (i.e., position in relation to the other person, comfortable eye contact, appropriate tone of voice for the setting, etc.)

- Demonstrate knowledge of and sensitivity to cultural differences

- Elicit information using effective counseling techniques (i.e., asking open-ended questions, summarizing the discussion, and providing emotional support)

- Make appropriate referrals to other health care professionals and community resources

---

* Jointly published by the International Board of Lactation Consultant Examiners (IBLCE) and the International Lactation Consultant Association (ILCA). Reprinted with permission from International Board of Lactation Consultant Examiners.

The student will provide individualized breast-feeding care with an emphasis on the mother's ability to make informed decisions.

The student will:

- Assess mother's psychological state and provide information appropriate to her situation
- Include those family members or friends the mother identifies as significant to her
- Obtain the mother's permission for providing care to her or her baby
- Ascertain the mother's knowledge about and goals for breastfeeding
- Use adult education principles to provide instruction to the mother that will meet her needs
- Select appropriate written information and other teaching aids

History Taking and Assessment Skills

The student will be able to:

- Obtain a pertinent history
- Perform a breast evaluation related to lactation
- Develop a breastfeeding risk assessment
- Assess and evaluate the infant's ability to breastfeed
- Assess effective milk transfer

Documentation and Communication Skills with Health Professionals

The student will:

- Communicate effectively with other members of the health care team, using written documents appropriate to the location, facility, and culture in which the student is being trained, such as consent forms, care plans, charting forms/clinical notes, pathways/care maps, and feeding assessment forms

- Use appropriate resources for research to provide information to the health care team on conditions and medications that affect breastfeeding and lactation
- Write referrals and follow-up documentation/letters to referring and/or primary health care providers that illustrate the student's ability to identify:
  - The mother's concerns or problems, planned interventions, evaluation of outcomes, and follow-up
  - Situations in which immediate verbal communication with the health care provider is necessary, such as serious illness in the infant, child, or mother
- Report instances of child abuse or neglect to specific agencies as appropriate or legally required

Skills for the First Two Hours after Birth

The student will:

- Identify events that occurred during the labor and birth process that may adversely affect breastfeeding
- Identify and discourage practices that may interfere with breastfeeding
- Promote continuous skin-to-skin contact of the term newborn and mother until the first breastfeed
- Assist the mother and family to identify newborn feeding cues
- Help the mother and infant to find a comfortable position for latch-on/attachment during the first breastfeed after birth
- Identify correct latch-on/attachment
- Reinforce to mother and family the importance of:
  - Keeping the mother and baby together
  - Feeding the baby on cue—but at least 8 times in each 24-hour period

APPENDIX A (cont.)

Postpartum Skills

Prior to a mother–baby dyad's discharge from care, the student will observe a breastfeed and effectively instruct the mother about:

- Assessment of adequate milk intake by the baby
- Normal infant sucking patterns
- How milk is produced and supply maintained, including discussion of growth/appetite spurts
- Normal newborn behavior, including why, when, and how to wake a sleepy newborn
- Avoidance of early use of a dummy/pacifier and bottle teat
- Importance of exclusive breast milk feeds and possible consequences of mixed feedings with cow's milk or soy
- Prevention and treatment of sore nipples
- Prevention and treatment of engorgement
- SIDS prevention behaviors
- Family planning methods and their relationship to breastfeeding
- Education regarding drugs (such as nicotine, alcohol, caffeine, and illicit drugs) and complementary remedies (such as herbal teas)
- Plans for follow-up care for breastfeeding questions, infant's medical, and mother's postpartum examinations
- Community resources for breastfeeding assistance

Problem-Solving Skills

The student will be able to:

- Identify problems
- Assess contributing factors and cause
- Develop an appropriate breastfeeding plan in consultation with the mother
- Assist the mother to implement the plan
- Evaluate effectiveness of the plan

Skills for Maternal Breastfeeding Challenges

The student will be able to assist mothers with the following challenges:

- Cesarean birth
- Flat/inverted nipples
- Thrush infections of breast, nipple, areola, and milk ducts
- Continuation of breastfeeding when mother is separated from her baby
  - Milk expression techniques
  - Maintaining milk production
  - Collection, storage, and transportation of milk
- Cultural beliefs that are not evidence based and may interfere with breastfeeding (i.e., discarding colostrum, rigidly scheduled feedings, necessity of formula after every breastfeeding, etc.)
- Medical conditions that may impact on breastfeeding
- Adolescent mother
  - Strategies for returning to school
  - Maintaining milk production
- Nipple pain and damage
- Engorgement
- Blocked duct and/or nipple pore
- Mastitis
- Breast surgery/trauma
- Overproduction of milk
- Postpartum psychological issues including transient sadness ("baby blues") and postpartum depression
- Appropriate referrals
- Medications compatible with breastfeeding
- Insufficient milk supply, differentiating between perceived and real

- Weaning issues
- Safe formula preparation and feeding techniques
- Care of breasts

Skills for Infant Breastfeeding Challenges

The student will be able to assist mothers who have infants with the following challenges:

- Traumatic birth
- 35–38 weeks' gestation
- Small for gestational age (SGA) or large for gestational age (LGA)
- Multiple births
- Preterm birth, including the benefits of kangaroo care
- High risk for hypoglycemia
- Sleepy infant
- Excessive weight loss, slow/poor weight gain
- Hyperbilirubinemia (jaundice)
- Ankyloglossia (short frenulum)
- Thrush infection
- Colic/fussiness
- Gastric reflux
- Lactose overload
- Food intolerances
- Neurodevelopmental problems
- Teething and biting
- Breast refusal/early baby-led weaning
- Breastfeeding a toddler
- Breastfeeding through pregnancy
- Tandem feeding

Management Skills

The student will demonstrate the ability to:

- Perform a comprehensive breastfeeding assessment

- Assess milk transfer
- Calculate an infant's caloric/kilojoule and volume requirements
- Increase milk production

Skills for Use of Technology and Devices

The student will have up-to-date knowledge about breastfeeding-related equipment and demonstrate appropriate use and understanding of potential disadvantages or risks of the following:

- A device to evert nipples
- Nipple creams/ointments
- Breast shells
- Breast pumps
- Alternative feeding techniques
  - Tube feeding at the breast
  - Cup feeding
  - Spoon feeding
  - Eyedropper feeding
  - Finger feeding
  - Bottles and artificial nipples/teats
- Nipple shields
- Pacifiers/soothers
- Infant scales
- Use of herbal supplements for mother and/or infant

Skills for Breastfeeding Challenges That Are Encountered Infrequently

The following issues are encountered relatively infrequently and might not be seen during the student's training. The entry-level lactation consultant would not be expected to be proficient in these situations, but should have the basic skills to assist the mother and infant while seeking guidance from a more experienced IBCLC.

APPENDIX A (cont.)

Infant:
- Infant with tonic bite/ineffective/dysfunctional suck
- Cranial-facial abnormalities, such as micronathia (receding lower jaw) and cleft lip and/or palate
- Down syndrome
- Cardiac problems
- Chronic medical conditions, such as cystic fibrosis, PKU, etc.

Mother:
- Induced lactation and relactation
- Coping with the death of an infant
- Chronic medical conditions, such as multiple sclerosis, lupus, seizures, etc.
- Disabilities that may limit mother's ability to handle the baby easily, such as rheumatoid arthritis, carpal tunnel syndrome, cerebral palsy, etc.
- HIV/AIDS: understanding of current recommendations

Skills for Meeting Professional Responsibilities

The student will demonstrate the following professional responsibilities:

- Conduct herself or himself in a professional manner, by complying with the IBLCE *Code of Ethics for International Board Certified Lactation Consultants* and the ILCA *Standards of Practice*; and by adhering to the *International Code of Marketing of Breast-Milk Substitutes* and its subsequent World Health Assembly resolutions.
- Practice within the laws of the setting in which she/he works, showing respect for confidentiality and privacy.
- Use current research findings to provide a strong evidence base for clinical practice, and obtain continuing education to enhance skills and obtain/maintain IBCLC certification.
- Advocate for breastfeeding families, mothers, infants and children in the workplace, community, and within the health care system.
- Use breastfeeding equipment appropriately and provide information about risks as well as benefits of products, maintaining an awareness of conflict of interest if profiting from the rental or sale of breastfeeding equipment.

Sites for Acquisition of Skills

The student may acquire clinical/practical skills in the following settings:

- Private practice IBCLC office
- Private obstetric, pediatric, family, or independent midwifery practice
- Public health department; Women, Infants and Children (WIC) Program (in the United States); maternal and child health services
- Hospital
  - Lactation services
  - Birthing center
  - Postpartum unit
  - Mother–baby unit
  - Level II and level III nurseries: special care nursery, neonatal intensive care nursery
  - Pediatric unit
- Home health (community nursing) services
- Outpatient follow-up breastfeeding clinics
- Breastfeeding telephone counseling services
- Prenatal and postpartum breastfeeding classes
- Home births (if legally permitted)
- Volunteer community support group meetings

SCOPE OF PRACTICE FOR

*International Board Certified Lactation Consultants (IBCLCs)**

International Board Certified Lactation Consultants (IBCLCs) have demonstrated specialized knowledge and clinical expertise in breastfeeding and human lactation and are certified by the International Board of Lactation Consultant Examiners (IBLCE).

This Scope of Practice encompasses the activities for which IBCLCs are educated and in which they are authorized to engage. The aim of this Scope of Practice is to protect the public by ensuring that all IBCLCs provide safe, competent, and evidence-based care. As this is an international credential, this Scope of Practice is applicable in any country or setting where IBCLCS practice.

IBCLCs have the duty to uphold the standards of the IBCLC profession by:

- Working within the framework defined by the IBLCE *Code of Ethics*, the *Clinical Competencies for IBCLC Practice*, and the International Lactation Consultant Association (ILCA) *Standards of Practice for IBCLCs*
- Integrating knowledge and evidence when providing care for breastfeeding families from the disciplines defined in the IBLCE Exam Blueprint
- Working within the legal framework of the respective geopolitical regions or settings
- Maintaining knowledge and skills through regular continuing education

IBCLCs have the duty to protect, promote and support breastfeeding by:

- Educating women, families, health professionals and the community about breastfeeding and human lactation
- Facilitating the development of policies which protect, promote, and support breastfeeding
- Acting as an advocate for breastfeeding as the child-feeding norm
- Providing holistic, evidence-based breastfeeding support and care, from preconception to weaning, for women and their families
- Using principles of adult education when teaching clients, healthcare providers and others in the community
- Complying with the International Code of Marketing of Breast-milk Substitutes and subsequent relevant World Health Assembly resolutions

IBCLCs have the duty to provide competent services for mothers and families by:

- Performing comprehensive maternal, child, and feeding assessments related to lactation
- Developing and implementing an individualized feeding plan in consultation with the mother
- Providing evidence-based information regarding a mother's use, during lactation, of medications (over-the-counter and prescription), alcohol, tobacco, and street drugs, and their potential impact on milk production and child safety

---

* Reprinted with permission from International Board of Lactation Consultant Examiners.

- Providing evidence-based information regarding complementary therapies during lactation and their impact on a mother's milk production and the effect on her child

- Integrating cultural, psychosocial and nutritional aspects of breastfeeding

- Providing support and encouragement to enable mothers to successfully meet their breastfeeding goals

- Using effective counseling skills when interacting with clients and other healthcare providers

- Using the principles of family-centred care while maintaining a collaborative, supportive relationship with clients

IBCLCs have the duty to report truthfully and fully to the mother and/or infant's primary healthcare provider and to the healthcare system by:

- Recording all relevant information concerning care provided and, where appropriate, retaining records for the time specified by the local jurisdiction

IBCLCs have the duty to preserve client confidence by:

- Respecting the privacy, dignity and confidentiality of mothers and families

IBCLCs have the duty to act with reasonable diligence by:

- Assisting families with decisions regarding the feeding of children by providing information that is evidence-based and free of conflict of interest

- Providing follow-up services as required

- Making necessary referrals to other healthcare providers and community support resources when necessary

- Functioning and contributing as a member of the healthcare team to deliver coordinated services to women and families

- Working collaboratively and interdependently with other members of the healthcare team

- Reporting to IBLCE if they have been found guilty of any offence under the criminal code of their country or jurisdiction in which they work or is sanctioned by another profession

- Reporting to IBLCE any other IBCLC who is functioning outside this Scope of Practice

INTERNATIONAL LACTATION CONSULTANT ASSOCIATION

*Standards of Practice for IBCLCs**

Introduction

This is the third edition of *Standards of Practice for International Board Certified Lactation Consultants (IBCLCs)* published by the International Lactation Consultant Association (ILCA). All individuals practicing as a currently certified IBCLC should adhere to ILCA's *Standards of Practice* and the International Board of Lactation Consultant Examiners (IBLCE) *Code of Ethics for International Board Certified Lactation Consultants* in all interactions with clients, families, and other healthcare professionals. ILCA recognizes the certification conferred by the IBLCE as the worldwide professional credential for lactation consultants.

Quality practice and service are the core responsibilities of a profession to the public. Standards of practice are stated measures or levels of quality that are models for the conduct and evaluation of practice. Standards of practice:

- Promote consistency by encouraging a common systematic approach.
- Are sufficiently specific in content to guide daily practice.
- Provide a recommended framework for the development of policies and protocols, educational programs, and quality improvement efforts.
- Are intended for use in diverse practice settings and cultural contexts.

Standard 1. Professional Responsibilities

The IBCLC has a responsibility to maintain professional conduct and to practice in an ethical manner, accountable for professional actions and legal responsibilities.

1.1 Adhere to these ILCA *Standards of Practice* and the IBLCE *Code of Ethics*.

1.2 Practice within the scope of the International Code of Marketing of Breast-milk Substitutes and all subsequent World Health Association resolutions.

1.3 Maintain an awareness of conflict of interest in all aspects of work, especially when profiting from the rental or sale of breastfeeding equipment and services.

1.4 Act as an advocate for breastfeeding women, infants, and children.

1.5 Assist the mother in maintaining a breastfeeding relationship with her child.

1.6 Maintain and expand knowledge and skills for lactation consultant practice by participating in continuing education.

1.7 Undertake periodic and systematic evaluation of one's clinical practice.

1.8 Support and promote well-designed research in human lactation and breastfeeding, and base clinical practice, whenever possible, on such research.

---

* Reprinted with permission from International Lactation Consultant Association.

APPENDIX C (cont.)

Standard 2. Legal Considerations

The IBCLC is obligated to practice within the laws of the geopolitical region and setting in which she/he works. The IBCLC must practice with consideration for rights of privacy and with respect for matters of a confidential nature.

2.1 Work within the policies and procedures of the institution where employed, or if self-employed, have identifiable policies and procedures to follow.

2.2 Clearly state applicable fees prior to providing care.

2.3 Obtain informed consent from all clients prior to:

- assessing or intervening.

- reporting relevant information to other health care professional(s).

- taking photographs for any purpose.

- seeking publication of information associated with the consultation.

2.4 Protect client confidentiality at all times.

2.5 Maintain records according to legal and ethical practices within the work setting.

Standard 3. Clinical Practice

The clinical practice of the IBCLC focuses on providing clinical lactation care and management. This is best accomplished by promoting optimal health, through collaboration and problem solving with the client and other members of the health care team. The role of the IBCLC includes:

- Assessment, planning, intervention, and evaluation of care in a variety of situations.

- Anticipatory guidance and prevention of problems.

- Complete, accurate, and timely documentation of care.

- Communication and collaboration with other health care professionals.

3.1 Assessment.

3.1.1 Obtain and document an appropriate history of the breastfeeding mother and child.

3.1.2 Systematically collect objective and subjective information.

3.1.3 Discuss with the mother and document as appropriate all assessment information.

3.2 Plan.

3.2.1 Analyze assessment information to identify issues and/or problems.

3.2.2 Develop a plan of care based on identified issues.

3.2.3 Arrange for follow-up evaluation where indicated.

3.3 Implementation.

3.3.1 Implement the plan of care in a manner appropriate to the situation and acceptable to the mother.

3.3.2 Utilize translators as needed.

3.3.3 Exercise principles of optimal health, safety, and universal precautions.

3.3.4 Provide appropriate oral and written instructions and/or demonstration of interventions, procedures, and techniques.

3.3.5 Facilitate referral to other health care professionals, community services, and support groups as needed.

3.3.6 Use equipment appropriately.

- Refrain from unnecessary or excessive use.

- Assure cleanliness and good operating condition.

- Discuss the risks and benefits of recommended equipment including financial considerations.

- Demonstrate the correct use and care of equipment.

- Evaluate safety and effectiveness of use.

3.3.7 Document and communicate to health care providers as appropriate.

- Assessment information.

- Suggested interventions.

- Instructions provided.
- Evaluations of outcomes.
- Modifications of the plan of care.
- Follow-up strategies.

3.4 Evaluation.
3.4.1 Evaluate outcomes of planned interventions.
3.4.2 Modify the care plan based on the evaluation of outcomes.

Standard 4. Breastfeeding Education and Counseling

Breastfeeding education and counseling are integral parts of the care provided by the IBCLC.

4.1 Educate parents and families to encourage informed decision-making about infant and child feeding.

4.2 Utilize a pragmatic problem-solving approach, sensitive to the learner's culture, questions and concerns.

4.3 Provide anticipatory guidance (teaching).

4.3.1 Promote optimal breastfeeding practices.

4.3.2 Minimize the potential for breastfeeding problems or complications.

4.4 Provide positive feedback and emotional support for continued breastfeeding, especially in difficult or complicated circumstances.

4.5 Share current evidence-based information and clinical skills in collaboration with other health care providers.

International Board of Lactation Consultant Examiners Candidate Information*

IBLCE, the International Board of Lactation Consultant Examiners, is a nonprofit organization that develops and administers the certification examination for International Board Certified Lactation Consultants (IBCLCs).

IBCLC requirements and achievements:

- Have experience providing lactation specific care to breastfeeding families including lactation assistance to pregnant and breastfeeding women and lactation education to breastfeeding families and/or professionals.

- Complete education in human lactation and breastfeeding that covers the disciplines and chronological periods shown on the *IBLCE Exam Blueprint* (see below) and/or training in the clinical skills listed on the *Clinical Competencies for IBCLC Practice* (See Appendix A of this book).

- Pass the IBLCE certification examination.

Pathways: Pathways are based on health care professional or lay breastfeeding support backgrounds and lactation education preparation. The pathways describe the minimum amount of education and experience the candidate must complete.

	Pathway 1	**Pathway 2**	**Pathway 3**
General Background for Pathway	Have experience as a health care professional working in maternal-child health or as a breastfeeding support counselor as defined by IBLCE.	Graduate from an accredited academic program in human lactation and breastfeeding that is at least one year in length and that includes clinical practice assignments above and beyond the required clinical practice experience.	Complete an approved lactation education plan under the supervision of one or more IBCLCs, all of whom have recertified at least once. The plan must be approved by IBLCE before the candidate begins the clinical practice component.

---

* Adapted from International Board of Lactation Consultant Examiners *2008 Candidate Information Guide.*

Health Disciplines Education (college level course in each of the following - human anatomy and physiology, sociology or cultural sensitivity, nutrition, psychology or counseling and communication skills, infant and child growth and development, and medical terminology)	*Recommended* For candidates who have not already studied these subjects as part of their university program.	*Required* A minimum of one course that is at least one semester in length in each of the six subjects. This requirement may be completed prior to or during the program.	*Recommended* For candidates who have not already studied these subjects as part of their education.
Lactation Specific Clinical Experience	**1000 hours** within 5 years prior to exam.	**300 hours** directly certified by IBCLC and before completion of program. Exam must be applied for within 5 years of completion.	**500 hours** directly supervised by IBCLC who is the plan supervisor and done within 5 years before exam application.
Education in Human Lactation and Breastfeeding	*Required 45 hours* Based on the IBLCE Exam Blueprint and completed within the 5 years immediately prior to exam application. *Recommended 80–150 hours*	*Required 90 hours* Based on the IBLCE Exam Blueprint and included in the academic program. Primary faculty must be recertified IBCLCs.	*Required 45 hours* Based on the IBLCE Exam Blueprint and completed within the 5 years immediately prior to exam application. *Recommended 80–150 hours*

Source: Adapted from International Board of Lactation Consultant Examiners *2009 Exam Application Guide.*

IBLCE Exam Blueprint

All exam questions have both *Discipline* and *Chronological* parameters. The range for the possible number of questions related to each *Discipline* or *Chronological Period* is indicated.

Disciplines

- **Maternal and Infant Anatomy** (19–33 questions)
- **Maternal and Infant Normal Physiology** and **Endocrinology** (19–33 questions)
- **Maternal and Infant Normal Nutrition and Biochemistry** (10–16 questions)
- **Maternal and Infant Immunology and Infectious Disease** (10–16 questions)
- **Maternal and Infant Pathology** (19–33 questions)
- **Maternal and Infant Pharmacology and Toxicology** (10–16 questions)
- **Psychology, Sociology, and Anthropology** (10–16 questions)
- **Growth Parameters and Developmental Milestones** (10–16 questions)

APPENDIX D (cont.)

- **Interpretation of Research** (4–8 questions)
- **Ethical and Legal Issues** (4–8 questions)
- **Breastfeeding Equipment and Technology** (10–16 questions)
- **Techniques** (19–33 questions)
- **Public Health** (4–8 questions)

Chronological Periods

1. Preconception (2–7 questions)
2. Prenatal (9–17 questions)
3. Labor/birth (Perinatal) (9–17 questions)
4. Prematurity (9–17 questions)
5. 0–2 days (19–31 questions)
6. 3–14 days (19–31 questions)
7. 15–28 days (19–31 questions)
8. 1–3 months (9–17 questions)
9. 4–6 months (9–17 questions)
10. 7–12 months (2–7 questions)
11. Beyond 12 months (2–7 questions)
12. General principles (40–53 questions)

Source: Adapted from *International Board of Lactation Consultant Examiners Exam Blueprint.* Accessed December 29, 2008, at http://www.iblce.org/examblueprint.php?region=am.

APPENDIX E

INTERNATIONAL BOARD OF LACTATION CONSULTANTS EXAMINERS

*Code of Ethics for International Board Certified Lactation Consultants**

Preamble

It is in the best interests of the profession of lactation consultants and the public it serves that there be a Code of Ethics to provide guidance to lactation consultants in their professional practice and conduct. These ethical principles guide the profession and outline commitments and obligations of the lactation consultant to self, client, colleagues, society, and the profession.

The purpose of the International Board of Lactation Consultant Examiners (IBLCE) is to assist in the protection of the health, safety, and welfare of the public by establishing and enforcing qualifications of certification and for issuing voluntary credentials to individuals who have attained those qualifications. The IBLCE has adopted this Code to apply to all individuals who hold the credential of International Board Certified Lactation Consultant.

Principles of Ethical Practice

The International Board Certified Lactation Consultant shall act in a manner that safeguards the interests of individual clients, justifies public trust in her/his competence, and enhances the reputation of the profession.

The International Board Certified Lactation Consultant is personally accountable for her/his practice and, in the exercise of professional accountability, must:

1. Provide professional services with objectivity and with respect for the unique needs and values of individuals.

2. Avoid discrimination against other individuals on the basis of race, creed, religion, gender, sexual orientation, age, and national origin.

3. Fulfill professional commitments in good faith.

4. Conduct herself/himself with honesty, integrity, and fairness.

5. Remain free of conflict of interest while fulfilling the objectives and maintaining the integrity of the lactation consultant profession.

6. Maintain confidentiality.

7. Base her/his practice on scientific principles, and on current research and information.

8. Take responsibility and accept accountability for personal competence in practice.

9. Recognize and exercise professional judgment within the limits of her/his qualifications. This principle includes seeking counsel and making referrals to appropriate providers.

10. Inform the public and colleagues of his/her services by using factual information. An International Board Certified Lactation Consultant shall not advertise in a false or misleading manner.

11. Provide sufficient information to enable clients to make informed decisions.

12. Provide information about appropriate products in a manner that is neither false nor misleading.

13. Permit use of her/his name for the purpose of certifying that lactation consultant services have been rendered only if she/he provided those services.

* Reprinted with permission from International Board of Lactation Consultant Examiners.

APPENDIX E (cont.)

14. Present professional qualifications and credentials accurately, using "IBCLC" only when certification is current and authorized by the IBLCE, and complying with all requirements when seeking initial or continued certification from the IBLCE. The lactation consultant is also subject to disciplinary action for aiding another person in violating any IBLCE requirements or aiding another person in representing herself/himself as an IBCLC when she/he is not.

15. Report to an appropriate person or authority when it appears that the health or safety of colleagues is at risk, as such circumstances may compromise standards of practice and care.

16. Refuse any gift, favor, or hospitality from patients or clients currently in her/his care that might be interpreted as seeking to exert influence to obtain preferential consideration.

17. Disclose any financial or other conflicts of interest in relevant organizations providing goods or services. Ensure that professional judgment is not influenced by any commercial considerations.

18. Present substantiated information and interpret controversial information without personal bias, recognizing that legitimate differences of opinion exist.

19. Withdraw voluntarily from professional practice if she/he has engaged in any substance abuse that could affect her/his practice; has been adjudged by a court to be mentally incompetent; or has an emotional or mental disability that affects her/his practice in a manner that could harm the client.

20. Obtain maternal consent to photograph, audiotape, or videotape a mother and/or her infant(s) for educational or professional purposes.

21. Submit to disciplinary action under the following circumstances: if convicted of a crime under the laws of the practitioner's country that is a felony or a misdemeanor, an essential element of which is dishonesty, and that is related to the practice of lactation consulting; if disciplined by a national, state, province, or local government or authority, and at least one of the grounds for the discipline is the same or substantially equivalent to these principles; if committed an act of misfeasance or malfeasance which is directly related to the practice of the profession as determined by a court of competent jurisdiction, a licensing board, or an agency of a governmental body; or if violated a Principle set forth in the Code of Ethics for International Board Certified Lactation Consultants that was in force at the time of the violation.

22. Accept the obligation to protect society and the profession by upholding the Code of Ethics for International Board Certified Lactation Consultants and by reporting alleged violations of the Code through the defined review process of the IBLCE.

23. Require and obtain consent to share clinical concerns and information with the medical practitioner or other primary health care provider before initiating a consultation.

24. Adhere to those provisions of the International Code of Marketing of Breast-Milk Substitutes and subsequent WHA resolutions that pertain to health workers.

25. Understand, recognize, respect, and acknowledge intellectual property rights, including but not limited to copyrights (which apply to written material, photographs, slides, illustrations, etc.), trademarks, service marks, and patents.

Effective December 1, 2004

To Lodge a Complaint

IBCLCs shall act in a manner that justifies public trust in their competence, enhances the reputation of the profession, and safeguards the interests of individual clients.

To protect the credential and to assure responsible practice by its certificants, the IBLCE depends on IBCLCs, members of the coordinating and supervising health professions, employers, and the public to report incidents that may require action by the IBLCE Discipline Committee.

Only signed, written complaints will be considered. Anonymous correspondence will be discarded. The IBLCE will become involved only in matters that can be factually determined, and will provide the accused party with every opportunity to respond in a professional and legally defensible manner.

Complaints that appear to fit the scope of the Discipline Committee's responsibilities should be sent to:

IBLCE, Chair of the Discipline Committee
7245 Arlington Boulevard, Suite 200
Falls Church VA 22042-3217 USA

Inquiries may be directed to ethics@iblce.org.

APPENDIX F

TABLES OF EQUIVALENCIES AND METHODS OF CONVERSION

METRIC

1 liter (L) = 10 deciliters (dl) = 1000 milliliters (ml) or 1000 cc
1 dl = 100 ml
1 ml = 0.001 L = 10^{-3} L = 1 cc = 1 gm (water)
1 kilogram (kg) = 1000 grams (gm)
1 gm = 100 milligrams (mg) = 0.001 kg
1 mg = 1000 micrograms (g or mcg) = 0.001 gm = 10^{-3} gm
1 g = 0.001 mg = 10^{-6} gm
1 nanogram (ng) = 0.001 g = 10^{-9} gm
1 picogram (pg) = 0.001 ng = 10^{-12} gm

VOLUME

Household Measure	Fluid Ounces (fl oz)	Metric Equivalent* (ml)	
1 cup (c)	8	240	1 c = 16 Tbsp
2 Tablespoons (Tbsp)	1	30	1 Tbsp = 3 tsp
1 Tbsp	not used	15	
1 teaspoon (tsp)	not used	5	
1 quart (qt)	32	960 ($\cong$ 1 L)	1 qt = 4 c = 2 pt
1 pint (pt)	16	480 ($\cong$ 500 ml)	1 pt = 2 c

WEIGHT

1 pound (1 lb or #) = 0.45 kg   1 oz = 28 gm $\cong$ 30 gm
1 kg = 2.2 lb
To convert lb to kg, divide lb by 2.2 *or* multiply lb by 0.45
To convert kg to lb, multiply kg by 2.2

LINEAR MEASURE

1 inch (in. or ″) = 2.54 centimeters (cm) ($\cong$ 2.5)
1 cm = 0.4 in.
To convert in. to cm, multiply in. by 2.5.
To convert cm to in., multiply cm by 0.4 *or* divide cm by 2.5.

TEMPERATURE

To convert Celsius (C) to Farenheit (F), $°C = \frac{5}{9} (°F - 32)$
(Subtract 32, then multiply by $\frac{5}{9}$)
To convert Fahrenheit to Celsius, $°F = \frac{5}{9} °C + 32$
(Multiply by $\frac{5}{9}$, then add 32)

---

* Equivalent is given to nearest multiple of five. Number given in parentheses may sometimes be used to simplify calculations.
$\cong$ means approximately equals.

APPENDIX G

INFANT WEIGHT CONVERSION TABLE

The nurse or lactation consultant can use the table below to convert an infant's weight from pounds/ounces to grams (metric). Example: An infant weighing 5 pounds and 4 ounces (find 5 pounds in left column and then 4 ounces in top row) weighs 2381 (intersecting number) grams. To convert grams to kilograms (kg), 1000 grams equal 1 kg, so the infant weighing 5 pound 4 ounces would weigh 2.38 kg. To convert from grams to pounds/ounces, find the gram number and read across the left (pounds) column and then read upward to the top (ounces) row to determine the infant's weight.

Ounces

Pounds	0	1	2	3	4	5	6	7	8	9	10	11	12	13	14	15
	Grams	28	57	85	113	142	170	198	227	255	283	312	340	369	397	425
1	454	482	510	539	567	595	624	652	680	709	737	765	794	822	850	879
2	907	936	964	992	1021	1049	1077	1106	1134	1164	1191	1219	1247	1276	1304	1332
3	1361	1389	1417	1446	1474	1502	1531	1559	1588	1616	1644	1673	1701	1729	1758	1786
4	1814	1843	1871	1899	1928	1956	1984	2013	2041	2070	2098	2126	2155	2183	2211	2240
5	2268	2296	2325	2353	2381	2410	2438	2466	2495	2523	2551	2580	2608	2637	2665	2693
6	2722	2750	2778	2807	2853	2863	2892	2920	2948	2977	3005	3033	3062	3090	3118	3147
7	3175	3203	3232	3260	3289	3317	3345	3374	3402	3430	3459	3487	3515	3544	3572	3600
8	3629	3657	3685	3714	3742	3770	3799	3827	3856	3884	3912	3941	3969	3997	4026	4054
9	4082	4111	4139	4167	4196	4224	4552	4281	4309	4337	4366	4394	4423	4451	4479	4508
10	4536	4564	4593	4621	4649	4678	4706	4734	4763	4791	4819	4848	4876	4904	4933	4961
11	4990	5018	5046	5075	5103	5131	5160	5188	5216	5245	5273	5301	5330	5358	5386	5415
12	5443	5471	5500	5528	5557	5585	5613	5642	5670	5698	5727	5755	5783	5812	5840	5868
13	5897	5925	5953	5982	6010	6038	6095	6095	6123	6152	6180	6209	6237	6265	6294	6322
14	6350	6379	6407	6435	6464	6492	6520	6549	6577	6605	6634	6662	6690	6719	6747	6776
15	6804	6832	6860	6889	6917	6945	6873	7002	7030	7059	7087	7115	7144	7172	7201	7228

Breastfeeding Weight Loss Table

Weight (grams)	5% Loss	10% Loss	Weight (grams)	5% Loss	10% Loss
2250	2138	2025	3250	3088	2925
2275	2161	2048	3275	3111	2948
2300	2185	2070	3300	3135	2970
2325	2209	2093	3325	3159	2993
2350	2233	2115	3350	3183	3015
2375	2256	2138	3375	3206	3038
2400	2280	2160	3400	3230	3060
2425	2304	2183	3425	3254	3083
2450	2328	2205	3450	3278	3105
2475	2351	2228	3475	3301	3128
2500	2375	2250	3500	3325	3150
2525	2399	2273	3525	3349	3173
2550	2423	2295	3550	3373	3195
2575	2446	2318	3575	3396	3218
2600	2470	2340	3600	3420	3240
2625	2494	2363	3625	3444	3263
2650	2518	2385	3650	3468	3285
2675	2541	2408	3675	3491	3308
2700	2565	2430	3700	3515	3330
2725	2589	2453	3725	3539	3353
2750	2613	2475	3750	3563	3375
2775	2636	2498	3775	3586	3398
2800	2660	2520	3800	3610	3420
2825	2684	2543	3825	3634	3443
2850	2708	2565	3850	3658	3465
2875	2731	2588	3875	3681	3488
2900	2755	2610	3900	3705	3510
2925	2779	2633	3925	3729	3533
2950	2803	2655	3950	3753	3555
2975	2826	2678	3975	3776	3578
3000	2850	2700	4000	3800	3600
3025	2874	2723	4025	3824	3623
3050	2898	2745	4050	3848	3645
3075	2921	2768	4075	3871	3668
3100	2945	2790	4100	3895	3690
3125	2969	2813	4125	3919	3713
3150	2993	2835	4150	3943	3735
3175	3016	2858	4175	3966	3758
3200	3040	2880	4200	3990	3780
3225	3064	2903	4225	4014	3803

APPENDIX I

NURSING BEST PRACTICE GUIDELINES*

Vaginal Birth—Newborn

		BIRTH DATE AND TIME	
	Addressograph	/YY /MM /DD at	
		C R I T I C A L P A T H	
	0–2 HOURS	**2–24 HOURS (DAY 1)**	**2–48 HOURS (DAY 2)**
Consults	**TM Sticker**	• Social Work prn • Home Care prn • Lactation Consult prn	• Social Work prn • Home Care prn • Lactation Consult prn
Medications	• IM Vitamin K 1 mg @ date/time _____ by _____ • Apply erythromycin ophthalmic ointment to each eye × 1 dose @ date/time _____ by _____		
Tests	• Venous cord blood if mother Rh neg by _____ • Venous cord blood prn by _____ • Arterial cord gases by _____ • Glucose meter prn	• Bilirubin meter reading prn (Civic) • Glucose meter prn • Initial total bilirubin test prn	• PKU, thyroid blood test @ date/time _____ by _____ • Bilirubin meter reading prn (Civic) • Glucose meter prn • Initial total bilirubin test prn
Assessments/ Treatments	<table><tr><td>Nursing</td><td>Normal</td><td>Abnormal</td></tr><tr><td>Head/Neck</td><td></td><td></td></tr><tr><td>Palate</td><td></td><td></td></tr><tr><td>Chest/Back</td><td></td><td></td></tr><tr><td>Abdomen</td><td></td><td></td></tr><tr><td>Extremities</td><td></td><td></td></tr><tr><td>Anus</td><td></td><td></td></tr><tr><td>Genitalia</td><td></td><td></td></tr><tr><td>Comments</td><td></td><td></td></tr></table> Time: Initial: • Weight • Vital signs q1h ×2	• Weight • **Head Circumference** _____ cm • Vital signs q1h ×2; then vital signs qshift • Temperature before initial bath • initial bath done @ date/time _____ by _____ • Cord care as per standard • Physician's physical exam completed by 24 hrs **Circumcision care:** • Time of circumcision _____ • Observe ×4 hours for bleeding and voiding • Routine circumcision care	• Weight • Vital signs qshift • Remove cord clamp @ date/time _____ by _____ **Circumcision care:** • Time of circumcision _____ • Observe ×4 hours for bleeding and voiding • Routine circumcision care
Nutrition	• Initiate breastfeeding • Initiate bottle feeding prn	• Breastfeeding on cue–minimum of 6 feeds/24 hrs • Bottle feeding on cue a minimum of 6 feeds/24 hrs (15–60 mls per feed)	• Breastfeeding on cue–minimum of 8 feeds/24 hrs • Bottle feeding on cue a minimum of 6 feeds/24 hrs (15–60 mls per feed)
Elimination	❑ Initial void ❑ Initial meconium	❑ Initial void ❑ Initial meconium ❑ Post circumcision void	❑ Post circumcision void
Discharge Planning	• OHIP Form: ❑ provided (General)	If discharged prior to 24 hours: • ❑ Discharge order • PKU, thyroid blood test & F/U information • F/U visit to physician/midwife within 2 days • ❑ Discharge forms • OHIP form: ❑ Provided ❑ Returned • **ID band #** _____ • **Mother's signature** _____ • **Nurse's initials** _____	❑ Discharge order • F/U visit to physician/midwife within 7 days • OHIP form: ❑ Returned • **ID band #** _____ • **Mother's signature** _____ • **Nurse's initials** _____
Discharge Date & Time		DATE (YY/MM/DD) & TIME INITIALS	DATE (YY/MM/DD) & TIME INITIALS
Patient progress corresponds with Clinical Pathway	0–2 hrs: ❑ Yes ❑ No Date (y/m/d) _____ Time _____ Initials _____	2–12 hrs: ❑ Yes ❑ No Date (y/m/d) _____ Time _____ Initials _____ 12–24 hrs: ❑ Yes ❑ No Date (y/m/d) _____ Time _____ Initials _____	24–36 hrs: ❑ Yes ❑ No Date (y/m/d) _____ Time _____ Initials _____ 36–48 hrs: ❑ Yes ❑ No Date (y/m/d) _____ Time _____ Initials _____

* Adapted from original developed by The Ottawa Hospital, Ottawa, ON, Canada.

Vaginal Birth—Newborn

PATIENT OUTCOMES			
Patient Problem List 1) Potential for hyperbilirubinemia 2) Potential for feeding difficulties 3) Potential for hypothermia (T < 36.5° C) or hyperthermia (T > 37.5° C)		4) Potential for cardiac and/or respiratory difficulties 5) Potential for sepsis 6) Potential for bleeding post circumcision	
	0–2 HOURS	**2–24 HOURS (DAY 1)**	**24–48 HOURS (DAY 2)**
Hyper Bilirubinemia	• Demonstrates no signs of jaundice	• Demonstrates no signs of jaundice	• Demonstrates jaundice WNL • Bilirubin meter WNL (Civic)
Nutrition/ Elimination	• Initiates breastfeeding: – *licks, nuzzles* – *Intermittent latch and suck* • Nomal skin turgor	• Initiates feeding: – *breast: effective latch, intermittent sucking* – *bottle: coordinated suck and swallow* • Normal skin turgor • Voids–minimum ×1 • Passes meconium/stool	• Demonstrates a minimum of 2 effective breastfeeding: – *effective latch, sustained sucking* • Demonstrates effective bottle feeding (suck and swallow) • Voids–minimum ×2 • Passes meconium/stool • Weight loss less than 10% from birth weight
Hypo/Hyper Thermia	• Maintains stable temperature between 36.5° C–37.5° C	• Maintains stable temperature between 36.5° C–37.5° C	• Maintains stable temperature between 36.5° C–37.5° C
Cardiac/ Respiratory Difficulties	• Shows no signs of cardiac or respiratory diffculties: – *HR 100–160/min* – *RR 40–60/min* – *respiratory rhythm and effort are normal* – *no cyanosis, nasal flaring or grunting*	• Shows no signs of cardiac or respiratory diffculties: – *HR 100–160/min* – *RR 40–60/min* – *respiratory rhythm and effort are normal* – *no cyanosis, nasal flaring or grunting*	• Shows no signs of cardiac or respiratory diffculties: – *HR 100–160/min* – *RR 40–60/min* – *respiratory rhythm and effort are normal* – *no cyanosis, nasal flaring or grunting*
Sepsis	• Temperature WNL • No apnea • Maintains colour WNL • No vomiting • Cord: moist and clamped	• Temperature WNL • No apnea • Maintains colour WNL • No vomiting • Cord: moist and clamped	• Temperature WNL • No apnea • Maintains colour WNL • No vomiting • Cord: drying
Bleeding Post Circumcision		• No evidence of bleeding	• No evidence of bleeding
Patient progress corresponds with Clinical Pathway	0–2 hrs: ❑ Yes ❑ No Date (y/m/d) _____ Time _____ Initials _____	2–12 hrs: ❑ Yes ❑ No Date (y/m/d) _____ Time _____ Initials _____ 12–24 hrs: ❑ Yes ❑ No Date (y/m/d) _____ Time _____ Initials _____	24–36 hrs: ❑ Yes ❑ No Date (y/m/d) _____ Time _____ Initials _____ 36–48 hrs: ❑ Yes ❑ No Date (y/m/d) _____ Time _____ Initials _____

Nutrition & Elimination

Criteria for assessment of newborn infant at the breast position:

- Mother states that she is comfortable: back, feet & arms supported (head supported in side-lying)
- Infant's head and body supported at the level of the breast (pillows usually helpful with cradle and football to support mother's arm that is holding infant's head and body)
- Infant turned completely on side with nose, chin, chest, abdomen and knees touching mother (cradle and side-lying)
- Infant's head in neutral position (hip, shoulder and ear aligned)
- Infant kept close by support from mother's arm and hand along the infant's back and buttocks
- Mother's breast supported with cupped hand; thumb and fingers well back from areola

Addressograph

			DAY																			
Year/Month ____																							
✓ First Side x Second Side			TIME																				
		Breast																					
RIGHT SIDE	POSITION	Reverse arm hold																					
		Cradle																					
		Football																					
		Sidelying																					
	BABY RESPONSE	Latch achieved																					
		Minimal sucking																					
		Sustained sucking																					
		Sucking & swallowing																					
		No latch achieved																					
		Too sleepy																					
		Reluctant																					
LEFT SIDE	POSITION	Reverse arm hold																					
		Cradle																					
		Football																					
		Sidelying																					
	BABY RESPONSE	Latch achieved																					
		Minimal sucking																					
		Sustained sucking																					
		Sucking & swallowing																					
		No latch achieved																					
		Too sleepy																					
		Reluctant																					
ASSISTANCE		Independent																					
		Minimum																					
		Moderate																					
		Maximum																					
		Feeding observed by nurse																					
		Feeding reported by patient																					
		Expressed breast milk (EBM)																					
		Formula:																					
		Nurse's initials																					
STOOLS		Meconium																					
		Transitional																					
		Curdy																					
		Yellow																					
		Green																					
		✓ for each stool																					
URINE		Normal																					
		Uric acid crystals																					
		✓ for each void																					

Criteria for assessment of newborn infant at the breast (con't)

Latch:

- Mouth wide open (like a yawn)
- Lips visible and flanged outward
- ¾–1" of areola covered by the infant's (usually most or all of areola)
- Tongue over lower gum line
- No clicking or smacking sounds

Suck and Swallow:

- Mother states she is comfortable (no persistent nipple pain)
- Chin moves in rhythmic motion
- Bursts of sucking, swallowing and rests

Addressograph

Year/Month _____	**DAY**																				
✓ **First Side** / **x Second**	**TIME**																				
	Breast																				
RIGHT SIDE — POSITION	Reverse arm hold																				
	Cradle																				
	Football																				
	Sidelying																				
RIGHT SIDE — BABY RESPONSE	Latch achieved																				
	Minimal sucking																				
	Sustained sucking																				
	Sucking & swallowing																				
	No latch achieved																				
	Too sleepy																				
	Reluctant																				
LEFT SIDE — POSITION	Reverse arm hold																				
	Cradle																				
	Football																				
	Sidelying																				
LEFT SIDE — BABY RESPONSE	Latch achieved																				
	Minimal sucking																				
	Sustained sucking																				
	Sucking & swallowing																				
	No latch achieved																				
	Too sleepy																				
	Reluctant																				
ASSISTANCE	Independent																				
	Minimum																				
	Moderate																				
	Maximum																				
	Feeding observed by nurse																				
	Feeding reported by patient																				
	Expressed breast milk (EBM)																				
	Formula:																				
Nurse's initials																					
STOOLS	Meconium																				
	Transitional																				
	Curdy																				
	Yellow																				
	Green																				
	✓ for each stool																				
URINE	Normal																				
	Uric acid crystals																				
	✓ for each void																				

Glossary

Acinus (Acini, pl.) Smallest division of a gland; a group of secretory cells arrayed around a central cavity. In the breast, an acinus secretes milk. *See also* Alveolus.

Acrocyanosis Bluish discoloration of the hands and feet in the newborn; also known as peripheral cyanosis. Normal after birth but should not persist beyond 24 hours.

Aerobic Requiring air for metabolic processes (e.g., aerobic bacteria). Normal skin, including the breast, is colonized with aerobic bacteria.

Allergen Any substance causing an allergic response. Foods, drugs, or inhalants may be allergens. Cow's milk protein is a common allergen of infants.

Alphalactalbumin The principal protein found in the whey portion of human milk; it assists the synthesis of lactose. The dominant whey protein in cow's milk and most artificial infant milks, betalactoglobulin, is not found in human milk. *See also* Noncasein protein.

Alveolar ridge The ridge on the hard palate immediately behind the upper gums. Movement of the infant's jaw during nursing compresses the areola between his tongue and alveolar ridge.

Alveolus (Alveoli, pl.) In the mammary gland, a small sac at the terminus of a lobule in which milk is secreted and stored. Groups of alveoli, organized in lobes, give the mammary gland the appearance of a "bunch of grapes." *See also* Acinus.

Anorectic abnormalities Anomalies of the rectum, the lower few inches of the large intestine, and the anus, the opening in the skin at the distal end of the rectum. An example is imperforate anus, in which the rectum ends in a blind pouch.

Ankyglossia Tongue-tie, condition of a thick, short, or tight frenulum beneath the tongue. Condition can lead to difficult or painful infant latch to the breast and nipple pain.

Antibody An immunoglobulin formed in response to an antigen, including bacteria and viruses. Antibodies then recognize and attack those bacteria or viruses, thus helping the body resist infection. Breastmilk contains antibodies to antigens to which either the mother or the infant has been exposed.

Antigen A substance that stimulates antibody production. It may be introduced into the body (as dust, food, or bacteria) or produced within it (as a by-product toxin).

Apoptosis Greek, *apo*, away, *ptosis*, falling. A form of programmed cell death. The sloughing off of a scab or other skin crust.

Applied research Research that focuses on solving or finding an answer to a clinical or practical problem.

Areola Pigmented skin surrounding the nipple. To suckle effectively, an infant should have his gums placed well back on the areola.

Artificial infant milk Any milk preparation, other than human milk, intended to be the sole nourishment of human infants.

Atopic eczema An inherited allergic tendency to rashes or inflammation of the skin. Exclusively breastfed infants are less likely to manifest this condition, as cow's milk protein is a common allergen.

Atresia, intestinal Congenital blockage or closure of any part of the intestinal tract.

Axilla The underarm area; in it lies the uppermost extent of the mammary ridge or milk line. Deep breast tissue (the axillary tail or tail

863

of Spence) extends toward and sometimes into the axilla. This tissue may engorge the axilla along with the rest of the breast in the early postpartum period.

B cell   A lymphocyte produced in bone marrow and peripheral lymphoid tissue; found in breastmilk. It attacks antigens and is one type of cell that confers cell-mediated immunity.

Bactericidal   Capable of destroying bacteria. Breastmilk contains so many bactericidal cells that the bacteria count of expressed milk actually declines during the first 36 hours following milk expression.

Bacteriostatic   Capable of inhibiting the proliferation of bacterial colonies.

BALT/GALT/MALT   Bronchus/gut/mammary-associated immunocompetent lymphoid tissue. A lymphocyte pathway that causes IgA antibodies to be produced in the mammary gland after a lactating woman is exposed to an antigen on her intestinal or respiratory mucosa. These antibodies are then transferred through breastmilk to the breastfeeding infant, who thus may possess antibodies to antigens to which he has not been directly exposed.

Banked human milk   *See* Donor milk.

Basic research   Research that generates knowledge for the sake of knowledge.

Bioavailable   That portion of an ingested nutrient actually absorbed and used by the body. Because the nutrients in breastmilk are highly bioavailable, low concentrations may actually result in more nutrients absorbed by the infant than do the higher, less bioavailable concentrations in cow's milk or artificial infant milks.

Bivariate   Statistics derived from the analysis of the relationship between two variables.

Buccal pads   Fat pads sheathed by the masseter muscles in young infants' cheeks. The buccal pads touch and provide stability for the tongue, which enhances the tongue's ability to compress breast tissue during suckling. Breastfed infants typically have a plump-cheeked appearance because of well-developed buccal pads.

Candidiasis   A fungal infection caused by *Candida albicans;* also called "thrush." Common in the maternal vagina, it may inoculate the infant during delivery and be transferred from the infant's mouth to the mother's nipple. Candidiasis of the nipple and breast may produce intense nipple and breast pain. In the infant it may produce white spots on the oral mucosa and a bright red, painful rash ringing the anus. Formerly termed *moniliasis.* Also referred to as *Candidosis.*

Caput succedaneum   Diffuse swelling or collection of serum under the scalp of the newborn caused by pressure during descent in the maternal pelvis. Differentiated from cephalhematoma by unrestriction by the sutures of the skull.

Casein   The principal protein in milks of all mammals. (The whey-to-casein ratio changes as lactation progresses).

Centers for Disease Control and Prevention (CDC)   An agency of the US Public Health Service established in 1973 to protect the public health of the nation by providing leadership and direction in the prevention and control of diseases and other preventable health conditions, and to respond to public health emergencies. The mission of the CDC is to promote health and quality of life by preventing and controlling disease, injury, and disability.

Cephalhematoma   A collection of blood due to an effusion of blood beneath the periosteum frequently seen in a newborn as a result of birth trauma; contrasted with caput succedaneum, in which the effusion overlies the periosteum and consists of serum.

Certification   The process by which a nongovernmental professional association attests that an individual has met certain standards specified by the association for the practice of that profession.

Chi-square   A statistical procedure that uses nominal level data and determines significant differences between observed frequencies in relation to data and expected frequencies.

Colic   A syndrome in early infancy characterized by episodic loud crying, apparent abdominal pain (legs drawn up and rigid abdomen) and irritability.

Colostrum　The fluid in the breast at the end of pregnancy and in the early postpartum period. It is thicker and yellower than mature milk, reflecting a higher content of proteins, many of which are immunoglobulins. It is also higher in fat-soluble vitamins (including A, E, and K) and some minerals (including sodium and zinc).

Concept　A word, idea, or phenomenon that generally has abstract meaning.

Conceptual framework　A structure of interrelated concepts that may be generated inductively by qualitative research to provide a base for quantitative study.

Congenital infection　An infection existing at birth that was acquired transplacentally. Infections that may be so acquired include HIV and TORCH organisms. *See also* Human immunodeficiency virus; TORCH.

Complementary food　Any food used as a complement to breastmilk or to a breastmilk substitute.

Conjunctivitis　Inflammation of the mucous membrane that lines the eyelid. In many traditional and some modern societies, fresh breastmilk is instilled into the eyes to alleviate this condition.

Construct　A higher order theoretical or empirical idea or phenomenon that has abstract meaning and requires multiple concepts to represent it more concretely.

Contraception　The prevention of conception. Breastfeeding provides significant contraceptive protection during the first few months postpartum—as long as the infant is fully breastfed and feeds during the night, and maternal menses have not resumed.

Cooper's ligaments　Triangular, vertical ligaments in the breast that attach deeper layers of subcutaneous tissue to the skin.

Cord blood　Blood remaining in the umbilical cord after birth. Recently cord blood storage and registry in public or private banks has become popular for the purpose of obtaining stem cells for transplantation.

Correlation coefficient　A statistic that indicates the degree of relationship between two variables. The range in value is +1.00 to -1.00; 0.0 indicates no relationship, +1.00 is a perfect positive relationship, and -1.00 is a perfect inverse relationship.

Creamatocrit　The proportion of cream in a milk sample, determined by measuring the depth of the cream layer in a centrifuged sample. An indicator of caloric content of milk, which must be used with care; the fat (and thus caloric) content of human milk varies between breasts, within a feeding, diurnally, and over the entire course of lactation.

Cross-nursing　Occasional wet-nursing on an informal, short-term basis, usually in the context of child care.

Cultural relativism　Recognition of the wide variation in beliefs and actions that pertain to given behaviors of humans living in different cultures.

Culture　The values, beliefs, norms, and related practices of a given group that are learned and shared by the group members and that guide both the thoughts and behaviors of that group.

Cytokines　Protein signals secreted by lymphocytes, monocytes, macrophages, neutrophils, and other cells. Proinflammatory cytokines cause inflammation, pain, tenderness, redness, and fever at infected site.

Cytoprotective　Any condition or factor that protects cells from inflammation or death.

Deductive reasoning　The process of reasoning from a general premise to the concrete and specific.

Dependent variable　The variable the investigator measures in response to the independent or treatment variable; the outcome variable that is affected by the independent variable.

Design　The blueprint or plan for conducting a study. The major categories of study design are quantitative and qualitative.

Diagnostic-related grouping (DRG)   A group of diagnoses for health conditions that result in similar intensity of hospital care and similar length of hospital stay for patients hospitalized with those conditions.

Diffusion   The process by which the molecules of one substance (e.g., a drug) are spread uniformly throughout a given substance (e.g., blood or plasma). *Passive diffusion* refers to movement from a higher to a lower concentration; *active diffusion* refers to movement from a lower to a higher concentration.

Disaccharide   A carbohydrate composed of two monosaccharides. The principal sugar in human milk is lactose, a disaccharide; its constituent monosaccharides are glucose and galactose.

Donor milk   Human milk voluntarily contributed to a human milk bank by women unrelated to the recipient.

Donor milk, pooled   A batch of milk containing milk from more than one donor.

Dopamine   The prolactin-inhibiting factor (PIF), or a mediator of the PIF, secreted in the hypothalamus. It blocks the release of prolactin into the bloodstream.

Drip milk   Milk that leaks from a breast that is not being directly stimulated. Because its fat content is low, this milk should not be used regularly for infant feedings.

Ductules   Small ducts in the mammary gland that drain milk from the alveoli into larger lactiferous ducts that terminate in the nipple.

Dyad   A pair (e.g., the breastfeeding mother and her infant).

Eczema   Skin inflammation or rash. *See also* Atopic eczema.

Eminences of the pars villosa   Tiny swellings on the inner surfaces of the infant's lips that help the infant to retain a grasp on the breast during suckling.

EMM   Expressed mother's milk.

Energy density   The number of calories per unit volume; caloric density. Mature human milk averages 65 calories/dl, controlled largely by the fat content of the milk.

Engorgement   Condition of breast fullness or swelling; occurs as a result of incomplete breast emptying or as a natural part of lactogenesis (physiological engorgement) in which there is generalized tissue edema in the breasts to the axillae and fullness from copious secretion of milk.

Envelope virus   A virus that cannot infect other cells without its coat (envelope). If the envelope is destroyed (e.g., by heat or soap and water) the ability of the virus to produce infection is destroyed. Cytomegalovirus and the human immunodeficiency virus are two envelope viruses.

Epidemiology   The study of the frequency and distribution of disease and the factors causing that frequency and distribution.

Epiglottis   Cartilaginous structure of the larynx. An infant's epiglottis lies just below the soft palate. It closes the larynx when the infant swallows, ensuring passage of milk to the esophagus.

Estrogen   A hormone that causes growth of mammary tissue during part of each menstrual cycle and assists in the secretion of prolactin during pregnancy; one of the hormones whose concentration falls sharply at parturition/birth.

Ethnocentrism   A view that one's own culture and how it defines appropriate behavior is used as the basis for assessing all other cultures and behaviors.

Ethnography   One research method that attempts to support an understanding of the beliefs, practices, and behavioral patterns within a culture or subculture from the perspective of the people living in that culture.

Exclusive breastfeeding   An infant receives only breastmilk and no other liquids or solids with the exception of drops or syrups consisting of vitamins, mineral supplements, or medicines.

Exogenous   Derived from outside the body—such as iron supplements that provide the infant with exogenous iron.

External validity The extent to which study findings can be generalized to samples and settings different from those studied.

Extraneous variable Variables that can affect the relationship of the independent and dependent variables (i.e., interfere with the effect of treatment). In experimental studies, strategies for controlling these variables are built into the research design.

Foremilk The milk obtained at the beginning of a breastfeeding. Its higher water content keeps the infant hydrated and supplies water-soluble vitamins and proteins. Its fat content (1–2 gm/dl) is lower than that of hindmilk.

Frenulum Fold of mucous membrane, midline on the underside of the tongue, that helps to anchor the tongue to the floor of the mouth. A short or inelastic frenulum, or one attached close to the tip of the tongue, may restrict tongue extension enough to inhibit effective breastfeeding. Also called the *frenum*.

Galactogogue Any food or group of foods thought to possess qualities that increase the volume or quality of milk produced by the lactating woman who eats such foods.

Galactopoiesis Maintenance of established milk synthesis that is controlled by the autocrine system of supply and demand.

Galactorrhea Abnormal production of milk. It may occur under psychological influences or be a sign of pituitary tumor.

Galactose A monosaccharide present in small quantities in human milk. It is derived from lactose and, in turn, helps to produce elements essential for the development of the human central nervous system.

Galactosemia Autosomal recessive disorder in which galactose-1-phosphate metabolism is impaired due to lack of liver enzyme that changes galactose to glucose. Because human breast milk contains galactose breastfeeding is contraindicated.

Gastroenteritis Inflammation of the stomach and intestines resulting from bacterial or viral invasion. Breastfed infants are at lower risk for this illness, as compared to nonbreastfed infants.

Gastroschisis A congenital malformation characterized by herniation of abdominal contents through a fusion defect.

Gestational age An infant's age since conception, usually specified in weeks. Counted from the first day of the last normal menstrual period.

Gigantomastia A rare, debilitating condition appearing in early pregnancy characterized by massive enlargement of breasts that results in tissue necrosis, ulceration, and infection. This breast hypertrophy resolves to near prepregnancy size in the postpartum period.

Half-life The length of time for half of a drug dosage to be eliminated; generally, it takes four to five half-lives for a drug to be considered completely or nearly completely eliminated. *Example:* Half-life of drug A is 12 hours; so 50 percent of the original drug dosage is eliminated in 12 hours; 25 percent of the drug remains after 24 hours; 12.5 percent remains after 36 hours; 6.25 percent remains after 48 hours; and only 3.12 percent remains after 60 hours (five half-lives from time of original dosage).

Harlequin sign Color change in which one side of the body is a deep color while the other side is light and pink; caused by vasomotor disturbances, which are usually transient.

Hematemesis Vomiting of blood. The bleeding is usually from the upper gastrointestinal (GI) tract. This means the bleeding may be from the upper small intestine (duodenum), the stomach, or the esophagus (the tube that connects the mouth and stomach).

Hindmilk Milk released near the end of a breastfeeding, after active letdown of milk. Fat content of hindmilk may rise to 6 percent or more, two or three times the concentration in foremilk.

Horizontal transmission Transmission of pathogens through direct contact. *See also* Vertical transmission.

Human immunodeficiency virus (HIV) A retrovirus that disarms the body's immune system, causing death from an opportunistic infection. The virus may be transmitted to unborn infants, and it is carried in the breastmilk, although not all breastfed infants born to HIV-positive mothers become ill themselves. The greatest risk to the infant is posed when a woman experiences her initial HIV-related illness while pregnant or breastfeeding.

Human milk Milk secreted in the human breast.

Human milk bank A service that collects, screens, processes, stores, and distributes donated human milk to meet the needs of infants, and sometimes adult recipients, for whom human milk has been prescribed by a physician.

Human milk fortifiers Nutrients added to expressed human milk to enhance the growth and nutrient balances of very low birth weight infants. Added protein may be derived from protein components of donor human milk or from cow's milk-based products. *See also* Lactoengineering.

Hydration The water balance within a body. Adequate hydration is necessary to maintain normal body temperature and for most other metabolic functions. Breastmilk is 90 percent water. Therefore, even in hot or dry climates, fully breastfed infants obtain all the water they require through breastmilk.

Hyperalimentation The intravenous feeding of an infant, commonly a very premature infant, with a solution of amino acids, glucose, electrolytes, and vitamins.

Hyperprolactinemia Higher-than-normal prolactin levels, which may result in spontaneous breastmilk production and amenorrhea. Causes include pituitary tumors and some pharmaceuticals. *See also* Prolactin.

Hypothalamus A gland that controls postpartum serum prolactin levels through release of dopamine. Inhibition of dopamine permits the release of prolactin, which controls the secretion of milk.

Hypoxia Inadequate oxygen at the cellular level, characterized by tachycardia, hypertension, peripheral vasoconstriction, dizziness, and mental confusion.

Immunity, active Immunity conferred by the production of antibodies by one's own immune system.

Immunity, passive Immunity conferred on an infant by antibodies manufactured by the mother and passed to the infant transplacentally or in breastmilk. Passive immunity is temporary but very important to the young infant.

Immunoassay Any method for the quantitative determination of chemical substances that uses the highly specific binding between antigen or hapten and homologous antibodies (e.g., radioimmunoassay, enzyme immunoassay, and fluoro-immunoassay).

Immunogen A Substance that stimulates the body to form antibodies. *See also* Antigen.

Immunoglobulin Proteins produced by plasma cells in response to an immunogen. The five types are IgG, IgA, IgM, IgE, and IgD. IgG is transferred *in utero* and provides passive immunity to infections to which the mother is immune; IgA is the principal immunoglobulin in colostrum and mature milk; IgM is produced by the neonate soon after birth and is also contained in breastmilk. *See also* Noncasein protein.

Immunomodulator An agent in human milk that changes the function of another defense agent and thus enhances the quality or magnitude of the immune response.

Incidence How much a particular behavior is practiced at a given time. *Example*: How many women are initiating breastfeeding from time A to time B?

Incubation period The period between exposure to infectious pathogens and the first signs of illness.

Independent variable The experimental or treatment variable that is manipulated by the investigator to influence the dependent variable.

Inductive reasoning   The process of reasoning from specific observations or abstractions to a general premise.

Infection control   Practices—in hospitals formalized by protocols—that reduce the chance that infection will be spread between patients or between patients and staff. Hand washing and wearing of disposable gloves are two such practices.

Internal validity   The extent to which manipulation of the independent variable makes a significant difference on the dependent variable, or the extent to which the independent variable, rather than extraneous variables, has caused the change in the dependent variable.

International Code of Marketing of Breast-Milk Substitutes   A set of resolutions that regulate the marketing and distribution of any fluid intended to replace breastmilk, certain devices used to feed such fluids, and the role of healthcare workers who advise on infant feeding. Intended as a voluntary model that could be incorporated into the legal code of individual nations in order to enhance national efforts to promote breastfeeding. Also referred to as the *WHO Code* or the *WHO/UNICEF Code*.

Intracellular   Occurring within cells. Viruses live within other cells during part of their reproductive lives. Although viruses within cells may be passed to the infant in breastmilk, other cells in breastmilk enhance the destruction of these infected cells.

Intrauterine   Within the uterus; *in utero*.

Intrauterine growth rate   The normal rate of weight gain of a fetus. It is considered by many, but not all, physicians to be the ideal growth rate for premature infants.

Involution   Refers to the return of the mammary gland to a nonproductive state of milk secretion.

Lactase   Enzyme needed to convert lactose to simple sugars usable by the infant. Present from birth in the intestinal mucosa, its activity diminishes after weaning.

Lactase deficiency   *See* Lactose intolerance.

Lactation   The secretion of milk from the mammary glands, the process of providing that milk to the child (breastfeeding or nursing), and the period of time that a mother lactates to feed her young. Lactation stages include mammogenesis, lactogenesis I and II, galactopoiesis, and involution.

Lactation, induced   Lactation that is stimulated through chemical, hormonal, and mechanical means in the woman who has not been pregnant for the intended nursling. The practice of inducing lactation is more common today among adoptive mothers.

Lactiferous ducts   Milk ducts; the 15 to 24 tubes that collect milk from the smaller ductules and carry it to the nipple. They appear similar to stems on a bunch of grapes, the alveoli being the "grapes." The ducts open into nipple pores.

Lactobacillus bifidus   Principal bacillus in the intestinal flora of breastfed infants. Low intestinal pH (5–6) of fully breastfed infants discourages the colonization of bacteria, which are common in feces of infants fed cow's milk-based infant milks.

Lactoengineering   The process of fortifying human milk with nutrients (especially protein, fat, calcium, and phosphorus) derived from other batches of human milk, in order to meet the special nutritional needs of very low birth weight infants. *See also* Human milk fortifiers.

Lactoferrin   A protein that is an important immunological component of human milk. It binds iron in the intestinal tract, thus denying it to bacteria that require iron to survive. Exogenous iron may upset this balance. *See also* Noncasein protein.

Lactogenesis   The initiation of milk secretion. The initial synthesis of milk components that begins late in pregnancy is termed *lactogenesis I*; the onset of copious milk production 2 or 3 days postpartum is termed *lactogenesis II*.

Lactose   The principal carbohydrate in human milk, forming about 4 percent of colostrum and 7 percent of mature milk. A disaccharide, it metabolizes readily to glucose, which is used for

comment on and attempt to influence UNICEF activities. La Leche League International and the International Lactation Consultant Association are NGOs.

NNS Nonnutritive suckling.

Nonparametric statistics Statistical procedures used when required assumptions for using parametric procedures are not met, especially assumptions regarding a normal probability distribution. Nonparametric statistics are appropriate for use with nominal and ordinal level data.

Nonprotein nitrogen (NPN) About one fourth of the total nitrogen in human milk is derived from sources, such as urea, other than protein. NPN contains several free amino acids, including leucine, valine, and threonine, which are essential in the young infant's diet because he cannot yet manufacture them.

Nutriment Any nourishing substance.

Oligosaccharide Carbohydrate, comprised of a few monosaccharides, present in human milk. Some oligosaccharides promote the growth of *Lactobacillus bifidus*, thus increasing intestinal acidity, which discourages the growth of intestinal pathogens.

OMM Own mother's milk.

Operational definition The explicit description of a concept or variable of interest in measurable terms.

Oxytocin A lactogenic hormone produced in the posterior pituitary gland. It is released during suckling (or other nipple stimulation) and causes ejection of milk as well as uterine contractions.

Pacing Periodically removing the nipple during a feeding to allow the infant to rest.

Palate, hard The hard, anterior roof of the mouth. A suckling infant uses his tongue to compress breast tissue against the hard palate.

Palate, soft The soft, posterior roof of the mouth, which lies between the hard palate and the throat. It rises during swallowing to close off nasal passages. Also called the *velum*.

Parametric statistics Statistical procedures used when a sample is randomly selected, represents a normal distribution of the target population, and is considered sufficiently large in size, and interval level data are collected.

Parenchyma The functional parts of an organ. In the breast, the parenchyma include the mammary ducts, lobes, and alveoli.

Parenteral The introduction of fluids, nutrients, or drugs into the body by an avenue other than the digestive tract (intravenous, intramuscular).

Pasteurization The heating of milk to destroy pathogens. Milk banks commonly heat donor milk to 62.5°C for 30 minutes.

Pathogen A substance or organism capable of producing illness.

Peristalsis An involuntary, rhythmic, wavelike action. Commonly thought of in relation to food and waste products moving along the gastrointestinal tract. To strip milk from the breast, an infant's tongue uses a peristaltic motion that begins at the tip of the tongue and progresses toward the back of the mouth.

Pharynx The muscular tube at the rear of the mouth, through which nasal air travels to the larynx and food from the mouth travels to the esophagus. During infant feeding, contraction of pharyngeal muscles moves a bolus of fluid into the esophagus.

Phenylketonuria Autosomal recessive inherited disorder in which phenylalanine (PHE) metabolism is impaired due to a defect in phenylanaline hydoxylase with resultant decreased conversion of phenylalanine to tyrosine. Abnormal metabolites accumulate in blood and tissue, including the brain. To prevent brain damage dietary PHE must be limited. Because breast milk contains low levels of PHE, breastfeeding can continue along with supplemental use of PHE formula.

Philtrum The midline region between the nose and the lips. In the newborn this region should be well defined and grooved. In fetal alcohol syndrome the philtrum is flat.

Pituitary An endocrine gland at the base of the brain that secretes several hormones. Prolactin, which is essential for production of milk, is secreted by the anterior lobe; oxytocin, which is essential for milk letdown, is secreted by the posterior lobe.

Placenta The intrauterine organ that transfers nutrients from the mother to the fetus. The expulsion of the placenta at birth causes an abrupt drop in estrogen and progesterone, which in turn permits the secretion of milk.

Polymastia The presence of more than two breasts. These additional structures, which usually contain only a small amount of glandular tissue, may occur anywhere along the milk line from the axilla to the groin.

Population The total set of individuals that meet the study criteria from which the sample is drawn and about whom findings can be generalized.

Power The probability that a statistical test will reject a null hypothesis when it should be rejected, or, in other words, detect a significant difference that does exist.

Premature infant One born before 37 weeks' gestational age, regardless of birth weight.

Primary infection The first incidence of illness after exposure to a pathogen.

Primiparous Having carried one pregnancy to viability.

Progesterone The hormone produced by the corpus luteum and placenta that maintains a pregnancy and helps develop the mammary alveoli.

Prolactin The hormone produced in the anterior pituitary gland that stimulates development of the breast and controls milk synthesis. Normal concentrations are 10–25 ng/ml in a nonpregnant woman; 200–400 ng/ml at birth.

Prone Lying on one's stomach.

Raynaud's phenomena Named for a French physician, a dermatological condition characterized by intense pain and pallor of the skin (usually of the fingers or toes, but in the breastfeeding woman the nipples), caused by vasospasm.

Reliability The degree to which collected data are accurate, consistent, precise, and stable over time.

Respiratory syncytial virus (RSV) Organism causing a respiratory illness; breastfed infants are at less risk for this illness than are non-breastfed infants.

Rickets Abnormal calcification of the bones and changes in growth plates that lead to soft or weak bones due to lack of Vitamin D. Risk is greatest for children not exposed to the sun and breastfed children of women who are vegetarians. The AAP advises that full-term breastfed infants receive vitamin D supplement beginning at 2 months of age.

Rotavirus A class of viruses that are a major cause of diarrheal illness leading to hospitalization of infants. Breastfed infants are at less risk for illness caused by this organism, as compared to nonbreastfed infants.

Rugae Corrugations on the hard palate behind the gum ridge that help the infant to retain a grasp on the breast during suckling.

Sample A subset of the population selected for study.

Sampling The procedure of selecting the sample from the population of interest.

Secretory IgA An immunoglobulin abundant in human milk that is of immense value to the neonate. It is synthesized and stored in the breast; after ingestion by the infant, it blocks adhesion of pathogens to the intestinal mucosa.

Secretory immune system The system that produces specific antibodies or thymus-influenced lymphocytes in response to specific antigens.

Sepsis The presence of bacteria in fluid or tissue.

Seroconvert A process by which serum comes to show the presence of a factor that previously has been absent, or vice versa. When antibodies to an infecting agent, such as cytomegalovirus, become present the person is said to have seroconverted.

Serological tests Tests performed on blood samples to ascertain the presence or absence of pathogens.

Seronegative Serum that does not demonstrate the presence of a factor for which tests were conducted; "tests negative."

Seropositive Serum that demonstrates the presence of a factor test for which tests were conducted; "tests positive."

Serum Clear fluid portion of blood that remains after coagulation.

Serum albumin A protein in serum. *See also* Noncasein protein.

SIDS Sudden infant death syndrome.

Smooth muscle The type of muscle that provides the erectile tissue in the nipple and areola.

Somatic Pertaining to the body, especially nonreproductive tissue.

Spontaneous lactation Secretion and release of milk unrelated to a pregnancy or to nipple stimulation intended to stimulate milk production.

STS Skin-to-skin (kangaroo) care.

Suck, suckle Used in this textbook interchangeably to mean the baby's milking action at the breast. In traditional usage, a baby at the breast *sucked*, whereas a mother *suckled*.

Sucking, nonnutritive Sucking not at the breast (e.g., as on a pacifier or on baby's own tongue); or, sucking at the breast characterized by alternating brief sucks and long rest periods during minimal milk flow. However, insofar as any milk is transferred, even this latter pattern of sucking may in fact be nutritive. *See also* Sucking, nutritive.

Sucking, nutritive Steady rhythmic sucking during full, continuous milk flow. Insofar as any milk is transferred, other sucking patterns also may be nutritive. *See also* Sucking, nonnutritive.

Supine Lying on one's back.

Switch nursing A simple intervention for low intake in an actively suckling infant in which baby is frequently switched from breast to breast, concurrent with breast massage, to facilitate more active swallowing and promote multiple letdowns during the feeding.

Symbiosis The intimate association of two different kinds of organisms. The breastfeeding dyad is considered by many to exemplify a mutually beneficial symbiosis.

Systemic immune system The nonspecific immune responses of the body.

Tachypnea An abnormally rapid rate of breathing.

Target population The population that is of interest to the investigator and about which generalizations of study results are intended.

T cells Any of several kinds of thymic lymphoid cells or lymphocytes that help to regulate cellular immune response. A subset of these cells (T4 cells) are preferentially attacked by the human immunodeficiency virus.

Teleological Describing the belief that all events are directed toward some ultimate purpose.

Thrombocytopenia Low levels of platelets in blood.

TORCH An acronym for organisms that can damage the fetus: toxoplasmosis, rubella, cytomegalovirus, herpes simplex.

Torticollis A condition of the neck in which the cervical muscles are contracted, producing twisting of the neck and an unnatural position of the head.

Transcutaneous bilimeter A device that estimates bilirubin concentrations in the blood by measuring intensity of yellowish skin coloration.

Transitional milk Breast fluid of continuously varying composition produced in the first 2 to 3 weeks postpartum as colostrum decreases and milk production increases.

Transplacental Transferred from mother to fetus through the placenta. Nutrients and certain immunoglobulins are transferred to the fetus transplacentally; some infections also may be transferred.

Univariate The statistics derived from the analysis of a single variable (e.g., frequencies).

Universal precautions Guidelines for infection control, based on the assumption that every person receiving health care carries an infection that can be transmitted by blood, body fluids, or genital secretions.

Vaccine An infectious agent, or derivatives of one, given to a person so that his or her immune system will produce antibodies to that infection without a preceding illness.

Validity The degree to which collected data are true and represent reality; the extent to which a measuring instrument reflects what it is intended to measure.

Variable Attributes, properties, and/or characteristics of persons, events, or objects that are examined in a study.

Vertical transmission Transmission of infection from mother to child transplacentally or through breastmilk.

Very low birth weight Term applied to infants weighing less than 1500 gm at birth.

Virus Very small organisms that rely on material in invaded cells to reproduce. Viruses identified in breastmilk include cytomegalovirus, *Herpes zoster*, *Herpes simplex*, hepatitis, and rubella.

Water-soluble vitamins The B vitamins and vitamin C, pantothenic acid, biotin, and folate. These vitamins are present in serum; concentrations in breastmilk approximate those in serum. Concentrations reflect current maternal diet more directly than do fat-soluble vitamins (A, D, E, K).

Wet nurses Women who breastfeed infants who are not their own.

Whey The liquid left after curds are separated from milk. Alphalactalbumin and lactoferrin are the principal whey proteins. Whey forms soft, easily digested curds in the infant stomach. *See also* Casein; Noncasein protein.

Witch's milk Colostrum, formed under the influence of maternal hormones, which may be expressed from temporarily enlarged mammary tissue in the neonate's breasts.

World Health Organization (WHO) An agency of the United Nations charged with planning and coordinating global health care and assisting member nations to combat disease and train healthcare workers.

Xerophthalmia Disease of the eyes caused by vitamin A deficiency; endemic in parts of Africa. Human milk is preventive.

Index

Note: *b* with page number indicates boxes, *f* indicates figures, *t* indicates tables.